HANDBOOK OF PHARMACEUTICAL GRANULATION TECHNOLOGY

DRUGS AND THE PHARMACEUTICAL SCIENCES
A Series of Textbooks and Monographs
Series Editor

Anthony J. Hickey
RTI International, Research Triangle Park, USA

The Drugs and Pharmaceutical Sciences series is designed to enable the pharmaceutical scientist to stay abreast of the changing trends, advances and innovations associated with therapeutic drugs and that area of expertise and interest that has come to be known as the pharmaceutical sciences. The body of knowledge that those working in the pharmaceutical environment have to work with, and master, has been, and continues, to expand at a rapid pace as new scientific approaches, technologies, instrumentations, clinical advances, economic factors and social needs arise and influence the discovery, development, manufacture, commercialization and clinical use of new agents and devices.

Recent Titles in Series

For more information about this series, please visit: www.crcpress.com/Drugs-and-the-Pharmaceutical-Sciences/book-series/IHCDRUPHASCI

HANDBOOK OF PHARMACEUTICAL GRANULATION TECHNOLOGY

Fourth Edition

Edited by
Dilip M. Parikh

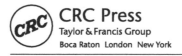

CRC Press
Taylor & Francis Group
Boca Raton London New York

CRC Press is an imprint of the
Taylor & Francis Group, an **Informa** business

Cover photo courtesy of L.B. Bohle Maschinen + Verfahren GmbH.

Fourth edition published 2021
by CRC Press
6000 Broken Sound Parkway NW, Suite 300, Boca Raton, FL 33487-2742

and by CRC Press
2 Park Square, Milton Park, Abingdon, Oxon, OX14 4RN

© 2021 Taylor & Francis Group, LLC

Second edition published by CRC Press 2005
Third edition published by CRC Press 2009

CRC Press is an imprint of Taylor & Francis Group, LLC

Library of Congress Cataloging-in-Publication Data
Names: Parikh, Dilip M., 1945- editor.
Title: Handbook of pharmaceutical granulation technology / edited by Dilip M. Parikh.
Description: Fourth edition. | Boca Raton, FL : CRC Press, 2021. | Series: Drugs and the pharmaceutical sciences | Includes bibliographical references and index.
Identifiers: LCCN 2020047289 (print) | LCCN 2020047290 (ebook) | ISBN 9780367334772 (hardback) | ISBN 9780429320057 (ebook)
Subjects: LCSH: Drugs--Granulation--Handbooks, manuals, etc.
Classification: LCC RS199.G73 H36 2021 (print) | LCC RS199.G73 (ebook) | DDC 615.1/9--dc23
LC record available at https://lccn.loc.gov/2020047289
LC ebook record available at https://lccn.loc.gov/2020047290

ISBN: 978-0-367-33477-2 (hbk)
ISBN: 978-0-367-74145-7 (pbk)
ISBN: 978-0-429-32005-7 (ebk)

Typeset in Times New Roman
by MPS Limited, Dehradun

Dedication

To my wife Leena, my son Neehar, his wife Joan, and my grandsons Kalyan and Tej for their support and love during this project

Contents

SECTION I PARTICLE FORMATION

SECTION II GRANULATION PROCESSES

SECTION III PRODUCT-ORIENTED GRANULATIONS

SECTION IV CHARACTERIZATION AND SCALE-UP

SECTION V   OPTIMIZATION STRATEGIES, TOOLS, AND REGULATORY CONSIDERATIONS

Preface

As we prepare this fourth edition of our book, all of us are going through a pandemic caused by Covid-19 worldwide. While we've all faced unprecedented challenges this year that we never imagined, this time has underscored the importance of relationships and connectivity, of humanity and kindness, and of strength and resilience. The disaster caused by this virus in terms of human lives lost and the economies of so many countries almost destroyed has affected all of us. Some of the authors were personally affected as well. Despite these difficulties created by the virus, most of the authors have spent valuable time updating or writing new chapters in time. I sincerely appreciate all the hard work of all the authors in making this fourth edition possible. My sincere thanks to all the authors and staff at the publisher Taylor and Francis (Informa Healthcare).

The first edition of this book was published in 1997. Before that, most pharmaceutics textbooks devoted a small portion to the granulation unit operation because they were generally focused on retail and hospital pharmacy students and academia. As granulation is a critical unit operation in the manufacture of solid dosage forms, the first edition of this book gave comprehensive treatment to the area of granulation from an industrial perspective. The book appealed not only to members of academia and students of pharmacy and pharmaceutics but also professionals in pharmaceutical and related industries, where agglomerating particles is one of the critical unit operations. Subsequent editions in 2005 and 2009 demonstrated that the book has been able to provide comprehensive coverage of this critical unit operation by updating and adding relevant technologies that provide a knowledge base essential for the pharmaceutics student, academia, researchers, and operational professionals in the industry. During these intervening years, the pharmaceutical industry has endured considerable changes and challenges. The industry is under intense pressure to accelerate the drug development process, shorten the development timelines, and launch new pharmaceutical products. Applications of continuous manufacturing, artificial intelligence (AI), additive printing, or 3D printing are starting to affect product development and manufacturing of pharmaceutical dosage forms. Concurrently, there have been rapid developments in the science of granulation, particle engineering, and process controls, that called for publication of this fourth edition.

The concept of design space, process optimization, and harmonization of regulations by the global health authorities are being implemented in the industry. The United States and international regulatory bodies are restructuring their oversight of pharmaceutical quality regulation by developing a product quality regulatory system that provides a framework for implementing quality by design, continuous improvement, and risk management. This edition addresses topics generated by these technologies as well as regulatory changes in the unit operation of particle generation and granulation.

After the introductory chapter, Chapter 2 provides a detailed theory of granulation with an emphasis on the engineering aspect.

Subsequent chapters are divided into the five following sections:

Section one "Particle Formation" contains chapter "Drug Substance and Excipient Characterization," which critically evaluates the techniques, ranging from common to state-of-the-art, employed to analyze individual and bulk properties of particles, (e.g., size, shape, surface area, density, solubility, crystal form, flow, sticking, and microstructure). For greater insight, drug substance-excipient physical (e.g., segregation and compaction) and chemical (e.g., compatibility) interactions are also discussed. The next chapter "Binders in Pharmaceutical Granulation" is important because to agglomerate the primary particles, particles must bond together. The selection and mechanism of binder functionality are detailed in this chapter. Because excipient functionality and their variability can affect the final product attributes as well as a batch-to-batch variability, a new chapter is added "Excipients and Their Attributes in Granulation," which I am sure the readers will find very helpful in selecting the right excipient for their formulation. The next updated chapter is on the spray drying technology, which is a critical particle formation technology. In keeping to provide the most comprehensive research and development and manufacturing led me to combine two chapters from the third edition on nanotechnology and supercritical technology to present a new chapter "Emerging Particle Engineering Technologies." This chapter addresses various newer approaches that already have started to have an impact on the pharmaceutical industry in general and the dosage form developments and manufacturing in particular. Electrospinning has emerged as the most viable approach for the fabrication of nanofibers with several beneficial features that are essential to various applications ranging from the environment to biomedicine. Along with the nanotechnology, supercritical fluid technology, the inclusion of 3-D printing, machine learning, and artificial intelligence (AI), and their impact are explored in this chapter. The nanoparticulate technology offers a potential path to the rapid preclinical assessment of poorly soluble drugs. It offers increased bioavailability, improved absorption, reduced toxicity, and the potential for drug targeting. Supercritical fluids have emerged as the basis of a system that optimizes the physicochemical properties of pharmaceutical powders. Three-dimensional printing has set off a true manufacturing transformation, and chemical and pharmaceutical industries are incorporating the technology in their research and development activity as well as commercial manufacturing as can be seen by the US Food and Drug Administration (FDA)-approved products on the market recently. Machine learning and artificial intelligence (AI) are in their infancy as far as how they affect particle generation, but I think it is just the beginning of their impact in pharmaceutical processing since these technologies are revolutionizing every facet of our life and have benefited other areas of the pharmaceutical industry immensely.

Section two "Granulation Processes" covers the well-established and revised granulation process chapters on roller compaction, fluid bed granulation, single-pot processing, extrusion spheronization as a granulation technique, and continuous granulation. The chapter on wet granulation was completely revised as "Advances in Wet Granulation of Modern Drugs" and includes small molecule granulations as well as therapeutic protein granulation, various formulation strategies, and process technologies involved in producing stabilized granules or powdered therapeutic proteins. The application of AI in the process modeling of high-shear granulation is presented via several case studies in the final section of this chapter.

Section three "Product-Oriented Granulation" covers technologies specifically addressing the technologies to produce the various dosage forms with specific quality attributes. For example, chapters "Effervescent Granulation," "Granulation of Plant Products and Nutraceuticals," Granulation Approaches for Modified Release Products," "Granulation of Poorly Water-Soluble Drugs," "Granulation and Production Approaches of Orally Disintegrating Tablets," and "Melt granulation" are included. All these chapters are updated by well-known researchers and revised to provide cutting-edge information in these areas.

Section four "Characterization and Scale-Up" provides a critical area of understanding the product. Chapter "Sizing of Granulation" discusses the technique of producing the right particle size for subsequent processing. Next chapter "Granulation Characterization" provides how to evaluate the properties of granulation and characterize it. Chapter "Bioavailability and Granule Properties" discusses the importance of the ideal properties of granules, including its composition and physical attributes, and their impact on the delivery of the active ingredient to the "site of action." Chapter "Granulation Process Modeling" was substantially rewritten to bring together the new material added into the chapter. There are several benefits from the use of process modeling, such as an increased understanding of the governing mechanisms through endeavoring to represent them in the model description, capturing of insight and knowledge in a mathematically usable form, an increased understanding of the relative importance of mechanistic contributions to the output of the process, and application of the models for improved control performance and process diagnostics. Chapter "Scale-Up Consideration in Granulation" discusses unique challenges in scaling up a process, from a chemical engineering perspective, and understanding through considering granulation as a combination of rate processes. Chapter "Advances in Process Controls and End-Point Determination" explores various approaches for monitoring the process. End-point determination of a granulation process is the most prominent concern of any practicing industry professional as well as an academician. Advances on both sensors and surface characterization of powder properties are presented in this chapter. Overall, this chapter provides an overview of the considerable refinement in our quantitative understanding of granulation, based on growing knowledge on materials functionality, advances in measurement science that have advanced process understanding, and granulation techniques used. The revised chapter discusses this very important topic and provides helpful guidance.

Section five "Optimization Strategies, Tools, and Regulatory Consideration" contains two chapters, namely, "Use of Artificial Intelligence and Expert Systems in Pharmaceutical Applications" and "Regulatory Issues in Granulation: Leading Next-Generation Manufacturing" both focused on optimizing the process. Future success in all areas of pharmaceutical science will depend entirely on how fast pharmaceutical scientists will adapt to the rapidly changing technology. It is common in most formulation development studies that the formulation scientist may have extensive knowledge of the active ingredients and yet still needs to know, which excipients to select, and their proportions. At this stage, a knowledge-based so-called an expert system can be helpful to the scientist in selecting suitable excipients. Another case where such an expert system could be of use in formulation studies is the determination of the design space for manufacturing conditions. Chapter "Use of Artificial Intelligence and Expert Systems in Pharmaceutical Applications" (titled as "Expert Systems and Their Use in Pharmaceutical Application" in the previous edition) discusses developments in this emerging field. As a complement to the US FDA regulations for Good Manufacturing Practices, chapter "Regulatory Issues in Granulation: Leading Next-Generation Manufacturing" (titled as "The Pharmaceutical Quality for the 21st Century – A Risk-Based Approach" in the previous edition), reflects the impact of these regulations. This important topic is critical in building and maintaining the desired quality of a pharmaceutical product. It covers current regulatory guidelines that dictate approaches one needs to take to optimize granulation processing, possibly using an expert system. Optimization of a process has a greater chance of success if the product is developed with Process Analytical Technology (PAT) tools (PAT)and the following Quality by Design (QbD), which the chapter on QbD and PAT addresses with current approaches in the industry

Over the past 10 years since the last edition of the book was published, there are several changes in regulations worldwide. This manuscript is completely revised to reflect these changes supporting next-generation manufacturing. Specifically:

- ICH Q12 covers pharmaceutical product life cycle management.
- FDA guidance on continuous manufacturing issued in Feb 2019 is new and ICH has also just embarked on a similar guideline.
- Data integrity is currently a hot topic with regulatory agencies from FDA, EMA, Japan PMDA, and others.
- The book includes references to guidance from regulatory agencies such as ANVISA (Brazil) and NMPA (China), indicating the importance of emerging economies in global trade and quality/regulatory expectations.

This book is designed to give readers comprehensive knowledge of the subject. As in the earlier editions, all chapters include an appropriate level of theory on the fundamentals of powder characterization, granulation, and state-of-the-art technologies, modeling, application of expert systems, and manufacturing optimization.

Pharmaceutical professionals, such as research and development scientists, manufacturing management professionals, process engineers, validation specialists, process specialists, quality assurance, quality control; regulatory professionals; and graduate students in industrial pharmacy and chemical engineering programs will find the level of theory appropriate and the wealth of practical information from renowned pharmaceutical professionals from respective industry and academia invaluable. The knowledge provided will help select the appropriate granulation technology while keeping in mind regulatory requirements and cost-effectiveness.

I feel very confident that the assembled experts in their respective field will give the readers fresh and updated information in their respective chapters and readers will be able to use this book as a text or reference or for troubleshooting process problems they may encounter.

I'd like to thank the authors who contributed to this book despite their busy schedules. All of them are recognized and respected experts in the areas they wrote about.

I am also thankful to all the equipment manufacturers who graciously granted permission to use their product information and photographs in this book.

The most appreciation goes to my wife, Leena, who endured many missing evenings and weekends while I worked alone in the office.

Finally, you, the readers are to be thanked for your support and comments. I trust you will find that the fourth edition of *Handbook of Pharmaceutical Granulation Technology* continues the high standards as set by its predecessors. As always, I welcome your comments and suggestions for new titles.

I am very thankful to Jessica Poile and Hillary LaFoe of Informa Healthcare for their guidance and constant inspiration during this endeavor. I am also thankful to Ms. Madhulika Jain Project Manager at MPS and her team for keeping this publication timeline on track with planning and hard work.

Dilip M. Parikh
Ellicott City, MD USA

Editor

Dilip M. Parikh is President, DPharma Group Inc., Ellicott City, Maryland, USA. As a chemical and pharmaceutical engineer, he has more than 45 years of hands-on experience in product development, manufacturing, process engineering, and executive operational management of various pharmaceutical facilities in Canada and the USA. He is an invited speaker globally on various solid dosage manufacturing technologies, process troubleshooting and optimization strategies, regulatory remediation, and PAT & QbD implementation strategies. Author of many scientific journal articles and book chapters, including the recently published book *How to Optimize Fluid Bed Processing Technology* and is the editor of the first, second, and third editions of *Handbook of Pharmaceutical Granulation Technology*.

Contributors

Fatemeh Bahadori
Bezmialem Vakif University Faculty of Pharmacy
Department of Pharmaceutical Biotechnology
Fatih-Istanbul, Turkey

Thomas De Beer
Laboratory of Pharmaceutical Process Analytical
    Technology
Ghent University
Ottergemsesteenweg Gent, Belgium

Guia Bertuzzi
IMA S.p.A.-IMA Active Division
Bologna, Italy

Gulsilan Binzet
University of New Mexico,
College of Pharmacy
Albuquerque New Mexico, USA
and Altinbaş University
Istanbul, Turkey

Albert W. Brzeczko
Acura Pharmaceuticals, Inc.
Palatine, Illinois, USA

Ian T. Cameron
The University of Queensland
Brisbane Australia

Anthony E. Carpanzano
JRS Pharma
Adjunct Professor of Pharmaceutics
Long Island University, USA

M. Teresa Carvajal
Purdue University
West Lafayette, Indiana, USA

Metin Çelik
Pharmaceutics International Inc.
Skillman, New Jersey, USA

Lai Wah Chan
GEA-NUS Pharmaceutical Processing Research
Laboratory Department of Pharmacy
National University of Singapore, Singapore

Shivang Chaudhary
QbD Expert
Ahmedabad, India

Keat Theng Chow
Roquette Asia Pacific Pte. Ltd.
Singapore

Tansel Comoglu
Ankara University
Faculty of Pharmacy
Department of Pharmaceutical Technology
Tandoğan-Ankara, Turkey

Parind M. Desai
GlaxoSmithKline (GSK) R&D Pharmaceutical
    Development
Collegeville Pennysylvania, USA

Thomas Dürig
Ashland LLC
Wilmington Delaware, USA

Brandon Ennis
E & G Associates Inc.
Chattanooga, Tennessee, USA

Bryan Ennis
E & G Associates Inc.
Chattanooga, Tennesse, USA

David F. Erkoboni
Cedar Consulting Corporation
Peddington, New Jersey, USA

Wen Chin Foo
Roquette Asia Pacific Pte. Ltd.
Singapore

Rajeev Gokhale
Roquette Asia Pacific Pte. Ltd.
Singapore

Yinghe He
College of Science and Engineering James
Cook University
Townsville, Queensland, Australia

Paul Wan Sia Heng
GEA-NUS
Pharmaceutical Processing Research Laboratory
Department of Pharmacy
National University of Singapore, Singapore

Sunil S. Jambhekar
School of Pharmacy
Lake Erie College of Osteopathic Medicine
Bradenton, Florida, USA

Naseem Jibrin
E & G Associates Inc.
Chattanooga, Tennessee, USA

Prasad Kanneganti
Tessa Therapeutics Ltd.
Singapore

Kapish Karan
Ashland LLC
Wilmington, Delaware, USA

Defne Kayrak-Talay
Pharmaceutical Consultant
California, USA

James Litster
Department of Chemical and Biological
   Engineering
The University of Sheffield
Sheffield, UK

Lian X. Liu
Department of Chemical and Process
   Engineering
The University of Surrey
Guildford, Surrey, UK

Kevin A. Macias
Bristol Myers Squibb
New Jersey, USA

Ronald W. Miller
Miller Pharmaceutical Technology Consulting
Travelers Rest, South Carolina, USA

Pavan Muttil
University of New Mexico, College of Pharmacy
Albuquerque, New Mexico, USA

Sree Nadkarni
Biopharmaceutical Consulting
USA

Vishwas Nesarikar
Takeda Pharmaceuticals
Cambridge, Massachussetts, USA

Dilip M. Parikh
DPharma Group Inc.
Ellicott City, Maryland, USA

Neelima V. Phadnis
Phadnis Consultancy Services
Texas, USA

Cecil W. Propst
Propst Consulting
Norton Shores, Michigan, USA

Gurvinder Singh Rekhi
University of Georgia College of Pharmacy
Athens, Georgia, USA

Firas El Saleh
Ashland Industries
Deutschland Gmbh
Düsseldorf, Germany

Richard Sidwell
Recro Gainesville LLC
Gainesville, Georgia, USA

Harald Stahl
GEA Group
Huerth, Germany

Shana Van de Steene
Laboratory of Pharmaceutical Process Analytical
   Technology
Ghent University
Ottergemsesteenweg Gent, Belgium

Bing Xun Tan
Roquette Asia Pacific Pte. Ltd.
Singapore

Hibreniguss Terefe
ExxPharma Therapeutics LLC
New Jersey, USA

Griet Van Vaerenbergh
GEA Group
Wommelgem, Belgium

Valérie Vanhoorne
Laboratory of Pharmaceutical Technology
Ghent University
Ottergemsesteenweg Gent, Belgium

Chris Vervaet
Laboratory of Pharmaceutical Technology
Ghent University
Ottergemsesteenweg Gent, Belgium

Fu Y. Wang
The University of Queensland
Australia

Susan C. Wendell
Johnson and Johnson
Spring House Pennsylvania
USA

Michael Winn
E & G Associates Inc.
Chattanooga, Tennesee, USA

1 Introduction

Dilip M. Parikh

CONTENTS

1.1 INTRODUCTION

Solid-dosage forms encompass the largest category of dosage forms that are clinically used. Several types of tablet solid dosage forms are designed to optimize the absorption rate of the drug, increase the ease of administration by the patient, control the rate and site of drug absorption, and mask the taste of a therapeutic agent. This also applies to the capsules of various sizes and various release profiles. The formulation of tablets and capsules involves the use of several components, each of which is present to facilitate the manufacture or to control the biological performance of the dosage form. The practice of delivering medicinal powder by hand rolling into a pill by using honey or sugar has been used for centuries. The delivery of some of the botanical and herbal extracts in homeopathic and ayurvedic branches of medicine by rolling into a pill is still practiced in India along with allopathic medicine.

1.2 NEED FOR GRANULATING POWDERS

Processing powders in the industry is a challenge. Particularly in the chemical and pharmaceutical industries as different powders are mixed there to make a solid dosage form such as tablets, capsules, and pellets. It becomes even more critical since the segregation of different ingredients can create a dosage form, which may result in variability in the final product quality attributes. Segregation of powders is due primarily to differences in the size or density or flow properties of the components of the mix. If the product composition has a desirable flow and non-segregating properties, it can be directly compressed or encapsulated. For powder mixture to be homogeneous, the composition of the mix should have complementary physical properties, such as flow, particle size, and morphology. Where drug substance dosage is high and has a poor flow property, and a larger quantity of excipients are needed to facilitate the direct compression, the resulting dosage form may be larger, and thus may not be normally unacceptable due to the difficulty of swallowing such a large tablet. The decision on whether to opt for a granulation operation should also be based on the knowledge of the potential disadvantages associated with employing the direct compression of the powdered mix. Failing these physical attributes, dry or wet granulation should be considered. Granulation is a process of size enlargement used primarily to prepare powders for tableting. It consists of homogeneously mixing the drug and excipients and then wetting them in the presence of a binder so that larger agglomerates or granules are formed. An ideal granulation should contain all the constituents of the mix in the correct proportion in each granule, thus the segregation of the ingredients will not occur.

An earlier mention of granulating medicine cited in 1773, by Thomas Skinner in Duncan's Elements of Therapeutics in 1862 as follows: "by the application of art, it is intended that medicines should be rendered more agreeable, more convenient, safer and more efficacious than they are in their natural state. To obtain these ends is the intention of pharmacy." Skinner further describes the earlier method of making granules by French pharmacists who had a form of medication that they call "poudres granules." Perry's Chemical Engineer's Handbook [1] defines the granulation process as "any process whereby small particles are gathered into larger, permanent masses in which the original particles can still be identified." This definition is appropriate to a pharmaceutical granulation where the rapid breakdown of agglomerates is important to maximize the available surface area and aid in the solution of the active drug. The granulated material can be obtained by direct size enlargement of primary particles or size reduction from dry, compacted material.

In the pharmaceutical field, solid dosage forms remain an important part of the overall drug market, despite the success and the development of new pharmaceutical forms. The high risk of failure in drug discovery and development throughout the pharmaceutical industry statistically shows that, on average, only 1 in 5000 compounds screened in research will reach the market. The new drug approvals for 2018 and 2019 show predominant approvals are for solid dosages. For example for 2018, out of 59 total approvals listed on the FDA website, 31 approvals are for either tablets, capsules, or powders, while for the year 2019, there were a total of 48 novel drug approvals, with 5 new formulations and 7 new dosage forms using the technologies described in this book. In 2019, The Center for Drug Evaluation and Research (CDER) approved 48 novel drugs. The ten-year graph below shows that from 2010 through 2018, CDER has averaged about 37 novel drug approvals per year. A number of these approvals are for the solid dosage forms [2], (Figure 1.1).

CDER identified 20 of the 48 novel drugs approved in 2019 (42%) as first-in-class, which is one indicator of the drug's potential for a strong positive impact on the health of the American people. These drugs often have mechanisms of action different from those of existing therapies.

Similarly, global spending on cancer medicines – both for therapeutic and supportive care use – rose to $133 billion globally in 2017, up from $96 billion in 2013. It is predicted that the global market for oncology therapeutic medicines will reach as much as $200 billion by 2022 [3].

1.3 GRANULATION OPTIONS

Several products cannot be directly compressed because of the low dosage of drug substance, or flow properties of the drug and excipient mixture. The formulation containing such a low dose could be challenging to meet the bioavailability or content uniformity. Several other reasons why

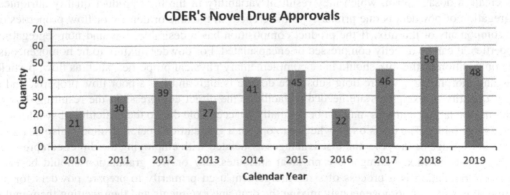

FIGURE 1.1   *FDA.* https://www.fda.gov/drugs/new-drugs-fda-cders-new-molecular-entities-and-new-therapeutic-biological-products/new-drug-therapy-approvals-2019.
Source: From Ref. [2].

direct compression may not be suitable for a wide array of products include the required flow properties; dissimilar ingredient physical attributes, such as particle size, morphology, moisture content and the content of each excipient in the formulation form; requirement of densification to reduce the size of the drug product, obtain the required hardness, friability, and disintegration/ dissolution; and others. The final quality attributes of the dosage form will be based on the process of technology to be employed. The selection of the process also entails ancillary equipment that could have an impact on the granule properties; hence, characterizing the granulation for its flowability, morphological properties, and impact on bioavailability is necessary.

Many researchers studied the influence of material properties of the granulating powders and process conditions on the granulation process in a rather empirical way. In the 1990s, a fundamental approach to research was started on various topics in the granulation process, looking into more detailed aspects of particle wetting, mechanism of granulation, material properties, and influence of mixing apparatus on the product. The overall hypothesis suggested that the granulation can be predicted from the raw material properties and the processing conditions of the granulation process. One of the major difficulties encountered in the granulation technology is the incomplete description of the behavior of powders in general. The ongoing fundamental research on mixing, segregation mechanisms of powder, surface chemistry, and material science is necessary to develop the theoretical framework of granulation technology. An excellent review of the wet granulation process was presented by Iveson and coauthors [4]. They have advanced the understanding of the granulation process by stating that there are three fundamental sets of rate processes that are important in determining wet granulation behavior. These are wetting and nucleation, consolidation and growth, and breakage and attrition. Once these processes are sufficiently understood, then it will be possible to predict the effect of formulation properties, equipment type, and operating conditions of granulation behavior, provided these can be adequately characterized according to the reviewers. The most widely used granulation technologies that are used in the industry are shown in Figure 1.2. As can be seen, making granules from powders provides several different options.

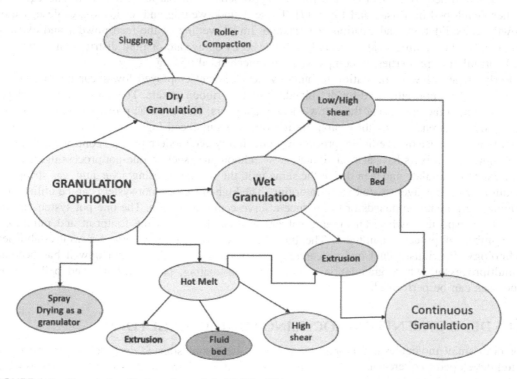

FIGURE 1.2 Granulation Options *(copyright DM Parikh).*

With the development of rotary tablet presses in the 19th century initially and the advent of high-speed compression and encapsulation machines requiring production rates, the demand for free-flowing powders and granules has increased substantially. In the pharmaceutical industry, the simplest form of solid dosage form employs granules prepared from the drug and other components in stable aggregates in sizes large enough to facilitate the accurate formulation and dispensing for the subsequent processing. For a pharmaceutical solid dosage form, the granulation process is the first unit operation that needs to be carefully planned. The excipient variability is well known in the industry. All of the excipients necessary for the robust formulation usually meet all the compendial requirements, but more often the particle size and morphology consistency from batch to batch do not. Physical properties of excipient, as well as API, should be consistent from batch to batch, as one of the requirements to develop a robust formulation that will reduce final dosage form variability. This requirement has become even more critical as the industry has started to adopt continuous granulation technology.

Dry compaction technique like roller compaction is experiencing a renewed interest in the industry. The roller compaction processes and equipment were adapted and modified from other industries like metal, mineral, and recycling industries. In the early 19th century, the process was utilized in the mining industry to crush rocks for easy extraction of desired precious material. In the mid-20th century, the process was used to compress pharmaceutical powders. Several drug substances are moisture sensitive. The roller compaction process provides suitable alternative technology for granulating these products. It offers advantages compared with wet granulation for processing physically or chemically moisture-sensitive materials since a liquid binder and thus drying of granulation is not required. This technology can also be used to produce effervescent granulations. The current offering of this technology is equipped with process analytical tools (PATs) that provide process monitoring and help in scale-up and optimization.

In the wet granulation process, primary particles of drug and excipient mixture granulated with either water, alcohol, or mixture of water and alcohol are the choice of binder. Four key mechanisms outlined by Ennis [5,6] are for the agglomeration of particles, that were subsequently further developed by Litster and Ennis [7]. These include wetting and nucleation, coalescence or growth, consolidation, and attrition or breakage. Initial wetting of the feed powder and existing granules by the binding fluid is strongly influenced by spray rate or fluid distribution as well as feed formulation properties, in comparison with mechanical mixing.

Early stages of wet granulation technology development employed low-shear mixers, or the mixers/blenders normally used for dry blending such as ribbon mixers. There are several products currently manufactured using these low-shear granulators. However, as process control and efficiency have increased over the years; the industry has embraced high-shear granulators for wet granulation because of its efficient process reproducibility and modern process control capabilities. The high-shear mixers have also facilitated new technologies, such as one-pot processing, that use the mixer to granulate and then dry in the same unit, the wet mass, using a vacuum, gas stripping/ vacuum, or microwave-assisted vacuum drying. The high-shear one-pot system can be utilized for granulating potent compounds or to produce effervescent granulation. The one-pot system has an advantage especially where an organic solvent is used. It reduces the footprint and minimizes the number of process equipment. The fluid bed processing of powders is a well-established technology. Previously fluid bed processors were used only as a dryer but now it has become a multiprocessor, where granulation, drying, particle coating, taste masking, and pelletization processes can be performed.

1.4 DEVELOPMENTS IN PROCESSING SOLID DOSAGE FORMS

For both small molecules and biopharmaceuticals, more sophisticated drug delivery systems are being developed to overcome the limitations of conventional forms of drug delivery systems (e.g., tablets and intravenous [IV] solutions), problems of poor drug absorption, noncompliance of patients, and inaccurate targeting of therapeutic agents. Futuristic drug delivery systems are being developed, which are hoped to facilitate the transport of a drug with a carrier to its intended destination in the body and then release it there. Liposomes, monoclonal antibodies, and modified viruses are being considered to deliver "repair genes" by IV injection to target the respiratory epithelium in the treatment of cystic fibrosis. These novel drug delivery systems not only offer clear medical benefits to the patient but can also create opportunities for commercial exploitation, especially useful if a drug is approaching the end of its patent life. *Particle engineering* is a term coined to encompass means of producing particles having a defined morphology, particle size distribution, and composition. Particle engineering combines elements of many others, including chemistry, pharmaceutics, colloid science, mass and heat transfer, aerosol and powder science, and solid-state physics.

Since the development in the classical granulation technologies mentioned earlier, there are numerous developments in the field related to the application of granulation processes to produce dosage form with a specific application such as modifying particles, impart higher solubility, modify the release mechanism, provide taste-masking, or produce orally disintegrating dosage form, among others. For producing modified-release products, several options are available, for example, matrix granulation with polymers, pelletization with extrusion spheronization technique, or pellets production in a fluid bed processor using powder, solution, or suspension layering of drug substance and subsequently coating with a functional coat.

Poorly water-soluble drugs present a challenge to formulators of pharmaceutical oral solid dosage forms to improve the drug's bioavailability while maintaining product stability, both physically and chemically, and providing a robust commercial process. The molecular structure of new chemical entities that researchers are discovering is becoming more complex, leading to drugs with low aqueous solubility and dissolution rate, and limited absorption after oral administration, thus resulting in decreased bioavailability. The reduction of particle size is widely used to improve the dissolution rate of such drugs. Approaches such as complexation, and hot-melt extrusion to improve the solubility are described in this book. Another approach for improving the solubility of poorly soluble drug substances is by a spray drying process. Compounds that are sparingly soluble due to its crystalline morphology can be converted to an amorphous form by spray drying, enabling greater solubility and hence enhanced bioavailability. This is possible because the hollow structure of the spray-dried particles increases the solubility and subsequent dissolution rate of the drugs by several folds. The rapid nature of the spray drying process improves the stability of otherwise unstable amorphous forms. With a polymer as a carrier, a molecular dispersion is formed, or so-called glass solution, and crystallization is avoided as the nucleation and growth slow down or even impede. A spray drying can be used to produce a granulated product from a composition of the starting material made with a suspension of drug and excipients. The desired attributes of the granule are controlled by a combination of the formulation and the process. Spray drying technique is now routinely used to prepare particles for inhalation dosage forms. Aseptic spray drying is now used to process vaccines or proteins. Recent interest in nanotechnology research has opened many avenues for creating newer drugs. Various development groups are working to enhance traditional oral delivery systems with nano-engineered improvements. There are some areas where nano-enhanced drugs could make a big difference in increasing oral bioavailability and reducing undesirable side effects. By increasing bioavailability, nanoparticles can increase the yield in drug development and more importantly may help treat previously untreatable conditions. Nanotechnology provides methods for targeting and releasing therapeutic compounds in very defined regions. Three-dimensional (3D) printing is a manufacturing method in which objects are made by fusing or depositing materials (e.g., plastic, metal, ceramics, powders, liquids, or even living cells) in layers to produce a 3D object. The 3D printing technology is expected to play an important role in the trend toward personalized medicine, through its use in customizing nutritional products, organs, and drugs. It is anticipated that 3D printing will continue to gain much attention in solid dosage forms as the most popular drug dosage form. Other emerging particle engineering approaches include supercritical fluid technology, co-crystallization, electrospinning, and microbiome-based therapeutics. One of the major areas on which the research and development of supercritical fluids are focused is particle design. There are different concepts such as "rapid expansion of supercritical solution," "gas antisolvent recrystallization," and "supercritical antisolvent" to generate particles, microspheres, microcapsules, liposomes, or other dispersed materials. When the supercritical fluid and drug solution make contact, a volume expansion occurs leading to a reduction in solvent capacity, an increase in solute saturation, and then supersaturation with associated nucleation and particle formation. Several advantages are claimed by using this platform technology such as particle formation from nanometers to tens of micrometers, low residual solvent levels in products, preparation of polymorphic forms of the drug, and so forth [8]. Similarly, machine learning and artificial intelligence (AI) are promising potentials for precision and personalized medicine in the coming years. All these emerging particle engineering technologies will change the way we develop and manufacture pharmaceutical dosage forms in the coming years.

Over these years of research, the pharmaceutical granulation process is still based on trial and error by the experience of scientists and production professionals. This constitutes problems for many and frequently changing formulations containing different compositions with widely varying properties. Thus, new formulations always need expensive and lengthy laboratory and pilot-scale testing. Moreover, even when pilot-scale testing is OK, there is still a significant failure rate during scale-up to commercial production [9]. Over the past decade, however, design, scale-up, and operation of granulation processes have been considered as quantitative engineering and significant advances have been made to quantify the granulation processes [10]. Expert systems and mathematical modeling approaches for the granulation process have been thus introduced with the aim both to understand and underline the observed physical phenomena, and to propose predictive tools able to forecast granulation results in terms of the size distribution of obtained granular materials. Expert system and process modeling is an area that has grown enormously over the past 50 years. Modeling is a vital activity across the life cycle of processes and products. It plays an important role in decision making around aspects of experimentation and the use of fundamental physicochemical phenomena that inform the design and operational decisions. Continuous granulation with roller compaction, fluid bed, twin-screw, and continuous drying is becoming common. Along with the availability of mature manufacturing technology, QbD and the successful implementation of PAT probes for process monitoring has promoted the adoption of continuous processing for the manufacturing of oral solid dosage forms.

1.5   SCOPE OF THIS BOOK

The significant advances that have taken place in pharmaceutical granulation technology are presented in this book to provide the readers with available choices. The various discussed techniques will further help the scientists in their understanding and selection of the granulation process most appropriate for the drug in question. With complete updated chapters from the previous edition, this book will provide current scientific practices in the industry and research labs worldwide. There is no substitute for good science. The characterization of the drug substance along with the knowledge of granulation theory, identification of the critical process parameters, process modeling capability, in-line or on-line PATs, process scale-up approaches, expert systems, and modeling of the granulation process will prepare the reader to explore the various options presented in this book. It can be used as a reference source and a guidance tool for those working in the pharmaceutical or related industries, for example, chemical, nutraceutical, or biopharmaceutical, as well as academia and the pharmacy students who will learn various technologies to produce particles and granules, or anyone seeking for an insight into this subject area. The information presented is essentially based on the extensive experiences of the editor and contributors who are all actively working in the industry or academia and have learned "best practice" from their subject matter expertise and experiences.

REFERENCES

1. Ennis B. J., Litster J. D. Particle enlargement. Perry R. H., Greens D., eds. *Perry's Chemical Engineer's Handbook*. 7th ed. New York: McGraw Hill, 1997:20-56–20-89.
2. FDA https://www.fda.gov/drugs/new-drugs-fda-cders-new-molecular-entities-and-new-therapeutic-biological-products/new-drug-therapy-approvals-2019.
3. Aitken M. Global Oncology Trends 2018. IQVIA Institute for Human Data Science, 2018. https://www.iqvia.com/insights/the-iqvia-institute/reports/global-oncology-trends-2018.
4. Iveson S. M., Litster J. D., Hopgood K, Ennis B. Nucleation, growth, and breakage phenomenon in agitated wet granulation process: a review. Powder Technol 2001; 117: 3–39.
5. Ennis, B. J. On the Mechanics of Granulation, PhD Thesis, The City College of the City University of New York, University Microfilms International (No.1416), 1990.
6. Ennis, B. J. Design & Optimization of Granulation Processes for Enhanced Product Performance, Nashville, TN: E&G Associates, 1990.
7. Litster, J. & Ennis, B. J. The Science & Engineering of Granulation Processes, Dordrecht, Netherlands: Kluwer Academic, 2004.
8. York P., et al. Supercritical fluids ease drug delivery. Manuf Chemist 2000; 71(6): 26–29.
9. Iveson S., Litster J. Growth regime map for liquid-bound granules. AIChE J. 1998; 44(7): 1510–1518
10. Hapgood K. P., Litster J. D., Smith R. Nucleation regime map for liquid bound granules. AIChE J 2003; 49(2): 350.

2 Theory of Granulation

An Engineering Perspective

Bryan J. Ennis, Michael Winn, Brandon Ennis,
and Naseem Jibrin

CONTENTS

2.1 INTRODUCTION

2.1.1 OVERVIEW

Granulation technologies, both wet and dry, are a subset of particle size enlargement production methods [1–8]. These technologies involve any process whereby small particles are agglomerated, compacted, or otherwise brought together into larger, relatively permanent structures in which the original particles can still be distinguished. Granulation technology and size enlargement processes have been used by a wide range of industries, ranging from pharmaceutical, agricultural chemical, consumer products, or detergent production to mineral and ceramics processing, as well as more recent advances in additive manufacturing. Particle size enlargement generally encompasses a variety of unit operations or processing techniques dedicated to particle agglomeration. These processes can be loosely broken down into agitation and compression methods.

Although the terminology is industry-specific, agglomeration by agitation will be referred to as granulation, specifically wet granulation. Here a particulate feed is introduced to a process vessel and is agglomerated in the presence of binding fluid, either batch-wise or continuously, to form a granulated product. Agitative processes include fluid bed, pan (or disk), drum, and mixer granulators. Such processes are also used as coating operations for controlled release, taste masking, and cases where solid cores may act as a carrier for a drug coating. The feed typically consists of a mixture of solid ingredients, referred to as a formulation, which includes an active or key ingredient, binders, diluents, flow aids, surfactants, wetting agents, lubricants, fillers, or end-use aids (e.g., sintering aids, colors or dyes, and taste modifiers). A closely related process of spray drying is also included here, but discussed in detail later (see Ref. 9 and chapter 6). It also includes in part recent advances in the use of additive manufacturing to produce pharmaceutical and other dosage forms. Product forms generally include agglomerated or layered granules, coated carrier cores, or spray-dried products consisting of agglomerated solidified drops.

An alternative approach to size enlargement is by agglomeration by compression, or compaction, where the mixture of particulate matter is fed to a compression device, which promotes agglomeration due to pressure. Both wet and dry compaction processes are possible. In dry processing, either continuous sheets of solid material or some solid form such as a briquette or tablet is produced. Typically in wet processing, wet extrudate is produced, as cylindrical or rounded granulate or as extruded monolithic structures. Compaction processes range from confined compression devices, such as tableting, to continuous devices, such as roll presses (chapter 8), briquetting machines, and extruders (chapter 12). Some processes operate in a semicontinuous fashion such as ram extrusion. Capsule filling operations would be considered a low-pressure compaction process.

In both agitative and compression granulation technologies, binding and carrier fluids can be introduced as aqueous or solvent solutions by spraying or pumping, or they may be created by heating a melt activated binder (chapter 19).

At the level of a manufacturing plant, size enlargement processes involve several peripheral unit operations such as milling, blending, drying or cooling, and classification. The combination of these unit operations is referred to generically as an agglomeration circuit (Figure 2.1). In addition, more than one agglomeration step may be present. In the case of pharmaceutical granulation, granulated material is almost exclusively an intermediate product form, which is then followed by tableting.

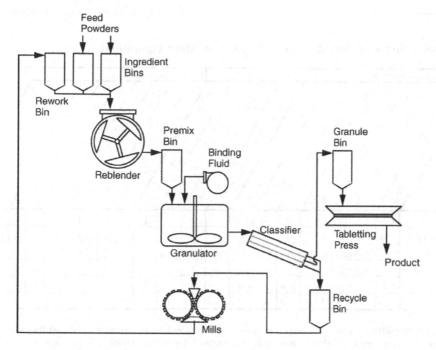

FIGURE 2.1 A Typical Agglomeration Circuit Utilized in the Processing of Pharmaceuticals Involving Both Granulation and Compression Techniques.
Source: From Refs. [1–3,5,6].

In addition, interactions of the unit operations are critical. In the context of granulation, it is important to understand compaction processes to establish desirable granule properties for tableting performance. In wet granulation, it is conceptually important to consider drying and cooling as an integral part of the granulation process. As another example, high recycling can readily destabilize an agglomeration circuit.

Numerous benefits result from size enlargement processes as summarized in Table 2.1. A wide variety of size enlargement methods are available; a classification of available equipment and initial criteria of process selection is given in Tables 2.2 and 2.3. A primary purpose of wet granulation, in the case of pharmaceutical processing, is to create free-flowing, nonsegregating blends of ingredients of controlled strength, which may be reproducibly metered in subsequent

TABLE 2.1

Objectives of Size Enlargement

Production of useful structural form

Provision of a defined quantity for dispensing, with improved flow properties for metering and tableting

Improved product appearance

A reduced propensity to caking

Increased bulk density for storage and tableting feeds.

Creation of nonsegregating blends with an ideally uniform distribution of key ingredients.

Control of solubility, and dissolution profiles.

Control of porosity, hardness, and surface to volume ratio and particle size

Source: From Refs. [1–3,5,6].

TABLE 2.2

Process Selection Considerations for Wet Granulation Equipment

Process	Product density	Production: [tn/hr] or [kg/batch]	Size range [mm]	Width of Size Distribution	Flowability for metering	Product form	Poor wettability / high viscosity	Able to process	Heat or pressure induction time	Sensitive to small feed variations	Stable non-deformable growth	Competing deformable growth	Simultaneous drying / reaction	Heat activated granulation	Typical Level of Recycle	Ease of cooling or heating	Ease of dust/toxicity containment	Typical Pre/post processing
Batch Fluid-bed	L-M	100-900	0.2-1	M	M-H	SG	✗	✓	✓	L	✓	✗	✓	✗	L	H	✓	C
Continuous Fluid-bed	L-M	50	0.1-3	M	M-H	SG	✗	✓	✓	L	✓	✗	✓	✗	L-M	H	✓	C,R
Continuous Disc	M	0.5-800	0.5-20	L	VH	VSG	✗	✗	✓	L	✓	?	✗	✗	L	L	✗	B,D,C,R
Continuous Drum	M	0.5-800	2-20	M	M-H	SG	✗	?	✓	L	✓	?	✓	✗	H	L	✗	B,D,C,G,R
Batch Mixer	M-H	100-500	0.1-3	M-H	M	IG	✓	✓	?	M	✗	✓	✓	✓	L-M	H	✓	D,C
Continuous Mixer	M-H	50	0.1-3	M-H	M	IG	✓(1)	?(1)	?	M	✗	✓	✓	✓	L-M	H	✓	D,C,T

Binder required. Either solvent required, or in some cases, heat-activated binder. A maximum feed of 500 µm, smaller preferred. Moisture no more than 80% pore saturation. Able to process brittle, abrasive, elastic, most plastic materials. Source: From Refs. [7,8]. Definitions: ✓=Yes, ✗=No, ?=Possible Product form: L=Low, M=Medium, H=High, V=Very, G=Granular, S=Spherical, I=Irregular, T=Tablet form, C=Cylindrical Processing: C=Classification, R=Recycle, B=Blending, D=Drying, G=Grinding, T=Two-stage Notes: (1) Dependent on contact time.

TABLE 2.3

Process Selection Considerations for Compaction Equipment

Process	Product density	Production: [tn/hr] or [kg/batch]	Size range [mm]	Width of Size Distribution	Flowability for metering	Product form	Can process low wall friction	Can process low permeability	Can process hard materials	Sensitive to small feed variations	Simultaneous reaction	Heat activated granulation	Solvent	Typical Level of Recycle	Ease of cooling or heating	Ease of dust/toxicity containment	Typical Pre/post processing
Roll Pressing (Smooth)	H	50	0.2-5	M-H	M	IG	✗	✓	✗	VH	✗	✗	✗	M-H	H	M	B,G,C,R,T
Roll Pressing (Pattern)†	H	50	5-50	VL	M	B	✓	?	✗	H	✗	✗	✗	L-M	M	M	T,B
Tabletting	H-VH	1	5-10	O	M	T	✓	✗	✗	H	✗	✗	✗	O	L	H	T,B
Ram/Piston Extrusion	H-VH	5	5-10	O	M	IT	✓	✗	✗	VH	✗	✗	✗	O	H	H	T,B
Pelleting Mills	H-VH	10	0.5-3	L	M	C-SG	✗	✓	✓	VH	✗	✓	✗	L	L	M-H	B,C,D,R
Radial Extrusion	M-H	5	0.5-3	L	M	C-SG	?	✓	✓	H	✓	✓	✓	L	H	H	B,C,D,R
Axial Extrusion	VH	5	0.5-3	L	M	C-SG	?	✓	✓	VH	✓	✓	✓	L	H	H	B,C,D,R

Binder not required except for some hard materials. Small levels of moisture common; must be low or compaction arrested. A minimum feed of 100 µm, unless deaeration/vacuum provided. Moisture no more than 80% pore saturation. Extrusion normally involves aqueous or solvent binders, or heat activated melt binders. Nonwettable material is acceptable. Source: From Refs. [7,8].

tableting or for vial or capsule filling operations. The wet granulation process must generally achieve desired granule properties within some prescribed range. These attributes depend on the application at hand. However, common to most processes is a specific granule size distribution and granule voidage. Size distribution affects flow and segregation properties, as well as compaction behavior. Granule voidage controls strength and impacts capsule and tablet dissolution behavior, as well as compaction behavior and tablet hardness.

Control of granule size and voidage will be discussed in detail throughout this chapter. The approach taken here relies heavily on attempting to understand interactions at a particle level and scaling to bulk effects. Developing an understanding of these micro-level processes of agglomeration allows a rational, engineering based approach to the design, scale-up, and control of agglomeration processes (Figures 2.2 and 2.3). Although the approach is difficult, qualitative trends are uncovered along the way, which aid in formulation development and process optimization, and which emphasize powder characterization as an integral part of product development and process design work.

2.1.2 Granulation Mechanisms

Four key mechanisms or rate processes contribute to wet granulation, as originally outlined by Ennis [4,5], and later developed further by Litster and Ennis [6]. These include *wetting* and nucleation, *coalescence* or growth, *consolidation*, and *attrition* or breakage (Figure 2.2). Initial wetting of the feed powder and existing granules by the binding fluid is strongly influenced by spray rate or fluid distribution, as well as feed formulation properties, in comparison with mechanical mixing. Wetting promotes nucleation of fine powders or coating in the case of feed particle size in excess of drop size. In the coalescence or growth stage, partially wetted primary particles and larger nuclei coalesce to form granules composed of several particles. The term *nucleation* is typically applied to the initial coalescence of primary particles in the immediate

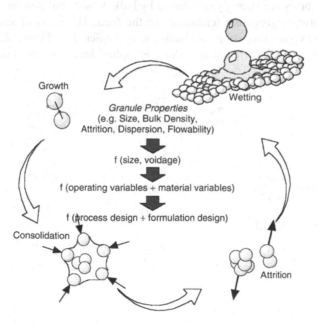

FIGURE 2.2 The Mechanisms or Rate Processes of Agitative Agglomeration, or Granulation, Which Include Powder Wetting, Granule Growth, Granule Consolidation, and Granule Attrition. These Processes Combine to Control Granule Size and Porosity, and They May Be Influenced by Formulation or Process Design Changes.
Source: From Refs. [4,5,7].

vicinity of the larger wetting drop, whereas the more general term of coalescence refers to the successful collision of two granules to form a new larger granule. In addition, the term of layering is applied to the coalescence of granules with primary feed powder. Nucleation is promoted from some initial distribution of moisture, such as a drop or from the homogenization of a fluid feed pumped to the bed, as with high-shear mixing. As granules grow, they are consolidated by compaction forces due to bed agitation. This consolidation stage strongly influences internal granule voidage or granule porosity, and therefore end-use properties such as granule strength, hardness, or dissolution. Formed granules may be particularly susceptible to attrition if they are inherently weak or if flaws develop during drying.

These rate mechanisms can occur simultaneously in all processes. However, certain mechanisms may dominate. For example, fluidized-bed granulators are strongly influenced by the wetting process, whereas mechanical redispersion of binding fluid by impellers and particularly high-intensity choppers diminish the wetting contributions to granule size in high-shear mixing. On the other hand, granule consolidation is far more pronounced in high-shear mixing than fluidized-bed granulation. These simultaneous rate processes are taken as a whole—and sometimes competing against one another—determine the final granule size distribution and granule structure and voidage resulting from the process and, therefore, the final end-use or product quality attributes of the granulated product.

2.1.3 COMPACTION MECHANISMS

Compaction is a forming process controlled by mechanical properties of the feed, in relationship to applied stresses and strains, as well as interstitial gas or carrier fluid interactions. Micro-level processes are controlled by particle properties, such as friction, hardness, size, shape, surface energy, elastic modulus, and permeability. Key steps, in any compaction process, include (i) powder filling, (ii) stress application and removal, and (iii) compact ejection. Powder filling and compact weight variability are strongly influenced by bulk density and powder flowability [2,3], as well as any contributing segregation tendencies of the feed. The steps of stress application and removal consist of several competing mechanisms, as depicted in Figure 2.3. Powders do not transmit stress uniformly. Wall friction impedes the applied load, causing a drop in stress as one

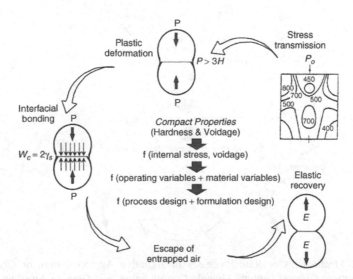

FIGURE 2.3 The Mechanisms or Micro-Level Processes of Compressive Agglomeration or Compaction. These Processes Combined Control Compact Strength, Hardness, and Porosity.
Source: From Refs. [5,7].

moves away from the point of the applied load (e.g., a punch face in tableting or roll surface in roll pressing). Therefore, the applied load and resulting density are not uniform throughout the compact, and powder frictional properties control the *stress transmission* and distribution in the compact [10]. The general area of study relating to compaction and stress transmission is referred to as powder mechanics [2,3,10–12]. For a local level of applied stress, particles deform at their point contacts, including *plastic deformation* for forces in excess of the particle surface hardness. This allows intimate contact at surface point contacts, allowing cohesion/adhesion to develop between particles, and therefore *interfacial bonding*, which is a function of their interfacial surface energy. During the short timescale of the applied load, any *entrapped air* must escape, which is a function of feed permeability, and a portion of the elastic strain energy will be converted into permanent plastic deformation. Upon stress removal, the compact expands because of the remaining *elastic recovery* of the matrix, which is a function of elastic modulus, as well as any expansion of remaining entrapped air. This can result in loss of particle bonding and flaw development, and this is exacerbated for cases of wide distributions in compact stress because of poor stress transmission. The final step of stress removal involves compact ejection, where any remaining radial elastic stresses are removed. If recovery is substantial, it can lead to the capping or delamination of the compact.

For wet compaction such as paste or melt extrusion, wall, and screw powder friction remain important, in addition to formulation high pressure rheology and yield properties of the binding fluid, which impacts solid-liquid phase separation and extrudate quality.

These micro-level processes of compaction control the final flaw and density distribution throughout the compact, whether it is a roll pressed, extruded, or tabletted product, and as such, control compact strength, hardness, and dissolution behavior. Compaction processes will not be discussed further here, with the remainder of the chapter focusing on wet granulation and agitative processes (for further discussion regarding compaction, see chapter 8 and 12 and Refs. 2,3,7,8,12,13).

2.1.4 FORMULATION VERSUS PROCESS DESIGN

The end-use properties of granulated material are controlled by granule size and internal granule voidage or porosity. Internal granule voidage (or porosity) $\varepsilon_{\text{granule}}$ and bed voidage ε_{bed}, or voidage between granules, are related by:

$$\rho_{\text{bulk}} = \rho_{\text{granule}}(1 - \varepsilon_{\text{bed}}) = \rho_e(1 - \varepsilon_{\text{bed}})(1 - \varepsilon_{\text{granule}}) \tag{2.1}$$

where ρ_{bulk}, ρ_{granule}, and ρ_e are bulk, granule and envelop primary particle density, respectively. Here, granule voidage and granule porosity will be used interchangeably. Granule structure may also influence properties. To achieve the desired product quality as defined by metrics of end-use properties, granule size and voidage may be manipulated by changes in either process operating variables or product material variables, which affect the underlying granulation and compaction mechanisms, as initially outlined by Ennis [4,5], and later developed further by Ennis and Litster [2,3,6]. The first approach is the realm of traditional process engineering, whereas the second is product engineering or quality by design. Both approaches are critical and must be integrated to achieve the desired end-point in product quality. Operating variables are defined by the chosen granulation technique and peripheral processing equipment, as listed for typical pharmaceutical processes in Figure 2.4. In addition, the choice of agglomeration technique dictates the mixing pattern of the vessel. Material variables include parameters such as binder viscosity or wet mass rheology, surface tension, feed particle size distribution, powder friction, and the adhesive properties of the solidified binder. Material variables are specified by the choice of ingredients or product formulation. Both operating and material variables together define the kinetic

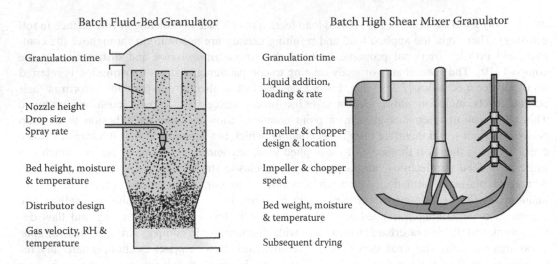

FIGURE 2.4   Typical Operating Variables for Pharmaceutical Granulation Processes. *Source*: From Refs. [2,5,8].

mechanisms and rate constants of wetting, growth, consolidation, and attrition. Overcoming a given size enlargement problem often requires changes in both processing conditions and in product formulation.

The importance of granule voidage to final product quality is illustrated in Figures 2.5 and 2.6 for a variety of formulations. Here, bulk density is observed to decrease, and granule attrition to increase. Similarly, the dissolution rate is known to increase with an increase in the granule voidage [1,5]. Bulk density is clearly a function of both granule size distribution, which controls bed voidage and the voidage or porosity within the granule itself. The data of Figure 2.5 is normalized with respect to its zero intercept, or its effective bulk density at zero-granule voidage. The granule attrition results of Figure 2.6 are based on a CIPAC test method, which is effectively the percentage of fines passing a fine mesh size following attrition in a tumbling apparatus. Granules weaken with increased voidage. All industries have their own specific quality and in-process evaluation tests. However, what they have in common are the important contributing effects of granule size and granule voidage in controlling granule quality.

The importance of distinguishing between the effects of process versus formulation changes can be illustrated with the help of Figure 2.6. Let us assume the particular formulation and current process conditions produce a granulated material with a given attrition resistance and dissolution behavior (indicted as "current product"). If one desires instead to reach a given "target," either the formulation or process variable may be changed. Changes to the process, or operating variables, generally readily alter granule voidage. Examples to decrease voidage might include increased bed height, increased processing time, or increased peak bed moisture. However, only a range of such changes in voidage is possible for a given formulation. The various curves are due to changes in formulation properties. Therefore, it may not be possible to reach a target change in granule properties without changes in formulation, or material variables. Examples of key material variables affecting voidage would include feed primary particle size, inherent formulation bond strength, and binder solution viscosity, as discussed in detail in the following sections. This crucial interaction between operating and material variables is crucial for the successful formulation and requires substantial collaboration between processing and formulation groups and a clear knowledge of the effect of scale-up on this interaction.

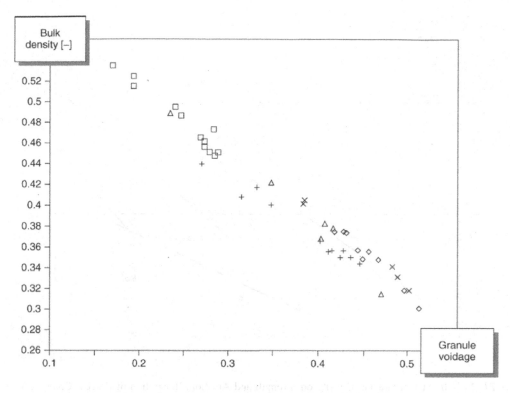

FIGURE 2.5 Impact of Granule Density on Bulk Density. Normalized Bulk Density as a Function of Granule Voidage.
Source: From Ref. [5].

2.1.5 Key Historical Investigations

A range of historical investigations has been undertaken involving the impact of operating variables on granulation behavior [4 6,14–23]. Two key pieces of historical investigation require mention, as the approach developed here stems heavily from this work. The first involves growth and breakage mechanisms that control the evolution of the granule size distribution [17] (Figure 2.7). There are strong interactions between these mechanisms. In addition, various forms have been incorporated into population balances modeling to predict granule size in the work of Sastry and Kapur [17–21] (see chapter 23 for details). Given the progress made in connecting rate constants to formulation properties, the utility of population balance modeling has increased substantially.

The second important area of contribution involves the work of Rumpf and colleagues [22–24], who studied the impact of interparticle force H, and in detail for capillary forces, on granule static tensile strength, or:

$$\sigma_T = \frac{9}{8}\left(\frac{1-\varepsilon}{\varepsilon}\right)\frac{H}{a^2} = A\left(\frac{1-\varepsilon}{\varepsilon}\right)\frac{\gamma\cos\theta}{a} \text{ with } \begin{cases} A = 9/4 \text{ for pendular state} \\ A = 9 \text{ for capillary state} \end{cases} \quad (2.2)$$

Forces of a variety of forms were studied, including viscous, semisolid, solid, electrostatic, and van der Waals forces

Of particular importance was the contribution of pendular bridge force arising from surface tension, and its contribution to granule tensile strength. Capillary pressure deficiency

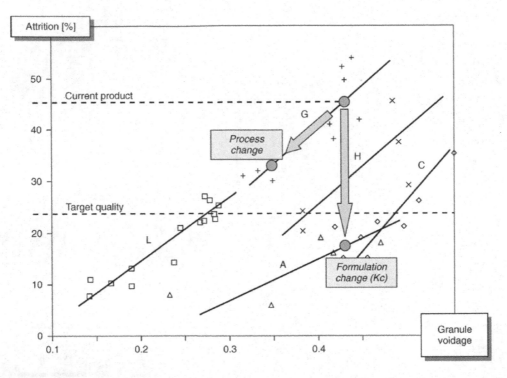

FIGURE 2.6 Impact of Granule Density on Strength and Attrition. Illustration of Process Changes Versus Formulation Changes. Individual Trendlines Represent the Processing Range for a Given Formulation. *Source*: From Ref. [5].

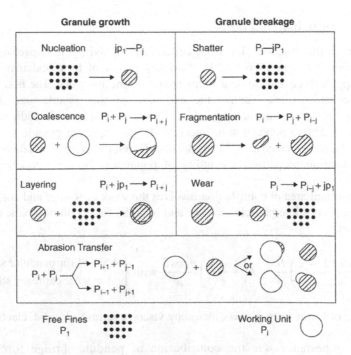

FIGURE 2.7 Growth and Breakage Mechanisms in Granulation Processes. *Source*: From Ref. [17].

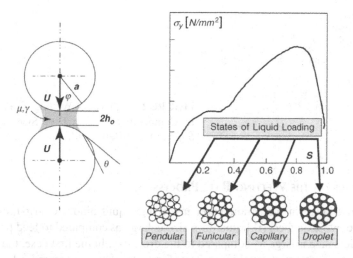

FIGURE 2.8 Static Yield Strength of Wet Agglomerates Versus Pore Saturation.
Source: From Refs. [21,22].

due to the curvature of the pendular bridge in addition to a contact line force results in an interparticle force, as highlighted in Figure 2.8 (here, interparticle velocity $U = 0$). This force summed over the granule area results in a granule static strength, which is a function of pore saturation S. The states of pore filling have been defined as pendular (single bridges), funicular (partial complete filling and single bridges), and capillary (nearly complete filling $S \sim$ 80–100%), followed by drop formation and loss of static strength. This approach will be extended in subsequent sections to include viscous forces and dynamic strength behavior ($U \neq 0$). The approach taken in this chapter follows this same vein of research as originally established by Rumpf and Kapur, namely, relating granule and particle level interactions to bulk behavior through the development of the rate processes of wetting and nucleation, granule growth and consolidation, and granule breakage and attrition. Each of these will now be dealt with in the subsequent sections.

2.2 WETTING

2.2.1 OVERVIEW

The initial distribution of binding fluid can have a pronounced influence on the size distribution of seed granules, or nuclei, which are formed from the fine powder. Both the final extent of and the rate at which the fluid wets the particulate phase are important. Poor wetting results in drop coalescence, fewer larger nuclei with ungranulated powder, and over-wetted masses, leading to broad nuclei distributions. Granulation can retain a memory, with nuclei size distribution impacting final granule size distribution. Therefore, initial wetting can be critical to uniform nuclei formation and often a narrow, uniform product. Wide nuclei distributions can lead to a wide granule size distribution. When the size of the particulate feed material is larger than drop size, wetting dynamics controls the distribution of coating material, which has a strong influence on the later stages of growth. Wetting phenomena also influence the redistribution of individual ingredients within a granule, drying processes, and redispersion of granules in a fluid phase. Other granule properties such as voidage, strength, and attrition resistance may be influenced as well. Preferential wetting of certain formulation ingredients can cause component segregation across granule size classes. An extensive review of wetting research may be found in Parfitt [25], Litster and Ennis [6], and Hapgood [26].

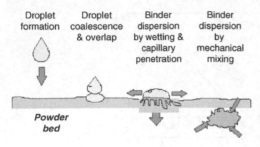

FIGURE 2.9 Stages of Wetting for Fine Powder as Wet by Comparatively Larger Drop Size.
Source: From Refs. [5,6].

2.2.2 MECHANICS OF THE WETTING RATE PROCESS

Wetting is the first stage in wet granulation involving liquid binder distribution onto the feed powder. There are two extremes: (i) liquid drop size is large as compared to feed particle or granule size, and (ii) particle size is large as compared to the drop size. In the first case, the wetting process consists of several important steps (Figure 2.9). First, droplets are formed related to spray distribution or spray flux defined as the wetting area of the bed per unit time. Both atomization and the rate of drops are critical. In addition to binder viscosity and rheology, important operating variables include nozzle position, spray area, spray rate, and drop size. Second, droplets impact and coalesce on the powder bed surface if mixing or wet-in time is slow, or the spray flux is low. Third, droplets spread and penetrate into the moving powder bed to form loose nuclei, again coalescing if wet-in is slow or mixing is slow. In the case of high-shear processes, shear forces breakdown over-wet clumps, also producing nuclei.

For the second case of small drop size compared with the primary particle size, the liquid will coat the particles. The coating is produced by collisions between the drop and the particle followed by the spreading of the liquid over the particle surface. If the particle is porous, then the liquid will also be sucked into its pores by capillary action, lowering the effective moisture content promoting growth [27]. Wetting dynamics control the distribution of coating material on large particles or formed granules, which has a strong influence on the later stages of growth as well as coating quality.

2.2.3 METHODS OF MEASUREMENT

Methods of characterizing wetting consist of four possible approaches: (i) drop spreading on powder compacts, (ii) penetration of fluid into powder beds, (iii) particle penetration into fluids, and (iv) interfacial characterization of powder surfaces [2,5,6]. In the first approach, the ability of a drop to spread is considered [25,28], and it involves the measurement of a contact angle θ of a drop on a powder compact, given by the Young-Dupré equation, or

$$\gamma^{sv} - \gamma^{sl} = \gamma^{lv}\cos\theta \tag{2.3}$$

where γ^{sv}, γ^{sl}, γ^{lv} are the solid-vapor, solid-liquid, and liquid-vapor interfacial energies, respectively, and θ is measured through the liquid. In the limit of $\gamma^{sv} - \gamma^{sl} \geq \gamma^{lv}$, the contact angle equals $0°$ and the fluid spreads on the solid and is often referred to as the spreading coefficient. The extent of wetting is controlled by the group $\gamma^{lv}\cos\theta$, which is referred to as adhesion tension. Sessile drop studies of contact angle can be performed on powder compacts in the same way as on planar surfaces. Methods involve (i) the direct measurement of the contact angle from the tangent to the air-binder interface, (ii) solution of the Laplace-Young equation involving the contact angle as a boundary condition, or (iii) indirect calculations of the contact angle from measurements of, for example, drop height. The compact can either be saturated with the fluid for static measurements, or dynamic measurements may be made through a computer imaging goniometer (Figure 2.10).

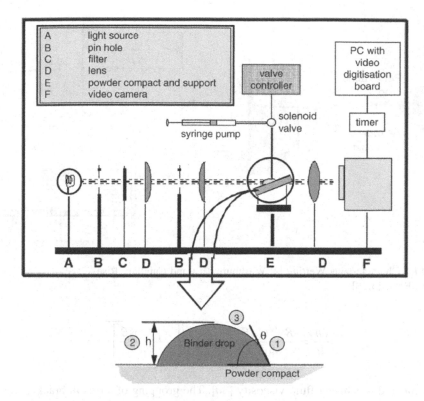

FIGURE 2.10 Characterizing Wetting by Dynamic Contact Angle Goniometry. *Source*: From Refs. [5,28].

For granulation processes, the dynamics of wetting are often crucial, requiring that powders be compared on the basis of a short timescale, dynamic contact angle. In addition, spreading velocity can be measured. Important factors are the physical nature of the powder surface (particle size, pore size, porosity, environment, roughness, pretreatment). The dynamic wetting process is, therefore, influenced by the rates of ingredient dissolution and surfactant adsorption and desorption kinetics [29].

The second approach to characterize wetting considers the ability of the fluid to penetrate into a powder bed (Figure 2.11). It involves the measurement of the extent and rate of fluid rise by capillary suction into a column of powder, better known as the Washburn test or the Bartell cell variant [30,31]. Considering the powder to consist of capillaries of radius R, the equilibrium height of rise h_e is determined by equating capillary and gravimetric pressures, or:

$$h_e = \frac{2\gamma^{lv}\cos\theta}{\Delta\rho g R} \tag{2.4}$$

where $\Delta\rho$ is the fluid density with respect to air, and g is gravity. In addition to the equilibrium height of rise, the dynamics of penetration are particularly important. Ignoring gravity and equating viscous losses with the capillary pressure, the rate (dh/dt) and dynamic height of rise h are given by:

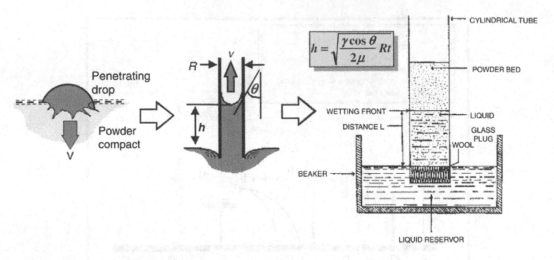

FIGURE 2.11 Characterizing Wetting by Washburn Test and Capillary Rise.
Source: From Refs. [5,28].

$$\frac{dh}{dt} = \frac{R\gamma^{lv}\cos\theta}{4\mu h}, \text{ or } h = \sqrt{\left[\frac{R\gamma^{lv}\cos\theta}{2\mu}\right]t} \qquad (2.5)$$

where t is time and μ is binder fluid viscosity [30]. The grouping of terms in brackets involves the material properties that control the dynamics of fluid penetration, namely average pore radius, or tortuosity R (related to particle size and void distribution of the powder), adhesion tension, and binder viscosity. The rate of capillary fluid rise, or the rate of binding fluid penetration in wet granulation, increases with increasing pore radius (generally coarser powders with larger surface-volume average particle size), increasing adhesion tension (increased surface tension and decreased contact angle), and decreased binder viscosity.

The contact angle of a binder-particle system itself is not a primary thermodynamic quantity, but rather a reflection of individual interfacial energies, which are a function of the molecular interactions of each phase with respect to one another. Interfacial energy may be broken down into its dispersion and polar components. These components reflect the chemical character of the interface, with the polar component due to hydrogen bonding and other polar interactions and the dispersion component due to van der Waals interactions. These components may be determined by the wetting tests described here, where a variety of solvents are chosen as the wetting fluids to probe-specific molecular interactions [32]. Interfacial energy is strongly influenced by trace impurities that arise in the crystallization of the active ingredient, or other forms of processing such as grinding. It may be modified by the judicious selection of surfactants [32,33].

Charges can also exist at interfaces, as characterized by electrokinetic studies [34]. The total solid-fluid interfacial energy (i.e., both dispersion and polar components) is also referred to as the critical solid surface energy of the particulate phase. It is equal to the surface tension of a fluid, which just wets the solid with zero contact angle. This property of the particle feed may be determined by a third approach to characterize wetting, involving the penetration of particles into a series of fluids of varying surface tension [33,35], or by the variation of sediment height [36].

The last approach to characterizing wetting involves chemical probing of properties, which control surface energy [34,37]. As just described, these methods include electrokinetic and surfactant adsorption studies. Additional methods are moisture or solvent adsorption studies and inverse gas chromatography (IGC). A distinct advantage of IGC is reproducible measurements of physical and chemical surface properties that control adhesion tension. IGC uses the same principles and equipment as standard gas chromatography [38], however, the role of the gas and solid phases are reversed. In the case of IGC, the mobile phase consists of probe gas molecules that move through a column packed with the powder of interest, which is now the stationary phase. As the probe molecules travel through the column, they adsorb onto and desorb off the powder. The rate and degree of this interaction are determined by the surface chemistry of the powder and the probe molecules. Since the surface chemistry of the probe molecules is known, this allows the calculation of the surface energies of the powder with the help of a series of plots of alkane and various polar probes. The strength of the solid/liquid interactions determines the average retention time of a probe, which is converted into net retention volume V_N.

The free energy of desorption is then given by:

$$\Delta G = RT \ln V_N + c = 2Na\left(\sqrt{\gamma_S^D \gamma_L^D} + \sqrt{\gamma_S^P \gamma_L^P}\right) \tag{2.6}$$

where R is the universal gas constant, T is the column temperature, c is a system constant, N is Avogadro's number, and a is the surface area of a probe molecule. As illustrated in Figure 2.12, a plot of $RT \ln V_N$ versus $a\sqrt{\gamma_L^D}$ should give a straight line for a series of alkanes, the slope of which allows determination of the solid's dispersive surface energy γ_S^D. Plotting $RT \ln V_N$ versus $a\sqrt{\gamma_L^D}$ for the polar probes will give a point that is generally somewhere above the alkane reference line. The polar solid energy γ_S^P is then found from a plot of these deviations.

2.2.4 GRANULATION EXAMPLES OF WETTING

Wetting dynamics have a pronounced influence on initial nuclei distribution formed from the fine powder. As an example, the initial nuclei size in fluid-bed granulation is shown to increase with

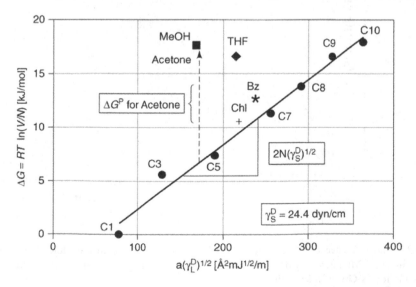

FIGURE 2.12 Characterizing Wetting by Inverse Gas Chromatography.
Source: From Ref. [5].

decreasing contact angle, and therefore increasing adhesion tension (Figure 2.13). The water contact angle was varied by changing the percentages of hydrophilic lactose and hydrophobic salicylic acid [39]. Aulton et al. [40] also demonstrated the influence of surfactant concentration on shifting nuclei size due to changes in adhesion tension.

Figure 2.14A illustrates an example of dynamic imaging of drop wetting, where a time series of drop profiles are imaged as a drop wets into a formulation. Note that the timescale of wetting, in this case, is two seconds, with nearly complete wet-in occurring in one second. This particular formulation was granulated on a continuous pan system in excess of 2 ton/hr. Figure 2.14B compares differences in lots of the formulation. Note that a second lot—referred to as problem active—experiences significantly degraded granule strength and required production rates to be substantially reduced. This is associated with nearly twice the initial contact angle (120°) and a slower spreading velocity when compared with the good active. Poor wetting in practice can translate into reduced production rates to compensate for increased time for drops to work into the powder bed surface. Weaker granules are also often observed, since poor wet phase interfacial behavior translates, in part, to poor solid bond strength and high granule voidage. Note that differences in the lots are only observed over the first one-fourth to half a second, illustrating the importance of comparing dynamic behavior of formulations, after which time surfactant adsorption/desorption reduces contact angle.

As an example of Washburn approaches, the effect of the rate and extent of fluid penetration on granule size distribution for drum granulation were shown by Gluba [41]. Increasing penetration rate, as reflected by (2.5) increased granule size and decreased asymmetry of the granule size distribution (Figure 2.15).

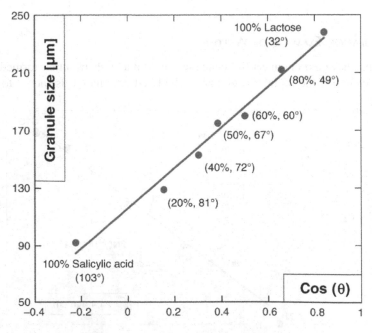

FIGURE 2.13 The Influence of Contact Angle on Nuclei Size Formed in the Fluid-Bed Granulation of Lactose/Salicylic Acid Mixtures. Powder Contact Angle Determined by Goniometry and Lactose Percentage of Each Formulation is Given in Parentheses.
Source: From Ref. [39].

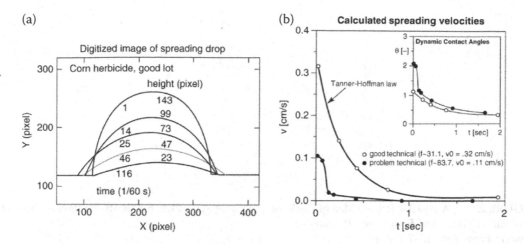

FIGURE 2.14 Dynamic Imaging of Drop Wetting and its Impact on Continuous Pan Granulation. (a) Dynamic Image of a Drop Wetting into a Formulation with a Good Active Ingredient. (b) Comparison of Surface Spreading Velocity and Dynamic Contact Angle Versus Time for Good and Problem Active Ingredients or Technical. Problem Active Required Reduced Production Rates.
Source: From Ref. [5].

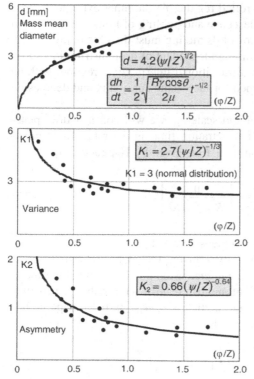

FIGURE 2.15 Influence of Capillary Penetration on Drum Granule Size. Increasing Penetration Rate, as Reflected by (2.5) Increases Granule Size and Decreases Asymmetry of the Granule Size Distribution.
Source: From Ref. [41].

2.2.5 REGIMES OF NUCLEATION AND WETTING

The mechanisms of nucleation and wetting may be determined from a wetting regime map (Figure 2.16), and is controlled by two key parameters. The first is the time required for a drop to wet into the moving powder bed, in comparison to the circulation time of the process. As

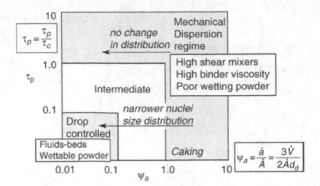

FIGURE 2.16 A Possible Regime Map of Nucleation, Relating Spray Flux, Solids Mixing (Solids Flux and Circulation Time), and Formulation Properties.
Source: From Refs. [5–7,26,42].

discussed previously, this wet-in time is strongly influenced by formulation properties [(2.5)]. The second parameter is the actual spray rate or spray flux, in comparison with solids flux moving through the spray zones. Spray flux is strongly influenced by process design and operation. If wet-in is rapid and spray fluxes are low, individual drops will form discrete nuclei somewhat larger than the drop size in a droplet-controlled regime. At the other extreme, if drop penetration is slow and spray flux is large, drop coalescence and pooling of binder material will occur throughout the powder bed. Shear forces due to solids mixing must then breakdown over-wet masses or clumps in a mechanical dispersion regime, independent of drop distribution. Drop overlap and coalescence occur to varying extents in a transitional intermediate regime, with an increasingly wider nucleation distribution being formed for increasing spray flux and decreasing wet-in time.

To better understand the impact of process design and scale-up, we will consider drop penetration time and spray flux in greater detail. Small penetration time is desirable for droplet-controlled nucleation. Dimensionless drop penetration time T_p is given by Hapgood [26]:

$$T_p = \frac{t_p}{t_c} \text{ where } t_p = 1.35 \frac{V_d^{2/3}}{\varepsilon_{eff}^2} \left[\frac{\mu}{R_{eff} \gamma \cos\theta} \right] \tag{2.7}$$

Note the similarity with the Washburn relation (2.5). Dimensionless drop wet-in time decreases with increasing pore radius R_{eff}, decreasing binder viscosity μ, increasing adhesion tension $\gamma \cos\theta$, decreasing drop volume V_d, increasing bed porosity ε_{eff}, and increasing process circulation time t_c. Circulation time is a function of mixing and bed weight and can change with scale-up. Effective pore radius R_{eff} is related to the surface-volume average particle size d_{32}, particle shape ϕ, bed porosity ε, tapped porosity ε_{tap}, and effective porosity ε_{eff} by:

$$R_{eff} = \frac{\varphi d_{32}}{3} \left(\frac{\varepsilon_{eff}}{1 - \varepsilon_{eff}} \right) \varepsilon_{eff} = \varepsilon_{tap} \left(1 + \varepsilon + \varepsilon_{tap} \right) \tag{2.8}$$

To remain within a droplet-controlled regime of nucleation, the penetration time t_p should be less than the characteristic circulation time t_c of the granulator in question.

Now turning attention to spray distribution, the dimensionless spray flux Ψ_d is the ratio of the rate at which drops cover a given spray area ψ_d to the rate at which solids move through this same zone ψ_s and is a measure of the density of drops falling on the powder surface. The volumetric spray rate V' and drop size d_d determine the number of drops formed per unit time, and, therefore, both the area occupied by a single drop and the total drop coverage area per unit time, or $\psi_d = 3V'/2d_d$. The dimensionless spray flux is then given as follows:

$$\Psi_d = \frac{\psi_d}{\psi_s} = \frac{3}{2}\frac{V'}{d_d\psi_s} \tag{2.9}$$

As with drop penetration time, spray flux plays a role in defining the regimes of nucleation (Figures 2.16 and 2.17) [5,6,26]. For small spray flux ($\Psi_d < 0.1$), drops will not overlap on contact and will form separate discrete nuclei if the drops also have fast penetration time. For large spray flux ($\Psi_d > .5$), however, significant drop overlap occurs, forming nuclei much larger than drop size, and in the limit, independent of drop size. Spray flux is strongly influenced by process design.

For the case of random drop deposition described by a Poisson's distribution (Figure 2.18), Hapgood [26] showed the fraction of surface covered by spray:

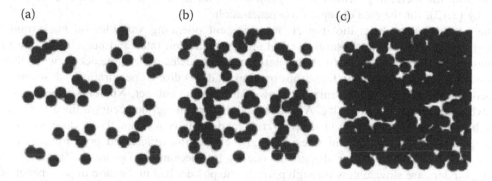

FIGURE 2.17   Monte-Carlo Simulations of Drop Coverage on a Powder Bed: (A) $\Psi_d = 0.26$, (B) $\Psi_d = 0.59$, and (C) $\Psi_d = 2.4$.
Source: From Refs. [6,24].

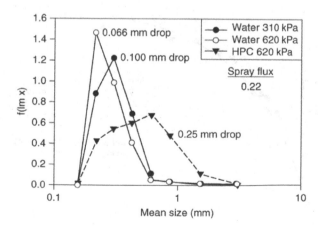

FIGURE 2.18   Effect of Spray Drop Distribution at Low Spray Flux on Nuclei Distribution. Lactose Feed Powder in the Spinning Granulator.
Source: From Refs. [33,42].

$$f_{single} = 1 - \exp(-\Psi_d) \qquad (2.10)$$

In addition, the fraction of single drops forming individual nuclei (assuming rapid drop penetration) versus the number of agglomerates formed was given as follows:

$$f_{single} = \exp(-4\Psi_d) \qquad (2.11)$$

and

$$f_{agglom} = 1 - \exp(-4\Psi_d) \qquad (2.12)$$

Examples of the above as applied to nucleation are described by Litster et al. [42]. Here, nuclei distribution was studied as a function of drop size and spray flux. For a moderate, intermediate spray flux of $\Psi_d = 0.22$, a clear relationship is seen between nuclei size and spray distribution, with nuclei formed somewhat larger than the drop size (Figure 2.18). In addition, the nuclei distribution widens with the increasing formation of agglomerates for increasing spray flux (Figure 2.19), as given by (2.12), for the case of rapid drop penetration.

The spray flux captures the impact of equipment operating variables on nucleation and wetting, and as such is very useful for scale-up if nucleation rates and nuclei sizes are to be maintained constant (Figure 2.16). A droplet-controlled nucleation regime occurs when there is both low spray flux—relatively few drops overlap; and fast droplet penetration—drops wet into the bed completely before bed mixing allows further drop contact. Nuclei will be formed of somewhat larger than the drop size. A mechanical dispersion regime occurs at the other extreme of high spray flux—giving large drop overlap and coalescence, and large drop penetration times, promoted by poor wet-in rates and slow circulation times, and poor mixing. In this regime, nucleation and binder dispersion occurs by mechanical agitation. Viscous, poorly wetting binders are slow to flow through pores in the powder bed in the case of poor penetration time. Drop coalescence on the powder surface occurs (also known as "pooling") creating very broad nuclei size distributions. Binder solution delivery method (drop size, nozzle height) typically has minimal effect on the nuclei size distribution, though interfacial properties may affect nuclei and final granule strength. An intermediate regime exists for moderate drop

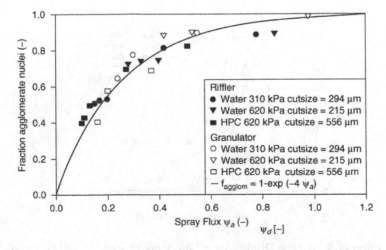

FIGURE 2.19 Agglomerate Formation with Lactose, Water, and HPLC Spray Solutions.
Source: From Refs. [42].

penetration times and moderate spray flux, with the resulting nuclei regime narrowing with decreases in both.

There are several implications with regard to the nucleation regime map in the troubleshooting of wetting and nucleation problems. If drop penetration times are large, making adjustments to spray may not be sufficient to narrower granule size distributions if remaining in the mechanical regime. Significant changes to wetting and nucleation occur only if changes take the system across a regime boundary. This can occur in an undesirable way if processes are not scaled with due attention to remaining in the drop controlled regime, or alternatively, within the mechanical dispersion regime. For example, scale-up may cause a granulation process to move from one regime of wetting to another, resulting in unexpected behavior and an entirely different dependence of atomization method and mixing.

2.2.6 EXAMPLE OF WETTING REGIME CALCULATION

As an example of wetting calculations [78], consider an idealized powder bed shown in Figure 2.20 of width $B = 0.10$ m, moving past a flat spray of spray rate $dV/dt = 100$ mL/min as a solids velocity of $w = 1.0$ m/sec. For a given spray rate, the number of drops is determined by drop volume or diameter $d_d = 100$ μm, which, in turn, defines the drop area a per unit time, which will be covered by the spray, giving a spray flux ψ_d of:

$$\psi_d = \frac{da}{dt} = \frac{dV/dt}{V_d}\left(\frac{\pi d_d^2}{4}\right) = \frac{3}{2}\frac{(dV/dt)}{d_d} = \frac{3}{2}\frac{(100 \times 10^{-6}/60 \text{ m/s})}{(100 \times 10^{-6} \text{ m})} = 0.025 \text{ m}^2/\text{s} \quad (2.13)$$

As droplets contact the powder bed at a certain rate, the powder moves past the spray zone at its own velocity, or at solids flux ψ_s given for this simple example by:

$$\psi_s = \frac{dA}{dt} = B_w = 0.1 \text{ m} \times 1.0 \text{ m/s} = 0.1 \text{ m}^2/\text{sec} \quad (2.14)$$

This gives a dimensionless spray flux of:

$$\Psi_d = \frac{\psi_d}{\psi_s} = \frac{0.025 \text{ m}^2/\text{sec}}{0.1 \text{ m}^2/\text{sec}} = 0.25 \quad (2.15)$$

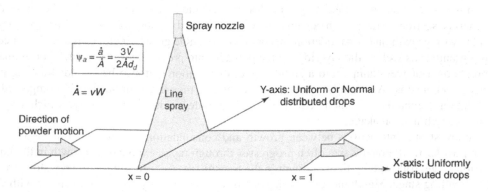

FIGURE 2.20 Idealized Flat Spray Zone in a Spinning Riffle Granulator.
Source: From Refs. [6,24].

This is at the limit of allowable spray flux to remain within a droplet-controlled regime. If double the spray rate is required, wetting and nucleation would occur within the mechanical dispersion regime, diminishing the need for spray nozzles. To lower the spray rate by a factor of two, as safety for droplet-controlled nucleation, either two nozzles spread well apart, double the solids velocity, or half the spray rate would be needed (e.g., doubling the spray cycle time). Alternately, smaller drops might prove helpful.

The last requirement for droplet-controlled growth would be a short drop penetration time. For a lactose powder of $d_{32} = 20$ μm, and loose and tapped voidage of $\varepsilon = 0.60$ and $\varepsilon_{tap} = 0.40$, the effective voidage and pore radius are given by:

$$\varepsilon_{eff} = \varepsilon_{tap}\left(1 - \varepsilon + \varepsilon_{tap}\right) = 0.4(1 - 0.6 + 0.4) = 0.32 \tag{2.16}$$

$$R_{eff} = \frac{\varphi d_{32}}{3}\left(\frac{\varepsilon_{eff}}{1 - \varepsilon_{eff}}\right) = \frac{0.9 \times 20}{3}\left(\frac{0.32}{1 - 0.32}\right) = 2.8 \text{ μm} \tag{2.17}$$

The penetration time should be no more than 10% of the circulation time. For water with a viscosity of $\mu = 1$, $cp = 0.001$ Pa/sec, and adhesion tension of $\gamma \cos\theta = .033$ N/m, we obtain a penetration time of

$$t_p = 1.35\frac{V_d^{2/3}}{\varepsilon_{eff}^2}\left[\frac{\mu}{R_{eff}\gamma\cos\theta}\right] = 1.35\frac{(100 \times 10^{-6}\pi/6)^{2/3}}{0.32^2}\left[\frac{0.001}{2.8 \times 10^{-6} \times 0.033}\right] = 0.0009 \text{ sec} \tag{2.18}$$

Note that the penetration time is a strong function of drop size ($\propto d_d^2$) and viscosity. For a 100-fold increase in viscosity representative of a typical binding solution and twice the drop size, the penetration time would increase to 0.4 seconds. This time could, in fact, be short when compared with the circulation times of high-shear systems, suggesting a move toward mechanical dispersion.

2.3 GRANULE GROWTH AND CONSOLIDATION

2.3.1 MECHANICS OF GROWTH AND CONSOLIDATION

The evolution of the granule size distribution is controlled by several mechanisms. The nucleation of fine powders and coating of existing granules by the fluid phase has already been discussed in the previous section. Breakage mechanisms will be treated in the following. Here, we focus particularly on growth and consolidation mechanisms. Granule growth includes the coalescence of existing granules as well as the layering of fine powder onto previously formed nuclei or granules. The breakdown of wet clumps into a stable nuclei distribution can also be included among coalescence mechanisms. As granules grow by coalescence, they are simultaneously compacted by consolidation mechanisms, which reduce internal granule voidage or porosity, which impacts granule strength and breakage.

There are strong interactions between growth and consolidation, as illustrated in Figure 2.21. For fine powder feed, granule size often progresses through rapid, exponential growth in the initial nucleation stage, followed by linear growth in the transition stage, finishing with very slow growth in a final balling stage. Simultaneously with growth, granule porosity is seen to decrease with time as the granules are compacted. Granule growth and consolidation are intimately connected;

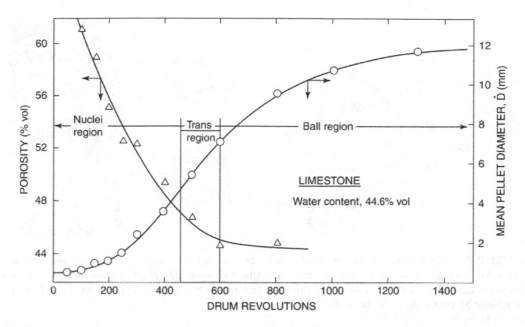

FIGURE 2.21 Granule Porosity and Mean (Pellet) Size. Typical Regimes of Granule Growth and Consolidation, Shown for Drum Granulation of Fine Limestone.
Source: From Refs. [18–21].

increases in granule size are shown here to be associated with a decrease in granule porosity. This is a dominant theme in wet granulation.

As originally outlined in Ennis [4], these growth patterns are common throughout the fluidized bed, drum, pan, and high-shear mixer processes for a variety of formulations. Specific mechanisms of growth may dominate for a process—sometimes to the exclusion of others, with the prevailing mechanisms dictated by the interaction of formulation properties, which control granule deformability, and operating variables, which control the local level of shear, or bed agitation intensity.

For two colliding granules to coalesce rather than break up, the collisional kinetic energy must first be dissipated to prevent rebound as illustrated in Figure 2.22. In addition, the strength of the bond must resist any subsequent breakup forces in the process. The ability of the granules to deform during processing may be referred to as the formulation's deformability, and deformability has a large effect on the growth rate, as well as granule consolidation. Increases in deformability increase the bonding or contact area, thereby dissipating and resisting breakup forces. From a balance of binding and separating forces and torque acting within the area of granule contact, Ouchiyama and Tanaka [43] derived a critical limit of size above which coalescence becomes impossible or a maximum growth limit is given by:

$$D_c = \begin{cases} (AQ^{3/2}K^{3/2}\sigma_{\mathrm{T}})^{1/4} \ \text{plastic deformation}\,(K \propto 1/H) \\ (AQK^{3/2}\sigma_{\mathrm{T}})^{1/3} \ \text{elastic deformation}\,(K \propto 1/E^{2/3}) \end{cases} \qquad (2.19)$$

Here, K is deformability, a proportionality constant relating the maximum compressive force Q to the deformed contact area, A is a constant with units of [L^3/F] and σ_{T} is the tensile strength of the granule bond. Depending on the type of collision, deformability K is a function of either hardness H, or reduced elastic modulus E^*. Granules are compacted as they collide. This expels pore fluid to

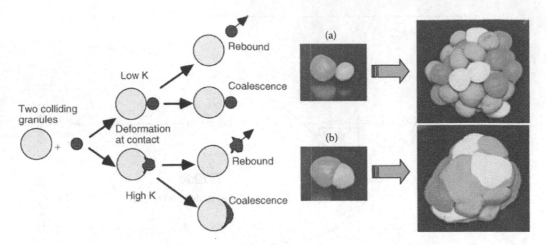

FIGURE 2.22   Mechanisms of Granule Coalescence for Low and High Deformability Systems. Rebound Occurs for Average Granule Sizes Greater than the Critical Granule Size D_c. K = Deformability. Granule Structures Resulting From (a) Low- and (b) High-Deformability Systems, Typical for Fluid-Bed and High-Shear Mixer Granulators, Respectively.
Source: From Refs. [1,2,4,5,7].

the granule surface, thereby increasing local liquid saturation in the contact area of colliding granules. This surface fluid (i) increases the tensile strength of the liquid bond σ_T, and (ii) increases surface plasticity and deformability K.

The degree of granule deformation taking place during granule collisions defines possible growth mechanisms (Figure 2.22). If little deformation takes place, the system is referred to as a low-deformability/low-shear process. This generally includes fluid bed, drum, and pan granulators. Growth is largely controlled by the extent of any surface fluid layer and surface deformability, which act to dissipate collisional kinetic energy and allow permanent coalescence. Growth generally occurs at a faster timescale than overall granule deformation and consolidation. This is depicted in Figure 2.22, where smaller granules can still be distinguished as part of a larger granule structure, or a popcorn-type appearance as often occurs in fluid-bed granulation. Note that such a structure may not be observed if layering or nucleation alone dominates. Granules may also be compacted, becoming smoother over time because of the longer-timescale process of consolidation. Granule coalescence and consolidation have less interaction than they do with high deformability systems, making low-deformability/ low-shear systems easier to scale-up and control, for systems without high recycling.

For high-shear rates, large granule deformation occurs during collisions, and granule growth and consolidation occur on the same timescale. Such a system is referred to as a deformable/high-shear process, and includes a continuous pin and plow shear-type mixers, as well as batch high-shear pharmaceutical mixers. In these cases, kinetic energy is dissipated through the deformation of the wet mass composing the granule. Rather than the sticking together mechanism of low-deformability processes such as a fluid-bed, granules are smashed or kneaded together, and smaller granules are not distinguishable within the granule structure (Figure 2.22). High-shear and high-deformable processes generally produce denser granules than their low-deformability counterpart. In addition, the combined and competing effects of granule coalescence and consolidation make high-shear processes difficult to scale-up.

Although these extremes of growth are still the subject of much research investigation, a general model has emerged to help process engineers unravel the impact of operating variables and process selection. Two key dimensionless groups control growth. As originally defined by Ennis [4] and

Tardos and Khan [44], these are the viscous and deformation Stokes numbers are given, respectively, by:

$$St_v = \frac{4\rho u_o d}{9\mu} \tag{2.20}$$

$$St_{def} = \frac{\rho u_o^2}{\sigma_y}(\text{impact}) \text{ or } \frac{\rho(du/dx)^2 d^2}{\sigma_y}(\text{shear}) \tag{2.21}$$

The viscous Stokes number St_v is the ratio of kinetic energy to viscous work due to binding fluid occurring during granule/particle collisions. Low St_v or low granule energy represents an increased likelihood of granule coalescence and growth, and this occurs for small granule or particle size (d is the harmonic average of granule diameter), low relative collision velocity u_o or granule density ρ, and high binder phase viscosity μ. The deformation Stokes number represents the amount of granule deformation taking place during collisions and is similarly a ratio of kinetic energy to wet mass yield stress, a measure of granule deformability.

Bed agitation intensity is controlled by mechanical variables of the process such as fluid-bed excess gas velocity or mixer impeller and chopper speed. Agitation intensity controls the relative collisional and shear velocities of granules within the process and therefore growth, breakage, consolidation, and final product density. Figure 2.23 summarizes typical characteristic velocities, agitation intensities, and compaction pressures, and product relative densities achieved for a variety of size enlargement processes.

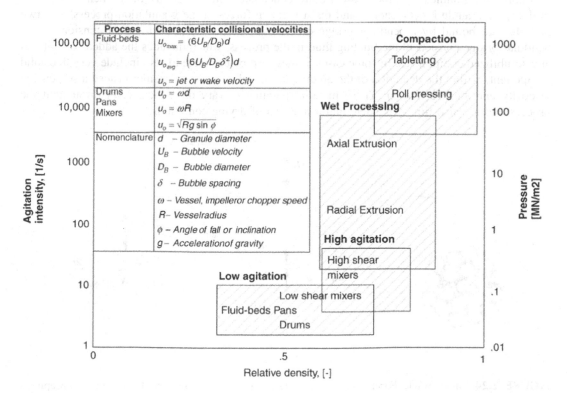

FIGURE 2.23 Classification of Agglomeration Processes by Agitation Intensity and Compaction Pressure. *Source*: From Refs. [1,3].

Note that the process or formulation itself cannot define whether it falls into a low or high agitation intensity process. As discussed more fully further, it is a function of both the level of shear as well as the formulation deformability. A very stiff formulation with low deformability may behave as a low-deformability system in a high-shear mixer, or a very pliable formulation may act as a high-deformable system in a fluid-bed granulator.

Granule consolidation or densification is also controlled by Stokes numbers, and typically increases for all processes with increasing residence time, shear levels, bed height, bed moisture or granule saturation, particle feed size or pore radius, surface tension, and decreasing binding fluid viscosity. Simultaneous drying or reaction usually acts to arrest granule densification.

2.3.2 INTERPARTICLE FORCES

Interstitial fluid and resulting pendular bridges play a large role in both, granule growth and granule deformability. As shown previously, they control the static yield stress of wet agglomerates [Figure 2.8, (2.2)]. Pendular bridges between particles of which a granule is composed give rise to capillary and viscous interparticle forces, which allows friction to act between point contacts (Figure 2.24). Interparticle forces due to pendular bridges and their impact on deformability warrant further attention. Note that capillary forces for small contact angles attract particles (but repel for $\theta > 90°$), whereas viscous and frictional forces always act to resist the direction of motion.

As originally developed by Ennis [4], consider two spherical particles of radius as separated by a gap distance $2h_o$ approaching one another at a velocity U (Figure 2.24). The particles could represent two primary particles within the granule, in which case we are concerned about the contribution of interparticle forces on granule strength and deformability. Or they could represent two colliding granules, in which case we are concerned with the ability of the pendular bridge to dissipate granule kinetic energy and resist breakup forces in the granulation process. The two particles are bound by a pendular bridge of viscosity μ, density ρ, and surface tension γ. The pendular bridge consists of the binding fluid in the process, which includes the added solvent and any solubilized components. In some cases, it may also be desirable to also include very fine solid components within the definition of the binding fluid, and, therefore, consider instead a suspension viscosity and surface tension. These material parameters vary on a local level throughout the process and are also time-dependent and a function of drying conditions.

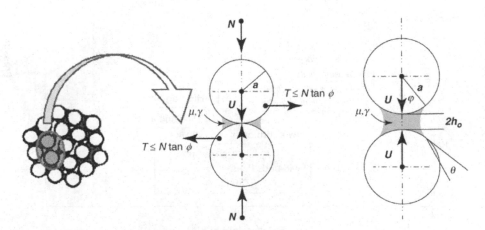

FIGURE 2.24 Interparticle Forces and Granule Deformability. Interparticle Forces Include Capillary Forces, Viscous Lubrication Forces, and Frictional Forces.
Source: From Ref. [4].

For the case of a static liquid bridge (i.e., $U = 0$) with perfect wetting, surface tension induces an attractive capillary force between the two particles due to a three-phase contact line force and a pressure deficiency arising from interfacial curvature. (For a poorly wetting fluid, the capillary pressure can be positive leading to a repulsive force.) The impact of this static pendular bridge force on static granule strength has been studied and reported extensively [3,22–24]. It is important to recognize that in most processes, however, the particles are moving relative to one another and, therefore, the bridging liquid is in motion. This gives rise to viscous resistance forces, which can contribute significantly to the total bridge strength. The strengths of both Newtonian and non-Newtonian pendular bridges have been studied extensively [4,45,46]. For Newtonian fluids [4,38,45], the dimensionless dynamic strength was shown to be given by:

$$\frac{F}{\pi\gamma a} = F_{\mathrm{cap}} + F_{\mathrm{vis}} = F_{\mathrm{o}} + \frac{3\mathrm{Ca}}{\varepsilon} \quad \text{where} \quad \begin{cases} F_{\mathrm{cap}} = (2 - 2H_{\mathrm{o}})\sin^2\varphi \\ \quad F_{\mathrm{vis}} = 3\mathrm{Ca}/\varepsilon \\ \quad\quad \mathrm{Ca} = \mu U/\gamma \end{cases} \quad (2.22)$$

Forces have been made dimensionless with respect to a measure of the capillary force, or $\pi\gamma a$. Ca is the capillary dimensionless group given as the ratio of viscous to static capillary forces. F_{cap} is the strength of a static capillary bridge, which is a function of air-fluid interfacial curvature H_{o} and the filling angle φ. In dimensional form, it is given by:

$$F_{\mathrm{cap}}^* = \pi\gamma a(2 - 2H_{\mathrm{o}})\sin^2\varphi \quad (2.23)$$

F_{vis} is the strength of a viscous, dynamic bridge, and is equivalent to the force between two spheres approaching one another in an infinite fluid. This force is a function of binder viscosity μ, and the collision velocity U. Here, $\varepsilon = 2h_{\mathrm{o}}/a$ is gap distance and not granule voidage. In dimensional form, the viscous force is given by:

$$F_{\mathrm{vis}}^* = 6\pi\mu U a/\varepsilon \quad (2.24)$$

From (2.22), one finds that the dynamic bridge force begins with the static bridge strength, which is a constant independent of velocity (or Ca), and then increases linearly with Ca, which is a capillary number representing the ratio of viscous (μUa) to capillary (γa) forces and is proportional to velocity. This is confirmed experimentally as illustrated in Figure 2.25 for the case of two spheres approaching axially. Extensions of the theory have also been conducted for nonNewtonian fluids (shear thinning), shearing motions, particle roughness, wettability, and time-dependent drying binders. The reader is referred to Ennis [4,45] for additional details.

For small velocities, small binder viscosity, and large gap distances, the strength of the bridge will approximate a static pendular bridge, or F_{cap}, which is proportional to and increases with increasing surface tension. This force is equivalent to the static pendular force previously given in (2.23) as studied by Rumpf [22–24]. On the other hand, for large binder viscosities and velocities, or small gap distances, the bridge strength will approximately be equal to F_{vis}, which increases with increasing binder viscosity and velocity. This viscous force is singular in the gap distance and increases dramatically for the small separation of the particles. It is important to note that as granules are consolidated, resulting in decreases in effective interparticle gap distance, and binders dry, resulting in large increases in binder viscosity, that the dynamic bridge strength can exceed the static strength by orders of magnitude.

Lastly, the role of interparticle friction can be large, though rigorous experimental studies of the interaction between particle friction, granule porosity, and binder viscosity, and surface tension in controlling bulk dynamic yield stress have not been undertaken.

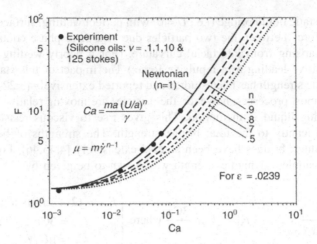

FIGURE 2.25 Maximum Strength of a Liquid Bridge Between Two Axial Moving Particles as a Function of Ca for Newtonian and Shear-Thinning Fluids.
Source: From Refs. [4,43].

2.3.3 DYNAMIC WET MASS RHEOLOGY AND GRANULE DEFORMABILITY

Granule deformability and the maximum critical size D_c are strong functions of moisture. Figure 2.26A illustrates the low-shear rate, stress-strain behavior of agglomerates during compression as a function of liquid saturation. Deformability K is related to both the yield strength of the material σ_y, that is, the ability of the material to resist stresses, and the ability of the surface to be strained without degradation or rupture of the granule, with this maximum allowable critical deformation strain denoted by $(\Delta L/L)_c$. In general, high deformability K requires low yield strength σ_y and high critical strain $(\Delta L/L)_c$, which is a measure of plastic versus brittle deformation. Increasing granule saturation increases deformability by lowering interparticle frictional. In most cases, granule deformability increases with increasing moisture (or granule saturation to be more precise), decreasing binder viscosity, decreasing surface tension, decreasing interparticle friction, and increasing average particle size (specifically d_{sv}, or the surface-volume mean size), as well as increasing bed agitation intensity.

Figure 2.26A illustrates yield stress behavior for slow yielding. However, the dependence of interparticle forces on shear rate impact wet mass rheology and, therefore, deformability. Figure 2.26B demonstrates that the peak flow or dynamic yield stress increases proportionally with compression velocity [47]. In fact, in a similar fashion to dynamic liquid bridge forces, the peak flow stress of wet unsaturated compacts is seen to also increase with bulk capillary number $\overline{Ca}$ (Figure 2.27 ahead):

$$\frac{\sigma_y^{Peak}}{\gamma/a} = \sigma_o + A\overline{Ca}^B \text{ where } \begin{cases} \sigma_o = 5.0 - 5.3 \\ A = 280 - 320, \quad B = 0.58 - 0.64 \\ \overline{Ca} = \mu\varepsilon\, a/\gamma \end{cases} \quad (2.25)$$

There are several important points worth noting. First is the similarity between the yield strength of the compact [(2.25)] and the strength of the individual dynamic pendular bridge [(2.22)]; both curves are similar in shape with a capillary number dependency. As with the pendular bridge,

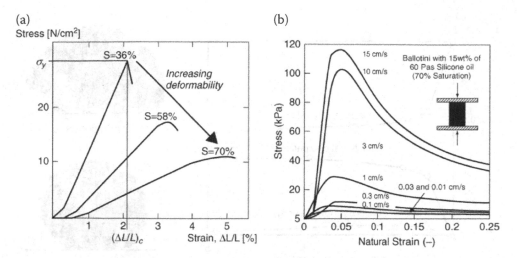

FIGURE 2.26 (**A**) The Influence of Sample Saturation S on Deformation Strain ($\Delta L/L$) and Yield Strength σ_y. Dicalcium Phosphate with 15 wt.% Binding Solution of PVP/PVA Kollidon® VA64. Fifty Percent Compact Porosity. (**B**) Typical Compact Stress Response for Fast Compression Versus Crosshead Compression Velocity for Glass Ballotini (d_{32} = 35 μm).
Source: From Refs. [45,47].

two regions may be defined. In region 1, for a bulk capillary number of $Ca < 10^{-4}$, the strength or yield stress of the compact depends on the static pendular bridge, and therefore on surface tension, particle size, and liquid loading. In region 2, for $Ca > 10^{-4}$, the strength depends on the dynamic pendular bridge, and therefore on binder viscosity and strain rate, in addition to particle size.

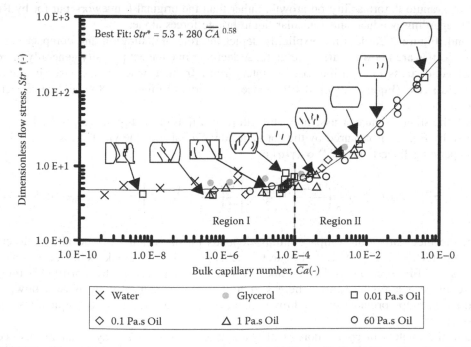

FIGURE 2.27 Dimensionless Peak Flow Stress of Figure 2.26B Versus Bulk Capillary Number, for Various Binder Solutions.
Source: From Ref. [40].

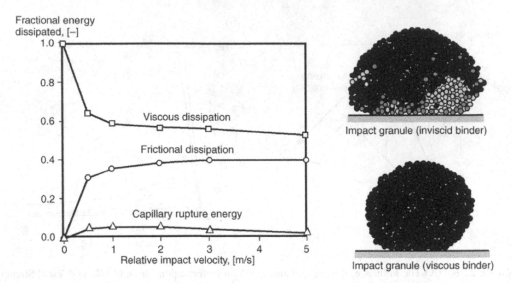

FIGURE 2.28 Distribution of Energy Dissipation During Agglomerate Collisions, with Granular Simulations of Wall Impact for 128 μsec Duration for Inviscid and Viscous Binder Agglomerates. *Source*: From Refs. [2,46].

The important contributions of binder viscosity and friction to granule deformability and growth are illustrated by fractions of energy dissipated during a granule collision as depicted in Figure 2.28. Note that 60% of the energy is dissipated through viscous losses, with the majority of the remainder through interparticle friction. Very little is lost because of capillary forces controlled by surface tension. Therefore, modern approaches to granule coalescence rest in understanding the impact of granule deformability on growth, rather than the original framework put for by Rumpf [22–24] regarding pendular and funicular liquid bridge forces alone.

Second, Figure 2.28 does not explicitly depict the role of saturation and compact porosity, these properties are known to affect strength. A decrease in compact porosity generally increases compact yield stress through increases in interparticle friction, whereas increases in saturation lower yield stress (Figure 2.26) [48,49]. Hence, the curve of Figure 2.28 should be expected to shift with these variables.

Third, the static granule or assembly strength [(Eq. 2)] as originally developed by Rumpf [22] and given by Eq. (2) is captured by the constant, low Ca value of the yield stress, with this yield stress depending linearly on $\sigma_y^{\text{Peak}} \propto (\gamma/a)$ or:

$$\sigma_y^{\text{Peak}} \approx \sigma_o(\gamma/a) \approx \frac{9}{8}\left(\frac{1-\varepsilon}{\varepsilon}\right)\frac{F_{\text{cap}}}{a^2} \approx \left[\frac{9}{4}\left(\frac{1-\varepsilon}{\varepsilon}\right)\cos\theta\right](\gamma/a) \text{ for } Ca < 10^{-4} \qquad (2.26)$$

Fourth, the mechanism of compact failure depends on the strain rate and allowable critical strain rate $(\Delta L/L)_c$. Figure 2.28 illustrates schematically the crack behavior observed in compacts as a function of capillary number. At low Ca, compacts fail by a brittle fracture with macroscopic crack propagation, whereas at high Ca, compacts fail by plastic flow. Large critical strain helps promote plastic flow without rupture, referred to as the squish test among process operators.

Within the context of granulation, small yield stresses at low Ca may result in unsuccessful growth when these yield stresses are small compared with breakup forces. With increased yield stress not only comes stronger granules but also decreased deformability. Therefore, high strength might imply a low-deformability growth mechanism for low-shear processes such as a fluid bed. On the other hand, it might imply smaller growth rates for high-shear processes that are able to overcome this yield stress and bring about kneading action and plastic flow in the process. Therefore, it is important to bear in mind that increased liquid saturation may initially lower yield stress, allowing more plastic deformation during granules collisions. However, as granules grow and consolidate and decrease in voidage, they also strengthen and rise in yield stress, becoming less deformable with time and withstanding shear forces in the granulator. Hence, the desired granule strength and deformability is linked in a complex way to granulator shear forces and consolidation behavior.

2.3.4 Low-Shear, Low-Deformability Growth

For those low-shear processes or formulations that allow little granule deformation during granule collisions, consolidation of the granules occurs at a much slower rate than growth, and granule deformation can be ignored to a first approximation. The growth process can be modeled by the collision of two nearly stiff granules, each coated by a liquid layer of thickness h, as illustrated in Figure 2.29. For the case of zero plastic deformation, as developed by Ennis [4,50], successful coalescence requires that the viscous Stokes number St_v be less than St^*, or:

$$St_v = \frac{4\rho u_0 a}{9\mu} < St^* \text{ where } St^* = \left(1 + \frac{1}{e_r}\right) \ln(h/h_a) \qquad (2.27)$$

where St^* is a critical Stokes number representing the energy required for a rebound, u_0 is the relative collisional velocity of the granules, and a is the harmonic average of granule diameter. The Stokes number is one measure of normalized bed agitation energy, representing the ratio of granule collisional kinetic energy to viscous binder dissipation. The binder layer thickness h is related to liquid loading, e_r is the coefficient of restitution of the granules, and h_a is a measure of surface roughness or asperities. This critical condition, given by (2.27), controls the growth of low-deformability systems. This criterion has also been extended to capillary coalescence [4], and for cases of small plastic deformation [51].

Binder viscosity, μ, is a function of local temperature, strain rate (for non-Newtonian binders), and binder concentration dictated by drying rate and local mass transfer and local-bed moisture. It can be controlled as discussed earlier through the judicious selection of binding and surfactant agents and measured by standard rheological techniques [52]. The collisional velocity is a function of process design and operating variables, and is related to bed agitation intensity and

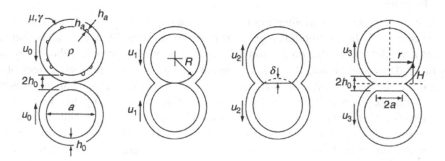

FIGURE 2.29 Collisions Between Surface Wet Granules, Beginning with Granule Approach, and Ending with Granule Rebound and Separation. Note that no Plastic Deformation Takes Place in the Original Stokes Model.
Source: From Refs. [4,50].

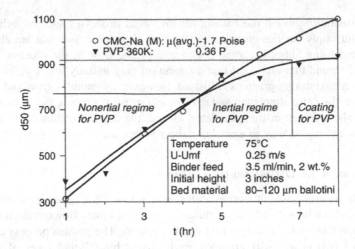

FIGURE 2.30 Median Granule Diameter for Fluid-Bed Granulation of Ballotini with Binders of Different Viscosity Indicating Regimes of Growth. CMC - Carboxymethyl Cellulose, PVP - Polyvinylpyrrolidone. *Source*: From Refs. [4,49].

mixing. Three regimes of granule growth may be identified for low-shear/low-deformability processes [4,50], as shown for fluid-bed granulation in Figure 2.30.

a) Noninertial Regime

For small granules or high binder viscosity lying within a noninertial regime of granulation, all values of St_v will lie below the critical value St^* and all granule collisions result in successful growth, provided binder is present. The growth rate is independent of granule kinetic energy, particle size, and binder viscosity (provided other rate processes are constant). Distribution of binding fluid and degree of mixing then control growth, and this is strongly coupled with the rate process of wetting described in the previous section. As shown in Figure 2.30, both binders have the same initial growth rate for similar spray rates, independent of binder viscosity. (Note that binder viscosity can affect atomization and therefore nuclei distribution through the wetting process.) Increases in bed moisture (e.g., spray rate and drop rate) and increases in granule collisions in the presence of binder will increase the overall rate of growth. Bear in mind, however, that there is a 100% success of these collisions since the dissipation of energy far exceeds the collisional kinetic energy required for breakup/rebound.

b) Inertial Regime

As granules grow in size, their momentum increases, leading to localized regions in the process where St_v exceeds St^*. In this inertial regime of granulation, granule size, binder viscosity, and collision velocity determine the proportion of the bed in which granule rebound is possible. Increases in binder viscosity and decreases in agitation intensity increase the extent of granule growth—that is, the largest granule that can be grown [D_c of (2.19)]. This is confirmed in Figure 2.30 with the carboxymethyl cellulose binder (CMC) continuing to grow whereas the polyvinylpyrrolidone binder (PVP) system with lower viscosity slows in growth. Note that the rate of growth, however, is controlled by binder distribution and mixing, and not binder viscosity. Increasing binder viscosity will not affect growth rate or initial granule size but will result in an increased growth limit.

Adetayo et al. [53] provides a detailed example of the limit or extent of granule growth as a function of binder viscosity and bed moisture, as well as granule growth versus drum revolutions for varying binder systems.

c) Coating Regime

When the spatial average of St_v exceeds St^*, growth is balanced by granule disruption or breakup, leading to the coating regime of granulation. Growth continues by the coating of granules by binding fluid alone. The PVP system with lower viscosity is seen to reach its growth limit and therefore coating regime in Figure 2.30.

The exact transitions between granulation regimes depend on bed hydrodynamics. As demonstrated by Ennis et al. [4,5,50], granulation of initially fine powder may exhibit characteristics of all three granulation regimes as time progresses, since St_v increases with increasing granule size. Implications and additional examples regarding the regime analysis are highlighted by Ennis [4,5,50]. Increases in fluid-bed excess gas velocity exhibit a similar but opposite effect on growth rate to binder viscosity; namely, it is observed to not affect growth rate in the initial inertial regime of growth, but instead lowers the growth limit in the inertial regime.

2.3.5 HIGH-SHEAR, DEFORMABLE GROWTH

For high agitation processes involving high-shear mixing or for readily deformable formulations, granule deformability, plastic deformation, and granule consolidation can no longer be neglected as they occur at the same rate as granule growth. Typical growth profiles for high-shear mixers are illustrated in Figure 2.31. Two stages of growth are evident, which reveal the possible effects of binder viscosity and impeller speed, as shown for data replotted versus impeller speed in Figure 2.32. The initial, nonequilibrium stage of growth is controlled by granule deformability and is of most practical significance in manufacturing for high-shear mixers. Increases in St due to lower viscosity or higher impeller speed increase the rate of growth since the system becomes more deformable and easier to kneed into larger granule structures. These effects are contrary to what is predicted from the viscous Stokes analysis based on rigid, low-deformability granules, where high viscosity and low velocity increase the growth limit.

Growth continues until disruptive and growth forces are balanced in the process. This last equilibrium stage of growth represents a balance between dissipation and collisional kinetic energy, and so increases in St decrease the final granule size. Note that the equilibrium granule diameter decreases with the inverse square root of the impeller speed, as it should be based on $St_v = St^*$, with $u_0 = a(du/dx) = \omega a$.

The viscous Stokes analysis is used to determine the effect of operating variables and binder viscosity on equilibrium growth, where disruptive and growth forces are balanced. In the early stages of growth for high-shear mixers, the Stokes analysis, in its present form, is inapplicable. Freshly formed, uncompacted granules are easily deformed, and as growth proceeds and consolidation of granules occur, they will surface harden and become more resistant to deformation. This increases the importance of the elasticity of the granule assembly. Therefore, in later stages of growth, older granules approach the ideal Stokes model of rigid collisions. In addition, the Stokes number controls, in part, the degree of deformation occurring during a collision since it represents the importance of collision kinetic energy in relation to viscous dissipation, although the exact dependence of deformation on St_v is presently unknown.

The Stokes coalescence criterion of (2.27) must be generalized to account for substantial plastic deformation occurring during the initial nonequilibrium stages of growth in high-shear systems. In this case, granule growth and deformation are controlled by a generalization of St_v, or a deformation Stokes number St_{def}, as originally defined by Tardos and colleagues [4,44,55]:

$$St_{def} = \frac{\rho u_0^2}{\sigma_y} \text{ (impact) or } \frac{\rho(du/dx)^2 d^2}{\sigma_y} \text{ (shear)} \qquad (2.28)$$

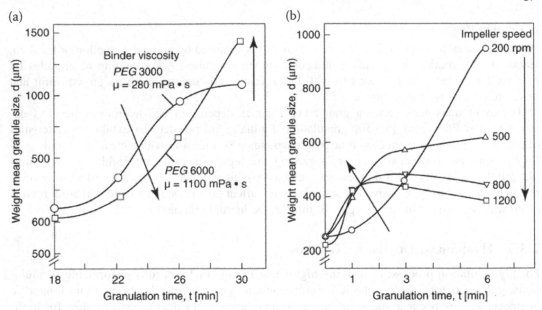

FIGURE 2.31 High-Shear Mixer Granulation, Illustrating the Influence of Deformability on Growth. Increasing Binder Viscosity and Impeller Speed Indicated by Arrows. (a) Ten-Liter Melt Granulation, Lactose, 15 wt.% Binder, 1400 rpm Impeller Speed, Two Different Viscosity Grades of Polyethylene Glycol Binders. (b) Ten-Liter Wet Granulation, Dicalcium Phosphate, 15 wt.% Binder Solution of PVP/PVA Kollidon® VA64, Liquid Loading of 16.8 wt.%, and a Chopper Speed of 1000 rpm for Varying Impeller Speed.
Source: From Refs. [53,54].

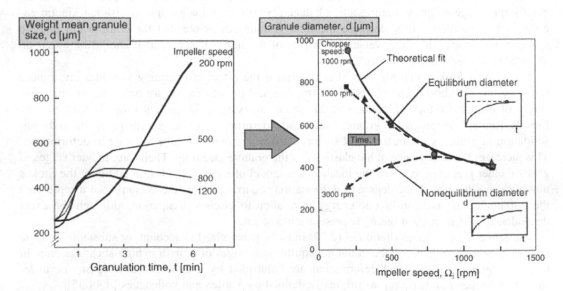

FIGURE 2.32 Granule Diameter Versus Impeller Speed for Both Initial Nonequilibrium and Final Equilibrium Growth Limit for High-Shear Mixer Granulation.
Source: From Ref. [14].

Viscosity has been replaced by a generalized form of plastic deformation controlled by the yield stress σ_y, which may be determined by compression experiments. As shown previously, the yield stress is related to the deformability of the wet mass and is a function of shear rate, binder viscosity, and surface tension, primary particle size and friction, and saturation and granule porosity. Critical conditions required for granule coalescence may be defined in terms of the viscous and deformation Stokes number, or St_v and St_{def}, respectively. These represent a complex generalization of the critical Stokes number given by (2.27) and are discussed in detail elsewhere [6,51]. In general terms, as the yield stress of a material decreases, there is a relative increase in St_{def}, which leads to an increase in the critical Stokes number St^* required for granule rebound, leading to an increase in maximum achievable granule size D_c.

An overall view of the impact of deformability of growth behavior may be gained from Figure 2.33, where types of granule growth are plotted versus deformability in a regime map, and yield stress has been measured by compression experiments [56]. The growth mechanism depends on the competing effects of high-shear promoting growth by deformation on one hand, and the breakup of granules giving a growth limit on the other. For high velocities and low yield stress (high St_{def}), growth is not possible by deformation due to high shear, and the material remains in a crumb state. For low pore saturation, growth is only possible by initial wetting and nucleation, with the surrounding powder remaining ungranulated. At intermediate levels of moisture, growth occurs at a steady rate for moderate deformability but has a delay in growth for low deformability. This delay or induction time is related to the time required to work moisture to the surface to promote growth. For high moisture, very rapid, potentially unstable growth occurs. The current regime map, as presented, requires considerable development. Overall growth depends on the mechanics of local growth, as well as the overall mixing pattern and local/overall moisture distribution. Levels of shear are poorly understood in high-shear processes. In addition, growth by both deformation and the rigid growth model is possible. Lastly, deformability is intimately linked to both granule porosity and moisture. They are not constant for a formation but depend on time and the growth process itself through the interplay of growth and consolidation.

2.3.6 EXAMPLE: HIGH-SHEAR MIXER GROWTH

An important case study for high deformability growth was conducted by Holm et al. [49] for high-shear mixer granulation. Lactose, dicalcium phosphate, and dicalcium phosphate/starch mixtures (15% and 45% starch) were granulated in a Fielder PMAT 25 VG laboratory-scale mixer. Granule size, porosity, power level, temperature rise, and fines disappearance were monitored during liquid addition and wet massing phases. Impeller and chopper speeds were kept constant at 250 and 3500 rpm, respectively, with 7.0 to 7.5 kg starting material. Liquid flow rates and the amount of binder added were varied according to the formulation. Power profiles and resulting granule size and porosity are depicted in Figures 2.34 and 2.35, respectively. Note that wet massing time (as opposed to total process time) is defined as the amount of time following the end of liquid addition, and the beginning of massing time is indicated in Figure 2.36.

Clear connections may be drawn between granule growth, consolidation, power consumption, and granule deformability. Noting from Figures 2.34 and 2.36 for lactose, there is no further rise in power following the end of water addition (beginning of wet massing), and this corresponds to no further changes in granule size and porosity. In contrast, dicalcium phosphate continues to grow through the wet massing stage, with corresponding continual increases in granule size and porosity. Lastly, the starch formulations have power increases for approximately two minutes into the wet massing stage, corresponding to the two minutes of growth; however, growth ceased when power consumption levels off. Therefore, power clearly tracks growth and consolidation behavior. Lastly, power levels and granule size also tracked the temperature rise of the bowl and the level of remaining ungranulated fine powder.

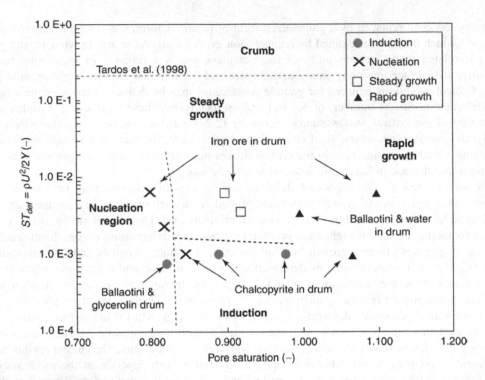

FIGURE 2.33 Regime Map of Growth Mechanisms, Based on Moisture Level and Deformability of Formulations.
Source: From Ref. [56].

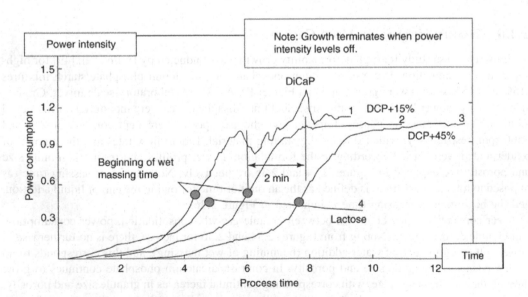

FIGURE 2.34 Power Consumption for Lactose, Dicalcium Phosphate, and Dicalcium Phosphate/Starch Mixtures (15% and 45% Starch) Granulated in a Fielder PMAT 25 VG.
Source: From Refs. [5,49].

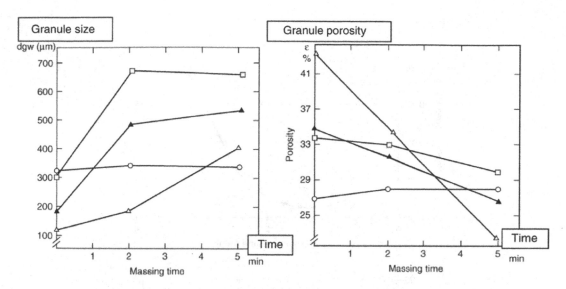

FIGURE 2.35 Granule Size and Porosity Versus Wet Massing Time for Lactose, Dicalcium Phosphate and Dicalcium Phosphate/Starch Mixtures (15% and 45% Starch) Granulated in a Fielder PMAT 25 VG. *Source*: From Refs. [5,49].

Further results connecting power and growth to compact deformability and rheology are provided in Holm [49]. The deformability of lactose compacts, as a function of saturation and porosity, is shown to increase with moisture in astable fashion toward reaching a large critical strain $(\Delta L/L)_c$ required for plastic deformation. Therefore, growth rates and power rise do not lag behind spray addition, and growth ceases with the end of spraying. Dicalcium phosphate compacts, on the other hand, remain undeformable until critical moisture is reached, after which they become extremely deformable and plastic. This unstable behavior is reflected by an inductive lag in growth and power after the end of spray addition, ending with unstable growth and bowl sticking as moisture is finally worked to the surface.

2.3.7 POWER, DEFORMABILITY, AND SCALE-UP OF GROWTH

In the work of Holm [49], split lots of lactose and dicalcium phosphate exhibited reproducible power curves, suggesting the use of power as a control variable. While it is true that power is reflective of the growth process, it is a dependent variable in many respects. For small variations in physical feed properties, specific power may be used for batch control, or scale-up, to the extent that the entire bowl is activated. In practice, however, different lots of a formulation can possess different yield properties and deformability, and a different dependence on moisture. Therefore, there may not be a unique relationship between power and growth, or more specifically, unique enough to use power level to compensate for physical property variations of the feed that the control rate processes. Specific power is required for scale-up, where power is normalized by the active portion of the powder bed. The impact of scale-up on mixing and distribution of power in a wet mass, however, is only partly understood at this point. In many commercial, vertical high-shear designs, the active portion of the bowl changes greatly with scale, and geometric similarity is not maintained with scale-up. This is much less of a concern with horizontal plow shear designs.

Growth by a high-deformable mechanism requires deformation of wet mass, and therefore work input. Work provides a more natural variable than time, demonstrated in Figure 2.35, for plant-scale wet granulation of an NSAID product with power curves versus time are replotted versus

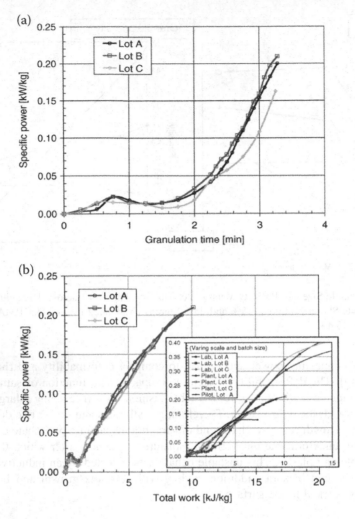

FIGURE 2.36 High-Shear Mixer Granulation of NSAID Product, Plant Scale, Nominal 300 kg Batches, 1000 L. Impeller Power Versus (a) Wet Mass Time, and (b) Total Work Input (*Inset*, Varying Batch Size and Scale, 1–1000 L).
Source: From Refs. [5,49].

work input. Power curves from mixer scales of 1–1000 L also collapse onto one curve when replotted versus specific work. This is consistent with the work of Holm [50], where granule size tracked thermodynamic temperature rise of the mixer bowl, a measure of work input.

The work concept is taken a step further by Ennis [80] and Cuitino and Bridgwater [57], by plotting growth curves versus specific energy (or work) normalized by yield stress of each formulation, again with growth profiles collapsing onto a common line (Figures 2.36 and 2.37). These trials used a high-shear horizontal pin mixer, of varying mixer speed, temperature, and moisture content. Note the equivalence between this normalized energy or work input, and the deformation number of Tardos, or $st_{def} = \rho u_0^2 / \sigma_y \sim \rho \, (E/M) / \sigma_y$.

2.3.8 DETERMINATION OF STOKES NUMBER, (ST*)

The extent of growth is controlled by some limit of granule size, either reflected by the critical Stokes number, St^*, or by the critical limit of granule size, D_c. There are several possible methods

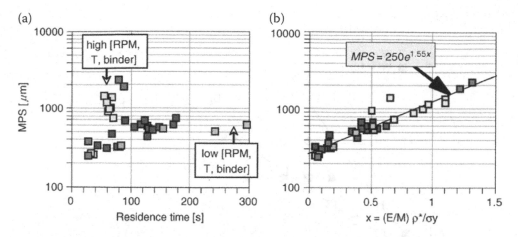

FIGURE 2.37 High-Shear Horizontal Mixer Granulation. Varying Binder Content, Mixer Speed, and Temperature. Initial Mean Particle Size 200 μm. (a) Mean Particle Size Versus Residence Time, and (b) Mean Particle Size Versus Normalized Specific Work. *E/M,* Specific Energy Input; σ_y, Yield Stress. Figure Courtesy Paul Mort [57].

to determine this critical limit. The first involves measuring the critical rotation speed for the survival of a series of liquid binder drops during drum granulation [5]. A second refined version involves measuring the survival of granules in a Couette-fluidized shear device [44,55]. Both, the onset of granule deformation and complete granule rupture are determined from the dependence of granule shape and the number of surviving granules, respectively, on shear rate. The critical shear rate describing complete granule rupture defines St^*, whereas the onset of deformation and the beginning of granule breakdown defines an additional critical value. The third approach is to measure the deviation in the growth rate curve from random exponential growth [58]. The deviation from random growth indicates a value of w^* or the critical granule diameter at which noninertial growth ends. This value is related to D_c (Figure 2.38). The last approach is through the direct measurement of the yield stress through compression experiments.

2.3.9 SUMMARY OF GROWTH PATTERNS

Figure 2.39 summarizes possible ideal profiles of the evolution of the granule size distribution and the impact of the discussed growth mechanisms [7]. For nondeformable growth typical of a fluid-bed or drum granulation, there is an increase in granule size, which is independent of energy and viscous dissipation, and primarily a function of spray rate and contacting (e.g., mixing frequency). For fluid beds, this increase is often linear; whereas, for drums, exponential growth is possible on the basis of contact frequency. The demarcation between linear and exponential growth likely depends on the spray rate versus the mixing rate. Here, attrition has been neglected. In addition, bimodal distributions are possible, with part of the distribution related to ungranulated powder, and the other portion to the granule phase.

For nuclei less than D_c, the granule size distribution starts at some nuclei distribution, which is a function of the wetting regime, and then widens with time in the nucleation regime. Variance increasing in proportion to average granule diameter under the conditions of self-preserving growth, as shown in the inset Figure 2.39a [59,60]. When the largest granules reach the limiting granule size D_c [(2.27) and (2.29)], they slow down substantially in their rate of growth as a balling regime is reached, now only able to grow by sticking to the smallest granules of the distribution (based on a harmonic average granule size less than D_c). However, the smaller size portions of granules may grow with all granule size classes. The distribution, therefore, narrows, as it pushes

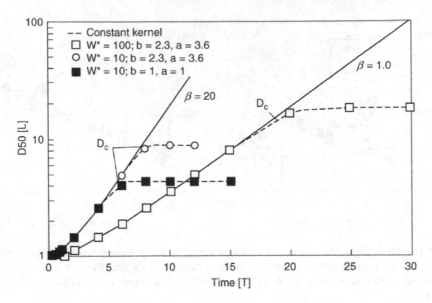

FIGURE 2.38 Determination of Critical Granule Growth Limit From Evolution Granule Size.
Source: From Ref. [58].

up against D_c, as shown in the inset Figure 2.39b. The limit of growth increases with lowering shear rates and collisional velocities or raising binder viscosity, or increasing bed moisture in this nondeformable growth regime governed by the viscous Stokes number St_v. (Here, we have assumed $St_{def} = 0$.)

As the yield stress of materials decreases, for example, by the introduction of more moisture, or shear rates increase, the deformation Stokes number St_{def} increases as we enter deformable growth.

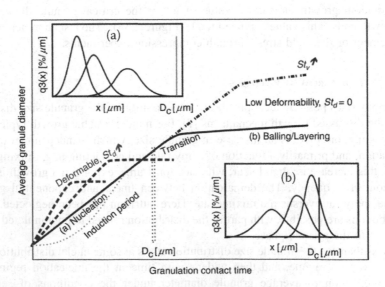

FIGURE 2.39 Typical Evolution of Mean Granule Size and Variance for Different Growth Mechanisms in Batch or Ideal Plug Flow Systems. (a) Shows Granule Size Distribution Variance Increasing in Proportion to Average Granule Diameter. (b) Shows Increase in Narrow Granule Size Distribution with Increase in Smaller Granules as It Pushes up Against Critical Granule Size Limit (Dc).
Source: From Ref. [7].

The growth rate increases as St_{def} increases, as illustrated in Figure 2.39. However, two features remain for this growth mechanism. First, a growth limit is to be expected, depending on the yield properties of the formulation. Second, both widening and narrowing regions for the granule variance are possible, depending on the critical growth limit for the process. Lastly, for the very stiff formulation, an induction period of no growth is possible, as discussed previously.

2.3.10 Granule Consolidation

Consolidation of granules determines granule porosity or voidage, and hence granule density [4]. Granules may consolidate over extended times and achieve high densities if there is no simultaneous drying to stop the consolidation process. The extent and rate of consolidation are determined by the balance between the collision energy and the granule resistance to deformation. The voidage ε may be shown to depend on time as follows:

$$\frac{\varepsilon - \varepsilon_{min}}{\varepsilon_0 - \varepsilon_{min}} = \exp(-\beta t) \text{ where } \beta = fn(y, \, St, \, St_{def}) \qquad (2.29)$$

Here, y is liquid loading, ε_0 and ε_{min} are, respectively, the beginning and final minimum porosity [61].

The effect of binder viscosity and liquid content are complex and interrelated. For low-viscosity binders, consolidation increases with liquid content as shown in Figure 2.40 [62]. This is the predominant effect for the majority of granulation systems, with liquid content related to peak bed moisture on average. Increased drop size and spray flux are also known to increase consolidation. Drying affects peak bed moisture and consolidation by varying moisture levels as well as binder viscosity. For very viscous binders, consolidation decreases with increasing liquid content [61]. As a second important effect, decreasing feed particle size decreases the rate of consolidation because of the high-specific surface area and low permeability of fine powders, thereby decreasing granule voidage. Lastly, increasing agitation intensity and process residence time increases the degree of consolidation by increasing the energy of collision and compaction. The exact combined effect of formulation properties is determined by the balance between viscous dissipation and particle frictional losses, and, therefore, the rate is expected to depend on the viscous and deformation Stokes numbers [61].

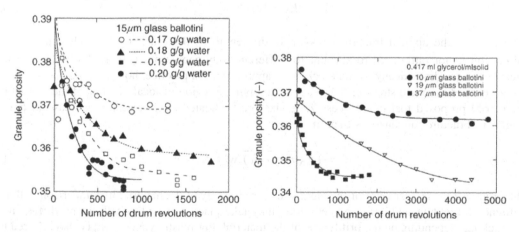

FIGURE 2.40 Effect of Binder Liquid Content and Primary Feed Particle Size on Granule Porosity for the Drum Granulation of Glass Ballotini. Decreasing Granule Porosity Corresponds to the Increasing Extent of Granule Consolidation.
Source: From Ref. [61].

2.4 GRANULE STRENGTH AND BREAKAGE

2.4.1 OVERVIEW

Dry granule strength impacts three key areas of pharmaceutical processing. These include physical attrition or breakage of granules during the granulation and drying processes, breakage of granules in subsequent material handling steps, such as conveying or feeding, and lastly, deformation and breakdown of granules in compaction processes, such as tableting. Modern approaches to granule strength rely on fracture mechanics [62]. In this context, a granule is viewed as a nonuniform physical composite possessing certain macroscopic mechanical properties, such as generally anisotropic yield stress, as well as an inherent flaw distribution. Hard materials may fail in tension, with the breaking strength being much less than the inherent tensile strength of bonds because of the existence of flaws, which act to concentrate stress.

Bulk breakage tests of granule strength measure both inherent bond strength and granule flaw distribution and voidage [3,4,63]. Figure 2.6, presented previously, illustrates granule attrition results for a variety of formulations. Granule attrition clearly increases with increasing voidage; note that this voidage is a function of granule consolidation discussed previously. Different formulations fall on different curves, because of inherently differing interparticle bond strengths. It is often important to separate the impact of bond strength versus voidage on attrition and granule strength. Processing influences flaw distribution and granule voidage, whereas inherent bond strength is controlled by formulation properties.

The mechanism of granule breakage is a strong function of the material properties of the granule itself, as well as the type of loading imposed by the test conditions [64]. Ranking of the product breakage resistance by ad hoc tests may be test specific, and in the worst-case differ from actual process conditions. Instead, material properties should be measured by standardized mechanical property tests that minimize the effect of flaws and loading conditions under well-defined geometries of internal stress, as described in the next section.

2.4.2 MECHANICS OF THE BREAKAGE

Fracture toughness, K_c, defines the stress distribution in the body just before fracture and is given by:

$$K_c = Y\sigma_f \sqrt{\pi c} \qquad (2.30)$$

Where is σ_f the applied fracture stress, c is the length of the crack in the body, and Y is a calibration factor introduced to account for different body geometries (Figure 2.41). The elastic stress increases dramatically as the crack tip is approached. In practice, however, the elastic stress cannot exceed the yield stress of the material, implying a region of local yielding at the crack tip. Irwin [65] proposed that this process zone size, r_p, be treated as an effective increase in crack length δ_c. Fracture toughness is then given by:

$$K_c = Y\sigma_f\sqrt{\pi(c + \delta c)} \text{ with } \delta c \sim r_p \qquad (2.31)$$

The process zone is a measure of the yield stress or plasticity of the material in comparison with its brittleness. Yielding within the process zone may take place either plastically or by diffuse microcracking, depending on the brittleness of the material. For plastic yielding, r_p is also referred to as the plastic zone size. The critical strain energy release rate $G_c = K_c^2/E$ is the energy equivalent to fracture toughness, first proposed by Griffith [66].

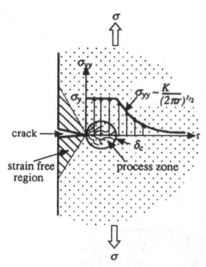

FIGURE 2.41 Fracture of a Brittle Material by Crack Propagation.
Source: From Ref. [63].

2.4.3 FRACTURE MEASUREMENTS

To ascertain fracture properties in any reproducible fashion, specific test geometries must be used as it is necessary to know the stress distribution at predefined, induced cracks of known length [4,63]. Three traditional methods are: (i) the three-point bend test, (ii) indentation fracture testing, and (iii) Hertzian contact compression between two spheres of the material. Figures 2.42 and 2.43 illustrate a typical geometry and force response for the case of a three-point bend test. By breaking a series of dried formulation bars under three-point bend loading of varying crack length, fracture toughness is determined from the variance of fracture stress on crack length, as given by (2.31) [63].

In the case of indentation fracture, one determines hardness, H, from the area of the residual plastic impression and fracture toughness from the lengths of cracks propagating from the indent as a function of indentation load, F [67]. Hardness is a measure of the yield strength of the material. Toughness and hardness in the case of indentation are given by:

$$K_c = \beta \sqrt{\frac{E}{H} \frac{F}{c^{3/2}}} \text{ and } H \sim \frac{E}{A} \tag{2.32}$$

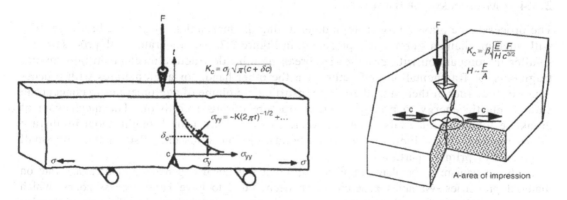

FIGURE 2.42 Three-Point Bend and Indentation Testing for Fracture Properties.
Source: From Ref. [63].

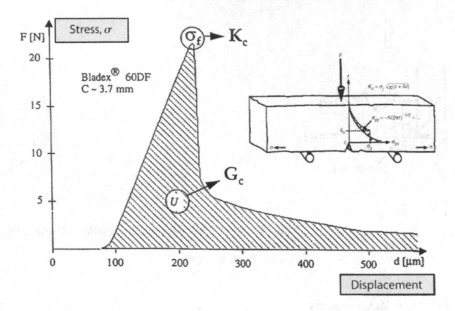

FIGURE 2.43 Typical Force-Displacement Curve for Three-Point Bend Semistable Failure.
Source: From Refs. [4,63].

Table 2.4 compares the typical fracture properties of agglomerated materials. Fracture toughness, K_c, is seen to range from 0.01 to 0.6 MPa/m$^{1/2}$, less than that typical for polymers and ceramics, presumably due to the high agglomerate voidage. Critical strain energy release rates G_c from 1 to 200 J/m^2, typical for ceramics but less than that for polymers. Process zone sizes, δc, are seen to be large and of the order of 0.1–1 mm, values typical for polymers. Ceramics, on the other hand, typically have process zone sizes less than 1 μm. Critical displacements required for a fracture may be estimated by G_c/E, which is an indication of the brittleness of the material. This value was of the order of 10^{-7} to 10^{-8} mm for polymer-glass agglomerates, similar to polymers, and of the order of 10^{-9} mm for herbicide bars, similar to ceramics. In summary, granulated materials behave similarly to brittle ceramics that not only have small critical displacements and yield strains but also are similar to ductile polymers that have large process, or plastic zone sizes.

2.4.4 MECHANISMS OF BREAKAGE

The process zone plays a large role in determining the mechanism of granule breakage [63], with such mechanisms previously presented in Figure 2.7. Agglomerates with process zones smaller in comparison with granule size break by a brittle fracture mechanism into smaller fragments, or fragmentation or fracture. On the other hand, for agglomerates with process zones of the order of their size, there is an insufficient volume of agglomerates to concentrate enough elastic energy to propagate gross fracture during a collision. The mechanism of breakage for these materials is one of wear, erosion, or attrition brought about by diffuse microcracking. In the limit of very weak bonds, agglomerates may also shatter into small fragments or primary particles.

Each mechanism of breakage implies a different functional dependence of breakage rate on material properties. Granules generally have been found to have large process zones, which suggests granule wear as a dominant mechanism or breakage or attrition. For the case of abrasive

TABLE 2.4
Fracture Properties of Agglomerated Materials

Material	Id	Kc (Mpa/m$^{1/2}$)	Gc (J/m^2)	δ_c (µm)	E (MPa)	G_c/E (m)
Bladex 60[*][a]	B60	0.070	3.0	340	567	5.29e–09
Bladex 90[*][a]	B90	0.014	0.96	82.7	191	5.00e–09
Glean[*][a]	G	0.035	2.9	787	261	1.10e–08
Glean[*] Aged[a]	GA	0.045	3.2	3510	465	6.98e–09
CMC-Na (M)[b]	CMC	0.157	117.0	641	266	4.39e–07
Klucel GF[b]	KGF	0.106	59.6	703	441	1.35e–07
PVP 360K[b]	PVP	0.585	199.0	1450	1201	1.66e–07
CMC 2% 1KN[b]	C2/1	0.097	16.8	1360	410	4.10e–08
CMC 2% 5KN[b]	C2/5	0.087	21.1	1260	399	5.28e–08
CMC 5% 1KN[b]	C5/1	0.068	15.9	231	317	5.02e–08

Notes

[a] DuPont corn herbicides.

[b] 50 µm glass beads with polymer binder.*Source*: From Ref. [63].

wear of ceramics due to surface scratching by loaded indentors, Evans and Wilshaw [68] determined a volumetric wear rate, V, of:

$$V = \frac{d_i^{1/2}}{A^{1/4} K_c^{3/4} H^{1/2}} P^{5/4} l \tag{2.33}$$

where d_i is indentor diameter, P is applied load, l is wear displacement of the indentor and A is an apparent area of contact of the indentor with the surface. Therefore, the wear rate depends inversely on fracture toughness.

For the case of fragmentation, Yuregir et al. [69] have shown that the fragmentation rate of organic and inorganic crystals is given by:

$$V \sim \frac{H}{K_c^2} \rho u^2 a \tag{2.34}$$

where a is crystal length, ρ is crystal density, and u is impact velocity. Note that hardness plays an opposite role for fragmentation than for wear, since it acts to concentrate stress for fracture. The fragmentation rate is a stronger function of toughness as well.

Drawing on analogies with this work, the breakage rates by wear, B_w, and fragmentation, B_f, for the case of fluid-bed granulation and drying processes should be of the form:

$$B_w = \frac{d_0^{1/2}}{K_c^{3/4} H^{1/2}} h_b^{5/4} (U - U_{mf}) \tag{2.35}$$

$$B_f \sim \frac{H}{K_c^2} \rho (U - U_{mf})^2 a \tag{2.36}$$

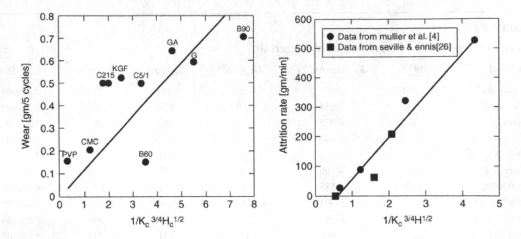

FIGURE 2.44   Bar Wear Rate and Fluid-Bed Erosion Rate as a Function of Granule Material Properties. K_c is Fracture Toughness and H is Hardness.
Source: From Ref. [63].

where d is granule diameter, d_0 is primary particle diameter, $(U - U_{mf})$ is fluid-bed excess gas velocity, and h_b is bed height. Figure 2.44 illustrates the dependence of erosion rate on material properties for bars and granules undergoing a wear mechanism of breakage, as governed by (2.31) and (2.35), respectively.

2.5   CONTROLLING GRANULATION PROCESSES

2.5.1   AN ENGINEERING APPROACH TO GRANULATION PROCESSES

Future advances in our understanding of granulation phenomena rest heavily on engineering process design. A change in granule size or voidage is akin to a change in chemical species, and so analogies exist between granulation growth kinetics and chemical kinetics and the unit operations of size enlargement and chemical reaction [5]. These analogies are highlighted in Figure 2.45, where several scales of analysis must be considered for successful process design. Let us begin by considering a small volume element of material A within a mixing process as shown in Figure 2.46, and consider either the molecular or the primary particle/single granule scale. On the granule scale of scrutiny, the design of chemical reactors and granulation processes differ conceptually in that the former deals with chemical transformations whereas the latter deals primarily with physical transformations controlled by mechanical processing[1] [70–72].

Here, the rate processes of granulation are controlled by a set of key physicochemical interactions. These rate processes have been defined in the proceeding sections, including wetting and nucleation, granule growth and consolidation, and granule attrition and breakage.

We now consider a granule volume scale of scrutiny, returning to our small volume element of material A of Figure 2.46. Within this small volume for the case of chemical kinetics, we generally are concerned with the rate at which one or more chemical species is converted into a product. This is generally dictated by a reaction rate constant or kinetic constant, which is, in turn, a local function of temperature, pressure, and the concentration of feed species, as was established from previous physicochemical considerations. These local variables are, in turn, a function of overall heat, mass, and momentum transfer of the vessel controlled by mixing and heating/cooling. The chemical conversion occurring within a local volume element may be integrated over the entire vessel to determine the chemical yield or extent of

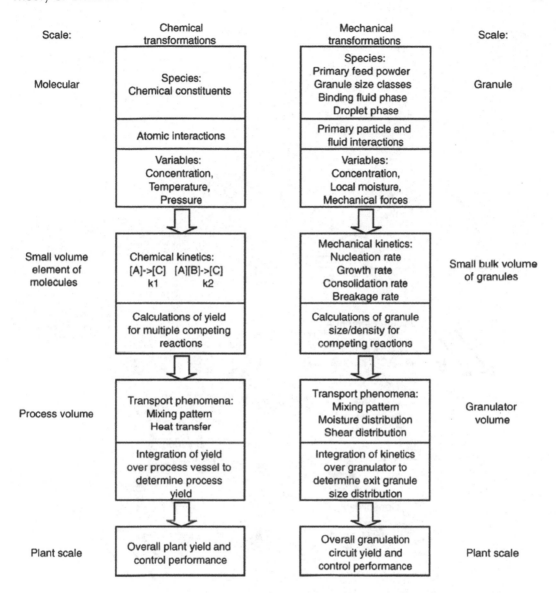

FIGURE 2.45 Changes in a State as Applied to Granulator Kinetics and Design.
Source: From Ref. [5].

conversion for the reactor vessel; the impact of mixing and heat transfer is generally considered in this step at the process volume scale of scrutiny. In the case of a granulation process, an identical mechanistic approach exists for design, where chemical kinetics is replaced by granulation kinetics. The performance of a granulator may be described by the extent of granulation of a species. Let $(x_1, x_2, ..., x_n)$ represent a list of attributes such as average granule size, porosity, strength, and any other generic quality metric and associated variances. Alternatively, $(x_1, x_2, ..., x_n)$ might represent the concentrations or numbers of certain granule size or density classes, just as in the case of chemical reactors. The proper design of a chemical reactor or a granulator then relies on understanding and controlling the evolution (both time and spatial) of the feed vector X to the desired product vector Y. Inevitably, the reactor or granulator is contained within a larger-plant-scale process chain, or manufacturing circuit, with overall plant performance being dictated by the interaction

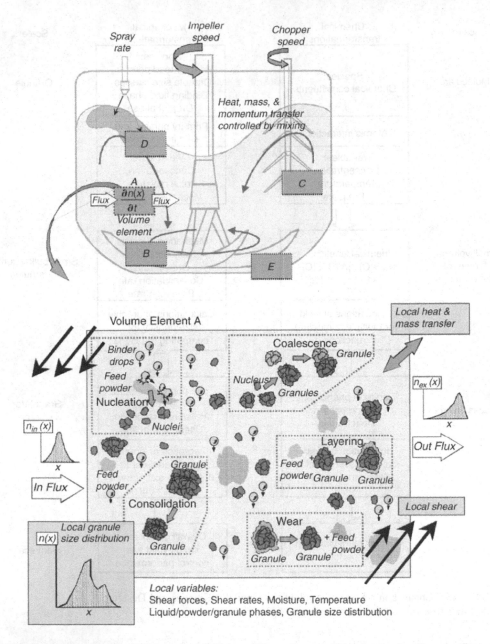

FIGURE 2.46 Granulation Within a Local Volume Element, as a Subvolume of a Process Granulator Volume, Which Controls Local Size Distribution.
Source: From Ref. [5].

between individual unit operations. At the plant scale of scrutiny, understanding interactions between unit operations can be critical to plant performance and product quality. These interactions are far more substantial with solids processing than with liquid-gas processing. Ignoring these interactions often leads processing personnel to misdiagnose sources of poor plant performance. Tableting is often affected by segregation or poor mixing. Segregation becomes vital for preferential wetting and drug assay variation per size class, which can be influenced by trace impurities in the production of drugs or excipients.

There are several important points worth noting concerning this approach. First, the engineering approach to the design of chemical reactors is well developed and an integral part of traditional chemical engineering education [73]. At present, only the most rudimentary elements of reaction kinetics have been applied to granulator design. Much more is expected to be gleaned from this approach over the coming decade. Examples might include staged addition of ingredients, micronization of processes, and tailored process designs based on specific formulation properties. Second, an appreciation of this engineering approach is absolutely vital to properly scale-up granulation processes for difficult formulations. Lastly, this perspective provides a logical framework with which to approach and unravel complex processing problems, which often involve several competing phenomena. Significant progress had been made with this approach in crystallization [74] and grinding [75].

Many complexities arise when applying the results of the previous sections detailing granulation mechanisms to granulation processing. The purpose of this section is to summarize approaches to controlling these rate processes by placing them within the context of actual granulation systems and granulator design. Additional details of modeling and granulator design can be found in chapters 23 and 24.

2.5.2 SCALE OF A GRANULE SIZE AND PRIMARY FEED PARTICLES

When considering a scale of scrutiny of the order of granules, we ask what controls the rate processes, as presented in detail in the previous sections. This key step links formulation or material variables to the process operating variables, and successful granulator design hinges on this understanding. Two key local variables of the volume element, A, include the local-bed moisture and the local level of shear (both shear rate and shear forces). These variables play an analogous role of species concentration and temperature in controlling kinetics in a chemical reaction, with the caveat that granulation mechanisms are primarily path functions in the thermodynamic sense, with work input as opposed to time controlling deformation mechanisms. In the case of chemical reaction, increased temperature or concentration of a feed species generally increases the reaction rate. For the case of granulation considered here, increases in shear rate and moisture result in increased granule/powder collisions in the presence of binding fluid, resulting in an increased frequency of successful growth events and increases in granule growth rate. Increases in shear forces also increase the granule consolidation rate and aid growth for deformable formulations. In the limit of very high shear (e.g., due to choppers), they promote wet and dry granule breakage or limit granule growth. In the case of simultaneous granulation and drying, bed and gas-phase moisture, temperature control, heat and mass transfer, and the impact of drying kinetics on currrent bed moisture should be considered.

2.5.3 SCALE OF A GRANULE VOLUME ELEMENT

Next consider a scale of scrutiny of the level of a small bulk volume of granules, or volume element of material, A, in Figure 2.45. This volume element has a particular granule size distribution controlled by the local granulation rate processes as shown pictorially in Figure 2.46. In the wetting and nucleation rate process, droplets interact with a fine powder to form initial nuclei, either directly or through the mechanical breakdown of pooled over-wetted regions. It is generally useful to consider the initial powder phase and drop phase as independent feed phases to the granule phase. In addition, the granule phase can be broken down into separate species, each species corresponding to a particular granule mesh size cut. Nucleation, therefore, results in a loss of powder and drop phases, and the birth of granules. Granules and initial nuclei collide within this volume element with each other and with the surrounding powder phase, resulting in both granule growth and consolidation due to compaction forces. Granule growth by coalescence results in the discrete birth of granules to a new granule size class or species, as well as loss or death of granules from the originating size classes. This is a rapid, often exponential mechanism, with a widening of the distribution when below the limiting granule size. On the other hand, granule growth by layering and granule consolidation results in a slow differential increase and decrease in granule size, respectively. Granule breakage by fracture and attrition (or wear) act in a similar, but opposite, fashion to granule coalescence and layering, increasing the powder phase and species of smaller granules. Lastly, this volume element of granules interacts with the surrounding material of the bed, as granulated, powder, and drop phases flow to and from surrounding volume elements. The rate processes of granulation and the flows or exchanges with surrounding elements combine to control the local granule size distribution and growth rate within this small volume element.

As illustrated in Figure 2.47, conducting an inventory of all granules entering and leaving a given size class $n(x)$ by all possible granulation mechanisms leads to a microlevel population balance over the volume element given by:

$$\frac{\partial n_a}{\partial t} + \frac{\partial}{\partial x_i}(n_a u_i) = G_a = B_a - D_a \tag{2.37}$$

where $n(x,t)$ is the instantaneous granule size distribution, which varies with time and position. G, B, and D are growth, birth, and death rates due to granule coalescence and granule fracture. The second LHS term reflects contributions to the distribution from layering and wear, as well as interchanges of granules from surrounding volume elements. The nucleation rate would be considered a boundary condition of (2.37), providing a source of initial granules. (2.37) governs the local growth rate within volume element A.

Solutions to this population balance are described in greater detail in chapter 23, as well as in Refs. [6,74,75]. Analytical solutions are only possible in the simplest of cases. Although actual processes would require specific examination, some general comments are warranted. Beginning

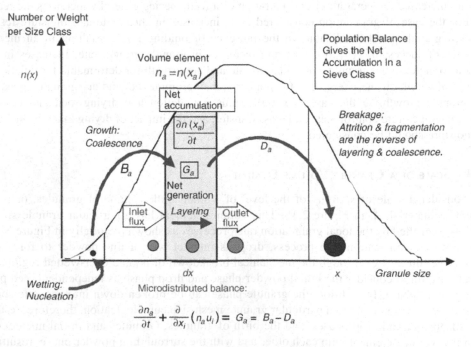

FIGURE 2.47 The Population Balance over a Sieve Class or Specific Granule Size Class.
Source: From Ref. [5].

with nucleation, in the case of fast drop penetration into fine powders and for small spray flux, new granules will be formed of the order of the drop size distribution, and contribute to those particular size cuts or granule species. If the spray is stopped at low moisture levels, one will obtain a bimodal distribution of nuclei size superimposed on the original feed distribution. Very little growth may occur for these low moisture levels. This should not be confused with induction type growth, which is a result of low overall formulation deformability. In fact, the moisture level of the nuclei themselves will be found to be high and nearly saturated. Moisture, however, is locked up within these nuclei, surrounded by large amounts of fine powder. Therefore, it is important not to confuse granule moisture, local moisture, and the overall average peak bed moisture of the process; they are very much not the same but all are influenced by proper vessel design and operation. As moisture levels increase and the concentration of the ungranulated powder phase decreases, the portion of the granule phase increases. As granules begin to interact more fully because of de-creased surrounding powder and greater chances to achieve wet granule interaction, granule coalescence begins to occur. This, in turn, results in a decrease in granule number, and a rapid often exponential increase in granule size as previously demonstrated. Coalescence generally leads to an initial widening of the granule size distribution until the granule growth limit is reached, discussed in detail in section "Summary of Growth Patterns" (Figure 2.39). As larger granules begin to exceed this growth limit, they can no longer coalesce with granules of similar size. Their growth rate drops substantially as they can only continue to grow by coalescence with fine granules or by layering with any remaining fine powder. At this point, the granule size distribution generally narrows with time. This provides a local description of growth, whereas the overall growth rate of the process depends greatly on mixing described next, as controlled by process design.

2.5.4 SCALE OF THE GRANULATOR VESSEL

The local variables of moisture and shear level vary with volume element, or position in the granulator, which leads to the kinetics of nucleation, growth, consolidation, and breakage being dependent on position in the vessel, leading to a scale of scrutiny of the vessel size. As shown in Figure 2.46, moisture levels and drop phase concentration and nucleation will be high at position D. Significant growth will occur at position B because of increased shear forces and granule deformation, as well as increased contacting. Significant breakage can occur at position C in the vicinity of choppers. Each of these positions or volume elements will have its own specific, local granule size distribution at any moment in time.

Solids mixing [3,76] impacts the overall granulation in several ways. First, it controls the local shear. Local shear rates and forces are a function of shear stress transfer through the powder bed, which is, in turn, a function of mixer design and bed bulk density, granule size distribution, and frictional properties. Local shear rates determine granule collisional velocities. This first area is possibly one of the least understood areas of powder processing and requires additional research to establish the connection between operating variables and local shear rates and forces. It is also a very important scale-up consideration, as discussed in chapter 24 [3,6,76].

Second, solids mixing controls the interchange of moisture, powder phase, and droplet phases among the local volume elements. Third, it controls the interchange of the granulated phase. Within the context of reaction kinetics [73], one generally considers extremes of mixing between well-mixed continuous, plug flow continuously, or well-mixed batch processes. The impact of mixing on reaction kinetics is well understood, and similar implications exist for the impact of mixing on granulation growth kinetics. In particular, well-mixed continuous pro-cesses would be expected to provide the widest granule size distribution (deep continuous fluidized beds are an example), whereas plug flow or well-mixed batch processes should result in narrower distributions.[2] In addition, it is possible to narrow the distribution further by purposely segregating the bed by granule size,[3] or staging the addition of ingredients, though this is a less explored area of granulator design. Lastly, it should be possible to predict the effects of dispersion, back-mixing, and dead/stagnant zones on granule size distribution on the basis of previous work regarding chemical reaction kinetics.

(2.37) reflects the evolution of granule size distribution for a particular volume element. When integrating this equation over the entire vessel, one is able to predict the granule size distribution versus time and position within the granulator. Lastly, it is important to understand the complexities of scaling rate processes on a local level to the overall growth rate of the granulator. If such considerations are not made, misleading conclusions with regard to granulation behavior may be drawn. Wide distributions in moisture and shear level, as well as granule size, and how this interacts with scale-up must be kept in mind when applying the detailed description of rate processes discussed in the previous sections. With this phenomenological description of granulation in place, we will now discuss controlling wetting, growth and consolidation, and breakage in practice, as well as the implications for two of the more common pharmaceutical granulation processes, namely fluid-bed and high-shear mixer granulation.

2.5.5 CONTROLLING PROCESSING IN PRACTICE

Table 2.5 summarizes operating variables and their impact on fluid-bed and high-shear mixer granulation [5]. From a processing perspective, we begin with the uniformity of the process in terms of solids mixing. Approaching a uniform state of mixing as previously described will ensure equal moisture and shear levels and, therefore, uniform granulation kinetics throughout the bed; on the other hand, poor mixing will lead to differences in local kinetics. If not accounted for in a design, these local differences will lead to a wider distribution in granule size distribution and properties than is necessary, and often in unpredictable fashions—particularly with scale-up.

Fluidized beds can be one of the most uniform processes in terms of mixing and temperature. Powder frictional forces are overcome as drag forces of the fluidizing gas support bed weight, and gas bubbles promote rapid and intensive mixing. Increasing fluid-bed excess gas velocity ($U - U_{mf}$) will increase solids flux and decrease circulation time. This can potentially narrow nuclei distribution for intermediate drop penetration times. Growth rates will be minimally affected because of increased contacting; however, the growth limit will decrease. There will be some increase in granule consolidation, and potentially a large increase in attrition. Lastly, initial drying kinetics will increase. With regard to bed weight, forces in fluid beds and, therefore, consolidation and granule density generally scale with bed height.

Impeller speed in mixers will play a similar role in increasing solids flux. However, initial growth rates and granule consolidation are likely to increase substantially with an increase in impeller speed. The growth limit will decrease, partly controlled by chopper speed.

In the case of mixers, impeller speed, in comparison with bed mass, promotes mixing, with choppers eliminating any gross maldistribution of moisture and overgrowth.

As a gross rule of thumb, ideally, the power input per unit mass should be maintained with mixer scale-up, related, in part, to swept volume per unit time, as studied by Kristensen and coworkers. However, cohesive powders can be ineffective in transmitting stress, meaning that only a portion of the bed may be activated with shear at a large scale, whereas the entire bowl may be in motion at a lab scale. Therefore, mixing may not be as uniform in mixers as it is in fluidized beds. Equipment design also plays a large role, including air distributor and impeller/chopper design for fluid bed and mixers, respectively.

Increasing bed moisture and residence time increases overall growth and consolidation. However, it also increases the chances of bed defluidization or over massing/bowl buildup in fluid beds and mixers, respectively. Increasing bed temperature normally acts to lower bed moisture due to drying. This acts to raise effective binder viscosity and lower granule consolidation and density, as well as initial growth rates for the case of high-shear mixers. This effect of temperature and drying generally offsets the inverse relationship between viscosity and temperature.

TABLE 2.5

Impact of Key Operating Variables in Pharmaceutical Granulation Source: From Ref. [5]

Effect of Changing Key Process Variables	Fluidized Beds (Including coating & drying)	High Shear Mixers
Increasing solids mixing, solids flux, and bed agitation	Increasing excess gas velocity: Improves bed uniformity Increases solids flux Decreases solids circulation time Potentially improves nucleation No effect on noninertial growth rate Lowers growth limit Some increase in granule consolidation Increases granule attrition Increases initial drying kineticsDistributor design: Impacts attrition and defluidization	Increasing impeller/chopper speed: Improves bed uniformity Increases solids flux Decreases solids circulation time Potentially improves nucleation Increases growth rate Lowers growth limit Increases granule consolidation Increases granule attrition impeller/chopper design: Improvements needed to improve shear transmission for cohesive powders.
Increasing bed weight	Increasing bed height: Increases granule consolidation, density, and strength	Increasing bed weight: Generally lowers power per unit mass in most mixers, lowering growth rate. Also increasing non-uniformity of cohesive powders, and lowers solids flux, and increases circulation time.
Increasing bed moisture (Note: Increasing bed temperature normally acts to lower bed moisture due to drying.) Increasing residence time	Increases rates of nucleation, growth, and consolidation giving larger, denser granules with generally a wider distribution. Distribution can narrow if the growth limit is reached. Increases chances of defluidization	Increases rates of nucleation, growth, and consolidation giving larger, denser granules with generally a wider distribution. Distribution can narrow if the growth limit is reached. Increases chances of over massing and bowl buildup.
Increasing spray distribution:Lower liquid feed or spray rateLower drop sizeIncrease number of nozzlesIncrease air pressure (2-fluid nozzles)Increase solids mixing (above)	Largely effected Wettable powders and short penetration times generally required for fast penetration: Decreases growth rate Decreases spread of size distribution decreases granule density and strength for slow penetration: Poor process choiceDefluidization likely	Less effectedPoorly wetting powders and longer penetration time possible for fast penetration: Decreases growth rate Decreases spread of size distribution decreases granule density and strength for slow penetration: Mechanical dispersion of fluid little effect of distribution, however, slowing rate of addition minimizes lag in growth rate.
Increasing feed particle size (Can be controlled by milling)	Requires increase in excess gas velocity minima effect of a growth rate increase in granule consolidation and density	Increase in a growth rate increase in granule consolidation and density

Spray distribution generally has a large effect in fluid beds, but in many cases, a small effect in mixers. In fact, fluid-bed granulation is only practical for wettable powders with short drop penetration time, since otherwise defluidization of the bed would be promoted by local pooling of fluid. Mechanical dispersion counteracts this in mixers. There may be a benefit, however, to slowing the spray rate in mixers for formulation with inductive growth behavior, as this will minimize the lag between spray and growth, as discussed previously.

In summary for the case of fluid-bed granulation, the growth rate is largely controlled by spray rate and distribution and consolidation rate by bed height and peak bed moisture. For the case of mixers, growth and consolidation are controlled by impeller and chopper speed. From a formulation perspective, we now turn to each rate process.

2.5.6 CONTROLLING WETTING IN PRACTICE

Typical changes in material and operating variables that improve wetting uniformity are summarized in detail elsewhere [1,3]. Improved wetting uniformity generally implies a tighter granule size distribution and improved product quality. (2.7) and (2.9) provide basic trends of the impact of material variables on wetting dynamics and extent, as described by the dimensionless spray flux and drop penetration time.

Since drying occurs simultaneously with wetting, the effect of drying can substantially modify the expected impact of a given process variable and this should not be overlooked. In addition, simultaneously drying often implies that the dynamics of wetting are far more important than the extent.

Adhesion tension should be maximized to increase the rate and extent of both binder spreading and binder penetration. Maximizing adhesion tension is achieved by minimizing the contact angle and maximizing the surface tension of the binding solution. These two aspects work against one another as a surfactant is added to a binding fluid, and in general, there is an optimum surfactant concentration for the formulation [33]. Surfactant type influences adsorption and desorption kinetics at the three-phase contact line. Inappropriate surfactants can lead to Marangoni interfacial stresses, which slow the dynamics of wetting [30]. Additional variables, which influence adhesion tension include (i) impurity profile and particle habit/ morphology typically controlled in the particle formation stage such as crystallization, (ii) temperature of granulation, and (iii) technique of grinding, which is an additional source of impurity as well.

Decreases in binder viscosity enhance the rate of both binder spreading and binder penetration. The prime control over the viscosity of the binding solution is through binder concentration. Therefore, liquid loading and drying conditions strongly influence binder viscosity. For processes without simultaneous drying, binder viscosity generally decreases with increasing temperature. For processes with simultaneous drying, however, the dominant observed effect is that lowering temperature lowers binder viscosity and enhances wetting due to decreased rates of drying and increased liquid loading.

Changes in particle size distribution affect the pore distribution of the powder. Large pores between particles enhance the rate of binder penetration, whereas they decrease the final extent. In addition, the particle size distribution affects the ability of the particles to pack within the drop as well as the final degree of saturation [77].

The drop distribution and spray rate of binder fluid have a major influence on wetting. Generally, finer drops will enhance wetting, as well as the distribution of binding fluid. The more important question, however, is how large may the drops be or how high a spray rate is possible. The answer depends on the wetting propensity of the feed. If the liquid loading for a given spray rate exceeds the ability of the fluid to penetrate and spread on the powder, maldistribution in the binding fluid will develop in the bed. This maldistribution increases with the increasing spray rate, increasing drop size, and decreasing spray area (due to, for example, bringing the nozzle closer to the bed or switching to fewer nozzles). The maldistribution will lead to large granules on one hand and fine ungranulated powder on the other. In general, the width of the granule size distribution will increase and generally the average size will decrease. Improved spray distribution can be aided by increases in agitation intensity (e.g., mixer impeller or chopper speed, drum rotation rate, or fluidization gas velocity) and by minimizing moisture losses due to spray entrainment, dripping nozzles, or powder caking on process walls.

2.5.7 CONTROLLING GROWTH AND CONSOLIDATION IN PRACTICE

Typical changes in material and operating variables, which maximize granule growth and consolidation, are summarized else in detail elsewhere [1,3]. Also discussed are appropriate routes to achieve these changes in a given variable through changes in either the formulation or in processing. Growth and consolidation of granules are strongly influenced by rigid (especially fluid beds) and deformability (especially mixers) Stokes numbers. Increasing St increases energy with respect to dissipation during the deformation of granules. Therefore, the rate of growth for deformable systems (e.g., deformable formulation or high-shear mixing) and the rate of consolidation of granules generally increases with increasing St. St may be increased by decreasing binder viscosity or increasing agitation intensity. Changes in binder viscosity may be accomplished by formulation changes (e.g., the type or concentration of binder) or by operating temperature changes. In addition, simultaneous drying strongly influences the effective binder concentration and viscosity. The maximum extent of growth increases with decreasing St and increased liquid loading, as reflected by (2.29). See the section "Summary of Growth Patterns" and Figure 2.40 for additional discussion. Increasing particle size also increases the rate of consolidation, and this can be modified by upstream milling or crystallization conditions.

2.5.8 CONTROLLING BREAKAGE IN PRACTICE

Typical changes in material and operating variables, which are necessary to minimize breakage, are summarized in detail elsewhere [1,3]. Also discussed are appropriate routes to achieve these changes in a given variable through changes in either the formulation or processing. Both fracture toughness and hardness are strongly influenced by the compatibility of the binder with the primary particles, as well as the elastic/plastic properties of the binder. In addition, hardness and toughness increase with decreasing voidage and are influenced by the previous consolidation of the granules. While the direct effect of increasing gas velocity and bed height is to increase the breakage of dried granules, increases in these variables may also act to increase the consolidation of wet granules, lower voidage, and, therefore, lower the final breakage rate. Granule structure also influences breakage rate, for example, a layered structure is less prone to breakage than a raspberry-shaped agglomerate. However, it may be impossible to compensate for extremely low toughness by changes in structure. Measurements of fracture properties help define expected breakage rates for a product and aid product development of formulations.

ACKNOWLEDGMENTS

This chapter is the result of many collaborative efforts. Support for initial granulation research was provided by the International Fine Particle Research Institute, G. Tardos and R. Pfeffer of the City College of the City University of New York, and E.I. du Pont de Nemours & Company. On the basis of earlier versions with A. Maraglou of Du Pont, the material was developed into a training course by E&G Associates and later refined in collaboration with J. Litster of the University of Queensland. All of these collaborations, as well as discussions with P. Mort, A. Adetayo, J. Seville, S. Pratsinis, S. Iveson, K. Hapgood, J. Green, P.C. Kapur, T. Schaefer, and H. Kristensen are acknowledged with great appreciation. Lastly, to the countless granulation and compaction course participants over the past three decades goes a special thank you.

NOTES

1 This approach was pioneered by Rumpf and others in the early 1960s at the Universitat Karlsruhe, leading to development of mechanical process technology within chemical engineering in Germany, or Mechanische Verfahrenstechnik. This was key to the founding of powder technology as a discipline.

2 All else being equal, plug-flow continuous and batch well-mixed processes should produce identical size distributions in the absence of back-mixing. It is very difficult to achieve uniform mixing in practice, with properly operating fluidized bed possibly coming the closest.
3 Pan granulation is a specific process promoting segregation by granule size. Since large granules interact less with smaller granule size classes, layering can be promoted at the expense of coalescence, thereby narrowing the granule size distribution.

REFERENCES

1. Ennis B. J. Chapter 2 Theory of granulation: An engineering perspective. In: Parikh D., ed. Handbook of Pharmaceutical Granulation. 3rd ed. New York USA: Informa Healthcare, 2010.
2. Ennis B. J., Litster J. Size enlargement and size reduction. In: Green D., Perry R., eds. Perry's Chemical Engineers' Handbook. Section 20 7th ed. New York: McGraw-Hill, 1997.
3. Ennis B. J., section ed. Solids-solids processing. In: Green D., Perry R., eds. Perry's Chemical Engineers' Handbook. Section 21 8th ed. New York: McGraw-Hill, 2008.
4. Ennis B. J. On the Mechanics of Granulation, PhD Thesis, The City College of the City University of New York, University Microfilms International (No.1416), 1990.
5. Ennis B. J. Design & Optimization of Granulation Processes for Enhanced Product Performance. Nashville: E&G Associates, 2006.
6. Litster J., Ennis B. J. The Science & Engineering of Granulation Processes. Dordrecht, Netherlands: Kluwer Academic, 2004.
7. Ennis B. J. Agglomeration technology: equipment election. Chem Eng Mag May 2010.
8. Ennis B. J. Agglomeration technology: mechanisms. Chem Eng Mag March 2020.
9. Masters K. Spray Drying Handbook. 3rd ed. Wiley, 1979; Spray Drying in Practice. ApS, Denmark: SprayDryConsult International, 2002.
10. Ennis B. J. Characterizing the impact of flow aids on flowability of pharmaceutical excipients by automated shear cell. AAPS Annual Meeting, Baltimore, MD, 2004.
11. Nederman R. Statics and Dynamics of Granular Material. Cambridge University Press, 1990.
12. Ennis B. J. Measuring Powder Flowability: Its Theory and Applications. Nashville: E&G Associates, 2009.
13. Stanley-Wood N. Enlargement and Compaction of Particulate Solids. London: Butterworth & Company Limited, 1983.
14. Ennis B. J. Agglomeration and size enlargement session summary paper. Powder Technol 1996; 88:203.
15. Turton R., Tardos G., Ennis B. Fluidized Bed Coating and Granulation. Yang W. C., ed. Westwood: Noyes Publications, 1999:331.
16. Pietsch W. Size Enlargement by Agglomeration. Chichester: Wiley, 1992.
17. Sastry K., Fuerstenau D. In: Sastry KVS, ed. Agglomeration 77. New York: AIME, 1977:381.
18. Kapur P. C. Balling and granulation. Adv Chem Eng 1978; 10:55.
19. Kapur P. C. The crushing and layering mechanism of granule growth. Chem Eng Sci 1971; 26:1093.
20. Kapur P. C, Fuerstenau DW. Size distributions and kinetic relationships in the nuclei region of wet pelletization. Ind Eng Chem Eng 1966; 5:5.
21. Kapur P. C. Kinetics of granulation by non-random coalescence mechanism. Chem Eng Sci 1972; 27:1863.
22. Rumpf H. The strength of granules and agglomerates. In: Knepper WA, ed. Agglomeration. New York: Interscience, 1962:379–414.
23. Rumpf H. Particle adhesion. In: Sastry KVS, ed. Agglomeration 77. New York: AIME, 1977:97–129.
24. Augsburger L, Vuppala M. Theory of granulation. In: Parikh DM, ed. Handbook of Pharmaceutical Granulation Technology. New York: Marcel-Dekker, 1997:7–23.
25. Parfitt G. ed. Dispersion of Powders in Liquids. London: Elsevier Applied Science Publishers Limited, 1986.
26. Hapgood K. Nucleation and binder dispersion in wet granulation, PhD thesis, University of Queensland, 2000.
27. Smith P. G. A study of fluidized bed granulation. London: University College, 1980.
28. Kossen NWF, Heertjes PM. The determination of the contact angle for systems with a powder. Chem Eng Sci 1965; 20:593.
29. Pan S. et al. Dynamic Properties of Interfaces & Association Structure. American Oil Chemists' Society Press, 1995.

30. Washburn E. W. The dynamics of capillary flow. Phys Rev 1921; 17:273.
31. Bartell F. E, Osterhof H. J. Determination of the wettability of a solid by a liquid. Ind Eng Chem 1927; 19:1277.
32. Zisman W. A. Relation of the equilibrium contact angle to liquid and solid construction. In: Fowkes F. M, ed. Contact Angle, Wettability, & Adhesion, Advances in Chemistry Series, 43. Washington, DC: American Chemical Society, 1964:1.
33. Ayala R. Critical parameters in the wetting of powder agglomerates by aqueous media, Ph.D. Thesis, Chemical Engineering, Carnegie Mellon University, 1986.
34. Shaw D. J., Williams R. Introduction to Colloid & Surface Chemistry. London: Butterworths & Company Limited, 1980:273.
35. Fuerstaneau D. W., Diao J, Williams M. C. Characterization of the wettability of solid particles by film flotation 1. Experimental investigation. Colloids & Surfaces, 1991; 60:127.
36. Vargha-Butler E. I. Chapter 2 Characterizations of coal by contact-angle and surface-tension measurements. In: Botsaris G. D., Glazman Y. M., eds. Interfacial Phenomena in Coal Technology, 1989: 33.
37. Aveyard R., Haydon D. A. An Introduction to the Principles of Surface Chemistry. London: Cambridge University Press, 1973:70.
38. Lloyd D. R., Ward T. C., Schreiber HP. eds. ACS Symposium Series 391. Washington DC: ACS, 1989.
39. Aulton M. E., Banks M. Proceedings of Powder Technology in Pharmacy Conference, Powder Advisory Centre, Basel, Switzerland, 1979.
40. Aulton M. E., Banks M., Smith D. K. The wetttability of powders during fluidized bed granulation. J Pharm Pharmacol 1977; 29:59.
41. Gluba T., Heim A., Kochanski B. Application of the theory of moments in the estimation of powder granulation of different wettabilities. Powder Hand Process 1990; 2:323.
42. Litster J. D., Hapgood K. P., Michaels J. N., Sims A, Roberts M, Kameneni S. K., Hsu T. Liquid distribution in wet granulation: dimensionless spray flux. Powder Technol 2001; 114:32.
43. Ouchiyama N., Tanaka T.. Kinetic analysis and simulation of batch granulation. Ind Eng Chem Proc Des Dev 1982; 21:29.
44. Tardos, G. I., Khan, M.I. Study of granulation in a constant shear granular flow couette device. AIChE Annual Meeting, Miami, 1995.
45. Ennis B. J., Li J., Tardos G., Pfeffer R. The influence of viscosity on the strength of an axially strained pendular liquid bridge. Chem Eng Sci 1990; 45(10):3071.
46. Mazzone D., Tardos G., Pfeffer R. The effect of gravity on the shape and strength of a liquid bridge between 2 spheres. J Colloid Interface Sci 1986; 113:544.
47. Iveson S. M., Breathe J. A., Page NW. The dynamic strength of partially saturated powder compacts: the effect of liquid properties. Powder Technol 2002; 127:149.
48. Holm P. et al. Granulation in high speed mixers. Part I. Effects of process variables during kneading. Powder Technol 1985; 43:213.
49. Holm P., Schaefer T., Kristensen H. G. Granulation in high-speed mixers. Parts V and VI. Powder Technol 1985; 43:213–233.
50. Ennis B., Tardos G., Pfeffer R. A microlevel-based characterization of granulation phenomena. Powder Technol 1991; 65:257.
51. Liu L. X., Litster J. D., Iveson S. M., Ennis B. J. Coalescence of deformable granules in wet granulation processes. AIChE J 2000; 46(3):529.
52. Bird R. B., Armstrong R. C., Hassager O. Dynamics of Polymeric Liquids, Vol.1. Wiley, 1977.
53. Adetayo A. A., Lister J. D., Pratsinis S. E., Ennis B. J. Population balance modeling of drum granulation of materials with wide size distribution. Powder Technol 1995; 82:37.
54. Schaefer T., Holm P., Kristensen H. G. Melt granulation in a laboratory scale high shear mixer. Drug Dev Ind Pharm 1990; 16(8):1249.
55. Tardos G. I., Khan M. I., Mort P. R. Critical parameters and limiting conditions in binder granulation of fine powders. Powder Technol 1997; 94:245.
56. Iveson S. M., Wauters P. A. L., Forrest S., Litster J. D., Meesters G. M. H., Scarlett B. Growth regime map for liquid-bound granules: Further development and experimental validation. Powder Technol 2001; 117:83.
57. Cuitino A. M., Bridgwater J. Personal communication and figure from Mort P (2005), and Forrest S, Bridgwater J, Mort PR, et al. Flow patterns in granulating systems. Proceedings of World Congress of Chemical Engineering, Melbourne, Australia 2001.

58. Adetayo A., Ennis B. A unifying approach to modeling granule coalescence mechanisms. AIChE J 1996; 43(4):927.
59. Sastry K. V. S., Fuerstenau DW. Mechanisms of agglomerate growth in green pelletization. Powder Technol 1973; 7: 97.
60. Matsoukas T., Friedlander S. K. Dynamics of aerosol agglomerate formation. J Colloid Interface Sci 1991; 146: 495–506.
61. Iveson S., Litster J. D., Ennis B. J. Powder Technol 1996; 88:15.
62. Lawn B. Fracture of Brittle Solids. 2nd ed. Cambridge: Cambridge University Press 1993.
63. Ennis B. J., Sunshine G. On wear mechanism of granule attrition. Tribiol Int 1993; 26:319.
64. Bemros C. R., Bridgwater J. A review of attrition and attrition test methods. Powder Technol 1987; 49:97.
65. Irwin G. R. Analysis of stresses and strains near the end of a crack traversing a plate. J Appl Mech 1957; 24:361.
66. Griffith A. A. The phenomena of rupture and flow in solids. Phil Trans Royal Soc 1920; A221:163.
67. Johnsson N. L., Ennis D. M. Proc First Int Part Technol Forum, Vol. 2, AIChE, Denver, 1994:178.
68. Evans A. G., Wilshaw T. R. Quasi-static solid particle damage in brittle solids. I. Observations analysis and implications. Acta Metal 1976; 24:939.
69. Yuregir K. R., Ghadiri M., Clift R. Impact attrition of sodium chloride crystals. Chem Eng Sci 1987; 42:843.
70. Rumpf H. Particle Technology. Translated Bull FA. New York: Chapman & Hall, 1975.
71. Ennis B. J., Green J., Davies R. Particle technology: The US legacy of neglect. Chem Eng Prog 1994; 90 (4):32.
72. Ennis B., Green J. Visualizing Pharmaceutical Manufacturing as an Integrated Series of Particle Processes. New York: Interphex, 1995.
73. Levenspiel O. Chemical Reaction Engineering. 2nd ed. New York: Wiley, 1972.
74. Randolph A. D., Larson M. A. Theory of Particulate Processes. San Diego: Academic Press, Inc., 1988.
75. Prasher C. L. Crushing and Grinding Process Handbook. New York: Wiley, 1987.
76. Weinekötter R., Gericke H. Mixing of Solids. Dordrecht, Netherlands: Kluwer Academic, 2000.
77. Waldie B. Growth mechanism and the dependence of granule size on drop size in fluidized-bed granulation. Chem Eng Sci 1991; 46:2781.
78. Adams M., Thornton C., Lian G. Agglomeration & Size Enlargement, Proc 1st Int Particle Technology Forum, Vol. 1, AIChE, Denver, 1994:155–286.
79. Schaefer T., Holm P., Kristensen G. Wet granulation in a laboratory scale high shear mixer. Pharm Ind 1990; 52(9):1147.

Section I

Particle Formation

3 Drug Substance and Excipient Characterization

Parind M. Desai, Lai Wah Chan, and Paul Wan Sia Heng

CONTENTS

3.1 INTRODUCTION

Characterization of drug substances and excipients is often considered to be in the realm of pre-formulation studies. It is recognized that the quality of finished products is dependent on process intermediates such as granules and certain properties of the raw materials employed. Thus, the characterization of drug substances and excipients is an integral pre-formulation step. Good knowledge of different test methods is necessary to select the most appropriate methods for the wide range of raw materials. The usefulness of the tests to give relevant information on the properties of the raw materials and their effects on the manufacturing, functionality, and esthetics of the intermediate and finished products should be carefully considered to avoid unnecessary testing and additional cost. This chapter aims to provide an overview of the more important properties of raw materials to granulation and the test methods that are available to evaluate these properties. Readers are strongly encouraged to refer to the appropriate references for an in-depth discussion of the related scientific theories.

3.2   PARTICLE SIZE, SHAPE, AND SURFACE AREA

Particle size is an important physical characteristic of the raw materials used in granulation. It has a significant influence on the dissolution and bioavailability of the drug in the granules, as well as the flow, packing, and compaction behavior of the bulk powder in the production of granules [1]. Segregation of different components in a powder mixture is often attributed to the variation in particle size between the components [2]. Particle shape is another important parameter that can have a significant effect on the bulk properties of the powder. Spherical particles are known to flow better, pack better, and have a lower surface area to volume ratio than non-spherical particles. There is an increasing interest to determine particle surface area due to its significant influence on drug-carrier interaction in dry powder inhalation formulations. Particles of the same size may not have the same surface area if the roughness of their surfaces differs significantly. The extent of interaction between particles may not be adequately accounted for by the size of the particles as their surface area also plays an important role. Increasingly, there is an interest to characterize particles based on three-dimensional (3D) characteristics as physical interactions encountered in pharmaceutical granulation are mainly surface-mediated. In view of the above effects of particle size, shape, and surface area, it is easy to understand their significant influence on the granulation process and properties of granules produced.

3.2.1   PARTICLE SIZE

Among the physical characteristics of particles, size is perhaps the most obvious descriptor. Also, particle size can influence many processing operations in product manufacturing as well as end-product quality. Thus, information on the particle size of the raw material is important and the various methods for assessment of particle size have been extensively studied.

3.2.1.1   Microscopy

One of the oldest methods for determining particle size involves the examination of the particles placed on a microscope slide using a light microscope with a calibrated scale in the eye-piece. The slide is moved in an orderly manner to avoid repetitive measurements of the same particles. Fine particles that tend to aggregate are usually dispersed in a non-solvent liquid medium for measurement. Popular liquids used are silicone and paraffin oils. It is better to prepare the dispersion directly on the microscope slide used for measurement, and care should be taken to minimize any change to the particle shape and agglomeration in the preparation of the dispersion. The liquid medium used should not cause any dissolution of the particles as this will result in underestimation of the particle size. For small particles, especially those in the micron range, the scanning electron microscope may be employed to produce sharper images. In the latter method, the sample is prepared by dispersing the particles on double-sided tape and sputter-coating with gold. Statistically, at least 625 particles should be measured for accurate results [3], but a larger number of particles has been recommended [4]. Thus, the microscopy method is tedious and less preferred unless it is used with an image analyzer capable of measuring the particle size from its projected image [5]. Examples of projected dimensions are shown in Figure 3.1. Commonly used particle

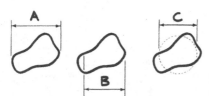

FIGURE 3.1 Commonly used particle diameters: (A) Feret's diameter, (B) Martin's diameter and (C) projected area diameter.

diameters are the Feret's diameter, which is the longest horizontal dimension of the particle image; Martin's diameter, which is the particle diameter that comprises a theoretical horizontal line that passes through the center of gravity of the particle image; and the projected area diameter, which is the diameter of a theoretical circle with the same projected area as the particle image.

The microscopy method has several intrinsic drawbacks. There is a natural tendency for the operator to pay greater attention to large particles as they are less likely to be missed. In addition, small particles tend to clump and this will cause an overestimation of particle size [6]. The problem with clarity of the image will occur as the particle size approaches the limits of the light microscope optics, which is about 1 μm. Depending on the quality of the lenses, particles may be oversized slightly due to fringe effects. Image resolution may, however, be improved by employing various microscope accessories and dyes to increase the contrast between the particle and its background. Besides the above, the measurement is taken from the top view of the particle, which normally rests in its most stable orientation. As such, it does not give an accurate assessment of the size of particles that deviate from the spherical shape.

The microscopy method is further improved (e.g., Morphologi, Malvern Panalytical, Malvern, UK) by adding a dispersion system along with better lenses and sophisticated analytical software [7]. The disperser uses a pulse of compressed air to disperse the particles on a glass plate placed on an automated sample stage. Particle imaging is further improved with vertical z-stacking, automated calibration of mean light intensity before the sample analysis and morphological filtering of captured data, to eliminate overlapping or partially captured particles.

Recent advances in the high-speed digital camera and computer systems have permitted the development of automated image analysis instruments. These instruments can capture two-dimensional images of particles that are either stationary or mobile when available in front of the detector. Two-dimensional particles in dynamic image analysis are distributed within a finite depth defined by the design of the instrument. The test powder is placed in a vibratory chute and then accelerated to a high-speed by a Venturi tube located in the sample dispersion line. Images of the particles are captured by a high-speed camera with a synchronized light source [8]. For imaging with sufficient optical contrast, the aperture is modified for the imaging objective to allow only light rays that are parallel to the optical axis to reach the camera. Motion blurring during image acquisition is minimized by the use of a pulsed light source with very short exposure time, of approximately one nanosecond. The images captured are analyzed and converted to the corresponding particle size distributions. Figure 3.2 provides a schematic diagram of the dynamic image analysis system [9,10].

3.2.1.2 Sieving

Sieving was initially employed for particle classification. Conceptually, particle sizing by sieving is easily understood as the different sieve meshes classify the particles to different weight-based size fractions giving rise to the weight percent frequency distribution. The typical dry sieving process involves a nest of sieves, usually five to eight, arranged from the coarsest mesh at the top to the finest at the bottom, followed by a receiving pan. The sample is placed in the topmost sieve which is covered with a lid. The whole assembly is then placed on a sieve shaker, which may gyrate, oscillate, or vibrate the sieves until there is no further change in the weight of material retained on each sieve. The amount of sample used should be sufficient in order that the size fraction collected on each sieve can be accurately weighed.

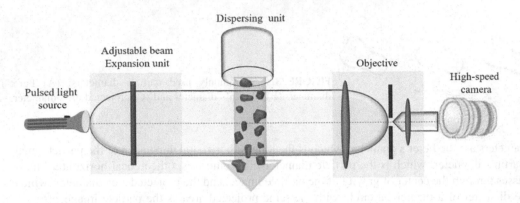

FIGURE 3.2 Schematic diagram of the dynamic image analysis system.
Sources: Adapted from Refs. [9,10].

The introduction of high-quality standardized woven-wire sieves, in a $\sqrt{2}$ progression starting from 75 µm, has helped to establish sieving as a widely used particle sizing method, especially for larger particles. Various types of sieves with different aperture sizes are available. These include sieves with aperture size down to about 30 µm, electroformed micromesh sieves (100 µm to a few µm) and sieves with screens that have accurately drilled or punched circular holes (about 500 µm and larger). Wet sieving is more suitable than the traditional dry sieving for sizing powders that are fine and cohesive. In this method, the sieving of the sample starts with the finest mesh to remove the fines with a volume of liquid. The particles retained are re-suspended in liquid, then classified using sieves with the largest to smallest aperture sizes. Wet sieving is very tedious as it requires additional drying of the size fractions collected. Air-jet sieving is preferred for sizing particles below 75 µm. It involves the use of a vacuum pump to remove air from the underside of a sieve. Air current is also supplied from the underside of the sieve through a rotating arm of jets, which helps to unclog the mesh. A collecting cyclone is usually attached in the vacuum line to collect the fines. The sample is sieved using a single mesh and the procedure repeated using fresh samples of the powder and sieves with different aperture sizes to obtain different size fractions.

Size analysis using sieves has several limitations. It is a relatively slow process and there may be problems with dust pollution. The safety of the operator has to be considered, particularly when drug actives are used. In addition, particles tend to pass through the apertures via their narrower cross-sectional area. Hence, the aperture size of a given sieve is not an absolute cut-off value for particle sizing. Inaccurate results will be obtained if the wire mesh used is stretched due to repeated use, the sieve apertures are blanked due to inadequate washing and small particles aggregate due to cohesive or electrostatic charge. Inadequate sieving time will also produce unreliable data while too vigorous sieving may cause size reduction, especially with weak agglomerates.

A common point of discontent with size analysis using sieves is that the process requires quite a bit of preparatory work, weighing, and subsequent washing. Due to the limited availability of sieves of various aperture sizes, a typical analysis would yield seven to eight points on the size distribution plot. This may not be sufficient to differentiate characteristics of powders. Nevertheless, sieving is a straightforward and robust technique for classifying powders and is suitable for a wide variety of fine to very coarse powders.

3.2.1.3 Sedimentation

The sedimentation technique for particle sizing is based on the settling of particles in a fluid under the influence of gravity, as described by Stokes' law. For a particle of diameter, d, and density, ρ_1, subjected to acceleration due to gravity, g, in a fluid of viscosity, η, and density, ρ_2, the gravitational force experienced at its terminal velocity, v, is balanced by the viscous drag and

$$v = \frac{d^2 g (\rho_1 - \rho_2)}{18\eta} \tag{3.1}$$

The Andreasen pipette introduced in the 1920s is commonly used for sampling from a sedimenting suspension of the test particles in a suitable liquid. Size determination is based on the following principle. As the terminal velocity of a particle varies with its size, the density of the sampled particle suspension will change with time, which enables the calculation of the size distribution of the particles. As Stokes' law applies only to spherical particles, the particle size is expressed as Stokes' equivalent diameter. The typical size range measurable by this method is from 2 to 60 μm. The upper limit depends on the viscosity of liquid used while the lower limit is due to the failure of very small particles to settle as these particles are kept suspended by Brownian motion.

Several innovations have improved the speed and sensitivity of the sedimentation sizing method. These involve sedimentation onto a sensitive weighing pan, turbidity measurements using light or x-ray as well as centrifugation to enhance sedimentation of smaller particles. In general, the sedimentation sizing method has limited use in pharmaceutical applications and remains more in academia, for understanding the principles of Stoke's law.

3.2.1.4 Electrical Sensing

The electrical sensing zone principle, which is more commonly known as the Coulter principle, is based on the phenomenon where the resistance at the aperture between two compartments containing an electrolyte is proportional to the electrical conducting area of the aperture (Figure 3.3). By drawing electrolyte from one compartment to the other, particles streaming through will decrease the conducting area of the aperture. Using fast time-based tracing of the resistance pulses, the number of particles passing through the aperture is obtained. The amplitude of the pulse is proportional to the volume of the particle. The electrical sensing zone sizer can analyze a large number of particles within a short time. Particle size range detectable depends on the aperture tube used. Each tube is effective over a size range of about 2–60% of its nominal aperture diameter. Apertures of sizes from 10 to 4000 μm are available. Before use, it is necessary to calibrate the equipment with standard latex-containing mono size spherical particles of mean size within 5–20% of the aperture diameter.

The blockage of small apertures is commonly encountered. Settling of large particles in the electrolyte will give rise to sizing errors, thus setting the upper limit for coarse particles. The material for sizing must be nonconductive and nonporous. The size of porous particles determined is much smaller than that derived by visual inspection. It is necessary to ensure a low background count of the electrolyte used. Care must be taken to ensure proper dispersion of the test particles,

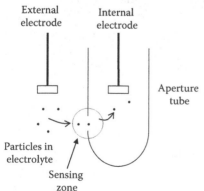

FIGURE 3.3 Schematic diagram of the electrical zone sensing sizer.

which should not flocculate or dissolve to any extent in the electrolyte [6]. The concentration of particles must be within the acceptable range (up to 10,000 particles per second) for the instrument.

3.2.1.5 Laser Scattering, Light Obscuration, and Photon Correlation Spectroscopy

In recent years, light scattering and light obscuration techniques have gained popularity as methods for determining particle size down to about 1 μm using Mie theory or Fraunhofer theory. The measurement of submicron particles had been difficult until the introduction of photon correlation spectroscopy for particle sizing. This latter technique enables particles from nanometers to a few microns to be measured.

As a small particle passes through a beam of light in a laser diffraction sizer, it will diffract light, which will be focused onto a diode array detector directly opposite the incident light (Figure 3.4). The detector has a series of photodiodes arranged outward from a central photodiode detector. Since the intensity of the light diffracted decreases as the scatter angle increases, photodiode elements are generally larger as they are further from the center. Calculations for particle size and size distribution involve rather complex mathematics. Simply put, the calculation is based on the angle of diffracted light, with smaller particles diffracting at wider angles than larger particles. Thus, from the scattered light angles and intensities, information on the size distribution of the particles can be obtained through a series of complex calculations.

In the light obscuration technique, the passage of each particle across the light beam reduces the amount of transmitted light, which is detected by a sensor directly opposite the incident light. The pulses are then classified to give the frequency of size distribution. The test sample in the light obscuration method is dispersed in an appropriate liquid medium for measurement.

Sizing by the laser diffraction technique may be carried out for powders using the dry powder module or as dispersions using the wet module. The dry powder module is used for free-flowing powders while the wet module is recommended for cohesive powders. The powder sample for the dry module is fed by a vibrating tray and purged by an air jet before entering the chamber for measurement. The powder sample for the wet module is dispersed in an appropriate liquid medium, such as alcohol or oil, and is sonicated just before measurement [11,12]. The complete dislodging of smaller particles adhering to larger ones can be an extremely difficult task and with different dispersing efforts, different results may be obtained. Moreover, particulate interactive forces, including electrostatic, intermolecular, and capillary forces, could hold particles together, acting as soft aggregates. This would lead to the overestimation of particle size and inaccurate size distribution measurement.

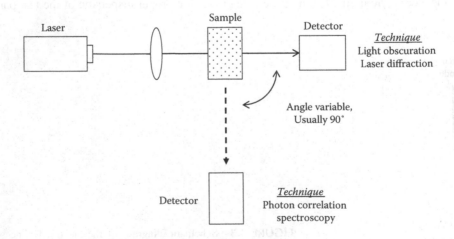

FIGURE 3.4 Schematic diagram of the light-scattering particle sizer.

Alteration in shape and size of particles should be avoided for powders to be measured, and thus, they are best measured in their dry state. This advantage is particularly important in the case of powders made up of a combination of hydrophilic and lipophilic components, one of which is likely to dissolve partially in the liquid medium used when sizing is carried out with the wet module. However, as previously discussed, the sizing of dry powders with laser diffraction sizer can be fraught with problems. Possible causes of poor reproducibility are the poor control of ambient humidity, cohesive nature of the powder, powder particles breaking down, large size distribution of the particles, variable rate of feed powder introduction during the measurement period, possible segregation of powders during the introduction and stray powder particles depositing on the lens. The sizing of a powder composed of very large and very small particles can be problematic as a portion of the small particles will adhere to the larger counterparts and not easily dislodged.

Detailed and reproducible particle size information can be obtained in a short measurement time for both the laser diffraction and light obscuration methods. Compared to the microscopy method, the laser diffraction method gives statistically more reliable data for the small particles especially at the end of the size distribution curve [13], provided that there is little agglomeration or flocculation of particles in the liquid. However, it tends to over-estimate the breadth of the size distribution for non-spherical particles. On the other hand, the results obtained by the light obscuration method can be affected by the degree of light diffraction, opacity, and orientation of the particles as they pass the beam of light.

In photon correlation spectroscopy, fluctuations in the scattered light intensity are determined. These fluctuations are due to the Brownian motion of the test particles suspended in a liquid medium. Larger particles will move more slowly than smaller ones and therefore, the rate of decay in intensity of the scattered light at a particular measuring point will depend on the size of the particle. The particle size distribution is computed using complex calculations based on the different intensity of scattered light (normally at 90° to the incident beam) and rate of decay. Multiple angle measurements are sometimes applied to improve the quality of the size parameters obtainable. Although there has been much development in the field of nanosizing, including real-time direct observation and measurements based on diffusion, these techniques determine particles that are not in the size range commonly encountered in larger scale product manufacture.

3.2.1.6 Time of Flight

In this method, the aerosizer is used to disperse the test sample in the air to create an aerosol beam. The resulting individual suspended particles are then accelerated in an airflow. The time-of-flight, which refers to the time taken by the particle to travel a specific distance, is then measured by triggering two laser beams and converted to the corresponding particle size [14]. The density should be taken into account when the size determined by the time of flight is converted to a geometric size. The results obtained have been reported to be affected by the feed rate and shear force exerted on the particles by the accelerating airflow. Thus, it is necessary to validate the measurement conditions employed [15].

3.2.1.7 Focused Beam Reflectance Measurement

This in-line particle sizing technology can be used to evaluate real-time changes in chord length (a geometric line segment whose endpoints lie within the surface of the particle) distribution and count of the particles. In the experimental setup, a probe is placed at an angle to the process stream. As particles pass across the probe window, the focused laser beam from the probe tube scans the particles at a fixed speed. The focal point position can be adjusted as per particle properties [16]. The distinct pulses of backscattered light returning from these particles will be propagated back through the probe, detected and counted by the detector. The chord length is determined by the product of the reflectance time and scan speed [17,18]. As can be imagined, particle size and orientation will impact the chord length measurements. Figure 3.5 shows the possible chord length measures for spherical and irregular shaped particles.

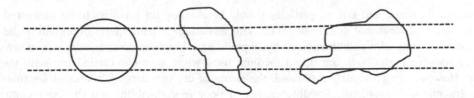

FIGURE 3.5 Illustration of chord length measurement (solid lines) when a laser beam (dashed lines) passes through different particle shapes.
Source: Adapted from Ref. [18].

3.2.1.8 Spatial Filtering Velocimetry

This is another in-line particle sizer technology, based on laser beams to acquire the particle chord lengths. When a laser beam crosses the particle, it casts a shadow, which further interrupts the flow of the light on a spatial filter detector (an array of the optical fibers). Particle velocity is obtained from the consecutive interruption of the neighboring fibers of the detector. The time required to block a single optical fiber is further used to determine the particle size. Raw chord length distributions can be further converted to the volume-based size distribution using the algorithm provided along with the spatial filtering velocimetry software system [18].

Focused beam reflectance measurement and spatial filtering velocimetry technologies can also be used in at-line and off-line modes if significant fouling of the probe window is experienced due to sticky or cohesive granules [19].

3.2.1.9 3D Imaging Using Photometric Stereo Imaging

Sizing by photometric stereo imaging is found suitable for moist, cohesive samples, as well as when the particle dispersion is difficult [20]. In this technique, multiple light sources are used to reconstruct 3D images. The direction of incident illumination between sequential images is changed while the viewing direction is kept constant. Sections 2.1.9.1 and 2.1.9.2 further discuss the examples of this technique (3D surface imaging and 3D particle characterizer) with their working principles in detail.

3.2.1.9.1 3D surface imaging

Sandler (2011) and Silva et al. (2013) used two lights sources (placed at 180 degree) for 3D surface imaging in their separate studies (e.g., Flashsizer FS3D, Intelligent Pharmaceutics, Helsinki, Finland) [18,20]. The instrument used also had a monochrome charge-coupled device (CCD) camera, a metal cuvette with a glass window, a sampling unit for online measurements, and a computer. The sample was illuminated with the two light sources to capture two digital images. Two-dimensional (2D) pixel matrices with gray value distributions were obtained from these images. The value of 0 represents black and 255 represents white and all values in-between represent shades of gray. Differences between these two matrices were further calculated resulting in values between −255 and +255. A value of zero indicates a smooth surface. The shades of gray, represented by different values, provide the information about the topography of the surface. Two-dimensional (2D) images were combined to acquire a 3D image from which the pertinent volume-based particle size information was obtained. Sandler (2011) has provided technical details describing the principle used by photometric stereo imaging to reconstruct 3D images from consecutive 2D images. Silva et al. (2013) concluded that FS3D underestimated particle size in comparison with laser diffraction (another volume-based) technique. It was further explained that the irregularities of rough particle surface could have cast shades which the software transcribed as the edges between the particles, resulting in underestimation of the particle size. Fines covering the measurement window could have further prevented the measurement of large particles.

3.2.1.9.2 3D particle characterizer

A 3D particle characterizer can be used off-line or as an in-process characterization tool (e.g. Eyecon, Innopharma Technology, Dublin, Ireland). From different angles, granules are illuminated using red, green, and blue LEDs and the system captures images of the granules in motion using brief (between 1 to 5 µs) pulses of illumination. Particle surface color is recorded in these images and the map of surface height is constructed. Thus, the system allows deducing 3D understanding from 2D images. In the next step, the ellipse is fitted on the particle edges to obtain the minimum and maximum diameters, which are further used to calculate the granule volume and sphericity [18,21,22]. The system evaluates the fully captured particles only and excludes partially captured and overlapping particles with unclear boundaries. The measurements are stored as a number-based density distribution. Since the working principle of this technique is based on diffuse reflected light, black or strongly reflecting or transparent particles may not suitable for this technique [23].

3.2.1.10 Laser Scanning Microscopy

One innovative advancement of the laser confocal technique is the development of laser microscopes capable of optical imaging of particles to provide highly accurate and resolved 3D images. Such microscopes use a high-resolution camera and a motorized X-Y stage to locate and move the area of interest in the sample. They also consist of a motorized lens turret that drives the objective lens in the z-axis direction, to provide highly resolved 3D information of particle surfaces (e.g., VK-X series, Keyence Corporation, Osaka, Japan). Measurement of particle size can be accurately carried out with a spatial resolution. Surface properties may also be derived using profilers, contact, and non-contact types. Profilers using non-contact white light interferometry can produce highly resolved surface characteristics and are particularly useful for surface roughness measurements.

3.2.1.11 Continuous Manufacturing and Material Sampling

With aims to improve the process efficiency and product quality, and to reduce space and energy footprints, the pharmaceutical industry has started manufacturing tablets from granules by continuous manufacturing [24,25]. Identical to batch manufacturing, key parameters of granules such as size need to be critically characterized during the continuous manufacturing operations. Representative size distributions are ensured by sampling granules when in motion. While a sample divider may be very useful in laboratory scaled or batch manufacturing operations, it is unsuitable for collecting the representative granule samples during continuous manufacturing [26]. Researchers have applied a specific in-line rotating tube sample divider to split the granules and determined their particle sizes in real time using dynamic image analysis [26]. This is an evolving field, and customization may be required, depending on the specifics of the manufacturing line for installing the appropriate in-line size characterizer.

There are many methods for measuring the size of particles. As discussed, the various methods are based on different principles and each has its merits and limitations. A preliminary microscopic examination of the test sample is recommended as it will provide useful information, such as approximate particle size range and extent of cohesiveness, for the selection of a method that is appropriate for the test sample. A comparison of different methods is shown in Table 3.1.

3.2.2 Particle Shape

Despite the well-recognized importance of particle shape, the method of shape determination has not been clearly defined owing to the complexity and variability of the 3D particles. In general, shape measurement methods are only able to define accurately the shape if the latter can be correctly predicted based on a 2D model. The shape of particles may be assessed descriptively by

TABLE 3.1

Comparison of Different Sizing Methods

Method	Suitable Shapes for Measurement	Sizing Range (μm)		Measurement Condition	Particle Concentration
		Lower	Upper		
Dynamic image analysis	Spherical, cubic, acicular	0.05	3500	Wet & dry	Low
Electrical sensing	Spherical, cubic, acicular	0.4	1600	Wet	Low
Laser diffraction	Spherical, cubic	0.01	5000	Wet & dry	Low
Light obscuration	Spherical, cubic	0.5	5000	Wet	Low
Photon correlation spectroscopy	Spherical, cubic, acicular, bladed, fibrous	0.001	10	Wet	Low
Sieve analysis	Spherical, cubic	5	10000	Wet & dry	High
Scanning electron microscopy	Spherical, cubic, bladed, fibrous	0.001	1000	Dry	Low
Light optical microscopy	Spherical, cubic, acicular, bladed, fibrous	1	10000	Wet & dry	Low
Time of flight	Spherical, cubic, acicular, bladed	0.3	500	Wet & dry	Low
Focused beam reflectance measurement	All shapes	3	3000	Wet	Low & high
Spatial filtering velocimetry	All shapes	50	6000	Wet* & dry	Depends on particle size[#]
Photometric stereo imaging - 3D surface imaging	All shapes	20	Relies on calibration	Wet* & dry	Low & high
Photometric stereo imaging - 3D particle characterizer	All shapes	50	3000	Wet* & dry	Low & high

Notes:
*Not suitable for suspensions; [#]Low & high, for particles < 1 mm, up to 12 vol.%; for larger particles, up to 30 vol.%.

terms such as spherical, elongated, acicular, angular, or a host of other terms. These descriptive terms convey a general idea of the particle shape. Without a comparative quantitative measure, it may be difficult to assess the effects of particle shape on a process or product.

The shape has been quantified using various descriptors based on measured dimensional attributes such as length, L, breadth, B, projected area, A, perimeter, P, and diameter, d, of the particle [5,27–30].

$$\text{Elongation ratio or aspect ratio} = L/B \tag{3.2}$$

$$\text{Circularity} = (4\pi A)/P^2 \tag{3.3}$$

$$\text{Roundness} = P^2/(4\pi A) \text{ or } (\pi d^2)/4A \tag{3.4}$$

$$\text{Bulkiness factor} = A/(L + B) \tag{3.5}$$

The elongation ratio or aspect ratio is very useful for assessing deviation from a spherical shape to an elongated form. The circularity, commonly also referred to as shape factor or form factor, on the other hand, gives a measure of sphericity, with a perfect sphere having a circularity value of unity. This shape descriptor provides the properties of shape. Roundness is the inverse of circularity. The bulkiness factor indicates solidity, with large indentations on the particle giving rise to low values.

Often, particle shape is predominantly determined by image analysis. Indirect methods using techniques such as laser diffraction and photon sedimentation have been studied [31–34]. However, these methods are seldom used in practice and hence will not be discussed here. Particle sizing by image analysis has already been discussed in an earlier section. Similar measurement procedures are employed to obtain the outlines of the particles for computing the various shape descriptors. Optical microscopy methods may be applied to evaluate various particle shape parameters such as elongation, aspect ratio, and circularity [35].

3.2.3 PARTICLE SURFACE AREA

Compared to particle size and shape, less attention has been paid to particle surface area. The methods for assessing this particle property are also relatively limited. Surface area measurement is usually carried out by either gas permeability or adsorption. In addition to surface area, surface roughness is another physical attribute of importance but measurement is considerably more difficult and variable due to the complex 3D roughness existence. Hence, it is best to just focus on surface area which also would take roughness into account.

3.2.3.1 Gas Adsorption

Gas adsorption is carried out by placing a powder sample in a chamber and evacuating the air within. The latter process is commonly referred to as degassing. Upon achieving a very high vacuum, known volumes of an adsorbing gas are introduced. From the knowledge of pressure and temperature before and after the introduction of the adsorbing gas, usually nitrogen, calculations of total sample surface area can be made. The surface area determined by gas adsorption is based on a simple principle. From Avogadro's number, a known volume of air at a certain temperature and pressure contains a determinable number of molecules. When various volumes of gas are introduced to a degassed sample, the small pressure changes in the chamber are recorded and using a calculation technique known as the Brunauer, Emmett, and Teller or BET method, the initial amount of gas molecules which are adsorbed onto the surface forming a monolayer can be calculated. Thus, the surface area covered by the gas molecules can be determined by multiplying the number of molecules needed with the surface area occupied per molecule. Samples are usually cooled to a low temperature using liquid nitrogen. There are variations in the technique for gas adsorption by different instrument manufacturers.

3.2.3.2 Gas Permeability

In the gas permeability method, the test powder is packed into a bed through which a gas, usually nitrogen, is passed. The bed must be uniformly packed. From the volumetric flow rate of the gas and the pressure drop across the bed, solid density, and packed bed porosity, the specific "envelope" surface area of the powder can be calculated using the Carman-Kozeny equation. The measurement of specific surface area by gas permeability does not take into account the very small pores or fissures since the flow of gas is not hindered as it passes over them. More accurate measurements can be made by measuring gas flow under reduced pressure but still, the accuracy cannot match that obtainable by gas adsorption if the total area to be determined includes those of the fine pores. Although gas permeability gives a lower specific area for a powder compared with gas adsorption, the value obtained is sometimes more useful in explaining factors like lubricity and flow, which would not involve the pores present within the particles. This measurement may be variously referred to as the Blaine method or methods using Fisher sub-sieve sizer or Rigden apparatus.

3.3 DENSITY

Density is an important parameter due to its influence on particle mechanical properties [36], powder porosity [37], and powder fluidization [38]. The bulk density of a mixed excipient powder used for tablet preparation has been found to affect the disintegration time of the tablet in a mouth [39]. Similarly, it can affect the disintegration of granules. On the other hand, the true density can serve to assure the formulator of the identity of the material. Determination of particle density is not straightforward as it can be carried out by many different techniques, with differing interpretations.

3.3.1 BULK DENSITY

A graduated cylinder is gently filled with the test sample, preferably through a sieve or mesh with apertures just larger than the largest particles. The sample is carefully leveled without compacting if required. The filled volume of the sample is noted and its mass determined by weighing. Bulk density is obtained by dividing the mass of the sample by its volume.

3.3.2 CONDITIONED BULK DENSITY

The operator may introduce packing errors in the aforementioned conventional bulk density measurement method. The measurement of conditioned bulk density was introduced in an attempt to minimize bulk density measurement errors. In this technique (Figure 3.6), an impeller with a twisted blade rotates at a specific tip speed and penetrates in and out of the powder bed filled in a cylindrical glass vessel under an extension vessel fitted with a splitting assembly. This first step of "conditioning methodology" removes the residual stress history, prepares a uniform, lightly packed sample, and brings the bed to a reproducible packing stage. The excess powder is removed by splitting the extension vessel from the cylindrical glass vessel and the weight of the conditioned sample, present in the cylindrical glass vessel, is recorded. The division of sample weight to the volume of the glass vessel is calculated as conditioned bulk density [40,41].

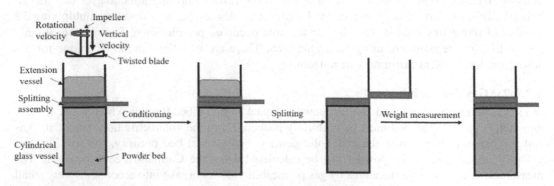

FIGURE 3.6 Schematic diagram for "conditioning methodology" and conditioned bulk density measurement.

3.3.3 TAP DENSITY

A graduated cylinder is filled with the test sample and tapped until the volume of the sample in the cylinder does not change. The mass of the sample is determined by weighing. Tap density is obtained by dividing the mass of the sample by its final tapped volume.

3.3.4 TRUE DENSITY

A calibrated pycnometer is used to determine the true volume of the test sample. The true density is obtained by dividing the mass of the sample by its true volume. Samples used for true density measurements should be very dry as the vapor pressure of volatiles at low pressure can introduce measurement errors [42,43].

3.4 SOLUBILITY

The solubility of drugs and excipients constitutes an important physicochemical property as it affects the rate of drug release into the dissolution medium, the bioavailability of the drug, and consequently, the therapeutic efficacy of the drug product. Factors affecting the solubility include the nature of the solvent, temperature, crystal characteristics, particle size, surface area of the material, pH, and presence of additives.

It must be borne in mind that a drug must first be in solution to be absorbed into the blood circulation. If the solubility of the drug is less than desirable, steps must be taken to improve its solubility or to use another more soluble drug form. Excipients that are poorly soluble in water might retard the release of a drug. Hence, the determination of drug and excipient solubility constitutes an important aspect of the formulation study.

The solubility of a material is usually determined by the equilibrium solubility method, in which a saturated solution of the material is obtained by stirring an excess of the material in the solvent for a prolonged period at a constant temperature until equilibrium is attained. The saturated solution can also be obtained by warming the solvent with an excess of the material and allowing the mixture to cool to the required temperature. This, however, may produce a supersaturated solution for some materials and therefore, this method is less desirable. A portion of the saturated solution obtained by either method is then removed with the aid of a syringe through a membrane filter at different time intervals for assay. The determination is completed only if at least two successive samples produce the same results. The final value thus obtained is the solubility of the material. The sample may be assayed by a variety of methods, such as ultra-violet spectrophotometry, electrical conductivity measurement, gravimetric or volumetric analysis, and chromatographic methods.

The solution-precipitation method is also employed to determine aqueous solubility. It is preferred when the amount of material available for use is low. In this method, a stock solution of the material in dimethyl sulfoxide is prepared. The solution is diluted by an aqueous medium until precipitation occurs. The material in the liquid mixture is then assayed. Precipitation is more accurately detected by the use of a nephelometer or polarized light microscope [44]. Solubility values obtained by the solution-precipitation method are often higher than the corresponding values obtained by the equilibrium solubility method. This could be attributed to the solubilization effect of dimethyl sulfoxide and inadequate equilibration time and the effect of solid-state in the equilibrium solubility method. A large discrepancy in the solubility values obtained is often due to the difference in the physical state of materials in the test. It was reported that the solubility of the crystalline state of a compound could be lower than that of the amorphous state by up to 100 folds [45], while the difference is two to fivefold among crystal polymorphs [46].

3.5 CRYSTALLINITY AND POLYMORPHISM

Materials may occur as amorphous substances without any internally ordered structure or as crystalline particles with a definite structure and somewhat regular external shape. Some materials may exist in more than one crystalline form (polymorph) and are described as exhibiting polymorphism. The type of crystal formed depends on the conditions, such as temperature and type of solvent, under which crystallization is induced. At a specific temperature or pressure, more than one polymorph can exist but only one will be thermodynamically stable. The less stable or metastable form will be converted to a stable form with time.

The different crystalline forms of a material generally differ in many physical characteristics, such as solubility, melting point, optical and electrical properties, density, hardness, and stability. The use of metastable polymorphs frequently results in higher solubility and dissolution rates while the stable polymorphs are often more resistant to chemical degradation. It is obvious that any change in the crystalline form will affect the therapeutic efficacy of a drug product. Drug polymorphism is especially important because it may affect the chemical stability, dissolution rate, bioavailability, efficacy, and safety of the drug. Therefore, knowledge of the crystalline form of the drug and changes to its crystalline form during processing is very important.

3.5.1 DISSOLUTION STUDY

An amount of the material in excess of its solubility is added to the dissolution medium and aliquot samples are removed and assayed at appropriate time intervals. The concentration of the material in solution as a function of time is then plotted. The crystalline form which constitutes the material is reflected by the shape of the dissolution curve (Figure 3.7). The concentration of the metastable polymorph typically increases much more rapidly in the initial period of the dissolution study and then drops to that of the stable polymorph. For the stable polymorph, the dissolution profile increases gradually to a plateau. The solubility of the metastable form is indicated by the peak of its dissolution curve. In some cases, the metastable polymorph does not revert readily to the stable form. The dissolution curve of such a metastable form lies above that of the stable form, indicating that the former is more soluble. The plateau of each curve indicates the solubility of the respective polymorph.

3.5.2 X-RAY DIFFRACTOMETRY

X-ray diffractometry may be carried out using a powder x-ray or a single crystal diffractometer. The latter is used to elucidate the crystal structure while the powder x-ray diffractometer is for general purpose. The polymorphs of material have different crystal packing arrangements and thus produce different x-ray diffractograms with characteristic peaks that are related to lattice distances (Figure 3.8a). The extent of conversion of a crystalline drug to the amorphous form during processing can be determined by comparing the magnitude of their characteristic peaks [47]. The sharp peaks (Figure 3.8a) indicate a crystalline component, whereas broad diffraction peak or features (also referred to as "halo") indicate an amorphous component (Figure 3.8b). The powder x-ray diffractometry method is non-destructive and requires a very small sample of the material, which can be examined without further processing. For structural determination, good single crystals are used in a single crystal diffractometer. Synchrotron sources have been employed to obtain high-resolution electron diffraction patterns for very small crystals or crystals of complex compounds. Very sensitive charge-coupled detectors have enabled electron diffraction patterns to be recorded in a few seconds using very low electron currents. In addition, micro-diffractometers with 2D area detectors have been developed for quick data acquisition [48].

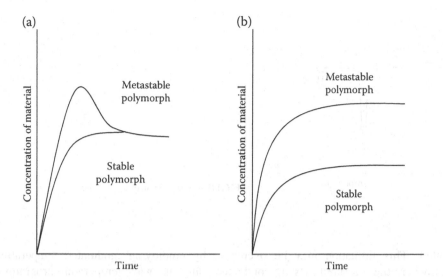

FIGURE 3.7 Typical dissolution profiles.

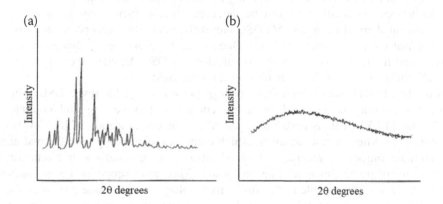

FIGURE 3.8 Typical x-ray diffractograms of (a) crystalline and (b) amorphous compounds.

3.5.3 THERMAL ANALYSIS

In this method, the polymorphs are identified by their thermal behaviors. The change in energy or related property of the polymorph as it undergoes a transformation when heated is recorded as a thermogram (Figure 3.9). The thermogram consists of characteristic peaks, including melting point (T_m) and glass transition temperature (T_g). The peaks pointing downward indicate endothermic changes, such as melting, sublimation, and desolvation. The different polymorphs of material will exhibit different thermograms, which allow them to be identified. Differential scanning calorimetry (DSC) and differential thermal analysis are two methods of thermal analyses that are commonly used. The sample is sealed in an aluminum pan and placed inside the test chamber where it is subjected to different heating rates. In DSC, the change in heat energy resulting from the crystalline transformation is recorded as a function of temperature. In the differential thermal analysis, the energy is expressed by differential temperature (sample vs. inert substance).

Conventional DSC has a major limitation; if a glass transition temperature occurs in the same temperature range as another transition, for example, water or solvent loss, the two events cannot

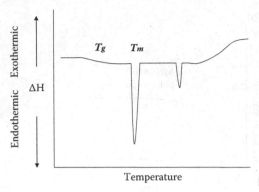

FIGURE 3.9 Example of a thermogram.

be separated. This limitation may be overcome by employing modulated temperature DSC (MTDSC), where the measurements are conducted using sine wave temperature programs defined by underlying heating rate, amplitude, and period. The heat capacity change associated with the glass transition temperature can be separated from the heat flow changes caused by melting, drying, and solvent loss. By use of the phase angle curve produced from the MTDSC data analysis, very small changes in specific heat can be detected, thereby increasing the sensitivity of the method. Based on thermal behavior, MTDSC can differentiate the amorphous and polymorphic forms of material with much greater clarity. One of the disadvantages of this method is that the data analysis and interpretation are more difficult than for DSC. Besides, the experiment process can be much prolonged as much lower heating rates are used.

One of the latest techniques is high-speed or high-performance DSC (hyperDSC) where higher measurement sensitivity is achieved by using controlled fast heating and cooling rates of 100–500 °C/min [49,50]. This is particularly useful for the quantification of low levels of amorphous content [51]. Microthermal analysis, which combines microscopy with thermal analysis, is another technique introduced recently. Mounted on a three-axis piezoelectric actuator, the microthermal analysis probe functions like an atomic force microscope probe in contact mode, scanning the surface of the sample to determine its topology. As the probe goes over the surface, changes in thermal properties will be recorded and converted to thermal conductivity images that are characteristic of the different polymorphs. The typical scanned surface is 100 μm by 100 μm because the z actuator only has a dynamic range of about 20 μm. As such, microthermal analysis requires relatively flat samples.

3.5.4 VIBRATIONAL SPECTROSCOPY

3.5.4.1 Infrared Spectroscopy

As mentioned earlier, the polymorphs of material show different crystal packing arrangements and produce different x-ray diffractograms. The crystal packing arrangement also affects the energy of molecular bonds and results in different infrared (IR) spectra that are characteristic of the polymorphs. IR analysis can be used for both qualitative and quantitative determinations, especially in the region of near-infrared (NIR). It is based on the principle that the peaks in the IR spectrum arise from the stretching or bending vibrations of a particular functional group [52]. The disappearance of a characteristic peak or the appearance of a new peak in the IR spectrum of the mixture can be attributed to chemical interaction between the components of the mixture. It is important to use only materials in the solid form as the polymorphs of a material in solution have identical IR spectra [53].

A combination of NIR spectroscopy and digital imaging technologies allows identification and quantification of the components present in a sample using the spectroscopy element, and visualization of the distribution of the components using the imaging capability (Figure 3.10). The technique is used to investigate the heterogeneity of the distribution within solid samples, visualizing both pharmaceutical excipients and the active. Thus, it is not only possible to gain information about the morphology of the particles or component domains within a sample, but using the NIR spectroscopy element of the data, it is possible to initially segregate the sample based on chemical differences and then calculate the morphological information for the separate species. This provides numerical metrics for the quantitative comparison of different samples.

3.5.4.2 Raman Spectroscopy

Raman spectroscopy provides molecular information about the crystalline, as well as the amorphous forms of a material. In this method, the material is subjected to a laser beam and a spectrum of the scattered light obtained. The spectrum shows vibrational bands of the material at their characteristic frequencies. The amorphous and polymorphic forms of a material can be distinguished by their characteristic spectra.

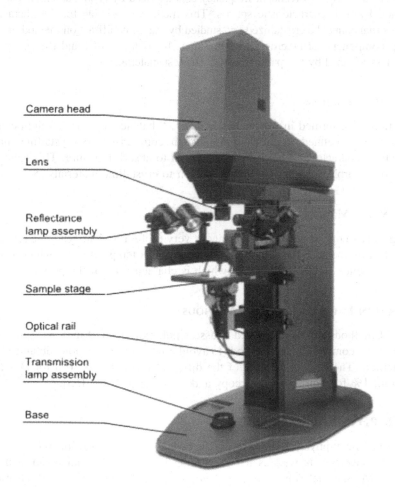

Camera head

Lens

Reflectance lamp assembly

Sample stage

Optical rail

Transmission lamp assembly

Base

FIGURE 3.10 Picture of NIR chemical imaging instrument.
Source: Courtesy by Malvern Instruments.

Raman spectroscopy and IR spectroscopy complement each other. The former measures a change in polarization, whereas the latter measures a change in dipole moment. IR-inactive vibrations can be strong in Raman spectra and vice versa. For example, vibrations in the wavenumber region of $10-400 \text{ cm}^{-1}$ are more easily studied by Raman than by IR spectroscopy. One advantage of the Raman spectroscopy method is that no sample preparation is required, thus the likelihood of inducing phase changes through sample preparation is avoided. However, representative sampling is critical for quantitative analysis. The results are affected by the particle size of the material. The use of Fourier transform Raman spectrometers with a longer wavelength laser of 1064 nm eliminates the problem of any fluorescent background. With the utilization of fiber optics, real-time crystallization can be monitored. Thus, this method is useful for in-line monitoring of pharmaceutical processes.

3.5.5 SOLID-STATE NUCLEAR MAGNETIC RESONANCE

Solid-state nuclear magnetic resonance (SSNMR) spectroscopy is a more advanced method for differentiating the polymorphs of a material. The sample is placed in a strong magnetic field and subjected to radiofrequency radiation. The individual nuclei experiences different magnetic environments and thus shows different changes in resonant frequency characterized by chemical shifts. The polymorphs are differentiated by their characteristic spectra. This method is suitable for the characterization of solid-state forms that cannot be crystallized and studied by the x-ray diffraction method. It is also useful for quantifying components of heterogeneous mixtures. In contrast to IR and Raman spectroscopies, the results are less affected by the particle size of the test material.

3.5.6 MOISTURE SORPTION

Moisture sorption is performed in a climatic chamber. A balance measures weight changes of the sample exposed to a defined humidity program. In comparison to crystalline materials, the amorphous state is characterized by a higher potential to absorb moisture. This leads to a higher mass increase of amorphous materials in comparison to crystalline materials [54].

3.5.7 HOT STAGE MICROSCOPY

The polarizing microscope fitted with a hot stage is very useful for identifying the crystalline forms of a material. In this method, the polymorph is heated to a temperature at which it undergoes a change in birefringence and/or appearance, which is characteristic of the polymorph.

3.5.8 DETECTION LIMITS OF DIFFERENT METHODS

A wide range of methods can be employed to assess polymorphism of materials. In some cases, it is necessary to use a combination of methods to avoid erroneous conclusions obtained from the use of a single method. The detection limits of the different methods are 10% for DSC, 1–10% for x-ray diffraction, 1% for Raman spectroscopy and 0.5% for SSNMR [55].

3.6 OTHER PHYSICAL PROPERTIES

Undoubtedly, the type of physical characterization tests for a drug or excipient depends very much on the material concerned as well as the processing involved. Material testing can be broadly divided into two types, namely physical testing, and functionality testing. Physical testing, which is used to determine properties, such as size, shape, surface area, solubility, and crystal form, is generally more direct and the procedures are better established. Functionality testing that evaluates properties, such as flowability, compressibility, tableting, segregation, sticking, and packing property is less direct. However, such tests may yield useful information about the raw materials, drug–excipient blends, and their potential effects on the processing.

3.6.1 Flow Properties

Powder flowability is important for the delivery of the powder from the hopper to the die during the tableting process. Flowability is influenced by numerous factors such as particle size, shape, size distribution, surface roughness, moisture content, and electrostatic charges [56]. The erratic flow of the powder will result in unacceptable variation in the weight of the tablets produced. In addition, uneven powder flow could lead to excess entrapped air within the powder, which in some high-speed tableting conditions may promote capping or lamination. Similarly, powders with poor flowability will move with greater difficulty in the granulation chamber and this will affect the granulation process and the properties of the granules produced. Knowledge of the flowability of powders, especially of the bulk excipients, is therefore important so that the necessary steps can be undertaken to avoid problems during processing. The Hausner ratio, Carr index, angle of repose, and angle of the slide are parameters that are commonly used to quantify the flowability of powders. For poorly flowing powders, the shear tests are used. The powder in motion can be studied (from flow perspective) by dynamic powder testing options.

3.6.1.1 Hausner Ratio and Carr Index

The tapped density (ρ_t) and bulk density (ρ_b) of the test sample are determined by the methods described previously.

$$\text{Hausner ratio} = \rho_t/\rho_b \tag{3.6}$$

$$\text{Carr index}(\%) = [(\rho_t - \rho_b)/\rho_t] \times 100 \tag{3.7}$$

Higher Hausner ratio and Carr index indicate poorer flow [57–59]. Table 3.2 provides an accepted scale of flowability based on the Hausner ratio and Carr index or compressibility Carr index [60–62].

TABLE 3.2
Flowability Scale Based on Hausner Ratio and Compressibility Carr Index

Hausner Ratio	Flow Character	Carr Index
1.00–1.11	Excellent	≤10
1.12–1.18	Good	11–15
1.19–1.25	Fair	16–20
1.26–1.34	Passable	21–25
1.35–1.45	Poor	26–31
1.46–1.59	Very poor	32–37
>1.6	Very, very poor	>38

3.6.1.2 Angle of Repose

A funnel is mounted vertically and at a distance from a horizontal plate. It is filled with the test sample, which is then allowed to flow down freely to form a conical heap on the plate. A metal tube may also be used in place of the funnel. The tube is placed vertically on the plate and filled with the test sample to a height of about 4 cm. It is then slowly lifted vertically, leaving a conical heap of powder on the plate [5]. Using either method, the height of the heap (h) is determined by measuring the distance between the plate and the tip of the heap. The radius of the heap (r) is determined by dividing the diameter of its circular base by 2. The angle of repose is obtained from the inverse tangential of the ratio between h and r [5,63]. A smaller angle of repose indicates better flow.

3.6.1.3 Angle of Slide

This is employed to quantify the flowability of a powder bed. A small amount (about 10 mg) of the sample is placed on a stainless-steel plane, which is then tilted by screwing a supporting spindle vertically upward until the powder slide occurs. The angle of the slide is equal to the angle between the tilted plane and the horizontal base at this point [5]. This method could be valuable in designing chutes. However, the measurement method and values are not standardized. Also, the measured angle will be highly influenced by the type of chute material, chute surface, amount of powder, humidity, and other factors.

3.6.1.4 Flowability Determined by Shear Tests

Originally, shear tests have been explored to understand soil mechanics. Around 1960, Andrew Jenike designed the first shear cell tester, referred to as translational shear cell tester, for bulk solids [64]. His work significantly contributed to the understanding of powder cohesivity and in hopper designs. The shear test has been applied widely for the analysis of powder flowability. Variants of the shear cell tester were developed, for example, Schulz ring shear tester, FT4 powder rheometer, Brookfield powder flow tester, Walker ring shear tester, Peschl rotational shear tester and others [65–67]. The general shear test method and principles are described here briefly. The shear cell is filled, the powder surface is leveled and consolidation stress (σ_1) is applied. Shear is produced in the sample using the appropriate shear lid under given consolidation stress. Failure of the powder bed (also called "incipient flow") is indicated by a sudden drop in shear stress and the stress responsible for this failure is called the unconfined yield strength (σ_c). The unconfined yield strength versus consolidation stress curve is known as the instantaneous flow function or flow function curve [68]. Flow function values (ffc) at specific consolidation stress can be calculated using the following equation.

$$ffc = \frac{\sigma 1}{\sigma c} \qquad (3.8)$$

The larger ffc values indicate better powder flow. Based on ffc values, Jenike provided the rough guide to classify the flowability of the powders. Schulze further elaborated on this classification (Table 3.3) with minor changes in ffc values [66]. Figure 3.11 provides an example of the flow function curve along with the flowability classification. Based on the flow function equation and the flowability classification, it is easy to understand that ffc values are influenced by the consolidation stress used to calculate them. Materials do not experience much consolidation stress during pharmaceutical unit operations and processing [69]. Therefore, it is advisable to evaluate and compare ffc values of pharmaceutical powders at a fixed and lower side of the consolidation stress values. For example, ffc data for the powders have been analyzed at 4 KPa [70] and 8 KPa consolidation stresses [71]. It is technically difficult to collect reproducible ffc values at very low consolidation stresses (particularly below 1 KPa). It has been reported that the lower limit for consolidation of the ring shear tester was approximately 0.5 KPa [69]. Clearly, the use of shear cell tester may be useful to characterize cohesive

TABLE 3.3
Flowability Classifications Based on *ffc* Values

ffc Values	Flowability
$ffc < 1$	Not flowing
$1 < ffc < 2$	Very cohesive
$2 < ffc < 4$	Cohesive
$4 < ffc < 10$	Easy-flowing
$10 < ffc$	Free-flowing

Source: From Ref. [66].

powders but is generally less effective for free-flowing powders. The need for the consolidation stress also presents particular issues as often, high consolidation stress does not represent the actual stress conditions encountered during product manufacture, and *ffc* comparison at high consolidation stress should be avoided.

Apart from rendering flow function curves and *ffc* values [56,72], various software can analyze the raw data and determine the angles of internal friction. Besides, by using appropriate lid design, shear testers can provide wall friction values and bin design parameters [73]. Compared to the angle of repose, compressibility Carr index, Hausner ratio, and flow through an orifice, the results of shear tests are more dependable for flow analysis [68].

3.6.1.5 Dynamic Flow Analysis

Traditional flow and bulk property evaluation techniques such as shear tests discussed earlier do not consider dynamic conditions experienced by powder passing through various unit operations. Techniques are now available (e.g., FT4, Freeman Technology - Micromeritics, Tewkesbury, UK) to analyze powder flow in dynamic conditions as a function of strain rate [41]. Dynamic flow analysis indicators, such as basic flow energy (BFE), stability index (SI), flow rate index (FRI), and specific energy (SE) can be derived on the basis of these tests. In this technique, an impeller with a twisted blade rotates at a specific tip speed and penetrates in and out of the powder bed filled in a vessel. The first step of "conditioning methodology" is discussed in section 3.2. In the next step, the blade penetrates again into the conditioned powder bed filled with force while rotating anti-

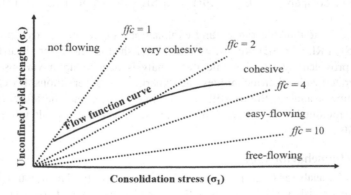

FIGURE 3.11   Flow function curve and flowability classification.
Source: Adapted from Ref. [66].

clockwise. This bulldozing blade action compacts the bed and applies normal stresses through the blade. Axial force (F) required for downward blade movement and torque required for blade rotation (T) are measured. Total input work (E), also called "flow energy," of the powder is computed using F and T values as shown below [74].

$$E = \int_0^H \left(\frac{T}{R \tan \alpha} + F \right) dH \tag{3.9}$$

where R is the radius of the blade, α is the helix angle, and H is the penetrated depth.

The steps (conditioning + testing) are repeated several times to obtain stabilized non-changing flow energy or BFE [75]. In short, BFE measures powder's flowability when it is forced to flow. BFE relies on density, compressibility, packing state, particle size, and shape [76]. Although reports claimed that BFE results can be correlated to flowability [40,41,75–77], researchers have also acknowledged that BFE evaluates different factors in combination and sometimes may show little correlation with shear test (flow) results [41].

Changes in the flow energy (as a result of the repeated conditioning + testing steps) are further used to calculate SI. Pharmaceutical powders are generally stable and have SI values in the range of 0.9–1.1 [76,78] with good repeatability. Phenomena like segregation, particle attrition, strong adhesion to the equipment, air release from the powder, or moisture uptake can impact SI values. Hence, a change in SI value can be an indicator of one of these phenomena.

FRI can be determined by sequentially decreasing the blade tip speed and sensitivity of the powder to the flow rate is evaluated. The instrument software determines the FRI by calculating the ratio of the flow energy when tip speed is reduced by a factor of 10. For example, in a study by Freeman, tip speed was reduced from 100 mm/s to 10 mm/s (factor of 10) and the ratio of flow energy between the corresponding speed tips was calculated to determine FRI [41]. Higher FRI values (>3) demonstrates that the powder is experiencing mechanical interlocking and could be cohesive in nature. FRI ~1 indicates that the powder is not sensitive to the flow rate. Generally, FRI is in the range of 1.5–3.

SE is another parameter that can be measured using the dynamic test analysis. This parameter represents powder flowability (and so cohesion) in an unconfined or low-stress condition [75]. Work required to bring the blade from bottom to top of the vessel through the powder bed is used to calculate SE. SE is significantly impacted by the shape of particles. Spherical or oval shapes have a low number of contacts and hence show a low SE value. Elongated particles provide a greater number of contacts, resulting in high SE values. Soft particle contacts may further lead to high SE values [78]. Generally, SE < 5 indicates low cohesion, 5 < SE < 10 shows moderate cohesion, and SE > 10 indicates high cohesion [76]. Researchers have critically evaluated and compared BFE, SI, FRI, and SE values obtained for different powders/ blends [41,75,76,78].

It is important to note that the ranges and explanations suggested for dynamic flow analysis indicators (BFE, SI, FRI, and SE) are not as well established as those for shear tests (*ffc* classification). Trends provided by the dynamic flow analysis depend upon various conditions and should be corroborated with other techniques and experimental observations. Based on the current literature information available, this is still an evolving science, and the aforementioned ranges may be updated or modified in the future. Utmost care should be taken while interpreting BFE, SI, FRI, and SE results.

3.6.1.6 Avalanche Behavior [56]

An avalanche powder analyzer (e.g., Revolution, Mercury Scientific, Newtown, CT, US) employs a transparent drum or disk partially filled with a powder and rotated to establish a consistent flowing powder mass. With a light source on one side, a camera on the opposite side captures

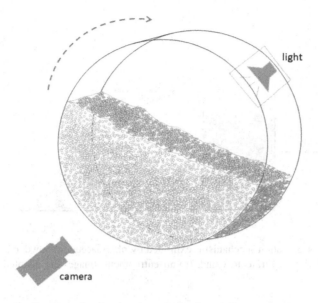

FIGURE 3.12 Schematic diagram of an avalanche powder flowability tester.

images of the avalanche behavior of the powder (Figure 3.12). A low disk rotational speed is usually preferred because it prevents the merging of powder avalanches and provides better discrimination of powders properties [79]. Qualitative visualization of the avalanching behavior can differentiate the powder flow, with free-flowing powders exhibiting slumping or rolling type of behavior while poorer flowing powders tend to cascade. From image processing, a variety of numerical descriptors together with visual observations can help to classify powder flow behaviors. Despite the versatility of the avalanche flow analyzer, interpretation of the derived descriptors may sometimes pose a challenge to inexperienced users, particularly with more cohesive powders. However, avalanche flow testing subjects the powder to a tumbling motion, which simulates the conditions during mixing. This attribute can be applied to studying mixing processes and powder flowability and mixability [80].

3.6.2 SEGREGATION

Segregation is the separation of the components of a powder blend from one another, which can lead to blend inhomogeneity. Differences in particle size, shape, density, texture, flowability, and adhesive forces are common physical factors responsible for segregation. In addition, external stimuli experienced by the powder blend during granulation, drying, blending, conveying, compression, and other unit operations also promote this phenomenon. Schulze described various segregation mechanisms (Figure 3.13) related to shifting and percolation, trajectory and air-entrapment [66]. Various modeling and small-scale prediction tools have been developed to evaluate segregation risk. Formulating blends with a similar particle size distribution, decreasing possible vibration, and avoiding large height free falls of blends during product manufacturing are possible ways to reduce the segregation risk.

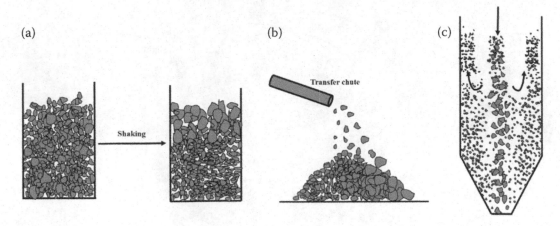

FIGURE 3.13 Major segregation mechanisms exhibited by pharmaceutical powder blends during handling: (a) shifting and percolation, (b) trajectory and, (c) air-entrapment. Images are adapted from Schulze [66].

3.6.3 TABLETING PROPERTIES

Mixtures of drugs and excipients are compressed directly from powder blends or via granules, to produce tablets that are the most widely used oral solid dosage form. Studying the capability of pharmaceutical powder blends to make the compacts of the required tensile strength is the fundamental requirement for the tablet dosage form. The tableting properties are often related to attributes of compressibility, compactability, and manufacturability [81]. Compressibility refers to the densification change of the powder when compressed [82], whereas compactability refers to the ability of the powder to form bonds and make robust compacts [83]. Various models and equations, including Heckel, Walker, Kawakita, and Gurnham equations, have been employed to study the relationship between applied pressure and porosity (compressibility) and deduce brittle versus plastic behavior of individual materials and blends [81–84]. Compactability may be quantified in different ways. One method is to determine the minimum compression pressure required to make the compact of required tensile strength. Compression pressure versus tensile strength, porosity or solid fraction versus tensile strength profiles is widely used to compare compactability of materials. It is desired to get compression pressure versus tensile strength profile linear. If the profile levels off or tensile strength decrease with an increase in compression pressure, it means that the solid fraction values are reaching the limit or there may be evidence of lamination or capping. Therefore, it is not advisable to produce tablets at those high compression pressure ranges. During tablet formulation development, it is necessary to develop a model to predict the compressibility and compactability of the tableting feed blends by appropriate characterization methods. In a study, three common pharmaceutical excipients were characterized using uniaxial compaction simulator, and models were developed with the capability to predict the compaction and compression properties of binary and ternary mixtures made from these excipients [82]. For good manufacturability, the blend should not experience significant friction when its compacted form is ejected from the die during tableting [81]. Ejection stress versus compression pressure profile is studied to evaluate the manufacturability.

3.6.4 STICKING

Punch sticking during compression is a challenging issue in tablet manufacturing, particularly for high drug load products (>30%, w/w) [85,86]. The material accumulates on the tooling surface over some time during the manufacturing run and this phenomenon can be observed by visual inspection of the tooling and tablets. Tableting process parameters (e.g., tableting speed, tooling designs, compression pressure, and tooling materials), material properties (e.g., particle size, mechanical properties, surface chemistry, hygroscopicity, and melting temperature), and granulation and lubrication (type, concentration, and blending time) have variously impacted this phenomenon. Higher tableting speed increases sticking propensity, whereas higher compression pressure decreases it. The degree of sticking for punch design can be ranked as follows: flat > bevel > concave [87]. Changing lubricant types, increasing lubricant levels, and blending time have also provided a solution to this problem in some cases. Sticking issues undetected during early stage and small-scale product manufacturing are often experienced after extended tablet manufacturing. Therefore, if detected at a late stage, it could significantly impact the product development timelines and cost [86]. To address this concern, researchers attempted various approaches and developed tools to evaluate the sticking propensity of materials. Some of these tools and approaches to predict punch sticking potential are discussed here briefly but the list of these tools/approaches is not exhaustive.

Surface roughness (R_A) measurement using atomic force microscopy was used to rank the work of adhesion among three model "profen" family compounds and iron (punch metal) [88]. Tablet take-off force, ejection force for "profen" family compounds, and their formulations were further measured using the compaction simulator. Punch face adhesion was then ranked using tablet take-off force and visual observation of the punch faces [89]. Through these studies, it was deduced that atomic force microscopy measurement of tablet take-off forces can be a good approach to evaluate drug-metal interaction. Leveraging on the influence of punch geometry on sticking, a material sparing approach of proactively using flat face and flat face bevel edge punch tip geometry was proposed in the early stage product development in a study. These flat-faced geometries provided an early indication of sticking problems compared to standard round concave geometry [86]. It is logical to postulate that sticking propensity will be more if the adhesive forces between tablet particles and punch surfaces are higher than the particles within the tablet. This postulation was substantiated, whereby shear test was used to predict the likelihood of sticking during tableting [90]. Particularly, the shear test was used to measure the angle of internal friction of powder blend (Φp, representing frictional forces between particle) and angle of wall friction of powder-punch surface (Φw, representing frictional forces between particle and punch surface). The sticking index was then calculated as follows:

$$Sticking\ index = \frac{\Phi w}{\Phi p} \tag{3.10}$$

Sticking was observed at sticking index > 0.3 and the suitability of the sticking index to predict sticking was further confirmed. In another study, an instrumented punch was developed to use along with the universal testing machine and measure adhesive forces between compact and punch surface [91]. Recently, an in-line material-sparing laser reflection-based tool was implemented to monitor sticking in real-time [92]. In this technique, a laser beam is targeted at the tip of the punch and the intensity of the reflected beam is quantified using a photosensor. The results confirmed that the area covered by sticking material correlated with the signal intensity. This simple, highly sensitive technique evaluates sticking during the actual tableting process without interrupting the manufacturing.

Sticking is a challenging issue in pharmaceutical product manufacturing particularly in tableting; researchers are continuously working in this field to further understand this phenomenon. Various approaches have been attempted to evaluate and mitigate the sticking propensity of materials but often, solutions are directed at changing the compression pressure or tableting rate, tool design or material, ambient or press temperature, and the use of anti-sticking agents.

3.6.5 COMPATIBILITY

Although excipients have traditionally been thought of as being inert, experience has shown that they can interact with a drug. Readers are encouraged to refer to the literature on drug–excipient interactions and their effects on drug absorption [93]. Incompatibility may occur between drug and excipient, as well as between the excipients themselves, and affect the potency, stability, and eventually, therapeutic efficacy of the product. It is therefore essential to avoid incompatibility and this can be achieved by carrying out studies to detect potential chemical interactions between the different components used in the formulation.

3.6.5.1 Stability Study

This is the traditional method of detecting incompatibility. Mixtures of the drug and excipients are prepared and stored under exaggerated conditions of heat, light, and humidity. The mixtures are examined for any physical change and aliquot samples are withdrawn for assay of the intact drug at various time intervals. Incompatibility is reflected by various signs such as the appearance of precipitate and a decrease in the concentration of the intact drug. Although this is a very important topic, it is better discussed separately as a topic on its own.

3.6.5.2 Chromatography

Chromatography was first used for the separation of leaf pigments. The operation of chromatography is based on the distribution of material between a stationary phase and a mobile phase. The stationary phase can be a solid or a liquid supported on a solid while the mobile phase can be a gas or a liquid, which flows continuously around the stationary phase. As a result of differences in their affinity for the stationary phase, the different components in a mixture can be separated and identified.

In addition to its application in the separation and identification of materials, chromatography is also employed to detect potential interactions between materials. Both thin-layer chromatography and liquid chromatography are commonly employed for this purpose. In thin-layer chromatography, the stationary phase consists of a powder adhered onto a glass, plastic, or metal plate. The powders commonly used are silica, alumina, polyamides, celluloses, and ion-exchange resins. Solutions of the drug, excipient, and drug–excipient mixture are prepared and spotted on the same baseline at one end of the plate. The plate is then placed upright in a closed chamber containing the solvent, which constitutes the mobile phase. As the solvent moves up the plate, it carries with it the materials. Those materials that have a stronger affinity for the stationary phase will move at a slower rate. The material is identified by its R_f value, which is defined as the ratio of the distance traveled by the material to the distance traveled by the solvent front. The position of the material on the plate is indicated by spraying the plate with certain reagents or exposing the plate to ultraviolet radiation. If there is no interaction between the drug and excipient, the mixture will produce two spots whose R_f values are identical to those of the individual drug and excipient. If there is interaction, the complex formed will produce a spot whose R_f value is different from those of the individual components.

In liquid chromatography, the affinity of the material for the solid stationary phase in a column governs the time taken by the material to elute from the column. The time of elution is used to identify the material. Solutions of the drug, excipient, and drug–excipient mixture are prepared and injected separately into the column. The concentration of the material that elutes from the column is detected and plotted against time to give a chromatogram. If there is interaction between the drug and excipient, the complex formed will exhibit an elution time different from those of the individual components (Figure 3.14). Similarly, gas chromatography may be used for volatile components.

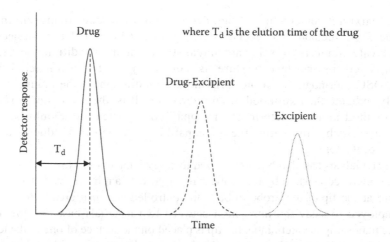

FIGURE 3.14 Chromatograms illustrating drug–excipient interaction.

3.6.5.3 Thermal Methods

DSC offers a relatively simple approach for the investigation of potential interaction between a drug and an excipient [94,95]. The drug, individual excipients, and binary mixtures of the drug and excipient are separately scanned at a standard rate over a temperature range that encompasses all the thermal features of the drug and excipients. Each mixture consists of equal proportions of drug and excipient in order to maximize the likelihood of an interaction. The thermograms of the mixtures and the individual components are compared (Figure 3.15). Interaction is deduced by changes in the thermal features such as the disappearance of characteristic peaks or the appearance of a new peak in the thermogram of the mixture. Changes in shape, onset, and relative height of the peaks may also indicate interaction. However, it should be cautioned that these changes could also arise from the physical mixing of the components or dissolution of components in the first molten substance.

A big advantage of the DSC method over the traditional stability test is the speed of determination. However, like all methods, DSC has its own limitations. It is not applicable if the test materials exhibit properties that make data interpretation difficult, such as the formation

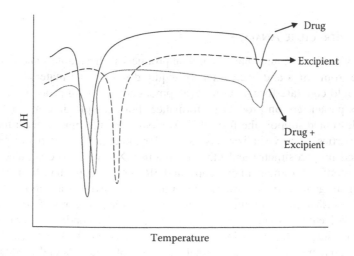

FIGURE 3.15 Thermograms indicating possible drug–excipient interaction.

of the eutectic mixture, coincident melting, and dissolution of one component in the melt of the other. The DSC method has received specific criticism [95] that it subjects drug and excipient to elevated temperatures that are unrealistically high. In addition, the ratio of drug to excipient employed in the test mixture is not likely to be encountered in practice. Furthermore, DSC thermograms do not provide information about the nature of the interaction; they only indicate the likelihood of an interaction. It is, therefore, not advisable to rely on the DSC method alone to determine incompatibility. Instead, it should be used to supplement stability tests by eliminating the incompatible excipients and reducing the number of samples for stability testing.

Microthermal analysis has also been employed to study interaction. This method is a derivative of atomic force microscopy whereby the probe is replaced with a miniaturized thermistor, allowing the temperature at the tip of the probe to be both controlled and measured. Different techniques have been employed to study the interaction between two materials based on the microthermal analysis. In the nanosampling technique, the tip is placed on the surface of one of the test materials, which is heated to soften the surface so that the tip is partially covered with the material. The tip, which is then withdrawn, retains some of the material in the nanogram to picogram range. In another technique, known as thermally assisted particle manipulation, the tip is used to pick up a particle of one of the test materials that have been softened by heat. By employing either technique, the tip (laden with the first test material) is placed on the surface of the second test material, which is then subjected to a heating program. Interaction between these two test materials is deduced from the thermal profiles obtained [96].

3.6.5.4   Other Methods

IR, particularly Fourier transform IR spectrometry, can also be employed to study interaction [95]. In the same way, modifications in the spectra obtained by Raman spectroscopy indicate that chemical interactions have occurred. The Raman spectra can be processed to give unambiguous identification of both drugs and excipients, and the relative intensity of the drug and excipient bands can be used for quantitative analysis. More information about the different Raman techniques can be obtained from the literature [97].

Unlike most other methods, SSNMR is applicable to materials of varying complexity, from pure drugs and excipients to their solid dispersions [98]. Selective investigation of the individual components of the solid dispersions does not usually require any chemical or physical treatment of the sample. However, the complexity and high cost of SSNMR restrict its application as a routine characterization method.

3.6.6   Internal Structure Analysis

Internal structure visualization and analysis of final products such as tablets and intermediates such as granules made from drugs and excipients are required to evaluate materials and products in a holistic way. It could correlate formulation development activity with process parameters and the impact of process parameters on product performance. For example, internal and external visualization of granules could support the formulation scientist to link binder performance to granule structure and properties. Such visualizations can render direct measurements of porosities, which are often estimated by porosimetry and other techniques. X-ray micro-computed tomography in conjunction with confocal Raman microscopy and IR spectroscopy has been successfully employed to investigate granule microstructure (3D) at micron level in a non-invasive way and to analyze chemical distribution within the granules [99]. Other applications of x-ray micro-computed tomography include identification of stress-induced micro-cracks, coating uniformity and thickness measurements, and drug distribution in granules and tablets. Optical coherence tomography is another non-destructive method to view internal structures of materials and products and has been used in medical and clinical practices for a few decades. Researchers in the past decade had used this interferometric method to evaluate tablet surfaces, mainly the coating [100–102]. Terahertz pulsed spectroscopy and 3D terahertz pulsed imaging are other technologies used in attempts to quantify crystallinity and polymorphism [103], calculate molecular mobility and crystallization of amorphous materials [104], detect porosity of compact [105], analyze coating structures and interfaces [106], quantify hardness, and map density distributions of tablets [107]. Working principles, advantages and applications of x-ray micro-computed tomography, optical coherence tomography, terahertz pulsed spectroscopy, and terahertz pulsed imaging are discussed in the review by Zeitler and Gladden [108] and can be referred for additional details. Another important process analytical technology (PAT) is NIR chemical imaging. The size of the drug particles or drug clusters in the process intermediates or final products can be detected using this imaging technology. This quick and efficient diagnostic technology renders a microscale/mesoscale imaging of the drug substance clusters during intermediate process steps, for example, before and after co-milling or before and after dry granulation. The tool can be used to confirm that the processing steps are robust enough to break agglomerates and provide content uniformity to the final tablet dosage form [109].

3.7   CONCLUSION

It can be challenging for any process technologist to decide on the type and extent of material characterization to be undertaken. The methods used should be able to provide accurate results, and yet easy to carry out and cost-effective. Often, it is the problem from the production run that necessitates further material characterization to be carried out either for the purpose of solving the problem or to prevent future occurrences. Comprehensive characterization of drug substances and excipients should be further linked to drug product formulation, process selections, and product critical quality attributes. This characterization workflow can provide a coveted starting point in pursuit of selecting suitable drug product processing and formulation development steps with a limited amount of drug substance in compressed development timelines. Risk analysis accomplished during this journey of the molecule to drug product development must include the material attributes. This chapter serves to identify the more commonly used, to advanced material characterization methods that can be carried out and could provide potentially useful information that can be inferred from the tests. It is hoped that the discussion of the many methods of material characterization could help in the judicious choice of characterization methods for material testing and the assessment of intermediates such as granules in the formulation or processing steps.

ABBREVIATIONS

Basic flow energy – BFE
Differential scanning calorimetry - DSC
Flow function values - *ffc*
Flow rate index - FRI
High-speed or high-performance DSC - hyperDSC
Infrared - IR
Modulated temperature DSC - MTDSC
Near infrared - NIR
Solid-state nuclear magnetic resonance - SSNMR
Specific energy - SE
Stability index - SI
Three-dimensional – 3D
Two-dimensional – 2D

SYMBOLS

Angle of internal friction of powder blend - Φp
Angle of wall friction of powder-punch surface - Φw
Axial force - F
Bulk density - ρ_b
Consolidation stress - σ_1
Flow energy (or total input work) - E
Glass transition temperature - T_g
Height of the heap - h
Helix angle - α
Melting point - T_m
Penetrated depth - H
Radius of the blade - R
Radius of the heap - r
Surface roughness - R_A
Tapped density - ρ_t
Torque required for blade rotation - T
Unconfined yield strength - σ_c

REFERENCES

1. Patel S., Kaushal A. M., Bansal A. K. Effect of particle size and compression force on compaction behavior and derived mathematical parameters of compressibility. Pharm Res. 2007; 24(1): 111–124.
2. Tang P., Puri V. M. Segregation quantification of two-component particulate mixtures: Effect of particle size, density, shape, and surface texture Particul Sci Technol. 2007; 25(6): 571–588.
3. British Standard 3406. Methods for determination of particle size distribution. Guide to microscope and image analysis method. Published: February 1993.
4. Jones M. D., Harris H., Hooton J. C., Shur J., King G. S., Mathoulin C. A., Nichol K., Smith T. L., Dawson M. L., Ferrie A. R., Price R. An investigation into the relationship between carrier-based dry powder inhalation performance and formulation cohesive–adhesive force balances. Eur J Pharm Biopharm. 2008; 69(2): 496–507.
5. Zeng X. M., Martin G. P., Marriott C., Pritchard J. Crystallization of lactose from carbopol gels. Pharm Res. 2000; 17(7): 879–886.
6. Bosquillon C., Lombry C., Preat V., Vanbever R. Comparison of particle sizing techniques in the case of inhalation dry powders. J Pharm Sci. 2001; 90(12): 2032–2041.
7. Gamble J. F., Ferreira A. P., Tobyn M., DiMemmo L., Martin K., Mathias N., Schild R., Vig B., Baumann J. M., Parks S., Ashton M. Application of imaging based tools for the characterisation of hollow spray dried amorphous dispersion particles. Int J Pharm. 2014; 465(1–2): 210–217.
8. Yu W., Hancock B. C. Evaluation of dynamic image analysis for characterizing pharmaceutical excipient particles. Int J Pharm. 2008; 361(1–2): 150–157.
9. Ben Abdelaziz I., Sahli A., Bornaz S., Scher J., Gaiani C. Dynamic method to characterize rehydration of powdered cocoa beverage: Influence of sugar nature, quantity and size. Powder Technol. 2014; 264: 184–189.
10. Kayser G., Graf-Rosenfellner M., Schack-Kirchner H., Lang F. Dynamic imaging provides novel insight into the shape and stability of soil aggregates. Eur J Soil Sci. 2019; 70(3): 454–465.
11. Yang J. Z., Young A. L., Chiang P.-C., Thurston A., Pretzer D. K. Fluticasone and budesonide nanosuspensions for pulmonary delivery: Preparation, characterization, and pharmacokinetic studies. J Pharm Sci. 2008; 97(11): 4869–4878.
12. Adi H., Larson I., Stewart P. Laser diffraction particle sizing of cohesive lactose powders. Powder Technol. 2007; 179(1): 90–94.
13. Stevens N., Shrimpton J., Palmer M., Prime D., Johal B. Accuracy assessments for laser diffraction measurements of pharmaceutical lactose. Meas Sci Technol. 2007; 18(12): 3697–3706.

14. Laitinen N., Juppo A. M. Measurement of pharmaceutical particles using a time-of-flight particle sizer. Eur J Pharm Biopharm. 2003; 55(1): 93–98.
15. Oskouie A. K., Wang H.-C., Mavliev R., Noll K. E. Calculated calibration curves for particle size determination based on time-of-flight (TOF). Aerosol Sci Technol. 1998; 29(5): 433–441.
16. Heath A. R., Fawell P. D., Bahri P. A., Swift J. D. Estimating average particle size by focused beam reflectance measurement (FBRM). Part Part Syst Char. 2002; 19(2): 84–95.
17. Greaves D., Boxall J., Mulligan J., Montesi A., Creek J., Dendy Sloan E., Koh C. A. Measuring the particle size of a known distribution using the focused beam reflectance measurement technique. Chem Eng Sci. 2008; 63(22): 5410–5419.
18. Silva A. F. T., Burggraeve A., Denon Q., Van Der Meeren P., Sandler N., Van Den Kerkhof T., Hellings M., Vervaet C., Remon J. P., Lopes J. A., De Beer T. Particle sizing measurements in pharmaceutical applications: Comparison of in-process methods versus off-line methods. Eur J Pharm Biopharm. 2013; 85(3, Part B): 1006–1018.
19. Närvänen T., Lipsanen T., Antikainen O., Räikkönen H., Heinämäki J., Yliruusi J. Gaining fluid bed process understanding by in-line particle size analysis. J Pharm Sci. 2009; 98(3): 1110–1117.
20. Sandler N. Photometric imaging in particle size measurement and surface visualization. Int J Pharm. 2011; 417(1–2): 227–234.
21. Naidu V. R., Deshpande R. S., Syed M. R., Wakte P. S. Real time imaging as an emerging process analytical technology tool for monitoring of fluid bed coating process. Pharm Dev Technol. 2018; 23(6): 596–601.
22. Kumar A., Dhondt J., De Leersnyder F., Vercruysse J., Vanhoorne V., Vervaet C., Remon J. P., Gernaey K. V., De Beer T., Nopens I. Evaluation of an in-line particle imaging tool for monitoring twin-screw granulation performance. Powder Technol. 2015; 285:80–87.
23. Treffer D., Wahl P. R., Hörmann T. R., Markl D., Schrank S., Jones I., Cruise P., Mürb R. K., Koscher G., Roblegg E., Khinast J. G. In-line implementation of an image-based particle size measurement tool to monitor hot-melt extruded pellets. Int J Pharm. 2014; 466(1–2): 181–189.
24. Desai P. M., Vaerenbergh G. V., Holman J., Liew C. V., Heng P. W. S. Continuous manufacturing: The future in pharmaceutical solid dosage form manufacturing. Pharm Bioprocess. 2015; 3(5): 357–360.
25. Desai P. M., Hogan R. C., Brancazio D., Puri V., Jensen K. D., Chun J. H., Myerson A. S., Trout B. L. Integrated hot-melt extrusion – injection molding continuous tablet manufacturing platform: Effects of critical process parameters and formulation attributes on product robustness and dimensional stability. Int J Pharm. 2017; 531(1): 332–342.
26. Wilms A., Knop K., Kleinebudde P. Combination of a rotating tube sample divider and dynamic image analysis for continuous on-line determination of granule size distribution. Int J Pharm: X. 2019; 1:100029.
27. Dickhoff B. H. J., de Boer A. H., Lambregts D., Frijlink H. W. The effect of carrier surface treatment on drug particle detachment from crystalline carriers in adhesive mixtures for inhalation. Int J Pharm. 2006; 327(1): 17–25.
28. Tee S. K., Marriott C., Zeng X. M., Martin G. P. The use of different sugars as fine and coarse carriers for aerosolised salbutamol sulphate. Int J Pharm. 2000; 208(1): 111–123.
29. Larhrib H., Martin G. P., Prime D., Marriott C. Characterisation and deposition studies of engineered lactose crystals with potential for use as a carrier for aerosolised salbutamol sulfate from dry powder inhalers. Eur J Pharm Sci. 2003; 19(4): 211–221.
30. Brewer E., Ramsland A. Particle size determination by automated microscopical imaging analysis with comparison to laser diffraction. J Pharm Sci. 1995; 84(4): 499–501.
31. Ma Z., Merkus H. G., de Smet J. G. A. E., Heffels C., Scarlett B. New developments in particle characterization by laser diffraction: Size and shape. Powder Technol. 2000; 111(1): 66–78.
32. Naito M., Hayakawa O., Nakahira K., Mori H., Tsubaki J. Effect of particle shape on the particle size distribution measured with commercial equipment. Powder Technol. 1998; 100(1): 52–60.
33. Borovoi A., Naats E., Oppel U., Grishin I. Shape characterization of a large nonspherical particle by use of its fraunhofer diffraction pattern. Appl Opt. 2000; 39(12): 1989–1997.
34. Mühlenweg H., Hirleman E. D. Laser diffraction spectroscopy: Influence of particle shape and a shape adaptation technique. Part Part Syst Char. 1998; 15(4): 163–169.
35. Das S. C., Behara S. R. B., Morton D. A. V., Larson I., Stewart P. J. Importance of particle size and shape on the tensile strength distribution and de-agglomeration of cohesive powders. Powder Technol. 2013; 249:297–303.
36. Sun C. Quantifying errors in tableting data analysis using the ryshkewitch equation due to inaccurate true density. J Pharm Sci. 2005; 94(9): 2061–2068.

37. Sun C. True density of microcrystalline cellulose. J Pharm Sci. 2005; 94(10): 2132–2134.
38. Hedden D. B., Brone D. L., Clement S., McCall M., Olsofsky A., Patel P. J., Prescott J., Hancock B. C. Development of an improved fluidization segregation tester for use with pharmaceutical powders. Pharm Technol. 2006(30):56–64.
39. Yamamoto Y., Fujii M., Watanabe K-i, Tsukamoto M., Shibata Y., Kondoh M., Watanabe Y. Effect of powder characteristics on oral tablet disintegration. Int J Pharm. 2009; 365(1): 116–120.
40. Mangal S., Gengenbach T., Millington-Smith D., Armstrong B., Morton D. A. V., Larson I. Relationship between the cohesion of guest particles on the flow behaviour of interactive mixtures. Eur J Pharm Biopharm. 2016; 102:168–177.
41. Freeman R. Measuring the flow properties of consolidated, conditioned and aerated powders – a comparative study using a powder rheometer and a rotational shear cell. Powder Technol. 2007; 174(1): 25–33.
42. Sun C. A novel method for deriving true density of pharmaceutical solids including hydrates and water-containing powders. J Pharm Sci. 2004; 93(3): 646–653.
43. Imamura K., Maruyama Y., Tanaka K., Yokoyama T., Imanaka H., Nakanishi K. True density analysis of a freeze-dried amorphous sugar matrix. J Pharm Sci. 2008; 97(7): 2789–2797.
44. Sugano K., Kato T., Suzuki K., Keiko K., Sujaku T., Mano T. High throughput solubility measurement with automated polarized light microscopy analysis. J Pharm Sci. 2006; 95(10): 2115–2122.
45. Hancock B. C., Parks M. What is the true solubility advantage for amorphous pharmaceuticals? Pharm Res. 2000; 17(4): 397–404.
46. Pudipeddi M., Serajuddin A. T. M. Trends in solubility of polymorphs. J Pharm Sci. 2005; 94(5): 929–939.
47. Dong W., Gilmore C., Barr G., Dallman C., Feeder N., Terry S. A quick method for the quantitative analysis of mixtures. 1. Powder x-ray diffraction. J Pharm Sci. 2008; 97(6): 2260–2276.
48. Yamada H., Suryanarayanan R. X-ray powder diffractometry of intact film coated tablets-an approach to monitor the physical form of the active pharmaceutical ingredient during processing and storage. J Pharm Sci. 2007; 96(8): 2029–2036.
49. Saunders M., Podluii K., Shergill S., Buckton G., Royall P. The potential of high speed dsc (hyper-dsc) for the detection and quantification of small amounts of amorphous content in predominantly crystalline samples. Int J Pharm. 2004; 274(1): 35–40.
50. Pijpers T. F. J., Mathot V. B. F., Goderis B., Scherrenberg R. L., van der Vegte E. W. High-speed calorimetry for the study of the kinetics of (de)vitrification, crystallization, and melting of macro-molecules. Macromolecules 2002; 35(9): 3601–3613.
51. Whiteside P. T., Luk S. Y., Madden-Smith C. E., Turner P., Patel N., George M. W. Detection of low levels of amorphous lactose using h/d exchange and ft-raman spectroscopy. Pharm Res. 2008; 25(11): 2650–2656.
52. Gombás Á., Antal I., Szabó-Révész P., Marton S., Erõs I. Quantitative determination of crystallinity of alpha-lactose monohydrate by near infrared spectroscopy (NIRS). Int J Pharm. 2003; 256(1): 25–32.
53. Blanco M., Valdés D., Llorente I., Bayod M. Application of nir spectroscopy in polymorphic analysis: Study of pseudo-polymorphs stability. J Pharm Sci. 2005; 94(6): 1336–1342.
54. Gorny M., Jakobs M., Mykhaylova V., Urbanetz N. A. Quantifying the degree of disorder in micronized salbutamol sulfate using moisture sorption analysis. Drug Dev Ind Pharm. 2007; 33(3): 235–243.
55. Young P. M., Chiou H., Tee T., Traini D., Chan H. K., Thielmann F., Burnett D. The use of organic vapor sorption to determine low levels of amorphous content in processed pharmaceutical powders. Drug Dev Ind Pharm. 2007; 33(1): 91–97.
56. Tay J. Y. S., Liew C. V., Heng P. W. S. Powder flow testing: Judicious choice of test methods. AAPS PharmSciTech. 2017; 18(5): 1843–1854.
57. Liu L. X., Marziano I., Bentham A. C., Litster J. D., White E. T., Howes T. Effect of particle properties on the flowability of ibuprofen powders. Int J Pharm. 2008; 362(1): 109–117.
58. Chawla A., Taylor K. M. G., Newton J. M., Johnson M. C. R. Production of spray dried salbutamol sulphate for use in dry powder aerosol formulation. Int J Pharm. 1994; 108(3): 233–240.
59. Steckel H., Markefka P., teWierik H., Kammelar R. Effect of milling and sieving on functionality of dry powder inhalation products. Int J Pharm. 2006; 309(1): 51–59.
60. United States Pharmacopeia 30/National Formulary 25. Chapter 1174 Powder Flow. Rockville, MD, USA 2006.
61. Carr R. L. Evaluating flow properties of solids. Chem Eng J. 1965; 72:69–72.
62. Hausner H. H. Friction conditions in a mass of metal powder. Int J Powder Met. 1967; 3(4): 7–13.
63. Joshi M., Misra A. Dry powder inhalation of liposomal ketotifen fumarate: Formulation and characterization. Int J Pharm. 2001; 223(1): 15–27.

64. Jenike A. W. Gravity Flow of Bulk Solids. Salt Lake City, Utah The University of Utah, October 1961. Report No.: 108 Contract No.: 29.
65. Schmitt R., Feise H. Influence of tester geometry, speed and procedure on the results from a ring shear tester. Part Part Syst Char. 2004; 21(5): 403–410.
66. Schulze D. Powders and bulk solids: Behavior, characterization, storage and flow 2008. Ed 1. Heidelberg: Springer-Verlag Berlin.
67. Freeman R. E., Cooke J. R., Schneider L. C. R. Measuring shear properties and normal stresses generated within a rotational shear cell for consolidated and non-consolidated powders. Powder Technol. 2009; 190(1–2): 65–69.
68. Salústio P. J., Inácio C., Nunes T., Sousa e Silva J. P., Costa P. C. Flow characterization of a pharmaceutical excipient using the shear cell method. Pharm Dev Technol. 2020; 25(2): 237–244.
69. Søgaard S. V., Pedersen T., Allesø M., Garnaes J., Rantanen J. Evaluation of ring shear testing as a characterization method for powder flow in small-scale powder processing equipment. Int J Pharm. 2014; 475(1): 315–323.
70. Megarry A. J., Swainson S. M. E., Roberts R. J., Reynolds G. K. A big data approach to pharmaceutical flow properties. Int J Pharm. 2019; 555:337–345.
71. Nalluri V. R., Puchkov M., Kuentz M. Toward better understanding of powder avalanching and shear cell parameters of drug–excipient blends to design minimal weight variability into pharmaceutical capsules. Int J Pharm. 2013; 442(1): 49–56.
72. Hou H., Sun C. C. Quantifying effects of particulate properties on powder flow properties using a ring shear tester. J Pharm Sci. 2008; 97(9): 4030–4039.
73. Garg V., Mallick S. S., Garcia-Trinanes P., Berry R. J. An investigation into the flowability of fine powders used in pharmaceutical industries. Powder Technol. 2018; 336:375–382.
74. Nan W., Ghadiri M., Wang Y. Analysis of powder rheometry of ft4: Effect of air flow. Chem Eng Sci. 2017; 162:141–151.
75. Jan S., Karde V., Ghoroi C., Saxena D. C. Effect of particle and surface properties on flowability of rice flours. Food Biosci. 2018; 23:38–44.
76. Allenspach C., Timmins P., Sharif S., Minko T. Characterization of a novel hydroxypropyl methylcellulose (HPMC) direct compression grade excipient for pharmaceutical tablets. Int J Pharm. 2020; 583:119343.
77. Osorio J. G., Muzzio F. J. Effects of powder flow properties on capsule filling weight uniformity. Drug Dev Ind Pharm. 2013; 39(9): 1464–1475.
78. Majerová D., Kulaviak L., Růžička M., Štěpánek F., Zámostný P. Effect of colloidal silica on rheological properties of common pharmaceutical excipients. Eur J Pharm Biopharm. 2016; 106:2–8.
79. Hancock B. C., Vukovinsky K. E., Brolley B., Grimsey I., Hedden D., Olsofsky A., Doherty R. A. Development of a robust procedure for assessing powder flow using a commercial avalanche testing instrument. J Pharm Biomed Anal. 2004; 35(5): 979–990.
80. Lee W. B., Widjaja E., Heng P. W. S., Chan L. W. The effect of rotation speed and particle size distribution variability on mixability: An avalanche rheological and multivariate image analytical approach. Int J Pharm. 2020; 579:119128.
81. Osamura T., Takeuchi Y., Onodera R., Kitamura M., Takahashi Y., Tahara K., Takeuchi H. Characterization of tableting properties measured with a multi-functional compaction instrument for several pharmaceutical excipients and actual tablet formulations. Int J Pharm. 2016; 510(1): 195–202.
82. Reynolds G. K., Campbell J. I., Roberts R. J. A compressibility based model for predicting the tensile strength of directly compressed pharmaceutical powder mixtures. Int J Pharm. 2017; 531(1): 215–224.
83. Ilić I., Kása P., Dreu R., Pintye-Hódi K., Srčič S. The compressibility and compactibility of different types of lactose. Drug Development and Industrial Pharmacy. 2009; 35(10): 1271–1280.
84. Khatri P., Katikaneni P., Desai D., Minko T. Evaluation of affinisol® hpmc polymers for direct compression process applications. J Drug Deliv Sci Technol. 2018; 47:461–467.
85. Chen H., Paul S., Xu H., Wang K., Mahanthappa M. K., Sun C. C. Reduction of punch-sticking propensity of celecoxib by spherical crystallization via polymer assisted quasi-emulsion solvent diffusion. Mol Pharm. 2020; 17(4): 1387–1396.
86. Simmons D. M., Gierer D. S. A material sparing test to predict punch sticking during formulation development. Drug Dev Ind Pharm. 2012; 38(9): 1054–1060.
87. Aoki S., Danjo K. Effect of tableting conditions on the sticking of tablet using ibuprofen. Yakugaku Zasshi. 1998; 118(11): 511–518.
88. Wang J. J., Li T., Bateman S. D., Erck R., Morris K. R. Modeling of adhesion in tablet compression. I. Atomic force microscopy and molecular simulation. J Pharm Sci. 2003; 92(4): 798–814.

89. Wang J. J., Guillot M. A., Bateman S. D., Morris K. R. Modeling of adhesion in tablet compression. II. Compaction studies using a compaction simulator and an instrumented tablet press. J Pharm Sci. 2004; 93(2): 407–417.

90. Nakamura S., Otsuka N., Yoshino Y., Sakamoto T., Yuasa H. Predicting the occurrence of sticking during tablet production by shear testing of a pharmaceutical powder. Chem Pharm Bull. 2016; 64(5): 512–516.

91. Swaminathan S., Ramey B., Hilden J., Wassgren C. Characterizing the powder punch-face adhesive interaction during the unloading phase of powder compaction. Powder Technol. 2017; 315:410–421.

92. Thomas J., Zavaliangos A. An in-line, high sensitivity, non-contact sensor for the detection of initiation of sticking. J Pharm Innov. 2020; 15(1): 66–72.

93. Jackson K., Young D., Pant S. Drug–excipient interactions and their affect on absorption. Pharm Sci Technolo Today. 2000; 3(10): 336–345.

94. Marini A., Berbenni V., Pegoretti M., Bruni G., Cofrancesco P., Sinistri C., Villa M. Drug–excipient compatibility studies by physico-chemical techniques; the case of atenolol. J Therm Anal Calorim. 2003; 73(2): 547–561.

95. Hartauer K. J., Guillory J. K. A comparison of diffuse reflectance ft-ir spectroscopy and dsc in the characterization of a drug–excipient interaction. Drug Dev Ind Pharm. 1991; 17(4): 617–630.

96. Harding L., Qi S., Hill G., Reading M., Craig D. Q. M. The development of microthermal analysis and photothermal microspectroscopy as novel approaches to drug–excipient compatibility studies. Int J Pharm. 2008; 354(1): 149–157.

97. Cîntă Pînzaru S., Pavel I., Leopold N., Kiefer W. Identification and characterization of pharmaceuticals using raman and surface-enhanced raman scattering. J Raman Spectrosc. 2004; 35(5): 338–346.

98. Geppi M., Mollica G., Borsacchi S., Veracini C. A. Solid-state NMR studies of pharmaceutical systems. Appl Spectrosc Rev. 2008; 43(3): 202–302.

99. Crean B., Parker A., Roux D. L., Perkins M., Luk S. Y., Banks S. R., Melia C. D., Roberts C. J. Elucidation of the internal physical and chemical microstructure of pharmaceutical granules using x-ray micro-computed tomography, raman microscopy and infrared spectroscopy. Eur J Pharm Biopharm. 2010; 76(3): 498–506.

100. Mauritz J. M. A., Morrisby R. S., Hutton R. S., Legge C. H., Kaminski C. F. Imaging pharmaceutical tablets with optical coherence tomography. J Pharm Sci. 2010; 99(1): 385–391.

101. Markl D., Hannesschläger G., Sacher S., Leitner M., Khinast J. G. Optical coherence tomography as a novel tool for in-line monitoring of a pharmaceutical film-coating process. Eur J Pharm Sci. 2014; 55(1): 58–67.

102. Lin H., Dong Y., Shen Y., Zeitler J. A. Quantifying pharmaceutical film coating with optical coherence tomography and terahertz pulsed imaging: An evaluation. J Pharm Sci. 2015; 104(10): 3377–3385.

103. Strachan C. J., Taday P. F., Newnham D. A., Gordon K. C., Zeitler J. A., Pepper M., Rades T. Using terahertz pulsed spectroscopy to quantify pharmaceutical polymorphism and crystallinity. J Pharm Sci. 2005; 94(4): 837–846.

104. Sibik J., Zeitler J. A. Direct measurement of molecular mobility and crystallisation of amorphous pharmaceuticals using terahertz spectroscopy. Adv Drug Del Rev. 2016; 100:147–157.

105. Bawuah P., Pierotic Mendia A., Silfsten P., Pääkkönen P., Ervasti T., Ketolainen J., Zeitler J. A., Peiponen K.-E. Detection of porosity of pharmaceutical compacts by terahertz radiation transmission and light reflection measurement techniques. Int J Pharm. 2014; 465(1): 70–76.

106. Zeitler J. A., Shen Y., Baker C., Taday P. F., Pepper M., Rades T. Analysis of coating structures and interfaces in solid oral dosage forms by three dimensional terahertz pulsed imaging. J Pharm Sci. 2007; 96(2): 330–340.

107. May R. K., Su K., Han L., Zhong S., Elliott J. A., Gladden L. F., Evans M., Shen Y., Zeitler J. A. Hardness and density distributions of pharmaceutical tablets measured by terahertz pulsed imaging. J Pharm Sci. 2013; 102(7): 2179–2186.

108. Zeitler J. A., Gladden L. F. In-vitro tomography and non-destructive imaging at depth of pharmaceutical solid dosage forms. Eur J Pharm Biopharm. 2009; 71(1): 2–22.

109. Scherholz M. L., Wan B., McGeorge G. A rational analysis of uniformity risk for agglomerated drug substance using NIR chemical imaging. AAPS PharmSciTech. 2017; 18(2): 432–440.

4 Binders in Pharmaceutical Granulation

Thomas Dürig and Kapish Karan

CONTENTS

4.1 INTRODUCTION

Granulation processes are among the most widely practiced unit processes in oral solid dosage form manufacturing. Granules are an important dosage form in and of themselves; however, most granules are prepared as an intermediate step during tablet and capsule manufacturing. Granulation (also referred to as agglomeration) can be used to improve powder flow properties and reduce fine dust through size enlargement and densification, thus improving tableting operations. Frequently, granulation provides the means to intimately combine a thermoplastic binder with other formulation components, thus improving the compactibility of tablet formulations [1]. In controlled release formulations, granulation is often used to embed the drug in release controlling polymers, thereby retarding dissolution more effectively than a dry blend would. Granulation is also used to prevent powder segregation, thereby ensuring uniform drug distribution. This is especially important in low-dose, high-potency drugs. Lastly, granulation is used to improve the solubility and dispersibility of powders and tablets in water. This may also be referred to as "instantizing" or "hydrophilizing."

Granulation may be practiced by only adding a solvent as a binder fluid, but in the majority of cases, binders (usually polymeric) are also included, either by being "fully activated," that is, pre-dissolved in a suitable granulating fluid, or by pre-blending ("dry addition") with the other formulation components. This step is followed by wet massing with a suitable granulation solvent. Dry binder addition is also the method of binder incorporation in dry granulation processes such as roller compaction and in the emerging field of hot melt granulation.

The general function of a binder is to promote bonding between the primary particles of the formulation, thereby assuring granule strength and density so that integrity is not compromised on further handling and processing. Additionally, for granules that are intended for compaction into tablets, it is equally important that the binder provides the necessary thermoplasticity and toughness to improve formulation compactibility without compromising tablet dissolution and disintegration times. Very frequently, drugs and other formulation components possess non-ideal compaction properties, such as excessive brittleness and elasticity, leading to capping tendencies, high friability, and generally poor tablet performance. This is especially true when compressed at the high strain rates that are typical of commercial, high-speed tablet presses. The ideal tablet and granule binder will, therefore, provide the necessary thermoplastic character to overcome the unfavorable mechanical properties of the formulation yielding a dense compact, while minimizing the amount of applied force. The various modes of consolidation during tablet formation are shown in Figure 4.1.

While binder selection has traditionally been empirical and often dependent on formulator experience and preference, significant progress has been made over the past two decades in bringing quantitative and mechanistic particle engineering and materials sciences approach to bear on this important aspect of pharmaceutical powder technology. The purpose of this chapter is therefore to review the major binders in current pharmaceutical use and to discuss practical considerations in binder selection and use in the context of their key physical and chemical properties. Recent advances in the understanding of granulation technology and particle design will be discussed in detail, specifically the importance of selecting binders with a focus on end-product stability, wetting and surface energetics of the granulation system, and thermomechanical properties.

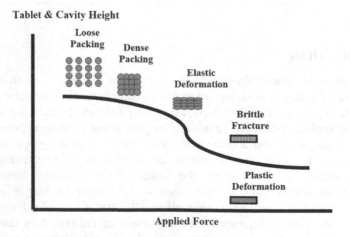

FIGURE 4.1 Mechanisms of Consolidation for Tableting Materials [1].

4.2 COMMONLY USED BINDERS IN CURRENT PHARMACEUTICAL PRACTICE

Many different types of materials have been used as binders in the past, including natural polymers such as gelatin, gum acacia, gum tragacanth, starch, and sugars, such as sucrose and glucose. Except for starch and acacia, these more traditional materials have for the most part been supplanted in current pharmaceutical practice by various derivatives of cellulose, polyvinylpyrrolidone (PVP), and modified starch. These binders have found increasing favor as they tend to be less variable and have presented fewer aging issues than some of the more traditional materials.

Among the most frequently used binders are povidone (PVP) and copovidone (PVA-PVP); modified starches such as partially pregelatinized starch (PGS); and various cellulose ethers such as hydroxypropylcellulose (HPC), methylcellulose (MC), hypromellose (HPMC), and less frequently ethyl cellulose (EC) and sodium carboxymethyl cellulose (NaCMC). These binders will be the focus of this chapter. Table 4.1 lists some of the most frequently used binders, typical use levels, and suitable solvents.

4.2.1 HYDROXYPROPYLCELLULOSE (HPC)

HPC is manufactured by reacting alkali cellulose with propylene oxide at elevated pressure and temperature. It is a highly substituted cellulose ether, with 3.4–4.1 moles of hydroxypropyl substituent per mole of anhydrous glucose backbone units [2]. The hydroxypropyl substituent groups, therefore, comprise up to 80% of the weight of HPC. This high level of substitution renders HPC more thermoplastic and less hygroscopic than other water-soluble cellulose ethers. HPC has compendial status in the National Formulary (USP/NF), European Pharmacopoeia (Ph. Eur.), Japanese Pharmacopeia (JP), and Food Chemicals Codex (FCC). HPC is fully soluble in water and polar organic solvents such as methanol, ethanol, isopropyl alcohol, and acetone. Water solubility is temperature-dependent with a cloud point around 45°C. HPC is a true thermoplastic polymer and has shown equivalent binder efficiency and good compactibility when added as a solution or in dry, powder form, before granulation [3]. Various molecular weight (MW) grades are available ranging from 60 to 1000 kDa; however, low MW grades are most typically used as binders (Table 4.2). Moreover, for dry addition, fine particle size grades (60–80 μm mean diameter) are preferred because of faster hydration and uniform mixing and distribution. Coarse grades are preferred for solution addition as they disperse more easily without lumping than dry grades. Lump-free aqueous solutions are best prepared by dispersing the powder in 30% of the required final volume of water at 65 °C. After 10 minutes of hydration, the remaining water can then be added cold while continuing to stir. Because of its high binder efficiency, HPC tends to be particularly well suited for high-dose, difficult-to-compress tablets, where only small amounts of binder can be added. In general, use levels above 8% are not recommended as they tend to cause excessive slowing of disintegration and dissolution times. HPC is also frequently used in film coating and melt extrusion.

4.2.2 METHYLCELLULOSE (MC)

MC is the reaction product of methyl chloride and alkali cellulose. In contrast to HPC, it is less heavily substituted, with methoxy groups comprising 27–32% by weight of the polymer. MC is soluble in hot water up to about 55°C and will reversibly gel at elevated temperatures. This indicates slightly higher water solubility than HPC. MC is also soluble in polar organic solvents like ethanol, methanol, and isopropyl alcohol, as long as a small amount of water (10%) is added as a cosolvent. Like all cellulose ethers, MC is available in a wide range of MW grades, but almost exclusively the low MW grade with nominal viscosity of 15 mPa.s at 2% concentration is used as a tablet binder (Table 4.2). Low-molecular weight MC is a versatile binder with the good thermoplastic flow and wetting ability. It is also a good film former. While MC can be added dry to a granulation blend before wet massing, it is generally more

TABLE 4.1

Commonly Used Binders

Binder	Typical Use Level	Comments	IID Limits*mg/ Dose
Hydroxypropylcellulose (HPC)	2–6%	Used with water, hydroalcoholic and neat polar organic solvents; equally effective in wet and dry addition because of high plasticity and wetting.	198.0
Methylcellulose (MC)	2–10%	Used with water or hydroalcoholic solvents; dry addition typically requires higher use levels than wet addition.	183.6
Sodium Carboxymethylcellulose (NaCMC)	2–5%	Used with water	119.8
Hypromellose (HPMC)	2–10%	Used with water or hydroalcoholic solvents; dry addition requires higher use levels.	445.0
Ethylcellulose (EC)	2–10%	Used with polar and nonpolar organic solvents; not soluble if water exceeds 20% of total solvent. Hydrophobic coating can slow down drug release for less soluble drugs; thus, it is best used for high-dose, highly soluble drugs, and moisture-sensitive drugs.	291.5
Povidone (PVP)	2–10%	Used with water, hydroalcoholic, and neat polar organic solvents; dry addition requires higher use levels. Ultra-low-viscosity grades allow for high solution concentrations (20%).	240.0
Copovidone (PVP-PVA)	2–8%	Used with water and hydroalcoholic solvents; more thermoplastic than PVP; dry addition requires higher use levels.	853.8
Polyethylene Glycol (PEG)	10–15%	Used dry as a meltable binder	400.0
Polymethacrylates	5–10%	Used as aqueous dispersions; powder grades used dry and with water and hydroalcoholic solvents	150.0
Polyvinyl alcohol (PVA)	5–10%	Can be used dry or only with water	40.0
Polyvinyl alcohol graft polyethylene glycol copolymer (PVA – PEG Graft)	2–10%	Used with water; dry addition requires higher use levels.	5.4
Pregelatinized starch (PGS)	5–15%	Can only be used with water; also acts as a disintegrant; effective use levels are mostly higher than other binders (8–20%).	346.0

Notes:
* Inactive Ingredient Database accessed in July 2020.
For the latest IID or IIG Limits: https://www.accessdata.fda.gov/scripts/cder/iig/.

TABLE 4.2
Selected Commercial Binder Grades

Binder	Trade Name/Grade/Supplier	Nominal Viscosity
Hydroxypropylcellulose (HPC)	Klucel™ hydroxypropylcellulose ELF, EF, and LF Pharm also available as fine particle grades EXF and LXF Pharm and Klucel EXF Ultra as an ultra-fine grade	2% viscosities at 5, 8, and 12 mPa.s
	Nisso® HPC SSL, SL and L select grades also available as fine and superfine grades	2% viscosities at 2.5, 5 and 8 mPa.s
Hypromellose (HPMC)	Methocel™ E3, E5, E6, and E15 Premium LV Hypromellose	2% viscosities at 3, 5, 6, and 15 mPa.s
	Pharmacoat® 603, 645, 605, 606, and 615 hypromellose	2% viscosities at 3, 4.5, 5, 6, and 15 mPa.s
	Tylopur® 603, 645, 605, 606, and 615 hypromellose	2% viscosities at 3, 4.5, 5, 6, and 15 mPa.s
	AnyCoat® AN3, AN4, AN5, AN6 and AN15	2% viscosities at 3, 4, 5, 6, and 15 mPa.s
Methylcellulose (MC)	Methocel™ A15 Premium LV methylcellulose	2% at viscosity 15 mPa.s
	Benecel™ A15 LV Pharm methylcellulose	2% viscosity at 15 mPa.s
	Metelose® SM 4 and 15 methylcellulose	2% viscosities at 4 and 15 mPa.s
Ethylcellulose (EC)	Aqualon™ ethyl cellulose N7, N10, N14, and N22 Pharm	5% viscosities at 4, 7, 10, 14, and 22 mPa.s
	Ethocel™ Standard Premium ethyl cellulose NF	5% viscosities at 4, 7, 10, and 20 mPa.s
Sodium carboxymethyl cellulose (NaCMC,)	Aqualon™ NaCMC 7L2P and 7LF Pharm	2% viscosities at 20 and 50 mPa.s
	Blanose™ NaCMC 7L2P and 7LF Pharm	2% viscosities at 20 and 50 mPa.s
Povidone (PVP)	Kollidon® 25, 30 and 90FPovidone	5% viscosities at 2, 2.5 and 55 mPa.s
	Plasdone™ K12, K17, K25, K29/32 and K90 povidone	5% viscosities 1, 1.8, 2.0, 2.5, and 55
Copovidone (PVP-PVA)	Kolidon® VA 64 copovidone	5% viscosity at 2.5 mPa.s
	Plasdone™ S630 copovidone, Plasdone™ S630 Ultra copovidone	5% viscosity at 2.5 mPa.s
Polyethylene Glycol (PEG)	Carbowax™ 4000 and 6000 polyethylene glycol	50% viscosities at 128 and 236 mPa.s
	Polyglykol® 4000 and 6000 polyethylene glycol	50% viscosities at 128 and 236 mPa.s
Polyvinyl alcohol (PVA)	Parteck® MXP PVA 4-88	4% viscosity at 5 mPa.s
	J-POVAL PE-05JPS polyvinyl alcohol	4% viscosity at 5 mPa.s
	GOHSENOL™ polyvinyl alcohol	4% viscosity at 5 mPa.s
Polyvinyl alcohol graft polyethylene glycol copolymer (PVA-PEG graft)	Kollicoat® IR	20% viscosity at 120 mPa.s

TABLE 4.2 (Continued)

Binder	Trade Name/Grade/Supplier	Nominal Viscosity
Polymethacrylates	Eudragit® E POEudragit® NE 30DEudragit® RS 30D	16% viscosity at 5 mPa.s20% viscosity at 5 mPa.s20% viscosity at 5 mPa.s
Pregelatinized starch (PGS)	Starch 1500® partially pregelatinized starch	N/A
	Prejel™ PA5 PH pregelatinized starch	N/A
	Lycatab® pregelatinized starch partially pregelatinized starch	N/A
	Superstarch® 200 partially pregelatinized starch	N/A

Klucel™, Benecel™, Aqualon™, Blanose™· and Plasdone™ are registered trademarks of Ashland LLC. Nisso® is a registered trademark of Nippon Soda Company. Pharmacoat® and Tylopur® is a registered trademark of Shin-Etsu Corporation. Methocel™ and Ethocel™ are trademarks of the DuPont Specialty Solutions. AnyCoat-C is a registered trademark of LOTTE Fine Chemical. Carbowax™ is a trademark of Dow Chemical Company. Polyglykol® is a registered trademark of Clariant. Eudragit® is a registered trademark of Evonik Industries. Kollidon® is a registered trademark of BASF Corporation. Parteck® MXP is a registered trademark of Millipore Sigma. Gohsenol™ is a registered trademark of Mitsubishi Chemical Corporation. Starch 1500® is a registered trademark of BPSI. Prejel™ PA5 PH and Superstarch® are trademarks of DFE Pharma. Lycatab® is a registered trademark of Roquette Frères.

---

effective when pre-dissolved and added as a solution [3]. Aqueous solutions can be prepared in an analogous fashion as described earlier for HPC. MC is listed in the USP/NF, Ph. Eur., JP, and FCC.

4.2.3 Hypromellose (HPMC)

HPMC is one of the most widely used excipients in general and is also frequently used as a tablet binder. It is also known as hydroxypropyl methylcellulose (HPMC) and is formed by reacting alkali cellulose with methyl chloride and propylene oxide to yield a mixed substitution cellulose ether. Various substitution ratios and MW grades are available. Primarily low-viscosity grades with substitution type "2910" (28–30% methoxy groups by weight and 4–12% hydroxypropyl groups) are used as tablet binders (Table 4.2). These grades are also very popular for film coating formulations. HPMC is listed in the USP/NF, Ph. Eur., JP, and FCC.

The properties of HPMC are largely similar to those of MC with the exception that HPMC is less thermoplastic and somewhat more hydrophilic. Although a good film former, unplasticized films are more brittle than MC and HPC and cloud points are higher. For example, HPMC type 2910 has a cloud point in the range of 65°C, which necessitates higher water temperatures for solution preparation. As with MC, HPMC is soluble in hydroalcoholic solvents with a minimum of 10% alcohol. It can be used in solution or added dry but is less efficient in the latter form (3).

4.2.4 Sodium Carboxymethyl Cellulose (NaCMC)

Sodium carboxymethyl cellulose (NaCMC) is the sodium salt of carboxymethyl cellulose, an anionic derivative. It's widely used in oral, ophthalmic, injectable, and topical pharmaceutical formulations. For solid dosage forms, it is primarily used as a binder or matrix former.

Pharmaceutical grades of NaCMC are available commercially at the degree of substitution (DS) values of 0.7, 0.9, and 1.2 – with a corresponding sodium content of 6.5–12 wt.%. It is also available in several different molecular weight grades, which influence the viscosity of the solution and its swelling properties. NaCMC is highly soluble in water at all temperatures, forming clear solutions. Its solubility is dependent on its degree of substitution.

NaCMC, when used as a binder, yields softer granules but has good compressibility – forming tough tablets of moderate strength. NaCMC, being highly hygroscopic, can absorb a large quantity of water (>50%) at elevated relative humidity conditions. Hence, the tablets tend to harden with age.

4.2.5 Povidone (PVP)

Povidone, which is alternately referred to as PVP, is recognized as a versatile excipient that is used in complexation, solubilization, and film applications in addition to being one of the most widely used granulations and tablet binders. PVP is manufactured by radical polymerization of *N*-vinylpyrrolidone and is available in multiple MW grades ranging from 2 to ~1500 kilodaltons (kDA). The high MW grades have been reported to have very high binder efficiency; however, medium and low MW grades are most often used as granulation and tablet binders since high MW grades may impede dissolution behavior (Table 4.2). PVP is listed in the USP/NF, Ph. Eur., and JP [4]. Much of its versatility derives from favorable solution behavior. Povidone is highly soluble in water and freely soluble in many polar organic solvents such as ethanol, methanol, isopropyl alcohol, and butanol. It is insoluble in nonpolar organic solvents. PVP is generally used in the form of a solution, where its low viscosity allows solids concentrations as high as 15–20%. PVP can also be added dry to a powder blend and then granulated with just the solvent, but as with MC and HPMC, binder efficiency is significantly lower in this case [3]. Although use levels in the literature are reported as 2% to 5% [4], higher levels up to 10% may have to be used in challenging, poorly compactable formulations. PVP is highly hygroscopic, and at 50% RH, typical equilibrium moisture content exceeds 15% by weight (Figure 4.2). It is therefore advisable to take precautions against uncontrolled and unnecessary exposure to atmospheric moisture.

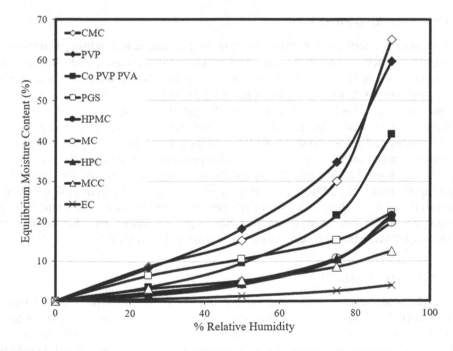

FIGURE 4.2   Equilibrium Moisture Contents at 25°C for Selected Polymeric Binders.

4.2.6 Copovidone (PVP-PVA)

Copovidone (PVP-PVA) is the 60:40, random, linear copolymer of N-vinyl-2-pyrrolidone and vinyl acetate. It is therefore a derivative of PVP. Vinyl acetate somewhat reduces the hydrophilicity and hygroscopicity of the PVP homopolymer. At 50% RH, the typical equilibrium moisture content is approximately 10% (Figure 4.2). The addition of vinyl acetate also increases the plasticity of the polymer, thus lowering the glass transition temperature and improving compactibility and adhesiveness. In addition to being used as a wet and dry binder, PVA-PVP can also be incorporated into film coating formulations together with HPMC [5]). PVA-PVP can be used in wet granulation either in dissolved form or added dry to the powder blend, followed by wet massing. Binder effectiveness is approximately equivalent to these two methods of incorporation. Copovidone is soluble in water and polar organic solvents and is listed in USP/NF and Ph. Eur., and also has a monograph in the Japanese Pharmaceutical Excipients (JPE).

4.2.7 Polyethylene Glycol (PEG)

Polyethylene Glycol is formed by the reaction of ethylene oxide and water under pressure in the presence of a catalyst. PEG is soluble in water and miscible with other grades of PEG. In tablet formulations, PEG's of higher molecular weight can enhance the effectiveness of tablet binders by imparting plasticity to the granule; however, they have limited binding action by themselves [6,7]. When used above 5% w/w, it may prolong tablet disintegration. Nowadays, PEG's are commonly used as binders in the melt granulation process. In this process, a powder blend containing 10–15% w/w of PEG 4000 or 6000 is heated to 70–75°C to obtain a paste-like mass that forms granules when mixed while cooling in an extruder. PEGs are versatile as low molecular or liquid PEG is mainly used as plasticizers while the higher molecular PEGs are used as tablet binders, polishing material, and as solid dispersion carriers to enhance the aqueous solubility of poorly soluble drugs [8].

4.2.8 Polyvinyl Alcohol (PVA)

Polyvinyl Alcohol is a well-established polymer in the pharmaceutical industry mainly due to its unique properties, such as excellent adhesive strength, film formation, and chemical stability (moisture and oxygen barrier properties). Its most widely used applications are tablet coating and wet granulation, but PVA also plays an important role in solubility enhancement, transdermal patches, and emulsions. This polymer is produced through the hydrolysis of polyvinyl acetate and typical pharmaceutical grades are partially hydrolyzed materials. PVA is available in a variety of viscosity grades and grades from 10 to 100 millipascal second (mPa.s) lend themselves for tablet granulation processes. PVA's are water-soluble polymers. It is reported that they form softer granulations, which yield tablets that do not harden with age [9]. They can also be used in melt granulation applications. In addition, polyvinyl alcohol-polyethylene glycol graft copolymer was also developed as a flexible, low viscosity, peroxide-free polymer for immediate release film-forming agent. Studies have found that this graft copolymer has the superior binding performance to HPMC while the performance was comparable to PVP [10].

4.2.9 Polymethacrylates

Polymethacrylates are used as immediate release binders as they provide excellent mechanical stability and flexibility. Select grades such as Eudragit E PO, NE 30D, and RS 30D can be used in aqueous and organic solvent-based wet granulation processes. Eudragit NE 30D and RS 30D are provided as 30% aqueous latex dispersions while Eudragit E PO is a powder [11]. Due to the low viscosity of the latex dispersions, granulations can be performed in a variety of granulation equipment; however, the fluid bed process has shown several advantages. The powdered grades of these polymers have also been evaluated in dry and melt granulation processes [12–14].

4.2.10 Starch and Modified Starches

4.2.10.1 Starch

Starch has traditionally been one of the most widely used tablet binders, although today PGSs are often preferred. Starch is a polysaccharide carbohydrate consisting of glucose monomers linked by glycosidic bonds. The main sources for excipient-grade starch are maize and potato starch. References to wheat, rice, and tapioca starch can also be found in the literature. Starch is a GRAS-listed material with monographs in the USP/NF, Ph. Eur., and JP. Starch is not cold water or alcohol soluble; traditionally, it is used by gelatinizing in hot water to form a paste. A starch paste can be prepared by heating a starch suspension to the boiling point with constant stirring. Binder use levels for starch are usually relatively high (5–25%). The high viscosity of starch paste can make granulation, efficient binder distribution, and substrate wetting somewhat problematic; however, an advantage of starch is that it tends to enhance tablet disintegration.

4.2.11 Pregelatinized Starch (PGS)

Pregelatinized starch is classified as modified starch. Chemical and mechanical treatment is used to rupture all or part of the native starch granules. Pre-gelatinization enhances starch cold-water solubility and also improves compactibility and flowability. PGS is marketed as a multifunctional excipient, providing binding, disintegration, good flow, and lubrication. PGS monographs can be found in the United States Pharmacopeia/National Formulary (USP/NF), European Pharmacopeia (Ph. Eur.), and JPE [15]. It is typically used from solution in wet granulation; it can also be dry added, but this reduces efficiency significantly. Furthermore, at 15% to 20%, use levels are usually higher for PGS relative to other binders. PGS is not compatible with organic solvents and thus is used only in aqueous binder systems. While it tends to have high equilibrium moisture levels (Figure 4.2), starch is known to hold water in different states, that is, only a portion of the sorbed water will be available as "free" water. This property can be exploited by using starch as a stabilizer or moisture sequestrant. Partially pregelatinized starch is the most frequently used form of PGS, but fully pregelatinized starch is also available. The degree of pre-gelatinization determines cold water solubility. Commercial partially pregelatinized starch typically has around 20% pregelatinized or water-soluble content. The cold-water soluble part acts as a binder, while the remainder aids tablet disintegration. For this reason, fully pregelatinized starches tend to have higher binder efficiency, but not necessarily good disintegrant properties.

4.2.12 Gum Acacia

Gum acacia is also known as gum arabic; it is a natural material made of hardened exudate from Acacia Senegal and Acacia Seyal. Commercial gum arabic is largely harvested from wild trees in the Sahel region of Africa. It is a complex mixture of polysaccharides and glycoproteins that is today used primarily in the food industry as an emulsion stabilizer. Acacia is a highly functional binder, in that it is known to form strong tablets and granules; however, dissolution times are often impeded. Additional reasons why today this binder is used rarely with exception of nutritional supplement applications where organic origin include solution susceptibility to enzymatic and bacterial degradation, large natural variability, and sporadic supply shortages.

4.3 PRACTICAL CONSIDERATIONS IN BINDER SELECTION AND USE

4.3.1 USE LEVELS AND BINDER EFFICIENCY

While the binder use levels in Table 4.1 serve as a general guide, the reader will appreciate that use levels tend to be drug and formulation specific and may deviate significantly from the typical values cited. In general, increased binder concentration leads to an increase in mean granule size and strength, and decreased granule friability. An increase in binder concentration strengthens bonds between the substrate particles as there is more binder per bond [16]. Binder efficiency may be defined as the minimum binder use level that is required to achieve a certain benchmark tablet crushing strength and friability [17]. Concerning binder efficiency, there is no absolute standard for these criteria. The strongest tablets and granulations may not always be the most desirable; rather the minimum amount of binder necessary to achieve a minimum acceptable strength or maximum acceptable friability is often chosen. This will minimize cost and tablet size because stronger granules and tablets tend to be correlated with slower drug release. In terms of maximum acceptable friability, as a general rule, friability needs to be low enough to allow handling and coating in commercial-scale tablet coating pans (e.g., 48- and 70-in diameter pans). The friability for smaller tablets (500 mg or less) should therefore be less than 0.8%. Larger tablets (1000 mg) should have friability's below 0.3% to allow for problem- and blemish-free handling and commercial-scale coating.

4.3.2 STABILITY AND COMPATIBILITY

It is well known that chemical or physical incompatibility between actives and excipients or their impurities can compromise drug stability and safety. Binders are brought into intimate contact with actives during mixing, wet massing, and co-drying; therefore, final formulation stability is a primary consideration in binder selection. Like all excipients, binders are generally designed to be "inert;" thus, direct chemical reactions between the functional groups of binder and drug molecules are relatively rare. More frequently, the interaction involves impurities that can be introduced into the final drug product by the drug, excipients, or packaging materials [18]. Most such impurity-induced incompatibilities in solid dosage forms can be attributed to a select group of small molecules including water, electrophiles such as aldehydes, and the often-related carboxylic acids and peroxides.

4.3.2.1 Aldehydes and Carboxylic Acids

Low molecular weight aldehydes and carboxylic acids are found in many excipients including sugars, polymers, and unsaturated fats [18]. The most common reactive species of concern in solid dosage forms tend to be formaldehyde and its corresponding acid, formic acid. Table 4.3 lists typical levels of these impurities for various binders, granulation aids, and tableting excipients. Others include acetaldehyde, glyoxal, furfural, glyoxylic, and acetic acid. Carboxylic acids could be introduced because of not only carryover from manufacturing but also autoxidation of excipients, which, for example, leads to the formation of formaldehyde, which is then further oxidized to form formic acid. The presence of these impurities needs to be considered in acid-labile drugs as well as drugs with nucleophilic functional groups, for example, primary and secondary amines and hydroxyl groups [18,19]. Formaldehyde and formic acid have been identified as being of particular concern when using polysorbate, povidone, and polyethylene glycol [20,21].

4.3.2.2 Peroxides

Peroxides are oxidizing materials. They can be found in several excipients including binders. Peroxides occur as "organically" bound peroxide (ROOH), where R is a carbon atom, or hydrogen peroxide (H_2O_2), which is the more mobile, freely available, and volatile form. Peroxides can react

TABLE 4.3

Levels of Formic Acid and Formaldehyde in Selected Binders and Tableting Excipients [19]

| Excipient | Supplier | Lot | Level (ppm) | |
			Formic Acid	Formaldehyde
Lactose	A	1	1.0	<0.2
Microcrystalline cellulose, 50 µm average size	D	1	9.3	<0.2
Microcrystalline cellulose, 100 µm average size	D	2	23.9	0.9
Microcrystalline cellulose, 100 µm average size	D	3	11.8	1.0
Starch 1500*	E	1	3.0	<0.2
Povidone K-25	H	1	3080.3	<0.2
Povidone K-90	H	2	630.0	<0.2
Povidone K-25	I	1	1990.5	0.4
Hypromellose	J	1	58.3	11.1
Hypromellose	J	2	86.4	15.7
Polyethylene glycol 4000	N	3	14.0	3.6
Polyethylene glycol 400	O	2	469.0	85.8

directly with drugs sensitive to oxidation as well as generate radicals, which initiate radical chain reactions, or themselves react with the active ingredient [18,22].

Excipients most often associated with peroxide impurities can be divided into two general groups, although peroxides may be found in many other excipients, albeit usually at lower levels. The first group comprises polymeric ethers, including polyethylene glycols, polyethylene oxides, and polysorbates. In general, only high molecular weight polyethylene glycol is occasionally used as a binder, although polysorbates are frequently used as wetting agents in binder solutions. These polymers frequently have some peroxide content as supplied but can also form greater amounts because of autoxidation. Frequently, these materials are supplied with small amounts of antioxidants added as stabilizers.

The second group chiefly consists of PVP and PVP-related polymers, such as crospovidone and copovidone. PVP-based excipients typically contain relatively high levels of peroxides. Table 4.4 lists total peroxide (hydrogen peroxide and organically bound peroxide) for a series of common tablet binders and related tableting excipients. PVP undergoes autoxidation, and greater amounts can form under high-shear conditions typical of granulation and tableting [18]. Several reports

TABLE 4.4

Total Peroxide Content in Selected Excipients [22]

Excipient	Number of Lots Tested	Average Level (nmol/g)
Povidone	5	7300
Polyethylene glycol 400	4	2200
Polysorbate 80	8	1500
Hydroxypropyl cellulose	21	300
Polyethylene glycol solid	4	20
Microcrystalline cellulose	5	<10
Lactose	5	<10

correlating drug-excipient incompatibilities to peroxide levels in PVP have been published [23–25]. In the case of raloxifene, peroxide impurities associated with PVP resulted in the formation of high levels of an *N*-oxide derivative of raloxifene. Hartauer et al. [23] were able to identify the critical destabilizing levels of peroxide, thus allowing for a peroxide limit test that assures product stability. Additionally, peroxides can also be formed, albeit at lower levels, in cellulose ethers such as HPC.

4.3.3 BINDER HYGROSCOPICITY AND WATER CONTENT

Water is ubiquitous in the manufacturing environment and is a major destabilizing factor for drug products. Water plasticizes the formulation components, thus lowering T_g and raising molecular mobility in the solid-state system [26].

This can accelerate oxidation and hydrolysis and additional physical changes such as recrystallization, tablet hardening or softening, and slower dissolution behavior [8,18,27–29]. Water can be found in most drugs and excipients and may be associated with solids in various states. These include loosely held surface water, intermediate bound water, which is not freely available, as well as very tightly bound water of crystallization, which can only be released as part of a transition in the crystal structure. Water is also the most frequently used solvent in granulation processing and film coating. Finally, adsorption of atmospheric moisture is a well-known pathway for water to enter finished dosage forms.

Binders with high equilibrium water content and high hygroscopicity (especially if used in quantities exceeding 5%) can, therefore, be problematic. The hygroscopicity of various binders is illustrated in Figure 4.2. Typically, manufacturing environments are humidity controlled to be at 50% relative humidity or less. At these levels, PVP and NaCMC equilibrium moisture levels are approximately 18 and 15 wt.%, respectively. Copovidone and PGS have equilibrium moisture levels of 10%, whereas the remaining cellulose ethers, HPMC, MC, HPC, and EC are at 5% moisture content or less. Most notably, EC is the least hygroscopic binder.

Examples of where hygroscopic binders are a problem include reports of tablet softening and reduction in disintegration time due to excessive moisture uptake by ranitidine tablets comprising PVP as a wet granulation binder [29]. It has been observed that PVP is predominately in the glassy state at room temperature and at a relative humidity below 55°C. At higher humidity, the glass transition temperature is significantly reduced, resulting in conversion to the rubbery state where molecular mobility is increased, resulting in the hardening of tablets prepared from glass ballotini and PVP [28]. In a further example, Fitzpatrick et al. [27] reported a significant decrease in the dissolution rate for a tablet formulation of a new chemical entity when wet granulated with PVP and stored at accelerated conditions (40°C and 75% relative humidity). Tablets stored at lower temperatures, for example, 30°C, and 60% relative humidity and tablets made with HPC as a wet binder remained stable and did not show the decreased dissolution rate. The change was correlated to a decrease in the glass transition temperature with increased moisture sorption.

Binder choice can also prevent API crystal transformation at high humidity. Paisana et al. [30] have reported that blends of HPC and PVP can inhibit polymorphic transformations of olanzapine at high humidity.

4.3.4 WETTABILITY AND SURFACE ENERGETICS

The ability to wet the porous powder substrate, to penetrate rapidly into the powder bed and spread across the surfaces of the host particles, and to distribute uniformly throughout the powder bed is important in granulation process control. Poor wettability and spreadability of the binder are frequently associated with porous, weak, low-density granules with nonuniform binder distribution and broad particle size distributions. During the initial wetting and nucleation phase, the binder fluid disperses mainly by wetting and capillary action. This crucial stage of

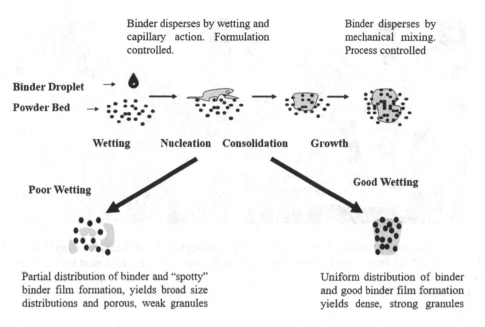

FIGURE 4.3 Schematic Showing Wetting, Nucleation, Consolidation, and Granule Growth Processes. *Source*: From Ref. [35].

granule formation is, therefore, strongly dependent on formulation and binder selection. It is the binder fluid characteristics (surface tension, viscosity) and the substrate characteristics (surface free energy) that determine the interaction between the binder fluid and the substrate, which can be characterized by substrate surface wetting (contact angles), spreading ability (spreading coefficients) of the binder over a substrate, and the resultant granule characteristics [31–34]. Once nuclei are formed, the binder is predominantly dispersed by the mechanical shear forces of the mixer during the consolidation and growth phases of the granulation. This phase is mainly dependent on process parameters, the amount of binder fluid added, and the rheological characteristics of the wet mass [35,36]. Depending on operating shear forces and strength and toughness of wet granules, granules break up and attrition can occur simultaneously with growth and consolidation in the later stages of a granulation process. Figure 4.3 depicts some of these key aspects.

The consequences of good and poor substrate wetting were highlighted in a seminal study by Cutt et al. [16] and further analyzed by Rowe [34], and are shown in Figure 4.4a,b and Table 4.5. Aqueous PVP solutions were able to spread easily over hydrophilic glass beads (positive or high spreading coefficient of the binder over the substrate), resulting in a continuous and strongly adhering film, which led to strong and dense granules with binder film bonds at all contact points between substrate particles. In these granules with good adhesion between binder and substrate, failure occurs within the binder film or bond (i.e., cohesive failure) (Figure 4.4a). By contrast, in the case of hydrophobically modified glass beads, where the spreading coefficient of the binder solution over the substrate was negative, no continuous binder film was formed; rather the binder is distributed in discontinuous "patches" [34]. This leads to a more open and porous granule structure and lower granule strength [37], as illustrated in Figure 4.3 and Table 4.5. The low binder-substrate adhesion in these weaker granules causes failure to occur at the interface between the substrate particles and the binder film as illustrated in Figure 4.4b.

Several techniques can be used to measure wetting and spreading abilities for binder solutions to ensure that an appropriate binder is chosen for a particular substrate. Figure 4.5 illustrates

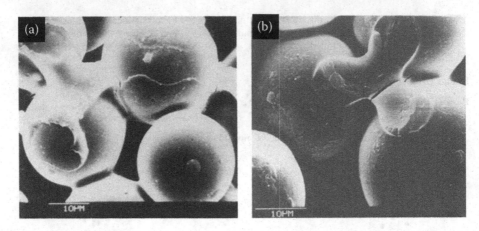

FIGURE 4.4 Broken PVP Bonds Within Granules of (a) Hydrophilic Glass Beads Showing Fracture Within the PVP Bonding Film and (b) Hydrophobic Glass Beads Showing Adhesive Failure at the Glass–PVP Film Interface.
Source: From Ref. [16].

TABLE 4.5
Properties of Glass Granules with 2.72% Polyvinylpyrrolidone Binder [16]

Glass Bead Type	Friability (%)	Strength (Load at Failure, g)
Hydrophilic	5.2	202
Hydrophobic	13.8	115

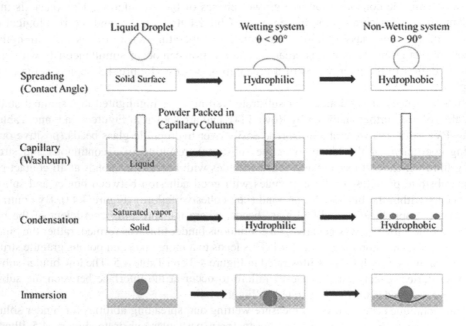

FIGURE 4.5 Different Wetting Measurement Methods.
Source: From Ref. [37].

various approaches, of which the direct measurement of spreading via the contact angle and the capillary rise or "Washburn" methods tend to be the most common.

Typically, this involves the calculation of surface free energies and the works of cohesion, adhesion, and spreading (also referred to as spreading coefficient) from measurements of solution contact angles on the substrate of interest and measurement of the liquid-vapor surface energy of the wetting liquid, which is usually referred to as surface tension.

The contact angle, θ, is a measure of the affinity of the fluid for a solid as described in the Young's equation:

$$\gamma_{sv} - \gamma_{sl} = \gamma_{lv} \cos \theta$$

where γ_{sv} is the solid-vapor surface or interfacial energy, γ_{sl} is the solid-liquid surface energy, and γ_{lv} is the liquid-vapor surface energy, which is more commonly referred to as the surface tension of the liquid. A fluid is said to wet a solid when the contact angle is less than 90°; this occurs when solid-vapor surface energy exceeds the solid-liquid surface energy. The extent of wetting is, therefore, determined by $\gamma_{lv} \cos\theta$, the product of the binder solution surface tension and the contact angle, which is known as adhesion tension [32].

Knowledge of the surface energies is important as it allows calculation of the works of adhesion, cohesion, and spreading. The work of cohesion for a solid can be written as:

$$W_{cs} = 2\gamma_{sv}$$

Similarly, for a liquid:

$$W_{cl} = 2\gamma_{lv}$$

The work of adhesion for a solid-liquid interface can be written as:

$$W_a = \gamma_{sv} + \gamma_{lv} - \gamma_{sl} = \gamma_{lv}(1 + \cos \theta)$$

W_a represents the work that is done when a particle adheres to a liquid surface, in the process replacing air-particle and air-liquid interfaces with a particle-liquid interface.

The work of spreading, W_s is also known as a spreading coefficient, can be calculated as:

$$W_s = W_a - W_{cl} = \gamma_{lv}(\cos \theta - 1)$$

The work of spreading represents the work that is done by a liquid spreading over a particle surface, thereby replacing the particle-air interface with a liquid-air and particle-liquid interface. The spreading coefficient is key. It has been demonstrated experimentally that positive W_s values are directly correlated with lower granule friability. The larger the W_s, the better the binder distribution and adhesion, and the stronger the granules [38]. In addition, it is possible to divide the respective surface energies into their polar and dispersive components [34].

Finally, Hapgood et al. [35] introduced the concept of liquid binder drop penetration time, t_p, as a measure of wetting and powder penetration kinetics for a liquid of viscosity, η, where:

$$t_P \propto \frac{\eta}{\gamma_{lv} \cos \theta}$$

Binder fluid drop penetration time can, therefore, be decreased by ensuring lower solution viscosity and by maximizing adhesion tension of the binder fluid, which, in practice, requires selection of a low-viscosity fluid that yields a contact angle as close to 0 as possible. For drop-controlled nucleation, both a fast (small) drop penetration time and a relatively low spray flux are required [35]. Readers who are interested in a more detailed review and treatment of the aforementioned topics are directed to references [32,34,35,39].

Direct measurement of contact angles on nonporous substrate surfaces can be made using the sessile drop technique and a contact angle goniometer. An important aspect of this technique is that the substrate needs to be rendered into a nonporous form, which often is done by sintering, or melting, or alternately forming very hard and smooth compacts by compression.

Alternatively, the penetration kinetics of liquid into a powder bed can be measured using the Washburn method [40,41], which has the advantage of mimicking the binder penetration by capillary action and wetting processes that occur in wet granulation. In this technique, the binder solution uptake by capillary action into a packed column of substrate powder is measured. The following equations describe this event:

$$t = Am^2, \quad A = \frac{\eta}{Cp^2\gamma_{lv}\cos\theta}$$

where t is the time after the solid and the liquid are brought into contact, m is the mass of the liquid drawn into the solid, A is a constant dependent on the liquid properties (viscosity η, density p, the liquid/vapor interfacial surface tension γ_{lv}, and the solid-liquid contact angle θ), and C is a material constant dependent on the porous architecture of the powder bed.

Additional techniques include floatation tests where the penetration kinetics of the substrate into liquid is measured and inverse gas chromatography, which allows calculation of surface energies by measuring preferential adsorption of various well-characterized probe gases onto the substrate particles [32,42].

4.3.5 WETTING STUDIES AS FORMULATION TOOLS

Krycer et al. [43] were among early workers to highlight the importance of binder fluid wetting and spreading abilities over the substrate in relation to granule friability and ultimately compressed tablet strength and capping tendencies. Studying relative binder efficiencies of HPMC, PVP, starch, acacia, and sugar for a model acetaminophen system, they concluded that important factors for optimum granulation included wetting of the substrate by the binder, binder-substrate adhesion, and binder cohesion. They also investigated the mechanical properties of binder films in detail. It is important to note that in addition to the surface interactions between binders and substrates, the mechanical properties of various binders will exert a strong influence on final granule and tablet strength. Granule and tablet characteristics are therefore a function of binder-substrate interactions and also mechanical properties of the binder and substrate mixture. The thermomechanical properties of binders will be discussed in more detail in the "Thermal and Mechanical Properties" section of this chapter. Table 4.6 shows the correlation between wetting characteristics and the acetaminophen granule friability and tablet crushing strength. In general, there is a good rank-order correlation between the surface tensions, contact angles and spreading coefficients, and granule friability and tablet strength, the exception being the friability of sucrose granules, which may be attributable to the significant brittleness of sucrose, which could result in reduced granule toughness and abrasion resistance.

Using independently measured and calculated values for surface free energies, Rowe [34] was able to also show a good correlation between the spreading coefficient and the experimental data of Krycer et al. [43] (Figure 4.6). A practical example where the spreading coefficients were used to select optimal binder solutions for a particular granulation substrate is illustrated in Figure 4.7, which shows spreading coefficients and granule friability's improving, for two experimental drug formulations, when PVP solutions are replaced with lower surface tension

TABLE 4.6

Properties of 4% (w/v) Binder Solutions and Resultant Granule and Tablet Properties in an APAP Model System

Binder Solution	Surface Tension (dyne/cm)	Contact Angle on APAP (o)	Work of Spreading (dyne/cm)	Granule Friability Index	Tablet Strength (N)[a]
Hypromellose	45.2	27.4	−5.07	14.8	180
Acacia	50.6	30.3	−6.92	19.8	162
Sucrose	50.4	32.8	−8.01	87. 6	98
Polyvinylpyrrolidone	53.6	42.2	−13.9	26.5	57
Starch	58.7	47.3	−18.9	45.3	37
Water	70.3	59.6	−110	–	–

Notes:
a Diametral crushing strength for tablets compressed at 120 MPa.
Source: From Ref. [43].
Abbreviation: APAP, acetaminophen.

HPC solutions. Further improvements occur when water is replaced by a less polar hydro-alcoholic solvent [44].

In a further example of the general applicability of wetting measurements to the selection of binder solutions, Lusvardi et al. [40] used the Washburn approach to study the wetting kinetics of selected binders on two low soluble drugs (ibuprofen and naproxen) and correlated these to final granulation and tablet characteristics. Figure 4.8 depicts the mass uptake of various binder

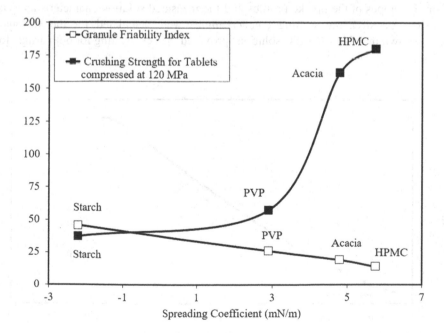

FIGURE 4.6   Relationship Between Spreading Coefficients Calculated by Rowe and Tablet and Granule Strength Data Reported by Krycer et al.
Source: From Refs. [34,43].

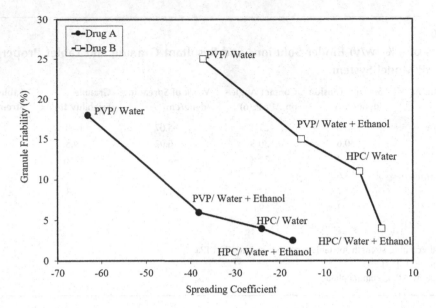

FIGURE 4.7 Effect of Spreading Coefficient on Granule Friabilities of Two Experimental Drug Formulations.
Source: From Ref. [44].

solutions into a column packed with ibuprofen powder. The HPC solution rapidly wets the ibuprofen as shown by the fast rate of adsorption. HPMC solution has an intermediate adsorption rate, while the PVP solution shows only a slight improvement over water, which was not absorbed at all.

Based on the slopes of the uptake profiles and the measured solution characteristics (viscosity, surface tension, density), the wetting contact angles were calculated for the various binder solutions. As shown in Table 4.7, HPC solutions provided the best wetting for both drugs, followed

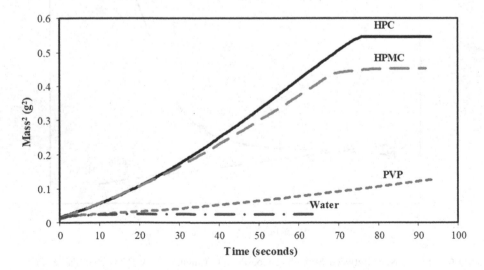

FIGURE 4.8 Binder Solution Uptake Profiles into an Ibuprofen Powder Bed.
Source: From Ref. [40].

TABLE 4.7

Binder Solution Wetting Characteristics on Drugs with Different Degrees of Hydrophobicity, Ibuprofen, and Naproxen

Wetting Solution	Surface Tension (mN/m)	Viscosity (mPa.s)	Contact Angle on Ibuprofen	Spreading Coefficient for Ibuprofen (mN/m)	Contact Angle on Naproxen	Spreading Coefficient for Naproxen (mN/m)
n-hexane	18.4	0.3	0°	0	0°	0
Hydroxypropyl cellulose	40.0	2.3	68°	−25.0	0°	0
Hypromellose	48.4	1.9	81°	−40.8	37°	−9.7
Polyvinylpyrrolidone	53.6	1.5	88°	−51.7	63°	−29.3
Water	72.1	1.0	>90°	>72.1	85°	−65.0

Source: From Ref. [40].

by HPMC and PVP. Naproxen was perfectly wetted by HPC solutions as indicated by the contact angle of 0.

Using Zisman's approach, one can estimate the surface energy of the solid from Young's equation and the contact angle data [45,46]. Figure 4.9 illustrates this approach. Extrapolating to the cosine of 1 (cos 0°) provides an estimate of ~40 mN/m for the surface energy of naproxen, which is consistent with the surface tension measured for HPC solutions. Extrapolating to 0 (cos 90°) indicates that liquids with surface tensions higher than ~75 mN/m can be expected to have contact angles greater than 90°, indicating that there will be no spontaneous wetting or penetration into the powder bed. Modification of the binder fluid through the selection of a binder with lower surface tension or use of a less polar solvent or surfactants is, therefore, necessary to ensure good binder distribution.

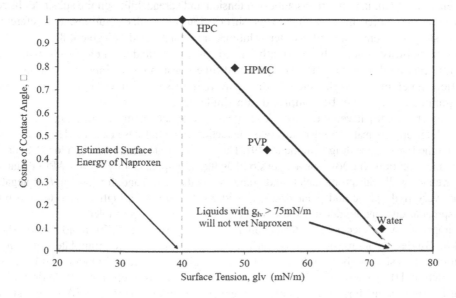

FIGURE 4.9 Zisman Surface Energy Plot for Naproxen.
Source: From Ref. [40].

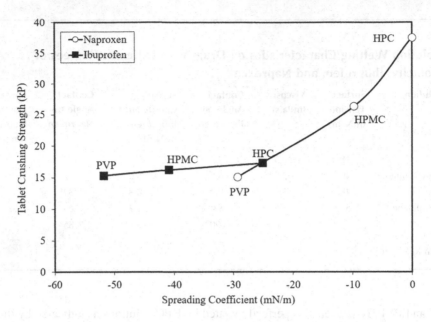

FIGURE 4.10   Relationship Between Spreading Coefficients of Binder Solutions of HPC, HPMC, and PVP over Ibuprofen and Naproxen and Tablet Crushing Strength. Ibuprofen and Naproxen were Granulated with HPC, HPMC, and PVP Solutions and Compressed at 15 kN Compression Force. Tablets Weighed 600 mg and were Compressed with 0.4375-inch Standard Concave Tooling.
Source: From Ref. [40].

The relevance of the wetting data to binder performance is shown in Figure 4.10, where the tablet strength of wet-granulated ibuprofen and naproxen tablets is plotted as a function of the calculated spreading coefficients.

The studies reviewed here allow the general conclusion that a binder choice is an important tool in assuring optimal wetting for granulation. The polarity of the binder directly affects binder solution surface tension, which, in turn, affects adhesion tension and spreadability on the substrate. In general, better wetting is assured by choosing lower surface tension binder solutions. For reference, the surface tensions for common binder-water solutions are summarized in Table 4.8.

While wettability studies have greatly aided in understanding key mechanisms in wet granulation, this methodology is too complex and time consuming for binder selection in routine formulation development work. Such studies may require several days of work, while multiple typical granulation trials can be completed in a single day.

Taflioglu et al. [48] have, therefore, developed an alternative, more practical, rapid screening method, which approximates binder-substrate interaction potential based on binder solution surface tension and the log P of the drug compound [49]. They demonstrated that for a high log P, hydrophobic drug, a binder solution with low surface tension has the best spreadability on the API crystal surface which correlates well with strong tablets and granules. On the other hand, for low log P or negative log P, that is, very hydrophilic and polar drugs, a binder solution with a high surface tension provided optimal spreadability and binder distribution and consequently stronger tablets.

This approach was successfully tested on four model drugs of different log P, as shown in Table 4.8. Binder solutions of varying surface tension were used to granulate the four model formulations. The studies showed that for APIs with high log P values, binders with lower surface tension, such as HPC, were indeed be more effective [47]. Conversely for very hydrophilic APIs (low log P), such as metformin HCl, polar binders such as PVP and PVP-PVA were significantly better (Figures 4.11 and 4.12).

TABLE 4.8
APIs of Varying Hydrophobicity (log *P*) and Binders of Various Surface Tension
Used to Measure Substrate Binder Interactions

API	Water Solubility	Lipophilicity (log P)	Flowability	Compactability	Plasticity
Metformin	>300 g/L	−0.50	Poor	Poor	*
Albendazole	2.28 mg/L	2.70	Poor	Good	***
Efavirenz	0.86 mg/L	4.60	Poor	Poor	*
Simvastatin	1.22 mg/L	4.68	Moderate	Moderate	**
Property		Klucel EXF HPC	Benecel E15 HPMC	Plasdone S-630 PVP/VA	PlasdoneK-29/ 32 PVP
Surface tension (mN/m)		40.00	45.90	49.50	53.60
Mean particle size (μm)		50.00	90.00	76.00	107.00
Surface area (m²/cm³)		0.32	0.15	0.21	0.37
Relative toughness		*****	*	****	**

Source: From Ref. [47].

For APIs with log *P* in the range of 2–3.5, binder choice and surface tension were less critical. These findings are summarized in Figure 4.13. This alternate method provides a good and often sufficient first approximation but ignores the fundamentals inherent in the more rigorous contact angle measurement techniques or inverse gas chromatography.

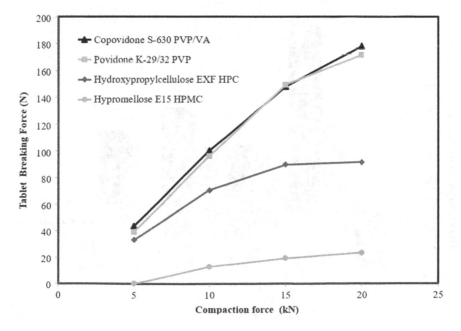

FIGURE 4.11 Compactibility of Metformin Formulations. More Polar, High Surface Tension Binders Such as Vinyl Pyrrolidones are Advantageous for this Low log P API.
Source: Ref. [47].

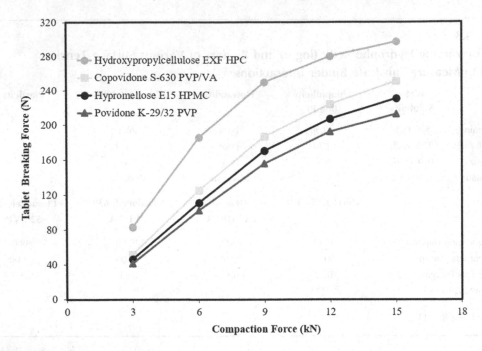

FIGURE 4.12 Compactibility of Efavirenz Formulations. Low Surface Tension, More Non-Polar Binders Such as HPC Provide Better Wetting for the High log P API.
Source: From Ref. [48].

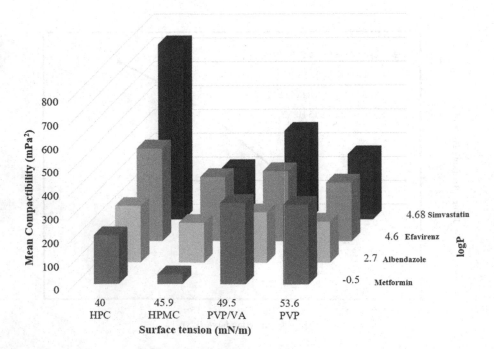

FIGURE 4.13 Effect of Binder Surface Tension and API log P on Tablet Compactibility.
Source: From Refs. [47–49].

4.4 THE ROLE OF SOLVENT

As indicated, a primary factor in good granulation is the wetting and spreading ability of the binder over the substrate. One of the obvious ways to modulate these properties is the modification of the solvent composition to influence polarity and wetting properties in the desired direction. In addition to choosing binders with lower surface tensions, one may add surfactants to reduce surface tension or alternately add a less polar organic solvent to water or completely replace the aqueous solution with a less polar, organic solvent. The report of Krycer et al. [43] was among the first reports that showed improved granule properties by adding a surfactant to PVP. Their work showed that the addition of sodium lauryl sulfate (SLS) markedly improved the spreadability coefficient of the PVP solution and with it granule friability was also significantly decreased. However, tablet crushing strength was only modestly influenced (Table 4.9). Surfactants such as sodium lauryl sulfate or polysorbate are now frequently added to binder solutions as wetting agents; however, caution needs to be exercised as an excessive film of surfactant on the granule surface can lead to poor binding. Most surfactants generally have poor compressibility and binding characteristics.

An alternate approach to modify the surface energies of the binding solution is to incorporate less polar, organic solvents. Among the frequently used solvents for granulation are hydroalcoholic solutions of methanol, ethanol, IPA, and acetone.

Figure 4.7 illustrates the effect of the granulation solvent on the granule friability for two experimental drugs granulated using either PVP or HPC and water or ethanol/water combinations. Granule friability decreases markedly as the spreadability coefficient increases by switching from water to ethanol: water blend. An obvious limitation of this approach to enhancing wetting is binder polymer solubility in the solvent system. For instance, starches and NaCMC are generally not soluble at all in organic solvents, and MC and HPMC require a minimum of about 10–15% water to be soluble in polar organic solvents such as methanol, ethanol, isopropyl alcohol, and acetone. HPC, PVP, PVA-PVP, and EC are fully soluble in these solvents. An additional complication that needs to be considered is that binder solutions with the same binder concentration may vary considerably in different solvent systems. Table 4.10 shows the variation in PVP solution viscosity when the water:alcohol ratio is varied. Similar behavior occurs for most polymers including HPC and HPMC.

Among the more detailed studies on solvent effects is the study by Wells and Walker [50]. These workers studied the effect of solvent choice on PVP acetylsalicylic acid granulations by varying the ratios of ethanol and water in the granulation fluid. In somewhat contradictory fashion, granule bulk density was found to decrease with decreased surface tension (increased ethanol).

TABLE 4.9

Properties of 4% (w/v) Binder Solutions and Resultant Granule and Tablet Properties for a PVP-Acetaminophen Model System

Binder Solution	Surface Tension (Dyne/cm)	Contact Angle on Acetaminophen (°)	Work of Spreading (Dyne/cm)	Granule Friability Index	Tablet Strength (N)[a]
PVP + sodium lauryl sulfate (90:10)	44.1	44.1	−0.9	20.8	58
PVP + glycerol (90:10)	43.8	40.1	−10.7	25.5	80
PVP	53.6	42.2	−13.9	26.5	48

Note
[a] Diametral crushing strength for tablets compressed at 120 MPa.
Source: From Ref. [43].

TABLE 4.10

Effect of Solvent Composition on PVP Binder Solution Properties and PVP Acetylsalicylic Acid Granulations and Tablet Strength

Binder Solution	Viscosity (mPa.s)	Surface Tension (Dyne/cm)	Wettability (r × cos θ × 10⁻⁴)	Bulk Density (g/mL)	Tablet Strength (kP)	Tablet Friability (%)
100% water	67	69.5	4.1	0.48	6.6	3.5
25% ethanol	194	42.6	12.16	0.44	6	4
50% ethanol	287	33.6	15.9	0.43	5.8	4.6
75% ethanol	240	30.1	18.68	0.425	8	3.4
100% ethanol	186	26.35	16.4	0.42	–	2.5

Source: From Ref. [50].

However, tablet crushing strength and tablet friability were found to be correlated with the lowest surface tension (100% ethanol). These results would indicate that a lower polarity and surface tension allow for stronger and denser tablets to be ultimately formed. The authors also pointed out that aspirin solubility is increased in this optimal solvent range, thus possibly contributing to the bond formation through greater dissolution and recrystallization of aspirin.

4.5   THERMAL AND MECHANICAL PROPERTIES

As indicated in subsection "Stability and Compatibility," the characteristics of granules and their resultant tablets are dependent on not only the interaction and surface energies of the binder solution and the substrate but also the mechanical properties of the binder films that are formed around and between the substrate particles. In their seminal study, Krycer et al. [43] concluded that in addition to having a favorable spreading coefficient on acetaminophen, HPMC also was a superior film former when compared with PVP, acacia, and starch in that it produced soft but tough films with those materials. Reading and Spring [51] investigated these concepts further using MC, PVP, starch, and gelatin as film-forming wet binders and sand as a hydrophilic, but otherwise inert, substrate. As shown in Table 4.11, MC film strength and deformation ability are significantly

TABLE 4.11

Selected Free Film, Granule, and Tablet Properties for MC, PVP, Gelatin, and Starch Binders. Sand Was Used as the Binder Substrate. Films Were Dried at 60°C

Property	MC	PVP	Gelatin	Starch
Film tensile strength (MPa)	70	18	27	33
Elongation percentage at break	37	5.3	3.1	3.2
Film toughness (J/m³ × 10⁵)	192	8	9	10
Film Brinell hardness,12% RH (MPa)	7.5	9.17	18.7	15.6
Granule friability percentage	5.0	11.0	14.6	20.4
Mean granule size (µm)	680	445	365	200
Tablet crushing strength[a] (kPa)	345	240	200	70

Note
[a]   Tablets compressed at 120 MPa compression force.
Source: From Ref. [51].

greater than those of the other binders. Simultaneously, MC films are softer, showing the lowest Brinell (indentation) hardness. These properties correlate with significantly larger, less friable granules, and stronger tablets.

The studies of Krycer et al. [43] and Reading and Spring [51] therefore suggest that binders that have good wettability, form films with high toughness (toughness is the work of failure as measured by the area under the stress-strain curve), and have high percentage of elongation at break, which together are indicators of plastic flow, will likely produce more robust granules and tablets. However, these studies do not directly address the compaction behavior of tablet binders when subjected to high-speed, uniaxial compaction, which occurs in commercial tableting.

Figure 4.14 shows the deformation behavior of pure binder tablets (100% polymer) when subjected to diametral compression on a universal testing machine. These binder tablets were prepared by compressing the dry binder powders, of similar fine particle size, on a rotary preformulation components in commercial tableting presses. HPC exhibits significantly greater plasticity and toughness (area under the curve) as compared with the other binders, which uniformly show an increased tendency to undergo brittle fracture. PVA-PVP, MC, and microcrystalline cellulose (MCC) tablets achieve high peak loads during compression testing, but these tablets fracture at very low deformation (0.28–0.46 mm). In contrast, HPC tablets do not show this brittle behavior. The HPC tablets were deformed beyond 2.6 mm without fracturing, while absorbing applied energy, providing much greater toughness. Relative to the other materials tested, the HPMC and PVP tablets were the least deformable and fractured at low peak loads.

The greater toughness and deformability of HPC also coincides with higher thermoplasticity as measured by thermal analysis. In contrast to other polymers, HPC at a typical equilibrium moisture content (~3%) exhibited a high-intensity glass transition in the low-temperature range (−3–0°C) (Table 4.12) [3,52]. Increased molecular mobility and plasticity are generally associated with lower glass transition. Overall, these results confirm a higher state of plasticization for HPC in relation to the other binders.

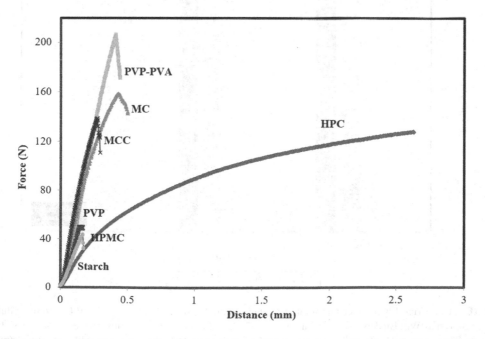

FIGURE 4.14 Load-Deformation Plots for Pure Polymer Tablets Subjected to Diametral Compression on a Universal Testing Machine (0.5 in/min Crosshead Speed). The 100% Polymer Tablets were Made on a Rotary Tablet Press [3].

TABLE 4.12

Glass Transition Temperature at Equilibrium Moisture Content as Received, Detected by Modulated Temperature Differential Scanning Calorimetry

Binder	Equilibrium Moisture Content (%)	Glass Transition Temperature (8 C)
Hydroxypropylcellulose	3.2	−2.6
Methylcellulose	4.7	145
Hypromellose (type 2910)	3.1	160
MCC	4.9	~105
Copovidone	4.8	101
Polyvinylpyrrolidone	8.0	164

Source: From Ref. [3].

Consistent with the results for pure polymer tablets and the earlier reports on binder film mechanical properties, Joneja et al. [53] showed that for wet-granulated acetaminophen formulations, binder toughness and a high degree of plastic flow were key determinants in assuring robust tablets. They studied four binders, HPC, MC, PVP, and PGS, at 6% use levels. HPC yielded stronger, more deformable, and therefore tougher tablets. The differences in terms of tablet friability and strength were further accentuated when the tablet press speed was increased to simulate the speeds typically encountered in commercial production (Figures 4.15 and 4.16). Further studies evaluated whether comparable properties could be achieved by varying the various binder levels.

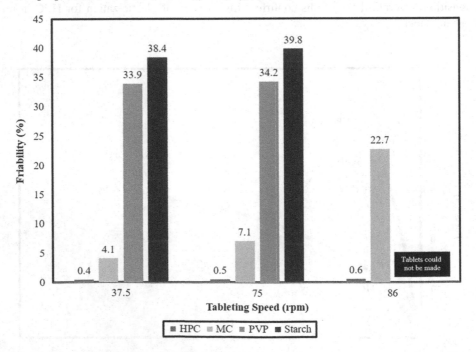

FIGURE 4.15   Friability for Wet-Granulated Acetaminophen Tablets Containing 6% HPC, Methylcellulose, PVP, or Starch as Wet Binders. 600-mg Tablets (0.4375 inch Standard Round Convex) were Compressed on a Manesty Betapress at 15 kN at Three Different Turret Speeds. HPC Comprising Tablets Showed Only a Negligible Increase in Friability. PVP and Starch Comprising Tablets Could not be Made at 86 rpm Because of Excessive Capping on Ejection from the Press.
Source: From Ref. [53].

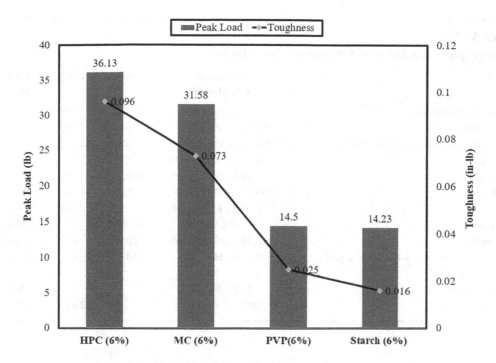

FIGURE 4.16 Tablet Strength and Toughness for Wet-Granulated Acetaminophen Tablets Comprising 6% Hydroxypropylcellulose, Methylcellulose, Polyvinylpyrrolidone, or Pregelatinized Starch Binder. Tablets were Compressed on a Manesty Betapress at 37.5 rpm Turret Speed at 15 kN Compression Force. Tablet Strength and Toughness were Assessed by Diametral Compression on a Universal Testing Machine at 0.05 in/min Crosshead Speed.
Source: From Ref. [53].

Notably, the results from this study are consistent with the studies of Krycer et al. [43], as also Lusvardi et al. [40] discussed in the subsection "Stability and Compatibility," and also correlate with the results of Reading and Spring [51] indicating that binder performance rank order can be predicted on the basis of thermal and mechanical properties such as binder plasticity and toughness.

However, it is important to recognize that the results also correlate well with measures of binder wettability and spreading such as aqueous surface tensions, binder solution contact angles on the substrate, and spreading coefficients. It is not possible to easily separate the contributions of surface interaction from those of the inherent mechanical properties of the binders. However, based on the consistent evidence from binder studies involving a variety of substrates, one can conclude that both binder solution-substrate wetting and the mechanical and compressive properties of the binder and binder films are key determinants of granule properties such as density and strength, as well as tablet strength and robustness. Furthermore, significant differences exist among currently available binders in terms of functionality, in particular wettability and surface tension, plasticity, and toughness.

4.6 REGULATORY ACCEPTANCE AND SUPPLIER RELIABILITY

Formulators and scientists are generally well attuned to focusing on technical aspects of a formulation development project, but regulatory acceptance and supplier reliability for the binders and formulation components that one chooses to work with are just as important to assure project success.

It is sometimes not appreciated that most excipients including binder polymers are manufactured in large chemical plants, rather than pharmaceutical manufacturing environments. Apart from the massive difference in scale compared with typical pharmaceutical manufacturing (a typical binder lot size maybe 20–30,000 kg), it is also important to understand that similar polymer grades may also be

TABLE 4.13

Monograph Compliance of Commonly Used Binders

Binder	Monograph Compliance	E Number	CFR	GRAS Status
Hydroxypropylcellulose	NF, FCC, Ph. Eur, JP,	E463	172.870	GRAS
Methylcellulose	USP, FCC, Ph. Eur., JP	E461	182.1480	GRAS
Sodium Carboxymethylcellulose (NaCMC)	NF, FCC, Ph. Eur., JP	E466	182.1745	GRAS
Hypromellose	USP, FCC, Ph. Eur., JP	E464	172.874	GRAS
Ethyl cellulose	NF, FCC, Ph. Eur., JP	E462	172.868	GRAS
Povidone	NF, FCC, Ph. Eur, JP	E1201	173.55	GRAS
PEG	USP, FCC, Ph. Eur., JP,	E1521	172.820	GRAS
Copovidone	NF, Ph. Eur, JP	E335	–	GRAS
Poly vinyl alcohol	USP, FCC, Ph. Eur., JPE	E1203	–	GRAS
Polyvinyl alcohol graft polyethylene glycol copolymer	NF, Ph. Eur., JPE	E1209	–	GRAS
Polymethacrylates	NF, Ph. Eur, JPE	–	–	N/A
Pregelatinized starch	NF, Ph. Eur., JP		182.90	GRAS

manufactured for industrial use. Frequently, pharmaceutical grades represent only a small portion of the output of a typical polymer plant. When working with a particular binder or excipient in general, it is therefore important to ensure that the chosen supplier has the necessary excipient Good manufacturing practice (GMP) manufacturing capabilities and has an audit history with the Food and Drug Administration (FDA) or similar authorities. It should also be understood that excipient GMP differs from drug product manufacturing GMP or API manufacturing.

In terms of choice of binders, it is important to work with materials that are well established as pharmaceutical excipients with established pharmacopeial monographs. Ideally, the binder will be represented in all the major pharmacopeias, that is, USP/NF, Ph. Eur., and JP. For nutritional supplements, it is also important that the binder has a monograph in the Food Chemicals Codex, or that the binder has GRAS status or is listed as a direct food additive by FDA or the relevant authorities in the country of interest. It is then also important for the formulator to ensure that the particular grade chosen to work is compliant with the relevant monographs and standards. Table 4.13 lists the monograph compliances of commonly used binders in granulation of oral solid dosage forms [54].

Last, to comply with the directives on quality by design, it will be important for the scientist to test the impact of varying the excipient quality parameters within and sometimes outside the specification limits. This is best accomplished by working with three to five lots of the chosen binder at an early stage to elucidate critical functional differences. Frequently, suppliers will also accommodate requests for samples made at the specification or process limits. Where possible and if available, it can also be useful to study multiyear lot histories for the various quality parameters.

REFERENCES

1. Rudnic, E. and J. B. Schwartz. 1995. Oral solid dosage forms. 19th ed. Vol. 2, Remington: The Science and Practice of Pharmacy. Easton: Mack Publishing Company, 1629.
2. Ashland. 2017. Klucel™ hydroxypropyl cellulose. Physical and Chemical Properties. In Ashland LLC, Wilmington, DE 19808. Wilmington: Ashland.
3. Skinner G. W. and W. W. Harcum. 1998. "Evaluation of Low-Viscosity Polymers in a Model High-Dose, Acetaminophen Formulation." Aqualon Pharmaceutical Technology Report PTR 11. http://www.herc.com/aqualon/product/data/ptr/ptr011. Accessed March 2009.

4. BASF. 2018. Pharma Solutions Product Overview 2018 – Technical Information. BASF SE. https://pharmaceutical.basf.com/global/en/drug-formulation.html - Portfolio Overview.

5. Porter, Stuart C., and Lana L. Terzian. 2008. Smooth, High Solids Tablet Coating Composition, edited by USPTO. USA:ISP Investments LLC.

6. Miller, Bernard, and Leonard Chavkin. 1954. "The Use of polyethylene glycol as a binder in tablet compression." Journal of the American Pharmaceutical Association (Scientific ed.) 43 (8):486–488. doi: https://doi.org/10.1002/jps.3030430813.

7. Shah, R. C., P. V. Raman, and P. V. Sheth. 1977. "Polyethylene glycol as a binder for tablets." Journal of Pharmaceutical Sciences 66 (11):1551–1552. doi: 10.1002/jps.2600661112.

8. Brady, James E., Thomas Dürig, and Sherwin S. Shang. 2009. "Polymer Properties and Characterization A2 - Qiu, Yihong." In Developing Solid Oral Dosage Forms, edited by Yisheng Chen, Geoff G. Z. Zhang, Lirong Liu, and William R. Porter, 187–217. San Diego: Academic Press.

9. Vandevivere, L., P Denduyver, C. Portier, O Häusler, T De Beer, C Vervaet, and V Vanhoorne. 2020. "Influence of binder attributes on binder effectiveness in a continuous twin screw wet granulation process via wet and dry binder addition." International Journal of Pharmaceutics 585:119466. doi: https://doi.org/10.1016/j.ijpharm.2020.119466.

10. Fouad, Ehab A., Mahmoud El-Badry, Steven H. Neau, Fars K. Alanazi, and Ibrahim A. Alsarra. 2011. "Technology evaluation: Kollicoat IR." Expert Opinion on Drug Delivery 8 (5):693–703. doi: 10.1517/17425247.2011.566266.

11. Evonik. 2015. "Technical Information EUDRAGIT® E 100, EUDRAGIT® E PO and EUDRAGIT® E 12,5." (INFO 7.1/E):1–6.

12. Batra, Amol, Dipen Desai, and Abu T. M. Serajuddin. 2017. "Investigating the use of polymeric binders in twin screw melt granulation process for improving compactibility of drugs." Journal of Pharmaceutical Sciences 106 (1):140–150. doi: https://doi.org/10.1016/j.xphs.2016.07.014.

13. Gohel, M. C., T. P. Patel, and S. H. Bariya. 2003. "Studies in preparation and evaluation of pH-independent sustained-release matrix tablets of verapamil HCl using directly compressible Eudragits." Pharm Dev Technol 8 (4):323–333. doi: 10.1081/pdt-120024686.

14. McGinity, James W., Claud G. Cameron, and George W. Cuff. 1983. "Controlled-release theophylline tablet formulations containing acrylic resins. I. Dissolution properties of tablets." Drug Development and Industrial Pharmacy 9 (1–2):57–68. doi: 10.3109/03639048309048545.

15. Colorcon. 2019. Starch 1500® Partially Pregelatinized Maize Starch Product Brochure. Westpoint, PA: Colorcon.

16. Cutt, Teresa, John T. Fell, Peter J. Rue, and Michael S. Spring. 1986. "Granulation and compaction of a model system. I. Granule properties." International Journal of Pharmaceutics 33 (1):81–87. doi: https://doi.org/10.1016/0378-5173(86)90041-4.

17. Iveson, S. M., and J. D. Litster. 1998. "Fundamental studies of granule consolidation part 2: Quantifying the effects of particle and binder properties." Powder Technology 99 (3):243–250. doi: https://doi.org/10.1016/S0032-5910(98)00116-8.

18. Waterman, Kenneth C., Roger C. Adami, and Jin Yang Hong. 2004. "Impurities in drug products." In Separation Science and Technology, edited by Ahuja Satinder and Alsante Karen Mills, 75–88. San Diego, California: Academic Press.

19. del Barrio, Mary-Anne, Jack Hu, Pengzu Zhou, and Nina Cauchon. 2006. "Simultaneous determination of formic acid and formaldehyde in pharmaceutical excipients using headspace GC/MS." Journal of Pharmaceutical and Biomedical Analysis 41 (3):738–743. doi: https://doi.org/10.1016/j.jpba.2005.12.033.

20. Nassar, M. N., V. N. Nesarikar, R. Lozano, W. L. Parker, Y. Huang, V Palaniswamy, W Xu, and N Khaselev. 2004. "Influence of formaldehyde impurity in polysorbate 80 and PEG-300 on the stability of a parenteral formulation of BMS-204352: identification and control of the degradation product." Pharm Dev Technol. 9 (2):189–195. doi: 10.1081/pdt-120030249.

21. Parker, M. D., P. York, and R. C. Rowe. 1990. "Binder-substrate interactions in wet granulation. 1: The effect of binder characteristics." International Journal of Pharmaceutics 64 (2):207–216. doi: https://doi.org/10.1016/0378-5173(90)90270-E.

22. Wasylaschuk, W. R., P. A. Harmon, G. Wagner, A. B. Harman, A. C. Templeton, H. Xu, and R. A. Reed. 2007. "Evaluation of hydroperoxides in common pharmaceutical excipients." J Pharm Sci 96 (1):106–116. doi: 10.1002/jps.20726.

23. Hartauer, K. J., G. N. Arbuthnot, S. W. Baertschi, R. A. Johnson, W. D. Luke, N. G. Pearson, E. C. Rickard, C. A. Tingle, P. K. Tsang, and R. E. Wiens. 2000. "Influence of peroxide impurities in povidone

and crospovidone on the stability of raloxifene hydrochloride in tablets: identification and control of an oxidative degradation product." Pharm Dev Technol 5 (3):303–310. doi: 10.1081/pdt-100100545.

24. Huang, T., M. E. Garceau, and P. Gao. 2003. "Liquid chromatographic determination of residual hydrogen peroxide in pharmaceutical excipients using platinum and wired enzyme electrodes." J Pharm Biomed Anal 31 (6):1203–1210.

25. ISP. Plasdone® S-630 Copovidone Product Guide. Wayne, NJ.: International Specialty Products.

26. Fassihi, T., and Durig, A. R. 1991. "Preformulation study of moisture effect on the physical stability of pyridoxal hydrochloride." International Journal of Pharmaceutics:315–319.

27. Fitzpatrick, S., J. F. McCabe, C. R. Petts, and S. W. Booth. 2002. "Effect of moisture on polyvinylpyrrolidone in accelerated stability testing." Int J Pharm 246 (1–2):143–151.

28. Kiekens, F., R. Zelko, and J. P. Remon. 2000. "Effect of the storage conditions on the tensile strength of tablets in relation to the enthalpy relaxation of the binder." Pharm Res 17 (4):490–493.

29. Uzunarslan, K., and J. Akbuğa. 1991. "The effect of moisture on the physical characteristics of ranitidine hydrochloride tablets prepared by different binders and techniques." Drug Development and Industrial Pharmacy 17 (8):1067–1081. doi: 10.3109/03639049109043845.

30. Paisana, M. C., M. A. Wahl, and J. F. Pinto. 2017. "Effect of polymers in moisture sorption and physical stability of polymorphic olanzapine." Eur J Pharm Sci 97:257–268. doi: 10.1016/j.ejps.2016.11.023.

31. Fowkes, Frederick M. 1964. Contact Angle, Wettability, and Adhesion. Vol. 43, Advances in Chemistry: American Chemical Society. doi:10.1021/ba-1964-0043.

32. Litster, Jim, and Bryan Ennis. 2004. "Wetting, Nucleation and Binder Distribution." In The Science and Engineering of Granulation Processes, 37–74. Dordrecht: Springer Netherlands.

33. Mills, P. J. T., J. P. K. Seville, PC Knight, and MJ Adams. 2000. "The effect of binder viscosity on particle agglomeration in a low shear mixer/agglomerator." Powder Technology 113 (1):140–147. doi: https://doi.org/10.1016/S0032-5910(00)00224-2.

34. Rowe, R. C. 1990. "Correlation between predicted binder spreading coefficients and measured granule and tablet properties in the granulation of paracetamol." International Journal of Pharmaceutics 58 (3):209–213. doi: https://doi.org/10.1016/0378-5173(90)90197-C.

35. Hapgood, Karen P., James D. Litster, Simon R. Biggs, and Tony Howes. 2002. "Drop Penetration into Porous Powder Beds." Journal of Colloid and Interface Science 253 (2):353–366. doi: https://doi.org/10.1006/jcis.2002.8527.

36. Ritala, M, O. Jungersen, P. Holm, T. Schæfer, and H. G. Kristensen. 1986. "A Comparison Between Binders in the Wet Phase of Granulation in a High Shear Mixer." Drug Development and Industrial Pharmacy 12 (11–13):1685–1700. doi: 10.3109/03639048609042603.

37. Lazghab, Mariem, Khashayar Saleh, Isabelle Pezron, Pierre Guigon, and Ljepsa Komunjer. 2005. "Wettability assessment of finely divided solids." Powder Technology 157 (1):79–91. doi: https://doi.org/10.1016/j.powtec.2005.05.014.

38. Planinšek, O., R. Pišek, A. Trojak, and S. Srčič. 2000. "The utilization of surface free-energy parameters for the selection of a suitable binder in fluidized bed granulation." International Journal of Pharmaceutics 207 (1):77–88. doi: https://doi.org/10.1016/S0378-5173(00)00535-4.

39. Wu, Souheng. 1973. "Polar and Nonpolar Interactions in Adhesion." Journal of Adhesion 5 (1):39–55. doi: 10.1080/00218467308078437.

40. Lusvardi K. M., Durig T., Skinner G. W. et al. 2003. "Fundamentals of Hydroxypropylcellulose Binders in Wet Granulation." Aqualon Pharmaceutical Technology Report PTR 26.

41. Washburn, Edward W. 1921. "The dynamics of capillary flow." Physical Review 17 (3):273–283.

42. Thielmann, F., D. Burnett, K. M. Lusvardi, and T. Durig. 2005. "Correlating drug-binder adhesive strengths measured using inverse gas chromatography with tablet performance." Journal of Pharmacy And Pharmacology 57:S91–S92.

43. Krycer, Ian, David G. Pope, and John A. Hersey. 1983. "An evaluation of tablet binding agents part I. Solution binders." Powder Technology 34 (1):39–51. doi: https://doi.org/10.1016/0032-5910(83)87026-0.

44. Zhang, D., J. H. Flory, S. Panmai, U Batra, and MJ Kaufman. 2002. "Wettability of pharmaceutical solids: its measurement and influence on wet granulation." Colloids and Surfaces A: Physicochemical and Engineering Aspects 206 (1):547–554. doi: https://doi.org/10.1016/S0927-7757(02)00091-2.

45. Fox, H. W., and W. A. Zisman. 1950. "The spreading of liquids on low energy surfaces. I. polytetrafluoroethylene." Journal of Colloid Science 5 (6):514–531. doi: https://doi.org/10.1016/0095-8522(50)90044-4.

46. Gould, Robert F. 1964. "Contact Angle, Wettability, and Adhesion, Copyright, Advances in Chemistry Series." In Contact Angle, Wettability, and Adhesion, edited by F. Gould Robert, i–iii. Washington D.C.: American Chemical Society.

47. Yu, Shen, Zhenyu Huang, Ian Gabbott, Firas El Saleh, Christian Muehlenfeld, Gernot Warnke, Edmont Styanov, marcel de matas, and Agba D. Salman. 2016. "Experimental Study of Biner Selection using Twin-Screw and Batch High-Shear Wet Granulation." 10th PBP World Meeting on Pharmaceutics, Biopharmaceutics and Pharmaceutical Technology, Glasgow.

48. Taflioglu, B., T. vago, G. Dere, T. Tuglu, Z. Oren, E. Stoyanov. 2014a. "Evaluating of Tablet Characteristics of Model Efavirenz Tablets in High-Shear Wet Granulation: The Role of the Binder." 9th PBP World Meeting on Pharmaceutics, Biopharmaceutics and Pharmaceutical Technology, Lisbon.

49. Taflioglu, B., T. vago, G. Dere, T. Tuglu, Z. Oren, E. Stoyanov. 2014b. "Evaluating Role of the Binders in Model Albendazole Formulation Done by High-Shear Wet Granulation." 9th PBP World Meeting on Pharmaceuticals, Biopharmaceuticals, and Pharmaceutical Technology, Lisbon.

50. Wells, James I., and Clive V. Walker. 1983. "The influence of granulating fluids upon granule and tablet properties: the role of secondary binding." International Journal of Pharmaceutics 15 (1):97–111. doi: https://doi.org/10.1016/0378-5173(83)90070-4.

51. Reading, Susan J., and M. S. Spring. 1984. "The effects of binder film characteristics on granule and tablet properties." Journal of Pharmacy and Pharmacology 36 (7):421–426. doi: 10.1111/j.2042-7158. 1984.tb04417.x.

52. Picker-Freyer, Katharina M., and Thomas Dürig. 2007. "Physical mechanical and tablet formation properties of hydroxypropylcellulose: In pure form and in mixtures." AAPS PharmSciTech 8 (4):82. doi: 10.1208/pt0804092.

53. Joneja, S. K., W. W. Harcum, G. W. Skinner, P. E. Barnum, and J. H. Guo. 1999. "Investigating the fundamental effects of binders on pharmaceutical tablet performance." Drug Dev Ind Pharm 25 (10):1129–1135. doi: 10.1081/ddc-100102279.

54. Sheskey, Paul J., Walter G. Cook, and Colin G. Cable. 2017. Handbook of Pharmaceutical Excipients. Eighth ed. London UK: Pharmaceutical Press.

5 Excipients and Their Attributes in Granulation

Anthony E. Carpanzano

CONTENTS

5.1 INTRODUCTION

Anyone who has ever tried to compress a powder or mixture of powders to form a hard compact probably discovered that not all powders are compactible. What they likely learned is that in many cases, the challenges of making these powders routinely flow into the compaction device, and form a cohesive monolithic structure, required some degree of manipulation of the physical characteristics of the powder. These characteristics ultimately affecting the flowability and compactability of the powder mixture include the deformations characteristics of the material, the density, and particle size distribution. Converting powders, which are typically finely divided, and may also be light and fluffy, into denser, larger granules enhances flow and depending on the material characteristics, may enhance compactability as well. The development of modern wet granulation techniques to enable processing of fine powders has opened a window of opportunity to include other benefits that add to the quality of the products produced, such as the inclusion of buffers to modulate the pH of the microenvironment of the tablet itself, or surfactants to enhance the solubility of the drug, as two examples. Many active ingredients used in the production of pharmaceuticals or nutraceuticals are so difficult to process due to their physical characteristics, that they are limited to granulation (wet or dry) as the best or maybe even the only choice for processing into a quality finished product. Just as some of these active ingredients can only be produced using some form of granulation, there are several commonly used inactive ingredients or excipients that have physicochemical characteristics making them perform well and in some cases even enhancing the wet granulation process and resulting product performance. This chapter attempts to cover the most widely used and effective excipients for pharmaceutical granulation applications, processed primarily by wet granulation (high-shear, low-shear, and fluid-bed processes) but also including melt granulation, or by dry granulation (roller-compaction and slugging).

5.2 WHY GRANULATE?

In addition to modifying the physical nature of the drug substance by densifying the powdered drug and increasing the particle size distribution (when fluffy, light, small particle size), wet granulation has been traditionally used as a reliable method of pharmaceutical processing whenever there are concerns or uncertainties about any of the following:

- API dose level
- API bioavailability
- API particle size variability, lot-to-lot
- API solubility
- Desired API release characteristics
- API content uniformity
- API stability

Experienced formulators know that by using tried-and-true processing like wet granulation, that produces a uniform, consistent product, they can overcome the variability that might exist due to the aforementioned concerns. While the focus of formulation is a finished dosage form with excellent integrity, sometimes we overlook the fact that the first step to an excellent finished dosage form is a final blend with the right characteristics. To enable trouble-free downstream processing during compression and coating, or encapsulation, and ultimately packaging, the primary prerequisite is to achieve a final blend that is uniform in its content, with good flow properties and good compactibility. The granulation process combined with the right excipients and processing techniques can provide these characteristics even when the active ingredient is lacking one or more of the desired traits. Providing a uniform distribution of the active ingredient in the final blend ensures that all dosages provide the same dose, rate of dissolution, and thus therapeutic effect. That therapeutic effect is a direct result of the disintegration and dissolution characteristics, and ultimately bioavailability of the drug from the dosage form. These characteristics are part of the overall performance of the dosage form, which can be affected and more importantly, manipulated by the excipients used, and must be reliable and repeatable within each lot, and lot-to-lot, and throughout the shelf life of the product.

The dose level of drug to be provided in the finished dosage form also impacts the selection of excipients. Naturally, if the dose is large, it will limit the number and amount of excipients that can be used in the product to keep the size (and swallow-ability) to a reasonable minimum. Conversely, if the dose is low, this will allow more freedom in the number and amount of excipients that can be used. The challenge with a low dose, however, is ultimately achieving uniformity of the drug in the finished dosage form, and in the case of poorly soluble drugs, achieving the desired dissolution rate. While the choice of certain excipients may enhance blending and dissolution, many times these challenges are the reasons for choosing granulation as the manufacturing process. The granulation process can also be used to incorporate excipients that enhance the disintegration and dissolution of a drug. Disintegrants and surfactants can be added in several ways to enhance the bioavailability of the drug, and the granulation process can ensure an intimate mixture of drug and surfactant merely by the mixing energy of the process, or by putting both the drug and surfactant in the liquid used for granulating (maybe a solution or a dispersion). In the same manner, adjustment of the pH of the granulation environment can be used to enhance the stability of the drug, protecting it from the conditions of the processing as well as throughout the shelf-life of the product.

5.3 PROCESSING OPTIONS

In-depth studies of the various process options used in granulation, the different types of equipment used, and the benefits and challenges they present are detailed very thoroughly elsewhere in

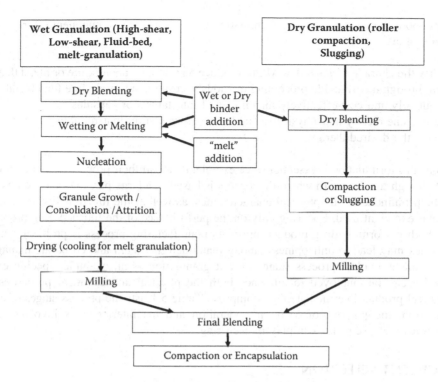

FIGURE 5.1 Typical flow chart for manufacturing solid dosage form.

this volume. Concerning the functionalities of the excipients, for the context of this chapter, a basic description of granulation processes used today is shown in the flow chart in Figure 5.1.

Wet granulation can be carried out by a high-shear mixer, low-shear mixer, fluid-bed, and by extrusion. In the case of melt-granulation, there are a number of similarities to conventional wet granulation. However, the granulating liquid or "binder" in this case is added either as a melted solid (usually of a fairly low, i.e., ~50–70°C, melting material) or as a powdered or granular solid, which melts during the process. During or at the end of the granulating process, instead of requiring drying to remove a solvent as in traditional wet granulation, the melted binder merely freezes, binding the particles together to form granules in the process. If the melted binder is sprayed into the process, droplet size can directly affect granule size and should be optimized for the best results. Managing heat transfer in the mix during the process is also an important factor, especially on scale-up.

(See chapter 19 for more information on melt granulation.)

Hot-melt extrusion granulation is similar; however, the process does not involve a conventional high-shear or low-shear mixer and utilizes an extruder to mix, melt, and consolidate the granulation ingredients. After cooling, the extrudate is milled/sized and may go through further blending with excipients (typically a disintegrant and lubricant) and then compressed or encapsulated.

5.3.1 From API to Processable Blend to Finished Product

While many young scientists starting their careers as formulators view most of the ingredients other than the API as "fillers," the best understanding of any pharmaceutical product/process comes from an in-depth understanding of the mechanistic behaviors or functionalities of the excipients being used. Excipients are not ingredients "along for the ride"; they do have an influence on the properties of the "product-in-process" as well as the performance of the finished product.

This brings about the need to view the formulation exercise as a two-component effort to achieve the following goals.

1. Modify the characteristics of the API to produce an intermediate mixture or blend that can be taken through the available processing methods to result in a trouble-free final blend that can be routinely and cost-effectively manufactured into tablets or capsules.
2. Create a chemically and physically stable final formulation that reliably and reproducibly delivers the desired therapy.

This approach to formulation is essential since excipients impart their properties to the product-in-process. Although the degree to which this occurs is based in a large part on the dose level of the API and the prominence of its physical characteristics, as well as the functionality and amount of the particular excipient used. Focusing only on the performance of the finished drug product may produce a high-performing drug product, but if its manufacturing process is problematic, the associated issues may lead to unhappiness among manufacturing team and corporate management. Considering the individual process stages of wet granulation as an example, specific excipient functionalities can be employed to influence both the physical and chemical properties of the pharmaceutical product intermediate they comprise. Table 5.1 lists the process stages of a typical wet granulation, the purpose of each unit operation and the intermediates involved, and the functional roles that excipients can play in each stage.

5.4 EXCIPIENT SELECTION

Excipients (traditionally lactose and microcrystalline cellulose [MCC]) seem to have been the most frequently used excipients, either singly or when combined in a specific ratio during the wet granulation to obtain best results selected based on their functionality. Since different formulations (and different APIs) pose different challenges, excipients should be chosen based on the functionalities that best mitigate the risks posed by the drug molecule. For example, one would not use lactose (a reducing sugar) in a formulation of phenylpropanolamine, a primary amine, which would react with the lactose to form a dark-colored degradation product (Maillard reaction). In this case, the selection of another excipient such as MCC would be the better choice.

Many times, the choice of whether or not to process by wet granulation is made based on some knowledge or experience with the active ingredient to be used, usually because of the predominance of some physical characteristics, such as low bulk density or poor compactibility. In the absence of such prior knowledge, pre-formulation studies conducted to characterize the compound are part of the routine course of development used in most all companies doing formulation work.

Pre-formulation studies typically include studies of the physicochemical characteristics of the active ingredient and its stability, including degradation pathways (thermal, oxidative, hydrolytic, photolytic, and catalytic). Also typically studied are the compound's morphology, solubility, particle size, and density. Of particular interest to formulators are the physical characteristics, which directly influence its flowability and compactibility. While there are several traditionally used instruments for determining powder flow, consolidation and compaction behavior, commonly used instruments such as the Flodex®, and other physical measurements, such as the angle of repose, Carr Index, and Hausner Index, are helpful basic tools. Fortunately, several new instruments have been developed to measure a multitude of characteristics falling under the scope of "powder rheometry" that measure many attributes and will no doubt provide tremendous insight in powder behaviors in continuous manufacturing applications. *(See Chapter 3 for characterizing the excipients and the APIs.)*

Conducting pre-formulation studies can arm the formulator with a thorough understanding of the physicochemical characteristics and behavior of the active ingredient. However, to achieve the best results in the formulation, it is just as important to have a similar understanding of the characteristics, that is, the *functionality* and limitations of the excipients under consideration.

TABLE 5.1

Excipient Functionalities for the Stages in a Wet Granulation Process in High/Low Shear Mixers

Process Stage	The Goal of Granulation Process Stage	Intermediate Composition	Excipient Functionalities Applicable to Each Process Stage
1 Dry mixing	Distribute API and excipient uniformly in the blend to be granulated	API + intra-granular excipients pre-granulation blend	Dry binder, diluent, filler, flow and compressibility enhancer, solubilizer, surfactant, pH modifier, disintegrant, wet binder (when added to dry blend)
2 Fluid addition/ mixing	Distribute liquid, nucleation, and agglomerate growth	Granulating liquid with or without binder + pre-blend	Solvent for binder and/or API, wet binder, pH modifier, surfactant, solubilizer
3 Wet massing	Granule growth, densify material	Wet-granules	Maintain some degree of physical integrity (may or may not absorb some liquid, may dissolve slightly)
4 Wet Milling	Create more uniform granules for better drying efficiency	Wet-milled granules	Maintain physical integrity while granules are wet milled and the solvent is removed (binder)
5 Drying	Remove solvent	Dried granules	
6 Milling	Achieve desired particle size distribution	Milled granules	Maintain physical integrity while granules are milled (binder)
7 Blending	Milled granulation: Enhance compactibility	Milled granulation	Active component granulated with excipients for enhanced flow and compactibility
	Running powders (dry add-ins): Enhance flowability, disintegration & compactibility	Extragranular excipients (dry add-ins)	Binder, disintegrant, surfactant,
8 Lubrication	Enhance flow and facilitate processing (ejection and capsule fill transfer)	Blend lubricant and glidant	Glidant to enhance flow, Lubricant for successful compaction or encapsulation
9 Discharge	Bulk blend for compression or encapsulation	Final blend	Provide bulk and integrity, maximize/maintain uniformity, enhance flow, compactibility, disintegration, and dissolution.

Note: For fluid bed granulation, granulating and drying are concurrent processes.

Excipients are chemicals, and though many may be chemically inert, some do react with certain materials, and knowing this before including a particular excipient in a formulation can save the formulator a lot of time and heartache. Having a thorough understanding of their functionality gives the formulator a well-equipped toolbox with many options to manipulate the manufacturing process and performance of a drug product. Moreover, from the standpoint of Quality by Design (QbD) the rationale for selection of an excipient and the level at which it is used must be justified in the development of any pharmaceutical product. The good news is that in today's market, there is extensive information regarding the properties and functionality of most excipients available, both in the literature and from reputable excipient manufacturers who routinely evaluate the functionality of their products as part of quality control.

Although there are many excipients used in granulation applications, only a few are commonly used. The selection of new excipients for granulation continues, as new challenges in formulation and processing are encountered, and this includes high-functionality, co-processed excipients. Table 5.2 shows common excipients categorized by process application. Many excipients are produced in different grades, each of which may be best suited for one specific mode of processing. Fortunately, however, many excipients have functionalities that are not limited to only one specific process.

5.4.1 Excipients in Wet Granulation, by Functionality

Terms "filler," "diluent," and "binder" are used somewhat interchangeably in the food and pharma industries and for this chapter, it will be used interchangeably together, but it would be good to set a clear definition of what they mean. A filler is an ingredient that only serves to add bulk or volume to a formulation, much like the gravel in concrete. It does not contribute to the overall physical integrity of the tablet or capsule structure other than to increase the volume of the dosage form. Similarly, the term "diluent" can be used interchangeably with "filler" in this analysis. A diluent is a material used to dilute another material to reduce the parent material's concentration and add volume. Fillers and diluents are used in direct compression and wet granulation and can be added to both the granulation mix as well as to the running powders. In the context of processing by granulation, the terms themselves imply the intent for the inclusion of the materials in a formulation, as described earlier. The term "binders" usually refers to excipients dissolved in the granulating fluid or added to the granulation pre-mix (dry) to serve as the "glue" that builds and holds the granules together.

At the same time, in the context of direct compression, materials having a mechanistic functionality of cohesion are in many cases referred to as binders, filler-binders, as well as diluents. In this application, binders usually make up a larger part of the formulation and are materials that can form a monolithic structure when compacted due to their cohesive nature.

(For a comprehensive review of binders see Chapter 4.)

5.4.1.1 Inorganic, Insoluble Excipients

For the most part, in wet granulation applications, the inorganic, insoluble filler/diluents, such as dibasic calcium phosphate (DCP), tribasic calcium phosphate (TCP), and calcium sulfate dihydrate, function as fillers so the physical strength of the granules produced relies largely on the binder used in the process. Their moderate to high density also helps to make granules that flow well and this is particularly important when the API to be granulated has low density and poor flow property. Their insoluble nature provides a benefit, in that it makes the powder mixture less prone to over-granulation. However, also because of their insoluble nature, these excipients can impair the dissolution of the drug from the granules by occlusion of the API within the granules, thus limiting the exposure of the drug to water. So, care should be taken when using an insoluble excipient in formulations where API solubility is limited. DCP is used widely in direct compression applications (more as the dihydrate) due to its moderately high density providing good flow and relative lack of lubricant sensitivity. These benefits also apply in wet granulation where the use of the anhydrous form is more prevalent since the dihydrate form will readily give off its water of crystallization under fairly moderate conditions of heat and physical stress. It is ideally suited for moisture-sensitive active ingredients. As used in wet granulation, it serves mostly as an

TABLE 5.2

Common Excipients Used for Granulation

Excipient	Dry Granulation (Roller-Compaction, Slugging)	Wet Granulation (High-Shear, Low-Shear, Fluid-Bed, and Extrusion)	Direct Compression
α-Lactose monohydrate (milled)	Filler/Diluent/Binder	Filler/Diluent/Binder	
α-Lactose monohydrate (agglomerated)			Filler/Diluent/Binder
α-Lactose monohydrate (spray dried)			Filler/Diluent/Binder
β-Lactose, anhydrous (β: α = 80:20)	Filler/Diluent/Binder		Filler/Diluent/Binder
Lactose, powdered	Filler/Diluent/Binder	Filler/Diluent/Binder	
Powdered cellulose	Filler/Diluent/Binder	Filler/Diluent/Binder	Filler/Diluent/Binder
Microcrystalline cellulose	Filler/Diluent/Binder	Filler/Diluent/Binder	Filler/Diluent/Binder
Calcium Phosphate, Dibasic (DCP)	Filler/Diluent/Binder	Filler/Diluent/Binder	Filler/Diluent/Binder
Calcium Phosphate, Tribasic (TCP)	Filler/Diluent/Binder	Filler/Diluent/Binder	Filler/Diluent/Binder
Calcium Sulfate, dihydrate	Filler/Diluent/Binder	Filler/Diluent/Binder	Filler/Diluent/Binder
Starch, unmodified	Disintegrant	Binder	Disintegrant
Starch, partially pregelatinized	Binder	Binder	
Sucrose		Filler/Diluent/Binder	Diluent
Dextrose		Filler/Diluent/Binder	
Dextrates		Filler/Diluent/Binder	
Povidone		Binder	
Co-povidone VA64	Binder	Binder	Binder
Ethylcellulose		Binder	
Methylcellulose		Binder	
Hydroxypropyl cellulose	Binder	Binder	Binder
Hydroxypropyl methylcellulose		Binder	
Mannitol	Binder	Binder	Binder
Sorbitol	Binder	Binder	Binder
Xylitol	Binder	Binder	Binder
Acacia		Binder	
Alginates		Binder	
Gelatin		Binder	
Guar gum		Binder	
Pectin		Binder	

insoluble filler-diluent but does have some binding properties upon compression due to its brittle nature. It is available in the powdered form, which is mostly used in wet granulation, or granular form, mostly used in direct compression applications. Although more true for the granular form, upon compaction, it fractures and the clean surfaces exposed are potential bonding sites, which may contribute to tablet hardness.

Figure 5.2 shows a scanning electron micrograph of granular DCP dihydrate (Emcompress). It clearly illustrates the agglomerated granular nature of this material and its crystallite morphology. From the image, one can imagine the interlocking of these granules upon interaction with a wet binder during the nucleation phase of granulation, and the fracturing and further interlocking of particles upon compaction.

TCP, another inorganic, insoluble filler/diluent, also known as hydroxyapatite, is also used in both direct compression applications as well as wet granulation. Surprisingly though, unlike DCP, TCP deforms by plastic deformation and therefore exhibits notably different characteristics in compression. Plastically deforming materials typically display strain-rate sensitivity, that is, the hardness of tablets produced can be increased by increasing the dwell time of compression (slowing the press speed). These materials are also more sensitive to lubricant over-blending since no fracturing occurs upon compression revealing binding surfaces free from exposure to lubricant.

TCP is available in powdered form, which like powdered DCP, is mostly used in wet granulation, or a granular form for direct compression applications. The powdered form is also used as an anti-caking agent in formulations where the active ingredient may be oily or sticky. Aside from the difference in deformation properties, the use of TCP in wet granulation is much the same as that of DCP, in that it is essentially another dense free-flowing filler of moderate compactibility, also insoluble in water. Calcium sulfate, dihydrate, also known as terra alba or gypsum, and available in both the powdered and granular form, is also a good filler for wet granulation

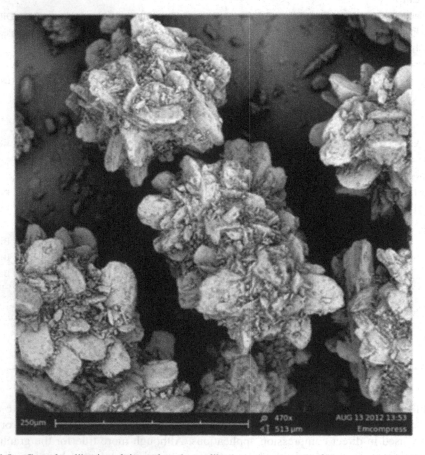

FIGURE 5.2   Granular dibasic calcium phosphate, dihydrate (emcompress®).
Source: JRS Pharma.

applications. Calcium sulfate is also slightly soluble and this has caused issues on stability in the past. It is a non-hygroscopic material and therefore good for use with moisture sensitive active ingredients. The material is quite dense, as well.

5.4.1.2 Organic, Insoluble Excipients

Cellulose is one of the most abundant organic compounds on earth. This polysaccharide is a chief constituent of plant fiber. Cotton fiber, for example, is composed of approximately 90% cellulose, and wood is composed of 40–50%. Cellulose, the main structural component of plant cell walls, helps make plants stable, elastic, and resilient to external influences. The basic building block of cellulose is glucose. Glucose monomers are connected through β1-4 glycosidic bonds. The degree of polymerization in cellulose ranges from 200 to 1500 glucose monomers. Powdered cellulose has been used as a filler, binder, and diluent in both wet granulation and direct compression for many years and is still used today in many legacy formulations. It deforms by plastic deformation and is available in various particle size ranges, with the smaller particle size material having the most compactibility but poorest flow and the large particle size material having the poorest compactibility but highest flow within the range. The functional performance of powdered cellulose for compactibility is relatively low and only 20–30% of that of Micro Crystalline Cellulose (MCC) [1]. Fortunately, by the processing of powdered cellulose to remove a large part of its amorphous content, it was discovered that the remaining MCC had a significantly greater functional performance with respect to compaction. The subsequent introduction of MCC as a tablet binder in the 1960s was a major advancement for the production of many solid dosage formulations. MCC enabled formulators to significantly enhance the wet granulation and dry granulation processes of the day and opened up the option of direct compression to many other formulations. MCC is a partially depolymerized cellulose, derived from high-quality, dissolving grade pulp from fibrous plant material, by processing with mineral acids using hydrochloric acid to reduce the degree of polymerization. Though MCC can be produced from several sources including cotton and many other plants, the majority of MCC used in the pharmaceutical industry is sourced from softwood pulp. After the hydrolysis process, which strips away most of the amorphous regions of cellulose, leaving a material high in crystallinity (roughly 60–90%), the cellulose is washed and typically spray dried. By varying process parameters during the spray drying process, different particle sizes and degrees of agglomeration can be achieved thus producing several different grades of MCC to address various challenges encountered in the formulation.

For wet granulation, MCC although insoluble in water, has some swelling tendencies and excellent water imbibing or wicking action. This property makes MCC an excellent excipient for wet granulation. When used as a filler in wet granulation, the wicking action of MCC promotes the rapid wetting of the powder mix. It also can retain the water absorbed in the process, which makes the wet mass, less sensitive to overwetting due to an excess of granulating fluid. MCC's moisture sorbing properties and resistance to overwetting make for a granulation texture that is less sensitive to variability in the process, the API, and other raw materials in the granulation mix. However, because MCC absorbs water during the process, it can make the granulation appear somewhat dry, and thus prompt further addition of water and continued mixing, in extreme cases, resulting in over-granulation and longer drying time.

A scanning electron micrograph of MCC in Figure 5.3 shows the fibrous, porous morphology.

When it comes to compaction of wet-granulated and dried MCC, however, the resulting tablet hardness is lower than the same tablets made by direct compression (not exposed to the wetting and drying cycle). This is why additional MCC or other binder is typically added to the granulation before compression into tablets. Figure 5.4 shows the comparative compaction profiles of MCC after wet granulation versus not granulated.

Researchers at the University of Bath and the Mendell division of the Penwest Pharmaceuticals Company conducted studies to determine the cause of this reduction in compactibility. After studying a process that occurs in papermaking, Professor John Staniforth coined the term for this

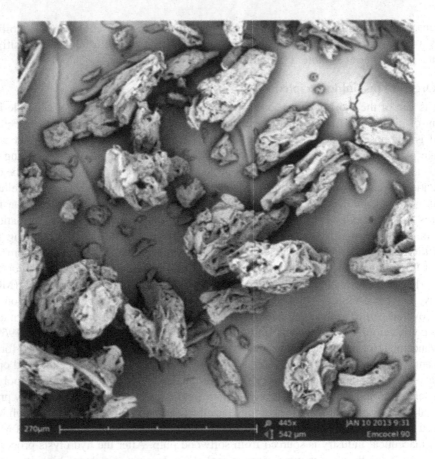

FIGURE 5.3 Microcrystalline cellulose (emcocel 50®).
Source: JRS Pharma.

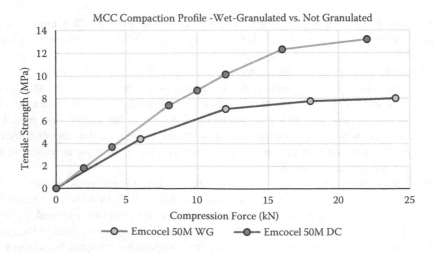

FIGURE 5.4 Comparative compaction profiles of MCC (emcocel 50 M®) before and after wet granulation.
Source: JRS Pharma.

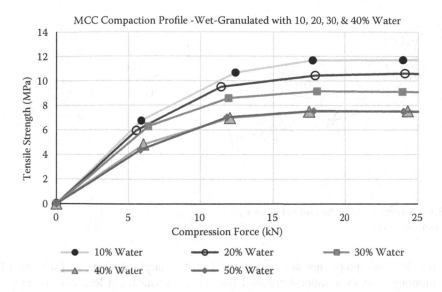

FIGURE 5.5 Compaction profiles of microcrystalline cellulose after wet granulating with various amounts of water.
Source: JRS Pharma.

phenomenon as *quasi-hornification* [2] to describe the reduced bonding capacity following wetting and drying of cellulose fibers. The conclusion was that the reduced bonding was the result of a high degree of lateral association of the cellulose fibers and microfibrils, which is facilitated by wetting, which promotes the formation of intra and inter-fiber hydrogen bonds during drying. The tenacity of this hydrogen bonding reduces the subsequent accessibility of water to the cellulose fibers and reduces the external surface area available for particle inter-locking and hydrogen bonding. Besides, as the amount of granulating water is increased, the resulting tablet hardness is also reduced (see Figure 5.5). This seems to level off, however, at around 40%.

Another study of the changes MCC undergoes during wet granulation with water in a high-shear mixer was conducted using x-ray diffraction. It was revealed that the hardness of the resulting MCC granules increased with granulation time and the amount of water added. The specific surface area (measured by the N_2 adsorption) was reduced during the process. Crystallite size of cellulose, calculated by Scherrer's equation adapted for wide-angle x-ray diffraction, decreased with granulation time and increasing amounts of water added. Debye plots for x-ray small scattering patterns suggested that the average magnitude of the continuous solid region in MCC granules became significantly greater, whereas the specific surface area of the MCC granules became smaller in comparison with that of intact MCC [3]. These findings suggested that the long-chain structures in MCC were disrupted, resulting in smaller units with shorter chain lengths due to the high shear forces of the impeller. These smaller units then form a network within the granules. Thus, MCC granules are strengthened with longer granulation time and greater amounts of water, resulting in a more intricate network, but may result in over granulation.

5.4.1.3 Organic Soluble Excipients

Lactose, or milk sugar, is a disaccharide composed of d-glucose and d-galactose, linked by a beta 1-4 glycosidic linkage. Crystalline lactose can exist in several forms. In pharmaceutical applications, lactose is used in two basic forms, α-lactose monohydrate and β-lactose. See Figure 5.6.

Both α-lactose monohydrate and β-lactose are available in several milled grades and spray dried grades from many producers. Milled α-lactose monohydrate is used in wet and dry granulation. While fine particle size milled α-lactose monohydrate produces fairly robust compacts in direct

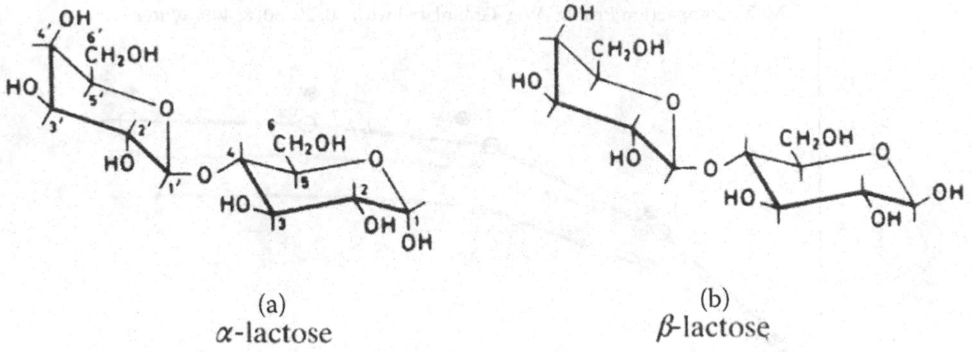

(a)
α-lactose

(b)
β-lactose

FIGURE 5.6 Structures of alpha and beta lactose.
Source: From Ref. [4].

compression, its flow properties are generally poor to marginal. Coarser fractions of milled α-lactose monohydrate show much-improved flow characteristics, but lose performance on compaction. For this reason, α-lactose monohydrate is also produced in spray agglomerated grades that combine the good compactibility characteristics of the fine milled material with the good flow of the coarser material.

By contrast, spray-dried lactose (FlowLac®, Meggle) is produced by spray-drying a suspension of fine milled α-lactose monohydrate crystals in a solution of lactose. During this spray drying process, where water is rapidly removed, some formation of amorphous lactose also occurs and can be controlled within the desired level. This content of amorphous lactose serves as a binder in the process, resulting in a finished excipient having a spherical morphology of α-lactose monohydrate crystals bound together by amorphous lactose. Naturally, the technological efforts and associated costs of producing such morphologies are geared primarily toward direct compression applications and would be largely wasted in wet granulation applications.

β-lactose, commonly referred to as anhydrous lactose, usually exists as a mixture of β-lactose and anhydrous α-lactose in a ratio of about 80:20. Anhydrous lactose (β-lactose) is also available in many different particle size grades (typically milled) and is used in wet and dry granulation. Because lactose is freely soluble in water (195 mg/ml), its behavior and functionality in wet granulation are different than that of the insoluble filler-diluent-binders reviewed previously in this text. Researchers found that when granulated with water, partial solubilization at the surface of the lactose crystals produces a sticky binder solution that promotes agglomeration and granule growth. Frequently granulated together in combination with MCC, in-process characteristics such as wet mass rheology, granule growth, and dried granule strength can be modulated by varying the relative ratios of lactose and MCC. The breaking force of tablets made by high shear granulation of lactose and MCC is most affected by the lactose/MCC ratio and the particle size of the lactose. Harder tablets are achieved by reducing the proportion of MCC, and by the use of finely milled lactose. The use of PVP K30 as a wet binder had only a small effect. When the MCC content is high, higher water amounts are needed to achieve sufficient wet massing and dry granule strength, presumably due to the high water sorption character of MCC.

In another study comparing twin-screw extrusion granulation for a continuous processing application with conventional high-shear granulation of lactose, researchers found that good granule properties could be obtained without the use of a wet binder (PVP) when using the extrusion process. This was not the case in the same formulation processed by high-shear granulation, where to produce robust granules, the PVP wet binder and additional water was required. This suggests that the shear properties encountered during extrusion are greater and produce more dissolution of the lactose resulting in a greater binding that would be the case under the shear conditions encountered in conventional high shear granulation. This suggests that for some formulations, extrusion granulation may be a more efficient wet granulation technique than high shear wet granulation. In still another study comparing roller compaction, fluid-bed, and high-shear granulation of lactose, the resulting granule strength was found to be variable depending on the process used. There was also an inverse relationship between granule strength and tablet hardness, with high-shear granulation producing the strongest granules but also the lowest resulting tablet hardness. Roller compaction showed moderately good tablets produced from robust granules. Tablets made from fluid-bed granulated lactose showed the highest tensile strength and least weight variation. Twin-screw granulation showed comparable results [5].

5.4.1.4 Sugar Alcohols

Sugar alcohols or polyols are polyhydric alcohols that occur naturally and can be synthetically produced from sugars and resemble sugars in that some exhibit significant sweetness but since they are polyols, they do not have the same incompatibilities as reducing sugars. They are also non-cariogenic and have a much lower glycemic index than sugar. These compounds are used in food products, confections, and pharmaceuticals. Most are available in different particle size grades in crystalline as well as granular form. As most manufacturers prefer to manufacture tablets by direct compression whenever possible, these products are positioned for direct compression applications through wet granulation of the sugar alcohols is not uncommon. In studying the granulation performance of three sugar alcohols – mannitol, sorbitol, and xylitol – in different amounts as compared to sucrose, researchers found that the increased viscosity of the liquid bridges formed, as a result of the partial dissolution of the sugars, strongly contributed to the agglomeration process. The viscosity influenced the liquid mobility and distribution of the solution. As with any soluble filler-diluent-binder, its solubility in the granulating fluid (typically water) is expected to have some influence in the process (visible in torque rheometry measurements) and the outcome of granule and tablet properties.

Mannitol is widely used in pharmaceutical applications both as an excipient and as an active ingredient, most notably as an osmotic laxative (also for modulation of osmotic pressure in several other therapeutic indications). The excipient is available from several sources in crystalline and granular form in several different particle sizes. It is a good replacement for lactose, in formulations containing a primary or secondary amine, that may react with lactose (Maillard Reaction).

Unlike sorbitol, which is very hygroscopic, mannitol exhibits very low hygroscopicity and because of this, it is well suited for wet granulation because it is easily dried. Also, because of its sweet taste and cooling effect in the mouth (due to a negative heat of solution), it is widely used in chewable tablets. The various granular grades of mannitol available, which exhibit good flow and compactibility properties, make it popular for direct compression applications. In wet granulation, mannitol is frequently used successfully in combination with MCC. Its good compactibility, offsets the loss in compactibility that MCC undergoes after the wetting and drying cycle. The solubility of mannitol, about 216 mg/ml,[1] [6] is about one-tenth that of lactose, and so when substituted for lactose in granulations where lactose is avoided due to incompatibility with the API, much less will dissolve and form binder bridges as compared to lactose. This may prompt the use of a dissolved liquid binder such as polyvinylpyrrolidone or hydroxypropylmethylcellulose. Mannitol can exist as three different polymorphs; an α-form, a β-form, and a δ-form. In a study where the δ-form of mannitol was wet granulated, it was determined that a moisture-induced polymorphic transition of mannitol to the β-form, with a concurrent change in particle morphology, occurred, and that the resulting granules exhibited significantly improved compactibility. Most commercially available mannitol is sold as the β-form polymorph and is available in several particle size grades to suit wet and dry granulation and direct compression applications.

Sorbitol, a structural isomer of mannitol, differs significantly in its physical properties, and although it is widely used in confections and the syrup form (70% w/w) in pharmaceuticals, it is mostly used in chewable tablets, usually in pediatric or vitamin applications. The primary reason for this is its very hygroscopic nature. It is also used as a humectant in syrups to prevent cap-locking. Like mannitol, it is also a hyperosmotic and similarly is used intravenously in some preparations and also produces laxation when given in gram quantities. Its water solubility is about 13 times that of mannitol and is widely used in foods as a non-nutritive sweetener. Because of its hygroscopic nature and humectant activity, it is not particularly well suited for wet granulation.

Xylitol, a five-carbon sugar alcohol that is also widely used as a sweetener in confections and foods, and in pharma, is also popular in direct compression applications. It is most comparable to sucrose in sweetness and taste and free from the aftertaste, with the usual cooling mouthfeel as is common with the sugar alcohols due to the negative heat of solution. It is also non-cariogenic and actually promotes dental health and so is used in many kinds of toothpaste and dental products where a sweetener is needed. It has a low glycemic index, which makes it a popular sugar sub-stitute for diabetic patients. As xylitol performs well in wet granulation, it is available in the granulated form in different particle size distributions for use in direct compression. This is common with the sugar alcohols since their compaction performance is improved by wet granulating.

Isomalt, a relatively new excipient is a mixture of polyols – glucopyranosyl-sorbitol and glucopyranosyl-mannitol – and by varying the relative ratios of the two components in the mixture as well as varying the particle size grades and granular grades, the resulting products are designed to address several formulation and processing challenges. Like the other polyols, isomalt is non-cariogenic, and has a negative heat of solution producing a cooling effect in the mouth. It has a sweetness level about half that of sucrose and is also used in preparations for diabetics because of its low glycemic index. It is used in tablets, capsules, coatings, sachets, and suspensions, and effervescent tablets and can be processed by direct compression and wet granulation depending on the grade. Isomalt is quite compactible, as can be seen in Figure 5.7. It is non-hygroscopic, re-latively inert, and quite stable, and therefore makes an ideal filler-diluent-binder regardless of the tablet manufacturing process to be used.

5.4.1.5 Starches and Sugar

Starch occurs as an odorless and tasteless, fine, white-colored powder, comprising very small spherical or ovoid granules or grains whose size and shape are characteristic for each botanical variety. Starch is a natural polymer consisting of amylose and amylopectin, two polysaccharides based on a-glucose. Starch is likely one of the most traditionally used excipients in the production of tablets and capsules. For pharmaceutical applications, most starch is sourced from corn (maize) and potatoes. Starch can serve as a wet-granulation binder when gelatinized by heating in water above 75°C and added as a starch paste dispersion in amounts ranging from about 5% to 25% of the formulation. Gelatinization ruptures the starch grains liberating the natural polymer, which like cellulose comprises both crystalline regions (about 45%) and amorphous regions [8]. Gelatinization reduces the crystalline content to about 5%. For many years, starch paste granu-lation has been carried out using both low- and high-shear mixer processes and is being used today for many old products. Determination of the optimal quantity of starch paste to use in any for-mulation is best determined experimentally through observation of parameters of granulated product such as granule friability, tablet hardness, and friability, disintegration rate, and ultimately drug dissolution rate. Starch (unmodified) is also used as a disintegrant (typically around 10% and up to 15%) due to its nature to swell upon hydration with a high-specific surface area for water sorption. High amounts of unmodified starch can cause capping and may negatively affect tablet friability.

When considering starch as a filler-diluent-binder as defined earlier in this text, there is a need for clarification due to the diverse functionality of starch. Dried pre-gelatinized starch, that is, what remains after the starch grains are ruptured (as is done in the starch paste preparation process) can serve as a binder in direct compression applications, when used at levels up to about 25% of the

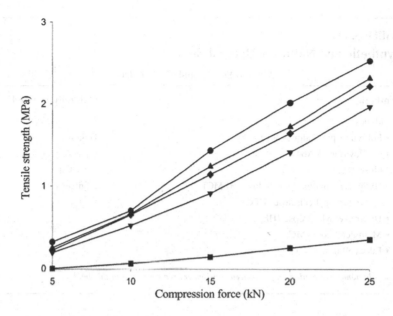

FIGURE 5.7   Tablet crushing strength of isomalt (palatinit® F and type C) profiles at different concentrations of magnesium stearate. keys: 0.25% (F;■); C: (•); 0.5% (▲); 0.75% (♦); 1% (▼) for only type C. *Source:* From Ref. [7].

formulation. Partially pre-gelatinized starch, in which a portion of the starch grains has been ruptured mechanically can be used as a filler-diluent-binder in direct compression or as a binder in wet granulation applications as well.

Sucrose, employed as an aqueous syrup of 50–67% by weight, has been used as a wet granulation binder. Unlike polymeric binders, sucrose is not a film-forming binder and generally results in tablets that are hard but brittle, and have greater friability than those made using polymeric film-forming binders. Also, tablets granulated with sucrose may harden upon aging. In a study comparing six wet granulation binders, sucrose was observed to compress by brittle fracture followed by plastic flow. This plastic flow and the resultant cold welding was, therefore, thought to be the major mechanism of cohesion. Sucrose can be found in many medical dosage forms such as chewable tablets, syrups, lozenges, or gums. Directly compressible sugar such as Di-Pac® has useful properties include high flowability, low hygroscopicity, sweetness, and nonreactivity with other tablet components.

5.4.1.6 Synthetic and Naturally Derived Binders

Many compounds have been used as binders for granulation and a number of these are described in detail elsewhere in this volume. It is important though to list a few of them and make mention of their types. Most of these compounds are polymers, either synthetic, semi-synthetic, or naturally derived materials. In general, they are very versatile compounds and some have many technical applications in the pharmaceutical, food, and textile industries as well.

Table 5.3 lists several of the most commonly used synthetic and naturally derived binders for granulation applications.

5.4.1.7 Excipients for Nutraceuticals

No discussion of solid dosage form formulation would be complete without mentioning "nutraceutical" products since many of them are produced by the same processes and utilize many of the same excipients. With a greater focus on the consumption of chemical derivatives and synthetic

TABLE 5.3

Synthetic and Naturally Derived Binders

Wet and Dry Granulation Binders

Synthetic	Naturally Derived
Povidones:	Starch
• Polyvinyl pyrrolidones K12-K90	Gelatin
• Co-Povidone VA64	Gum Acacia
Cellulose ethers:	Guar Gum
• Hydroxypropyl methylcellulose (HPMC)	Alginates
• Hydroxypropyl cellulose (HPC)	Pectin
• Hydroxyethylcellulose (HEC)	
• Methylcellulose (MC)	
• Ethylcellulose (EC)	

(For additional Information on pharmaceutical Binders see Chapter 4 in this book.)

polymers, the nutraceutical industry has undertaken a quest for the "clean label" (sometimes regardless of the true nature of the contents) and therefore taken on more use of naturally derived components. This trend is most prevalent in the production of vitamins and health-food supplements and is a significant market trend, getting considerable attention. Despite the trend, there are many excipients carried over from the pharmaceutical industry that regardless of their "chemical-sounding" names (a taboo in the Nutraceutical industry) are mainstays in providing the physical functionalities needed to make robust products. This point is evident when looking at just about any multivitamin or mineral supplement label, where a multitude of active ingredients (most of which do not flow or compact well) makes up tablet formulations, which are ultimately held together by tried and true pharma excipients such as DCP, MCC, and in the most challenging formulations, silicified microcrystalline cellulose (SMCC). The nutraceutical companies using DCP caught on quickly realizing that they could claim its calcium content as one of the active ingredients in their formulation and capitalize on both its functionality and therapeutic benefit. Although nutraceutical producers generally try to keep their excipient costs as low as possible, many have had their issues with granulation processing and try to avoid it whenever possible, even if it means spending more on high-functionality excipients and using direct compression processing. In this respect, they have followed much the same path as the pharmaceutical industry, and will likely continue to do so until more high-functionality "natural-ish" excipients are developed.

5.5 HIGH FUNCTIONALITY CO-PROCESSED EXCIPIENTS

Although wet granulation has been a traditional method of processing pharmaceutical solid dosage forms for many years, despite the development of newer techniques, it is still a routine practice and maybe the best or only approach for some otherwise very challenging drug compounds. Wet granulation as a process has presented formulators, quality control personnel, and corporate management with challenges of managing a train of unit operations that is at times difficult to control from the standpoint of variability and operate cost-effectively. The regulatory views on wet granulation (especially where operator judgment involved in the process was a critical factor in achieving finished product quality) were no doubt a strong driving force in the development of the QbD initiative that now drives the disciplines of drug product development. So, although the wet granulation remains an option, it is mostly viewed as the least preferred method of processing due to its cost and complexity.

Having a clear understanding of the issues around wet granulation, excipient manufacturers sought to bring greater functionality to excipients than what was available using traditional excipients, and thus arm formulators with excipients that may enable the use of simpler, less costly and less complex processing than wet granulation. In general, the simplification of pharmaceutical solid dosage form manufacturing was the driving force behind the development of co-processed higher-functionality excipients.

In the case of the development of silicified microcrystalline cellulose (SMCC), however, that's not how it started. Given the general high performance of MCC in direct compression applications, and in light of the previously mentioned phenomenon of *quasi hornification*, researchers at the Edward Mendell Co. enlisted the help of Professor John Staniforth of the University of Bath, U.K. to seek a way to improve this shortcoming by co-processing MCC with various other components. The result of this work was the development of Prosolv®, silicified microcrystalline cellulose (SMCC). Although the original intent, in this case, was to provide that would not lose compactibility during wet granulation, SMCC was later found to have exceptional functionality compared to MCC in direct compression applications, not only in higher compactibility but also in lower sensitivity to overlubrication. In addition, it was also discovered that SMCC enhances flow and promotes interactive blending, reducing the cohesive forces that exist between particles, therefore enhancing blend uniformity, especially effective when blending micronized drugs. Having seen the benefits co-processing brought to a single entity excipient like MCC, excipient manufacturers have since focused their efforts on seeking greater functionality through co-processing traditional mono-functional excipients, again, primarily for direct compression applications. Thus, formulators could avoid wet granulation, and use the direct compression process for more challenging compounds that otherwise previously might have only been produced by more complex processing means. SMCC is a co-processed, high-functionality excipient made in much the same way as MCC is made with an exception in the spray drying process. At this stage of the process, a slurry of colloidal silicon dioxide (CSD) is combined, and spray dried together with the slurry of MCC, creating an intimate mixture of the two ingredients. This degree of mixing is one that cannot be achieved through even the most vigorous dry blending. Figures 5.8a–5.8d show several electron micrographs of SMCC and MCC at similar magnifications. In the first series (5.8a and 5.8b) the morphology of SMCC and MCC does not appear different. Upon a closer look in the second series (5.8c and 5.8d), however, when comparing the two products, the SMCC micrograph clearly shows the relatively tiny particles of CSD, which are thoroughly distributed on the surface and in the pores of the MCC particles. Though there is no chemical interaction between the two compounds, the silica is believed to be held on the surface of the MCC through hydrogen bonding.

In a study assessing the effects of silicification on the performance of SMCC in wet granulation [9], MCC and SMCC were each wet granulated in a high-shear granulator with 42% by weight of water, wet screened through a 12 mesh sieve and tray dried to a moisture of 5%. The dried granules were sieved and reconstituted to form a standard distribution in the range of 74–177 microns. The granulations were lubricated with 0.25% sodium stearyl fumarate and compressed using flat-faced tooling. As can be seen in Figure 5.9, the wet granulated (co-processed) SMCC has significantly greater compactibility than that of the wet granulated MCC, and that of the physically blended and wet granulated MCC/CSD mixture, indicating that silicification of MCC prevents the loss of compactibility that MCC otherwise will undergo after wet granulation.

In addition, to elucidate the effects of co-processing on functionality, a physical blend of MCC and CSD was prepared in the same proportions as used in SMCC, and wet granulated and processed in the same manner (Figure 5.10). This demonstrated that co-processing is crucial to the performance of the excipient and this level of performance is not achievable through simple blending.

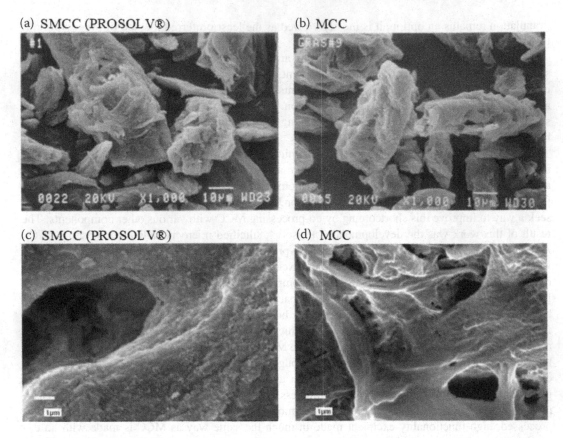

(a) SMCC (PROSOLV®)   (b) MCC

(c) SMCC (PROSOLV®)   (d) MCC

FIGURE 5.8 Comparative scanning electron micrographs of SMCC and MCC at different magnifications. *Source:* JRS Pharma.

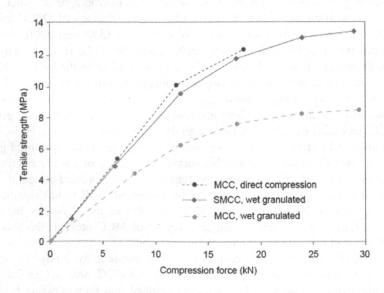

FIGURE 5.9 Comparative compaction profile of directly compressed MCC and wet granulated MCC and SMCC.
Source: From Ref. [9].

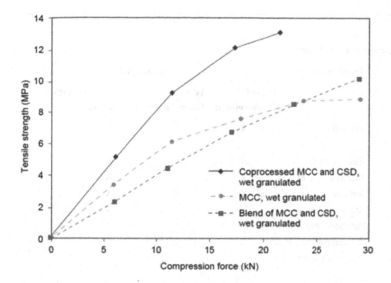

FIGURE 5.10 Comparative compaction profile of wet granulated MCC, Co-processed SMCC, and a physical blend of MCC and CSD.
Source: From Ref. [9].

The increased compactibility of SMCC over MCC also holds true in direct compression. Along with the increased flow, lower sensitivity to over-lubrication improved blending characteristics with micronized active ingredients, and this has enabled formulators to choose direct compression in many cases where wet granulation may have otherwise been the only option.

Since the development of SMCC, many co-processed high functionality excipients have been developed, leaving wet granulation behind, mostly as a last resort in choice of processing. Though it may seem counter-intuitive, there are benefits in using co-processed excipients in wet granulation applications as well.

- Since co-processed excipients are excipient composites, their uniformity of composition remains largely intact throughout the rigors of processing (blending, encapsulation, or tableting) ensuring finished product uniformity than might be achieved using the component materials.
- Co-processed excipients still may offer greater performance as compared to the physical mixtures of their component parts even if after the granulation process.
- Using a co-processed excipient in any process reduces the number of process steps, reduces the chances for error, and assures better mixing and content uniformity, as opposed to using the component parts.

This has become most evident in the recent past as more companies switch from batch processing to continuous processing. In a continuous process, mono-functional excipients must be added through individual feeders, possibly resulting in multiple sources of variability. Alternatively, a single high-functionality co-processed excipient can accomplish the same task using only one feeder, thus enhancing finished product performance while keeping variability to a minimum.

Table 5.4 lists some of the co-processed excipients available today, with their trade names, manufacturers, and generally recommended applications. As can be seen, many of the components are common, monofunctional excipients that have been augmented by the addition of another functional component. It is safe to say that in most or all cases, co-processing brings a greater synergy of the individual components to the functionality of the co-processed product. The

TABLE 5.4

Select Co-Processed Excipients

Co-Processed Components	Trade Name	Applications				Manufacturer
		Direct Compression	Wet Granulation	Dry Granulation	Other	
Lactose, MCC & Starch	Combilac	X		X		Meggle
Lactose, MCC	Cellactose 80	X		X		Meggle
Lactose, MCC	Microcelac 100	X		X		Meggle
Lactose, HPMC	Retalac	X	X	X		Meggle
Lactose, starch	Starlac	X		X		Meggle
Mix of polyols	Advantol 300	X				SPI Polyols
Fructose, starch	Advantose FS 95	X				SPI Polyols
Calcium carbonate, starch	Barcroft CS 90	X				SPI Polyols
Sorbitol, mannitol	Compressol SM	X				SPI Polyols
Mannitol, CSD, sorbitol, crospovidone	Pharmaburst	X			Orally disintegrating tablets	
MCC, CSD	Prosolv SMCC 50LD, 50, 90, 90HD, 90LM	X	X	X		JRS Pharma
	Avicel SMCC	X	X	X		DuPont
MCC, CSD, sodium starch glycolate, sodium stearyl fumarate	Prosolv EasyTab SP	X	X	X		JRS Pharma
MCC, CSD, croscarmellose sodium, palm fat, DATEM	Prosolv EasyTab Nutra	X	X	X		JRS Pharma
MCC, CSD, croscarmellose sodium, magnesium stearate	Prosolv EasyTab Nutra CM	X	X	X		JRS Pharma
MCC, CSD, sodium starch glycolate, magnesium stearate	Prosolv EasyTab Nutra GM	X	X	X		JRS Pharma
MCC, CSD, croscarmellose sodium, sodium stearyl fumarate	Prosolv EasyTab Nutra CP	X	X	X		JRS Pharma
MCC, NaCMC	Vivapur MCG				Liquids	JRS Pharma
	Avicel RC				Liquids	DuPont
MCC, DCP	Avicel DG			X		DuPont

(Continued)

TABLE 5.4 (Continued)

Co-Processed Components	Trade Name	Applications				Manufacturer
		Direct Compression	Wet Granulation	Dry Granulation	Other	
MCC, mannitol	Avicel HFE 102	X		X		DuPont
MCC, guar gum	Avicel CE-15	X			Chewables	DuPont
Calcium carbonate, sorbitol	Formaxx	X				Merck
Mannitol, starch, sorbitol	Pearlitol Flash	X			Orally disinte-grating tablets	Roquette
Lactose, PVP, crospovidone	Ludipress	X		X		BASF
Lactose, PVP	Ludipress LCE	X		X		BASF
Mannitol, PVA, crospovidone	Ludiflash	X	X	X		BASF
Mannitol, xylitol, MCC, calcium phosphate, crospovidone	F-Melt C	X			Orally disinte-grating tablets	Fuji
Mannitol, xylitol, MCC, crospovidone, Neusilin®	F-Melt M	X			Orally disinte-grating tablets	Fuji
Calcium phosphate, waxed starch, MCC	F-Melt F1	X			Orally disinte-grating tablets	Fuji
Mannitol, croscarmellose sodium	Partek ODT	X			Orally disinte-grating tablets	Merck
Sucrose, dextrin	DiPac	X		X		Domino foods
Mannitol, LHPC, PVA	Smartex QD50 a100	X		X	Orally disintegrating tablets	ShinEtsu

majority of co-processed excipients are specifically designed for direct compression, and by nature of that functionality, this makes them suitable for dry granulation as well. As previously stated, where wet granulation is used, there may be advantages in using co-processed excipients, though the primary intent of co-processing is to bring greater functionality to the excipient and thus avoid wet granulation.

5.6 EXCIPIENT VARIABILITY

One of the major challenges faced in our industry and one that many formulators do not realize is that most excipients are not produced by an industry born out of the need to produce these products for the pharmaceutical industry alone. In most cases, pharmaceutical ingredients are by-products of much larger-scale industrial products [10]. This puts the pharmaceutical industry at an unusual disadvantage when it comes to managing the supply, quality, pedigree, continuity, and costs of excipients. Many excipient manufacturers are chemical companies who manufacture a small portion of their total output for the pharmaceutical industry. The reality is that very often the amount sold into pharmaceutical companies is less than 10% of the output of these materials. Another key point regarding excipients is that many of them are derived from natural products, and natural products vary. They vary due to changes in the climate, length of the growing season, storage conditions and time, source location, transportation, and many other factors. Formulators need to understand that although the variability inherent in an excipient's source material may ultimately not impact the performance of their drug product, QbD studies required as a part of development may need to make the study of excipient variability part of their developmental design space. Ultimately, understanding and identifying the variability in the critical material attributes (CMAs) of all components in a formulation, and the variability that may exist in the manufacturing process and how these factors interact and impact the critical quality attributes (CQAs) of the finished drug product, is all part of the QbD design space. Unfortunately, there are many other sources of variability that may or may not impact a drug product's performance. They include the drug substance, excipients, process (equipment and unit operations), and how each of these factors interacts. Lastly, the variability in operators has to be considered as well.

Incorporating all of the sources of variability into a design space is no doubt challenging. If we look at excipients alone as a source of variability, there is a two-part question most important for the formulator. That is, does the variability existing in any of the critical material attributes (CMAs) of the excipient(s), have an impact on the critical quality attributes (CQAs) of my finished drug product, and if so, what are excipient manufacturers doing to minimize variability around those CMAs? Finding the answer to the first part of that question is the responsibility of the formulator. As for what excipient companies are doing to minimize variability, we need to look at this historically. As the pharmaceutical industry has evolved, so has the excipients industry, and many excipient manufacturers today are better tuned in to the needs of the pharmaceutical industry with the help of the International Pharmaceutical Excipients Council (IPEC). However, there are some suppliers of the excipients who do not track the variability of their products as they could. Excipients are used based on their functionality, and the aspects of their functionality, that is, CMAs are best evaluated in the context of each specific formulation and its resulting finished product performance, or CQAs. CMAs are formulation specific, that is, one attribute that may be critical in one formulation may have little impact in another. It is therefore difficult for the excipient manufacturers to know specifically which CMA is most important, and how much variability around that CMA is too much. The best approach an excipient manufacturer can choose is to

- understand the functionality and the most likely CMAs of their excipients;
- understand the sources of variability that impact their excipient CMAs (both in raw materials and manufacturing processes); and
- put control systems in place that minimize such variability.

It is up the formulator to come up with a robust formulation, that is, one in which sizeable variability in the excipients used have little or no impact on manufacturability or finished product performance. This is where QbD becomes part of the product development process. Struggling formulators should always feel free to seek the help of excipient manufacturers. Many excipient manufacturers are eager to work with their customers and provide support. They can help customers understand the complexities of manufacturing and control around variability and clear up miscommunications around the effects or understanding of chemical processing. One excipient manufacturer, when questioned about possible variability associated with an excipient,

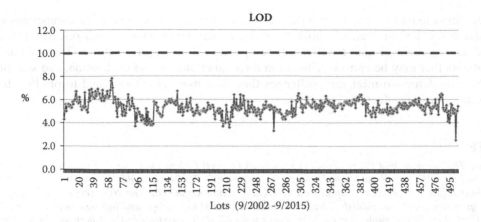

FIGURE 5.11 Historical variability around one specification (LOD) for a specific excipient as part of a data package provided to customers in support of QbD product development.
Source: JRS Pharma, LP.

successfully addresses the issue by providing (under a confidentiality disclosure agreement) an extensive QbD support presentation consisting of the following.

1. The raw material source for the excipient
2. Physical and chemical properties of the excipient
3. Typical use levels of the excipient
4. Scanning electron micrographs of the excipient
5. Manufacturing process flow diagram of the excipient
6. Manufacturing sites of the excipient
7. The molecular structure and chemistry around the manufacture of the excipient
8. The particle size distribution of the excipient
9. The functionality of the excipient
10. Current and past specifications of the excipient
11. Indication of which specifications may be considered as CMAs of the excipient
12. The historical variability around those CMAs presented in control chart format for several years representing a minimum of 40 lots of the excipient (an example is shown in Figure 5.11)
13. A historical data compilation supplied electronically to the customer to allow for their multivariate analysis or principle component analysis in support of a QbD submission.

The last point in the aforementioned list (#13) allows the formulator to study the variability around the specifications and specifically those specifications that may be CMAs for his product. Providing the raw data also allows the formulator to apply multivariate and principle component analysis techniques specifically in the context of their product in development. This has proved to be more helpful to formulators than merely providing samples of the excipient.

5.7 CONCLUSIONS

When considering excipients for any granulation process, formulators have a multitude of information available regarding the properties and functional behaviors of these ingredients. Understanding these characteristics will no doubt simplify the challenges of drug product development. The presence of other factors such as the processing used, the physical and chemical characteristics of the API, and the desired in-vivo performance of the finished drug product serve to underscore the fact that despite knowing these relatively few compounds well, the best outcomes are realized through careful experimentation and good science. The continued development of high-functionality, co-processed excipients is sure to bring about new ingredients that may be narrow or broad in their functionality and application, and will likely enable formulators to meet the challenges they face more effectively and to produce better performing drug products.

NOTE

1 *Note: The International Pharmaceutical Excipients Council Federation is pleased to announce that it has revised the IPEC Excipient Composition Guide (Version 2, 2020). The guide was originally published in 2009 and has been revised to update the references contained therein. The 2009 version of the Excipient Composition guide was published by IPEC-Americas and IPEC Europe and has now been converted into an IPEC Federation guide, representing inputs from all IPEC members in the Americas, China, Europe, India, and Japan.*

REFERENCES

1. S. Kothari, V. Kumar, G.S. Banker Comparative evaluations of powder and mechanical properties of low crystallinity celluloses, microcrystalline celluloses, and powdered celluloses. Iowa City, USA: College of Pharmacy, the University of Iowa, 24 January 2001.
2. High-Functionality Excipients: Silicified Microcrystalline Cellulose, Bob E. Sherwood, PhD, John W. Becker, PhD, Penwest Pharmaceuticals Co., now JRS Pharma.
3. T. Suzuki, H. Kikuchi, S. Yamamura, K. Terada, K. Yamamoto The change in characteristics of microcrystalline cellulose during wet granulation using a high-shear mixer. J Pharm Pharmacol 2001 May; 53(5): 609–16v.
4. Lactose, Some basic properties and characteristics, DFE Pharma. https://www.dfepharma.cn/Excipients/Certified-Knowledge/Knowledge-Base/Documentation/Technical-Documents/Technical-Papers.
5. O. Arndt, R. Baggio, A. Kira, J. Hartig, E. Francheschinis, P. Kleinbudde Impact of different dry and wet granulation techniques on granule and tablet properties: a comparative study. J Pharm Sci 2018; 107(12): 3143–3152.
6. Mannitol, PubChem, Yalkowsky, SH., Dannenfelser, RM (1992). https://pubchem.ncbi.nlm.nih.gov/compound/6251.
7. F. Ndindayino, D. Henrist, F. Kiekens, C. Vervaet, J.P. Remon Characterization and evaluation of isomalt performance in direct compression. Int J Pharm 1999; 189: 113–124.
8. J. Michaud Starch based excipients for pharmaceutical tablets. J Pharma Chem 2002; 42–44.
9. A New Class of High-Functionality Excipients: Silicified Microcrystalline Cellulose, Bob E. Sherwood, PhD, John W. Becker, PhD, Penwest Pharmaceuticals Co., now JRS Pharma.
10. R. Christian Moreton Functionality and performance of excipients in a quality-by-design world Part 2: Excipient variability, QbD and robust formulations excipients. Amer Pharm Rev 2009; 12(2). http://www.finnbrit.com/SubPages/Background/PDF%20Files/QbD%20APR_ExcipientSupplement%202010.pdf.

ADDITIONAL READING

• Comparison of Granules Produced by High-Shear and Fluidized-Bed Granulation Methods, Garett Morin, 1 and Lauren Briens, 1,2 Received 16 December 2013; accepted 24 April 2014; published online 17 May 2014, AAPS PharmSciTech, Vol. 15, No. 4, August 2014 (# 2014).
• A review of co-processed directly compressible excipients. J Pharm Pharmaceut Sci 8(1):76–93, 2005, M. C. Gohel Lallubhai Motilal College of Pharmacy, Navarangpura, Ahmedabad, India, Pranav D Jogani, USV Limited, B. S. D. Marg, Govandi, Mumbai,

India, Received 16 November 2004, Revised 28 January 2005, Accepted 31 January 2005, Published April 16, 2005.

- A review on co-processed excipients: current and future trend of excipient technology, Liew Kai Bin, Anand Gaurav, Uttam Kumar Mandal International Journal of Pharmacy and Pharmaceutical Sciences, Received: 21 Aug 2018 Revised and Accepted: 23 Nov 2018.
- An Evaluation of Tablet Binding Agents, Part I. Solution Binders, IAN KRYCER, DAVID G. POPE, Powder Technology, 34 (1983) 39 – 51, Department of Pharmacy. University of Sydney. Sydney. N.S.W., 2006 (Australia) and JOHN A. HERSEY*, Institute of Drug Technology Ltd., 391 Royal Parade. Pariwilie, ITic, 3052 (kstratia), (Received February 33,19SZ).
- Continuous twin screw extrusion for the wet granulation of Lactose, E.I. Keleb, A. Vermeire, C. Vervaet, J.P. Remon, International Journal of Pharmaceutics 239 (2002) 69–80, Laboratory of Pharmaceutical Technology, Faculty of Pharmaceutical Sciences, Ghent University, Harelbekestraat 72, B-9000 Ghent, Belgium, 24 September 2001.
- Co-processed excipients for direct compression of tablets, Čes. slov. Farm. 2018; 67, 175–181, Aleš Franc, David Vetchý, Pavlína Vodáčková, Roman Kubaľák, Lenka Jendryková, Roman Gončc, September 19, 2018.
- Co-Processed Excipients for Dispersible Tablets – Part 2: Patient Acceptability, Karolina Dziemidowicz, Felipe L. Lopez, Ben J. Bowles, Andrew J. Edwards, Terry B. Ernest, Mine Orlu,1 and Catherine Tuleu, AAPS PharmSciTech (# 2018).
- Coprocessed Excipients for Solid Dosage Forms, Satish K. Nachaegari and Arvind K. Bansal, Pharmaceutical Technology, January 2004.
- Effect of binder on the relationship between bulk density and compactibility of lactose granulations, K. Zuurman, G.K. Bolhuis, H. Vromans, International Journal of Pharmaceutics 119 (1995) 65–69, 4 July 1994.
- Effect of Crospovidone Particle Size on Tablet Properties Prepared via Wet Granulation, o Maschke (angelika.maschke@basf.com), F. Bang, K. Meyer-Böhm, and K. Kolter.
- BASF SE, R&D Project Management Excipients, 67056 Ludwigshafen, Germany.
- Effect of processing methods on xylitol-starch base co-processed adjuvant for orally disintegrating tablet application. Bin LK1, Helaluddin ABM2, Islam Sarker MZ2, Mandal UK3, Gaurav A4. Pakistan journal of pharmaceutical sciences March 2020, DOI: 10.36721/PJPS.2020.33.2.REG.551-559.1.
- Form conversion of anhydrous lactose during wet granulation and its effect on compactibility, Keyur R. Shah, Munir A. Hussain, Mario Hubert, Sherif I. Farag Badawy, International Journal of Pharmaceutics 357 (2008) 228–234, Bristol-Myers Squibb Research and Development, One Squibb Dr, 85/257, New Brunswick, NJ 08903, United States, November 21, 2007.
- Formulation of chlorpheniramine maleate tablets using co-processed excipient as a filler and binder, Yandi Syukri, Romdhonah, Anisa Nur Fazzri, Rio Fandi Sholehuddin, Aris Perdana Kusuma, Jurnal Farmasi Sains Dan Komunitas, May 2019, 29–35 Vol. 16 No. 1 p-ISSN 1693-5683; e-ISSN 2527-7146 doi: JURNAL FARMASI SAINS DAN KOMUNITAS, May 2019, 29–35 Vol. 16 No. 1, p-ISSN 1693-5683; e-ISSN 2527-7146, doi: http://dx.doi.org/10.24071/jpsc.001717. Department of Pharmacy, Islamic University of Indonesia, January 30, 2019.
- High shear mixer granulation using food grade binders with different thickening power, E. Franceschinis, A.C. Santomasob, A. Trotter, N. Realdona, Food Research International 64 (2014) 711–717.
- Introduction to tableting by wet granulation, DFE Pharma.
- Kollidon®, Polyvinyl pyrrolidone excipients for the pharmaceutical industry, Volker Buhler, BASF SE, Pharma ingredients and services, 67056 Ludwigshafen, Germany, 9th edition.
- Multifunctional coprocessed excipients for improved tabletting performance, Saha S1, Shahiwala AF., Expert Opinion on Drug Delivery March 2009 DOI: 10.1517/17425240802708978.

- Pharmaceutical applications of various natural gums, mucilages and their modified forms Vipul D. Prajapati, Girish K. Jani, Naresh G. Moradiya, Narayan P. Randeria, Carbohydrate Polymers, Volume 92, Issue 2, February 15, 2013, Pages 1685–1699.
- Pharmaceutical excipients – the continuing paradox(es) of pharmaceutical formulation science Richard Christian Moreton FinnBrit Consulting.
- Physicochemical comparison between microcrystalline cellulose and silicified microcrystalline cellulose, Michael J. Tobyn, Gerard P. McCarthy, John N. Staniforth, Stephen Edge, International Journal of Pharmaceutics 169 (1998) 183–194, Pharmaceutical Technology Research Group, Department of Pharmacy, University of Bath, Claverton Down, Bath, BA2 7AY, UK, 5 January 1998.
- Rheology, granule growth and granule strength: Application to the wet granulation of lactose–MCC mixtures, T.M. Chitu, D. Oulahna, M. Hemati, Powder Technology 208 (2011) 441–453.
- Roll compaction of granulated mannitol grades and the unprocessed crystalline delta-polymorph, Carl M.Wagner, Miriam Pein, Jörg Breitkreutz, Powder Technology 270 (2015) 470–475.
- Starch as a Pharmaceutical Excipient, Barmi Hartesi1, Sriwidodo, Marline Abdassah, Anis Yohana Chaerunisaa, Int. J. Pharm. Sci. Rev. Res., 41(2), November–December 2016; Article No. 14, Pages: 59-64 ISSN 0976-044X.
- Starch Source and Its Impact on Pharmaceutical Applications, Olobayo O. Kunle, IntechOpen, 2019.
- Strength and morphology of solid bridges in dry granules of pharmaceutical powders, D. Bikaa, G.I. Tardosb, S. Panmaia, L. Farbera, J. Michaelsa, Powder Technology 150 (2005) 104–116.
- Tableting functionality evaluation of Prosolv Easytab in comparison to physical mixtures of its individual components, A. Aljaberi1, A. Ardakani, A. Khdair1, S.A. Abdel-Rahim, E. Meqdadi, M. Ayyash, G.M. Alobaidi, N. Al-Zoubi, J. DRUG DEL. SCI. TECH., 23 (5) 499-504 2013.
- The effect of wet granulation on the physico-mechanical characteristics of microcrystalline cellulose, Meena Chatrath, Department of Pharmacy & Pharmacology, Doctoral Thesis, 1992.
- The improved compaction properties of mannitol after a moisture-induced polymorphic transition, Tomohiro Yoshinari, Robert T. Forbes, Peter York, Yoshiaki Kawashima, International Journal of Pharmaceutics 258 (2003) 121–131.
- Using spray-dried lactose monohydrate in wet granulation method for a low-dose oral formulation of a paliperidone derivative, Wan Huang, Yanan Shi, Chenhui Wang, Kongtong Yu, Fengying Sun, Youxin Li, Powder Technology 246 (2013) 379–394.
- Utilization of date syrup as a tablet binder, comparative study, Fars Kaed Alanazi, Saudi Pharmaceutical Journal (2010) 18, 81–89.
- Variability in the α and β anomer content of commercially available lactose, Mohamad Jamal Altamimia, Kim Wolffa, Ali Nokhodchic, Gary P. Martina, Paul G. Royalla, International Journal of Pharmaceutics 555 (2019) 237–249.

6 Spray Drying and Pharmaceutical Applications

Metin Çelik, Pavan Muttil, Gülşilan Binzet, and Susan C. Wendell

CONTENTS

6.1 INTRODUCTION

Spray drying is one of the oldest forms of drying and one of the fewest technologies available for the transforming of a liquid, slurry, or low-viscosity paste to a dry solid (free-flowing powder) in one-unit operation. The idea of spray drying, consisting of the transformation of feed from a fluid state into a dried particulate form by spraying the feed into a gaseous drying medium, has been expounded for a very long time. The first detailed description of the drying of products in spray form was mentioned in a patent of 1872 entitled "Improvement of Drying and Concentration Liquid Substances by Atomizing" [1]. The spray dryers of that time were primitive devices, and there were problems with the process efficiency, continuous process performance, and process safety, all of which stood in the way of the successful utilization of the spray drying process. However, this process found its first significant applications in the milk and detergent industries in the 1920s [2]. At that time, spray dryer devices underwent a degree of evolution that enabled their use in milk powder production. This was the first industrial application of the spray drying method,

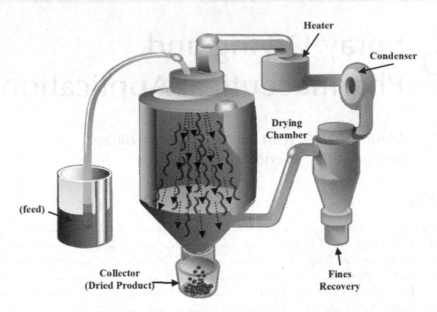

FIGURE 6.1 A schematic representation of a typical spray dryer with primary and secondary product separations.

and it remains one of the most important even today. The true boom in spray drying technology was driven by World War II, during which a necessity for the transport of huge amounts of food emerged, causing a search for new methods to reduce food's weight and volume, as well as a search for better conservation techniques. Spray drying proved to be the ideal technique for satisfying these requirements. During the postwar period, the application of the spray drying method was also directed toward the pharmaceutical industry. During the following years, the focus was transferred from the construction of spray dryer machines to the product characteristics. Almost 150 years of research into the spray drying method's principles has resulted in this method being a powerful technological tool and one of the most frequently used ways of drying [3].

In current times, spray drying is utilized extensively in many aspects of our daily life, from food products, cosmetics, and pharmaceuticals to chemicals, fabrics, and electronics. Typical pharmaceutical examples include spray dried enzymes (e.g., amylase, protease, lipase, and trypsin), antibiotics (e.g., sulfathiazole, streptomycin, penicillin, and tetracycline), and many other active pharmaceutical ingredients, vitamins (e.g., ascorbic acid and vitamin B12), and excipients for direct compression (e.g., lactose, mannitol, and microcrystalline cellulose). This method still presents a wide field for research and development for interested scientists. Recent books and review articles have reported the advances in spray drying technology and its applications [4–6].

A typical spray dryer is shown schematically in Figure 6.1.

6.1.1 Advantages and Limitation

There are several reasons why the technology of spray drying has found many applications in numerous industries. Advantages and challenges of this method for the production of pure drug particles and drug-loaded polymeric particles and the potential of this technique and the more advanced equipment to pave the way toward reproducible and scalable processes that are critical to the bench-to-bedside translation of innovative pharmaceutical products were discussed in a recent review [6,7].

The main advantages of spray drying with respect to other conventional methods can be summarized as follows:

Continuous process: It is a continuous process. As long as liquid feed can continue to be supplied to the drying system, the spray dried product will continue to be produced. In some instances, this process has been operated for months without interruption.

Speed and suitability of heat-sensitive APIs: The actual spray drying process is almost instantaneous as the major portion of the evaporation takes place in a short time as milliseconds or a few seconds, depending on the design of the equipment and process conditions. This makes spray drying well suited for heat-sensitive products with low risk of degradation.

Versatility: The process is versatile and adaptable to a wide range of industries and their feedstock and product specifications. Virtually any feedstock that can be pumped – solutions, suspensions, slurries, melts, pastes, and gels – can likewise be spray dried. It is possible to formulate nanocapsules with various encapsulating excipients. Also, open and closed cycle design allows the spray drying of aqueous and organic solvents.

Automation: The spray drying process can be fully automated as the process operates on basic principles and all of the associated process variables can be continuously and simultaneously monitored and recorded. Commercial-scale spray dryers are controlled by programmable logic controllers (PLCs) or solid-state controllers. These control systems monitor exhaust air temperature or humidity and provide an input signal that, by way of a set point, modulates the energy supplied to the process.

Particle characteristics: The physical properties of the resulting product (e.g., particle size and shape, degree of crystallinity, moisture content, and flow properties) and its overall quality can be controlled through the selection of equipment choices and the manipulation of process variables. Spray dried particles with unique morphology of predominantly spherical particles and with uniform size and hollow structure can be produced thus reducing the bulk density of the product. Also, this process allows the design of particles with controlled drug release properties. Being able to control physical properties makes the spray drying process desirable for industries like pharmaceuticals, where the optimum absorption of a drug depends greatly on particle size. The food industry puts a premium on moisture content, which determines a product's shelf life.

Cost-effectiveness: The initial installation cost of a spray drier could be high. However, because the operational requirements of small and large dryers are the same and it is a simple, one-step and easy to operate, easy to scale up process, the spray drying method is overall a highly cost-effective process. This makes spray drying a labor cost-effective process, especially for high-volume products. The actual spray drying process is almost instantaneous as the major portion of the evaporation takes place in as short time as milliseconds or a few seconds, depending on the design of the equipment and process conditions. This makes spray drying well suited for heat-sensitive products with low risk of degradation.

Miscellaneous:

- Corrosive and abrasive materials can be readily accommodated because the contact between the mechanical parts and materials is minimal as compared with other granulation processes.
- Spray dryers have few moving parts. In fact, careful selection of various components can result in a system having no moving parts in direct contact with the product.

Like all other granulation processes, spray drying has some limitations, as well:

Thermal efficiency: Spray drying process has poor thermal efficiency at lower inlet temperatures, and the exhaust air stream contains heat, which often requires sophisticated heat exchange equipment for removal. Because of the need to provide specific heat for evaporation in a short period of time, the energy consumption is high while a considerable amount of heat is lost with the exhaustion of air.

Capital and overhead cost: The installation cost of spray dryers could be very high because of the equipment required and its continuous operation. Main and auxiliary equipment are equally expensive, regardless of atomizer type and dryer capacity. Additionally, spray dryers that utilize two-fluid nozzles require compressed gas for atomizing. Without factoring in labor and maintenance costs, the high energy and pressure requirements already add greatly to the overhead costs.

Maintenance issues: Spray dryer maintenance mostly involves issues with the nozzle used. One-fluid and two-fluid nozzles are particularly prone to clogging and abrasion at the nozzle mouth. Rotary disc atomizers, due to the number of moving parts in direct contact with the powders, suffer from internal corrosion. Finally, issues with powders sticking to the internal chamber walls further contribute to cleaning costs and profit losses.

6.2 SPRAY DRYING PROCESS STAGES

The spray drying mechanism is based on moisture elimination using that a heated atmosphere to which the feed product is subjected. The process may be described by three major phases as shown schematically in Figure 6.2 [8], although some authors use four or five minor steps to describe it in

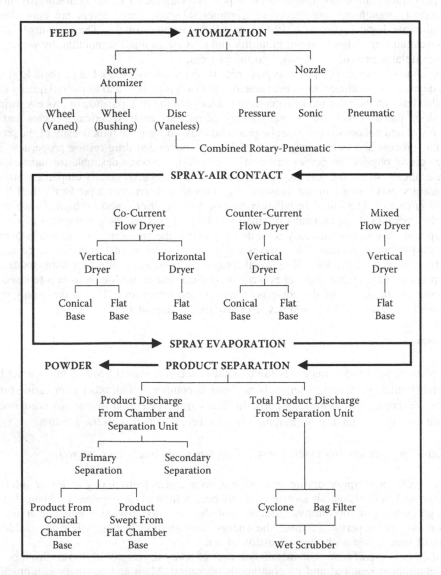

FIGURE 6.2   Schematic of spray drying process shown in stages: stage 1: atomization; stage II: spray air contact and evaporation; and stage III: product separation.
Source: From Ref. [8].

more detail [5]. The first stage is the atomization of a liquid feed into fine droplets. In the second stage, spray droplets mix with a heated gas stream, and the dried particles are produced by the evaporation of the liquid from the droplets. The final stage involves the separation of the dried powder from the gas stream and the collection of this powder in a chamber. The second stage (i.e., the mixing and drying step) has also been considered as separate steps [8]. The following section details each of these stages, their process parameters, and related equipment details.

6.2.1 ATOMIZATION

Atomization is the process by which a liquid feed is disintegrated into many fine droplets. The liquid feedstock is atomized into droplets by means of a nozzle or rotary atomizer. Nozzles use pressure or compressed gas to atomize the feed while rotary atomizers employ an atomizer wheel rotating at high speed. The breakup of the liquid feed into a large number of droplets reduces the internal resistance to moisture transfer from the droplet to the surrounding medium. This is because of the enormous increase in surface area of the bulk fluid as the liquid breaks up proceeds. Particle sizes are influenced by the liquid properties and choice of nozzles and atomizers as well as the feed rates. Typical particle distribution with different atomization systems under comparable conditions are given in Figure 6.3 [9] and for reference purpose, a diagrammatic representation of particle size and feed rate relation is shown in Figure 6.4 [10].

The formation of a spray with a high surface/mass ratio is highly critical for optimum liquid evaporation conditions and, consequently, the desired properties of the resulting product. Although ideally, the sizes of all droplets should be the same, in practical terms, the formation of droplets with a narrow size distribution would be satisfactory. A cubic meter of liquid forms approximately 2×10^{12} uniform 100 micron-sized droplets, offering a total surface area of over 60,000 m^2 [6].

This greater surface-to-volume ratio enables spray drying to achieve a faster drying rate (as drying time is proportional to the square of the particle dimension). Consequently, there is minimal loss of heat-sensitive compounds and, eventually, particles of the desired morphology and physical characteristics are obtained.

6.2.1.1 Atomizer Types and Designs

The formation of the atomized spray requires the application of a force. In the commercially available systems, the atomization process into droplet form may be accomplished by centrifugal energy, pressure energy, kinetic energy, ultrasonic energy, or electrostatic energy using specific devices called

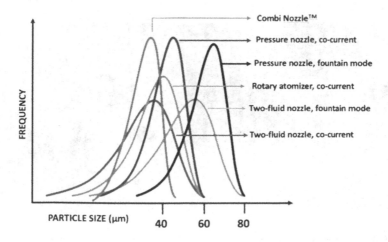

FIGURE 6.3 Typical particle distribution with different atomization systems under comparable conditions. *Source*: From Ref. [9].

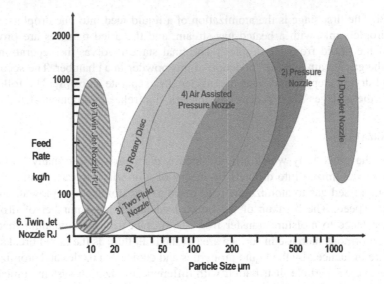

FIGURE 6.4 Range of particle sizes achievable by control of feed rate and the choice of nozzles and atomizers.
Source: From Ref. [10].

atomizers. There are different atomizers (Figure 6.5) that are used according to the desired product characteristics (shape, structure, and size) as well as depending on the nature of the feed solution. The most common devices used in the majority of atomization processes are explained ahead.

Centrifugal atomizers. Centrifugal atomizers utilize either a rotating disk or wheel to disintegrate the liquid stream into droplets [11]. Examples of rotary atomizers are shown in Figure 6.5. These devices form a low-pressure system, and a wide variety of spray characteristics can be obtained for a given product through combinations of feed rate, atomizer speed, and atomizer design. The droplet size distribution is fairly narrow for a given method and process conditions, but the mean droplet size can be varied from as small as 15 mm to as large as 250 mm, depending on the amount of energy transmitted to the liquid. Larger mean sizes require larger drying chamber diameters. Wheels are well suited for producing sprays in the fine- to medium-coarse size range while disks are used to produce coarse sprays.

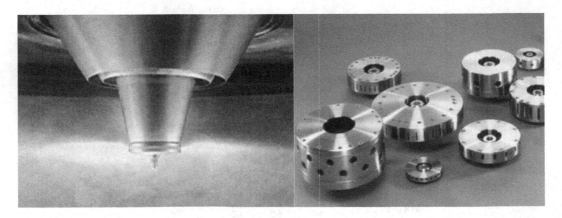

FIGURE 6.5 Common rotary atomizers.
Source: GEA pharma systems.

Rotary atomizers normally operate in the range of 5000 to 25,000 rpm with a wheel diameter of 5 to 50 cm. The mean size of the droplet produced is inversely proportional to the wheel speed and directly proportional to the feed rate and its viscosity. Solid content and surface tension are other factors having minor effects on the droplet size. For example, an increase in feed rate may slightly increase the particle size, but the use of a variable-speed drive on the centrifugal atomizer facilitates correction to the specified size.

Centrifugal atomizer designs include wheels with vanes or bushings and vaneless disks. Vaned atomizer wheels produce sprays of high homogeneity and are the most commonly used as compared with other designs. In this type of atomizer, liquid fed onto a wheel moves across the surface until contained by the rotating vane. The liquid flows outward under the influence of centrifugal force and spreads over the vane, wetting the vane surface as a thin film. At very low liquid vane loadings, the thin film can split into streams. No liquid slippage occurs on a wheel once the liquid has contacted the vanes. Whether radial or curved, the vanes prevent the transverse flow of liquid over the surface. Abrasive materials are best handled using atomizer wheels with bushings. Since the feed material is in direct contact with rotating parts, the bushings feature wear-resistant surfaces and require additional maintenance. Vaneless (disk) designs are often applied when coarse powders are required at high production rates.

Centrifugal atomizers have the advantage of handling large feed rates using single rotating wheels or disks and being suitable for abrasive feeds. Also, the clogging problem is minimized and particle size distribution can be controlled by changing the wheel rotary speed. Bulk pharmaceutical excipients and fine chemicals, such as antacids, are often produced using centrifugal atomizers. The particles produced by this technique are generally free-flowing and unless intentionally produced with very fine atomization, dust-free. The porous structure of the particles provides increased solubility, and the relatively low density and friability of these particles result in generally good compaction properties. Also, the batch-to-batch reproducibility and dryer-to-dryer transferability of this technique are excellent. The disentangles of centrifugal atomizers are their high cost, high energy consumption, and the requirement for a large drying chamber due to the broad spray pattern compared to pressure nozzles.

6.2.1.2 Droplet Formation Using Rotary Atomizer

During rotary atomization, a bulk liquid feed is accelerated to a high centrifugal velocity. During this acceleration, the liquid feed forms a thin film over the rotating surface. For smooth disk atomizers, the film or liquid feed disintegrates into droplets at the edge of the wheel by one of three mechanisms: (i) direct droplet formation, (ii) ligament formation, and (iii) sheet formation, respectively. The type of droplet formation mechanism that occurs during processing is a function of the surface tension and viscosity of the feed as well as the wheel speed and feed rate [11]. Direct droplet formation occurs at low wheel speeds when surface tension and viscosity dominate the atomization mechanism. The other variables that could potentially affect direct droplet formation are inertia and air friction. However, because of liquid slippage on the surface of the wheel, inertia is limited, and the low release velocities minimize air friction effects so that the effect of these variables is minimized at low wheel speeds. As wheel speeds and feed rates increase, the amount of feed-in each vane increases, giving rise to ligaments instead of droplets on the periphery of the wheel. These ligaments disintegrate into droplets with larger droplets forming from feeds with higher viscosity and higher surface tension. While the first two atomization mechanisms are partially controlled by the physical properties of the feed, sheet formation is a result of inertial forces becoming predominant over these properties. At high wheel speeds and feed rates, the ligaments join to form a liquid sheet that extends beyond the edge of the wheel. The liquid sheet disintegrates into a broad droplet distribution as it extends from this edge. To produce a narrow droplet distribution from this mechanism, high wheel speeds are combined with low wheel loading, which is often achieved with a decreased feed rate.

In contrast, a vaned wheel directs the flow of the liquid feed across the surface of an inner liquid distributor in which liquid slippage over the surface of the distributor occurs until there is contact with the vane or channel. The feed then flows outward because of centrifugal force and forms a thin film across the surface of the vane. As the liquid film leaves the edge of the vane, droplet formation occurs as a result of the radial and tangential velocities experienced. Atomizer wheel characteristics that influence droplet size include the speed of rotation, wheel diameter, and wheel design, for example, the number and geometry of the vanes.

Kinetic energy nozzles. Kinetic energy is applied in the form of two-fluid or pneumatic atomization. This is the most commonly used atomization technique within the pharmaceutical industry. Here, atomization is accomplished by the interaction of the liquid with a second fluid, usually compressed air. High air velocities are generated within the nozzle for effective feed contact, which breaks up the feed into a spray of fine droplets. Neither the liquid nor the air requires very high pressure, with 200 to 350 kPa being typical. Particle size is controlled by varying the ratio of the compressed air flow to that of the liquid. The main advantage of this type of atomization is that the liquid has a relatively low velocity as it exits the nozzle; therefore, the droplets require a shorter flight path for drying. Because many pharmaceutical applications use relatively small spray dryers, pneumatic nozzles are often used. Another advantage is the simple design that lends itself to easy cleaning, sterile operation, and minimal contamination. Pneumatic nozzles can be designed to meet the most stringent requirements for sterile or aseptic applications. Special consideration must be given to supplying a sterile source of compressed air for atomization. Kinetic energy nozzles are simple, compact, cheap, and have no moving parts. They can handle high viscosity feeds and can produce very small size particles. However, their energy consumption is high, and they have a low capacity feed rate. Also, they have a high tendency to be clogged.

There are various nozzle designs and nozzle sizes available to produce optimum conditions of liquid-air contact for atomization. Overall, it is reasonable to divide the two-fluid nozzles into the following categories [12]:

  i. Contacting of air and liquid within the nozzle head (internal mixing).
 ii. Contacting of air and liquid outside the nozzle head (external mixing).
iii. Contacting air and liquid at the rim of a rotating nozzle head (pneumatic cup atomizer).
 iv. The fourth type of nozzle combines internal and external mixing by using two air flows within the nozzle head. Such types of nozzles are commonly known as three-fluid nozzles.

As can be seen from the difference between a simple internal and external mixing nozzle shown schematically in Figure 6.6 [13], there is some overlap with respect to performance for the internal and the external mixing two-fluid nozzles, and the choice between the two types is often based on several things. All two-fluid nozzles have either limited gas flow rates, high specific gas consumption, modest liquid capacities, a wide droplet size distribution, or a combination of these limitations [14].

The external mixing nozzle has the liquid supply in the center and the atomizing gas supplied concentrically. Scaling this principle to larger liquid and gas flows shows typically an increasing gas-to-liquid rate for a given mean droplet diameter.

Internal mixing nozzles in general require less air than external mixing nozzles in order to produce droplets with the same mean droplet diameter. This is due to a higher energy transfer between the air and the liquid, as the atomization takes place under pressure difference inside the mixing chamber because the air and liquid pressures become equal first at the mixing chamber outlet. This is especially an advantage during nozzle scale-up where the increase in gas-to-liquid flow rate with scale is much less than for external mixing nozzles. The downside is, however, that over time, the impact surface becomes eroded and affects the spray droplet size pattern.

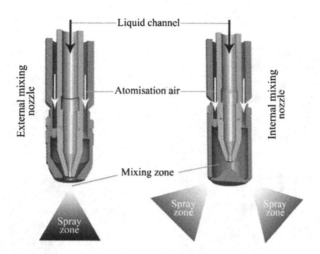

FIGURE 6.6 Schematic presentation of two-fluid nozzle designs. left: simple external mixing nozzle. right: simple internal mixing nozzle.
Source: From Ref. [13].

The lifetime of an internal mixing nozzle can be very short if the liquid has solid impurities in it. External mixing nozzles require more air, but the advantage is that it is possible to atomize a liquid that otherwise would have evaporated inside the mixing chamber of an internal mix nozzle [12].

The spray characteristics obtained by two-and three-fluid nozzles are similar when atomizing low-viscosity feeds at up to intermediate feed rates. The use of the second air stream with three-fluid nozzles causes a waste of energy, except for high feed rates of low-viscosity feeds.

The scheme of a commercially available spray drier with three-nozzle and scheme of droplet structures produced by 2-fluid and the 3-fluid nozzle is shown in Figure 6.7 [15].

6.2.1.3 Droplet Formation Using a Pneumatic Nozzle

Using a pneumatic nozzle, atomization is achieved by impacting the liquid feed with high-velocity air, which results in high frictional forces that cause the feed to disintegrate into droplets. To achieve optimal frictional conditions, this high relative velocity between liquid and air can be accomplished by either expanding the air to sonic velocities or destabilizing the thin liquid film by rotating it within the nozzle prior to spray air contact.

In general, two-fluid nozzles are capable of producing small droplet sizes over a wide range of feed rates. These droplets are then carried away from the nozzle by the momentum of the spray and the expanding atomizing air. The most important variable involved in the control of droplet size is the mass ratio of airflow to feed rate, which is also known as the air-to-feed ratio. An increase in this ratio causes a decrease in droplet size. This ratio generally ranges from 0.1 to 10. At ratios approaching 0.1, atomization is difficult even for low-viscosity feeds while a ratio of 10 approaches the limit above which atomization occurs using excess energy without an appreciable decrease in particle size [11].

Sprays formed by two-fluid nozzles are symmetrical with respect to the nozzle axis and have a cone-shaped pattern. The angle of this cone is called the spray angle, and, for two-fluid nozzles, it is narrow and cannot be varied greatly by adjusting the air-to-feed ratio. The maximum spray angle available is 708 to 808, which can be obtained by employing the maximum feed rate and airflow in a high-throughput nozzle. In general, an increase in air pressure will increase the spray angle if the feed rate is maintained at a constant level as long as the maximum angle has not been obtained. Spray angles are maintained if an increase in airflow is accompanied by an increase in feed rate, resulting in a similar air-to-feed ratio.

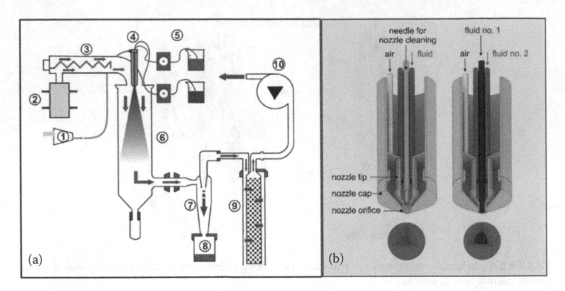

FIGURE 6.7 (a) Schematic diagram of spray drier buchi B-290 with 3-fluid nozzle (1 – compressor; 2 – inlet filter; 3 – heating coil; 4 – nozzle; 5 – stock solutions; 6 – drying chamber; 7 – cyclone; 8 – dry product; 9 – outlet filter; 10 – aspirator); (b) schematic diagram of droplet structures produced by 2-fluid (left) and 3-fluid (right) nozzle.
Source: From Ref. [15].

Pressure nozzles. The second most common form of atomization for pharmaceutical applications is hydraulic pressure nozzle atomization. Here the feed liquid is pressurized by a pump and forced through a nozzle orifice as a high-speed film that readily disintegrates into fine droplets. The feed is made to rotate within the nozzle, resulting in a cone-shaped spray pattern emerging from the nozzle orifice. Rotary motion within the nozzle can be achieved by the use of swirl inserts or spiral grooved inserts (Figure 6.8). The swirl inserts have comparatively larger flow passages and enable such nozzles to handle high-solid feeds without causing any wear or clogging.

Because the liquid spray exits the nozzle with a relatively high velocity, a spray drying chamber of at least 2.5 m in diameter and 3.0 m in cylinder height is usually required to operate with pressure nozzles.

The differential pressure across the orifice determines the mean droplet diameter. The distribution of the mean is similar to, but in most cases is narrower than, two-fluid atomization. In contrast, sprays from pressure nozzles handling high feed rates are generally less homogeneous and coarser than sprays from vaned wheels. At low feed rates, spray characteristics from nozzles and wheels are comparable. The mean size of the spray is directly proportional to the feed rate and inversely proportional to pressure.

Pressure nozzles are generally used to form coarse spray dried particles (120 to 300 mm mean particle size) with good flow properties. Antibiotics are a typical application for such a dryer.

Pressure nozzles are simple, compact, and cheap. They have no moving parts and their energy consumption is low. However, they have a low capacity feed rate for a single nozzle, their erosion can have an undesirable impact on spray characteristics, and they have a high tendency to be clogged.

Sonic energy atomizers. The use of sonic energy and vibrations for atomization in spray drying has found a growing interest in the past two decades. Ultrasonic atomization relies on an electromechanical device that vibrates at a very high frequency. Two piezoelectric disks, tightened between a mechanical amplifying element and a support element, constitute the electromechanical device of the ultrasonic atomizer (Figure 6.9).

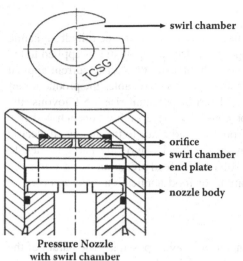

swirl chamber

orifice
swirl chamber
end plate

nozzle body

**Pressure Nozzle
with swirl chamber**

FIGURE 6.8 Schematic presentation of pressure nozzles.
Source: Courtesy of GEA Pharma Systems.

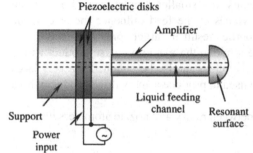

Piezoelectric disks

Amplifier

Liquid feeding
channel

Resonant
surface

Support

Power
input

FIGURE 6.9 Ultrasonic atomizer.
Source: [From Ref. 16]

Ultrasonic atomization is a two-stage process: first square waves develop on the liquid film surface, then, when resonance is reached, the amplitude growth causes droplet detachment from wave crests. An ultrasonic spray characteristic depends on resonant wave parameters (frequency) and liquid properties (surface tension, density). Liquid flow rate is not involved in this analysis and in fact recent studies showed that it will not affect droplet size [16]. But there is a maximum flow rate allowed above which no more droplet ejection occurs. This may be explained by the following reasoning: ultrasonic atomization relies on wave growth and crests breakup. When the liquid film depth increases damping becomes more and more important preventing wave growth and limiting the resonance amplitude [6,16].

The advantages of sonic nozzles operating at low pressure and having wide flow channels suggest they may be suitable for abrasive and corrosive materials, but it is most likely that sonic nozzles will continue to be developed as atomizers for special applications, such as very fine sprays of mean size 20 mm, where the nature of the spray angle and cone minimizes droplet coalescence [17]. However, ultrasonic atomization technology is effective only for low-viscosity Newtonian fluids. Since reduced pressure acts as the driving force for moisture evaporation from the atomized droplets, the use of the ultrasonic spray head demands large quantities of hot air. Nevertheless, the use of a sterile and hot drying medium would render this method appropriate for aseptic manufacturing of spray dried particles [18].

6.2.2 ELECTROHYDRODYNAMIC ATOMIZERS

A recent technique for atomizing the feed liquid is the use of electrospray or electrohydrodynamic sprays created by electrostatic charging. In the electrospray, an electrical potential is applied to the needle to introduce free charge at the liquid surface. The high intensity of electric current applied between the two oppositely charged electrodes of an electrospray system enables the production of droplets of narrow particle size distribution. When the electrical potential rises to kilovolts, the liquid meniscus develops into a conical shape (Taylor cone), having a highly concentrated free charge. The free charge accelerates the droplets away from the needle due to the generated electric stress. Monodispersed particles will be formed when the jet breaks into fine particles due to varicose instabilities (Figure 6.10). The requirement of solvents for feed preparation and extremely low flow rates limit the usage of electrospray atomization for food applications and commercial exploitation, respectively [6].

6.2.2.1 Atomizer Selection

The function of any atomizer is to produce as homogeneous a spray as possible. The nature of the feed, the characteristics of the spray, and the desired properties of the resulting dried product play very important roles in the selection of the atomizer type. With proper design and operation, nozzles and rotary atomizers can produce sprays having similar droplet size distribution. In all atomizer types, the size of droplets can be altered by either increasing or decreasing the atomization energy (e.g., increased atomization energy results in a smaller droplet size). For a given amount of energy, the viscosity and surface tension values of the feed influence the size of the droplet (e.g., higher values of these feed fluidity properties result in larger spray droplets).

In general, rotary atomizers are utilized to produce a fine to the medium-coarse product with a mean size of 20–150 μm, although larger spray dried particles can also be obtained if a very large drying chamber is used. Pressure nozzle atomizers are used to produce a spray dried product with a coarse mean particle size of 150–300 μm [20].

For a given spray drying application, the selection between rotary and nozzle atomizers involves the following considerations [6,21].

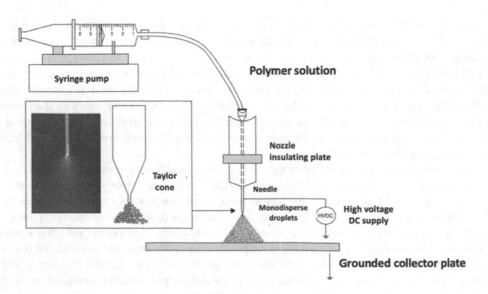

FIGURE 6.10 Mechanism of electro-spraying.
Source: From Refs. [6,19].

a. Energy utilized for atomization
b. Feed capacity range of the atomizer for which complete atomization is attained
c. Physical properties of the feed that can be handled by the atomizer
d. Atomization efficiency
e. Droplet size distribution at identical feed rates
 f. Relationship between the mean size of droplets and atomization parameters
g. Required final size range of droplets
h. Spray homogeneity
 i. Operational flexibility
 j. Suitability of dryer chamber design for atomizer operation
k. Atomizer experience available for the product in question

Comparison of conventional atomizers based on the aforementioned considerations is summarized in Table 6.1.

6.2.3 SPRAY AIR CONTACT AND EVAPORATION

Once the liquid is atomized, it must be brought into intimate contact with the heated gas for evaporation to take place equally from the surface of all droplets. This contacting step takes place within a vessel called the drying chamber. The heated gas is introduced into the chamber by an air dispenser, which ensures that the gas flows equally to all parts of the chamber.

6.2.3.1 Spray Air Contact

How spray contacts the drying air is a critical factor in spray drying operations. Spray air contact is determined by the position of the atomizer in relation to the air inlet.

Inlet air is introduced to the drying chamber via an air disperser, which uses perforated plates, or vaned channels through which the gas is equalized in all directions. It is critical that the air entering the disperser is well mixed and has no temperature gradient across the duct leading into it; otherwise, the drying will not be even within the chamber. The air disperser is normally built into the roof of the drying chamber and the atomization device is placed in or adjacent to the air disperser. Thus, instant and complete mixing of the heated drying gas with the atomized clouds of droplets can be achieved.

Spray droplet movement is classified according to the dryer chamber layout and can be designated as cocurrent, countercurrent, or mixed flow, although this designation is not a true representation of actual conditions.

1. Cocurrent flow is the configuration in which the spray and drying air pass through the dryer in the same direction. This arrangement is widely used and is ideal for heat-sensitive products. Spray evaporation is rapid, the drying air cools accordingly, and overall evaporation times are short. The particles are not subject to heat degradation. In fact, low-temperature conditions are achieved throughout the entire chamber despite very hot air entering the chamber.
2. Countercurrent flow is the configuration in which the spray and air enter at the opposite ends of the dryer. This arrangement has excellent heat utilization. Countercurrent flow is used with nozzle atomization and is well suited for meeting the final spray dried properties of non-heat-sensitive materials.
3. Mixed flow is the configuration in which both co-and counter-current flows are incorporated. The advantage of this type of arrangement is that coarse free-flowing products can be produced in relatively small drying chambers. In mixed-flow systems, the powder is subjected to higher particle temperature. A mixed-flow system can be integrated with a fluid-bed drying chamber when lower particle temperatures are necessary.

TABLE 6.1

Conventional Atomizers Used in Spray Drying (Refs. 6,20,22–24)

	Rotary Atomizer	Pressure Nozzle Atomizer	Pneumatic Nozzle Atomizer
Method of atomization	Motor	Pressurizing pump	Compressed gas
Atomization energy	Centrifugal, low	Pressure, low	Kinetic, high
Atomization uniformity	Even	Slightly uneven	Uneven
Atomization parameters	Disc speed 10,000–30,000 rotations per minute (rpm)	Nozzle pressure 250–10,000 PSI	Nozzle pressure 250–10,000 PSI
Process liquid capacity per nozzle	High	Medium	Low
Mean droplet particle diameter	Fine, medium, coarse (6)	Coarse, less homogeneous (6)	Medium coarseness, poor homogeneity (6)
	Coarse	Coarse	Fine
	Medium-coarse (20).	Coarse (20).	
	30–120 µm (6)	120–250 µm (6)	30–150 µm (6)
	10–200 µm [22]	30–350 µm [22]	5–100 µm [22]
		20–600 µm [23]	10–200 µm [23]
	10 – 100 µm [24]	0 – 150 µm [24]	5 – 30 µm [24]
	20–150 µm [20]	150–300 µm [20]	
The relation between droplet diameter and the feed solution properties	Droplet diameter is inversely proportional to disc speed and diameter. Droplet diameter is inversely proportional to disc speed and diameter.		
Spray angle	180°	Under 60°	Under 30°
Spray shape	Hollow cone	Full cone fine	Hollow cone fine
The relation between droplet diameter and atomization	Droplet diameter is inversely proportional to disc speed and diameter	Droplet diameter is inversely proportional to atomization pressure	Droplet diameter is inversely proportional to atomization pressure
Advantages	Handle high feed rates without clogging; formation of uniform size particles; low-pressure operation; high efficiency	Low price; formation of particles with little occluded air (i.e., particle production of higher density); enables the use of narrow drying chambers	Better control over particle size than in the hydraulic nozzle; useful for feeds of high viscosity; ideal to laboratory-scale since it requires a small drying chamber; good efficiency
Drawbacks	High price; not suitable to viscous feed; Inability to use a horizontal and small spray dryer chamber	Not suitable to high viscous feed; high feed rates cause coarse and less homogeneous sprays (i.e., broad particle size distribution)	High operation costs due to the need for high amounts of compressed gas for atomization; production of particles with high occluded air; downstream turbulence

The spray air contact design can be selected according to the required particle size and the temperature to which the dried particle can be subjected. For example, if a low product temperature is maintained at all times, a cocurrent rotary atomizer is selected for producing fine particles while a countercurrent pressure atomizer is preferred for obtaining coarser particles. If coarse particles with predetermined porosity and bulk density properties are desired, a countercurrent pressure nozzle atomizer is well suited as high product temperature can be maintained for obtaining the desired porosity and bulk density of the resulting product. For obtaining coarse spray dried particles of heat-sensitive materials, a mixed-flow nozzle system can be selected. Integration with a fluid bed is recommended for agglomerated or granulated powders.

6.2.3.2 Drying

The largest and most obvious part of a spray drying system is the drying chamber. This vessel can be tall and slender or have a large diameter with a short cylinder height. Selecting these dimensions is based on two-process criteria that must be met. First, the vessel must be of adequate volume to provide enough contact time between the atomized cloud and the heated gas. This volume is calculated by determining the mass of air required for evaporation and multiplying it by the gas residence time, which testing or experience dictates.

The second criterion is that all droplets must be sufficiently dried before they contact a surface. This is where the vessel shape comes into play. Centrifugal atomizers require larger diameters and shorter cylinder heights. In contrast, nozzle atomizer systems must have narrower and taller drying chambers. Most spray dryer manufacturers can estimate, for a given powder's mean particle size, what dimensions are needed to prevent wet deposits on the drying chamber walls.

6.2.3.3 Drying Gas

In pharmaceutical applications of spray drying, the feedstock can be prepared by suspending or dissolving the product to be spray dried in water. However, the utilization of a wide variety of organic solvents in feedstock preparations is also common. Alcohols, such as ethanol, methanol, and isopropanol, are preferred organic solvents in spray drying of pharmaceuticals, although other organic solvents such as ketones are also used in other industries; often the synthesis process upstream from the drying step determines the solvent selection. The drying characteristics of the solvents are also important. For example, a solvent with a low boiling point may be the only choice for heat-sensitive materials.

Although evaporating organic solvents by a spray drying process is very efficient because of the resulting shorter residence time, as compared with the evaporation of water, the risk of the explosion makes the use of these solvents very hazardous. Therefore, an inert gas, usually nitrogen, instead of air must be used as drying gas for the evaporation of the solvents. The use of inert gas requires the use of a closed-cycle system for spray drying to recover the solvent and to limit the gas usage. However, for small drying tests and laboratory work, the nitrogen can be used without recirculation, using a carbon bed on the exhaust gas to collect the solvent.

6.2.4 Dried Powder Separation

Powder separation from the drying air follows the drying stage. In almost every case, spray drying chambers have cone bottoms to facilitate the collection of the dried powder.

Two systems are utilized to collect the dried product. In the first type of system, when coarse powders are to be collected, they are usually discharged directly from the bottom of the cone through a suitable airlock, such as a rotary valve. The gas stream, now cool and containing all of the evaporated moisture, is drawn from the center of the cone above the cone bottom and discharged through a side outlet. In effect, the chamber bottom is acting as a cyclone separator. Because of the relatively low efficiency of collection, some fines are always carried with the gas stream. These must be separated in high-efficiency cyclones followed by a wet scrubber or in a fabric filter (bag collector). Fines collected in the dry state (bag collector) are often added to the larger powder stream or recycled. When very fine powders are being produced, the side outlet is often eliminated and the dried product together with the exhaust gas is transported from the chamber through a gooseneck at the bottom of the cone. The higher loading of entrained powder affects cyclone design but has little or no effect on the bag collector size.

In the second type of system, the total recovery of dried products takes place in the separation equipment. This type of system does not need a product-conveying system; therefore, the separation efficiency of the equipment becomes very critical. Separation of dried product from air influences powder properties by the mechanical handling involved during the separation stage. Excessive mechanical handling can produce powders with a high percentage of fines.

6.3 PROCESS LAYOUTS

The most widely used spray drying process layout is an open-cycle layout in which the air is drawn from the atmosphere, passed through the drying chamber, and exhausted back to the atmosphere. This layout is used for aqueous feedstock and employs air as the drying gas. There are numerous variations of open-cycle layout systems. The most common and cost-effective layout utilizes a high-efficiency cyclone and scrubber. In this layout, the loss of very fine particles to the atmosphere cannot be prevented. If the desired particle size of the spray dried product is too small to be recovered by cyclone and scrubber systems, then the use of a layout employing a bag filter is recommended.

Closed-cycle layouts are mainly used for nonaqueous (i.e., organic solvents) feedstock and generally require the use of inert gas as the drying medium. This type of spray dryer is operating in gaseous nitrogen as an inert medium circulating in a closed cycle within all the equipment. As the feed medium from the feed pump is atomized by the rotary atomizer or a nozzle that forms a fine droplet of liquid particles, further heat from the heater vaporizes the liquid droplets to vapor phase and the product is left as powder form in the cyclone separator. The drying process can be adjusted by the temperature controller of the heater. The evaporation of the solvent is to be recovered through the condensation unit. The success of closed-cycle spray drying washing and cooling operation requirements will be part of accurate temperature control. For a high boiling point of alcohol generally cooling water or saltwater is employed, whereas for the low boiling point solvents, such as dichloromethane, hexane, and acetone, the refrigeration cycle is incorporated in the design [25].

The advantages of closed-cycle spray dryers can be summarized as follows:

i. Prevent the products from oxidization and improve the quality of products.
ii. Provide dust free and aseptic operation.
iii. Recover solvent in the material liquid.
iv. Improve the preservation of fragrant composition.
v. Capable to dry flammable material liquid or do the cooling granulation.
vi. Capable to dry the material with strong heat sensitivity.
vii. Avoid public hazards.
viii. Capable of low-temperature application below $100°C$.

In addition to open-and closed-cycle systems, there are semi closed-cycle layouts that are not strict in terms of the type of drying medium and are operated under slight vacuum conditions.

Typical layout of the open-cycle, closed-cycle, and semi-closed-cycle spray dryers are shown schematically in Figures 6.11–6.13, respectively.

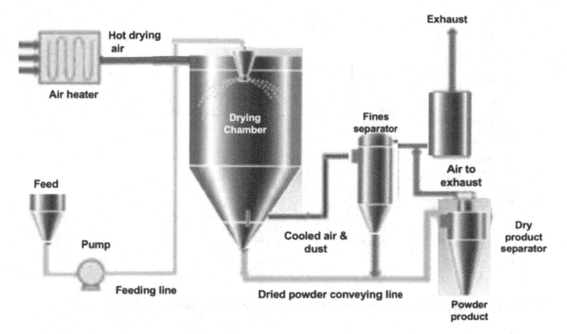

FIGURE 6.11 Typical layout of the open-cycle spray dryer systems.

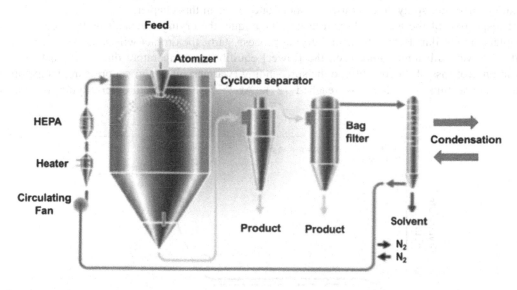

FIGURE 6.12 Typical layout of the closed-cycle spray dryer systems.

6.4 THEORY OF SPRAY DRYING FUNDAMENTALS

6.4.1 DROPLET DRYING MECHANISMS

Evaporation of water from a spray is often characterized using a curve that describes the change in drying rate as a function of time. This drying rate curve or evaporation history is a function of temperature, humidity, and the transport properties of the droplet formulation, as well as the air surrounding the droplet. The general drying rate curve has three main phases: an initial drying

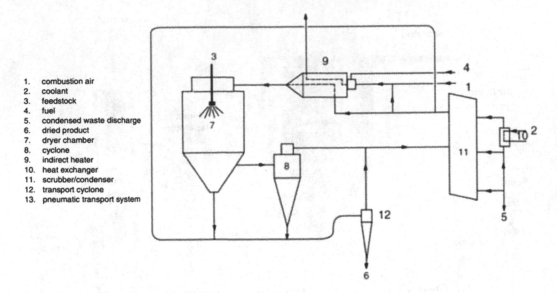

1. combustion air
2. coolant
3. feedstock
4. fuel
5. condensed waste discharge
6. dried product
7. dryer chamber
8. cyclone
9. indirect heater
10. heat exchanger
11. scrubber/condenser
12. transport cyclone
13. pneumatic transport system

FIGURE 6.13 Typical layout of the semi closed-cycle spray dryer systems.

phase, a phase in which the rate of drying is mainly constant, and a final phase during which the rate of drying decreases (falling-rate phase) [26]. A schematic diagram of the general droplet drying process is depicted in Figure 6.14. It must be noted that the drying curve would be different if an electrostatic spray dryer is used as mentioned later in this chapter.

Irrespective of the applied droplet drying technique, the drying mechanisms for free solution droplets are similar. Before the actual drying process starts, the droplet will be heated (or cooled) until the wet-bulb temperature (i.e., the [lower] equilibrium temperature due to a constant evaporation heat loss of the solvent into the surrounding (warmer) air at a given pressure, temperature and relative humidity [RH]) is reached [27]. At this phase, the droplet drying is mainly

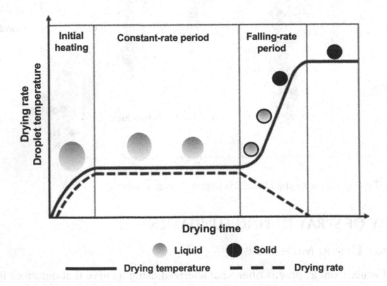

FIGURE 6.14 Schematic diagram of the different stages of droplet experiences during the drying rate process.
Source: From Ref. [27].

characterized by the solvent, similar to the evaporation of a pure solvent droplet. The driving force for solvent evaporation is the difference between the vapor pressure of the solvent and its partial pressure in the surrounding environment. However, the drying rate (generally expressed in kg/m^{2}s) is limited and controlled by the energy required for solvent evaporation and thus by the heat transport toward the surface of the droplet. After heating of the droplet to the wet-bulb temperature, drying will start from the surface of the droplet. As drying continues, solvent molecules will keep migrating from the center toward the surface. The migration of the solvent molecules can be mediated through molecular diffusion relative to the solute, convection of fluid within the droplet, or capillary solvent flow through a solid porous matrix. At this stage, drying that is analogous to free solvent evaporation results in droplet shrinkage. If the ambient parameters remain unchanged, the droplet temperature remains equal to the wet-bulb temperature and the drying rate is constant and only controlled by the heat transfer toward the surface of the droplet. For this reason, this stage is named the constant-rate drying stage [27]. This stage is followed by a falling-rate period, which is defined by the solutes present in the droplet. As solvent evaporation takes place from the surface of the droplet, the solute concentration at the surface increases and the growing concentration gradient causes a diffusional solute flux away from the droplet surface toward the center of the droplet. The diffusional motion of the dissolved components is a complex phenomenon that needs to be understood correctly to explain the final distribution of the different substances. Eventually, the diffusional motion of the solutes toward the center of the droplet becomes lower than the reduction rate of the droplet diameter due to the constant rate of solvent loss. At this point, crust formation will occur due to solute enrichment at the droplet surface, leading to decreased drying rate and introducing the second drying stage. This point is referred to as the critical point or locking point. At the start of this stage, a porous solid crust and an internal wet core can be distinguished in the drying droplet. The drying rate is now controlled by the diffusion or capillary flow rate of the solvent from the wet core through (the pores of) the crust. The slowed solvent evaporation still results in shrinkage of the wet core and substantial growth of the crust toward the center of the droplet. The thickening of the crust will lead to an increasing resistance for mass transfer and thereby a gradual reduction of the drying rate. Hence, this second stage is named the falling-rate stage of drying. During this stage, the droplet's surface dries and its surface temperature increases until the dry-bulb temperature (i.e., the temperature of the surrounding gas) is reached and a non-evaporating solid sphere is developed. This implies that a particle with the lowest possible amount of residual solvent is present, which can either be an equilibrium amount, or residual solvent that cannot be removed by the drying process. In some cases, a clear subdivision of the falling-rate period based on the degree of drying rate decrease can be observed: a first stage, where unsaturated surface drying occurs, and a second stage, where the diffusion of fluid from the center of the droplet toward the surface is the rate-limiting factor. Hence, the drying rate over time in the falling-rate period can take on different shapes depending on the system and the drying conditions [27].

While the general evaporation history is representative of the processes occurring during spray drying, the actual rate of moisture migration is affected by several factors including the temperature of the surrounding air. If the inlet temperature is so high that the evaporation rate is higher than the moisture migration rate needed to maintain surface wetness, then the constant rate drying phase is very short. This is because a dried layer forms instantaneously at the droplet surface that acts as a barrier to additional moisture transfer and retains moisture within the droplet causing the surface temperature to be much higher. In contrast, lower inlet temperatures yield a lower initial drying rate with a surface temperature equal to wet bulb temperature for a longer period of time.

It is important to note that the drying curve is the only representative. In reality, there are no defined points during an evaporation history. Some phases may not even occur or will be very short depending on the process conditions. One example of this is a spray drying process for a heat-sensitive material where the inlet temperature is low. In this case, the initial phase may extend until a critical point where moisture migration becomes rate limiting, effectively eliminating the constant rate drying period. In reality, the actual evaporation rate is dependent on several factors, including the droplet shape, composition, physical structure, and solid concentration. The actual drying time is a sum of the constant-rate period and the falling-rate period until the desired moisture content is achieved.

6.4.2 Effect of Formulation on Droplet Drying Mechanisms

Droplet composition also plays a significant role in droplet evaporation history. Typically, sprays are differentiated into three main types: pure liquids feeds containing undissolved solids and feeds containing dissolved solids [28].

6.4.2.1 Pure Liquid Sprays

For sprays comprising pure liquids, the droplet evaporates away completely. While this type of spray is not useful for pharmaceutical formulations, its behavior is representative of very dilute feed materials. The evaporation of pure liquids is dependent upon the dryer configuration. For low-velocity sprays in a low-velocity air stream (countercurrent dryer) or for low-velocity sprays in a high-velocity air stream (cocurrent dryer), the evaporation of the pure liquid spray causes the air temperature and evaporation rate to decrease. Pure liquid sprays having a wide droplet distribution evaporate more quickly than narrow distributions having the same mean droplet size because of the smaller droplets in the wide distribution. In addition, the size distribution of the droplet changes during evaporation. If the initial spray is homogeneous or there is a very narrow distribution, the mean droplet diameter decreases during evaporation. In contrast, if the initial spray is non-homogeneous or has a wide distribution, then the mean droplet diameter initially increases prior to decreasing. In general, a distribution is the best representation of a spray since the mean of this distribution may not adequately describe all characteristics of the distribution. For dryer configurations of high relative velocities such as coarse atomization in cocurrent or fountain-type dryers, the droplets travel farther before a given fraction is evaporated. The relative velocity between droplet and drying air affects evaporation rates more significantly at higher velocities and higher drying temperatures.

6.4.2.2 Feeds Containing Insoluble Solids

For droplets containing insoluble solids, the droplet temperature is equal to the wet-bulb temperature of the pure liquid droplet during the constant-rate phase since insoluble solids have negligible vapor pressure lowering effects. The total drying is the sum of the two drying periods. The drying time for the first period is short compared with the falling-rate period. The falling-rate period depends on the nature of the solid phase and can be estimated given the specific gravity of the feed slurry, the density of the dried product, and the thermal conductivity of the gaseous film around the droplet, where gaseous film temperature is the average between the exhaust temperature and droplet surface temperature. The droplet surface temperature is equal to the adiabatic saturation temperature of the suspension spray.

6.4.2.3 Feeds Containing Dissolved Solids

Droplets containing dissolved solids have lower evaporation rates than pure liquid droplets of equal size. The dissolved solids decrease the vapor pressure of the liquid, thus reducing the driving forces for mass transfer. Drying results in the formation of a solid crust on the droplet surface, which does not occur for pure liquid droplets. Vapor pressure lowering causes droplet temperature to increase over wet bulb temperature from the previous two examples. The formation of dried solid during evaporation has a significant effect on the subsequent evaporation history. During evaporation, spray air contact and constant-rate period occur but may be shorter. The main effect of dissolved solids is seen when the first period of drying ends and droplet moisture content falls to a critical value representing the formation of the solid phase on the surface. During the falling-rate

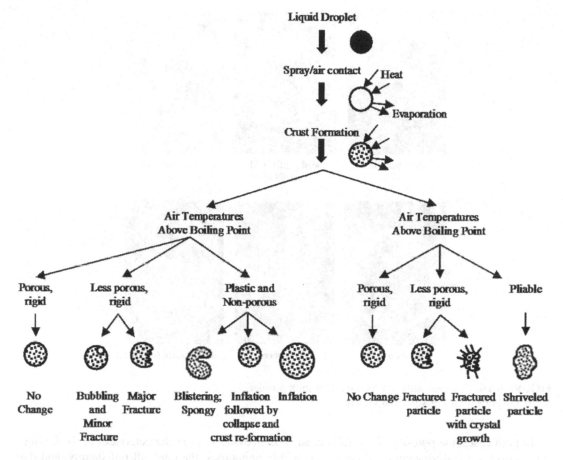

FIGURE 6.15 Potential spray dried particle morphologies about process conditions and material characteristics.
Source: From Ref. [29].

period, the migration of moisture decreases because of the resistance to mass transfer caused by an increasing solid phase. Lastly, the heat transfer is greater than the mass transfer, and the droplet temperature increases. Vaporization of the moisture within the droplet during this phase may occur if the transfer is sufficiently high.

The relationship between mass transfer and heat transfer for droplets containing dissolved solids can lead to the formation of many different particle morphologies depending on process conditions and material characteristics. Charlesworth and Marshall [29] have defined these morphologies as falling into two groups dependent on the temperature of the drying air relative to the boiling point of the droplet solution during the majority of the evaporation period (Figure 6.15).

If the air temperature exceeds the boiling point of the droplet solution, then vapor is formed. As the solid crust forms around each droplet, vapor pressure within the droplet is formed and the resultant effect of this pressure is dependent on the nature of the crust. A porous crust will release the vapor, but a nonporous crust may rupture resulting in fractured particles or fines from disintegrated particles.

Alternately, the droplet temperature may not reach boiling point levels because of cocurrent airflow or because the residence time of droplets in the hottest regions of the dryer is often very short. In this case, moisture migration occurs through diffusion and capillary mechanisms.

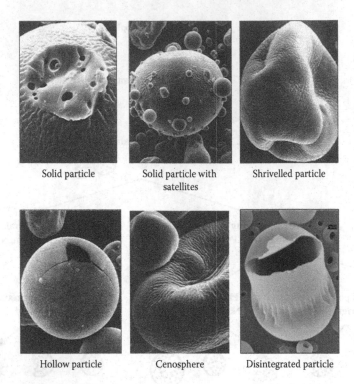

Solid particle	Solid particle with satellites	Shrivelled particle
Hollow particle	Cenosphere	Disintegrated particle

FIGURE 6.16   Various particle forms of skim milk powder.
Source: Courtesy of GEA pharma systems.

In both cases, the porosity of the solid crust is often evident in the characteristics of the falling-rate period of the drying curve. If the film is highly nonporous, the rate will fall sharply, and the evaporation time will be prolonged. However, if a highly porous film exists, then the vapor is easily removed from the droplet-air interface and the drying rate is similar to that found during the first period of drying.

These drying mechanisms result in a range of particle shapes including solid, hollow, shriveled, and disintegrated, examples of which are shown in Figure 6.16. However, it is important to note that particle morphology is also dependent on several material characteristics including solubility, the temperature of crystallization, melting point, and thermal conductivity since they will also impact the rate of crust formation, the porosity of the crust, and the subsequent drying rate.

It is also possible to influence particle density and size distribution through the modification of process parameter settings, such as atomizer settings, temperature levels, and feed rates [30]. For example, an increased feed rate while maintaining a constant inlet temperature results in particles that have higher moisture content and a resultant increased bulk density. By increasing the temperature of the feedstock, the ability of the feed to be atomized is often improved because of the reduction in ligament formation causing an increase in the bulk density of the dried particles. Also, an increase in the concentration of the feed solids often increases the bulk density of the dried particle as does the use of a rotary atomizer since many wheel designs reduce air entrapment. Alternatively, bulk density may be decreased through feed aeration or an increase in inlet temperature. Also, cocurrent spray air contact is often effective for a reduction in bulk density because the wettest droplets encounter the hottest air facilitating rapid evaporation and air entrapment. It is important to note that the outlined process modifications are generally applicable, but that exceptions to each can be found based on material characteristics.

Similarly, it is often possible to influence spray dried particle size distribution by changing process parameter settings. As mentioned earlier, the size of the droplets formed during atomization is affected by process parameters such as atomization type, atomizer settings, feed solids concentration, feed physical properties, and drying temperatures. The size of the resultant particles following evaporation is a function of the initial droplet size as well as the material characteristics such as solid-state and film formation mechanisms.

The research on the properties of droplet continues. In a recent study, the surface stickiness of droplets, subjected to a spray drying environment, to their surface layer and powder recovery in spray dryers was investigated. A model was proposed by introducing a dimensionless time as an indicator of spray drying ability and correlating this time parameter with the recovery of powders in practical spray drying. Droplets with initial diameters of 120 mm were subjected to simulated spray drying conditions, and their safe drying regime and dimensionless time values were generated. The model predicted the recovery in a pilot-scale spray dryer reasonably well [31].

6.4.2.4 Spray Drying Parameters

The final properties of the dried products are directly influenced by such equipment parameters as the atomization devices, the drying chamber configuration, and the collector type choice. Additionally, a variety of feedstock specificities and process parameters also play a crucial role in the final particle characteristics, resulting in different sized morphologies, or residual moisture content. It is thus fundamental to realize how these variables influence the spray drying mechanism in order to achieve an optimized operation [5].

Atomization pressure: The atomization stage is carried under pressure, namely when nozzle atomizers are used. The pressure involved during this process has an impact on droplet size. For a given atomizer device and feed solution, droplet size decreases with increasing pressure. In the case of rotary atomizers, droplet size exhibits an inverse relationship with wheel rotation speed and wheel diameter [3,6].

Feed flow rate: The feedstock solution is pumped into the atomizer at a controllable rate. Keeping the atomization pressure constant, there is an increase in the droplet size with increasing feed flow rates. This is easily understandable bearing in mind that the nozzle would have the same energy amount to spend in the atomization process of higher feeding volumes. Thus, the droplet fissions are minimized, provoking a small reduction of its size [6].

Feed viscosity: When feed viscosity is increased, a great percentage of atomization energy supplied to the nozzle is used to overcome the large viscous forces of the solution. Hence, a small amount of energy is left for the droplet fission, resulting in larger droplet sizes [6].

Feed surface tension: Atomization occurs due to the disruption of the feed surface tension. This means that a feedstock solution with higher surface tension hinders the atomization process. In that sense, before starting the spray drying process, feedstocks are usually emulsified and homogenized in order to reduce their surface tension [6].

Inlet temperature: The inlet temperature refers to the heated drying gas temperature and it is measured in front of the drying air entry into the drying chamber. This parameter affects the product properties in a feed-dependent manner. The thermal charge of inlet drying gas reflects its capacity to dry the humid atomized droplets and thereby, higher inlet temperatures enable higher solvent evaporation rates. Nevertheless, the inlet temperature should not just be increased to achieve better drying performances because it also has an impact on the wet-bulb temperature of the surrounding air. In fact, lower inlet temperatures lead to lower surrounding air wet-bulb temperature, preventing therefore thermal degradation of the final product. Hence, a wise choice of inlet temperature, balanced on these factors, should be done according to the feedstock properties [3,6].

Outlet temperature: This temperature is the temperature of the air containing the dried particles just before such content to be piped into the collection devices. Theoretically, it is the highest temperature to which the product may be heated, although, in the counter-current dryers, the final product may present a higher temperature than the outlet air [6]. Outlet temperature results from all heat and mass exchanges inside the drying chamber, and thus is not directly regulated by the operator. However, this is a function of parameters like the inlet temperature, the drying gas flow rate, as well as the feed properties such as solvent evaporation enthalpy and droplet solid concentration [3,6].

Drying gas flow rate: The drying gas flow rate can be described as the amount (volume) of drying air supplied to the system per unit of time. The dryer may operate in drying air suction or in injection mode. In suction mode, a slight under-pressure occurs in the system. The drying air supply rate also determines the drying level of the product and its separation in the cyclone. The lower the drying air feed rate, the slower the movement of the product particles through the system, and the longer the action of the drying air upon them. This means that the drying gas flow rate should be low enough to ensure a complete particle moisture removal, but on the other hand, it should be suitable for the subsequent separation procedure. Compressed gas is supplied through the nozzle simultaneously with the feed to ensure the feed's atomization. Higher amounts of gas result in better atomization of the liquid stream (smaller droplets) and, as a consequence, smaller product particles. The pressure under which the gas is supplied depends on the requirements imposed by the nozzle's construction. The possibility of supplying the atomizing device with the feed is dependent on the properties of the feed itself and is also related to the pumping device and pipes through which it is supplied. Considering the drying process stability, the possibility of continuous control over the mixture feed rate is necessary, and any feeding rate changes should happen smoothly [3].

Residence time inside the drying chamber: Residence time refers to the exposition period of the atomized droplets inside the drying chamber, being another important factor with a direct influence on the final product quality. Residence time should be long enough to guarantee that the main goal of the drying stage is accomplished, that is, to obtain dried particles. On the other hand, it is fundamental to keep the product characteristics and when the dried particles are subjected to longer residence times, thermal degradation may occur, especially upon heat-sensitive materials. In one of the earliest studies on drying kinetics and particle residence time in spray drying the experimental results proved that spray residence time was controlled by atomization ratio and airflow rate [32]. This study revealed that the drying gas temperature has some influence on particle residence time, but the atomization ratio and airflow rate appeared to be definitively the most important parameters impacting the residence time. It was shown that particle residence time is always shorter than average drying gas residence time due to high initial particle velocity. Smaller particles from the given spray stay longer in the drying chamber than bigger particles. For example. fraction up to 8 mm remains in the chamber for 3.1 s while fraction 112–120 mm for only 2.0 s. The study also revealed that an increase of atomization ratio decreased particle residence time (2.5 s for atomization ratio 39/5 to 4 s for 8/10. In this case, initial spray velocity controls the residence time of particles (higher for higher atomization ratio). An increase in gas velocity decreases the particle residence time. However, there is no simple relation between gas and particle residence time. In another study [33], the particle residence time distribution of the laboratory-scale spray dryer was characterized by a median residence time $\tau 50$ of 6 s as well as by $\tau 10$ and $\tau 90$ values of 0.2 s and 55 s, respectively. In contrast, longer particle residence times were measured in the pilot-scale dryer, where, a median particle residence time $\tau 50$ of 17 s was obtained, the $\tau 10$ and $\tau 90$ values being 4 s and 1 min 22 s, respectively. The last particles left the dryer after about 6 min. These long particle residence times indicate recirculation flows inside the drying chamber and possible wall deposition of particles. This hypothesis was confirmed by the comparison of the mean residence time of air with the mean residence time of particles. Assuming plug flow inside the spray dryer, the mean residence time of the air could be estimated by dividing the volume of the spray dryer by the air volume flow rate. Using this approach, the calculated mean residence time of air was 1.1 s for the laboratory-scale spray dryer and 12 s for the pilot-scale dryer. In contrast to that, the mean particle residence times are 24.8 s for the laboratory-scale dryer and 90.2 s for the pilot-scale spray dryer, respectively. Consequently, the particle mean-residence-time is longer than the mean residence time of air. This divergence can be explained by the presence of recirculation zones and powder backflow inside the drying chamber as well as by temporary particle deposition on the dryer walls. It was concluded in this study that particle residence time distribution in the laboratory-scale dryer differs significantly from particle residence time distribution in the pilot-scale spray dryer. As a consequence, the temperature-concentration-time-history of the particles would not be equal in both dryers. Because of the difficulties in experimentally predicting the minimum residence time to be used, some researchers calculated the approximate residence time theoretically [34]. Notwithstanding, it should be remarked that the residence time is usually in the order of a few seconds (e.g., in general, fine particles should not stay more than 10–15 s inside the drying chamber) [6,34].

Glass transition temperature (Tg): Glass transition temperature is an important thermophysical property of amorphous polymers. Above *Tg*, the material changes from a rigid glassy state to a more rubbery state. Hence, this could be related somehow with the material stickiness on the drying chamber, being, therefore, an obstacle to the spray drying process.

In summary, the importance of processing parameters on the spray drying efficiency is clear. Therefore, the advantages and drawbacks of each parameter must be weighed in order to produce products with desirable characteristics especially when the QbD approach is used for this process. Table 6.2 presents the network of mutual interrelationships among the spray drying parameters, nevertheless, it cannot be taken as a simplified list of instructions for drying. The heterogeneity of behaviors in substances subjected to the drying process usually forces the operator to work following the rule of trials and errors.

6.5 SPRAY DRYING APPLICATIONS

6.5.1 FEASIBILITY ASSESSMENTS

Before any spray drying application work begins, it may be advantageous to conduct following simple, qualitative tests at the laboratory bench using very little material to determine the feasibility of the application [35]. A rheological profile of the solution or suspension should be evaluated, or a small sample can be tested to see if droplets from a stirring rod can be readily formed. In the latter test, if the liquid strings from the surface or forms peaks, then high viscosity is indicated, and the product may not be a candidate for spray drying without formulation changes. The behavior of non-Newtonian fluids (pseudoplastic, thixotropic, dilatant, etc.) has been found to influence atomization and resultant droplet size [36]. However, while it is expected that Newtonian and non-Newtonian fluids atomize differently, this difference was not found to be as important as the more significant effect of the wheel speed on droplet size. It is also important to note that highly viscous materials cannot be atomized by pressure nozzles.

Once the effect of viscosity has been evaluated, it may be advisable to dry a few drops of product on a glass slide using a heated air gun. During this bench drying test, the air temperature is recorded, and the material is observed for the presence of stickiness, color changes, or other physical changes. If the dried powder is found to be suitable at the air temperature applied, it can be placed on a variable-temperature hot bench to determine the temperature at which the powder becomes tacky. For spray drying to be successful, this temperature must be higher than the outlet temperature of the dryer.

If the initial feasibility evaluation is successful, it is reasonable to commit additional materials for a spray drying trial. A laboratory dryer of at least 500 mm in diameter is recommended for such tests. Bench-scale spray dryers are available but limited in their ability to provide adequate atomization or sufficient process airflow for the successful production of dried particles. The laboratory unit, however, combined with very fine atomization (two-fluid or rotary) will often produce an acceptable product for further testing. A series of tests can be performed at different

TABLE 6.2

Interrelationships Among the Spray Drying Parameters (Adapted from Refs. 3,5)

	Outlet Temperature		Particle Size		Final Product Moisture		Efficiency
Drying Airflow Rate(↑)	↑↑	Lower heat losses on the basis of total energy	----------		↓↓	The lower partial pressure of water vapor	↑↑ Better separation in a cyclone
Air Humidity(↑)	↑	More energy contained in the moisture	----------		↑↑	The higher partial pressure of drying air	↓ More moisture may lead to adherence of the product to the chamber walls
Inlet Temperature(↑)	↑↑↑	Direct proportion	----------		↓↓	Lower relative humidity of the air	↑ Eventually, dryer product percent adhering
Atomizing airflow(↑)	↓	A higher amount of cold air to be heated	↓↓↓	A higher amount of available energy for atomization	----------		----------
Feed Rate(↑)	↓↓	More solvent to be evaporated	↑	More liquid to be dispersed	↑↑	A higher amount of water leading to its higher partial pressure	↑↓ Depending on application
Solid Concentration Feed(↑)	↑↑	Less water to be evaporated	↑↑↑	More solid available for particle formation	↓	Less water evaporation, lower partial pressure	↑ Bigger particles are easier to separate in cyclone
Organic Solvent (Instead of Water)	↑↑↑	Less energy required for evaporation	↓	Lower surface tension, more available energy to spend on particle fission	↓↓↓	Lack of water in feed leading to very dry product	↑↑ Lack of hygroscopicity results in easier drying
	(↑) Minor increase (↑↑) Moderate increase (↑↑↑) High increase				(↓) Minor decrease (↓↓) Moderate decrease (↓↓↓) High decrease		

inlet-outlet temperature combinations using small quantities of material and these samples can be tested for chemical stability to evaluate thermal effects from process air contact. The relationship between outlet temperature and final product moisture can also be established for this scale. While samples produced in a laboratory dryer are suitable for evaluating the effect of spray drying on the product, they are not suitable for use in downstream processing because the fine particle distribution produced as a result of the small drying chamber dimensions may not be representative of the final spray dried product.

Production of coarser particles requires a larger, pilot-scale dryer, which, in turn, requires larger feed volumes. This pilot-scale work is often conducted at a spray drying development center since many companies have laboratory dryers, but few have the sizes and variety of process types needed to fully develop a spray dried product from the pilot-scale through one-tenth commercial scale and into final production. These facilities are usually found at spray drying manufacturers or custom processing companies. In addition to having the equipment, manufacturers and custom processors often have the expertise to more quickly optimize product characteristics.

6.5.2 SPRAY DRYING TO PRODUCE A SPECIFIC TYPE OF PARTICLE

Because of its inherent costs, spray drying is not always considered as a processing option for many conventional formulations. However, when a specialized particle type is required by the active ingredient or dosage form, spray drying can become a feasible alternative to more conventional manufacturing processes. Such particle types include microcapsules, controlled-release particles, nanoparticles, and liposomes. The application of spray drying to pharmaceuticals has been extensively discussed in review articles [37,38].

6.5.2.1 Granulation

Spray drying is a unique process in several ways as compared to other granulation methods. The feedstock is a homogeneous liquid, which results in the uniform distribution of all components of the spray dried product in the same ratio in the powder blend; this eliminates the concerns of uniformly granulating dry components with a liquid. While granule characteristics may exhibit batch-to-batch variation, which, in turn, may influence the compaction behavior of the formulation or the post-compaction properties of the tablet, granules produced using spray drying are extremely consistent in terms of particle size, bulk density, and compaction behavior. These features make spray drying a suitable process for the production of directly compressible excipients such as lactose, microcrystalline cellulose, and mannitol [39]. Spray dried lactose is by far the most commonly encountered spray dried excipient [37,40,41].

Many granulation methods utilize mechanical energy to transform very fine particles into granules. Although shear forces are employed in the nozzle and centrifugal atomizer to create sprays, this form of energy will not destroy microencapsulated material as can happen in high-shear granulation. In spray drying, some trial and error are encountered in establishing the nozzle combinations and liquid pressures to obtain equivalent particle size distribution during scale-up; however, the resultant powder will have similar physical properties such as bulk density and compaction. Also, it is important to note that, within the spray dryer, the product is never in contact with moving parts, which facilitates the proper cleaning process greatly.

If the granulation size is a critical criterion for a given formulation, then the selection of the granulation process may be determined based on the desired particle size and feasible operating temperatures. Figure 6.17 compares the general particle size limitations of numerous granulation techniques. As seen in this figure, the spray drying process results in smaller size particles as compared to some other granulation methods such as fluid bed granulation or high shear (high intensity) granulation. One option for producing larger agglomerates using spray drying technology is to employ fluidized spray drying, which combines the features of the spray drying process with fluid bed granulation (Figure 6.18). The result of this process is particles similar to those obtained from a fluid bed granulation operation, and yet the process is a continuous type in contrast to the batch operation of a fluid bed granulator.

A variation of this system is the integrated fluid bed dryer (Figure 6.19). This system includes integrated filter bags, which are suspended from the chamber roof. This roof is perforated and serves a dual purpose as a gas disperser. The chamber above the roof contains clean gas that supplies the inlet process drying air and also has an exhaust point for clean gas since any remaining fines are entrapped in the filters.

Products produced using fluidized spray drying have a broader particle size distribution and lower bulk density than the particles produced by conventional spray dryers with a typical mean size particle size range of 150–400 microns. This process is not meant to replace conventional spray drying processes but instead is a feasible alternative for spray drying applications that require larger mean particle sizes.

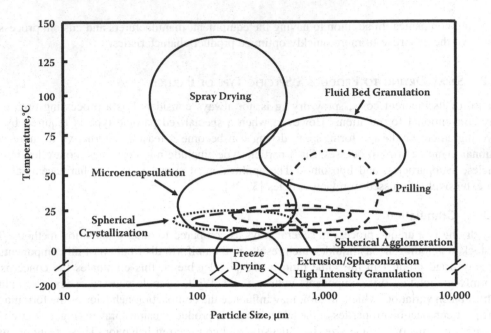

FIGURE 6.17 Particle size range of the methods utilized in particle growth.
Source: From Ref. [42].

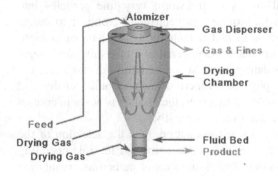

FIGURE 6.18 Schematic of fluidized spray drying system (FSD™).
Source: Courtesy of GEA Pharma Systems.

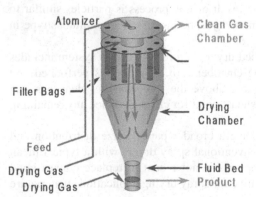

FIGURE 6.19 Schematic of an integrated fluid-bed dryer (IFD™).
Source: Courtesy of GEA Pharma Systems.

6.5.2.2 Modification of Solid-State Properties

Characterization and modification of solid-state properties of drug substances are profoundly important in developing pharmaceutical products with desired drug release properties. The importance of the process understanding and improvement of the dissolution rate for poorly water-soluble drugs has been known for decades [43]. The majority of the new drug entities have low aqueous solubility and potentially low bioavailability. Availability for absorption may decrease in magnitude or become more variable under the influence of factors such as poor wetting of the compound by gastrointestinal fluids leading to particle agglomeration, low solubility about dose and permeability, slow dissolution concerning gastrointestinal residence time, or precipitation of, for example, weak bases upon entry into the small intestine [44]. Dispersion of the drug as very fine particles increases the surface area available for dissolution and thus dissolution rate. However, very fine hydrophobic particles also lend themselves to agglomeration in the presence of GI fluid; this leads to larger particle size and ultimately lower dissolution.

Particle size reduction methods (e.g., grinding, micronization, and ball milling), precipitation, the formation of inclusion compounds, making solid dispersions by quench cooling, melt extrusion, rotary vacuum evaporation, freeze-drying, spray drying, and other process techniques have been used extensively for improving the solubility and dissolution rate of poorly water-soluble materials [4,45–51]. These processes generally impart a polymorphic change by transforming a low energy crystalline form into an amorphous form.

Particle size reduction may go to the nano-scale; however, this reduction will not lead to concentrations above the maximum solubility of the drug in the intestinal fluids. Alternatively, solid dispersions can be used to increase the dissolution rate of poorly water-soluble drugs and they increase the amount of drug at the absorption site, sometimes to supersaturated concentrations and consequently improved bioavailability. Such amorphous solid dispersions (ASDs) have been prepared using different techniques such as hot-melt extrusion (HME), freeze-drying, supercritical methods, and spray drying. Amorphous to the crystalline transition of an API is thermodynamically driven due to the lower free energy of the crystalline form; however, for crystalline to amorphous transition, external energy is required. Spray drying is an energy-intensive process where the energy-mass transfer occurs at the droplet surface when the droplets are transiting through the drying chamber.

Due to the large specific surface area offered by the droplets during spray drying, the solvent rapidly evaporates and the ASDs are formed within seconds, which is usually fast enough to prevent phase separation. Moreover, the ASDs prepared by spray drying allows particle size optimization by changing spray drying parameters such as drying gas flow, feed rate, and atomization parameters. This allows spray dried particles for applications such as pulmonary delivery or as free-flowing particles suitable for direct compression [4]. Spray drying usually produces low-density particles that are either porous or hollow [52]. The porous or hollow structure of the spray dried particles increases the surface area and subsequently the solubility and dissolution rate of the drugs by several folds. For example, the dissolution rate of poorly water-soluble salicylic acid was found to be almost instantaneous and 60 times faster when spray dried as compared to that of the original powder [45]. These spray dried particles also allow for pulmonary delivery based on their favorable aerodynamic diameter [53].

However, the energy of the amorphous state depends, to some extent, on the method of preparation [48]. The dissolution behavior of ASDs must remain unchanged during storage, especially at extreme conditions since partially or fully amorphous particles are thermodynamically unstable. For optimal stability, the molecular mobility of ASDs should be as low as possible. However, the recrystallization of the ASDs during storage (at high humidity and temperatures) is a challenge that has been documented in the literature [53,54,55]. The rapid drying during the spray drying process (i.e., the short residence time of the droplets during drying) improves the stability of otherwise-unstable amorphous forms. The drying rate can thus be a critical factor in determining whether the sprayed material is completely amorphous or not. Also, the time for which the droplets are exposed to high temperature is important for the stability of ASDs, which are usually susceptible to extreme temperature exposures. Therefore, adequate care should be taken to monitor the drying kinetics for generating ASDs [56]. The stabilization of the amorphous material can be accomplished by incorporating polymers with a high glass transition temperature (Tg). The choice of the solvent system is also critical as some combinations can result in different ASD morphology that can negatively influence drug release properties [57]. ASDs consisting of Naproxen-PVP had better miscibility when DCM-acetone solvent mixtures were used compared to methanol-acetone or DCM-methanol mixture [58]. Therefore, spray drying from the solvent/anti-solvent mixture may result in ASDs with greater drug-polymer miscibility, lower crystallinity, and higher physical stability of the formulation. The spray drying process is suitable for the integration of polymers as stability agents (e.g., PVP and PEG) into spray dried particles. Other polymers used for ASDs include, but are not limited to HPMC, HPMCP, HPMC-AS, ethylcellulose, various grades of Eudragit, poly (ethylene oxide), carbopol, pectin, and chitosan [56]. The choice of polymers for ASDs affect properties such as drug-polymer miscibility (discussed earlier), intermolecular interactions, and various relaxations that are associated with amorphous materials. Polymer characteristics such as their chemical composition, molecular weight, structure, solution/melt viscosity, kinetic and thermodynamic solubility of API in the polymer, solubility in solvents, solubility parameter, melting point, Tg, and hydrogen donor/acceptor count should be taken into consideration [57]. For example, spray drying of the poorly soluble drug with 50% PVP resulted in enhanced dissolution when compared to a physical mixture of micronized drug with PVP. A physically stable amorphous form of ibuprofen, which has a low melting point, was obtained when spray dried in the presence of 50–75% PVP [49]. In another study on the effect of spray drying varying lactose/PEG compositions, the most amorphous particles were obtained when PEG was present at 10% w/w concentration. Conversion to the crystalline form occurred over time and the crystallization of lactose appeared to be slowed at low PEG concentrations [50]. In another work, the authors showed an increased amount and molecular weight of PVP to increase the physical stability of amorphous lactose [51].

6.5.2.3   Microencapsulation

The preparation of microcapsules involves the coating of particles or liquid droplets with a biodegradable polymer. Applications for microspheres in the pharmaceutical industry include controlled release, particle coating, flavor stabilization, taste masking, and physical or chemical stabilization. Microencapsulation can be achieved through several processes, but, in general, an API is trapped within a reservoir and is usually coated by a polymer. This process often begins with the preparation of a three-phase, immiscible system containing a liquid vehicle, a core particle, and a coating material or polymer. Several manufacturing techniques can be employed to deposit the polymer around the particle and cause this coating to become rigid. These methods include spray drying, Wurster fluid-bed coating, pan coating, coacervation, and emulsion evaporation. In the spray drying process, the encapsulation process is achieved in one step in which desolvation and thermal cross-linking occur concurrently, and the particle is coated. A review of the main factors involved in the application of spray drying for achieving microencapsulation references many works that detail pharmaceutical applications, especially drug delivery systems [59].

Microencapsulation or microparticle (matrix) formation is a process that is often used to provide controlled release of a protein or drug. Several authors have studied microencapsulation formulations manufactured from a spray drying process as a means to achieve controlled release. In one case, the effect of polymer hydrophilicity on API release was evaluated and the most hydrophilic polymer was found to gel faster and retard drug release the most [60]. The size and cohesiveness of the resultant spray dried particles were found to be a function of the polymer and also affected drug release with the smaller, more cohesive particles tending to agglomerate and delay drug release. In another case, the release of a model drug was controlled using a spray dried, water-activated, pH-controlled microsphere [61]. Water influx into the microcapsule caused the buffer to dissolve and thus adjusted the inner pH causing the fraction of unionized drug to increase resulting in drug release.

One specific polymer type that has been employed in the spray drying of drugs to modify its release is acrylic resin. A commercial blend of neutral methacrylic acid esters was used for the preparation of spray dried controlled-release microcapsules containing model drugs [62]. The dissolution results of tablets compressed from these microspheres showed successful controlled release with advantages over a matrix system. In a similar study, sustained release and enteric tablets were prepared by directly compressing spray dried microspheres produced using different types of acrylic resins [63]. Complete enteric properties were observed for tablets made from pH-dependent, anionic acrylic polymers while a sustained release profile was observed for tablets made from microspheres containing pH-dependent, cationic acrylic polymers.

Two common biodegradable polymers used in microparticle formation using spray drying are polylactide (PLA) and polylactide-co-glycolide (PLGA). The efficacy of spray drying as a method for PLA and PLGA microsphere preparation was investigated using a model lipophilic drug [64]. The spray drying process parameters were tailored to each polymer and the microspheres obtained were evaluated for shape, size, drug content, and polymer influence on these characteristics. Polymer type, molecular weight, and concentration were the greatest contributing factors to these characteristics. In-vitro dissolution testing revealed different release profiles depending on the polymer type and microsphere morphology.

6.5.2.4   Inhalation and Nasal Dosage Forms

In recent years, spray drying has been increasingly used for manufacturing inhalable dry powders. Being a bottom-up approach, it is well suited for particle engineering that is critical for delivering drugs into the respiratory tract. Further, spray drying is a scalable process that enables fine control over multiple process parameters. For inhalation dosage forms to be clinically effective, the drug should deposit in the lower airways. The site of drug deposition in the lungs depends on the particle size and size distribution of the drug particles or droplets, the inhaler device and formulation, the patient's breathing patterns, and airway geometry [65]. The aerosol particles or droplets must be of size 1–3 μm in aerodynamic diameter to be deposited into the lower respiratory tract. This has been achieved by different nozzle designs that can be adapted with spray drying to achieve the appropriate particle size for inhalation. The two-fluid nozzle is the most commonly used nozzle for inhalable powders; however, in recent years, three-fluid and four-fluid nozzles have been used for manufacturing dry powders for inhalation [66–69]. Some of these nozzles are capable of microencapsulation of proteins that ultimately could potentially reduce the burst release observed using a conventional two-fluid nozzle.

Due to its known ability to tailor powders with the appropriate aerodynamic size and good flow properties, spray drying is a useful method for manufacturing particles for dry powder inhalers (DPIs). Spray drying for inhalation delivery has advantages not only in terms of powder particle size and flowability but also for drug uniformity. In a study, spray drying Salbutamol sulfate, a widely used drug in inhaler products, with lactose, which is amorphous when spray dried alone, resulted in amorphous composites. Spray drying salbutamol sulfate with PEG 4000 and PEG 20,000, which do not form amorphous systems when spray dried alone, resulted in systems of varying crystallinity; the crystallinity of the powders depended on the mass ratio of polymer to the drug. Feed concentration is also an important factor determining the particle size of the spray dried powders. The formation and physical stability of amorphous composites formed by spray drying was shown to be dependent on whether the Tg of one of the components was high enough to result in a Tg of the final powder mixture sufficiently high that the Kauzmann temperature of the mix is greater than the temperature of storage [70].

A formulation of mucoadhesive microspheres for nasal administration was examined containing active and one of two polymer types using a spray drying procedure [71]. The mean diameter of the spray dried particles was 3–5 microns, and surface morphology was dependent on polymer type. Microspheres containing active and either polymer were more mucoadhesive than any of the starting materials alone. The authors also showed that the dissolution rate of the spray dried formulation decreased with increasing polymer content.

As mentioned in the previous section, spray drying could formulate low-density powders with significant porosity. Low-density particles will have a lower aerodynamic diameter, despite having a large volumetric diameter, and thus allow for deep lung delivery [52]. Peclet number (Pe) is used to describe the powder formation process using spray drying and to explain low-density particle morphology [72,73]. A low Pe leads to the generation of dry powders with particle density close to the true density of the dry components used. This happens since the solutes remain evenly distributed in the droplet during the evaporation process. Conversely, a high Pe generates solid hollow particles due to the rapid evaporation or the slow diffusion of the solute from the drying particles. This leads to the surface enrichment of the powders with the components associated with high Pe.

The ability to control the particle size and density for inhalation were investigated using lactose solutions atomized with a two-fluid nozzle and a laboratory-scale spray dryer. The droplet size during atomization was affected by the nozzle orifice diameter and atomization airflow but not significantly by the feed concentration; however, the dried particle size was influenced by feed concentration. The authors suggested that the shell thickness of the hollow particles increased with increasing feed concentration [74].

An alternative method of atomization for the formation of respirable particles is the airblast atomizer. This type of two-fluid nozzle introduces a liquid feed pumped at a slow rate into a high-velocity gas stream via single or multiple jets. This atomizer type was utilized at a laboratory scale to evaluate the effect of grounded versus electrostatically charged tower configurations on the median particle size of the spray dried product. This study found significant differences between the two configurations with the latter producing small particles but compromising collection efficiency [75].

In recent years, spray drying has been used to deliver dry powders for inhalation for infectious diseases. This has necessitated the delivery of large powder doses since many of the antibiotics are low potency and thus require large quantities to achieve efficacy [76]. In the past two decades, many researchers have shown the efficacy of spray dried powders containing antibiotics for the treatment of tuberculosis (TB) by the pulmonary route [77–83]. Muttil et al. had shown high drug loading of two first-line anti-TB drugs, isoniazid and rifabutin, using spray drying for pulmonary delivery [84]. In a clinical trial published in 2013, Dharmadhikari et al. showed the safety of dry powder capreomycin for multi-drug resistant TB when delivered by the pulmonary route [85]. This opened the door for dry powders for inhalation for other infectious diseases and led to the FDA approval of dry powder tobramycin for cystic fibrosis patients [86]. Tobramycin dry powders are manufactured using an emulsion-based spray drying process that allowed the production of large porous particles [87]. This novel formulation, called PulmoSphere™, exhibited improved flow and dispersion from passive dry powder inhalers; a critical requirement for high drug dosing. Further, PulmoSphere™ tobramycin dry powders substantially improved lung deposition efficiency, faster delivery, and more convenient administration over nebulized formulations.

6.5.2.5 Liposomes

Another particle type capable of being produced by spray drying is liposomes. Traditional preparation of liposomes begins with the preparation of a solution containing the lipids in a volatile organic solvent mixture. Following filtration of the solution, the solvent mixture is removed under conditions that ensure phase separation does not occur. The dry lipid mixture is then hydrated by an aqueous mixture containing the drug to be entrapped. Lastly, this mixture is dried. Spray drying is one method for accomplishing one or both of these drying steps. For example, lipid vesicles were produced using a spray drying process instead of the first step of the traditional process [88]. Vesicles containing phosphatidylcholine (soybean lecithin) were produced by extruding the phospholipid through a 0.2-micron polycarbonate membrane followed by spray drying with 10% lactose. The particle size, vesicle size distribution, and stability of the multilamellar vesicles were measured. The mean particle diameter after spray drying with a rotary atomizer was seven microns and the dry particles could be reconstituted in water to form liposomes without any major change to the vesicle size distribution. Besides, the chemical stability of the liposomes was not significantly affected by the spray drying process. In subsequent work, the same authors utilized spray drying for the hydration step of the traditional process [89].

Although Arikace® (liposomal amikacin for inhalation) was recently approved by the FDA for non-tuberculous mycobacterial treatment, there are no spray dried liposomal formulations in the market yet. In recent years, liposomes (called proliposomes) have been spray dried into dry powders for inhalation. Two anti-tubercular drugs (rifapentine and isoniazid) have been spray dried to form proliposome powders for inhalation [90,91]. Spray drying was also utilized to encapsulate liposomal ciprofloxacin [92]. In this study, ciprofloxacin nanocrystals were made inside liposomes; this novel liposomal-nanocrystal formulation was spray dried into dry powders for inhalation. The authors concluded that this spray dried liposomal formulation was stable and was able to release the drug in a controlled manner.

6.5.2.6 Peptides, Proteins, and Vaccines

Recent advances in biotechnology have made it possible to use macromolecules such as peptides, proteins, and vaccines as therapeutic agents. Spray drying has been used for processing antibiotics, vaccines, and recently, for macro-molecular drugs. The effect of spray drying process parameters (such as heat and shear) on the activity of peptides and proteins has shown to affect their potency. Enzymes are sometimes used as model protein due to the ease with which their activity can be determined after spray drying.

Many proteins, peptides, and vaccines may be susceptible to degradation due to relatively high temperatures used during spray drying. However, it is to be noted that the drug substance is exposed to the heat only for a short duration (millisecond range) during the drying process. Many studies have shown the successful formulation of sensitive peptides and proteins using spray drying. In a study, the effects of inlet and outlet temperatures on spray dried peptides and proteins were reported [93]. In another study, enzyme activity was susceptible to the high temperature and only half of its activity remained after spray drying without additives at outlet temperatures below 50°C [94]. The authors found that the activity of a formulation comprising enzyme and mannitol was maintained at outlet temperatures below 50°C, however, was compromised above 50°C. Replacing mannitol with trehalose stabilized the spray dried enzyme and its activity was maintained at 100% at an outlet temperature of 100°C. Similar studies have shown the stabilizing effect of sugars in the spray drying of vaccines, which are generally formulated as liquids. Most vaccines are unstable as liquids due to their susceptibility to chemical (hydrolysis) and physical degradation [95]. For this reason, almost all currently approved vaccines require cold-chain storage, requiring them to be kept at 2°C–8°C, during storage and transportation [96]. Saboo et al. [97] showed the long-term stability of virus-like particles (VLPs) after spray drying. They showed that the VLPs remained stable for more than a year at room temperature after spray drying with sugar mixtures, such as trehalose, mannitol, dextran, and leucine (amino acid). The same group showed the stability of the marketed human papillomavirus vaccine (HPV; Gardasil 9) after spray drying using stabilizing excipients [98]. The authors also showed the preclinical efficacy of the spray dried vaccine after three months of storage at extreme conditions. Spray drying has also been used to stabilize live bacterial vaccines. Kunda et al. [99] showed the long-term stability of live Listeria monocytogenes vaccines after spray drying. They also showed the importance of excipients used to stabilize the live vaccine, as well as the role of storing the powder vaccines in an inert environment. Recently, Price et al. [100] showed similar stabilization of the live bacterial TB vaccine (BCG) after spray drying. In their study, they showed a minimal loss in immunogenicity of the dry powder BCG vaccine in a preclinical model after storing it at extreme storage conditions. Therefore, spray drying has been used to stabilize different types of vaccines; the goal of such stabilization is to prevent the vaccines from requiring a cold chain during storage and transportation. This becomes critical since the lack of a robust cold chain prevents vaccines from reaching remote regions of the world. According to the World Health Organization (WHO), one in five children, especially in low- and middle-income countries (LMICs), are not vaccinated against preventable infectious diseases due to the lack of availability of vaccines [101]. Also, the requirement of a cold chain for transporting vaccines usually leads to wastage of approximately half of the vaccine supply, potentially due to exposure to temperatures outside the recommended 2°C–8°C [102].

Another method of producing protein powders is the spray freeze-drying process. This process involves spraying the solution into a freezing environment, such as liquid nitrogen, causing the resultant droplets to immediately freeze. The frozen droplets are subsequently sublimed under vacuum to produce a dry product. Spray drying and spray freeze-drying were compared to produce protein inhalation powders and spray drying was found to be superior in scalability, operational cost, and product yield than spray freeze-drying [103]. In another study, comparisons of freeze-drying with spray drying to produce dry powder dispersions for non-viral gene delivery showed that spray drying produces stable, efficient, and potentially respirable particles [104]. This is mostly because spray freeze drying cannot optimize the particle size unlike spray drying, a critical requirement for pulmonary delivery. Also, spray drying does not involve a freezing step, thus any damage to proteins related to this aspect is avoided.

Several methods, including as spray drying, lyophilization, pulverization, precipitation, and some other techniques, currently available for protein powder preparation were evaluated in a review article based on the following criteria: control on particle size and size distribution, efficiency (yield), powder flowability, scalability, and long-term protein biochemical stability [105]. Based on these criteria, spray drying had advantages over other manufacturing methods for its convenience and simplicity as well as for controlling the particle size (< 5 μm) and shape (spherical) of proteins.

Although several vaccines have been spray dried into stable formulations and evaluated in preclinical models, both small and large animals, for their immunogenicity and efficacy when delivered by the pulmonary route, the number of vaccines evaluated in human trials are very limited. One of the major reasons for the lack of translation of these spray dried vaccine formulations from preclinical to the clinical realm is the use of delivery devices (inhalers) in general used for animals and humans. A recent review has captured the differences in the inhalers used for animal studies versus those used in humans [100]. This review discusses how researchers can overcome the variability in preclinical testing, to improve the translation success and ultimately bring the spray dried aerosol vaccines to the market.

6.5.2.7   Microparticles and Nanoparticles

Despite the availability of numerous crystal engineering techniques, generating drug-rich microparticles with a predetermined size, morphology and crystallinity still represent a challenge. Among many techniques, spray drying, due to its ability to control the size, shape, and other properties of the resulting particles, has become a versatile technology for the preparation of microparticles and more importantly, nanoparticles for the pharmaceutical/biotech applications. For example, in a study, it was shown that the adsorption of excipients onto micron size drug substrates using a spray drying process was found to be an attractive approach to engineer drug-rich microparticles with characteristics suitable for drug delivery [106]. In another recent study, a fast-dissolving mucoadhesive microparticulate delivery system was developed using a spray drying method for piroxicam, which is a drug with low water solubility and high membrane permeability [107]. It is known that such delivery systems intended for sublingual administration could be a suitable alternative to fast-dissolving tablets because the sublingual adsorption can be improved as a consequence of prolonging residence time on the mucosa and reducing the amount of swallowed drug [108].

Aranaz et al. prepared chitosan-based microparticles to study the effect of chitosan physico-chemical properties, TPP concentration, and chitosan-TPP ratio on the controlled release of venlafaxine hydrochloride [109]. They showed that chitosan physico-chemical properties had some effect on the practical yield and encapsulation efficiency but little effect on drug release pattern. The parameter with the main effect on venlafaxine release was the chitosan-TPP ratio. A formulation based on chitosan with low viscosity and chitosan: TPP ratio of 1:1 showed the most moderate controlled release, with a maximum release at 6 h in SIF of 60%.

Strob et al. [110] modified a conventional spray dryer by combining an internal mixing two-fluid nozzle with a cyclone droplet separator as a conventional spray drying process for the preparation of submicron-sized particles were found to be limited regarding small droplets and efficient precipitation. The precipitation of particles was realized with an electrostatic precipitator. Considering the difficulty of electrostatic precipitation concerning explosion risks and making it capable of using organic solvents, the spray dryer was integrated into a pressure-resistant vessel. The new design was compact and fit in a pressure-resistant vessel. Hence, spray drying experiments with pharmaceuticals that were dissolved in organic solvents are possible. Here, the spray dryer was characterized by the model substance mannitol in an aqueous solution for the simplicity of the operation. Compared to the previous design, slightly smaller droplets (d50; 3 < 1:7 μm) in the conditioned aerosol were produced. Nevertheless, a yield loss was recorded.

Attempts have been made to manufacture particles on the nanometer scale for applications such as controlled release and intravenous delivery systems. A comparison evaluating the processability and solid dosage performance of spray dried nanoparticles and microparticles were conducted [111]. In this study, nanoparticle suspensions were prepared by wet comminution in the presence of stabilizers and converted into dried particles using a spray drying process and subsequently compressed. Compacts prepared from microparticles and nanoparticles were found to differ in their internal structure and micromechanical deformations.

In another study, solid, lipid nanoparticles were produced using high-pressure homogenization and loaded with a drug, using hot or cold methods for lipophilic or hydrophilic drugs, respectively [112]. Surfactant addition was investigated and stability and entrapment efficiency were evaluated. Long-term sterile storage of these dispersions was difficult and spray drying was investigated as a potential, feasible technique.

The feasibility of developing nanoparticles for aerosol delivery has also been investigated [113]. The spray dried nanoparticles produced using one carrier type were found to be hollow while others had a continuous matrix. Particle size was measured before spray drying and after the spray dried powder was redissolved. Both carrier types resulted in an increase in particle size after spray drying although both were found to remain in the nanometer range after drying and were suitable for efficient lung delivery.

Demir and Degim employed a nano-spray (B-90) drying technology based on the piezoelectric spray head, laminar airflow, and electrostatic particle collector to produce chitosan nanoparticles [114]. The results indicated that the orifice, spray capacity, and polymer concentration played a crucial role to obtain satisfactory performance. According to the results of particle characteristics and operation capacity, a smaller orifice leads to a smaller particle size for the final product but a lower operation capacity. On the other hand, the sprayed volume showed a linear proportion with operational capacity but no effect on particle size. As the orifice directly had an impact on the particle characteristics, spray capacity affected total process time. Besides, both product yield and polymer concentration showed their effect on the process yield. Moreover, using small caps to get smaller particles required to use diluted samples in order to obtain the optimum manufacturing process. Increased polymer concentration improved the yield of dry powder and showed more positive zeta potentials as it exhibited decreased operation capacity.

Tewa-Tagne et al. [115] investigated the influence of formulation parameters (nanocapsules and silica concentrations) and spray drying process variables (inlet temperature, spray flow air, feed flow rate, and drying airflow rate) on spray dried nanocapsules when using silica as a drying auxiliary agent. Nanocapsules and silica concentrations were found to be the main factors influencing the yield, particulate density, and particle size. None of the studied variables had a major effect on the moisture content while the interaction between nanocapsules and silica in the feed was of first interest and determinant for both the qualitative and quantitative responses. The particle morphology depended on the feed formulation but was unaffected by the process conditions.

In order to overcome the stability problem encountered with the suspension of nanocapsules of poly ε-caprolactone and Eudragit S90, Müller et al. [116] added silicon dioxide (Aerosil 200) to the suspension and then spray dried the mixture using a mini spray dryer with the inlet and outlet temperatures of 138°C and 90°C, respectively. The morphological analysis of the surface at the powders showed that nanocapsules remained intact, and no change in particle size was detected after the spray drying process. The results suggested that nanocapsule suspensions could be spray dried to overcome the stability problem as an alternative method.

Using Nano Spray Dryer B-90 and spray mesh, a piezoelectric spray drying process was used to engineer CyA and DEX PLGA nanoparticles with spherical shape and porous surface [117]. The spray drying process parameters, such as spray mesh diameter, sample flow rate, spray rate, and sample concentration, were found to play key role in particle engineering and the produced yield. CyA was found to be molecularly dispersed within the PLGA nanoparticles while DEX's crystallinity varied according to the lactide/glycolide ratio. The drug-loaded nanoparticles showed sustained release profiles over several days with low MW PLGA grades presenting faster release rates. In conclusion, this novel spray drying process can be effectively used as an alternative process for nanoparticle engineering by optimizing the spraying parameters.

The concept of nanospray drying in the laboratory-scale and the influence of the main process parameters on how powder properties of nano-sized spray dried powders like particle size, morphology, encapsulation efficiency, and drug loading are influenced by the main process parameters are reviewed by Cordin [118].

Chitosan nanoparticles have strong antibacterial activity, and the efficiency of the loading of amoxicillin is high. It was shown that chitosan nanoparticles prepared by spray drying have much potential as an antibacterial agent and as a novel means of delivery for amoxicillin [119].

Sun et al. [120] spray dried an itraconazole nanosuspension, to generate a dry nanocrystal powder, which was subsequently formulated into a tablet formulation for direct compression. The nanosuspension was prepared by high-pressure homogenization and characterized by particle-size distribution and surface morphology. In this study, it was demonstrated that the spray drying of a nanosuspension with a mannitol-to-drug mass ratio of 4.5 and at an inlet temperature of 120 °C resulted in a dry powder with the smallest increase in particle size as compared with that of the nanosuspension. X-ray diffraction results indicated that the crystalline structure of the drug was not altered during the spray drying process. The tablet formulation was identified by determining the micromeritic properties, such as flowability and compressibility of the powder mixtures composed of the spray dried nanocrystal powder and other commonly used direct compression excipients. The dissolution rate of the nanocrystal tablets was significantly enhanced and was found to be comparable to that of the marketed Sporanox. No statistically significant difference in oral absorption between the nanocrystal tablets and Sporanox capsules was found. It was concluded that the nanosuspension approach is feasible to improve the oral absorption of a BCS Class II drug in a tablet formulation and capable of achieving oral bioavailability equivalent to other well-established oral absorption enhancement methods.

6.5.2.8 Dry Elixirs and Emulsions

A dry elixir is a novel dosage form developed by spray drying APIs and excipients dissolved or suspended in ethanol and water mixtures. One example is a dry elixir in which the feed solution contained API, dextrin, and sodium lauryl sulfate in a mixture of ethanol/water [121]. The spray dried product was spherical in shape with a smooth surface and a mean diameter of 13 mm. A comparison with the API in powder form revealed a major decrease in dissolution time from over 60 to 2 minutes.

A dosage form similar to dry elixir is a dry emulsion. In this case, the emulsified drug or oily drug solution with additives is spray dried to produce dry emulsion particles. A dry emulsion of a water-insoluble nutrient was studied, and release from the spray dried particle was found to be dependent on the type and amount of oily carrier and surfactant used [122]. Differences in release among the different formulations were attributed to the differences in the physical state of the drug and surfactant in the dried particle.

In a study to develop the long-acting nifedipine oral delivery with bioavailability enhancement, a nifedipine dry elixir (NDE) containing nifedipine ethanol solution in dextrin shell was prepared using a spray dryer and then coated nifedipine dry elixir (CNDE) was prepared by coating NDE with Eudragit acrylic resin. The authors concluded that CNDE, which could lower the initial burst-out plasma concentration and maintain the plasma level of nifedipine over a longer period with bioavailability enhancement, might be one of the potential alternatives to the marketed long-acting oral delivery system for nifedipine [123].

6.5.2.9 Effervescent Products

Spray dried particles have also been incorporated into effervescent products for decades even though this is not the most common method for the preparation of effervescent products. In one of the early studies, spray drying was used to protect a degradation-sensitive API by coating fine particles of the drug with a sugar alcohol solution [124]. In vivo results of tablets made using the spray dried particles combined with coated citric acid and sodium bicarbonate revealed that the API was rapidly absorbed from the tablet.

In another early study [125], sodium bicarbonate, a common carbon dioxide source indirectly compressible effervescent tablet formulation, was produced using spray drying in order to overcome the bad flowability and low compressibility of this material. Some additives such as polyvinylpyrrolidone and silicon oil were found to be essential to obtain direct compressible spray dried sodium bicarbonate. The spray dried sodium bicarbonate showed excellent compression characteristics compared to the non-spray dried one; this makes it a future candidate for a source of carbon dioxide in the manufacture of effervescent tablets by direct compression.

Ely et al. developed a new type of respiratory drug delivery carrier particle that incorporates an active release mechanism [126]. Spray drying was used to manufacture inhalable powders containing polybutylcyanoacrylate nanoparticles and ciprofloxacin as model substances for pulmonary delivery. The carrier particles incorporated effervescent technology, thereby adding an active release mechanism to their pulmonary route of administration. The effervescent activity of the carrier particles was observed when the carrier particles were exposed to humidity. This study revealed that effervescent carrier particles can be used to deliver a large range of substances to the lungs with possibly a faster release compared to conventional carrier particles. However, it was noted that further studies would be required to evaluate how the effervescent particles will behave at the lung surfactant air interface.

In a recent study that was aimed to determine the physical properties of probiotic effervescent tablets with two different coatings that are tapioca and maltodextrin to improve water quality in shrimp farming ponds, liquid probiotics suspended into 20% maltodextrin or 20% tapioca in water and, then spray dried after 30 minutes incubation at 370 °C. The Probiotic powder was ready to be used after coming out of the dryer [127]. This method facilitates the distribution of probiotics that are liquid and difficult to transport.

6.5.2.10   Other Process Variations

Two variations of the spray drying process have been developed in response to product require-ments. The first variation is the spray congealing. In this process, solids such as wax or mono-glycerides are melted. Other ingredients such as drugs, flavors, or fragrances are dissolved or suspended in the molten material. This molten feed is sprayed using the same basic spray drying equipment except that no heat source is required. Depending on the freezing point of the feed, ambient or chilled air may be used during the drying process. This process has been described in more detail and a comparison between particles produced by both the spray drying and spray congealing techniques has also been drawn [128]. One study compared microcapsules produced using both methods and found that the solvent used, the lipid type, and the chain length were variables that influenced the surface properties of both particle types [129,130].

A second variation of the spray drying process is spray freeze-drying. In this process, the feed is sprayed into freezing air causing the droplets to freeze. The frozen droplets are subsequently sublimed under vacuum conditions producing a dry product. One study investigated this method further by eliminating the use of vacuum conditions for sublimation [131]. In this study, the feasibility of spraying pharmaceutical solutions at atmospheric pressure was investigated using very low air temperatures and desiccated air for the removal of the water from the frozen particles. The process resulted in fine, free-flowing powder with high surface area, good wetting, and good solubility characteristics.

Another type of atomization employed for pharmaceuticals is supercritical fluid nebulization. The process uses carbon dioxide as an aerosolization aid, which permits drying at lower tem-peratures than usually needed in conventional spray drying [132]. Within the atomization system, supercritical carbon dioxide is intimately mixed with aqueous solutions containing API, often proteins or peptides. The outcome is the formation of microbubbles, which are rapidly dried in less than five seconds, resulting in dried particles predominately less than 3 mm in diameter [133,134]. This method is generally applied for the production of materials for pulmonary use or to achieve increased bioavailability [135].

6.6   ADVANCES IN SPRAY DRYING TECHNOLOGY

6.6.1   Electrostatic Spray Dryer

The incorporation of electrostatic technology is another significant recent advance in spray drying technology. An electrostatic spray dryer stratifies the components of the droplet during atomiza-tion, based on the polarities of the materials and hence creates the ideal drying conditions, leading to a near-perfect encapsulation of the active component without the use of high evaporation temperatures. Fluid Air's PolarDry electrostatic spray dry technology for solid dosage powder production is more energy-efficient, cost-effective, emission-reducing, and sustainable, and sig-nificantly improves the quality, stability, and shelf life of the final product [136]. For example, In the traditional spray dry process, a slurry is fed into a spray chamber where it is exposed to heated air and converted into a powder. This requires very high heat (+200°C), which contributes to active ingredient loss, degradation, or denaturalization. Conversely, electrostatic spray dry systems use significantly lower evaporation temperatures (ambient to 80°C), which protect active in-gredients [137].

Due to the intense heat required in traditional spray drying, APIs are lost, degraded, or denaturalized. To compensate, more of the API must be used in the formulation. For example, to formulate vitamin tablets, more of the raw ingredient—such as Vitamin B or Vitamin D—must be used at the start in order to retain potency for the final product to be effective.

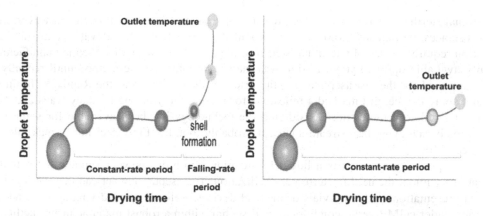

FIGURE 6.20 Drying curve of droplet temperature in: (left) conventional spray drying, and (right) electrostatic spray drying.
Source: From Ref. [138].

Because of the lower heat factor in electrostatic spray drying, more of the API is retained. In testing involving volatile components, approximately 20% of the active ingredient was lost during traditional spray drying. With electrostatic technology, processing of the same formula, a 98% active ingredient retention rate could be achieved. Requiring less raw materials, which results in considerable cost savings [137].

Beyond the obvious energy-saving factor resulting from highly reduced operating temperatures, a low-energy recirculating process minimizes emissions with safe non-reactive processing; nitrogen inertation. In traditional spray drying, the solvent becomes a vapor that cannot be released into the atmosphere without violating regulatory regulations designed to protect the environment. The vapor exhaust must be properly handled and is often burned off using a thermal oxidizer that requires a great deal of natural gas, not to mention the capital, operational, regulatory, and maintenance expense that is associated with this type of solvent handling equipment.

When spray drying is used to microencapsulate active or other components where, ideally, the carrier surrounds the active entirely as the solvent is dried off with the heated drying gas. The carrier acts as a protective layer around the active, protecting it from the outside environment, particularly oxygen, which keeps it from oxidizing. Traditionally, atomization in the spray dryer is achieved using a nozzle or rotary atomizer. An electrostatic spray dryer stratifies the components of the droplet during atomization, based on the polarities of the materials. Hence creates the ideal drying conditions, leading to a near-perfect encapsulation of the active component without the use of high evaporation temperatures [138].

Electrostatic spray drying allows water evaporation at significantly lower processing temperatures (from ambient to 80°C) compared to traditional spray drying. The comparison of the drying curves for the electrostatic and traditional spray dryers is shown schematically in Figure 6.20.

6.6.2 Aseptic Spray Dryer

Parenteral formulations are increasingly capturing a bigger share of the pharmaceutical market, driven by the booming biologics sector. The production of these injectables is, nonetheless, complicated and requires specialized equipment and facilities. The biggest challenge in aseptic processing is to maintain sterility especially if the manufacturing process involves novel or complex steps [139]. FDA, the European Medicines Agency (EMA), and the World Health Organization have laid out well-defined regulatory requirements for parenteral drug products.

Terminal sterilization is currently the preferred approach in drug manufacture. However, many drug substances, particularly biologics, cannot withstand exposure to the elevated temperatures or irradiation required as part of a terminal sterilization process. In such cases, aseptic manufacture is the only available option. Lyophilization was mainly the only aseptic method until recently the FDA's approval for the first aseptically spray dried product, which was the Raplixa® (fibrin sealant) and spray device, that marked a milestone for aseptic spray drying in many ways and was a significant regulatory milestone. Considering the technology has been available for some years without really achieving mainstream status, it probably took the FDA decision to make the real difference [140].

Aseptic spray drying converts a liquid formulation into a dry powder suitable for parenteral applications without the need for terminal sterilization. The aseptic powder can then be filled into different presentations including vials or medical devices. Reliable spray drying systems adopted to operate under cGMP sterile conditions are essential within a robust manufacturing facility. In-depth knowledge of aseptic manufacturing techniques will be essential to successfully maintain such a facility. However, in the spray drying of sterile powders, there are some concerns. These include the sterilization of the spray dryer, the source of air and its quality, the chamber temperatures, and the particle residence or contact time. In some cases, charring and product degradation have been found for small portions of a batch [139].

An example of aseptic spray drying is Nova's experience in scaling up the manufacturing process for Raplixa® (fibrin sealant), a spray dried product as mentioned earlier. This process was initially converted from a low-bioburden spray drying process to a fully aseptic spray drying process. It was subsequently scaled up from clinical trial manufacturing scale to commercial scale at our facilities. One of the main reasons for the cost difference is the mode of processing, (i.e., continuous processing helped to bring the unit cost down).

The particle-engineering capability of spray drying is an advantage over freeze-drying. Advances in liquid atomization and powder-collection technologies have enabled us to manufacture sterile powder with the desired characteristics. For example, by manipulating the surface area or morphology of spray dried particles, dissolution rates can be improved. This capability is, however, not available for a lyophilized product. If required, encapsulation or particle coating is another feature of spray drying that can facilitate different drug-release or dissolution profiles.

A spray dried product is by nature a powder. This characteristic allows the formulation to be powder-filled into final containers without further processing. A lyophilized product, on the other hand, will have to be milled or sieved first before undergoing the powder-filling step. Spray drying eliminates the need for additional milling or sieving step, thus reducing manufacturing costs. Quality concerns such as product uniformity can also be solved by spray drying. Spray dried powders can be engineered to have good flowability and compactability, which then enable easy filling into various containers including vials, pouches, and medical devices.

The stabilized products, using spray drying, are stable at 2°C–8°C or at room-temperature storage. This stability could be achieved because the drying method used was gentle to the product. During spray drying process optimization, the drying temperature can be adjusted to suit the sensitivity of the product. Other process parameters such as drying gas rate, atomization pressure, and product holding temperatures should be optimized to yield the best results.

6.6.3 Nanoscale Spray Dryers

In order to produce nanoscale particles via spray drying technology, some modifications to the experimental set-up of traditional spray dryers are necessary. A major constraint with the traditional spray dryers is the limited efficiency of separation and collection of submicron particles by cyclone separators. Typical cyclones are unable to collect particles below 2 μm. The median particle size cannot be reduced below 1.4 μm. In other words, submicron-sized particles cannot be collected using traditional spray dryers. The only feasible option for the collection of nanoparticles

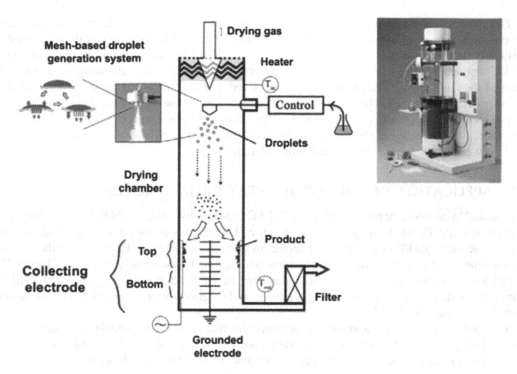

FIGURE 6.21   Schematic of the nano spray dryer B-90.
Source: From Ref. [141].

is to use electrostatic particle collectors. Another limitation is the turbulent gas flow in the drying chamber, which results in particle depositions on the chamber wall. Furthermore, traditional atomizers do not allow the fine droplets being generated to reach submicron particle sizes [141].

With the recent advances in nanospray drying technology, particles <1 μm can now be generated. The Nano Spray Dryer B-90 was introduced in 2009 to extend spray drying to the submicron scale. This laboratory spray dryer is based on a fundamentally new concept of spray drying technology, involving the fabrication of submicron particles from a solution, nano-emulsion, or nanosuspension. Its technological novelty lies in the gentle flow of laminar drying gas, the vibrating mesh spray technology to form fine droplets, and the highly efficient electrostatic precipitator to collect nanoparticles. A schematic of the Nano Spray Dryer B-90 is shown in Figure 6.21.

The droplet generation in the nanospray dryer is based on vibrating mesh technology which is incorporated in a spray head for nanospray drying. It includes a piezoelectric actuator driven by an electronic circuit. A small exchangeable spray cap is screwed onto the lower part of the spray head at a defined torque. This cap is made of a thin stainless steel mesh that is perforated with an array of precisely micron-sized holes. Spray meshes are available with orifice diameters of 4.0, 5.5, and 7.0 μm. A large number of holes are made in the thin membrane by laser drilling. These holes have a conical shape with a larger diameter toward the liquid supply side and the narrow diameter facing the droplet release side. By appropriate adjustment of the parameters during the drilling process, the mesh can be optimized for the production of droplets of a certain size. The drilling procedure determines the number and position of the nozzles, their tapered shape, and orifice size. The shape of the holes has been optimized for the creation of individual droplets. Plastic tubes connect the spray head to the feed reservoir. A peristaltic pump with variable speed circulates the fluid uniformly from the reservoir through the spray head to the spray mesh and back to the reservoir. This circulation mode enables efficient and continuous atomization.

The particle collection mechanism in the nanospray dryer is based on electrostatic charging, which, unlike cyclones, is independent of particle mass. The working principle of the electrostatic particle collector consists of the following basic steps: (1) generation of an electrical field of about 15 kV voltage between the discharge and collecting electrodes, (2) generation of negatively charged ions in the gas, (3) charging of the spray dried particles and (4) deflection of the particles to the collection electrode. The electrostatic particle collector in the nano spray dryer has a tubular shape. It comprises a stack of star-shaped discharge electrodes and a smooth cylindrical collecting electrode. A high voltage of about 15 kV is applied to the metallic cylinder to generate an electrical field between the discharge and the collecting electrodes.

6.7 APPLICATION OF QBD/PAT TO SPRAY DRYING PROCESS

The Scale-Up and Post-Approval Changes (SUPAC), Quality by Design (QbD)/Process Analytical Technology (PAT) are the subject matter of entire chapter 28, therefore, the focus of discussion here is not what QbD/PAT is but how it applies to spray drying process. However, for the sake of completeness of this section, there may be some overlapping between this section and Chapter 28.

"SUPAC: Manufacturing Equipment Addendum" states that although spray dryers may differ from one another in geometry, operating pressures, and other conditions, no spray dryer subclasses have been identified [142].

The QbD is a systematic approach to development that begins with predefined objectives and emphasizes product and process understanding and process control, based on sound science and quality risk management. QbD is emerging to enhance the assurance of safe, effective drug supply to the consumer, and also offers promise to significantly improve manufacturing quality performance. On the other hand, the PAT is defined as a system for designing, analyzing, and controlling manufacturing through timely measurements (i.e., during processing) of critical quality and performance attributes of raw and in-process materials and processes with the goal of ensuring final product quality [143]. It is important to note that the term "analytical" in PAT is viewed broadly to include chemical, physical, microbiological, mathematical, and risk analysis conducted in an integrated manner.

QbD normally starts in development and progresses through to manufacturing, with the intent of producing a control strategy for commercial-scale production. Sometimes, say, with a legacy product, QbD may start with an existing manufacturing process, for example, where a rich history of product and process knowledge is available. QbD can be applied to small and large molecules, to drug substance and drug product, to vaccines, to combination products, to all or parts of a process, to novel drugs, or generics. It can be used by leading companies, by contract research or contract manufacturing companies, or "virtual" companies. It is up to the particular organization to decide an appropriate level and application of QbD QbD can be applied nationally or internationally [144].

Understanding the science underpinning a product and its associated risks helps prioritize what is important for manufacturing and so normally leads to efficiency gains and cost benefits [145]

A typical systematic QbD approach to pharmaceutical product development should include the following phases as summarized as step-by-step algorithm in Figure 6.22:

- Begin with a target product profile that describes the use, safety, and efficacy of the product.
- Define a target product quality profile that will be used by formulators and process engineers as a quantitative surrogate for aspects of clinical safety and efficacy during product development.
- Gather relevant prior knowledge about the drug substance, potential excipients, and process operations into a knowledge space. Use risk assessment to prioritize knowledge gaps for further investigation.

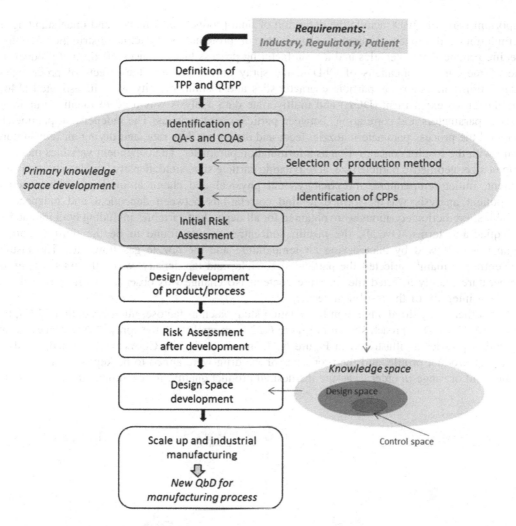

FIGURE 6.22 Overview of phases and elements a typical QbD approach.
Source: From Ref. [145].

- Design a formulation and identify the critical material (quality) attributes of the final product that must be controlled to meet the target product quality profile.
- Design a manufacturing process to produce a final product having these critical material attributes.
- Identify the critical process parameters and input (raw) material attributes that must be controlled to achieve these critical material attributes of the final product. Use risk assessment to prioritize process parameters and material attributes for experimental verification. Combine prior knowledge with experiments to establish a design space (DS) or other representation of process understanding.
- Establish a control strategy for the entire process that may include input material controls, process controls and monitors, DSs around individual or multiple unit operations, or final product tests. The control strategy should encompass expected changes in scale and can be guided by a risk assessment.
- Continually monitor and update the process to assure consistent quality.

Important parts of QBD include the definition of final product performance and understanding of formulation and process parameters. Inhalation of proteins for systemic distribution requires specific product characteristics and a manufacturing process that produces the desired product. In one of the early applications of QbD in the spray drying process, the effects of process and formulation parameters on particle characteristics and insulin integrity were investigated [146]. The design of experiment (DOE) and multivariate data analysis was used to identify important process parameters and correlations between particle characteristics. The independent parameters included the process parameters nozzle, feed, and drying air flow rate, and drying air temperature along with the insulin concentration as a formulation parameter. The dependent variables included droplet size, geometric particle size, aerodynamic particle size, yield, density, tap density, moisture content, outlet temperature, morphology, and physical and chemical integrity. The principal component analysis was performed to find correlations between dependent and independent variables. Prediction equations were obtained for all dependent variables including both interaction and quadratic terms. Overall, the insulin concentration was found to be the most important parameter, followed by inlet drying air temperature and the nozzle gas flow rate. The insulin concentration mainly affected the particle size, yield, and tap density, while the inlet drying air temperature mainly affected the moisture content. No change was observed in the physical and chemical integrity of the insulin molecule.

In another spray dried inhalation formulation study such as lactose, microcrystalline [149], the phases of the QbD approach shown in Figure 6.22 were applied to the spray drying process of an inhalation powder as illustrated in Figure 6.23. In this study, the CQAs were defined based on the target product profile, and the properties of the drug were aimed to be kept within an appropriate limit or range in order to assure the desired product quality, for example, purity, solid-state,

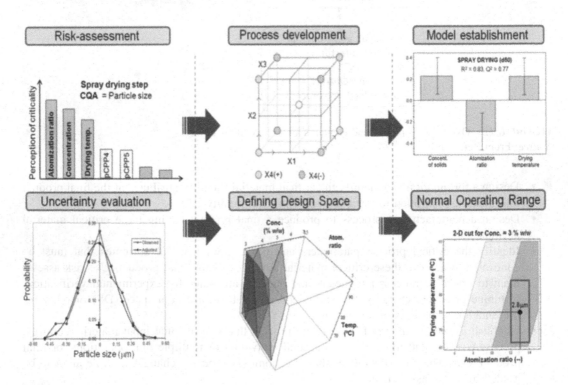

FIGURE 6.23 Application (main steps) of the general QbD approach to a spray drying process of an inhalation powder.
Source: From Ref. [147].

moisture content, and particle size. During the first risk assessment, and for each CQA, an analysis of the potential critical process parameters (pCPPs) and potential critical material attributes (pCMAs) was conducted with the aim to evaluate, in each process step, which operating parameters / raw materials have the potential to impact a CQA (within the known ranges) and, therefore, should be monitored or controlled. Since the number of parameters is usually high, this risk-assessment (based on prior knowledge of product/process) was used to rank the parameters in terms of the perception of criticality. The ultimate goal was to keep the development process as lean as possible, by focusing the studies on those parameters with a higher likelihood of being critical (atomization ratio, feed concentration, and drying temperature).

Often a statistical approach is followed through a sequence of designs of experiment (DoEs) with different objectives such as screening/ optimization and robustness studies. This development stage constitutes the core of the QbD methodology since most of the process knowledge is generated here and, although not mandatory, a statistical or mechanistic model is a usual outcome of this step.

Once the impact of the pCPPs/pCMAs is quantified on the CQAs, a feasible DS can be defined. The DS will consider the interactions between operating parameters and material attributes and will often be a multidimensional space as shown in Figure 6.23. Within the DS, the normal operating range (NOR) is established. This is the part of the DS where the process typically operates. When setting both these spaces, the error distributions that are associated with each prediction model should be considered in order to define statistical confidence levels. So, in Figure 6.23, the light gray shaded regions consider 90% of the error distribution, while darker shaded ones correspond to 95%, the latter being more constrained but also found to be more reliable (Figure 6.24).

Baldinger et al. [149] also utilized Ishikawa diagrams in a study to illustrate the influence of the processing parameters, inlet temperature, atomization air flow rate, and feed flow rate, on critical quality attributes of spray dried powders using DOE and concluded that although the particle size was influenced by both inlet temperature as well as atomization air flow rate, the yield mainly depended on the inlet temperature (Figure 6.25).

Maltesen et al. in their study of the spray drying process of insulin intended for pulmonary administration investigated, in particular, the effects of process and formulation parameters on particle characteristics and insulin integrity [146]. The DOE and multivariate data analysis were used to identify important process parameters and correlations between particle characteristics. The investigated process parameters were nozzle gas flow rate, feed flow rate, drying air flow rate, inlet drying air temperature, and insulin concentration. Insulin concentration was found to be the most important parameter for the powder characteristics, followed by the inlet drying air temperature and the nozzle gas flow rate. Feed flow rate and aspirator rate were not found significant. Insulin integrity was analyzed by RP-HPLC and SEC-HPLC, but no relationship was found between process parameters and degradation products. The results indicated that formulation parameters are at least as important as process parameters when spray drying proteins. In particular, parameters affecting the critical concentration are important when designing a proper process for spray drying proteins. The DOE and multivariate data analysis proved to be useful tools for QBD and was able to identify important parameters and variable correlations.

In a study to demonstrate the applicability of a Bayesian statistical methodology to identify the DS of a spray drying process [150], a predictive risk-based approach was set up in order to account for the uncertainties and correlations found in the process and in the derived critical quality attributes, such as the yield, the moisture content, the inhalable fraction of powder, the compressibility index, and the Hausner ratio. This allowed quantifying the guarantees and the risks to observe whether the process shall run according to specifications. These specifications describe satisfactory quality outputs and were defined a priori given safety, efficiency, and economical reasons. Within the identified DS, validation of the optimal condition was effectuated. The optimized process was shown to perform as expected, providing a product for which the quality is

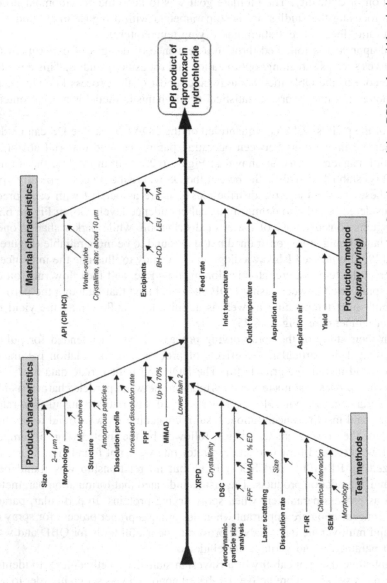

FIGURE 6.24 Ishikawa diagram illustrating the parameters influencing the quality of the ciprofloxacin containing DPI product. Abbreviations: DPI, dry powder inhalation; FPF, fine particle fraction; MMAD, mass median aerodynamic diameter; LEU, l-Leucine; FT-ir, Fourier-Transform infrared spectroscopy; PVA, polyvinyl alcohol.

Source: From Ref. [148].

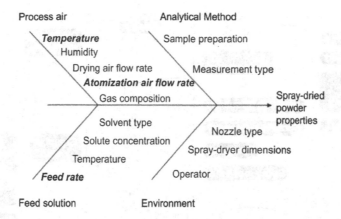

Process air   Analytical Method

Temperature   Sample preparation
    Humidity
    Drying air flow rate   Measurement type
    Atomization air flow rate
        Gas composition   Spray-dried
                                           powder
        Solvent type   properties
        Solute concentration   Nozzle type
        Temperature   Spray-dryer dimensions
    Feed rate   Operator

    Feed solution   Environment

FIGURE 6.25 Ishikawa diagram presenting causes that may affect the quality of the spray dried powder. *Source*: From Ref. [149].

built-in by the design and controlled setup of the equipment, regarding identified critical process parameters: the inlet temperature, the feed rate, and the spray flow rate.

It was concluded that when determining DS for a process such as spray drying, the use of the mean response surface optimization methodology is not recommended due to the inevitable uncertainties and interactions that are encountered. Accordingly, the data gathered through a well-designed experimental plan have been analyzed using a risk-based Bayesian predictive approach allowing the uncertainties and interactions to be integrated into a multivariate statistical model. These variabilities result in a minimum quality level that has been kept relatively low in order to be able to define a DS, that is, the guarantee of jointly observing the critical quality attributes within their acceptable limits is low. Even with this situation, these guarantees are quantified along with the risks of not observing such quality, jointly or marginally. The specifications have been designed such as providing a minimal satisfying quality for the whole process.

Kumar et al. [151] used the QbD approach to understand the spray drying process for the conversion of liquid nanosuspensions into solid nano-crystalline dry powders using indomethacin as a model drug. The effects of critical process variables, such as inlet temperature, flow, and aspiration rates on CQAs of particle size, moisture content, percent yield, and crystallinity, were investigated employing a full factorial design. Inlet temperature was identified as the only significant factor (p-value < 0.05) to affect dry powder particle size. Higher inlet temperatures caused drug surface melting and hence aggregation of the dried nano-crystalline powders. Aspiration and flow rates were identified as significant factors affecting yield (p-value < 0.05). Higher yields were obtained at higher aspiration and lower flow rates. All formulations had less than 3% (w/w) moisture content. Formulations dried at higher inlet temperatures had lower moisture compared to those dried at lower inlet temperatures.

Arpagaus et al. [150] recommended a framework use of a nanospray drying. In nano spray drying technology, the properties of the fabricated powder depend on the correlation and interdependency of the process parameters and formulation variables. Figure 6.26 illustrates the main adjustable process parameters and formulation variables for a nanospray dryer, as well as the outputs. The most important input parameters identified were the spray mesh size, the spray rate intensity, the solid concentration, the polymer and surfactant concentrations, the drying gas inlet temperature, the solvent type, and the drying gas flow rate. The effects on the particle size, product yield, and the amount of output produced per second are of primary importance. Other output parameters of interest are particle morphology, bioactive loading, controlled release profile, encapsulation efficiency, and stability. Table 6.3 also provides an overview of the main nanospray drying process parameters and presents their influence on the final powder characteristics. The

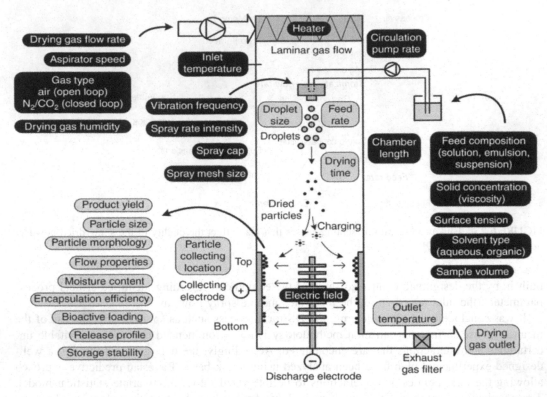

FIGURE 6.26 The main adjustable process parameters and formulation variables for a nano spray dryer (black), as well as the outputs (gray).
Source: From Ref. [152].

network of mutual interrelationships among the spray drying parameters for the conventional spray driers was also provided earlier in this chapter (Table 6.2).

In one of the early studies in applying PAT in the spray drying process, an in-line and at-line laser diffraction system was employed for monitoring the particle sizing during spray drying, and the particle size data were compared with those determined with offline laser diffraction and light microscopy [153].

The in-line laser diffraction system comprised the optical head, interface box, computer, and data analysis software. The optical head was directly connected in-line to the process stream. The main components used for the at-line laser diffraction system were the same as those used in the in-line system, except that for the at-line system, the laser module was not physically connected to the product flow stream. Instead, it was positioned adjacent to the spray dryer and worked as a separate system. Sampling and sizing were performed after the product had left the process stream (Figure 6.27). The system was found to be a rapid and convenient method, which provided instantaneous information about the particle size distribution of the microspheres (of maltodextrin and modified starch) as they were made. The at-line setup was reported to be superior to the in-line set up in this particular application. The workers pointed out the need for taking into account the cohesiveness of material measured and cautioned about the importance of the judicious data management and interpretation of results from PAT-enabled instruments to make valid conclusions.

In a recent study, a qualitative method of online NIR was developed to monitor the multi-component dissolution process and define the endpoint of spray drying solution preparation [154]. In this study, the NIR method was found to be capable of determining the endpoint of spray drying

TABLE 6.3
Nanospray Drying Process Parameter (Ref. 152)

Parameter	Drying gas flow rate ↑	Drying gas humidity ↑	Inlet temperature ↑	Spray mesh size ↑	Spray rate intensity ↑	Circulation pump rate ↑	Solid concentration (viscosity) ↑	Surfactant/ stabilizer in feed ↑	Solvent instead of water
Outlet temperature	⬆	↑	⬆	↑	⬇	—	↑	—	⬆
Droplet size	—	—	—	⬆	↑	↑	—	↓	↓
Particle size	—	—	↑	⬆	↑	↑	⬆	↓	↓
Feed rate	—	—	—	⬆	⬆	↑	⬇	↑	↑
Moisture content	⬇	⬆	↓	—	↓	—	↓	—	⬇
Yield Stability	—	↓	⬇	↑	⬇	↑	—	⬆	↑

⬆/⬇, Strong increasing/decreasing influence; ↑/↓, weak increasing/decreasing influence; —, minimal or no influence.

solution preparation with real-time NIR monitoring, and it was suggested that the qualitative method could be used for troubleshooting if an incorrect amount of material was added. Also, the quantitative NIR model demonstrated its capability of measuring the final solution composition based on the weight of materials added, accurately predicting the API concentration, which had also been verified by HPLC analysis of the resulting solid dispersion. The real-time measurement

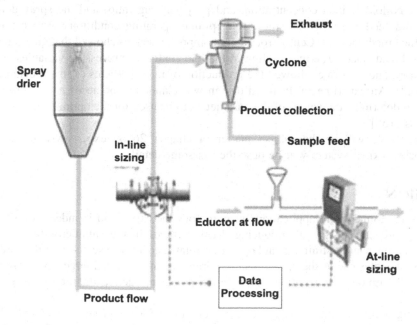

FIGURE 6.27 The layout of the spray dryer with the In-Line and At-Line laser diffraction setup. *Source*: From Ref. [154].

of batch composition via online NIR methods could improve the process control and quality as-surance of the spray drying solution preparation process.

One must bear in mind that the goal of PAT is to understand and control the manufacturing process and quality cannot be tested into products, but it should be built-in or should be by design. Therefore, the real-time monitoring (on-line or at-line measurements) or increase of process sample size or automated end-product testing alone does not qualify as PAT. The critical issue is the understanding of the spray drying process by applying the science and not regarding that as an art. Otherwise, what will be monitored in real-time will not necessarily ensure a quality product.

A process is generally considered well understood when all critical sources of variability are identified and explained; variability is managed by the process; and product quality attributes can be accurately and reliably predicted over the ranges of acceptance criteria established for materials used, process parameters, and manufacturing environmental and other conditions. The ability to predict reflects a high degree of process understanding.

In spray drying, some of the critical formulation and process factors are

1. material and feed properties (e.g., melting point of the material, feed type, solid content in the feed, and additives),
2. process variables (e.g., feed rate, atomizer type and speed, air pressure, and inlet and outlet gas temperatures), and
3. product specifications (e.g., moisture content, particle size, particle density, and flow characteristics).

The knowledge acquired for these factors during the structured product and process development studies can assure the quality of the spray dried product as one would expect an inverse re-lationship between the level of process understanding and the risk of producing a poor-quality product. In this respect, there were studies conducted before the publication of the FDA's PAT guidelines. An example of such a study involved the use of experimental factorial designs to investigate the effects of a number of formulation and process parameters on production yields and moisture contents of spray dried products. These factors concerned both the solution feed (drug concentration, colloidal silica concentration, and polymer/drug ratio) and the spray dryer (inlet temperature and feed rate). In this study, the optimal operating conditions were estimated by response surface methodology. Central rotational composite designs showed that quadratic models were found to be adequate. The results showed that the control of processing variables, especially inlet temperature and feed rate, allowed the production of microparticles of low moisture content with high yields. An experimental factorial design was claimed to be necessary before new pro-duction runs to determine the values of the parameters to be used for the optimization of the spray drying process [155].

Another example will be the subject matter of chapter 26 on expert systems in which a knowledge-based expert system will be described in some detail.

CONCLUSION

Spray drying has found many applications in numerous industries and is indeed a cost-effective manufacturing process capable of producing dried particles in the submicron-to-micron range despite its initial installation, training, and operation-related costs. The scale-up of the spray drying process is less troublesome as the operational requirements of small and large dryers are the same when compared with other conventional granulation processes such as the high-shear granulation method.

Spray drying, being a continuous process, is well suited for the production of bulk drug sub-stances and excipients. Using this process, the physical properties of the resulting product (e.g., particle size and shape, moisture content, and flow properties) can be controlled through the selection of equipment choices and manipulation of process variables; thus, the final spray dried particulate matter may not need further processing (wet or dry granulations) before compaction. Moreover, the ability to use different feedstocks and the high productivity and broad applications of this technique makes it more and more attractive to the scientific community.

Spray drying processes offer several advantages when solid-state properties of drug substances need to be modified. Using this process, solubility and dissolution rates of properties of poorly soluble materials can be increased by several folds and the stability of the amorphous form of the materials can be improved significantly. However, the advantages and drawbacks of spray drying parameters should be weighed in order to produce products with desirable characteristics. Such parameters should not be analyzed separately, but rather looked like a complex model, which as a whole contributes to the success of the spray drying process.

Because of its initial inherent costs, spray drying is not always considered as a processing option for many conventional formulations, especially for small batch size operations. However, when a specialized particle type is required by the active ingredient or dosage form, spray drying can become a feasible alternative to more conventional manufacturing processes. Such particle types include microcapsules, controlled-release particles, nanoparticles, and liposomes. The scalability and the cost-effectiveness of this manufacturing process in obtaining dried particles in submicron-to-micron scale favors an increasing variety of applications within the food, chemical, polymeric, pharmaceutical, biotechnology, and medical industries, as well.

The recent technological advances in spray drying process, such as nano-spray dryers, aseptic spray dryers, and electrostatic spray dryers, is contributing to the expansion of the spray drying to the areas that would not be possible or easy with the traditional spray dryers.

Lastly, the spray drying process matches the directives outlined in the QbD/PAT initiative currently being guided and championed by the FDA, and is well suited for continuous manufacturing, which is becoming more and more popular in the pharmaceutical industry.

ACKNOWLEDGMENT

We gratefully acknowledge the extensive contribution of Keith Masters whose handbook was referenced extensively as a leading text in the field. Also, one of the authors (Metin Çelik) appreciates the contribution of all coauthors to this chapter and assumes that any errors are his own and should not tarnish their reputation.

REFERENCES

1. Percy SR Improvement in drying and concentrating liquid substances by atomizing U.S. Patent 125,406. 9 April 1872.
2. Masters K Introduction. Spray Drying Handbook. 5th ed. Essex: Longman Scientific Technical, 1991:1–20.
3. Cal K, Sollohub K Spray drying technique. I: Hardware and process parameters. *Journal of Pharmaceutical Sciences* 2010; 99(2): 575–586. doi:10.1002/jps.21886
4. Parikh DM Advances in spray drying technology: new applications for a proven process. Am Pharm Rev 2008; 11(1):34–41.
5. Santos D, Maurício AC, Sencadas V, Santos JD, Fernandes MH, Gomes PS Spray drying: an overview. In Biomaterials – Physics and Chemistry, new edition. London: InTech, 2018.
6. Anandharamakrishnan C, Padma Ishwarya S *Spray-Drying for Food Ingredient Encapsulation*, 1st edition, John Wiley & Sons, 2015.
7. Sosnik A, Seremeta KP Advantages and challenges of the spray-drying technology for the production of pure drug particles and drug-loaded polymeric carriers. Advances in Colloid and Interface Science 2015; (223): 40–54. doi:10.1016/j.cis.2015.05.003.
8. Masters K Spray drying fundamentals: process stages and layouts. In: Spray Drying Handbook, 5th ed. Essex: Longman Scientific Technical, 1991:24.

9. GEA. GEA spray drying. https://www.gea.com/en/binaries/spray-drying-small-scale-pilot-plants-gea_tcm11-34874.pdf

10. https://www.freund-vector.com/technology/spay-drying/

11. Masters K Spray drying fundamentals: process stages and layouts. In: Spray Drying Handbook. 5th ed. Essex: Longman Scientific Technical, 1991:Pages 26, 199, 255.

12. Hede PD, Bach P, Jensen AD Two-fluid spray atomisation and pneumatic nozzles for fluid bed coating/agglomeration purposes: a review. Chemical Engineering Science 2008; 63(14): 3821–3842. doi:10.1016/j.ces.2008.04.014.

13. Salman AD, Hounslow MJ, Seville JPK Handbook of Powder Technology, Granulation. Amsterdam: Elsevier Publishing, 2007

14. Lefebvre AH Atomisation and Sprays. Washington: Hemisphere Publishing Corporation, 1989.

15. Kašpar O, Tokárová V, Nyanhongo GS, Gübitz G, Štěpánek F Effect of cross-linking method on the activity of spray-dried chitosan microparticles with immobilized laccase. Food and Bioproducts Processing 2013; 91(4): 525–533. doi:10.1016/j.fbp.2013.06.001

16. Dobre M, Bolle L Practical design of ultrasonic spray devices: experimental testing of several atomizer geometries. Experimental Thermal and Fluid Science 2002; 26:205–211.

17. Masters K The process stages of spray drying. In: Spray Drying Handbook, 5th ed. Essex: Longman Scientific Technical, 1991:268.

18. Dalmoro A, Barba AA, Lamberti G, d'Amore M Intensifying the microencapsulation process: Ultrasonic atomisation as an innovative approach. European Journal of Pharmaceutics and Biopharmaceutics 2012; 80: 471–477.

19. Anu Bhushani J, Anandharamakrishnan C Electrospinning and electrospraying techniques: Potential food based applications. Trends in Food Science and Technology 2014; 38(1): 21–33.

20. Masters K Spray drying fundamentals: process stages and layouts. In: Spray Drying Handbook. 5th ed. Essex: Longman Scientific Technical, 1991:31.

21. Masters K The process stages of spray drying. In: Spray Drying Handbook. 5th ed. Essex: Longman Scientific Technical, 1991:271.

22. Jain Manu S, Lohare Ganesh B, Chavan Randhir B, Barhate Shashikant D, Shah CB Spray drying in pharmaceutical industry: a review. Research Journal of Pharmaceutical Dosage Forms and Technology 2012; 4: 74–79.

23. Patel R, Patel M, Suthar A Spray drying technology: an overview. Indian Journal of Science and Technology 2009; 2(10): 44–47.

24. Fuzisaki Electric. Micro mist spray dryer. http://www.fujisaki-hest.com/product-description.html

25. Malchem. Closed cycle spray dryer. http://malchem.com.my/eng/10/a/np/products/dryer/closed-cycle-spray-dryer.html

26. Masters K Drying of droplets/sprays. In: Spray Drying Handbook, 5th ed. Essex: Longman Scientific Technical, 1991:309.

27. Boel, E, Koekoekx, R, Dedroog, S, Babkin, I, Vetrano, MR, Clasen, C, & Van den Mooter, G Unraveling particle formation: from single droplet drying to spray drying and electrospraying. Pharmaceutics 2020; 12(7): 625. doi:10.3390/pharmaceutics12070625

28. Masters K Drying of droplets/sprays. Spray Drying Handbook. 5th ed. Essex: Longman Scientific Technical, 1991:326.

29. Charlesworth DA, Marshall WR Evaporation for drops containing dissolved solids. AIChE J 1960; 6(1): 9–23.

30. Masters K Drying of droplets/sprays. Spray Drying Handbook. 5th ed. Essex: Longman Scientific Technical, 1991:345.

31. Adhikari B, Howes T, Lecomte D, Bhandari BR (2005). A glass transition temperature approach for the prediction of the surface stickiness of a drying droplet during spray drying. Powder Technology 2005; 149(2–3): 168–179. doi:10.1016/j.powtec.2004.11.007

32. Zbicinski I, Strumillo C, Delag A Drying kinetics and particle residence time in spray drying. Drying Technology 2002; 20(9): 1751–1768. doi:10.1081/drt-120015412

33. Iris Schmitz-Schug, Petra Foerst, Ulrich Kulozik. Impact of the spray drying conditions and residence time distribution on lysine loss in spray dried infant formula. Dairy Science & Technology, EDP sciences/Springer 2013; 93(4): 443–462. ff10.1007/s13594-013-0115-8ff. ffhal-01201427

34. Nandiyanto ABD, Okuyama K Progress in developing spray-drying methods for the production of controlled morphology particles: from the nanometer to submicrometer size ranges. Advanced Powder Technology 2011; 22(1): 1–19.

35. Shaw F Spray drying as a granulation technique. In: Parikh D M, ed. Handbook of Pharmaceutical Granulation Technology. New York: Marcel Dekker, 1997:93–96.
36. Filkova I, Weberschinke J Apparent viscosity of non-Newtonian droplet on the outlet of wheel atomizers. In: Mujumdar AS, ed. Drying '82. New York: McGrawHill, 1982:165–170.
37. Broadhead J, Rouan SK, Rhodes CT The spray drying of pharmaceuticals. Drug Dev Ind Pharm 1992; 18(11–12): 1169–1206.
38. Wendel SC, Çelik M An overview of spray-drying applications. Pharm Technol 1997; 21(10): 124–156.
39. Littringer, EM, Paus, R, Mescher, A, Schroettner, H, Walzel, P & Urbanetz, NA The morphology of spray dried mannitol particles – The vital importance of droplet size. Powder Technology 2013; 239: 162–174. doi:10.1016/j.powtec.2013.01.065 (2013)
40. Patel BB, Patel JK, Chakraborty S Review of patents and application of spray drying in pharmaceutical, food and flavor industry. Recnt Patents on Drug Delivery and Formulation 2014; 8: 63–78.
41. Sou T, Kaminskas LM, Nguyen TH, Carlberg R, McIntosh MP, Morton DA The effect of amino acid excipients on morphology and solid-state properties of multi-component spray-dried formulations for pulmonary delivery of biomacromolecules. European Journal of Pharmaceutics and Biopharmaceutics. doi:10.1016/j.ejpb.2012.10.015
42. Kadam KL Granulation Technology for Bioproducts. Boca Raton: FL CRC Press, 1990.
43. Fincher JH Particle size of drugs and its relationship to absorption and activity. J Pharm Sci 1968; 57(11): 1825–1835.
44. Kostewicz ES, Wunderlich M, Brauns U, Becker R, Bock T, Dressman JB. Predicting the precipitation of poorly soluble weak bases upon entry in the small intestine. J Pharm Pharmacol. 2004; 56(1): 43–51. doi:10.1211/0022357022511 PMID: 14980000.
45. Kawashima Y, Satio M, Takenaka H Improvement of solubility and dissolution rate of poorly water-soluble salicylic acid by a spray-drying technique. J Pharm Pharmacol 1975; 27: 1–5.
46. Pikal MJ, Lukes AL, Lang JE, Gaines K Quantitative crystallinity determinations for beta-lactam antibiotics by solution calorimetry: correlations with stability. J Pharm Sci. 1978; 67(6): 767–773. doi:10.1002/jps.2600670609.
47. Morris KR, Griesser UJ, Eckhardt CJ, Stowell JG Theoretical approaches to physical transformations of active pharmaceutical ingredients during manufacturing processes. Advanced Drug Delivery Reviews 2001; 48(1): 91–114. doi:10.1016/s0169-409x(01)00100-4
48. Junginger H, Wedler M Acta Pharm Technol 1984; 30(1): 68.
49. Corrigan OI, Holohan EM, Reilly MR Physicochemical properties of indomethacin and related compounds co-spray dried with polyvinyl-pyrrolidone. Drug Dev Ind Pharm. 1985; 11(2–3): 677–695.
50. Corrigan DO, Healy AM, Corrigan OI The effect of spray drying solutions of polyethylene glycol (PEG) and lactose/PEG on their physicochemical properties. Int J Pharm. 2002; 235(1–2): 193–205.
51. Berggren J, Alderborn G Effect of polymer content and molecular weight on the morphology and heat- and moisture-induced transformations of spray-dried composite particles of amorphous lactose and poly (vinylpyrrolidone). Pharm Res 2003; 20: 1039–1046.
52. Edwards DA, Hanes J, Caponetti G, Hrkach J, Ben-Jebria A, Eskew ML, Mintzes J, Deaver D, Lotan N, Langer R, Large porous particles for pulmonary drug delivery. Sci. 1997; 20;276(5320): 1868–1871. doi:10.1126/science.276.5320.1868. PMID: 9188534.
53. Xie T, Taylor LS. Effect of Temperature and Moisture on the Physical Stability of Binary and Ternary Amorphous Solid Dispersions of Celecoxib. J Pharm Sci. 2017; 106(1): 100–110. doi:10.1016/j.xphs.2016.06.017. Epub 2016 Jul 29. PMID: 27476771.
54. Sarode AL, Sandhu H, Shah N, Malick W, Zia H, Hot melt extrusion for amorphous solid dispersions: temperature and moisture activated drug-polymer interactions for enhanced stability. Mol Pharm 2013; 10(10): 3665–3675. doi:10.1021/mp400165b. Epub 2013 Sep 3. PMID: 23961978.
55. Lehmkemper K, Kyeremateng SO, Heinzerling O, Degenhardt M, Sadowski G. Long-Term Physical Stability of PVP- and PVPVA-Amorphous Solid Dispersions. Mol Pharm 2017; 14(1): 157–171. doi:10.1021/acs.molpharmaceut.6b00763. Epub 2016 Dec 7. PMID: 28043133.
56. Singh A, Van den Mooter, G Spray drying formulation of amorphous solid dispersions. Advanced Drug Delivery Reviews 2016; 100: 27–50. doi:10.1016/j.addr.2015.12.010
57. Paudel A, Worku ZA, Meeus J, Guns S, Van den Mooter, G Manufacturing of solid dispersions of poorly water soluble drugs by spray drying: formulation and process considerations. International Journal of Pharmaceutics 2013; 453: 253–284. doi:10.1016/j.ijpharm.2012.07.015
58. Paudel A, Van den Mooter G Influence of solvent composition on the miscibility and physical stability of naproxen/PVP K 25 solid dispersions prepared by cosolvent spray-drying. Pharmaceutical Research 2012; 29(1): 251–270.

59. Re MI Microencapsulation by spray drying. Drying Technol. 1998; 16(6): 1195–1236.
60. Wan LS, Heng PW, Chia CG Spray drying as a process for microencapsulation and the effect of different coating polymers. Drug Dev Ind Pharm. 1992; 18(9): 997–1011.
61. Sutinen R, Laasanen V, Paronen P, Urtti A pH-controlled silicone microspheres for controlled drug delivery. J Control Release 1995; 33: 163–171.
62. Palmieri GF, Wehrle P, Stamm A Evaluation of spray-drying as a method to prepare microparticles for controlled drug release. Drug Dev Ind Pharm. 1994; 20(18): 2859–2879.
63. Takeuchi H, Handa T, Kawashima Y Controlled release theophylline with acrylic polymers prepared by spray drying technique. Drug Dev Ind Pharm. 1989; 15(12): 1999–2016.
64. Pavanetto F, Genta I, Giunchedi P, Conti B Evaluation of spray drying as a method for polylactide and polylactide-co-glycolide microsphere preparation. J Microencapm. 1993; 10(4): 487–497.
65. Gonda I Targeting by deposition. In: Hickey AJ, ed. Pharmaceutical Inhalation Aerosol Technology. New York: Marcel Dekker, 1992:61–82.
66. Wan F, Maltesen MJ, Andersen SK, Bjerregaard S, Foged C, Rantanen J, Yang M One-step production of protein-loaded PLGA microparticles via spray drying using 3-fluid nozzle. Pharmaceutical Research 2014; 31: 1967–1977. doi:10.1007/s11095-014-1299-1.
67. Kauppinen A, Broekhuis J, Grasmeijer N, Tonnis W, Ketolainen J, Frijlink HW, Hinrichs, WLJ Efficient production of solid dispersions by spray drying solutions of high solid content using a 3-fluid nozzle. European Journal of Pharmaceutics and Biopharmaceutics 2018; 123: 50–58. doi:10.1016/j.ejpb.2017.11.009
68. Leng D, Thanki K, Foged C, Yang, M Formulating inhalable dry powders using two-fluid and three-fluid nozzle spray drying. Pharmaceutical Research 2018; 35: 247. doi:10.1007/s11095-018-2509-z
69. Kondo K, Niwa T, Danjo K Preparation of sustained-release coated particles by novel micro-encapsulation method using three-fluid nozzle spray drying technique. European Journal of Pharmaceutical Sciences 2014; 51: 11–19. doi:10.1016/j.ejps.2013.09.001
70. Corrigan DO, Corrigan OI, Healy AM Predicting the physical state of spray dried composites: salbutamol sulphate/lactose and salbutamol sulphate/polyethylene glycol co-spray dried systems. Int J Pharm 2004; 273(1–2): 171–182.
71. Vidgren P, Vidgren M, Pronen P, Vainio P, Nuutinen J. Nasal distribution of radioactive drug administered using two dosage forms. Eur J Drug Metab Pharmacokinet. 1991; 3:426–432.
72. Vehring R Pharmaceutical particle engineering via spray drying. Pharmaceutical Research 2008; 25: 999–1022. doi:10.1007/s11095-007-9475-1
73. Vehring R, Foss WR, Lechuga-Ballesteros D Particle formation in spray drying. Journal of Aerosol Science 2007; 38: 728–746. doi:10.1016/j.jaerosci.2007.04.005
74. Elversson J, Millqvist-Fureby A, Alderborn G, Elofsson U. Droplet and particle size relationship and shell thickness of inhalable lactose particles during spray drying. J Pharm Sci. 2003; 92, 900–910.
75. Dunbar CA, Concessio NM, Hickey AJ Evaluation of atomizer performance in production of respirable spray-dried particles. Pharm Dev Technol. 1998; 3(4): 433–441.
76. Sibum I, Hagedoorn P, de Boer AH, Frijlink HW, Grasmeijer F Challenges for pulmonary delivery of high powder doses. International Journal of Pharmaceutics 2018; 548: 325–336. doi:10.1016/j.ijpharm.2018.07.008
77. O'hara P, Hickey AJ Respirable PLGA microspheres containing rifampicin for the treatment of tuberculosis: manufacture and characterization. Pharmaceutical Research 2000; 17(8): 955–961.
78. Verma RK et al. Inhaled microparticles containing clofazimine are efficacious in treatment of experimental tuberculosis in mice. Antimicrobial Agents and Chemotherapy 2013; 57(2): 1050–1052.
79. Suarez S Airways delivery of rifampicin microparticles for the treatment of tuberculosis. Journal of Antimicrobial Chemotherapy 2001; 48(3): 431–434. doi:10.1093/jac/48.3.431
80. Misra A et al. Inhaled drug therapy for treatment of tuberculosis. Tuberculosis 2011; 91(1): 71–81.
81. Kaur J et al. A hand-held apparatus for "nose-only" exposure of mice to inhalable microparticles as a dry powder inhalation targeting lung and airway macrophages. European Journal of Pharmaceutical Sciences 2008; 34: 56–65. doi:10.1016/j.ejps.2008.02.008
82. Garcia-Contreras L et al. Inhaled large porous particles of capreomycin for treatment of tuberculosis in a guinea pig model. Antimicrobial Agents and Chemotherapy 2007; 51(8): 2830–2836. doi:10.1128/aac.01164-06
83. Sharma R et al. Inhalable microparticles containing drug combinations to target alveolar macrophages for treatment of pulmonary tuberculosis. Pharmaceutical Research 2001; 18(10): 1405–1410.
84. Muttil P et al. Inhalable microparticles containing large payload of anti-tuberculosis drugs. European Journal of Pharmaceutical Sciences 2007; 32: 140–150. doi:10.1016/j.ejps.2007.06.006

85. Dharmadhikari AS et al. Phase I, single-dose, dose-escalating study of inhaled dry powder capreomycin: a new approach to therapy of drug-resistant tuberculosis. Antimicrob Agents Chemother 2013; 57: 2613–2619. doi:10.1128/AAC.02346-12

86. Parkins, Michael D, Elborn JS. Tobramycin Inhalation Powder™: a novel drug delivery system for treating chronic Pseudomonas aeruginosa infection in cystic fibrosis. Expert Review of Respiratory Medicine 2011; 5(5): 609–622.

87. Geller DE, Weers J, Heuerding S Development of an inhaled dry-powder formulation of tobramycin using PulmoSphere technology. Journal of Aerosol Medicine and Pulmonary Drug Delivery 2011; 24: 175–182 doi:10.1089/jamp.2010.0855

88. Goldbach P, Brochart H, Stamm A Spray-drying of liposomes for a pulmonary administration. Part 1. Chemical stability of phospholipids. Drug Dev Ind Pharm. 1993; 19(19): 2611–2622.

89. Goldbach P, Brochart H, Stamm A Spray-drying of liposomes for a pulmonary administration. Part 2. Retention of encapsulated materials. Drug Dev Ind Pharm. 1993; 19(19): 2623–2636.

90. Patil-Gadhe A, Pokharkar V Single step spray drying method to develop proliposomes for inhalation: a systematic study based on quality by design approach. Pulm. Pharmacol. Ther. 2014; 27: 197–207.

91. Rojanarat W et al. Isoniazid proliposome powders for inhalation-preparation, characterization and cell culture studies. Int. J. Mol. Sci. (2011) 12: 4414–4434.

92. Khatib I et al. Formation of ciprofloxacin nanocrystals within liposomes by spray drying for controlled release via inhalation. International Journal of Pharmaceutics 2020; 578: 119045.

93. Costantino HR et al. Effect of mannitol crystallization on the stability and aerosol performance of a spray-dried pharmaceutical protein, recombinant humanized anti-IgE monoclonal antibody. Journal of Pharmaceutical Sciences 1998 87(11): 1406–1411. doi:10.1021/js9800679

94. Broadhead J, Ruan SK, Rhodes CT The effect of process and formulation variables on the properties of spray dried b-galactosidase. J Pharm Pharmacol. 1994; 46: 458–467.

95. Kumru OS et al. Vaccine instability in the cold chain: mechanisms, analysis and formulation strategies. Biologicals: Journal of the International Association of Biological Standardization 2014; 42, 237–259. doi:10.1016/j.biologicals.2014.05.007

96. Price DN, Kunda NK, McBride AA, Muttil P Vaccine preparation: past, present, and future. In: Hickey AJ, Misra A, Fourie PB, ed. Delivery Systems for Tuberculosis Prevention and Treatment. United Kingdom: John Wiley & Sons, 2016; 67–90.

97. Saboo S et al. Optimized formulation of a thermostable spray-dried virus-like particle Vaccine against human papillomavirus. Molecular Pharmaceutics 2016; 13: 1646–1655. doi:10.1021/acs.molpharmaceut.6b00072

98. Kunda NK et al. Evaluation of the thermal stability and the protective efficacy of spray-dried HPV vaccine, Gardasil(R) 9. Hum Vaccin Immunother 2019. doi:10.1080/21645515.2019.1593727

99. Kunda NK, Wafula D, Tram M, Wu TH, Muttil, P A stable live bacterial vaccine. European Journal of Pharmaceutics and Biopharmaceutics 2016; 103: 109–117. doi:10.1016/j.ejpb.2016.03.027

100. Price DN, Kunda N, Muttil P Challenges associated with the pulmonary delivery of therapeutic dry powders for preclinical testing. KONA Powder and Particle Journal 2019: 1–16. doi:10.14356/kona.2019008

101. Subaiya S et al. Global routine vaccination coverage, 2014. Morbidity and Mortality Weekly Report 2015; 64(44): 1252–1255.

102. World Health Organization (WHO). Monitoring vaccine wastage at country level: guidelines for program managers. Geneva, 2005.

103. Maa Y, Nguyen P, Sweeney T, Shire SJ, Hsu CC Protein Inhalation Powders: Spray Drying vs Spray Freeze Drying. Pharm Res. 1999; 16: 249–254. https://doi.org/10.1023/A:1018828425184

104. Sevelle PC, Kellay LW, Birchall JC Preparation of dry powder dispersions for non-viral gene delivery by freeze-drying and spray-drying. J Gene Med. 2002; 4: 428–437.

105. Maa YF, Prestrelski SJ Biopharmaceutical powders: particle formation and formulation considerations. Curr Pharm Biotechnol. 2000; 1: 283–302.

106. Buttini F, Soltani A, Colombo P, Marriott C, Jones SA Multilayer PVA adsorption onto hydrophobic drug substrates to engineer drug-rich microparticles. European Journal of Pharmaceutical Sciences 2008; 33(1), 20–28. doi:10.1016/j.ejps.2007.09.008

107. Cilurzo F et al. Fast-dissolving mucoadhesive microparticulate delivery system containing piroxicam. Eur J Pharm Sci. 2005; 24:355–361.

108. Ahuja A, Khar RP, Ali J Muchoadhesive drug delivery systems. Drug Dev Ind Pharm. 1997; 23: 489–515.

109. Aranaz I, Paños I, Peniche C, Heras Á, Acosta, N Chitosan spray-dried microparticles for controlled delivery of venlafaxine hydrochloride. Molecules 2017; 22(11): 1980. doi:10.3390/molecules22111980
110. Strob R et al. Preparation and characterization of spray-dried submicron particles for pharmaceutical application, Advanced Powder Technology 2018; 29: 2920–2927.
111. Lee J Drug nano-and microparticles processed into solid dosage forms: physical properties. J Pharm Sci. 2003; 92(10): 2057–2068.
112. Muller-Mehnert RH, Lucks JS, Schwarz C Solid lipid nanoparticles (SLN)-alternative colloidal carrier system for controlled drug delivery. Eur J Pharm Biopharm. 1995; 41(1): 62–69.
113. Sham JO-H, Zhang Y, Finlay WH, Roa WH, Löbenberg, R Formulation and characterization of spray-dried powders containing nanoparticles for aerosol delivery to the lung. International Journal of Pharmaceutics 2004; 269(2): 457–467. doi:10.1016/j.ijpharm.2003.09.041
114. Demir MG, Degim IT Preparation of Chitosan Nanoparticles by Nano Spray Drying Technology. FABAD J. Pharm. Sci. 2013; 38(3): 127–133.
115. Tewa-Tagne P, Degobert G, Briançon S et al. Spray-drying nanocapsules in presence of colloidal silica as drying auxiliary agent: formulation and process variables optimization using experimental designs. Pharm Res. 2007; 24: 650–661. https://doi.org/10.1007/s11095-006-9182-3
116. Müller et al. Preparation and characterization of spray-dried polymeric nanocapsules. Drug Development and Industrial Pharmacy 2000; 26(3): 343–347. doi:10.1081/ddc-100100363
117. Schafroth N, Arpagaus C, Jadhav UY, Makne S, Douroumis D Nano and microparticle engineering of water insoluble drugs using a novel spray-drying process. Colloids and Surfaces B: Biointerfaces 2012 90: 8–15. doi:10.1016/j.colsurfb.2011.09.038
118. Cordin A Pharmaceutical particle engineering via nano spray drying – process parameters and application examples on the laboratory-scale. International Journal of Medical Nano Research 2018; 5: 026.
119. Ngan LTK et al. Preparation of chitosan nanoparticles by spray drying, and their antibacterial activity. Research on Chemical Intermediates 2014; 40(6): 2165–2175. doi:10.1007/s11164-014-1594-9
120. Sun W, Ni R, Zhang X, Li LC, Mao S. Spray drying of a poorly water-soluble drug nanosuspension for tablet preparation: formulation and process optimization with bioavailability evaluation. Drug Dev. Ind. Pharm. 2015; 41: 927–933. doi:10.3109/03639045.2014.914528.
121. Kim DCK, Soon YS Development of digoxin dry elixir as a novel dosage form using a spray-drying technique. J Microencap. 1995; 12(5): 547–566.
122. Takeuchi H et al. Design of redispersible dry emulsion as an advanced dosage form of oily drug (vitamin E nicotinate) by spray-drying technique. Drug Development and Industrial Pharmacy 1992. 18(9): 919–937. doi:10.3109/03639049209069307
123. Choi J-Y et al. Development of coated nifedipine dry elixir as a long acting oral delivery with bioavailability enhancement. Archives of Pharmacal Research 2011; 34(10): 1711–1717. doi:10.1007/s12272-011-1015-1
124. Timmington H Improved aspirin. Chem Drug 1973; 63: 482–483.
125. Saleh SI, Boymond C, Stamm, A Preparation of direct compressible effervescent components: spray-dried sodium bicarbonate. International Journal of Pharmaceutics 1998; 45(1-2): 19–26. doi:10.1016/0378-5173(88)90030-0.
126. Ely L, Roa W, Finlay WH, Löbenberg, R Effervescent dry powder for respiratory drug delivery. European Journal of Pharmaceutics and Biopharmaceutics 2007; 65(3): 346–353. doi:10.1016/j.ejpb.2006.10.021
127. Oktavia DA, Ayudiarti DL, Febrianti D. Physical properties of the probiotic effervescent tablet from tapioca and maltodextrin coatings. E3S Web of Conferences 2020; 147: 03024. doi:10.1051/e3sconf/202014703024
128. Killen MJ Process of spray drying and spray congealing. Pharm Eng. 1993; 13: 58–62.
129. Eldem T, Speiser P, Altorfer H Polymorphic behavior of sprayed lipid micropellets and its evaluation by differential scanning calorimetry and scanning electron microscopy. Pharm Res. 1991; 8: 178–184.
130. Eldem T, Speiser P, Hincal A Optimization of spray-dried and -congealed lipid micropellets and characterization of the surface morphology by scanning electron microscopy. Pharm Res. 1991; 8(1): 47–54.
131. Mumenthaler M, Leuenberger H Atmospheric spray-freeze drying: suitable alternative in freeze dry technology. Int J Pharm. 1991; 72: 97–110.
132. Sievers RE et al. Low-temperature manufacturing of fine pharmaceutical powders with supercritical fluid aerosolization in a Bubble Dryer®. Pure and Applied Chemistry 2001; 73(8): 1299–1303. doi:10.1351/pac200173081299

133. Sievers RE, Karst U Methods for fine particle formation. U.S. Patent 5,639,441, June 1997.
134. Sievers RE, Karst U Methods and apparatus for fine particle formation. U.S. Patent 6,095,134, August 2000.
135. Sievers, RE Formation of aqueous small droplet aerosols assisted by supercritical carbon dioxide. Aerosol Science and Technology 1999; 30(1): 3–15. doi:10.1080/027868299304840
136. Fluid Air. Electrostatic spray drying. https://www.fluidairinc.com/encapsulation.html#undefined2
137. Szcza, JP The future is now: cooling the spray dry & microencapsulation process. Pharmaceutical Processing World. May 12, 2017. https://www.pharmaceuticalprocessingworld.com/the-future-is-now-cooling-the-spray-dry-microencapsulation-process/
138. Dokmak A, Barton B, Zisu B, Le, NL and Maudhuit, A, Gentle drying for probiotics products. https://www.vitafoodsinsights.com/sites/vitafoodsinsights.com/files/Spraying%20Systems%20-%20Fluid%20Air%20Poster.pdf
139. Siew A Exploring the use of aseptic spray drying in the manufacture of biopharmaceutical injectables. Pharmaceutical Technology 2016; 40(7): 24–27.
140. De Costa, S A green light for cGMP aseptic spray drying. 2016. https://www.manufacturingchemist.com/news/article_page/A_green_light_for_cGMP_aseptic_spray_drying/114844
141. Li X, Anton N, Arpagaus C, Belleteix F, Vandamme, TF Nanoparticles by spray drying using innovative new technology: the Büchi Nano Spray Dryer B-90. Journal of Controlled Release 2010; 147(2): 304–310. doi:10.1016/j.jconrel.2010.07.113
142. Department of Health and Human Services. SUPAC: manufacturing equipment addendum. 2014. https://www.fda.gov/media/85681/download
143. U.S. Department of Health and Human Services, Food and Drug Administration, Center for Drug Evaluation and Research (CDER), Center for Veterinary Medicine (CVM), Office of Regulatory Affairs (ORA). Guidance for industry: PAT—a framework for innovative pharmaceutical development, manufacturing, and quality assurance. September 2004.
144. Davis, B and Schlindwein, WS Introduction to quality by design (QbD) in Schlindwein, WS and Gibson M eds. Pharmaceutical Quality by Design: A Practical Approach. John Wiley & Sons Ltd, 2018:7–8.
145. Pallagi E, Karimi K, Ambrus R, Szabó-Révész P, Csóka, I New aspects of developing a dry powder inhalation formulation applying the quality-by-design approach. International Journal of Pharmaceutics 2016; 511(1): 151–160. doi:10.1016/j.ijpharm.2016.07.003
146. Maltesen MJ, Bjerregaard S, Hovgaard L, Havelund S, van de Weert M Quality by design – spray drying of insulin intended for inhalation. European Journal of Pharmaceutics and Biopharmaceutics 2008; 70(3): 828–838. doi:10.1016/j.ejpb.2008.07.015
147. Costa E, Neves F, Andrade G, Winters C Scale-up & QBD approaches for spray-dried inhalation formulations. ONdrugDelivery Magazine June 2014; Issue 50: 3–8.
148. Karimi K, Pallagi E, Szabó-Révész P, Csóka I, Ambrus, R Development of a microparticle-based dry powder inhalation formulation of ciprofloxacin hydrochloride applying the quality by design approach. Drug Design, Development and Therapy 2016; (10): 3331–3343. doi:10.2147/dddt.s116443
149. Baldinger A, Clerdent L, Rantanen J, Yang M, Grohganz H Quality by design approach in the optimization of the spray-drying process. Pharmaceutical Development and Technology 2011; 17(4): 389–397. doi:10.3109/10837450.2010.550623
150. Lebrun P et al. Design space approach in the optimization of the spray-drying process. European Journal of Pharmaceutics and Biopharmaceutics 2012; 80(1): 226–234. doi:10.1016/j.ejpb.2011.09.014
151. Kumar S, Gokhale R, Burgess DJ Quality by Design approach to spray drying processing of crystalline nanosuspensions. International Journal of Pharmaceutics 2014; 464(1–2): 234–242. doi:10.1016/j.ijpharm.2013.12.039
152. Arpagaus C, John P, Collenberg A, Rütti D Nanocapsules formation by nano spray drying. Nanoencapsulation Technologies for the Food and Nutraceutical Industries 2017; 346–401. doi:10.1016/b978-0-12-809436-5.00010-0
153. Chan L, Tan L, Heng P Process analytical technology: application to particle sizing in spray drying. AAPS Pharm Sci Technol. 2008; 9(1): 259–266.
154. Lee Y-C, Zhou G, Ikeda C, Chouzouri G, Howell, L Application of online NIR for process understanding of spray-drying solution preparation. Journal of Pharmaceutical Sciences. doi:10.1016/j.xphs.2018.10.022
155. Billon A, Bataille B, Cassanas G, Jacob, M Development of spray-dried acetaminophen microparticles using experimental designs. International Journal of Pharmaceutics 2000; 203(1–2): 159–168. doi:10.1016/s0378-5173(00)00448-8

7 Emerging Technologies for Particle Engineering

Dilip M. Parikh

CONTENTS

7.1 INTRODUCTION

Particles are an important part of many dosage forms and viewed as a carrier of drugs. Their size, shape, crystalline form, and structure directly affect the stability and releasing pattern of drugs. The constant requirement for the targeted delivery of therapeutically active agents has been the key driver in particle engineering and processing within the pharmaceutical sector. Particles are making particular advances in the area of human healthcare where they are being used to diagnose illnesses, cure cancer, deliver drugs, and retard aging. Particle science is becoming recognized as an enabling technology that helps us create new energy sources, clean our air and water, and build stronger and lighter materials. These increasingly complex agents are posing greater challenges to formulators because of their solubility, stability, and other physicochemical properties.

'Particle engineering' is a term coined to encompass means of producing particles having a defined morphology, particle size distribution, and composition. Generally, particle engineering is associated with particle size reduction techniques, such as media milling and homogenization, and micro- or nanoparticle formation techniques, such as spray-drying, supercritical fluid technologies, and precipitation. Recent additions to the pharmaceutical particle engineering technology include spray-freezing into cryogenic liquids, template emulsion, and self-assembly. Particle characterization and engineering can identify optimal particle size, provide a more thorough understanding of the drug, and point to bioavailability enhancement options through particle reduction processes. While advanced technologies for enhancing the delivery of poorly soluble drugs have included using polymorphic engineering, solid-dispersions, microemulsions, self-emulsifying systems, complexation, and liposomes, a truly particle engineering-based solution remains particularly desirable to the pharmaceutical industry. Nanoparticles fall into a size range similar to proteins and other macromolecular structures found inside living cells. As such, nanomaterials are poised to take advantage of existing cellular machinery to facilitate the delivery of drugs. Effective particle engineering depends on the achievement of three primary activities: target identification, knowledge gathering, and process control. Appropriate target identification ensures a high yield of a high-quality product that is produced as the desired polymorph with the desired particle properties. Successful knowledge gathering generates information about various particle characteristics, solubilities, the metastable zone, and the supersaturation properties of an active pharmaceutical ingredient (API). Implementation of appropriate controls leads to the development of an optimal solvent system, crystallization or milling/micronization processes, and the establishment of appropriate physical analytics. In this chapter, we will review current technologies and upcoming particle engineering technologies that may change the way we produce solid dosage forms.

7.2 NANOTECHNOLOGY

7.2.1 INTRODUCTION

Nanotechnology is the science and technology at the nanoscale, which is about 1 to 100 nanometers and it can be used across the entire spectrum of scientific fields including life sciences and healthcare [2] The prefix "nano" means 10^{-9}, or one-billionth and is about a thousand times smaller than a micron. Depending on the atom, approximately three to six atoms can fit inside of a nanometer. Nanoparticles possess many special physical, chemical, and biological properties. They have found applications in diverse fields, including materials synthesis and processing, dispersions and coatings, fuel cells and sensors, biotechnology and health effects, energy and environment, instruments and probes, and studies of fundamental transfer processes. Recent developments in nanoscience, combining physics, chemistry, material science, theory, and biosciences, have brought us to another level of understanding of "nanotechnology." The systems provide methods for targeting and releasing therapeutic compounds in very defined regions. These vehicles have the potential to eliminate or at least ameliorate many problems associated with drug distribution. Below 100 nm, materials exhibit different, more desirable physical, chemical, and biological properties. Given the enormity and immediacy of the unmet needs of therapeutic areas such as CNS disorders, this can lead to drugs that can extend the life and save untimely deaths [3].

The nanosystems are providing a viable alternative for drugs such as liposomes, polymeric micelles, and Nanoparticulate Drug Delivery Systems (NPDDSs). With recent advances in polymer and surface conjugation techniques as well as microfabrication methods, perhaps the greatest focus in drug-delivery technology is in the design and applications of nanoparticulate systems because of its ability for site-specific delivery of drugs such as proteins, peptides, and oligonucleotides. Many nanoparticulate systems provide both hydrophobic and hydrophilic environments, which facilitate drug solubility.

Recent advances in the ability to structure material on the nanometer size scale offer the pharmaceutical industry a new toolset: (i) high potency drugs can be made into small controlled release spheres, which can survive in the body for a long period and slowly release their payload keeping a steady safe concentration in the body; (ii) low solubility (lipophilic) compounds can be made into nano-sized spheres, which will have a very high surface area to volume ratio for improved solubility; (iii) nano-sized drug carriers can be surface modified with specific proteins to target specific areas of uptake and greatly reduce the occurrence of side effects. One of the most promising applications of nanoparticles is their use for the transport of drugs across the blood-brain barrier. This barrier represents an insurmountable obstacle for a large number of drugs, including anticancer drugs, antibiotics, and a variety of central nervous system (CNS)-active drugs, especially neuropeptides. The constant requirement for the targeted delivery of therapeutically active agents has been the key driver in particle engineering and processing within the pharmaceutical sector. Table 7.1 details representative examples of nanocarrier-based drugs in the market.

The commercialization of nanotechnology in pharmaceutical and medical science has made great progress. Taking the USA alone as an example, at least 15 new pharmaceuticals approved since 1990 have utilized nanotechnology in their design and drug delivery systems. Table 7.1 shows different drugs and indications of the drugs with the incorporation of nanotechnology.

TABLE 7.1
Representative Examples of Nanocarrier-Based Drugs in the Market

Type of Nanostructure	Brand Name	Active Ingredient	Indications
Nanocrystalline drugs	Rapamune®	Rapamycin	Immunosuppressive
	Emend®	Aprepitant	Anti-emetic
	Tricor®	Fenofibrate	Hypercholesterolemia
	Megace®	Megestrol	Anti-anorexia
Liposomes	AmBisome®	Amphotericin B	Fungal infections
	Doxil®	Doxorubicin	Ovarian cancer, Kaposi's sarcoma, and breast cancer
	Caelyx®	Doxorubicin	Ovarian cancer, Kaposi's sarcoma, and breast cancer
	Depocyt®	Cytarabine	Lymphomatous meningitis
	Daunoxome®	Daunorubicin	Kaposi's sarcoma
Polymer-drug conjugates	Adagen®	Adenosine deaminase	Adenosine deaminase enzyme deficiency
	Onscaspar®	L-asparaginase	Acute lymphoblastic leukemia
	Pegasys®	PEGylated IFN-α-2a	Hepatitis C
Polymeric micelles	Genexol-PM®	Paclitaxel	Cancer chemotherapy
Protein (albumin) nanoparticles	Abraxane®	Paclitaxel	Metastatic breast cancer
Lipid colloidal dispersion	Amphotec®	Amphotericin B	Fungal infections

Source: From Ref. [1].
PEG: Polyethylene glycol.

Research in the use of nanotechnology for regenerative medicine spans several application areas, including bone and neural tissue engineering. For instance, novel materials can be engineered to mimic the crystal mineral structure of human bone or used as a restorative resin for dental applications. Researchers are looking for ways to grow complex tissues with the goal of one-day growing human organs for transplant. Researchers are also studying ways to use graphene nanoribbons to help repair spinal cord injuries; preliminary research shows that neurons grow well on the conductive graphene surface.

7.2.2 Manufacture of Nanoparticles

Nanoparticles manufacturing is a field of science, which aims to control individual atoms and molecules to create material that has a size of only a few nanometers. The systems provide methods for targeting and releasing therapeutic compounds in very defined regions. There are wide varieties of techniques that are capable of creating nanostructures with various degrees of quality, speed, and cost. These approaches fall under two categories bottom-up and top-down. Both the processes just like dry and wet granulations generate materials with different properties. Broadly, there are two basic methods to manufacture nanoparticles:

1. A "bottom-up approach" (i.e., precipitation of drug from a solvent to an antisolvent system) [4]
2. A "top-down approach" (i.e., milling/grinding of the particles to achieve the required size)

The bottom-up process has significant similarities with the granulation process, which includes the building of nanostructures molecule by molecule. This can be accomplished by chemical synthesis, self-assembly, and positional assembly. These processes allow customizing the molecular granulation process to produce nano-material with surface-enhanced properties. The bottom-up approach is less time consuming and usually leads to amorphous particles due to fast evaporation of the solvent and thus precipitation of the API as amorphous particles.

Top-down manufacturing process requires a larger piece of material and etching, milling, or machining a nanostructure from it by removing material. Top-down methods offer reliability and device complexity. These processes are higher in energy usage, and usually lead to crystalline product and produce more waste than the bottom-up methods and limit surface modifications of nanomaterials. Currently, amorphous drugs are formulated in the form of solid dispersions, which are in the micron-size range, using different techniques such as spray drying, freeze-drying, or hot-melt extrusion. Stabilization of amorphous drug nanoparticles can be achieved by the presence of stabilizers such as polymers, surfactants, and sugars. These excipients are adsorbed on the surface of the nanoparticles via electrostatic or hydrophobic interactions. Excipient adsorption occurs instantaneously following the production of amorphous nanoparticles, inhibiting recrystallization of the high energy sites on the particles, as well as preventing particle growth due to Ostwald ripening [5]. Jog et al. describe various techniques that have been used to prepare amorphous nanoparticles, such as ultrasonication, drug-polyelectrolyte complexation, antisolvent precipitation, solvent evaporation, sonoprecipitation, flash nanoprecipitation, and nanoporous membrane extrusion [6].

Several different strategies have been proposed to modify the physicochemical characteristics of the nanoparticles, and thus their interactions within the biological systems. For example, it is possible to change the chemical nature of the polymeric matrix of the nanoparticles and thereby alter certain biological phenomena such as biorecognition, biodistribution, bioadhesion, biocompatibility, or biodegradation. Another approach to modifying the biological response is based on the incorporation of suitable adjuvants in the nanoparticles, like proteins such as albumin, invasins, and lectins; and polymers such as poloxamers and poloxamines. For enhancing ocular drug absorption, and prolonging the drug residence time, non invasive approaches such as the use of prodrug and colloidal systems or viscosity enhancers are used. Polymeric nanoparticles are attractive colloidal systems because they demonstrate increased stability and have a long elimination half-life in tear fluid (up to 20 min), than do conventional drugs applied topically to the eye, which have half-lives of just one to three minutes. Nanoparticle drug delivery system has been evaluated for ocular applications to enhance absorption of therapeutic drugs, improve bioavailability, reduce systemic side effects, and sustain intraocular drug levels. The first commercial nanoparticle product containing a drug (Abraxane™, human serum albumin nanoparticles containing paclitaxel) appeared in the market at the beginning of 2005. Nanoparticles have been fabricated using biodegradable synthetic polymers – such as polylactide-polyglycolide copolymers, polyacrylates, and polycaprolactones – or natural polymers, such as albumin, gelatin, alginate, collagen, and chitosan [7]. Various methods, such as solvent evaporation, spontaneous emulsification, solvent diffusion, salting out/emulsification-diffusion, use of supercritical CO_2, and polymerization, have been used to prepare the nanoparticles (NPs) [8].

7.2.3 NANOSUSPENSIONS

Nanosuspension is a technological tool applied mainly to unravel the problem of poor solubility and bioavailability of drugs and occasionally to improve drug safety and efficacy by altering their pharmacokinetics. It is used as an alternative approach to lipid systems, when the drug is insoluble in both aqueous and organic media. The reduced particle size of a poorly water-soluble drug to nano range enormously increases surface area leading to an increased rate of dissolution or an increase in saturation solubility due to an increased dissolution pressure. For example, the solubility and dissolution rate and consequently the bioavailability of crystalline simvastatin was increased significantly by preparation of nanosuspension employing nanoprecipitation technique at a laboratory scale [9]. A pharmaceutical nanosuspension is a biphasic liquid system in which insoluble solid drug particles of the submicron range are uniformly dispersed in an aqueous vehicle. The dosage forms are colloidal and usually stabilized using surfactants and polymers, and meant to be administered through various routes, such as oral, parenteral, topical, nasal, ocular, and more [10]. Similarly, the oral bioavailability of olmesartan Medoxomil was enhanced by improving its solubility and dissolution rate by preparing nanosuspensions [11]. Nanosuspension may also be used to improve the pharmacokinetic and pharmacodynamic profile of the drug and thus therapeutic efficacy of a drug, following oral administration. This has been illustrated in the case of atovaquone nanosuspension for improved oral delivery in the treatment of malaria [12] and the case of 1,3-dicyclohexylurea, by subcutaneous route in the treatment of hypertension [13]. Nanosuspensions are prepared to enhance the bioavailability of poorly soluble drugs by enhancing their solubility. "Nevirapine, a BCS class II, non-nucleoside reverse transcriptase inhibitor (NNRTI) with undesirable solubility and dissolution kinetics from the dosage form was formulated as nanosuspension by nano edge method which increased its solubility several times as also chemical stability" [14]. Similarly, nanocrystalline suspension of poorly soluble drug itraconazole prepared by pearl milling method was found to be promising for oral drug delivery for the treatment of fungal infection [15]. Other applications of nanosupension approach are utilized to formulate products for parenteral drug delivery [16], ocular drug delivery, [17] pulmonary drug delivery [18], CNS drug delivery [19], and enzymes delivery [20]. Junghans et al. [21] evaluated Protamine, a polycationic peptide as a potential penetration enhancer for phosphodiester antisense oligonucleotides (ODNs) and formed unique complexes in the form of nanoparticles called "Proticles". Nanoparticle drug delivery applications in cancer treatment [22], gene therapy [23] have been reported. An excellent paper reviews the application of nanotechnology in medicine [24].

7.2.4 NANOPARTICULATE DRUG DELIVERY SYSTEMS FOR PROTEINS AND PEPTIDES

Large numbers of new therapeutic proteins and peptides are being discovered, thus protein drug-delivery technologies are of ever-increasing importance. Traditionally, the protein is delivered parenterally via solutions that are injected subcutaneously, intramuscularly, and intravenously. Although such injections benefit from high bioavailability, they fail to provide sustained plasma concentrations and suffer from poor patient compliance due to the required frequency of injections. Targeted delivery of proteins and DNA requires a carrier system in submicron size or nanosize. This carrier needs to be the target site (cell or tissue) specific. Often, the actual target site location is intracellular, and the delivery of the carrier payload at this intracellular target site is a prerequisite for therapeutic success. Nanoparticle drug delivery systems are designed to provide the drug release over an extended period, thereby minimizing the need for frequent injections. These can be used for systemic or oral delivery, and the biodegradable nature of the nanoparticulate materials alleviates the need for surgical removal. Biodegradable nanoparticulate delivery for protein requires encapsulation of proteins with a high loading efficiency, which remains stable throughout the manufacturing process and during their intended dosing period. The nanoparticles having a size of around 200 nm could be used for delivering proteins [25].

7.2.5 PULMONARY DRUG DELIVERY

Pulmonary drug delivery for both systemic and local treatments has many advantages over other delivery routes because the lungs have a large surface area (43–102 m^2), a thin absorption barrier, and low enzymatic activity. An enormous diversity of therapeutic agents is currently administered to the patients via aerosol inhalation, and the number of potential drug candidates for pulmonary application increases daily. Insulin-loaded poly(n-butyl cyanoacrylate) (PBCA) nanoparticles were studied by Zhang et al. They demonstrated that the pulmonary administration of these nanoparticles could significantly prolong the hypoglycemic effect of insulin. It was reported that the bioavailability of insulin nanoparticles was relatively higher than that of a solution when administered by a pulmonary route to normal rats, but when nanoparticles were administered subcutaneously, the bioavailability was comparatively low as compared to the solution administered the same way [26].

7.2.6 DRUG DELIVERY

Particle engineering has become a hot topic in the field of modified-release delivery systems during the past decades. It includes a bridge linking drugs and drug delivery systems and has a wide range of pharmaceutical applications. One of the major challenges in drug delivery is to get the drug at the place it is needed in the body thereby avoiding potential side effects to non-diseased organs. This is especially challenging in cancer treatment where the tumor may be localized as distinct metastases in various organs. In the case of nanospheres, where the drug is uniformly distributed, drug release occurs by diffusion or erosion of the matrix. If the nanoparticle is coated by polymer, the release is then controlled by diffusion of the drug from the polymeric membrane. Membrane coating acts as a drug release barrier; therefore, drug solubility and diffusion in or across the polymer membrane becomes a determining factor in drug release. Furthermore, the release rate also can be affected by ionic interactions between the drug and auxiliary ingredients. For drug delivery, not only engineered particles may be used as a carrier, but also the drug itself may be formulated at a nanoscale, and then function as its own "carrier" [27–30]. The composition of the engineered nanoparticles may vary. Source materials may be of biological origin like phospholipids, lipids, lactic acid, dextran, chitosan, or have more "chemical" characteristics like various polymers, carbon, silica, and metals. Table 7.2 summarizes some of the drug delivery formulations with nanotechnology.

TABLE 7.2

Application of Nanotechnology for the Drug Delivery Formulations

Nanotechnology Systems	Formulation Application
Addressing the drug-delivery problems	• Solving the issues related to solubility • Overcoming the poor bioavailability of the drugs • Issues with fed/fasted variability • Pharmacokinetic variability
Finding solutions with nanoparticulate drugs	• Technology advances • Reduction in particle size of the poorly water-soluble drugs • Increased active agent surface area
Benefits for faster dissolution	• Greater bioavailability • Smaller drug doses • Diminished toxicity • Decreased dosing variability
Pharmacodynamic factors: applicable to peptides and other drugs	• These can be formulated as receptor-specific • These can be more resistant to unspecific degradation • They can deliver the drug in the encapsulated form to delay the degradation, set a depot form for prolonged signaling, and increase the treatment efficacy as compared to the substitution of the natural form of a peptide

Source: Modified from Ref. [31].

Nanoparticle-mediated drug delivery is especially useful for targets within endosomes because of the endosomal transport mechanisms of many nanomedicines within cells. Recently authors reported the design of a pH-responsive, soft polymeric nanoparticle for the targeting of acidified endosomes to precisely inhibit endosomal signaling events leading to chronic pain [32]. *(Endosomes are membrane-bound structures within a cell that we call vesicles. They are formed through a complex establishment of processes, which are known collectively as endocytosis. Endosomes are essential for the control of substances in and out of a cell and act as temporary vesicles for transportation.)*

One of the therapeutics under intensive study is paclitaxel (taxol). For paclitaxel, the nanoparticle formulation resulted in enhanced cytotoxicity for tumor cells in vitro, and at the same time an increased sustainable therapeutic efficacy in an in vivo animal model [33]. The paclitaxel was encapsulated in vitamin E TPGS-emulsified poly(D, L-lactic-co-glycolic acid) (PLGA) nanoparticles, and this system resulted in a higher and prolonged level above the effective concentration in vivo, reflected in an increased area under the curve (AUC). Kocbek et al. using polylactic-co-glycolic acid (PLGA) nanoparticles, having the ability to recognize and target-specific antigens on breast epithelial cancer cell lines, which were prepared by attaching monoclonal antibody (mAb) on the nanoparticle surface via the adsorption process. Monoclonal antibody (mAb) was used as a homing ligand and was attached to the nanoparticle surface. These immuno-nanoparticles were prepared for targeting invasive epithelial breast tumor cells [34]. Some of the polymer-based nanoparticle products on the market are listed in Table 7.3 and lipid-based nanoparticles are listed in Table 7.4.

7.2.7 ADVERSE EFFECTS OF NANOPARTICLES

Some engineered nanoparticles (NPs), which get airborne, will pose inhalation hazards, while cosmetics with NPs provide dermal exposures. For parenteral use, interactions with blood components, systemic distribution and kinetics are of importance, when engineered NPs are being used as devices to

TABLE 7.3

Polymer-Based Nanoparticle Products in the Market

Clinical Products	Formulation	Indication	Company	Year
Renagel	Poly(allylamine hydrochloride	Chronic kidney disease	Sanofi	2000
Eligard	Leuprolide acetate and polymer PLGA (poly(DL-lactide-co-glycolide	Prostate Cancer	Tolmar	2002
Estrasorb	Micellar estradiol	Menopausal Therapy	Novavax	2003
Cimzia/certolizumab pegol	PEGylated antibody fragment (certolizumab)	Crohn's disease, rheumatoid arthritis, psoriatic arthritis, and ankylosing spondylitis.	UCB	2008-2013
Genexol-PM	m PEG-PLA micelle loaded with paclitaxel	Metastatic breast cancer	Samyang Corp. (S. Korea)	2007
Adynovate	Polymer protein conjugate (PEGylated factor VCIII)	Hemophilia	Baxalta	2015

Source: Ref. [35].

target drugs to specific tissues, to increase their biological half time, or for imaging purposes. The healthy growth of this field depends on establishing a toxicology database to support safety determinations and risk assessments. The database should include toxicity as a function of material, size, shape, cell type or animal, duration of exposure, and the methods used to assay toxicity. Nanoparticles may cause the same effects as "traditional" particles (e.g., inflammation and lung cancer), but they may be more potent because of their greater surface area. Nanoparticles could also cause new types of effects

TABLE 7.4

Lipid-Based Nanoparticles Products in the Market

Clinical Products	Formulation	Indication	Company	Year
Doxil/Caelyx	Liposomal doxorubicin	Ovarian, breast cancer, Kaposi's sarcoma, and multiple myeloma	Janssen	1995–2008
DaunoXome	Liposomal daunorubicin	AIDS-related Kaposi's sarcoma	Galen	1996
Myocet	Liposomal doxorubicin	Combination therapy with cyclophosphamide in metastatic breast cancer	Elan Pharmaceuticals	2000
Marqibo	Liposomal vincristine	Acute lymphoblastic leukemia	Talon Therapeutics Inc.	2012
AmBisome	Liposomal amphotericin B	Fungal /protozoal infections cryptococcal meningitis in HIV-infected patients,	Gilead Sciences	2000–2008
Visudyne	Liposomal verteporfin	Choroidal neovascularization, macular degeneration, wet age-related myopia, and ocular histoplasmosis	Bauch and Lomb	2000
Onivyde	Liposomal irinotecan	Pancreatic cancer	Merrimack	2015

Source: Ref. [35].

not previously seen with larger particles or bulk chemicals. Each nanoparticle formulation should be tested on a case-by-case basis in the requisite ways focusing on their portal of entry. In this respect also, the potential adverse (toxic) effects of empty particles should be considered [36].

7.2.8 Summary: Nanotechnology

The small size, customized surface, improved solubility, and multi-functionality of nanoparticles will continue to open many doors and create new biomedical applications. Indeed, the novel properties of nanoparticles offer the ability to interact with complex cellular functions in new ways. This rapidly growing field requires cross-disciplinary research and provides opportunities to design and develop multifunctional devices that can target, diagnose, and treat devastating diseases such as cancer. The ultimate goal of nano-drug delivery systems is to develop clinically useful formulations for treating diseases. As nanomedical applications for personalized medicine become more advanced and multifunctional, they may increasingly challenge, and perhaps eventually invalidate traditional regulatory categories and criteria [1].

The type of hazards that are introduced by using nanoparticles for drug delivery are beyond that posed by conventional hazards imposed by chemicals in delivery matrices. However, so far, the scientific paradigm for the possible (adverse) reactivity of nanoparticles is lacking and we have little understanding of the basics of the interaction of nanoparticles with living cells, organs, and organisms. A conceptual understanding of biological responses to nanomaterials is needed to develop and apply safe nanomaterials in drug delivery in the future [36]. Nanoparticles do have great potential for anticancer drug delivery and tumor targeting. Another very promising area for nanoparticles is the possibility to deliver drugs that normally cannot cross the blood-brain barrier to the brain after intravenous injection [37].

Recently during the COVID-19 pandemic, a water repellent coating was developed by the University of Houston researcher based on nanotechnology. The product is marketed by a Houston-based company (https://www.integricote.com/) [38A]. The hydrophobic coating works on masks, fabrics, personal protective equipment, and vent filters made from fiberglass and fabrics.

7.3 SUPER CRITICAL FLUID TECHNOLOGIES

Supercritical fluid technology is a relatively novel technique for the micronization of drugs. Different supercritical fluid processes are being developed to design particles with several purposes in the drug delivery system. These include the super critical fluid (SCF), the rapid expansion of supercritical solutions (RESS), the gas antisolvent process (GAS), supercritical antisolvent process (SAS) and its various modifications, and the particles from gas saturated solution (PGSS) processes. Super critical fluid (SCF), supercritical anti solvent (SAS) and particles from gas saturated solutions (PGSS) are three families of processes that lead to the production of fine and monodisperse powders, including the possibility of controlling crystal polymorphism.

7.3.1 Super Critical Fluid (SCF)

Since the mid-1980s, a new method of particle generation has appeared involving crystallization with supercritical fluids. The rapid expansion of supercritical solutions (RESS) is the most simple process in supercritical fluid technology used for particle production. For this process, the drug has to be dissolved in the supercritical fluid. Carbon dioxide is the most widely used solvent. The hereby formed supercritical solution is then expanded through a nozzle into an expansion chamber. The expansion leads to supersaturation and particle precipitation. In pharmaceutical technology, the primary choice of SCF is scCO2, trifluoromethane, and Norflurane. ScCO2 is the preferred fluid due to its inert behavior, easy to handle supercritical parameters, and non-toxicity. Apart from the rapid disappearance of the "solute" at the end of the processes caused by depressurization,

TABLE 7.5
Examples of Critical Pressure and Temperature of Supercritical Fluids

Type of Fluid	P_c [MPa]	T_c [K]
Trifluoromethane	4.7	299
CO_2	7.4	304.1
Ethane	4.8	305.3
N_2O	7.2	309.6
Propane	4.2	369.8
Norflurane (R134a)	4.0	374.2
n-Hexane	3.0	507.5
Water	22.1	647.1

Source: Refs. [39–43].
P_c: *critical pressure*; T_c: *critical temperature*.

remaining residues in the product would not be seen as critical. The low reactivity, even under high pressure, makes it suitable to be used for sensible drug molecules. The organic solvent is rapidly extracted by and dissolved in the supercritical fluid, and ultra-fine, crystalline micron-sized particles precipitate rapidly. By changing the processing conditions, particle engineering and tuning of particle characteristics can be achieved. Gases or liquids, which were used under pressure and temperature above the critical point, reach an aggregate state, which is called the supercritical fluid state. Under these conditions, which are typical for individual substances (Table 7.5), the fluid possesses properties that are unique and different from the liquid or gaseous state.

Several issues can be addressed through innovative processes using supercritical fluid technology:

- Very low solubility of active molecules in biological fluids
- Alteration along the digestive tract
- Delivery of very unstable bio-molecules
- Substitution of injection delivery by less invasive methods, like pulmonary delivery (inhalation)
- Need for controlled release due to high toxicity or long-term delivery

Rapid expansion of supercritical solutions (RESS) consists in atomizing a solution of the product in a supercritical fluid into a low-pressure vessel [44].

After almost 20 years of active research, and more than 10 years of process development, this technology is reaching maturity, and very soon commercial drugs produced by these techniques are likely to enter the market [45].

7.3.2 RAPID EXPANSION OF SUPERCRITICAL SOLUTIONS (RESS)

Particle formation processes using supercritical fluids [46–48] are now subjected to increasing interest, especially in the pharmaceutical industry with three aims: increasing the bioavailability of poorly soluble molecules, designing sustained-release formulations, and preparing drug delivery less invasive than parenteral (oral, pulmonary, transdermal). The characteristics of the product obtained are dependent on the working conditions. Particles may occur as amorphous or crystalline products, depending on the working conditions applied [49]; however, most authors report the occurrence of crystalline products. Particle size normally appears to be in the range of about 20–200 nm, with a narrow distribution, due to the short time available for crystallization during expansion, based on the jet-stream through the nozzle with ultrasonic speed range [50]. To overcome poor solubility of drugs in scCO2, modifiers or co-solvents can be added. During the past two decades, industrial applications of supercritical fluids have been mostly developed for natural product extraction/fractionation, both for food and pharmaceutical products. Extraction (SFE) from solid materials is the most developed application, mainly for natural products processing: food products (coffee, tea, low-fat cholesterol-free egg yolk powder, etc.), food ingredients, and supplements (hops and aromas, colorants, carotenoids, and vitamin-rich extracts, specific lipids, etc.). Fractionation (SFF) of liquid mixtures are designed to take advantage of the high selectivity of supercritical fluids with attractive costs related to continuous operation. Rapid expansion of supercritical solutions (RESS) consists of atomizing a solution of the product in a supercritical fluid into a low-pressure vessel [45]. This process could find valuable applications at a commercial scale only when the product solubility in the supercritical fluid is not too small (≥10-3 kg/kg), limiting the process application to non-polar or low-polarity compounds when CO2 is used as the solvent.

A different technique the particles from gas-saturated solutions/suspensions (PGSS) makes use of the fact that compressed gases sometimes show better solubility in liquid or dispersed drugs than these drugs in the compressed gases. Melts of drugs are, therefore, saturated with the supercritical fluid and this mixture is expanded through a nozzle.

7.3.3 DIRECT PARTICLE PRODUCTION: ANTISOLVENT TECHNIQUES

If the drug of interest is insoluble in SCF, antisolvent techniques can help for the production of particles. The drug, which should be insoluble in the SCF, must, therefore, initially be dissolved in a suitable solvent, which has to be soluble in the supercritical fluid used. The solution is then mixed with the SCF. Due to the dissolution of the solvent in the SCF and hereby reduced solvent strength, the drug particles will start to crystallize and precipitate and can be collected from the mixture. With careful control of the working parameters, the morphology of the obtained product can be designed to either crystalline or amorphous [51] as can be the particle size and shape [52]. The nucleation and crystal growth is induced by dissolving of the drug's solvent in the supercritical fluid (atmosphere). Both methods are used for the preparation of insulin microparticles in the range of 1–5 μm [53,54]. The supercritical assisted atomization (SAA) uses a drug solution that is mixed with the SCF, and the mixture subsequently expanded through a nozzle into an expansion chamber. The antisolvent techniques, which are in use for pure drug processing, can also be employed for the preparation of composites. Here, however, again the solubility criteria are valid not only for the drug but for the functional excipients.

7.3.4 SUPERCRITICAL ANTI-SOLVENT (SAS)

SAS applies to most molecules that can be dissolved in a very wide range of organic solvents. Recent development opens a bright future for "engineering" new types of particles of different morphologies leading to nanoparticles (50–500 nm) or micro-particles (0.5–5 μm) or empty "balloons" (5–50 μm) made of nano-particles, permitting a very significant increase in bioavailability of poorly water-soluble drugs, or preparation of drug with a narrow particle size distribution dedicated to pulmonary delivery.

7.3.5 FLUID-ASSISTED MICROENCAPSULATION

Fluid-assisted microencapsulation uses the concept known as particle generation from supercritical solutions or suspensions (PGSS), consisting in atomizing a solution of compressed gas or supercritical fluid with the coating agent in which the particles of active are dispersed in form of a slurry, which by decompression in a low-pressure vessel; the rapid fluid demixing induces solidification of the coating agent, leading to very small core-shell microcapsules of active inside the excipient. This process could be suitable for encapsulating protein molecules. Fei Han and colleagues applied supercritical fluid (SCF) technology to prepare reliable solid dispersions of pharmaceutical compounds with limited bioavailability using ibuprofen (IBU) as a model compound [55]. The dissolution performance of the SCF-prepared IBU dispersions was significantly improved compared to that of the physical mixtures of crystalline IBU and a polymer. In addition, the PK results revealed that the SCF-prepared IBU dispersions produced remarkably high blood drug concentrations (both the AUC and C_{max}) and a rapid absorption rate (T_{max}). The variety of methods to micronize particles utilizing SCF is large. Compounds that are soluble or insoluble in SCF can be handled by either solvent or antisolvent techniques, with good efficiency. All these methods suffer from the difficulties to collect and handle very small particles, separation, agglomeration, dust formation, or bad flowability cause problems.

7.4 THREE DIMENSIONAL PRINTING (3DP) OR ADDITIVE MANUFACTURING (AM)

Conventional methods for designing the dosage form for drug delivery include multiple manufacturing steps, such as granulation, extrusion, or coating [56]. Three-dimensional (3D) printing is a manufacturing method in which objects are made by fusing or depositing materials (e.g., plastic, metal, ceramics, powders, liquids, or even living cells) in layers to produce a 3D object. In 3D printing, additive processes are used, in which successive layers of material are laid down under computer control, thus also called additive manufacturing (AM). 3DP is a unique and powerful technology, first described by Charles Hull in 1986 who called it "stereolithography" [57]. In the past 30 years, researchers have utilized 3D printing technologies to address the current limitations in the manufacturing of drug products and challenges in the treatment of patients. The shift from bulk manufacturing of drugs, toward the design and production of personalized medication and dose tailoring, requires the optimization of different 3D printing technologies and the processing of suitable materials. Three-dimensional printing includes a wide variety of manufacturing techniques, which are all based on digitally controlled depositing of materials (layer-by-layer) to create freeform geometries. Therefore, three-dimensional printing processes are commonly associated with free-form fabrication techniques. 3DP is revealing its potential in the pharmaceutical industry as it turns personalized medicine into reality. It has the unique ability to deliver quickly, flexibly, and economically set amounts of patient-specific drugs with customizing properties, such as formulations, dosages, or geometries. Several 3D printing technologies are available to design and manufacture oral dosage tablets. The most commonly used technologies are fused deposition modeling (FDM), selective laser sintering (SLS), stereolithography (SLA), semi-solid extrusion (SSE), and inkjet printing technologies [58]. The requirements for critical excipient attributes are different for each of the individual 3DP technologies, [59] with some 3DP technologies requiring polymers with good flexibility and mechanical strengths, but others may require different strategies like laser sintering or heating or cold extrusion or inkjet printing [60]. The methods used to produce 3D-printed drugs, or "printlets," conform to conventional additive manufacturing technologies, such as inkjet printing or *fused deposition modeling* (FDM). In these systems, the product is often built by depositing highly accurate doses of material layer by layer, until a 3D shape is formed. As a result, reproducibility is a key feature and conventional pharmaceutical manufacturing operations, such as milling, granulating, or compressing, do not take place in additive manufacturing. The advantages of 3DP include precise control of droplet size and dose, high reproducibility, and the ability to produce dosage forms with complex drug-release profiles [61]. Drug release can be easily controlled and targeted by 3D printing. It can be adopted by printing a binder in the layers of the matrix powder. This creates a barrier between the layers of API and allows variation, in the release profile. Various modified release dosage forms, such as diclofenac, endoephedrine hydrochloride, and acetaminophen and guaifenesin, have been prepared using 3D printing technology [62].

Fused deposition modeling (FDM) and pressure assisted microsyringe (PAM) extrusion printing methods make use of solid filaments, semi-solids, or viscous liquids that may be heated to different degrees, pushed through one, up to three nozzles, and deposited on a solid and sometimes heated platform, layer upon layer, a process that shows similarities to traditional pharmaceutical wet and hot-melt extrusion techniques [63].

A 2016 patent offered a printing technology, specifically fused filament fabrication (FFF) 3D printing, to produce solid dosage forms such as a tablet. The production process utilizes novel printing filaments, typically on a spool, which contains the active ingredient and provides access to a variety of viable formulations directly from a 3D printer. The invention also relates to purpose-built software for operating the printing apparatus, as well as local, national, and global systems for monitoring the real-time operation [64].

Various polymers have been investigated for 3D printing technologies, including fused deposition model, selective laser sintering, semi-solid extrusion, stereolithography, and inkjet printing. An excellent review by Ali et al. evaluated various polymers that can be used and their advantages and limitations. They describe different 3D printing models, namely, the fused deposition model and selective laser sintering (SLS). The fused deposition model is a two-step process where the main element is the melt extrusion at the processing temperatures that typically reach >100 °C. The extruded cooled filaments are then subjected to heating and melting during printing through a nozzle at much higher temperatures than used in extrusion [65]. Fina et al. investigated Kollidon® VA 64 and HPMC in SLS 3DP technology. By employing slow and faster laser scanning speeds, the authors fabricated the *printlets* with faster release characteristics [66]. Another 3D printing technology semi-solid extrusion (SSE) is used for sensitive APIs to avoid exposure to higher temperatures. This is a pressure-driven cold extrusion process requiring the use of a paste of drugs and excipients.

For sustained release dosage forms, stereolithography 3D printing technology can be used. Sustained release of drugs can also be achieved by cross-linking of polymers within the matrix by stereolithography (SLA) 3D printing technology. For example, Wang et al. investigated the modified release properties of two model drugs in PEG-based polymers by SLA 3DP technology. The two model drugs, 4-amino salicylic acid (4-ASA) and paracetamol, (acetaminophen) were successfully printed in 3D tablets [67]. Optimization of the process to develop 3D-printed dosage forms will require employing an appropriate method and selecting excipients. 3D printing also holds tremendous promise for orphan drugs, which are designed to treat rare diseases that are sometimes not developed by the pharmaceutical industry due to economic reasons. The number of such rare diseases is estimated to be between 4,000 and 5,000 worldwide [68]. Vithani et al. showed that a self-micro emulsifying drug delivery system (SMEDDS) can be produced with a 3DP process and solid and semi-solid lipid excipients. The proof of concept is established with cinnarizine and fenofibrate as model drugs [69]. Xiaowen Xu et al. studied the feasibility of using different 3D-printed internal geometries as tablet formulations to obtain controlled release profiles. To obtain controllable release profiles, three types of tablet models (Cylinder, Horn, and Reversed Horn), fabricated three types of tablets by a fused deposition modeling with a three-dimensional (3D) printer and injected with paracetamol (APAP)-containing gels. The results of in vitro drug release demonstrate that tablets with three kinds of structures can produce constant, gradually increasing, and gradually decreasing release profiles, respectively. The release attributes can be controlled by using different 3D-printed geometries as tablet formulations [70].

Shaban et al. used extrusion-based printing technology to fabricate multi-active tablets (Polypill) containing three drugs molecules (captopril, nifedipine, and glipizide) to treat patients suffering from diabetics and hypertension [71]. Deng et al. developed a complex matrix tablet with ethylcellulose gradients to achieve zero-order acetaminophen release using 3D printing processes.

The tablet showed linear drug release via a two-dimensional surface erosion mechanism up to 12 hours [72].

Wiebke Kempin et al. studied 3D printed pantoprazole sodium sesquihydrate, using a hot-melt extrusion process. Filaments obtained from hot-melt extrusion were used as the feedstock material for fused deposition modeling for printing that utilizes the layer-wise deposition of extruded material on to a build plate to form the requested object. Thus, researchers showed that five different polymers (PVP K12; PEG 6000; Kollidon®VA64; PEG20,000; poloxamer 407) could be successfully extruded and printed to tablets containing the thermo-sensitive drug pantoprazole sodium at temperatures below 100 °C [73]. 3D printers can print binder onto a matrix powder bed in layers typically 200 micrometers thick, creating a barrier between the active ingredients to facilitate controlled drug release. 3D-printed dosage forms can also be fabricated in complex geometries that are porous and loaded with multiple drugs throughout, surrounded by barrier layers that modulate release [74].

The medical use of 3DP includes the creation of custom prosthetics, body tissue, organ fabrication, anatomical models, dental implants, pharmaceutical research regarding drug dosage forms, drug delivery, and discovery [75]. In December 2015, the Food and Drug Administration (FDA) approved more than 85 3D-printed medical devices [76]. Moreover, the FDA also approved the first 3D-printed tablet, Spritam (levetiracetam), manufactured by Aprecia Pharmaceuticals in 2015 [77]. This innovative development was achieved through a proprietary powder bed and inkjet 3D printing technology known as ZipDose. In manufacturing, an initial powdered layer containing the drug itself is laid down. That first layer then passes under an inkjet printhead, and a binding liquid is printed at specified locations along with the powdered sheet. Successive layers are then printed up to 40 times, depending on the size of the tablet. Printing the layers allows the drug to be packed more tightly. A single tablet that would normally hold 200 mg can be layered to hold 1,000 mg. The result is a high-dose medicine that is easy to swallow for epileptic patients and breaks down inside the body to administer a steady dose over time. Arkema (www.arkema.com) recently inaugurated a Global Center of Excellence for 3D printing in Normandy, France. The center will be dedicated to additive manufacturing by powder fusion, based on high-performance polymers. Moreover, Lonza Group (www.lonza.com) and Allevi (www.allevi3d.com) and some of the universities are collaborating on 3D bioprinting for engineering complex tissues needed for pharmaceutical research. During the recent COVID-19 pandemic, many organizations and individuals with access to 3D printers are deploying the technology to help medical professionals. For example, HP has developed a 3D-printed nasopharyngeal test swabs, facemasks, and ventilator components, and, an Australian supplier of metal-based additive manufacturing technology, SEED3D, has developed a way to 3D print anti-microbial copper proven to kill the COVID-19 virus called ACTIVAT3D copper [78A].

In summary, 3D printing technology is expected to play an important role in the trend toward personalized medicine, through its use in customizing nutritional products, organs, and drugs. It is anticipated that 3D printing will continue to gain much attention in solid dosage forms as the most popular drug dosage forms. Although 3D printing technology showed promising results in drug delivery applications, it is still under the developing stage. The challenges include optimization of the process, performance improvement of the device for versatile use, selections of appropriate excipients, post-treatment method, and so on. These challenges need to be addressed to improve the 3D-printed products' performance and to expand the application range in novel drug delivery systems. Table 7.6 summarizes the most common 3-D printing technologies currently used in the industry.

7.5 ARTIFICIAL INTELLIGENCE (AI)

Artificial intelligence (AI) is defined as the ability of a machine to learn and "think" for itself from experience and perform tasks normally attributed to human intelligence, for example, problem-solving, reasoning, and process understanding. AI also has many subsets like machine learning

TABLE 7.6

Summary of the Most Common 3D Printing Technologies Currently Used in the Indutry

Type of 3DP Technology	Details
Inkjet printing	In the technique, different combinations of active ingredients and excipients (ink) are precisely sprayed in small droplets (via drug on demand) or continuous jet method) in varying sizes layer by layer into a non-powder substrate. The technique encompasses powder-based 3D printing that uses a powder foundation (powder substrate) for the sprayed ink where it solidifies into a solid dosage form.
Direct-write	Uses a computer-controlled translational stage that moves a pattern-generating device to achieve, layer-by-layer, 3D microstructure.
Thermal inkjet (TIJ) printing	TIJ system consists of a micro-resistor that heats a thin film of ink fluid (located in the ink reservoir) forming a vapor bubble that nucleates and expands to push the ink drop out of a nozzle. TIJ affords the opportunity of dispensing extemporaneous preparation/solution of the drug onto 3D scaffolds (drug carriers/films).
Zip dose	Provides a personalized dose in addition to the delivery of a high drug-load with high disintegration and dissolution levels by manufacturing highly porous material.
Fused deposition modeling (FDM)	The process can be applied to multiple dosage forms that apply polymers as part of the framework such as implants, zero-order release tablets, multi-layered tablets, and fast-dissolving devices. In the process, the polymer of interest is melted and extruded through a movable heated nozzle. The layer by layer ejection of the polymer is repeated along the x-y-z stage, followed by solidification to create a shape previously defined by the computer-aided design models.

Source: Modified from Ref. [79].

(ML), which describes the ability of an algorithm to learn with experience. It is the application of targeted statistical techniques that enable machines to improve upon tasks with experience. Machine learning has been used in combination with well-established techniques such as "fuzzy logic" to build a set of rules that allow the equipment to consistently improve its performance against a predefined set of objectives as it gathers data. Deep learning, another subset of AI, is composed of algorithms that permit software to train itself to perform tasks, such as speech and image recognition, by exposing multilayered neural networks to vast amounts of data. AI technologies are widely used in situations where tasks are multidimensional, and where relationships are nonlinear and extremely complex; for example, the underlying relationships between formulation ingredients, process conditions, and drug product quality. AI integrates many branches of statistical and machine learning, pattern recognition, logic, and probability theory as well as biologically motivated approaches, such as neural networks, evolutionary computing, or fuzzy modeling, collectively described as "computational intelligence" [80].

Fuzzy logic is a powerful problem-solving technique based on the mathematical theory of fuzzy sets. It is a method of reasoning that resembles human reasoning. This approach is similar to how humans perform decision making. And it involves all intermediate possibilities between YES and NO. The conventional logic block that a computer understands takes precise input and produces a definite output as TRUE or FALSE, which is equivalent to a human being's YES or NO. The Fuzzy logic was invented by Lotfi Zadeh in the 1960s, who observed that unlike computers, humans have a different range of possibilities between YES and NO such as "certainly yes, possible yes, cannot say, possibly no, certainly no." It has applications in control and decision making and derives its power from being able to draw conclusions and generate responses based on vague, ambiguous, incomplete, and imprecise information. On the other hand, neuro-fuzzy logic systems incorporate the neural network and the power of fuzzy logic. These have been useful in predicting the interactions between the formulation, analyzed process parameters, and target product properties. With the recent advances in computing power, data-based modeling approaches have been utilized to model the granulation process, where the main aim is to find a mapping between a set of inputs and outputs instead of deriving the real physical equations [81].

Linear regression models have been employed to predict the properties of granules and to find the optimal set of input parameters [82,83].

For AI to be useful in drug discovery, the availability of big data is essential. The term "big data" describes large data sets that can be used to find new associations and patterns. In medicine, this includes "omics" data that give vast amounts of information on genes, proteins, metabolites, and their biological functions. Additionally, the combinatorial chemistry and high-throughput screening capabilities developed in the 1990s have generated numerous public and proprietorial databases of molecular structures, pharmacological and biological activity and, safety data. Artificial intelligence is being widely used in pharmaceutical researches due to the ability to predict how process parameters or material properties affect the final product. The concept of artificial intelligence is designed to find the most adequate solution for an existing problem [84,85]. AI presents a software or a machine, which is capable of solving different kinds of problems that are usually solved by humans using our natural intelligence [86].

AI is of crucial importance in granulation processes. Various models are showing its influence in this field. Different machine learning methods suitable for optimizing granulation processes include artificial neural network (ANN), cubist, random forests (RF), k-nearest neighbors algorithm (k-NN), and machine learning tools, such as enetic programing (GP) and particle swarm optimization (PSO) [84,87]. AI encompasses many branches of statistical and machine learning, pattern recognition, clustering, similarity-based methods, logics, and probability theory, as well as biologically motivated approaches, such as neural networks and fuzzy modeling, collectively described as "computational intelligence." The main goal of ANN is to learn the relationship between the independent and dependent variables, which is achieved through repeatedly presenting training set formulations to the neural network in many training cycles. ANNs work by building up a network of interconnecting processing units or nodes, which are the artificial equivalents of biological neurons. The ANN can discover knowledge (e.g., cause-effect relationships) that is hidden in experimental data and generate predictive models linking important factors to key measurable outputs; for example, the effect of drug particle size and wet granulation conditions on tablet dissolution. Manufacturing of solid-dosage pharmaceutical formulations is aspiring to be continuous, which means that every step is interconnected. Model predictive control (MPS) represents an advanced control strategy [88]. To facilitate a more advanced approach to formulation development, machine learning can be used to make data-driven predictions with existing experimental data for efficient formulation development. Table 7.7 summarizes the recent progress of formulation design with machine learning [89].

TABLE 7.7
Recent Progress in Formulation Design with Machine Learning

Machine Learning Techniques	Formulation	References
Hybrid expert system with ANNs	Hard gelatin capsule formulations	[90]
Expert System (SeDeM Diagram)	Orally disintegrating Tablets	[91,92]
Expert System with ANNs	Osmotic pump tablets	[93,94]
Ontology-based expert system	Immediate-release tablets	[95]
ME_expert 2.0	Microemulsion formulations	[96]
Fuzzy logic-based expert system	Freeze-dried formulations	[97]
Cubist and random Forest	Cyclodextrin formulations	[98]

Source: Ref. [89].

Artificial neural network (ANN). Neural networks have been used by scientists for optimizing formulations as an alternative to statistical analysis because of its simplicity for use and the potential to provide detailed information. The neural network builds a model of the data space that can be consulted to ask "what if" kinds of questions. Recently, there has been an interest in using (ANN) for process control. Similar to the human brain, an ANN predicts events or information based upon learned pattern recognition. ANNs are computer systems developed to mimic the operations of the human brain by mathematically modeling its neurophysiological structure (i.e., its nerve cells and the network of interconnections between them). In ANN, the nerve cells are replaced by computational units called neurons and the strengths of the interconnections are represented by weights [99]. This unique arrangement can simulate some of the neurological processing abilities of the brain, such as learning and concluding experience [100]. Several researchers have published papers detailing the use of ANN for different applications [101–103]. An integrated network as a data-driven model has been proposed by AlAlaween et al. [104] to predict the properties of the granules produced by high shear granulation. The integrated network predicts the outputs by modeling and training the data in two consecutive phases. Such a structure can extract relevant information from a conservative number of data points; it can also capture the complex input/output relationships in the original data because of the number of basic functions and weights involved.

AI models are capable of predicting potential problems as well as find solutions for them. During the optimization of process parameters or formulation AI is capable of showing the correlation of these two. AI can be utilized to scale up the granulation process. Researchers used artificial intelligence tools to predict the endpoint of the granulation process in high-speed mixer granulators through adequate predictions of the impeller power [105]. Neuro-fuzzy logic was used to predict critical variables for every step of the process. The combination of neuro-fuzzy logic and gene expression programing was used to obtain a transparent model that could properly predict the impeller power values as a function of the diameter and speed of the impeller, the amount of granulation liquid and the characteristics of the wet mass. Researchers demonstrated that this experimental model has worked for granulators of similar and dissimilar shapes and sizes (PMA 25 L, 100 L, 600 L). Hossam M. Zawbaa [106] applied bio-inspired optimization algorithms for feature selection and prediction of different pharmaceutical properties while granulating with the roller compaction process. After that, he uses machine learning techniques (artificial neural network, k-nearest neighbor, extreme learning machine, etc.) to predict the different pharmaceutical properties (e.g., true density, porosity, tensile strength, and fines). The AI-assisted approach will increase successful drug discovery to drug development through commercialization. AI may provide the initial intelligence/molecule identification essential to the discovery process, but the incubation necessary to migrate into the development phase will likely continue to be the output of a techno-human hybrid effort.

The two firms are joining forces to develop AI-based technology for the continuous manufacturing of critical APIs necessary for producing crucial small-molecule drugs [107].

7.6 OTHER APPROACHES

7.6.1 Spray Drying Particle Engineering for Inhalation

Spray drying has been used over the past 30 years to produce particles for inhalation applications. Particle size is crucial for pulmonary delivery because particles that are too large (> 5 microns) will not go deep into the lungs and those that are too small (< 1 micron) may be exhaled. Spray drying can be used to engineer particles with specific densities and particle sizes. Because the process uses heat, it is not suitable for some thermally sensitive materials. The most common means of delivering inhalation particles to the lungs are dry powder inhalers or DPI. Emulsion, supercritical antisolvent, and spray drying are three examples of particle engineering systems adopted for the generation of inhalation powder [108].

A detailed discussion of spray drying is presented in Chapter 6 of this book.

7.6.2 PARTICLE REPLICATION IN NON-WETTING TEMPLATES (PRINT)

Liquidia Technologies has applied a mold-based particle engineering platform called PRINT. This platform achieves uniform particle shape, size, and morphology defined by the input mold features. The typical process described by the authors as the drug or drug mixed with excipients flows into a fluoropolymer micro mold of a precise size and shape. The molded particles, taking on the geometric dimensions of the mold cups, are isolated as stable dispersions of particles or free-flowing powders [109–111].

7.6.3 CO-CRYSTALLIZATION

Co-crystallization is a new technology that uses novel excipients and processes to create particles of the required size while incorporating excipients to enhance delivery to the lung. It is the supramolecular phenomenon of aggregation of two or more different chemical entities in a crystalline lattice through non-covalent interactions. Their application goes way beyond pharmaceuticals. Solvates, solid solutions, eutectics, salts, ionic liquids, solid dispersions, supramolecular gelators, and so forth are among the multifarious products of co-crystallization [112]. Among the earliest pharmaceutical co-crystals reported are of sulfonamides [113]. The area of pharmaceutical co-crystals has thus increased based on interactions between APIs and co-crystal formers. Most commonly, APIs have hydrogen-bonding capability at their exterior, which makes them more susceptible to polymorphism, especially in the case of co-crystal solvates, which can be known to have different polymorphic forms. While some co-crystallization processes use available equipment, other processes use novel equipment.

7.6.4 LIQUI-PELLET

Liqui-pellet is an emerging novel oral dosage form, which improves the bioavailability of poorly water-soluble drugs via increasing drug release rate in the GIT. The concept of the liquid-solid system comprises an active pharmaceutical ingredient (API), which is solubilized in a liquid vehicle, forming the liquid medication. This liquid medication is then incorporated into a carrier, which is coated with a nano-sized coating material to give the admixture of API and excipients a dry, free-flowing, and readily compressible property "liquipellet," which has the inherent advantages from both liquid-solid and pelletization technologies. The extrusion-spheronization technique can improve flow property, and the inherent advantages from the liquid-solid aspect can enhance the drug release rate. The authors have termed this next-generation oral dosage form as "liquipellets" [114].

7.6.5 MICROENCAPSULATION USING POLYLACTIC-CO-GLYCOLIC ACID (PLGA) [115]

Encapsulation of APIs can be delivered in a controlled way in the body. This encapsulation technique offers protection to an API from enzymatic or acidic degradation in the stomach, improves diffusion of the drug across the digestive tract, and offers a way to introduce hydrophobic molecules into the body. To perform drug encapsulation, a solution of PLGA in an organic solvent is mixed with the chosen API, and the polymer is then solidified into a particle. However, the efficiency of entrapment and release depends on the physicochemical properties of API and the particle. The author provides an example of an approach taken at the University of Manchester, where researchers are formulating the PLGA drug delivery system, using microfluidics to produce nanoparticles capable of a sustained release in oncology applications. Such a delivery system aims to accumulate the API at the tumor site, localizing the therapeutic effect, and controlling and sustaining drug release over time [115].

Multidrug-resistant (MDR) cancer may be treated using combinations of encapsulated cytotoxic drugs and chemosensitizers. To optimize the effectiveness of this combinational approach, poly(D, L-lactide-co-glycolic acid) (PLGA) nanoparticles formulations capable of delivering a cytotoxic drug, vincristine, a chemosensitizer, verapamil, or their combination were prepared via combining oil in water emulsion solvent evaporation and salting-out method [116].

7.6.6 ELECTROSPINNING

Electrospinning is a fiber production method that uses electric force to draw charged threads of polymer solutions or polymer melts up to fiber diameters in the order of some hundred nanometers. Electrospinning shares characteristics of both electrospraying and conventional solution dry spinning of fibers. Its applications in the pharmaceutical industry are rapidly being explored. In this technology, a solution of a polymer and an API is prepared in a volatile solvent. This then is injected in a collector using the syringe fitted with spinneret (needle). A pump is used to extrude the solution through the needle at a controlled rate. The power supply is used to apply a high voltage between the spinneret and a collector evaporating the solvent forming a mat of one-dimensional fiber. These fibers have a nanoscale diameter and comprise amorphous solid dispersion of drug in the polymer [117]. Electrospinning can be used to prepare formulations using polymers containing various APIs ranging from small molecules through the peptides and protein cells. A range of drug-loaded polyvinylpyrrolidone(PVP)-based fibers have been reported, containing irbesartan [118], mebeverine hydrochloride [119], and isosorbide dinitrate [120]. These fiber mats can be cut into various shapes and dissolve readily. Thus, this technique can be used to make solid dispersions as well as the development of oral fast dissolving films. Production of fiber mats with carvacrol and polylactic acid [121] the immobilization of the antibiotic gentamicin sulfate (GS) in electrospun fiber mats composed of poly(lactic acid) (PLA), poly(ε-caprolactone) (PCL) and the copolymer poly(lactic-co-glycolic acid) (PLGA) was reported recently [122]. Also, a comprehensive review was published summarizing the effect of electrospinning parameters and potential applications of nanofibers in biomedical and biotechnology [123].

7.6.7 MICROBIOME-BASED THERAPEUTICS

The microbial population in the human body numbers in the trillions; estimates range from 10 to 100 trillion, and knowledge is emerging on its role in human health and diseases. The influence of the microbiome on drug response has only been investigated in detail for the past 10 years. Microbiome-based therapies, such as prebiotics and probiotics, are often aimed at proliferating specific microbial species that are known to produce beneficial metabolites (e.g., butyrate). Instead of enriching or depleting such bacterial producers, another strategy that has been developed recently is the use of postbiotics (i.e., supplements of bacteria-derived metabolites either to restore the depleted microbial pool or inhibition of specific metabolites) [124]. Ingestion of prebiotics or probiotics has been used to treat a range of conditions including constipation, allergic reactions and infections in infancy, and Irritable Bowel Syndrome (IBS).. Fecal microbiota transplantation (FMT) highly effective in treating recurrent *Clostridium difficile* infections [125], in Rhinosinusitis [126] plays a regulatory role in people with ALS [127], and is effective for cirrhotic patients [128]. The contribution of the modified or engineered microbiome to the drug development process and drug pharmacokinetics can be explored for an efficacious, tolerable, and personalized drug delivery [129]. In May 2016, the USA announced the National Microbiome Initiative with $121 million in federal and $400 million in private funds to promote the study and use of the microbiome. The National Institute of Health (NIH) in the USA established Common Fund Human Microbiome

Project (HMP) to generate research resources to enable the characterization of the human microbiota and the analysis of their role in human health and disease, with goals of supporting interdisciplinary research; developing platform technologies; and expanding the microbiome workforce [130]. In 2018 alone, over 2400 clinical trials were testing therapies based on microbiome science. That number is growing quickly, as in comparison, there were just 1600 the previous year. As microbiome research has grown, more and more health conditions have been linked to having an unbalanced microbial composition – something known as dysbiosis. The gut microbiome has emerged as an important target in cancer therapy to repair the microbiome following harsh chemotherapy and antibiotic treatment regimens to improve patient survival [131]. The majority of microbiome-based therapies under development today target either diseases of the gastrointestinal tract, such as ulcerative colitis and irritable bowel syndrome, or conditions where a strong link between the gut microbiome and disease has been established, as is the case for psoriasis and diseases that involve the gastrointestinal-brain axis, such as Parkinson's and other neurological disorders [132]. Microbiome research looks set to continue as the next area of growth. This research could provide us one more avenue toward precision and personalized medicine.

7.7 SUMMARY

As can be seen from this chapter, the scientific pursuit of modification of particles is gaining momentum as the commercial exploitation propels the scientific community more intent on delivering the particles, especially for the pharmaceutical industry. Particle engineering, a young discipline, combines elements of many others, including chemistry, pharmaceutics, interface and colloid science, mass and heat transfer, aerosol and powder science, and solid-state physics. Considering that the current level of development of pharmaceutical particle technologies is relatively limited, and the understanding of the relationships between such materials and processes in the development and manufacturing of pharmaceutical products is at an early stage, there remains an onerous path for the successful development and implementation of particle-based technologies in the pharmaceutical industry. Several emerging technologies such as electrospinning, microbiome, PLGA, additive manufacturing (3D), and artificial intelligence are revolutionizing how we create therapeutic dosage forms. All these emerging engineering technologies will change the way we develop and manufacture pharmaceutical dosage forms in the coming years.

REFERENCES

1. Bamrungsap S. et al. Nanotechnology in therapeutics: a focus on nanoparticles as a drug delivery system. Nanomedicine 2012; 7(8): 1253–1271.
2. Kwon K., Kim S., Park K., Kwon I. C. Nanotechnology in drug delivery: past, present, and future. AAPS 2009; 10: 581.
3. Willis R. C. Good things in small packages. Modern Drug Discov. 2004; 7:1.
4. Merisko-Liversidge E., Liversidge G. G., Cooper E. R. Nano sizing: a formulation approach for poorly-water-soluble compounds. Eur J Pharm Sci 2003; 18(2): 113–120.
5. Lindfors L., Skantze P., Skantze U., Rasmusson M., Zackrisson A., Olsson U. Amorphous drug nanosuspensions. 1. Inhibition of Ostwald ripening. Langmuir 2006; 22(3): 906–910.
6. Rajan Jog, Diane J. Burgess. Pharmaceutical amorphous nanoparticles. J Pharma Sci 2017; 106: 39–65.
7. Panyam J., Labhasetwar V. Biodegradable nanoparticles for drug and gene delivery to cells and tissue. Adv Drug Deliv Rev 2003; 55: 329–347.
8. Soppimath K. S., Aminabhavi T. M., Kulkarni A. R., Rudzinski W. E. Biodegradable polymeric nanoparticles as drug delivery devices. J Control Release 2001; 70(1–2): 1–20.
9. Pandya V. M., Patel J. K., Patel D. J. Formulation, optimization, and characterization of Simvastatin nanosuspension prepared by nanoprecipitation technique. Der Pharmacia Lettre 2011; 3(2): 129–140.
10. Prabhakar C., Krishn K. B. A review on nanosuspensions in drug delivery. IJPBS 2011; 2(1): 549–558.

11. Thakkar H. P., Patel B. V., Thakkar S. P. Development and characterization of nanosuspensions of olmesartan Medoxomil for bioavailability enhancement. J Pharm Bioallied Sci. 2011; 3(3): 426–434.

12. Borhade V., Pathak S., Sharma S., Patravale V. Formulation and characterization of Atovaquone nanosuspension for improved oral delivery in the treatment of malaria. Nanomed 2013; 8(7): 1031–1033.

13. Chiang P. C., Ran Y., Chou K. J., Cui Y., Wong H. Investigation of utilization of nanosuspension formulation to enhance the exposure of 1, 3-dicyclohexylurea in rats: Preparation for PK/PD study via subcutaneous route of nanosuspension drug delivery. Nanoscale Res Lett 2011; 6(1): 413.

14. Raju A., Reddy A. J., Satheesh J., Jithan A. V. Preparation and characterization of nevirapine oral nanosuspensions. Indian J Pharm Sci 2014; 76(1): 62–71.

15. Nakarani M., Misra A. K., Patel J. K., Vaghani S. S. Itraconazole nanosuspension for oral delivery: Formulation, characterization and in vitro comparison with the marketed formulation. Daru 2010; 18(2): 84–90.

16. Wang Z., Li Z., Zhang D., Miao L., Huang G. Development of Etoposide-loaded bovine serum albumin nanosuspensions for parenteral delivery. Drug Deliv 2014: 79–84.

17. Ahuja M., Verma P., Bhatia M. Preparation and evaluation of chitosan-itraconazole co-precipitated nanosuspension for ocular delivery. J Exp Nanosci 2013. doi:10.1080/17458080.2013.822108#.Uz7d6KiSw4U (Accessed October 13, 2014).

18. Yang J. Z., Young A. L., Chiang P. C., Thurston A., Pretzer D. K. Fluticasone and budesonide nanosuspensions for pulmonary delivery: preparation, characterization, and pharmacokinetic studies. J Pharm Sci 2008; 97(11): 4869–4878.

19. Koziara J. M., Lockman P. R., Alen D. D., Mumper R. J. In situ blood-brain barrier transport of nanoparticles. Pharm Res 2003; 20: 1772.

20. Dziubla T. D., Karim A., Muzykantov V. R. Polymer nanocarriers protecting active enzyme cargo against proteolysis. J Control Release 2005; 102: 427.

21. Junghans M., Kreuter J., Zimmer A. Antisense delivery using protamine-oligonucleotide particles. Nucleic Acid Res 2000; 28: e45.

22. Chawla J. S., Amiji M. M. Biodegradable poly(epsilon-caprolactone) nanoparticles for tumor-targeted delivery of tamoxifen. Int J Pharm 2005; 249: 127.

23. Zhao Z., Wang J., Mao H. Q. Polyphosphoesters in drug and gene delivery. Adv Drug Deliv Rev 2003; 55: 483.

24. Nikalje A. P. G. Nanotechnology and its applications in medicine. Med Chem 2015; 5(2): 081–089.

25. Rodrigues J. S., Magalhaes N. S. S., Coelho L. C. B. B., Couvreur P., Ponchel G., Gref R. Novel core (polyester)-shell (polysaccharide) nanoparticles: protein loading and surface modification with lectins. J Control Release 2003; 19(1-2): 103–112.

26. Zhang Q., Shen Z., Nagai T. Prolonged hypoglycemic effect of insulin loaded poly butyl cyanoacrylate nanoparticles after pulmonary administration to normal rats. Int J Pharm 2001; 218: 75.

27. Cascone M. G., Lazzeri L., Carmignani C., Zhu, Z. Gelatin nanoparticles produced by a simple W/O emulsion as a delivery system for methotrexate. J Mat Sci Mat in Med 2002; 13: 523–526.

28. Kipp J. E. The role of solid nanoparticle technology in the parental delivery of poorly water-soluble drugs. Int J Pharm 2004; 284: 109–122.

29. Baran E. T., Özer N., Hasirci V. In vivo half-life of nano encapsulated L-asparaginase. J Mat Sci Mat in Med 2002; 13: 1113–1121.

30. Duncan R. The dawning era of polymer therapeutics. Nat Rev Drug Disc 2003; 2: 347–360.

31. Thassu et al. Pharmaceutical Applications of Nanoengineering: Chapter 7, Handbook of Pharmaceutical Granulation Technology 3rd edition, D. M. Parikh (Editor), New York, USA: Informa Health (Publ.), 2009.

32. Paulina D., Ramírez García et al. A pH-responsive nanoparticle targets the neurokinin 1 receptor in endosomes to prevent chronic pain. Nat Nanotechnol 2019. doi:10.1038/s41565-019-0568-x.

33. Win K. Y., Feng S. S. In vitro and in vivo studies on vitamin E TPGS-emulsified poly(D, L-lactic-co-glycolic acid) nanoparticles for paclitaxel formulation. Biomaterials 2006; 27: 2285–2291.

34. Kocbek,P. Targeting cancer cells using PLGA nanoparticles surface modified with monoclonal antibody. J Control Release 2007; 120: 18–26.

35. Lombardo D. Kiselev M.A., Caccamo, M.T. Smart nanoparticles for drug delivery application: development of versatile nanocarrier platforms in biotechnology and nanomedicine. J Nanomater 2019. doi:10.1155/2019/3702518.

36. De Jong W. H., Borm P.J.A. Drug delivery and nanoparticles: applications and hazards. Int J Nanomed 2008 Jun; 3(2): 133–149.

37. Kreuter J. Nanoparticles – a historical perspective. Int J Pharm (2007); 331: 1–10.

38. Integricote. University of Houston and Integricote company announcement.April 3, 2020. https://www.integricote.com/news-events-1.

39. Arai Y., Sako T., Takebayashi Y. Supercritical Fluids. Berlin, Heidelberg, New York: Springer, 2002: 71–126.

40. Martinez J. L. Supercritical Fluid Extraction of Nutraceuticals and Bioactive Compounds. Boca Raton, London, New York: CRC Press; 2008: 1–24.

41. Cabanas A., Renuncio J. A. R., Pando C. Thermodynamic study of the N2O + CO2 and N2O + CO2 + cyclohexane systems in the near-critical and supercritical regions. Ind Eng Chem Res 2000; 39(10): 3566–3575.

42. Tillner-Roth R., Baehr H. D. Measurement of liquid, near-critical, and supercritical (p, r, T) of 1,1,1,2-tetrafluoroethane (R 134a) and of 1,1-difluoroethane (R 152a). J Chem Thermodyn 1993; 25(2): 277–292.

43. Wahl M.A. Supercritical Fluid Technology" Chapter 6, Handbook of Pharmaceutical Granulation Technology 3rd edition, D. M. Parikh (editor), New York, USA: Informa Health, 2009.

44. Fages J. Particle generation for pharmaceutical applications using supercritical fluid technology. Powder Technol 2004; 141(3): 219–226.

45. Ya-Ping Sun, Ed. New York: Marcel Dekker, 2002, pp. 387–437.

46. Kompella U. D. and Koushik K. Preparation of drug delivery systems using supercritical fluids. Crit Rev Therapeutic Carrier Syst 2001; 18(2): 173–199.

47. Jung J. and Perrut, M. Particle design using supercritical fluids: literature and patent review. J Supercrit Fluids 2001; 20: 179–219.

48. Palakodaty S., Sloan R., Kordikowski A. and York P. "Pharmaceutical and biological materials processing with supercritical fluids," In: Supercritical Fluid Technology in Materials Science and Engineering, Ya-Ping Sun, Ed. New York: Marcel Dekker, 2002, pp. 439–490.

49. Gosselin P. M., Thibert R., Preda M., Mcmullen, J. N. Polymorphic properties of micronized carbamazepine produced by RESS. Int J Pharm. 2003, 252(1–2): 225–233.

50. Tuerk M. Manufacture of submicron drug particles with enhanced dissolution behavior by rapid expansion processes. J Supercrit Fluids 2009; 47(3): 537–545.

51. Martin A., Scholle K., Mattea F. Meterc D., Cocero M. J. Production of polymorphs of ibuprofen sodium by supercritical antisolvent (SAS) precipitation. Cryst Growth Des 2009; 9(5): 2504–2511.

52. Shekunov B. Y., York P., Baldyga J. Particle formation using supercritical antisolvent: influence of flow velocity and supersaturation. Int Symp Ind Cryst 1999: 1112–1126.

53. Snavely W. K., Subramaniam B., Rajewski R. A. et al. Micronization of insulin from halogenated alcohol solution using supercritical carbon dioxide as an antisolvent. J Pharm Sci 2002; 91(9): 2026–2039.

54. Amidi M., Pellikaan H. C., de Boer A. H., Defelippis, M. R. Preparation and physicochemical characterization of supercritically dried insulin-loaded microparticles for pulmonary delivery. Eur J Pharm Biopharm 2008; 68(2): 191–200.

55. Han F. Applying supercritical fluid technology to prepare ibuprofen solid dispersions with improved oral bioavailability. Pharmaceutics 2019; 11: 67. doi:10.3390/pharmaceutics11020067.

56. Maraie N. K., Salman Z. D., Yousif N. Z. Design and characterization of oroslippery buoyant tablets for ranitidine hydrochloride. Asian J Pharm Clin Res 2018; 11: 143–149.

57. Maulvi F. A., Shah J. M., Solanki B. S., Patel A. S., Soni T. G., Shah D. O. Application of 3D printing technology in the development of novel drug delivery systems. Int J Drug Dev Res 2017; 9: 44–49.

58. Rahman Z., Barakh Ali S. F. Ozkan T., Charoo N. A., Reddy I. K., Khan M. A. Additive manufacturing with 3D printing: progress from bench to bedside. AAPS J 2018; 20: 101. doi:10.1208/s12248-018-0225-6

59. T. Huang, Wang S., He K. (Editors). Quality control for fused deposition modeling based additive manufacturing: current research and future trends. In Reliability Systems Engineering (ICRSE), First International Conference, 2015, Beijing: IEEE.

60. Maulvi F. A., Shah M. J., Solanki B. S., Patel A. S., Soni T. G., Shah D. O. Application of 3D printing technology in the development of novel drug delivery systems. Int J Drug Dev 2017; 9: 44–49.

61. Lee H., Cho D.-W. One-step fabrication of an organ-on-a-chip with spatial heterogeneity using a 3D bioprinting technology. Lab Chip 2016;16(14): 2618–2625.

62. Bala R., Madaan R., Kaur A., Mahajan K. 3D printing: basic role in pharmacy. Eur J Biomed Pharm Sci 2017; 4: 242–247.

63. On-Bogdan Dumitrescu et al. The age of pharmaceutical 3d printing: technological and therapeutical implications of additive manufacturing. Farmacia 2018; 66: 3.

64. International Patent WO 2016/038356 Al, March 17, 2016.
65. Ali S., Kolter K., Karl, M. Evaluation of different polymers in 3D printing technologies. Ame Pharm Rev 2019; 166–175.
66. Fina F., Madla C. M., Goyanes A., Zhang J., Gaisforda S., Basit A. W. Fabricating 3D printed orally disintegrating printlets using selective laser sintering. Int J Pharm 2018; 541: 101–107.
67. Wang J., Goyanes A., Gaisford S., Basit A. W. Stereolithographic (SLA) 3D printing of oral modified-release dosage forms. Int J Pharm 2016; 503: 207–212.
68. Orphanet. What is an orphan drug. https://www.orpha.net/consor/cgi-bin/Education_AboutOrph anDrugs.php.
69. Vithani K. Goyanes A., Jannin V., Basit A. W., Gaisford S., Boyd B. J. A proof of concept for 3D printing of solid lipid-based formulations of poorly water-soluble drugs to control formulation dispersion kinetics. J Pharm Res. May 16, 2019; 36(7): 1.
70. Xiaowen Xu, Zhao J., Wang M., Wang L., Yang J. 3D printed polyvinyl alcohol tablets with multiple release profiles. Sci Rep 2019; 9: 12487. doi: 10.1038/s41598-019-48921-8.
71. Khaled S. A., Burley J. C., Alexander M. R., Yang J., Roberts C. J. 3D printing of tablets containing multiple drugs with defined release profiles. Int J Pharm 2015; 494: 643–650.
72. Yu D. G., Yang X. L., Huang W. D., Liu J., Wang Y. G., Xu, H. Tablets with material gradients fabricated by three-dimensional printing. J Pharm Sci 2007; 96: 2446–2456.
73. Wiebke Kempin et al. Immediate release 3D-printed tablets produced via fused deposition modeling of a thermo-sensitive drug. Pharm Res 2018; 35: 124. doi:10.1007/s11095-018-2405-6
74. Ventola C. L. Medical applications of 3D printing: current and projected use. P&T (2014); 39(10): 704–711.
75. Schubert C., Van Langeveld M. C., Donoso L. A. Innovations in 3D printing: a 3D overview from optics to organs. Br J Ophthalmol 2014; 98: 159–161.
76. Gosnear T., Brettler D. Three big risks in 3D printing pharmaceuticals are the risks of leveraging this new technology outweighing the benefits for drug makers? Ran Pharma Manuf 2016. 10/31/2016 https://www.pharmamanufacturing.com/articles/2016/three-big-risks-in-3d-printing-pharmaceuticals/.
77. Acosta-Velez G. F., Wu B. M. 3D pharming: direct printing of personalized pharmaceutical tablets. Polym Sci 2016; 2: 1–10.
78. Daniel E. 3D printing used to make coronavirus-killing copper surfaces. April 15, 2020. https://www.verdict.co.uk/3d-printing-copper-coronavirus/.
79. Jassim-Jaboori, A. H. Oyewumi M. O. 3D printing technology in pharmaceutical drug delivery: prospects and challenges. J Biomol Res Ther 2015; 4(4): 1000e141.
80. Prital Sable, Khanvilker V. V. Pharmaceutical applications of artificial intelligence. Int J Pharma Res Health Sci. 2018; 6(2): 2342–2345. doi:10.21276/ijprhs.2018.02.01.
81. Bishop C. Neural Networks for Pattern Recognition. Oxford: Clarendon Press, 1995.
82. J. Westerhuis, Coenegracht P., Lerk C. Multivariate modelling of the tablet manufacturing process with wet granulation for tablet optimization and in-process control. Int J Pharm 1997; 156: 109–117.
83. Miyamoto Y., Ogawa S., Miyajima M., Matsui M., Sato H., Takayama K., Nagai T. An application of the computer optimization technique to wet granulation process involving explosive growth of particles. Int J Pharm 1997; 149: 25–36.
84. Hessler, G., Baringhaus, K.-H. Artificial intelligence in drug design. Molecules 2018; 23(10): 2520.
85. Kazemi, P. et al. Effect of roll compaction on the granule size distribution of microcrystalline cellulose-mannitol mixtures: computational intelligence modeling and parametric analysis. Drug Des Dev Ther 2017; 11: 241–251.
86. Shabbir, J., Anwer, T. Artificial intelligence and its role in the near future. CoRR 2015; 14(8): 1–11.
87. Barrett, S., Langdon, W. Advances in the application of machine learning techniques in drug discovery, design, and development. Appl Soft Comput 2006; 99–110.
88. Shirazian, S., Kuhs, M., Darwish, S., Croker, D., Walker, G. Artificial neural network modelling of continuous wet granulation using a twin-screw extruder. Int J Pharm 2017; 521(1–2): 102–109.
89. Yang Y. Ye Z. Su Y. Zhao Q., Li X, Ouyang D. Deep learning for in vitro prediction of pharmaceutical formulations. Acta Pharm Sinica B. 2019; 9(1): 175–185.
90. Wilson W. I., Peng Y., Augsburger, L. L. Generalization of a prototype intelligent hybrid system for hard gelatin capsule formulation development. AAPS PharmSciTech 2005;6: E449–E457.
91. Edward A-D. J., García-Montoya E., Suñe-Negre J. M., Pérez-Lozano P., Miñarro M., Grau J. R. T. Predicting orally disintegrating tablets formulations of ibuprofen tablets: an application of the new SeDeM-ODT expert system. Eur J Pharm Biopharm 2012; 80(3): 638–648.

92. Edward A-D. J., García-Montoya E., Suñe-Negre J. M., Pérez-Lozano P., Miñarro M., Grau J. R. T. "New odt expert system for formulation of orodispersible tablets obtained by direct compression," Formulation Tools for Pharmaceutical Development, Anguilar JE Amsterdam: Elsevier Ltd., 2013, pp. 137–154.

93. Zang Z. H., Pan W. S. "Expert system for the development and formulation of pull-push osmotic pump tablets containing poorly soluble drug," In: Formulation Tools for Pharmaceutical Development Anguilar JE, Ed. Amsterdam: Elsevier Ltd., 2013, pp. 73–108.

94. Zang Z. H. et al. Design of an expert system for the development and formulation of push-pull osmotic pump tablets containing poorly water-soluble drugs. Int J Pharm May 30, 2011; 410(1–2): 41–47.

95. Charoltham N., Ruangrajitpakorn T., Supnithi T., Leesawat P. "Oxpirt: Ontology based expert system for production of the generic immediate-release tablet," In: Formulation Tools for Pharmaceutical Development, Anguilar JE, Ed. Amsterdam: Elsevier Ltd., 2013, pp. 203–228.

96. Mendyk A., Szlęk J., Jachowicz R. "Heuristic decision support system for microemulsions formulation development," In: Anguilar JE, Ed. Formulation Tools for Pharmaceutical Development.Amsterdam: Elsevier Ltd., 2013, pp. 39–71.

97. Trnka H., Wu J. X., Van De Weert M., Grohganz H., Rantanen J. Fuzzy logic-based expert system for evaluating cake quality of freeze-dried formulations. Journal of Pharmaceutical Sciences December 2013; 102(12): 4364–4374.

98. Merzlikine A., Abramov Y. A., Kowsz S. J., Thomas V. H., Mano T. Development of machine learning models of β-cyclodextrin and sulfobutylether-β-cyclodextrin complexation free energies. Int J Pharm 2011, October 14; 418(2): 207–216.

99. Jha B. K., Tambe S. S., Kulkarni B. D. Estimating diffusion coefficients of a micellar system using an ANN. J Colloid Interface Sci 1995; 170: 392–398.

100. Bourquin J., Schmidt H., Van Hoogevest P., Leuenberger H. Basic concepts of ANN modeling in the application to pharmaceutical development. Pharm Dev Technol. 1997; 2(2): 95–109, 111–121.

101. Vandel D., Davari A., Famouri P. Modeling of fluidized bed neural networks. Proceedings of 32nd IEEE SSST. Florida: FAMU-FSU Tallahassee, 2000.

102. Quantrille T. E., Liu Y. A. Artificial Intelligence in Chemical Engineering. San Diego: Academic Press, 1991.

103. Leane M. M., Cumming I., Corrigan O. I. The use of artificial neural networks for the selection of the most appropriate formulation and processing variables in order to predict the in vitro dissolution of sustained-release mini tabs. AAPS PharmSciTech 2003; 4(2): E26.

104. AlAlaween, W. H. Predictive modelling of the granulation process using a systems-engineering approach. Powder Technol 2016; 302: 265–274. doi:10.1016/j.powtec.2016.08.049.

105. Landin, M. Artificial intelligence tools for scaling up of high shear wet granulation process. J Pharm Sci 2017; 106(1): 273–277.

106. Zawbaa H. M. Computational Intelligence Modeling of Pharmaceutical Properties. Carretero J., Blas J. G., Petcu, D. (Editors). Proceedings of the First Ph.D. Symposium on Sustainable Ultrascale Computing Systems (NESUS Ph.D. 2016) Timisoara, Romania, February 8–11, 2016.

107. https://www.outsourcing-pharma.com/Article/2020/05/11/Collaboration-to-use-AI-to-produce-critical-pharmaceutical-ingredients#.

108. Chow A. H., Tong H. H. Y., Chattopadhyay P., Shekunov, B. Y. Particle engineering for pulmonary delivery. Pharm Res 2007, March; 24(3): 411–437.

109. Mack P., Harvath K., Garcia A., Tully J., Maynor B. Particle engineering for inhalation formulation and delivery of biotherapeutics. Inhalation, August 2012.

110. Rolland J. P. et al. Direct fabrication and harvesting of monodisperse, shape-specific nano biomaterials. J Ame Chem Soc. 2005 July; 127(28): 10096–10100.

111. Garcia A. et al. Microfabricated engineered particle systems for respiratory drug delivery and other pharmaceutical applications. J Drug Del. 2012; 6: 941243.

112. Cherukuvada S., Kaura R., Row, T. N. G. Co-crystallization and small molecule crystal form diversity: from pharmaceutical to materials applications. CrystEngComm 2016;18:8528–8555.

113. Blagden, N. et al. Current directions in co-crystal growth. New J Chem 2008; 32(10): 1659. doi:10.1039/b803866j.hdl:10454/4848.

114. Lam M., Ghafourian T., Nokhodchi A. Liqui-pellet: the emerging next-generation oral dosage form which stems from liquisolid concept in combination with pelletization technology. AAPS PharmSciTech 2019; 20: 231. doi:10.1208/s12249-019-1441-9.

115. Fray R. Microfluidic encapsulation: controlling drug delivery with PLGA. Drug Dev Deliv October 2019; 19(7).

116. Song X. R., Cai Z., Zheng Y., He G., Cui F. Y., et al. Reversion of multidrug resistance by co-encapsulation of vincristine and verapamil in PLGA nanoparticles. Eur J Pharm Sci 2009; 37: 300–305.

117. Williams G. R., Nagy Z. K., Lagaron J. M. Electrospinning from benchtop to bedside? American Pharma Review January-February 2020; 20–25.

118. Adeli E. Irbesartan-loaded electrospun nanofibers-based PVP-K90 for the drug dissolution improvement fabrication, in vitro performance assessment and in vivo evaluation. J Appl Polym Sci. 2015; 132 (27): 42212.

119. Illangakoon U. E., Nazir T., Williams G. R., Chatterton N. P. Mebeverine-loaded electrospun nanofibers: physicochemical characterization and dissolution studies. J Pharm Sci 2014; 103(1): 283–292.

120. Chen J. et al. A novel application of electrospinning technique in the sublingual membrane: characterization, permeation and in *vivo study*. Drug Dev Ind Pharm 2016; 42(8): 1365–1374.

121. Scaffaro R., Maio A., Gulino E. F., Micale, G. D. M. PLA-based functionally graded laminates for tunable controlled release of carvacrol obtained by combining electrospinning with solvent casting. React Funct Polym March 2020; 148: 104490.

122. Coimbra P., Freitasbc J. P., Gonçalves T., Gil, M. H., Figueiredo, M. Preparation of gentamicin sulfate eluting fiber mats by emulsion and by suspension electrospinning. Mater Sci Eng C January 2019; 94(1) 86–93.

123. Haider A., Haider S., Kanga I.-K. A comprehensive review summarizing the effect of electrospinning parameters and potential applications of nanofibers in biomedical and biotechnology. Arab J Chem 2018; 11: 1165–1188.

124. Sharma A., Das P., Buschmann M., Gilbert J. A. The future of microbiome-based therapeutics in clinical applications. Clin Pharmacol Ther Jan 2020; 107(1): 123–128.

125. Mohajeri M. H., Brummer R-J., Rastall R. A., Weersma R. K. The role of the microbiome for human health: from basic science to clinical applications. Eur J Nutr May 2018; 57(Suppl 1): 1–14.

126. Cope E. K. Novel microbiome-based therapeutics for chronic rhinosinusitis. Rhinosinusitis March 2015; 15(3): 504.

127. Terry M. The brave new world of microbiome-based therapies. Biospace Feb 11, 2020. https://www.biospace.com/article/the-brave-new-world-of-microbiome-based-therapies/.

128. Fukui H. Gut microbiome-based therapeutics in liver cirrhosis: basic consideration for the next step. J Clin Transl Hepatol Sep 28, 2017; 5(3): 249–260. doi:10.14218/JCTH.2017.00008.

129. Sanghvi G. et al. Microbiome as therapeutics in vesicular delivery. Biomed Pharmacother August 2018; 104: 738–741.

130. Jones L. The human microbiome – a new frontier in drug discovery. DDW 2016; Summar issue. https://www.ddw-online.com/the-human-microbiome-a-new-frontier-in-drug-discovery-528-201608/.

131. Fernández C. R. No guts, no glory: how microbiome research is changing medicine. January 22, 2019. https://www.labiotech.eu/in-depth/gut-microbiome-research/#.

132. Bamforth M. Supporting commercialization of live biotherapeutic products for microbiome-based therapies. Pharma's Almanac December 6, 2019. https://www.pharmasalmanac.com/articles/supporting-commercialization-of-live-biotherapeutic-products-for-microbiome-based-therapies.

Section II

Granulation Processes

8 Roller Compaction Technology

Ronald W. Miller and Vishwas Nesarikar[1]

CONTENTS

8.1 INTRODUCTION

Since the publication of *Handbook of Pharmaceutical Granulation Technology*, third edition, the world's economy has picked up, as well as a capital expansion is witnessed in the worldwide biopharmaceutical industry. However, oral solid dosage forms have lagged [1]. Several pharmaceutical drug companies, large and small, have reduced staff, sold manufacturing sites, or merged. CenterWatch.com tracks approved FDA drug approvals and has shown an increase in large molecule drug product approvals in the past few years. Despite the apparent pharmaceutical industry economic outlook, I do believe, the important need for dry granulation technology keeps growing in the pharmaceutical industry, as well as in other industries.

The legacy pharmaceutical roller compaction technology and scale-up book chapters, by this author, previously published in *Handbook of Pharmaceutical Granulation Technology*, first, second, and third editions; *The Encyclopedia of Pharmaceutical Technology*; and *The Pharmaceutical Process Scale-Up*, second edition covered a very wide range of useful related topics [1–5]. The learnings and findings expressed in these chapters reviewed and discussed roller compaction theory, equipment design features, for example, feed screw and specifically the importance of vacuum deaeration theory and equipment designs of different manufacturers. New findings by Guigon and his team were expressed about their advanced roll sensor instrumentation his work showed that the pressure variance applied to powder across the roll surface was caused by the feed screw position.

Miller presented the first at-line near-infrared (NIR) roller compaction evaluations of compacts manufactured at different roll pressures, vacuum deaeration pressures, power consumptions, and compared different processing effects. Later, he teamed with Purdue University Industrial Physical Pharmacy School faculty and graduate students, in a series of noninvasive real-time NIR dynamic-mode roller-compacted powder blend property (e.g., content uniformity, moisture content, compact density, tensile strength, and Young's modulus), evaluations that were published [6].

The beginning section of this book chapter describes the industrial perspective of the value of roller compaction technology, its importance, and some technical aspects. While the primary focus of this chapter is related to the pharmaceutical industry, other industrial viewpoints are illustrated for comparison and reference. Modeling techniques were developed to predict compactor process parameters for scale-up.

8.2 ACTIVE PHARMACEUTICAL INGREDIENT POWDERS

In the pharmaceutical industry, brand name innovator companies aim to develop formulations and processes to convey new therapeutic benefits of active pharmaceutical ingredients (APIs), in oral solid dosage forms for patients.

Typically, the morphology of newly invented synthesized API powders is very fine, with low density and not uniform in shape; with powder particle physical attributes not free-flowing. Ultimately, the API is a poor actor regarding powder property behaviors for formulation and process development considerations and downstream drug product manufacturing. Similar situations arise in the battery, beverage, cement, chemical, and food industries, where synthesized processes produce powders that have poor powder physical properties for next-step downstream processing operations.

When manufacturing solid oral dosage forms, there must be successful powder rheology performance. This means it is often necessary to modify the morphology characteristics of fine API powders, typically those powders that are less than 150 μm in size, to obtain a better powder properties for tableting, encapsulation, and powder for oral suspensions (PFOSs) drug product manufacturing.

Emphasizing the key considerations of powder technology properties for pharmaceutical oral solid dosage forms, which are given further, cannot be understated.

- Powder flowability
- Powder compactibility
- Chemical stability

Controlling these three key powder properties will assure achieving critical oral solid dosage form specifications and efficacy. Without the proper physical properties of powder flowability and powder compactibility, meeting worldwide pharmacopeia requirements—such as a tablet or capsule content uniformity, assay, dissolution, weight, and dosage form physical robustness—hardness and friability are virtually impossible.

The third powder property, chemical stability, is very important for any manufactured drug product. The effects of moisture and dry heat from processing powder granulations can be problematic and stressful for drug products manufactured by non-dry granulation technologies. There is significantly less product stability risk from latent moisture and heat liable degradation products when manufacturing by a dry granulation processing method. The author admits that from a stability standpoint, it has been his observation that the most robust drug product granulation manufacturing is by roller compaction dry granulation technology. Anecdotal proof of this assertion can be surveyed online in the pharmaceutical "The Pink Sheets" or "The Pink Sheets Daily," publisher FDC Reports, where product recall information identifies which commercial oral solid dosage form product failed specifications and why it failed, and describes the general drug process method. Reviewing these two published resources since 2000, there have been no cited dry granulated recalled products [7].

8.3 GRANULATION TECHNOLOGIES

There are three key technology drug product processing methods that are most widely used to enable modifying API physical properties to formulate pharmaceutical oral solid dosage forms: direct compression, wet agglomeration, and dry agglomeration. Direct compression is a process by which tablets are compressed directly from powder blends containing the API and suitable excipients, for example, disintegrants, binders, glidants, and lubricants, without any preprocessing treatment. For some time now, many new API powder substances in the pharmaceutical industry cannot be directly compressed into tablets or encapsulated into hard gelatin capsules or even filled into PFOS bottles. Typically, a successful direct compression blend must be designed and developed to meet drug product specification requirements when operating high-speed compression machines, for example, filling a die cavity in 12 msec; anecdotally, not a trivial task [8].

The majority of new active pharmaceutical powder ingredients are small, needle-like habit morphology that is very heterogeneous in size and very potent. Oral solids formulations of these drugs are usually low dosage strengths that are generally well under 100 mg per dose. Achieving active uniform distribution to guarantee correct drug product uniformity in each unit dose is paramount and not easy, requiring an optimal processing technology.

The demanding robustness of such formulations and drug product processes must imperatively withstand API and excipients' additional physical property variances, for example, lot-to-lot granulometry and morphology differences, which affect potential segregation of powder blend transfers from one manufacturing floor to another, or the transfer of the product's process to multiple drug product manufacturing sites. Illustrating the point, potential powder segregation can occur during the conveyance of a final blend from a holding vessel through a long tube or chute (possibly as long as two to four meters) from one processing floor to another where compressing or encapsulating machines are located. Variable API and excipient raw material physical properties and the potential rigorous handling of drug product blend throughout the drug product manufacturing process requires that the successful drug product be undisturbed by potential segregation mechanisms or influences. Thus, the author contends that it is less likely that brand name innovator companies would want to develop and manufacture new oral solid drug formulations via direct compression technology.

The increasingly important reason for pretreatment of active pharmaceutical powders is the necessity to attain acceptable powder flowability and powder compactibility, and minimize powder segregation after mixing during downstream process handling.

The wet granulation pretreatment technologies, low shear, high shear, and fluid bed have two common processing technology requirements: a liquid to granulate the batch and a drying cycle to dry the granulated mass. The author has observed that the new APIs developed today are more potent and much more sensitive to non-dry preprocessing treatments and environments. The pharmaceutical risk is that in aqueous drug product manufacturing environments, the API can be potentially modified, and new degradants formed or a known degradant level abnormally increased.

Pharmaceutically, this is unacceptable for stability, efficacy, and potential safety reasons and can delay or doom a promising API for potential patient therapeutical use. It is the author's opinion that the risk is so great that it can over-ride all other attributes regarding wet agglomeration development and product manufacturing. Other issues that compare and illustrate additional wet granulation differences versus dry granulation roller compaction drug product technologies are given further.

- Typically, there are more machines and plant space requirements to maintain aqueous granulation processes than dry granulation technology.
- Equipment sunken costs are greater for wet granulation equipment cross-contamination issues than with dry granulation technology requirements.
- Variable operating costs are higher for wet granulator and dryer systems than with dry granulation technology.
- Cleaning cycles are more frequent with wet granulation equipment trains than dry granulation manufacturing equipment.
- Initial operating and recovery safety issues are very costly with solvent granulating systems, there are none with roller compaction.
- Scale-up is less complicated with dry granulation compared with wet granulation [5].
  - Wet granulation scale-up has many more major and minor variables to monitor during wet granulation and drying processes than a dry granulation roller compaction process [9].
  - Scale-up using wet granulation equipment requires a larger bowl and batch sizes—manufacturing capacity is a function of bowl size volume and manufacturing time.
  - Scale-up using roller compaction can be accomplished with development sized equipment—it only requires longer equipment operating hours as manufacturing capacity is primarily a function of operating time providing more capacity and operational flexibility.
- Wet granulation endpoints can change as the granulator power consumption profile can change when manufacturing multiple consecutive batches during a shift or campaign-requiring more sensor controls to understand the process.
- The wetting of raw material is more influenced by raw material property changes, for example, particle size distribution (PSD), and density than raw material changes affecting roller compaction.
- In the case of manufacturing a wet granulation batch, if an electrical outage occurs, the probability of losing the batch is high if there is no backup battery system to quickly start and continue the process; this is not an issue with a roller compaction process.
- Massing effects and drying capacity issues are key concerns in scale-up for drying granulations produced in separate steps for high-or low-shear wet granulation technologies [9].

A word regarding solvent granulation processing technology: while the solvent granulation technology generally eliminates the issues and the pharmaceutical risks that are associated with aqueous drug product manufacturing environments as aforementioned, the manufacturing equipment and ancillary supporting equipment costs; environmental, U.S. government, and OSHA safety issues; and public concerns with solvent manufacturing technologies have become significantly more intense, complex, and costly, particularly for a startup. Lastly, it is highly questionable that this technology, in general, does not reduce pharmaceutical drug product manufacturing costs for the potential drug product manufacturing gains.

8.3.1 SUMMARY

The aforementioned concerns and issues, which are associated with the development of new APIs transformed into pharmaceutical drug product processes, direct compression, wet and solvent granulation technologies, and improved drug product granulation processes, make use of dry granulation technology, roller compaction. A schematic picture depicts basic dry agglomeration processing stages (Figure 8.1).

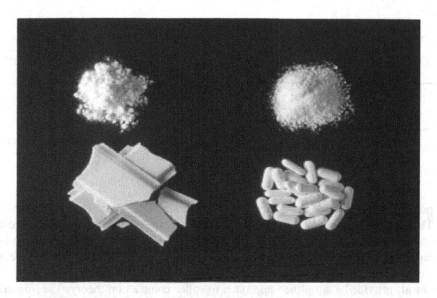

FIGURE 8.1 Dry agglomeration processing steps; API powder (upper left), compacted API blend (lower left), milled and blended compacts (upper right), and compressed tablets (lower right).

8.4 COMPACTION THEORY

The bonding forces in a dry aggregate are important for granulation properties such as granule integrity, flowability, friability, density, compressibility, and size for downstream manufacturing process steps. Pietsch and coworkers [10] described the bonding mechanisms occurring during dry granulation as a mixture of van der Waals forces, mechanical interlocking, recombination of bonds established between freshly created surfaces, and solid bridges, created because of solidification during compression.

A general theory describes particle bonding related to roller compaction in *The Handbook of Pharmaceutical Granulation Technology* [3]. The process of dry granulation relies on inter particulate bond formation. Granule bond formation is characterized in different stages, which usually occurs in the following order:

1. Particle rearrangement
2. Particle deformation
3. Particle fragmentation
4. Particle bonding

Particle rearrangement occurs initially as powder particles begin filling void spaces. The air begins to leave the powder blend's interstitial spaces, and particles begin to move closer together. This action increases the powder blend's density. Particle shape and size are key factors in the rearrangement process. Spherical particles will tend to move lesser than other shaped particles because of their close initial packing to one another. Particle deformation occurs as compression forces are increased. This deformation increases the points of contact between particles where bonding occurs and is described as plastic deformation [3]. Particle fragmentation follows as the next bonding stage. This occurs at increased compression force levels. At this stage, particle fracturing creates multiple new surface sites, additional contact points, and potential bonding sites. Particle bonding occurs when plastic deformation and fragmentation happen. It is generally accepted that bonding takes place at the molecular level and that this is due to the effect of van der Waals forces [3].

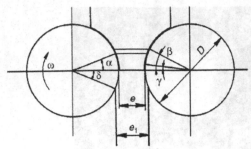

FIGURE 8.2   Front view of rolls in the horizontal plain.
Source: From Ref. [11].

When powder granules undergo an applied force or stress, a stress force is released from the granules. The granules attempt to return to their original shape or form; this is described as elastic deformation. A deformation that does not totally recover after the stress is released is a plastic deformation. Elastic and plastic deformations can occur simultaneously, but one effect usually predominates.

Dehont et al. provided a simplified approach to roller compaction theory. They described that powder granules move through stages in the feed area. The material is drawn into the gap by rubbing against the roll surfaces. The densification that occurs in this area is particle rearrangement. At this stage, the speed of the powder is slower than the peripheral speed of the rollers. Figure 8.2 represents compactor rolls in the horizontal plane; the powder is pushed vertically downward into the compaction area [11].

Note that in Figure 8.2, α is the nip angle and β is the material in volume space. The material is located in the compaction area between α and the horizontal axis (Figure 8.2). At this stage, the material undergoes additional compaction forces.

The particles undergo plastic deformation and are bonded. Dehont's team noted that the nip angle varies according to the material characteristics of particle size and density and the angle is about 12° [11]. They defined the neutral angle, γ, which corresponds to the point where the pressure applied by the rollers is the greatest on the material. They also defined elastic deformation, δ, and that occurs after the compact begins leaving the compression roll area. Compacted flakes may increase in size because of material elastic deformation and actually may have a larger thickness than the roll gap, e, [11]. Dehont et al. developed Equation (8.1) for the linear variation of flake thickness at a specific roll diameter [11].

$$e_1 = D\left(\frac{d_0}{d_1 - d_0}\right)(1 - \cos \alpha) \tag{8.1}$$

Equation (8.1) defined:
  e_1 = flake thickness
  D = roll diameter
  d_0 = material density at angle α
  d_1 = flake density

Dehont et al. assumed that the material in the compaction area remains horizontal and moves at the peripheral speed of the rollers. They also considered that the angle, α, is independent of the roller diameter size and noted that the flake thickness, e_1, depends on the roller speed, the roller surface, and the compaction pressure. All these parameters influence the density of the flake, d_1. Dehont et al. concluded that if the same flake thickness were obtained with different roller diameters, the flake density would be greater with larger diameter rollers [11]. This is due to the greater nip angle formed with the larger rolls allowing more material to be compacted.

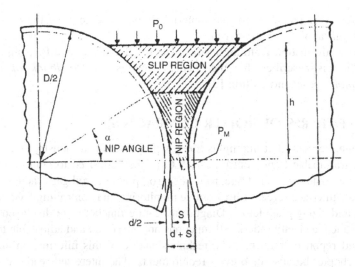

FIGURE 8.3 Front view of compactor rolls in horizontal plain depicting powder regions under different compaction forces. Abbreviations: P_o, horizontal pressure between rolls; θ, angular position of roll bite; α, nip angle; $2d$, roll diameter D; h, height above the roll centerline at which feed pressure P_o is applied; P_m, horizontal pressure at $\theta = 0$; S, roll gap.
Source: From Ref. [12].

Johanson identified, through very comprehensive mathematical models and relationships, material properties, press dimensions, and operating conditions for roll compactors. For more information, the interested person should read the entire reference [12]. In short, he described that roller compaction involves a continuous shear deformation of the granules into a solid mass.

To satisfy the theory's assumption, it was postulated that the material be isotropic, frictional, cohesive, and compressible. Figure 8.3 depicts material in a roll press that undergoes shear deformation into a solid mass [12].

Johanson pointed out that no roller compactor theories at that time determined the angle of the nip and the bulk density at $\theta = \alpha$, except by actually rolling the granular solid in a roll press. He also provided a method to calculate the nip angle and the pressure distribution between the rolls. His calculations determined the pressure distribution above the nip area and the pressure in that area [12].

He provided the technical rationale to calculate the nip pressures in the nip region. He showed that the material trapped in a volume, V_α, between arc-length segments ΔL, must be compressed to volume, V_θ, between the same arc-length segments. The relationship requires that the bulk densities, γ_α and γ_θ in volumes, V_α, and V_θ, be related by Eq. (8.2) [12]

$$\frac{\gamma_\alpha}{\gamma_\theta} = \frac{V_\theta}{V_\alpha} \tag{8.2}$$

Johanson stated that the pressure, σ_θ, at any $\theta < \alpha$ can be determined as a function of the pressure σ_α, at $\theta = \alpha$, by the pressure-density relationship. It was understood that, for increasing pressures, log density was a linear function of log pressure [13].

Johanson found that the nip angle does not depend on the magnitude of the roll force or the roll diameter. He demonstrated that the nip angle was affected very little by the geometry of the press or the cut grooves on the roll surface. It was mostly influenced by the nature of the materials that were compressed. The very compressible materials, with small K values, had very large nip angles. On the other hand, incompressible materials, with large K values, had very small nip angles.

Ultimately, Johanson's results showed that material properties determine the maximum pressure that a roller press can apply to the material.

Note that further information from authorities, Heckel, Johanson, and Pietsch, on bonding and compaction theories is described for the readers' interest in *Handbook of Pharmaceutical Granulation Technology*, second edition [2].

8.5 DESIGN FEATURES OF ROLLER COMPACTORS

Certainly, a key enhancement that highlights today's pharmaceutical industry state-of-the-art roller compactors is programmable logic controllers (PLCs). They are used to control and monitor mechanical parts that regulate screw feed rate, roll speed, roll pressure, roll gap, vacuum deaeration, and mill speed. Operator interface screens allow online monitoring and controlling feed screw speed, roll gap and pressure, and sizing granulators. Diagnostic feature functions are displayed online, such as operation, maintenance, and calibration. All functions are interfaced and adjustable through PLC for process control and report monitoring. The technical nature of this information and discussion is precluded in this chapter because of brevity requirements. The interested reader can contact roller compactor manufacturing vendors and get information on the same subject.

Briefly, a key machine innovation, vacuum deaeration, was a new important feature design added by some roller compactor vendors in the early-mid-1990s. The design feature has been shown to help premodify raw material density before compacting and increase throughput [14]. Other equipment features, such as multiple horizontal or angled feed screws, assist manufacturing a uniform powder feed across the rolls [14,15].

Newly designed roll machine blocks, featuring cantilever roll systems, offer more efficient ways to clean, handle, and facilitate product and equipment changeovers. Newly designed storage hoppers and various screw feeder designs have improved delivering poor powder flowing materials to the rolls. A history of the hopper and feed screw designs showed that each design evolved to facilitate and improve powder flow to the compactor feed screw conveyance system. Innovatively designed feed screw systems are used commercially in roller compactors worldwide to improve powder feed to the rolls. These systems can be seen in reference [4]. Sizing mills are now trimly fitted to the compactor body and controlled by variable-speed drives. Most compactors no longer require a second machine (mill) in tandem to size compacts as required by slugging technology. Roller compactors have clean-in-place (CIP) systems that offer environmental and safety features. These systems minimize human exposure to chemicals and improve cleaning efficiencies.

Compactor design features have evolved over the years. By the mid-1970s, research revealed a number of roll design improvements that increased compacting efficiency. Three key conditions were identified, at that time, which optimized the roll compact throughput and minimized leakage of noncompacted powder [16].

- Adequate powder supply must enter the gripping zone.
- Powder must be conveyed fully into the narrowest part of the roller gap.
- Compaction pressure must be distributed as uniformly as possible across the whole roller-gripped powder mass.

Equipment engineers and researchers worked on improving feeding-equipment systems and roll designs to satisfy and maximize the aforementioned conditions. Some of the key advances are identified in reference [14] and are reemphasized here.

Because of powder feed variability at the nip and in the roll gap regions, powder leakage is produced during the compVaction process. This situation produces excessive fines and possible undesirable processed material. Usually, this problem is caused by uneven powder flow and compact formed when the powder is fed toward the middle of the roll width. Granules produced under these conditions are sometimes not optimal for further pharmaceutical processing.

This leads to some questions; what is the optimum roll speed for a compaction process? What factors does the formulating scientist or process engineer need to consider to maximize compact quality and compaction throughput? Johanson [17] attempted to answer these questions by predicting roll-limiting speeds for briquetting presses. He developed mathematical expressions considering even the gas and liquid effects as they can theoretically be squeezed from a solid mass. Solid properties, press dimensions, and operating conditions were evaluated to predict optimum roll speeds. The results necessary for a quality briquette are most critical for low-density fine particles. Johanson's work showed the relation between feed pressure and roll speed to essentially be proportional to the material's permeability (porosity). For additional information, the interested reader should peruse the reference list.

Sheskey and Hendren, in 1999, studied the effect of roll surface configuration on the drug release and physical properties of an HPMC matrix controlled-release dosage form [18]. Smooth and axial-grooved roll surface designs were studied using a Vector Model TF-Mini roller compactor (Vector Corporation, Marion, IA). They hypothesized that the greater the depth of the roll concavity surface, the less evenly the powder would displace on the roll surface compared to a smooth non-concave roll surface. Thus, as with tablet-tooling design, the top of the crown area of the compacted ribbon would theoretically be softer than the rest of the ribbon. However, the results of a particle size distribution test performed on milled ribbons generated using both smooth and axial-grooved roll pairs, showed similarity between tested samples. Besides, results showed little difference in tablet-crushing strength values between samples manufactured using either type of (smooth or axial grooved) roll surface designs. Drug release profiles of tablets prepared from roller-compacted granulations using both roll surface configurations were also similar.

The consistency and evenness of the powder feed, largely determined by powder flow properties and by the feed screw conveyance into the roll pair determines to a large extent, how complete a compact is made and ultimately the success of a compaction process. Most roller compacting systems suffer the disadvantage of leakage, that is, 20% to 30% powder particles (depending on the formulation) that are not uniformly compacted. This primarily occurs because of uneven powder feed and powder slippage between individual loose particles and the roll surfaces. Under these conditions, it is usually necessary to recycle the uncompacted powder or fines. Recycling a compaction process is a significant drawback because of additional capital expenditure, labor costs, and increased throughput time.

Operationally, the key goal of a compactor is to maintain a range of pressure on the powder feedstock, independent of the fluctuating powder granulometry and powder flow fed to the rolls, so that a consistent compact is made. Historically, the compaction process was managed by controlling the input material, the quantity per unit of time, the roll speed, and the roll gap. Allowing the roll gap to float unchecked can influence the production rate and compact quality. Therefore, it is important to control the compaction process by setting a constant powder feed rate during the compaction operation. Design innovations on the powder feed input side of the roller compactor are complex. It is suggested that the interested readers read *Handbook of Pharmaceutical Granulation Technology*, first edition, for additional details.

8.5.1 Deaeration Theory

A key factor limiting compaction throughput and quality is air entrapment in powder materials. During compression, air-occupying voids between particles are compressed and squeezed. The gas pushes through the powder causing powder fluidization and a nonuniform level of powder at the roll gap. It is best described in Figure 8.4a. This situation limits compact throughput and creates a nonuniform compact density. It also creates excess fines prior to sizing because of "spidering" compact edges [19].

The spidering condition occurs when gases rush across the inside of a compact to thinly and weakly formed flaked edges. The flake edges break apart perpendicular to the compaction

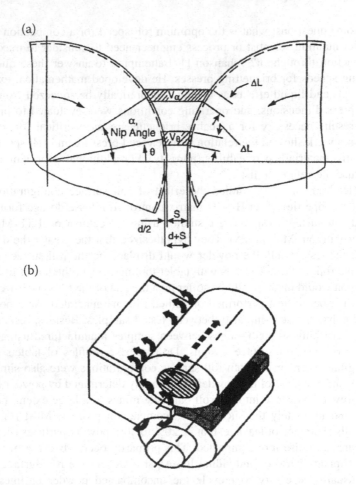

FIGURE 8.4 (a) Front view of compactor rolls in a horizontal plain depicting nip angle. (b) pattern of gas escape from the roll nip region. Abbreviations: P_o, horizontal pressure between rolls; θ, angular position of roll bite; α, nip angle; $2d$, roll diameter D; h, height above the roll centerline at which feed pressure P_o is applied; P_m, horizontal pressure at $\theta = 0$; S, roll gap; ΔL, arc-length segments; V_α, material trapped in volume space described by arc lengths; V_θ, compressed volume space described by arc lengths; γ_α and γ_θ, respective powder bulk densities in volume spaces V_α and V_θ; K, a material property constant for given moisture content, temperature, and time of compaction.
Source: From Refs. [12,19].

direction. The compact edge breakage appears "saw tooth" in structure and varies in length depending on the nature of the powder binding properties, the amount of air entrainment and the roll dwell time.

Both Johanson and Pietsch reported that expanding gas in a compact is detrimental to the compaction process: by reducing the compaction throughput and increasing the amount of fine particles. The effects of roll speed and powder porosity on air pressure in a compacted sheet are illustrated in Figure 8.5 by Pietsch [20]. This graphic shows a relatively larger roll speed operating range when compacting a permeable (porous) powder. Air entrainment does not limit roller speed for coarse granular powders. On the other hand, when compacting very fine powders, the operating roll speed range is significantly reduced because of air entrainment.

Miller indicated that the evenness of the powder feed into the rolls determines, to a large extent, the success of compaction. Roller compactor systems suffer from two disadvantages: as the

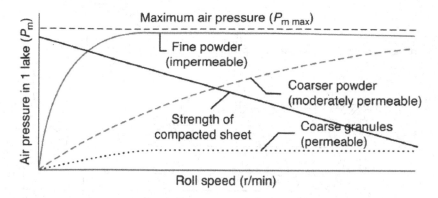

FIGURE 8.5 Effects of roll speed and permeability on air pressure in a compact.
Source: From Ref. [20].

powder feed bulk density approaches 0.3 g/cm^3 or less, the compaction throughput efficiency decreases. Secondly and concurrently, the uncompacted powder leakage generally increases around the rolls [14]. Miller, in 1994, described a new machine design improvement that used vacuum deaeration to remove air entrainment from the powder just before the nip angle during roller compaction. The multiple benefits of such an action are significant, and remarkable efficiency results have been observed when compacting low-density raw materials [14].

- More uniform powder feed to the rollers
- Less voltage and amperage variability for the roll pair
- More uniform and strong compact
- Less powder leakage
- Greater yield
- Less powder adhering to the compact prior to sizing
- Higher compact throughput
- Less airborne particles

The newly designed equipment involved a compactor fitted with two horizontal feed screws, which featured vacuum deaeration. Specifically, the roll compactor was equipped with a conical storage hopper containing a variable-speed agitator. The bulk powder was fed directly from the top of the hopper to the top of twin horizontal auger feed screws, which directly transported the powder to the nip roll area. A side view of the design features is shown in Figure 8.6.

The design is described as a novel stainless steel encasing that leads to the compactor rolls that enclose the variable-speed auger screws. Just before the nip area, a pair of sintered stainless steel segments are assembled within the horizontal auger feed system, which can operate under a partial vacuum. A small, self-contained vacuum pump draws negative pressure through a dry filter and a stainless steel line to the sintered assembly plates. The partial vacuum is adjustable from −0.1 to −0.8 bars. The compaction rolls operate at different speeds and are supported on heavy-duty bearings in such a way that the lower roll is fixed and the upper roll is slightly movable in the vertical plane. The deaerated material passes through the roll pair, which is under infinitely variable hydraulic pressure. The deaeration, auger feed screws' design and speed, roll speed, and hydraulic roll pressures are the main factors in producing a compact with specified properties.

In several experiments, Miller studied the effects of using horizontal twin auger feed screws under partial vacuum (Alexanderwerk, Inc., Horsham, Pennsylvania, U.S., model 50/75 compactor). The powder feed was deaerated just before roller compaction. The experimental design

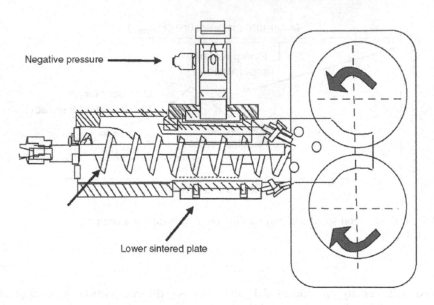

FIGURE 8.6   Side view of feed screw system and vacuum deaeration with sintered plate segments. *Source*: From Ref. [3].

showed that the compactor's deaeration feed system significantly increased compaction output and minimized powder leakage when compacting very low-density blends (< 0.35 g/cm^3) [14].

In several other trials, Miller also studied the effects of using two different compactor's vacuum deaeration systems. His experiments evaluated the effects of powder density, screw feed speed, roll speed, roll pressure, vacuum deaeration pressure, compaction rate, and compaction-leakage rate. Test results demonstrated that the first compactor's deaeration and feed system designs significantly increased compaction output. The new equipment design and process provided high compact yields and virtually eliminated powder leakage, obviating the need for expensive powder recirculation equipment. Vacuum deaeration design of the compactor 1 (Figure 8.7) proved to be superior to the second compactor design (Figure 8.8) when compacting an active bulk drug with a density of approximately 0.2 g/cm^3. In summary, a new critical condition, vacuum deaeration, had been identified in optimizing roller compacting effectiveness and efficiency [3,14].

Miller concluded that four key processing conditions must exist to optimize roller compaction throughput and minimize powder leakage around the rolls [3,14].

- Adequate powder supply must enter the gripping zone.
- Powder must be fully conveyed into the narrowest part of the roller gap.
- Compaction pressure must be distributed as uniformly as possible over the whole of the roller-gripped powder mass.
- Sufficient vacuum deaeration must be effectively distributed prior to the nip roll region, particularly for low bulk density powder feedstock.

Today most compactor companies have designed deaeration systems and have engineered improvements in their deaeration operational effectiveness.

8.6 FORMULATION CONSIDERATIONS

There has not been much published about which ingredients are typically used and at what percentages in the pharmaceutical industry as well as in other industries. This is a very sensitive

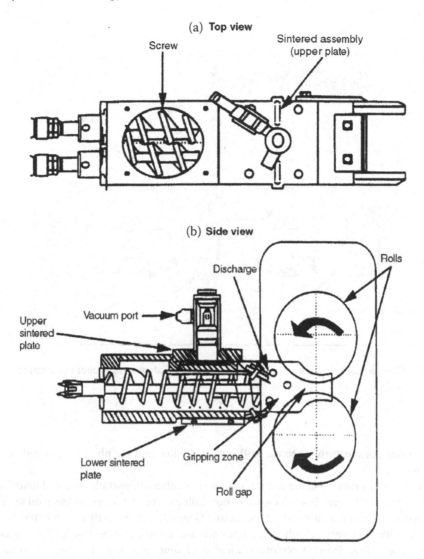

FIGURE 8.7 Horizontal twin-screw vacuum deaeration feed system.
Source: From Ref. [21].

subject as it goes to patentability, competitive business advantages, and privileged information. The author, while reviewing previous book chapters that he wrote, noted there was no mention of this subject matter and thus brief remarks are made here.

The nature of a dry granulated formulation is directly tied very closely to API, the intended therapeutical use and its physical characteristics. Looking at the intended drug use, we need to determine if the dosage form is for immediate-or extended-release therapy. Both dosage forms are uniquely different and require a different formulation approach in the selection of pharmaceutical excipients to make drug products.

The percentage of the API in a formulation is usually dependent on its potency and therapeutical effect, for example, a highly potent API, usually requires a smaller percentage of active drug substance, by weight, to be formulated. On the other hand, a lower potent API, usually requires a larger percentage of the active drug substance, by weight, to be formulated into a dosage form. Thus, the physical characteristics of the API generally come more into play when developing a

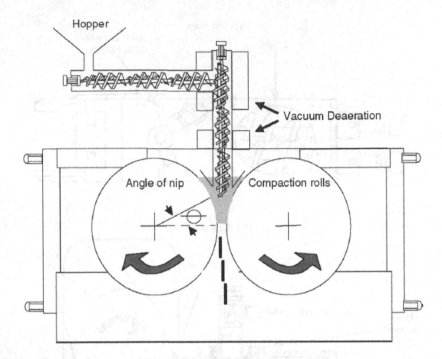

FIGURE 8.8 Compactor front view of a vertical feed screw system with vacuum deaeration. *Source*: From Ref. [3].

roller compaction formulation when the API potency is low and the physical amount of the API is greater by weight.

The API physical property characteristics, cohesive/adhesive, particle size and distribution, low density—typically less than 0.4 g/cc—and morphology are the keys to determine if the API powder property behavior is a good or bad actor. Generally, if the API powder has poor powder properties, then more or very specific excipients are needed to enhance powder flow to assist roller compaction processing. Typical pharmaceutical excipient selections for roller compaction formulations are cited here. Specific ingredients and concentrations vary depending on the aforementioned drug product release discussion. Useful formulation starting points are noted here.

- Filler/diluents/binders—microcrystalline cellulose, mannitol, corn starch, povidone, tribasic calcium phosphate, lactose, HPC, HPMC ~10% to 90%.
- Disintegrants—sodium starch glycolate, (all; half intra and half extra), ~ 1% to 1.5%.
- Lubricants—magnesium stearate, PEGs, SSF, stearic acid, calcium stearate ~1%.
- Glidants—colloidal silicon dioxide ~ 0.5%.
- Surfactant—sodium lauryl sulfate ~ less than 0.5%.

8.6.1 COMPACTION FORMULATION TECHNOLOGY NEEDS

Year 2001 survey findings concluded that companies worldwide using roller compaction manufactured less than 25% of their products. More pharmaceutical innovator companies used roller compaction for a larger percentage of their product line than other industry segments, Figure 8.9. It was speculated by the authors that the innovator industry may be more likely to prefer a

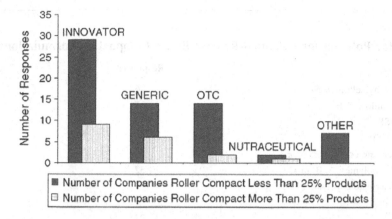

FIGURE 8.9 Companies' approximate percentage of products roller compacted worldwide. *Source*: Ref. [22].

granulation of one type versus another because of long lead times from discovery to market and to minimize the risk of the uncertainty of API chemical properties [22].

In the same survey, Table 8.1 illustrates the preferences for different polymer types used to roller compact immediate-release formulations. Pharmaceutical formulators, in general, appeared to have a similar formulating mindset when it came to developing solid dosage forms. The authors speculated that roller compaction, in the mind of a pharmaceutical formulator, is a combination of a direct compression choice for a polymer (e.g., microcrystalline celluloses) and a granulation choice for a polymer (e.g., the wet granulation polymers chosen by formulators such as poly-vinylpyrrolidone, hydroxypropyl methylcellulose, and starch) [22].

When developing an immediate-release tablet formulation, the tablet must release the drug quickly while maintaining good physical characteristics. To achieve fast drug dissolution properties, it is useful to incorporate a portion of the disintegrant excipient within the powder mix prior to roller compaction. A remaining portion of the disintegrant should be added extra granular to the final blend just before the lubricant addition. This intra-and extra granular disintegrant placement is quite important to maintain minimal tablet disintegration and fast dissolution times. This concept is

TABLE 8.1
Preferences for Polymer for Immediate-Release Roller Compaction Formulations

Polymer	Responses	Average Rating
Microcrystalline cellulose, PH 101 or PH 102, USP	48	3.8
Polyvinylpyrrolidone, USP	41	3.7
Hydroxypropyl methylcellulose, NF	40	3.4
Starch, USP	45	3.2
Methylcellulose, USP	38	2.8
Hydroxypropyl cellulose, NF	36	2.8
Methacrylic acid copolymer, A, B, or C	20	2.3
Ammonio methacrylate copolymer, A or B	29	1.7
Wax	28	1.5
Others	8	1.9

Source: From Ref. [22].
5, high preference; 1, low preference.

TABLE 8.2

Preferences for Polymer for Extended-Release Roller Compaction Formulations

Polymer	Responses	Average Rating
Hydroxypropyl methylcellulose, NF	46	4.5
Hydroxypropyl cellulose, NF	37	3.6
Ethylcellulose, USP	37	3.5
Methylcellulose, USP	38	3.0
Ammonio methacrylate copolymer, A or B	29	2.5
Methacrylic acid copolymer, A, B, or C	32	2.5
Aminoalkyl methacrylate copolymer, E	29	2.1
Others	9	2.3
Wax	27	2.1

Source: From Ref. [22].
5, high preference; 1, low preference.

described in U.S. patent 4609695 (Franz and Guyer). They described tablet disintegration, and drug release of ibuprofen from a high dose drug formulation was enhanced through the use of intra-and extra granular placement of a disintegrant excipient.

Table 8.2 shows that hydroxypropyl methylcellulose is the preferred polymer for use in extended-release roller compaction formulations. Hydroxypropyl cellulose and ethylcellulose polymers are also significantly preferred, followed by methylcellulose and various methacrylate polymers. The polymer preferences for extended-release formulations, using roller compaction technology, appeared to reflect polymer usage that is associated with matrix extended-release systems.

Survey information ranked compaction formulations containing API and lubricant only versus compacting formulations containing API with small amounts of lubricant and excipients. The combination of API + lubricant + excipients was more preferred in formulations. This process preference may be due, in part, to improved efficiencies of technical operations, from minimizing subsequent processing and less cumbersome handling steps downstream before encapsulating and or tableting.

Table 8.3 indicates that the binder class is slightly more likely to be used than other excipient classes when a roller compaction formulation is developed. The preferred usage of the other excipient classes is about the same.

Table 8.4 shows that the most preferred excipient filler for pharmaceutical roller compaction is the microcrystalline celluloses followed by lactoses. Microcrystalline celluloses and lactoses are popular in solid-dose formulations because of their compactibility, compatibility, functionality, uniformity of

TABLE 8.3

Excipient Class Preferences

Excipient Class	Responses	Average Rating
Binder	54	3.6
Disintegrant	51	3.2
Lubricant	53	3.0
Filler	53	2.9
Glidant	52	2.5

Source: From Ref. [22].
5, high preference; 1, low preference.

TABLE 8.4
Excipient Filler Preferences

Excipient Filler	Responses	Average Rating
Microcrystalline cellulose, PH 101	54	4.0
Microcrystalline cellulose, PH 102	53	3.6
Lactose	48	3.2
Lactose, anhydrous	43	3.1
Dibasic calcium phosphate	48	2.5
Starch	52	2.4
Others	6	2.7

Source: From Ref. [22].
5, high preference; 1, low preference.

supply, and their long withstanding use in the industry. A comment about the "other" excipient category is warranted; a number of survey write-ins included sucrose as an excipient filler of choice.

Regarding the use of disintegrants, Table 8.5 shows the most highly rated disintegrants used in roller compaction, croscarmellose sodium, and sodium starch glycolate.

It is useful to incorporate half of the total lubricant in the powder mix before the roller compaction step and incorporate the remaining portion of the lubricant post granulation.

The idea is to have sufficient lubricity in the powder mix to adequately lubricate the surfaces of the roller compaction equipment (interior of the powder feed area, feed screws, and roll surfaces) and secondly, also for the tablet press tooling and dies. Figure 8.10 describes lubricant usage levels in roller-compacted formulations. Seventy-five percent of the roller-compacted formulations containing magnesium stearate are formulated at 0.5% to 1.0% level. Stearic acid, hydrogenated vegetable oil, and talc are formulated primarily at 1% or higher levels in roller compaction formulations. Sodium stearyl fumarate, at this time, appears to be used sparingly in roller compaction formulations [22].

Sheskey et al. conducted studies demonstrating the enhancement of material flow properties of the niacinamide controlled-release matrix. The excipients used consisted of methylcellulose, hydroxypropyl methylcellulose, and magnesium stearate. Using roller compaction technology, the

TABLE 8.5
Disintegrant Preferences

Disintegrant	Responses	Average Rating
Croscarmellose sodium	36	3.7
Sodium starch glycolate	44	3.4
Pregelatinized starch 1500	34	3.3
Crospovidone	30	2.8
Starch	37	2.5
Other	6	1.3

Source: From Ref. [22].
5, high preference; 1, low preference.

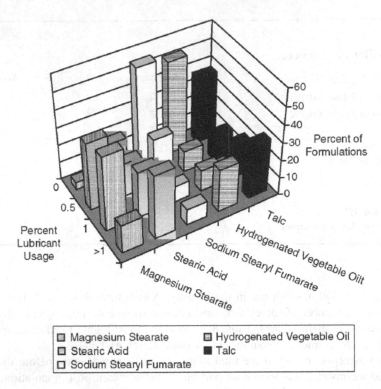

FIGURE 8.10 Lubricant usage in roller-compacted formulations.
Source: From Ref. [22].

authors successfully demonstrated the processing of high molecular weight polymers with niacinamide into free-flowing granules that were compressed into controlled-release tablets [23].

They also roller-compacted powder blends at low, intermediate, and high-pressure levels and
selectively sized the compacts. The granule portions were evaluated for the following process
attributes: recompactibility, content uniformity, and tablet characteristics. Evaluations of the selective granule portions indicated that the smaller granules were produced at lower compaction
pressures and the larger granules were produced at higher compaction pressures. The relationship
is explained by higher compactor pressures producing a stronger, more resilient powder mass,
which, when subsequently milled, resists sizing. This, in turn, produced a coarser particle size
distribution. Compressed tablets from the three different pressure compacts demonstrated consistently higher hardness values and lower friability results from granulations compacted at the
lowest compaction pressures. These findings parallel other authors' results [24,25] pertaining to
reworking compressed tablets into sized granules that were then recompressed into tablets.

Sheskey et al. [25] also found that extensive recycling coarse and fine materials with the original feedstock produced poor tablet content uniformity results. The subsequent tablet compression
produced lower tablet hardness values than were observed in the original tablet compression. This
situation is explained by the production of robust granules that exhibit increased resistance to
deformation during recompression. This effect is known as the work hardening principle. Sheskey
and the team found no apparent relationship between the compaction pressure level applied to the
polymers in the matrix system and the resultant drug tablet dissolution. Also, no relationship was
observed between the tablet hardness levels and the drug tablet dissolution. In their studies, they
observed that the granulation densities increased because of roller compaction. The interested
reader will find more information per the reference.

8.7 INSTRUMENTED ROLLER COMPACTOR TECHNOLOGY FOR PRODUCT DEVELOPMENT, DESIGN OF EXPERIMENTS, AND SCALE-UP

In the mid-1990s, I mentioned, "There is no such thing as a standard approach to solving compactor scale-up or compactor equipment changes in the pharmaceutical production process" [3]. At that time, it appeared that was very much the case history of roller compaction scale-up in the pharmaceutical industry. This understanding was based on the fact that there were no pharmaceutical industrial journal articles published at the time on the subject. On the other hand, it was also true that considerations, approaches, and examples presented in that chapter were experienced by others and were not all-inclusive.

The Pharmaceutical Process Scale-Up, second edition, roller compaction scale-up chapter, published in 2006 offers specific compaction process scale-up and equipment technology transfer concepts experienced by the author and others that were published since 1997. To those who contributed and are advancing roller compaction technology, it is gratifying to see a paradigm shift and an expansion to dry granulation roller compaction technology in our industry. Additionally, with process analytical technology tools, significant opportunities to standardize roller compaction design of experiments and scale-up exist. It is my view that process analytical technology tools will drive roller compaction scale-up for years to come.

Factors of scaling-up a pharmaceutical compaction process or equipment technology transfer involve a number of issues and technologies. Numerous considerations go beyond the specific process and technology that evolve from the pilot plant to the manufacturing technical operations center. Most of these concerns are centered on the plant's current operations, and its previous use or manufacture of dry granulations using roller compaction technology. See Ref. [22], which cites a comparative study summary.

Some scale-up factors that go beyond specific formulation technical aspects follow: What type of equipment manufacturer support is expected? What is the reputation and reliability of the equipment manufacturer in the country where the start-up will occur? What is the equipment manufacturer's customer service record worldwide? How many days will it take to replace a broken or worn out part? Does the equipment manufacturer carry a reliable stock parts inventory? *Note*: A survey evaluated industrial practices and preferences that addressed some of these questions [22].

Professionals in pharmaceutical manufacturing science understand that no single written journal article could hope to provide universal guidance on roller compaction scale-up. On the one hand, the best way to solve these types of challenges is to attack them systematically. This usually can be achieved through appropriate process qualifications and validation efforts: trial and error approach before start-up, knowledge of equipment processing capabilities and limitations, and understanding raw materials' variability. On the other hand, process analytical technology tools and approaches will offer different pathways to attack the scale-up and the validation process [26].

Discussion about roller compaction solid dosage form scale-up, specifically here, does not imply compliance with suggested scale-up and post-approval change (SUPAC) guidelines. The described approaches do not necessarily provide ideas/recommendations that meet tests and filing requirements for changes in manufacturing processes and equipment. Scale-up guidance for immediate-release solid dosage forms and post-approval changes have been published. Readers are suggested to familiarize themselves with the referenced material [27].

FDA CDER has issued significant new changes for good manufacturing practices for process validation when advanced pharmaceutical science and engineering principles and manufacturing control technologies provide a high level of process understanding and control capability [28,29]. The Agency, for example, indicates that manufacturers using such procedures and controls may not necessarily have to manufacture multiple conformance batches to complete process validation [28]. One can readily see how the times are changing and how I believe roller compaction technology for the pharmaceutical industry, because of its simplicity, is primed for additional manufacturing technology advancement.

8.7.1 Technology and Physics Understanding

The compacted ribbon characteristics emerging from a roller compactor depend on the force time profile imparted to the entering powder by the rollers. A central key for drug product development and scale-up is, therefore, to quantitatively characterize the loading profile across the roller width that the powder is subjected to during the compaction process.

Knowing the force-time profile, the compact density can be determined and modeled in real-time. Generating real-time compaction density provides not only a compact process footprint but the compactor vendor can initiate control with an electronic signal to equilibrate compaction density, for example, adjusting feed screw speed, roll gap, and roll pressure. Also important is that the sized-compacted granulate can be modeled from the force-time profile relationship to understand and predict the granulometry and particle size distribution.

This temporal loading profile is a signature of the process that can be directly linked to the characteristics of the ribbon from the fed powder blend, as schematically described in Figure 8.11.

Three elements, powder blend, ribbon property, and final blend characterizations, are necessary to understand the process characterization. These sources of information are necessary to build an experimental database, which contains the information for the development of physically based models that link the properties of the input (powder blend) with the compactor output (compact ribbon and sized granules).

This type of model is desired for designing products attendant to the powder and process characteristic, and thus, central to the quality by design initiative. These models are also necessary for developing robust scaling-up guidelines using numerical simulations that account for the material characteristics as well as boundary and initial conditions, such as techniques that include discrete particle dynamics and finite element method. The predictive capabilities of these numerical techniques rest on the accuracy of the constitutive relations for the evolving properties, in this case, the roller-compacted material, which starts as a loose powder and is transformed into solid-ribbon compact and is then converted back to loose powder.

The instrumented roll provides a new dimension in the translation from R&D to scale-up and routine manufacturing, which is a model-independent approach. The central idea is to instrument two different rolls, one typically for R&D environments (small roll) and one for manufacturing environments (large roll). The strategy is that once a successful roller compaction process is achieved in the R&D lab, the load-time signature is recorded, as well as the sized granulometry

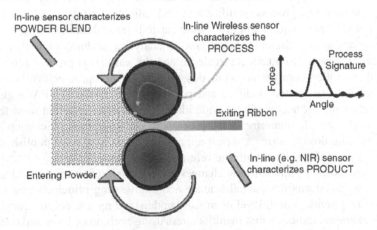

FIGURE 8.11 Schematic of roller compaction in-line sensor approach. Powder blend (input) and compacted ribbon properties (output) are monitored, as well as the force-time profile (process). This approach allows for the control and optimization of the final product as a function of process and input materials. Details of the roll sensor technology are shown in Figure 8.12.

measured. When in the manufacturing site, the conditions of the production compactor are tuned to produce the same load-time signature using the larger instrumented roll as the one obtained from the R&D compactor. From an operational point, there is no need for constant use of the instrumented roll in the laboratory or in the manufacturing plant after the specific process has been validated by this technology. The sensor-roll will be used only to develop and record the load-time profile during the design of experiments. Similarly, the sensor-roll on the production compactor will be used only during scale-up and validation. Process parameters are stored in the compactor's control memory for real-time process monitoring and control.

Figure 8.12 shows pictorially the development of an instrumented roll with small inserted load cells across the roll face that measure $F = P \times A$ on the compact in real-time. Real-time information is generated by this device that enables the development of the design of experiments, modeling, and scale-up strategies to larger roll compactors (with more of the same sensors on the larger roll).

Wireless communication instrumented from the roll facilitates the sensor information to software that statistically interprets the data real-time. The scale-up and compaction control through real-time statistical feedback goes to a monitor where the information is processed, displayed, and stored.

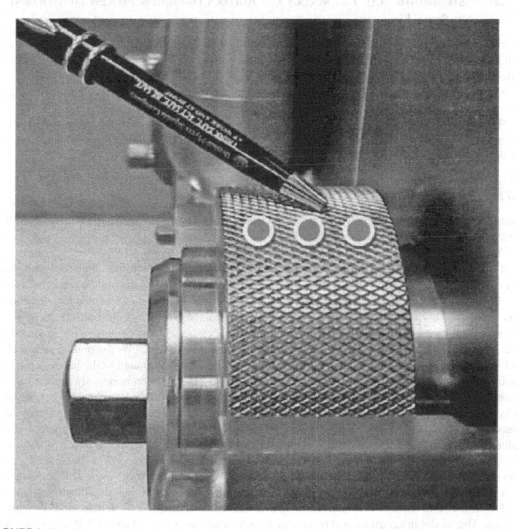

FIGURE 8.12 Using embedded load cells the temporal force profile across the roll is measured in real-time on an alexanderwerk wp120 roll. Wireless technology transports signals to a control monitor where statistical analysis determines compact density in real-time.

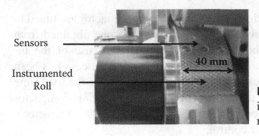

Sensors

Instrumented
Roll

40 mm

FIGURE 8.13 Instrumented roll with three load cells installed on the lower shaft of the Alexanderwerk WP120 roller compactor.

This applied instrumented roll approach goes to the heart of process analytical technology, by providing real-time data to expand the processing knowledge, to shorten the drug product development time, to shorten drug product scale-up time, to reduce raw material loses, and to reduce drug product manufacturing risks due to processing failures that originate from noncontrolled processes.

8.7.2 INSTRUMENTED ROLL TECHNOLOGY FOR ROLLER COMPACTION PROCESS DEVELOPMENT AND SCALE-UP

Instrumented roll technology was developed and applied successfully for process development and scale-up. The instrumented roll was installed on the bottom shaft of the Alexanderwerk® WP120 roller compactor. Three subminiature load cells were installed linearly across the width of on knurled roll as shown in Figure 8.13. The side sensors are located at 6.75 mm from the outer edge. The middle sensor is equidistant from the edges (i.e., 20 mm from each edge).

The nip angle was measured using an optical encoder. The subminiature load cells measure the pressure developed by compacted material in the nip zone. The details of instrumentation are provided in references [30,31].

8.7.3 PLACEBO MODEL

During the initial phase of this work [30], a placebo blend was used to understand the relationship between normal force and ribbon properties.

Placebo pre-blend composition is shown in Table 8.6.

Ribbon densities were measured for ribbon samples manufactured at various combinations of feed screw speed, roll speed, and roll pressure. The normal stress measured by the middle sensor was used for developing statistical models. For the top knurled roll and bottom instrumented knurled roll, it was noted that normal stress values recorded by the middle sensor (P2) were uniform for a given setting of roll speed, feed screw speed, and hydraulic roll pressure. Normal stress values recorded by side sensors (P1) and (P3) were lower than normal stress values recorded by the middle sensor (P2) and showed greater variability than the middle sensor (P2). This is attributed to the heterogeneity of feeding pressure in the last flight of the feed screw and this has also been previously reported in the literature [32]. The tip of the Alexanderwerk® feed screw is approximately 10 mm and is consistently delivering a uniform flow of the powder blend into the nip zone and hence it is applying steady feed pressure resulting in steady normal stress (P2) at the center of the roll. Therefore, normal stress values (P2) recorded at various combinations of roll speed, feed screw speed, and hydraulic roll pressure were used for data analysis. The normal stress (P2) was analyzed as a function of screw speed to roll speed ratio (SR), hydraulic roll pressure (HP), and roll speed (R) using JMP® 8.0 (SAS). Roll speed and its interaction with remaining factors were found to be not significant and not included in the final model. The final linear model included only significant factors and their interactions. The model fit summary and parameter estimates are provided in Table 8.7. R-square for this model was equal to 0.996.

TABLE 8.6

Placebo Composition

Ingredient	% w/w
Intragranular	
Microcrystalline Cellulose PH102	47.75
Anhydrous Lactose	47.75
Magnesium Stearate	0.5
Colloidal Silicon dioxide	0.25
Croscarmellose sodium	1.5
Extra granular	
Magnesium Stearate	0.5
Colloidal Silicon dioxide	0.25
Croscarmellose sodium	1.5

As can be seen from Figure 8.14, the normal stress (P2) correlated well with hydraulic roll pressure (HP) and Feed screw to roll speed ratio (SR). Normal stress (P2) increased as hydraulic roll pressure (HP) increased, with factor (SR) fixed at the center point of the data set. Normal stress (P2) decreased as feed screw speed to roll speed ratio (SR) increased, with factor (HP) fixed at the center point of the data set. As screw speed to roll speed ratio (SR) increased at a given hydraulic roll pressure, more material is passed through the rolls and upper roll is pushed upward, thus resulting in a decrease in normal stress (P2). For the ribbon density measurements, full-width ribbon samples were collected, and density was measured using a GeoPyc instrument. Ribbon density of the placebo blend was found to be mainly function of normal stress (P2) as shown in Eqn (8.3) and Rsquare for the model was equal to 0.884.

$$Ribbon\ density = 0.9014067 + 0.0020673\ (P2) \ldots\ldots\ldots\ldots\ldots \tag{8.3}$$

True density data and Porosity versus compaction pressure data of the placebo blend was used to estimate average ribbon density and compared against the experimental data. The tip of the Alexanderwerk® WP120 feed screw is approximately 10 mm and delivers a uniform flow of the powder blend into the nip zone. Therefore, the feed screw applies steady feed pressure resulting in steady normal stress (P2) at the center of the ribbon. The normal stress values recorded by side sensors (P1 and P3) were smaller than P2 for the top knurled and bottom knurled roll combination.

TABLE 8.7

Summary of Fit for Normal Stress (P2) vs. Hydraulic Roll Pressure (HP) and Screw Speed to Roll Speed Ratio (SR) for Placebo Blend

RSquare	0.99608
RSquare Adj	0.99581
Root mean square error	1.55153
Mean of response	96.03396
Observations (or Sum Wgts)	48

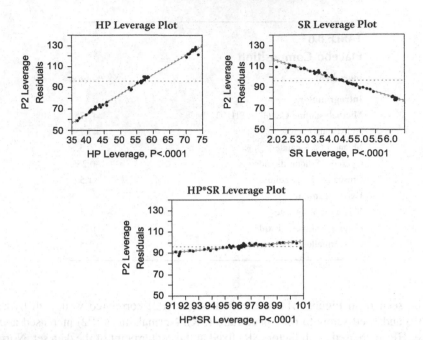

FIGURE 8.14 Leverage plots of normal stress (P2) versus screw speed to roll speed ratio (SR), and hydraulic roll pressure (HP) for placebo formulation.

Using the true density of pre-blend (1.5587 gm/cc) and compaction data (i.e., out of die porosity vs. compaction pressure), and normal ribbon stress data (P1, P2, and P3), the ribbon density across the ribbon width is calculated for each placebo run using profile shown in Figure 8.15. The average ribbon density across ribbon width is calculated by trapezoidal rule using MATLAB®. As shown in Figure 8.16, the estimated ribbon densities compared well against experimentally measured ribbon densities. This methodology may be used for online estimation of ribbon densities on a roller compactor equipped with instrumented roll and thus can be a valuable process analytical tool.

8.7.4 Application of Placebo Model to Predict Ribbon Densities of Active Blends

The authors of this study [30] also demonstrated the application of statistical models developed for placebo blend to predict ribbon densities of low drug load blends. The normal stress data (P2) of active blends was used in Eqn. (8.3) to estimate ribbon densities.

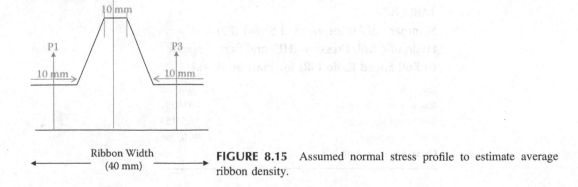

FIGURE 8.15 Assumed normal stress profile to estimate average ribbon density.

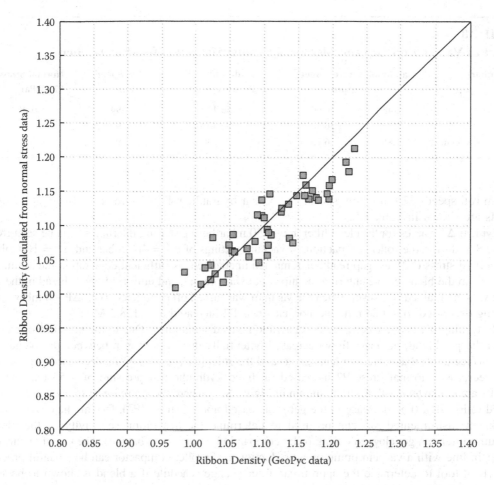

FIGURE 8.16 Average ribbon density of placebo runs. Comparison of experimentally measured (GeoPyc) versus calculated using normal stress data and normal stress profile. RMSE = 0.030498 (%RSD = 2.77).
Source: From Ref. [30].

The root mean square errors (RMSE) for placebo model-predicted density versus experimental ribbon densities of active blends with various percentage of drug load were calculated. The RMSE decreased as the internal angle of friction and compressibility (K) values of active blends approached those of the placebo blend. For low drug load formulations, a formulator may be able to use the placebo models to determine the ribbon densities of low drug load active blends thus minimizing API consumption during development.

8.7.5 Effect of Deaeration on Normal Stress (P2) Measurements and Gap

Miller [14] described vacuum deaeration technology to remove air entrainment from the powder just before the nip angle during roller compaction. The numerous benefits and efficient results were observed when compacting low-density raw materials [14]. Nesarikar et al. [30] studied the effects of vacuum levels using an instrumented roll. Alexanderwerk® WP120 is equipped with a vacuum pump for the deaeration of pre-blend. Deaeration of blend consolidates the powder blend before its entry in the nip region. The vacuum pump pulls air from pre-blend as it enters the nip zone. The authors [30] studied the effect of vacuum level settings on normal stress (P2) and gap measurements using an instrumented roll. In this experiment, placebo pre-blend was roller compacted at

TABLE 8.8

Effect of Vacuum on Gap and Measured Normal Stress (P2) for Placebo Blend

ΔP (mbar)	Gap (mm)	Screw Speed (rpm)	Hydraulic Roll Pressure (bar)	Roll Speed (rpm)	Normal Stress P2 (MPa)
160	2.48	36.60	56.40	7.94	101.40
460	2.46	36.60	56.50	7.94	99.70
0 (i.e., no vacuum)	1.86	36.70	57.70	7.94	128.20

8 rpm roll speed; 37 rpm screw speed, and 55 bar hydraulic roll pressure. The effects of vacuum levels are shown in Table 8.8.

Typical ΔP values for the clean filter are ~ 750 mbar before starting the run. As can be seen from Table 8.8, during the roller compaction, at vacuum settings of ΔP = 460 mbar and ΔP = 160 mbar, the normal stress (P2) and gap readings remained unchanged, as sufficient de-aeration (i.e., removal of air from the blend before entering the nip zone) was present, and uniform flow of blend in the nip zone was maintained. However, when the vacuum was turned off completely (i.e., ΔP ~ 0 mbar), gap reading decreased to ~ 1.86 mm and normal stress P2 increased to ~ 128.2 MPa.

By turning off vacuum completely, deaeration was discontinued. Due to the presence of excess air in the pre-blend, net mass flow decreased potentially due to poor grip between pre-blend and roll surface as well as increased leakage around the rolls [21], resulting in a decreased gap. As the gap decreased, normal stress P2 increased (at fixed hydraulic roll pressure of ~ 55 bar). These results are consistent with findings shown in Figure 8.14 where the decrease in screw speed to roll speed ratio (SR), (i.e., decrease in the gap), increased normal stress (P2). During the development work, an instrumented roll can be used to determine the deaeration sensitivity of the blend. Vacuum filter can get clogged during roller compaction of large-size batches. The use of an airflow meter in line with a vacuum pump on a production scale roller compactor can be a useful process analytical tool to determine the appropriate filter change schedule if a blend is shown to be sensitive to deaeration during development work.

In summary, the use of instrumented roll technology provided an in-depth understanding of the impact of machine parameters on normal stress experienced by the ribbon and ribbon density. The use of instrumented roll during development work may be helpful to reduce experimental work and API consumption of low drug load formulations.

8.7.6 . USE OF INSTRUMENTED ROLL TECHNOLOGY FOR SCALE-UP USING MODIFIED JOHANSON MODEL

During scale-up or transfer of roller compaction process, it is critical to maintaining comparable average ribbon densities at each scale in order to achieve similar tensile strengths and subsequently similar particle size distribution of milled material [33]. By maintaining comparable average ribbons densities across different scales, similar tensile strengths and subsequently similar particle size distribution can be obtained when milled under identical conditions [33]. Comparable average ribbon densities can be achieved by maintaining analogous normal stress applied by the rolls on ribbon for a given gap between rolls. However, measurements of normal stress applied on a ribbon at a given roll pressure is not possible without the use of instrumented roll technology either on a laboratory scale or production scale roller compactor. Therefore, roller compaction scale-up in the pharmaceutical industry has been traditionally done by trial and error approach using the design of experiments on both laboratory and large scales. The statistical models for ribbon density as a function of roll pressure and the gap from laboratory-scale machine typically do not correlate well to the ribbon density model on large scale machine, due to differences in roll width, roll diameter, and feed screw dimension differences. In a simpler term, for a given gap, the hydraulic roll pressure used on a laboratory scale and the hydraulic roll pressure used on a production-scale machine will be different to achieve similar average ribbon density. Therefore, during the technology transfer stage, a statistical model for ribbon density is typically developed using the design of experiments on a production-scale machine, which can result in a significant consumption of API.

Johanson [12] developed a model to predict normal stress profile using material properties and roll diameter. However, the practical utility of the Johanson model is limited due to its requirements of nip pressure at the nip angle. Johanson model assumes a fixed angle of wall friction, which leads to a fixed nip angle. The offline static measurements of wall friction may not truly represent wall friction experienced during the dynamic mode. In addition, Johanson model assumes a flat normal stress profile across the roll width, which is not true as shown by Nesarikar et al. [30] where normal stress applied on the ribbon, P1 and P3 were lower than the P2 values.

Nesarikar et al. [31] demonstrated a novel scale-up approach using instrumented roll data collected during development work at a laboratory scale. A set of calibration runs are performed on WP120 roller compactor equipped with instrumented roll to obtain normal stress profile across ribbon width on WP120 by regressing model predicted ribbon densities to match experimental ribbon density data. Once, normal stress profile is estimated, design space for ribbon density as a function of gap and roll pressure on WP120 is obtained. Nesarikar et al. [31] utilized instrumented roll data to directly measure nip angles using pressure peak data as using the procedure by Bindhumadhavan et al. [34]. The roll force equation derived by Johanson [12] was used to correlate roll force (using hydraulic roll pressure) as a function of normal stress (P2), gap, and nip angle.

As a first step of the modeling work, the validation of the roll force approach was demonstrated using measured normal stress, gap, and nip angle data of the placebo runs collected using instrumented roll [31]. The subset of placebo runs data (roll speed = 8 rpm) was used for validation (Table 8.9). The nip angle for each run was calculated as the intersection of tangents drawn through ascending and descending parts of the pressure peak as shown in Figure 8.17. The measured values of normal stress (P2), gap (S), nip angle (α), and average ribbon density along with corresponding process parameters are given in Table 8.9. The compressibility (K) of the placebo pre-blend was determined to be equal to 4.34 using uni-axial compaction data as shown in Figure 8.18. The pre-blend compressibility (K) is determined from the reciprocal of the slope of an initial linear portion of the logarithmic plot of density as a function of pressure data obtained in uniaxial compaction. The roll force value for each placebo run was calculated using Eqs. (8.4) and (8.5) with corresponding values of process parameters, normal stress (P2), gap (S), and nip angle (α) from Table 8.9. The roll width (W) is equal to 40 mm and roll diameter (D) is equal to 120 mm for the WP120 roller compactor. As shown in Figure 8.19, the model calculated roll force values using Eqn. (8.5) compared well with those determined using roll force equation (i.e., Eqn. 8.7) available for the Alexanderwerk® WP120 roller compactor. These findings are consistent with those reported by Dec et al. [35].

Thus, calculation procedure developed by Johanson [12] to correlate normal stress (P2) to RFU (roll force per unit roll width), gap, and nip angle was verified using instrumented roll data of placebo blend. In addition, directly measured nip angle data eliminated the need for calculation of nip angles as well as pre-requisite of nip pressure values, as required by Johanson's original model [12].

After demonstrating validation of roll force calculations from the Johanson model, the calculation approach is reversed to estimate normal stress and corresponding ribbon density as a function of gap and RFU. A calibration experimental set consists of a limited number of roller compaction runs on Alexanderwerk® WP120 roller compactor equipped with an instrumented roll. A typical two-factorial design of experimental design is used (gap and RFU as two factors). Nip angle data measured for each run is then expressed as a function of gap and RFU as shown in Eqn. (8.4) where coefficients a, b, and c are determined for a given formulation.

TABLE 8.9
Actual Parameters, Ribbon Densities, Nip Angle, and Normal Stress Data of Placebo Runs

RUN #	Feed Screw (S) (rpm)	Roll Pressure (bar)	Roll Speed (R) (rpm)	S/R	Gap (mm)	P2 (MPa)	Measured Nip Angle (rad)	Exp Ave Density GeoPyc (gm/cc)
16	18.70	41.15	7.97	2.35	1.16	81.3	0.155997	1.0716
17	24.70	41.02	7.97	3.10	1.64	74.83	0.177987	1.0546
18	30.60	41.22	7.97	3.84	2.11	71.4	0.198613	1.0296
19	36.63	41.63	7.97	4.60	2.60	67.95	0.215289	1.0296
20	42.56	41.95	7.96	5.35	3.07	62.75	0.233195	1.0144
21	24.71	56.52	7.97	3.10	1.53	108.05	0.175556	1.1393
22	30.60	57.63	7.96	3.84	1.98	102.75	0.195775	1.0818
23	36.64	57.82	7.96	4.60	2.42	96.05	0.213439	1.0867
24	36.64	56.83	7.96	4.61	2.41	94.5	0.212449	1.1119
25	42.56	57.09	7.95	5.35	2.87	88.65	0.230763	1.0772
26	48.54	55.83	7.95	6.11	3.32	80.45	0.248685	1.0635
27	24.71	71.61	7.96	3.10	1.46	138.1	0.172229	1.1931
28	30.60	71.58	7.96	3.85	1.87	131.2	0.192821	1.1394
29	36.64	73.15	7.95	4.61	2.29	124.6	0.209587	1.1414
30	42.54	73.09	7.94	5.36	2.73	115.5	0.227488	1.1439
31	48.51	72.37	7.93	6.12	3.17	105.05	0.243255	1.1203

Source: The above data is a subset of data from Ref. [31].
Compressibility (K) =4.34

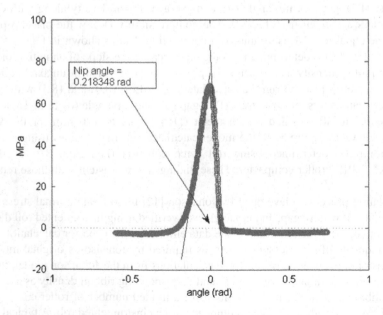

FIGURE 8.17 Nip angle calculation for placebo pressure profile (roll speed = 4 rpm, screw speed = 19 rpm, roll pressure = 40 bar, and Gap = 2.65 mm).
Source: From Ref. [31].

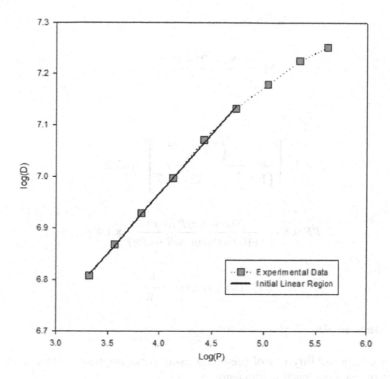

FIGURE 8.18 Compressibility (k) determination for placebo blend using uni-axial compaction data.
Source: Refs. [31,36].

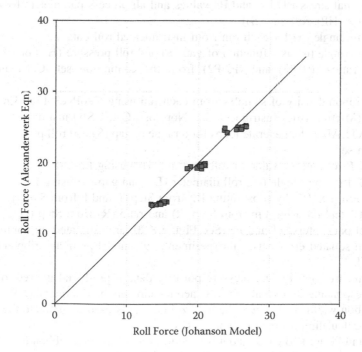

FIGURE 8.19 Comparison of roll force values calculated using Johanson model versus Alexanderwerk®
equation.
Source: From Ref. [31].

$$\propto = a + b * (gap) + c * (RFU). \ldots \tag{8.4}$$

$$RF = \frac{Pm * W * D * F}{2} \ldots \ldots \tag{8.5}$$

Where

$$F = \int_0^\alpha \left[\frac{\left(\frac{S}{D}\right)}{\left(1 + \frac{S}{D} - cos\theta\right)cos\theta} \right]^K cos\theta d\theta \ldots \ldots \tag{8.6}$$

$$RF\,(kN) = \frac{0.86 \times HP\,(bar)}{(10\,bar)(cm\,roll\,width)} \times (W)\ldots \tag{8.7}$$

$$RFU\,(kN\,per\,cm) = \frac{RF}{W} \ldots \tag{8.8}$$

The modeling steps are described as follows:

a. Estimate compressibility (K) of pre-blend using porosity-pressure data from uni-axial die compaction on a compaction simulator.

b. Conduct set of calibration runs on a roller compactor with instrumented roll (2^2 factorial DOE with gap and roll pressure as factors).

c. Record normal stress P1, P2, and P3 values and all process parameters for each run (e.g., roll pressure (HP), roll gap (S)).

d. Estimate nip angle (α) for each run from instrumented roll data.

e. Express nip angle (α) as a function of gap (S) and roll pressure (HP) or RFU (Eqn. (8.4))

f. Calculate ratios (P1/P2) and (P3/P2) from the calibration set. Calculate the average ratio (R).

g. Measure ribbon density of samples from each run using GeoPyc® 1360 Envelope Density Analyzer (Micromeritics Instrument Co., Norcross, GA, USA) instrument.

h. Using MATLAB code, generate loops for a range of gap (S) and roll pressure (HP) from the calibration set.

i. Estimate RF for a given value of roll pressure (HP) using Eqn. (8.7).

j. Estimate F from nip angle (α), roll diameter (D), and gap (S) using Eqn. (8.6).

k. Calculate Pm (i.e., P2) by substituting RF from Step (i) and F from Step (j) into Eqn. (8.5).

l. Estimate P1 and P3 using Pm from Step (k) and ratio (R) from Step (f).

m. The model parameters, x1 and Pe (See Figure 8.20) are estimated by nonlinear regression where sum squared error between experimental vs. model predicted ribbon density data is minimized.

n. In Step (m), true density and pressure-porosity data of pre-blend is used to calculate densities corresponding to normal stress at each location on the ribbon. Once the density profile across ribbon width is obtained, the trapezoidal rule is used to estimate the area under the curve for calculating average ribbon density.

o. Once x1 and Pe are known, a model is used to estimate average ribbon densities for a given range of gap (e.g., 1.8–3 mm) and roll pressures (or RFU).

As shown in Figure 8.20, Pe is normal stress at the ribbon edge and x1 is the distance from the center on both sides over which P2 (i.e., Pm) is effective. Note that sensors 1 and 3 are located 6.75 mm each from the roll edge.

Once x1 and Pe values are determined for a given formulation on the WP120 roller compactor with instrumented roll, these values were used along with feed screw dimensions and roll width data of Alexanderwerk W200 to create an initial estimate of normal stress profile as shown in Figure 8.21. Using this initial approximate of profile across roll width, ribbon density versus gap and RFU surface plot was generated and thus obtaining initial estimates of RFU and hydraulic roll pressures (for a desired gap range) to obtain target and lower and upper limits of ribbon density.

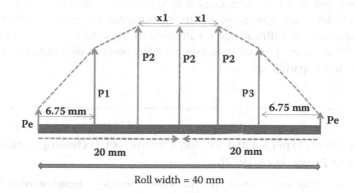

FIGURE 8.20 Assumed pressure profile across the roll width on WP120. The distance (*x1*) and normal stress (Pe) at the edge are optimized to match the experimental ribbon density of the calibration runs. *Source*: From Refs. [31,36].

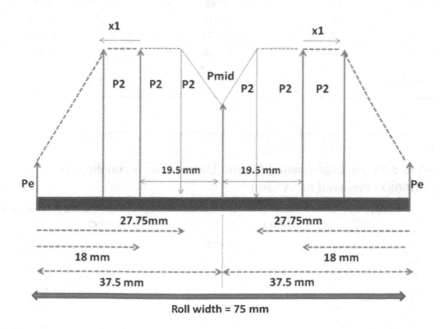

FIGURE 8.21 Assumed pressure profile across roll width on WP200 with distance (x1) and normal stress (Pe) at the edge, (Pmid/P2) ratio obtained from WP120 analysis. *Source*: From Ref. [36].

This scale-up approach was successfully applied for scale-up of drug product C. The model predicted ribbon densities and experimental ribbon densities matched well as shown in Tables 8.10 and 8.11 for two separate large-scale batches made on Alexanderwerk WP200. In addition, the compaction properties of final granulations from WP120 and WP200 compared well as shown in Table 8.12, thus further confirming successful scale-up.

The modeling approach was also applied for the placebo blend scale up (to simulate low drug load formulations) on WP200. The model predicted ribbon densities compared well with experimentally measured ribbon densities as shown in Figure 8.22. The normal stress profile for placebo was similar to the one shown in Figure 8.21, except values of x1, Pe, and the ratio (Pmid/P2) were different than those of the drug product C blend (data not shown).

In summary, instrumented roll technology was successfully used to gain a fundamental understanding of the roller compaction process. The instrumented roll data of calibration runs on the WP120 compactor was used with roll force equations of the Johanson model to predict process parameters on WP200. Use of this technology-enabled process development and scale-up on WP200 using a material sparing approach.

TABLE 8.10
Model Predicted Versus Experimental Ribbon Densities of Technology Transfer Batch 1 (2G9016X) Prepared on WP200

Run	Roll Pressure (bar)	Gap (mm)	Model Predicted Ribbon Density (gm/cc)	Experimental Ribbon Density (gm/cc)
1	55	2.5	1.0482	1.0111
2	65	2.5	1.0778	1.0594
3	75	2.5	1.1027	1.0984
4	80	2.5	1.1135	1.0963
5	70	2.5	1.0908	1.0731
6	60	2.8	1.0538	1.0354
7	80	2.1	1.1273	1.1041
8	70	2.5	1.0908	1.0706

Source: From Ref. [36].

TABLE 8.11
Model Predicted Versus Experimental Ribbon Densities of Technology Transfer Batch 2 (2H9008X) Prepared on WP200

Run	Roll Pressure (bar)	Gap (mm)	Model Predicted Ribbon Density (gm/cc)	Experimental Ribbon Density (gm/cc)
1	60	2.2	1.0748	1.0526
2	60	2.8	1.0538	1.0336
3	75	2.5	1.1027	1.0819
4	90	2.2	1.1415	1.1198
5	90	2.8	1.1236	1.1110

Source: From Ref. [36].

TABLE 8.12

Compactibility Data of Final Granulations. Comparison of Development Versus Scale-Up Batches

Batch	Process Parameters	Ribbon Density (gm/cc)	Compactibility (Mpa/Mpa)	Std Error
Laboratory batch (5 kg)WP120 [Center point]	50 bar/ 2.5 mm gap (WP120)	1.0864	0.013366	0.000396
Large-scale batch (120 kg) WP200 [Center point]	75 bar/ 2.5 mm gap (WP200)	1.0819	0.013566	na

Source: From Ref. [36].

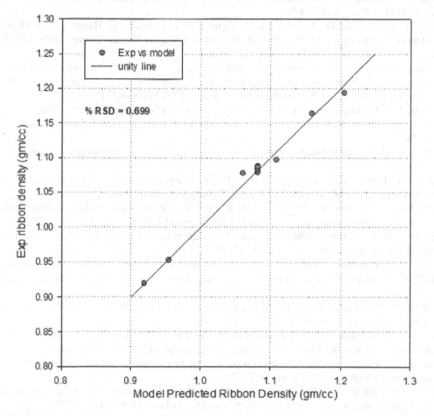

FIGURE 8.22 Experimental versus model predicted ribbon densities of placebo batch (3C9007X).
Source: From Ref. [36].

NOTE

1 Work described by this author in this chapter was completed at Bristol Myers Squibb Company, New Brunswick, New Jersey.

REFERENCES

1. Miller, R. W. Roller compaction technology. In: Parikh D.M., ed. Handbook of Pharmaceutical Granulation Technology. Vol 198. 3rd ed. New York, NY: Informa Healthcare, 2010: 163–182.
2. Miller, R. W. Roller compaction technology. In: Parikh DM, ed. Handbook of Pharmaceutical Granulation Technology. Vol 154. 2nd ed. Boca Raton: Taylor Francis Group, 2005: 159–190.
3. Miller, R. W. Roller compaction technology. In: Parikh DM, ed. Handbook of Pharmaceutical Granulation Technology. Vol 81. 1st ed. New York: Marcel Dekker, Inc., 1997: 99–150.
4. Miller, R. W. Roller compaction technology for the pharmaceutical industry. Encyclopedia of Pharmaceutical Technology. New York: Marcel Dekker, Inc., 2003 (online).
5. Miller, R. W., Morris, K. R., Gupta, A. Roller compaction scale-up. In: Levin, M Ed. Pharmaceutical Process Scale-Up. Vol 157. 2nd ed. Boca Raton: Taylor and Francis Group, 2006: 237–266.
6. Gupta, A., Peck, G., Miller, R. W., Morris, K. R. Real-time NIR monitoring of content uniformity, moisture content, compact density, tensile strength and Young's modulus of roller-compacted powder blends. J Pharm Sci. 2005; 94: 1589–1597. doi:10.1002/ JPS20375.
7. FDC Reports: the pink sheets. Published online. https://pink.pharmaintelligence.informa.com/PS015344/FDC-RReports-Inc.
8. Pietsch, W. Agglomeration in industry. In: Pharmaceutical Applications. Vol 1. Weinheim: Wiley-VCH Verlag GmbH & Company, 2005.
9. Parikh, D. In: Parikh, D. M., ed. Roller Compaction Technology. Handbook of Pharmaceutical Granulation Technology. Vol 154. 2nd ed. Boca Raton: Taylor Francis Group, 2005: 247–309.
10. Pietsch, W. Roll Pressing. London: Heyden, 1976.
11. Dehont, F. R., Hervieu, P. M., Jerome, E., Delacourte, A., Guyot, J. C. Briquetting and granulation by compaction: a new granulator-compactor. In: Wells J., Rubinstein M., eds. Pharmaceutical Technology, Tableting Technology. Vol 2 (Compression). London: Ellis Horwood, 1993: 1–11.
12. Johanson, J. R. Rolling theory for granular solids. Trans Am Soc Mech Eng 1965; Dec. 1965: 842–848.
13. Jenike, A. W., Shield, R. T. Plastic flow of coulomb solids beyond original failure. J Appl Mech 1959; 26:599–602.
14. Miller, R.W. Advances in pharmaceutical roller compactor feed system designs. Pharm Technol 1994; 18: 154–162.
15. Shileout, G., Lammens, R. L., Kleinebudde, P. Dry granulation with a roller compactor. Part 1. The function units and operational modes. Pharm Technol Eur 2000; 24–35.
16. Funakoshi, Y., Asogawa, T., Satake, E. Use of a novel roller compactor with a concavo-convex roller pair to obtain uniform compacting pressure. Drug Dev Ind Pharm 1977; 3(6):555–573.
17. Johanson, J. R. Predicting limiting roll speed for briquetting presses. Proceedings of the 13th Institute for Briquetting and Agglomeration, 1975, 13: 89–99.
18. Sheskey, P. J., Hendren, J. The effects of roll compaction equipment variables, granulation technique, and HPMC polymer level on a controlled-release matrix model drug formulation. Pharm Technol 1999; 23(3): 90–106.
19. Dec, R. T. Problems with processing of fine powders in roll press. Proceedings of the 24th Institute for Briquetting and Agglomeration, 1995, 24: 199–210.
20. Pietsch, W. Size enlargement by agglomeration. In: Fayed M., Otten L., eds. Handbook of Powder Science, and Technology. 2nd ed. New York: Chapman and Hall, 1997: 347–364.
21. Miller, R. W. Using vacuum-deaeration feed system to minimize powder leakage during roll compaction. Powder Bulk Eng 1997; 11(2): 71–75.
22. Miller, R. W., Sheskey, P. J. A survey of current industrial practices and preferences of roller compaction technology and excipients year 2000. Am Pharm Rev 2001; 4(1): 24–35.
23. Sheskey, P. J. et al. Use of roller compaction in preparation of controlled-release hydrophilic tablets containing methylcellulose and hydroxypropyl methylcellulose polymers. Pharm Technol 1994; 18: 132–150.
24. Malkowska, S., Khan, K. Effect of recompression on the properties of tablets prepared by dry granulation. Drug Dev Ind Pharm 1983; 9: 331–347.
25. Sheskey, P. J., Cabelka, T. Reworkability of sustained-release tablet formulation containing HPMC polymers. Pharm Technol 1992; 16: 60–74.
26. Miller, R. W. Process analytical technologies (PAT). Part 2. Am Pharm Rev 2003; 6(2): 52–61.
27. Guidance for industry immediate release solid oral dosage forms scale-up and post approval changes, SUPAC: chemistry, manufacturing, and controls in vitro dissolution testing and in vivo bioequivalence

documentation. Coordinating Committee (CMC CC) of the Center for Drug Evaluation and Research at the Food and Drug Administration, November 1997.

28. U.S. Department of Health and Human Services, Food and Drug Administration, Center for Drug Evaluation and Research (CDER), Center for Veterinary Medicine (CVM), and Office of Regulatory Affairs (ORA). PAT—a framework for innovative pharmaceutical development, manufacturing, and quality assurance. Available at: https://www.fda.gov/regulatory-information/search-fda-guidance-documents/pat-framework-innovative-pharmaceutical-development-manufacturing-and-quality-assurance.

29. Www.fdagov.com. Innovation and continuous improvement in pharmaceutical manufacturing pharmaceutical CGMPs for the 21st Century. September 29, 2004. Available at: https://www.gmp-compliance.org/gmp-news/fda-white-paperinnovation-and-continuous-improvement-in-pharmaceutical-manufacturing.

30. Nesarikar, V., Vatsaraj, N., Patel, C., Early, W., Pandey, P., Sprockel, O., Gao, Z., Jerzewski, R, Miller, R., Levin, M. Instrumented roll technology for the design space development of roller compaction process. Int J Pharmaceutics 2012; 426: 116–131.

31. Nesarikar, V., Patel, C., Vatsaraj, N., Early, W., Pandey, P., Sprockel, O., Jerzewski, R. Roller compaction process development and scale up using Johanson model calibrated with instrumented roll data. Int J Pharmaceutics. 2012; 436: 486–507.

32. Simon, O., Guigon, P. Correlation between powder-packing properties and roll press compact heterogeneity. Powder Tech 2003; 130: 257–264.

33. Zinchuk, A. V., Mullarney, M. P., Hancock, B. C. Simulation of roller compaction using a laboratory scale compaction simulator. Int J Pharm 2004; 269: 403–415.

34. Bindhumadhavan, G., Seville, J. P. K., Adams, M. J., Greenwood, R. W., Fitzpatrick, S. Roll compaction of a pharmaceutical excipient: Experimental validation of rolling theory for granular solids. Chem Eng Sci 2005; 60: 3891–3897.

35. Dec, R., Zavaliangos, A., Cunningham, J. Comparison of various modeling methods for analysis of powder compaction in roller press. Powder Technol 2003; 130: 265–271.

36. Nesarikar, V. Application of Johanson model calibrated with instrumented roll data for roller compaction process development and scale-up. AIChE Annual Meeting, San Francisco, CA, 2013.

9 Advances in Wet Granulation of Modern Drugs

Bing Xun Tan, Wen Chin Foo, Keat Theng Chow, and Rajeev Gokhale

CONTENTS

9.1 INTRODUCTION

The granulation process converts powders into granules to impart desirable properties such as adequate flow, density and compressibility, and segregation prevention. These properties ensure dose uniformity in the final dosage form, usually tablets, capsules, or granules, and are especially crucial in products with a low dose, or small volume.

This chapter aims to provide an overview of various advancements associated with low- and high-shear wet granulation technologies.

In wet granulation process, granules are produced via the aqueous or organic solvent liquid binder. The various low- and high-shear granulation equipment and technologies currently used in product manufacturing will be covered at the beginning of this chapter. Under the realm of these extensively used traditional granulation technologies, various innovations have emerged to address the issues such as limitation of batch processes, or moisture and heat sensitivity of the products. Continuous granulation is one of the advancements of low/high-shear processes, which has gained significant adoption by the industry. Other advanced granulation technologies include moisture activated dry granulation, melt/thermoplastic granulation, foam binder granulation, effervescent granulation, and steam granulation [1]. In this chapter, the advances in granulation for small molecular drugs will be discussed in the context of the aforementioned granulation technologies.

Since their pioneering development in the early 1980s, biologics have grown into an indispensable class of therapeutic agents today. The need for improved drug stability has driven major efforts to convert biologics from their original solution form into powders. This is potentially achieved through the mechanisms of granulation. The formulation and process technologies for granulation of biologics with an emphasis on drug stability will be discussed.

In parallel with the advances in computing power, adoption of big data and artificial intelligence (AI) is evident in the pharmaceutical industry, notably in the areas of new drug discovery, chronic disease management, and clinical trial processes. The application of AI in pharmaceutical product development and manufacturing is gaining importance amid the constant need of the industry to reduce cost and increase speed to market. The granulation process is an ideal juncture for AI implementation as it has a direct impact on downstream processes (e.g., tableting and encapsulation), and the eventual product quality. The application of AI in the process modeling of high-shear granulation will be presented via several case studies in the final section of this chapter.

9.2 SMALL MOLECULE DRUG GRANULATION

9.2.1 LOW-SHEAR GRANULATORS

Low-shear granulators, namely mechanical agitator granulators and rotating-shape granulators, operate on the principle of mechanical agitation or tumbling with a low power per unit mass. The granulators' agitator speed, sweep volume, or bed pressure result in lesser shear, which generally produces less dense, and more porous granules when compared to granules produced from a high-shear granulation process. Fluid bed granulators or fluidized bed spray granulators may also qualify as low-shear granulation equipment, and these processes will be discussed separately.

a) Mechanical Agitator Granulators

The common underlying mechanism of mechanical agitator granulators is the rotation of blades or paddles to create powder movement for initial dry mixing, followed by wet granulation through the addition and distribution of a granulating liquid. Examples of mechanical agitator granulators include ribbon, paddle, z-shaped or sigma blade mixers, planetary mixers, and orbiting screw granulators (Figure 9.1a and b). The ribbon, paddle, or sigma blade mixers are all top-loaded mixers with a side-driven agitator of either ribbon-shaped blades, paddles, or intermeshing sigma-shaped blades, respectively. The ribbon mixer is a popular dry powder mixer and is capable of wet granulation with the addition of granulating liquid. However, this equipment tends to produce non-homogeneous mixing due to material sticking on the walls and the creation of dead spaces at the ends and in the corners of the mixer. Besides, the torque required during granulation may sometimes exceed the threshold of the ribbon mixer. These limitations are overcome by the paddle mixer, which has less sticking problems and requires less torque. Paddle mixers may also be used in a continuous low-shear wet granulation process, which will be discussed later in this chapter. Sigma blade mixers are compressive or kneading mixers commonly used for formulations with a more pasty or dough-like consistency. This mixer has minimum dead space and also a good distribution of the granulating liquid within the powder bed due to the pressure generated by the intermeshing blades.

Similarly, planetary mixers are top-loaded mixers but with a top-driven agitator. In this case, the agitator not only rotates on its own axis but the entire agitator shaft also rotates simultaneously in a planetary motion opposite to that of the agitator. Powder mixing and granulation occur in a bowl that can be removed easily. While there is minimal dead space, this mixer has a limited vertical mixing ability and is also limited in batch size.

If a very gentle process is required, the orbiting screw granulator enables reduced attrition of granules formed. In this granulator, the agitator is in the form of a screw that rotates and conveys the material at the bottom of the cone-shaped vessel to the top. At the same time, this screw rotates around the periphery of the vessel. Granulating liquid can be introduced through the center of the

(a)   (b)

(c)   (d)

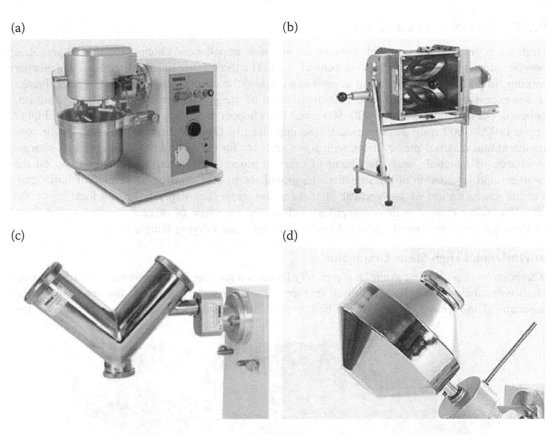

FIGURE 9.1 Low-Shear Granulator Attachments for Use with an R&D Multipurpose Drive Unit (AR 403, ERWEKA). (a) Planetary Mixer, (b) z-Blade Mixer, (c) V-Shaped Mixer, (d) Double Cone Mixer. *Source*: Courtesy of ERWEKA GmbH.

agitator and additional elements such as a chopper may be added to the sidewall if required for granulation.

b) Rotating-Shape Granulators

Rotating-shape granulators operate through a single-axis rotation of its vessel containing the powder to be granulated. The design of the vessel varies and often gives rise to the name of the equipment, for example, a double cone or a V-shaped mixer granulator (Figure 9.1c and d). Within the vessel, a bar, rotating on the same axis as the vessel but at a much higher speed, imparts more energy to the system, enabling efficient convective mixing, while potentially doubling-up as a delivery device for the granulating liquid. This bar is also known as an agitator or intensifier bar and can be supported at one or both ends. The speed, size, and design of the bar are all important factors in the optimization of the set-up. Other important process parameters to consider include the peripheral speed of the vessel, the vessel loading, mixing time, and conditions of granulating liquid addition (e.g., spray droplet size, rate, and quantity). For example, during scale-up, the peripheral rotation speed (typically ranging from 72.2 to 106.7 m/min) should be maintained, which consequently correlates to lowered revolutions per minute [2].

Generally, these granulators are easy to clean, scalable, and create little attrition due to its gentle mixing. Furthermore, the enclosed system may be jacketed for process temperature manipulation and/or designed for operation with a vacuum or inert gases to facilitate in situ drying or granulation with solvents, respectively.

9.2.2 HIGH-SHEAR GRANULATORS

High-shear granulators commonly involve the use of an impeller and chopper to mix and granulate powder blends inside a cylindrical or conical bowl. The three-blade impeller performs dry powder mixing, imparting shear force and compression, while the chopper, as its name suggests, breaks down excessive agglomerates and aids distribution of the granulation liquid. Generally, the impeller is operated at speeds of 100–500 rpm. The chopper is always operated at a much higher speed (1000–3000 rpm) as compared to the impeller [3]. Overall, the bowl is enclosed for containment and material preservation, with some accesses for the addition of liquid binders, charge/discharge of materials, and attachment of other in-process monitoring tools. Depending on the position and orientation of the impeller, the granulator may be considered vertical or horizontal. Further classification of the vertical high-shear wet granulator depends on the location of the impeller motor (top or bottom driven) as well as the inclusion of other functionalities such as process temperature control (jacketed systems) or integrated drying (single pot).

a) Horizontal High-Shear Granulator

The horizontal high-shear granulator typically features a rotating impeller in the form of a mixing shaft with blades in a cylindrical drum (Figure 9.2). The rotation of the mixing shaft creates the mechanical movement of the powder bed, maximizing mixing and creating a separation of the

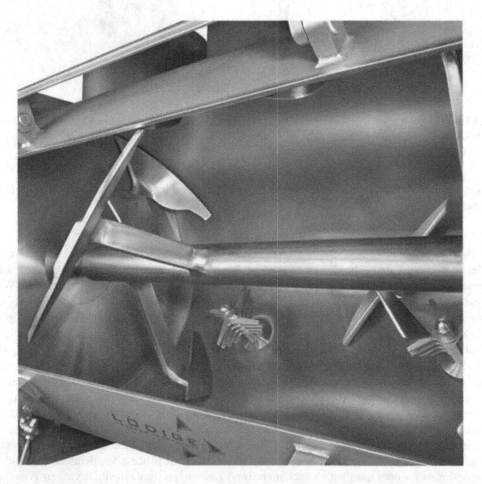

FIGURE 9.2 Lödige's Ploughshare® Mixer Type FKM 300 Hygienic Design for Batch Operation. *Source*: Courtesy of Gebrüder Lödige Maschinenbau GmbH.

particles. This allows for the optimal wetting of the particles with a dispersion of the granulation liquid, reducing the risks of lumps and non-uniform wetting. Choppers may also be added to increase agitation of the powder bed and to ensure the formation of uniform agglomerates.

b) Vertical High-Shear Granulator

Vertical high-shear granulators are commonplace in the pharmaceutical industry due to their versatility, high containment, integrated wash-in-place or clean-in-place capabilities, compliance to Good Manufacturing Practice, ease of use, and advanced endpoint detection technologies. Relative to low-shear methods, granules produced in the vertical high-shear granulators require less granulating liquid and are generally denser, less friable, and consistent in size between batches. However, the granules may be relatively less compressible. Both bottom-driven (Figure 9.3) and top-driven (Figure 9.4) vertical high-shear granulators are available with some studies reporting no significant dissimilarity in the products obtained from both types of equipment. Minor differences observed in the produced granules were attributed to the differences in the design of the equipment.

Different designs of impeller and chopper are available depending on the equipment supplier. For example, GEA offers a M8 impeller and Fir-tree chopper in addition to its standard offer for improved functionality (Figure 9.5). Studies demonstrate that the design of the impeller has a significant effect on the flow of the powder bed and also the properties of the final product. In one example, curved blades generated more spherical granules versus irregularly shaped granules with the use of flat blades. A specially designed two-blade impeller had also been proposed as an improvement to a standard three-blade impeller with advantages in larger granule size, reduced

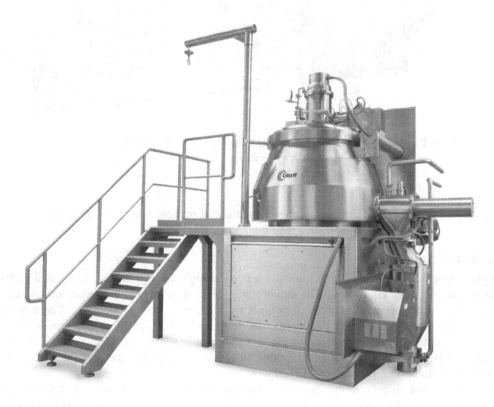

FIGURE 9.3 A Bottom-Driven Vertical High-Shear Granulator (VG Pro 1200, Glatt).
Source: Courtesy of Glatt GmbH.

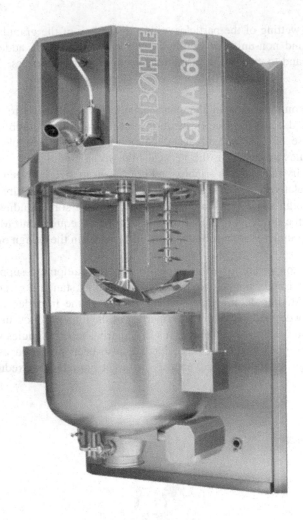

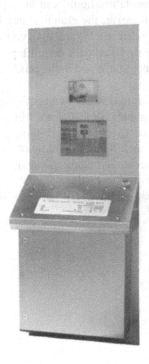

FIGURE 9.4 A Top-Driven Vertical High-Shear Granulator (GMA 600, Bohle).
Source: Courtesy of L.B. BOHLE Maschinen + Verfahren GmbH.

heat generation, larger drive torque, and desensitization of particle growth to the impeller rotation speed [4].

c) Single-Pot Granulators

A single-pot or one-pot granulator is typically a vertical high-shear granulator that has the ability for drying in the same equipment. The single-pot granulator eliminates the problems associated with the manual or pneumatic transfer of product from the granulator to the dryer. These benefits include reduced risk of product contamination, improved safety due to containment, ease of cleaning, validation, and compliance to Good Manufacturing Practice (Figure 9.6). However, optimization is required to avoid the formation of clumps during granulation as the wet milling step is not available in this case.

In the single-pot granulator, drying may be accomplished by direct heating via elevation of the bowl temperature, often coupled with a vacuum to lower the evaporation temperature of the granulation liquid. Sometimes, a stripping gas or carrier gas is also introduced from the bottom of

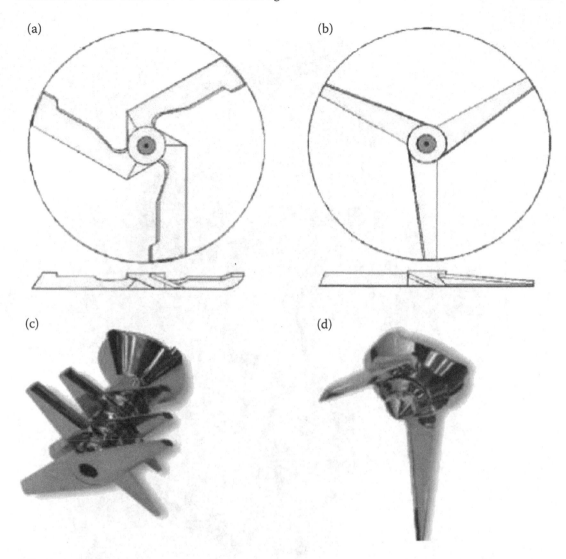

FIGURE 9.5   Impeller and Chopper Options for a Bottom-Driven Vertical High-Shear Granulator (PMA™, GEA). (a) M8 Impeller, (b) Tapered Blade Impeller, (c) Fir-Tree Chopper, (d) U-Shaped Chopper. *Source*: Courtesy of GEA.

the equipment, passing through the product bed to enhance vapor removal, which enables very low final moisture content. However, this conductive heating method is limited by the efficiency of heat transfer for drying. For example, the surface area of the inner bowl wall and the batch size affects the surface/volume ratio. Hence, a higher temperature and extended time may sometimes be required, which is less ideal, and this method is better suited for small-scale granulation using organic solvents or low amounts of granulation liquid.

One advancement of the single-pot granulator is the use of microwave-assisted drying instead of the conventional heating mechanism. This drying method offers several advantages. Firstly, a faster and more efficient rate of heating and drying is possible with microwaves [5]. Heat can be rapidly generated through direct interactions between the waves and molecules of the granulated material with favorable dielectric properties. Also, as microwaves interact preferentially with strongly dipolar water molecules in the granules, the energy efficiency of drying is improved

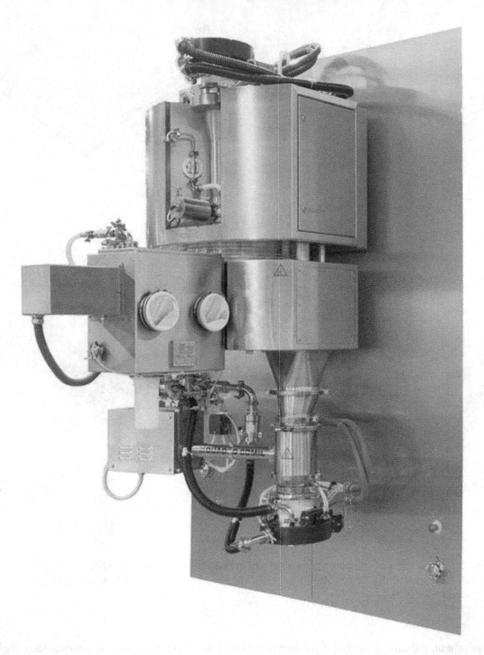

FIGURE 9.6 Single-Pot Granulator Equipped with Full Containment Capabilities (UltimaPro™ HC 75, GEA).
Source: Courtesy of GEA.

versus conventional conduction drying, which is non-selective [6]. This can lead to better energy utilization and hence, cost-savings. Furthermore, the drying in the product bed will be more uniform.

In sub-optimized processes using conduction drying, the temperature of the product increases at the end of drying due to the accumulation of excess heat energy. This is not desirable for heat-sensitive products. The use of microwaves in this scenario can help to minimize the unnecessary exposure of the product to heat as the reduction of free moisture in the product results in a corresponding decrease in dielectric loss and hence, a reduced rate of heating as the product dries. Loh et al. also reported the correlation of drying time on the stability of acetylsalicylic acid where prolonged exposure to moisture and heat led to increased drug degradation [7]. The drying efficiency was found to be affected by material and process factors, such as batch size, filler particle size, and quantity of granulating liquid added. Differences observed in size and structural properties of the granules produced consequently impacted microwave-assisted drying, which could be attributed to the volumetric generation of heat.

Another process advantage of microwave-assisted drying in high-shear granulators can be seen in processes utilizing organic solvents. For conventional fluid bed drying systems, a mixture of solvent and process gases will be exhausted, whereas in microwave-assisted drying systems, only pure organic vapors need to be treated on the exhaust side [8].

(For additional reading on the single pot processing refer to Chapter 11 in this book.)

9.2.3 ADVANCED APPLICATIONS OF LOW- AND HIGH-SHEAR WET GRANULATION

This section provides an overview of advanced applications of wet granulation via high- or low-shear granulators for small molecule drug products. These advances mainly address the optimization of granulating liquid quantity and distribution, as well as the transition from batch to continuous process in light of its associated benefits. Optimization of granulating liquid quantity and distribution is often used to enable the granulation of formulations, which may contain moisture-sensitive or thermolabile actives or ingredients. As less granulating liquid or alternative non-liquid binders are used, the drying step can be adjusted to accommodate challenging formulations. Some of these approaches are briefly described next.

a) Moisture Activated Dry Granulation

Moisture activated dry granulation (MADG) was developed in order to provide a simple, cost-effective alternative that can overcome challenges in end-point sensitivity, drying, and milling associated with the traditional wet granulation process [9]. This technique is also sometimes referred to as moist aqueous granulation. The process begins with an agglomeration step where dry mixing of the formulation (comprising at least one binder) is performed, followed by slow addition of a limited amount of granulating liquid to hydrate the dry binder. This creates nuclei, which, in turn, leads to moist agglomerates as the fine powder starts to adhere and layer on the tacky nuclei. The second stage of this process is moisture distribution and an absorbent excipient is added to the blend at this time to further distribute the moisture and "dry" the granules. Further ingredients may also be added at this stage if required [10]. Depending on the amount of granulating liquid added, post-process drying may or may not be required. The resultant granules are typically small and uniform.

MADG is a relatively faster process with greater versatility for heat and moisture sensitive formulations. As it uses traditional wet granulation equipment, the technology is also more accessible for manufacturers. Typically, high-shear granulators are used, but MADG had also been successfully demonstrated in low-shear granulators such as planetary mixers or fluid bed granulators [11,12]. Some variables to be considered during the development of a MADG process include the binder and moisture content effect, the impact of granulating liquid amount, as well as choice of extragranular excipients for moisture absorption during the moisture distribution step [13–15]. Christensen et al. demonstrated the effectiveness of a 1:1 microcrystalline cellulose (MCC) and potato starch mixture as a moisture absorbing material to produce MADG granules in a vertical high-shear granulator. The resultant tablets had high crushing strength, low friability, short disintegration time, and low mass variation on a rotary tablet press. Considering the significant impact of water quantity on granule flowability, tablet strength and disintegration time, the optimal water requirement for granulation was reported in this study to be in the range of 1.5–2.5% w/w [16].

The MADG technology had also been shown to be useful for high drug load formulations, which require granulation. In a study by Moravka et al., formulations containing more than 80% of either acetaminophen, metformin hydrochloride, or ferrous ascorbate were successfully granulated using MADG. Three different binders, polyvinylpyrrolidone (PVP), hydroxypropyl cellulose (HPC), and maltodextrin DE16, were evaluated and the choice of binder contributed to differences observed in granule strength, flow and tablet hardness [17].

b) Steam Granulation

Steam granulation involves the injection of steam as a granulating liquid to induce granulation of a bed of fluidized particles. The main process benefits of this technology are improved distribution uniformity, greater penetration, or diffusion into the powder bed and favorable thermal balance during the drying step. For the product, freshly distilled steam can provide better microbial control, and there is no risk of residual solvents since solvents are not required.

Steam granulation may be performed using traditional high-shear granulators or fluid bed granulators with additional precautions or modifications required to prevent the accidental introduction of condensation droplets, which can cause lumping or sticking to the vessel walls [18]. The vessel also has to be kept at an elevated temperature (e.g., 60–70 °C) to prevent condensation on the vessel walls.

Steam granulation is already used at a commercial level, for example, in granulation of fertilizers containing nitrogen, phosphorus, and potassium (NPK). However, the use of steam granulation in pharmaceutical applications appears limited and has been mainly reported in research studies. Several authors had reported the application of steam granulation technology in complexation processes for drug dissolution modifications. Albertini et al. successfully prepared controlled release granules containing a 1:1 drug-resin complex of potassium diclofenac and cholestyramine as the drug and ion exchange resin, respectively. The complexation was completed in situ using a high-shear granulator with steam as the granulating liquid. Compared to the conventional multi-step process, this proposed single-step process with steam granulation was found to be effective. This process was fast, taking only 35 minutes to complete and produced granules of desirable physical properties and dissolution kinetics [19]. Similarly, the complexation of piroxicam and β-cyclodextrin for enhancement of drug dissolution was demonstrated by Cavallari et al. using steam granulation technology. Compared to traditional wet granulation, only half the amount of water was required for granulation with steam, hence significantly reducing the overall process time. The granules obtained with steam granulation were also reported to have a higher surface area for faster dissolution and lower moisture content despite a shorter drying time [20].

Steam granulation was also employed by Vialpondo et al. to investigate the use of mesoporous silica as a dissolution enhancer for the poorly water-soluble drug, itraconazole. As mesoporous silica possesses poor powder flow, granulation is required to improve its physical properties for tableting. However, the use of traditional wet granulation and dry granulation negatively impacts the performance of mesoporous silica. Hence, steam granulation was evaluated as one potential alternative [21]. Factors such as binder content, steam amount, mixing time, impeller speed, spray pause time, and filler content were varied in the design of experiment (DOE). The significance of these parameters was reported with respect to the choice of binder, namely polyvinylpyrrolidone (PVP) or hydroxypropylmethylcellulose (HPMC). Overall, granules prepared from PVP in steam granulation were desirable, possessing higher bulk density, granule size, improved flow properties, better compression and compaction behavior, and with premature drug release less than 5%. The process parameters and binder properties were found to influence the risk of drug extraction from the pores of mesoporous silica and should be optimized during steam granulation [22].

c) Effervescent Granulation

The wet granulation of an effervescent formulation may be conducted in a two-step process (granulating the acidic and alkaline components separately and then blending them) or in a single-step process (granulating the acidic and alkaline components together). The single-step granulation is more technically challenging as the addition of aqueous granulating liquid can initiate an effervescent reaction that must be controlled. The effervescent reaction produces carbon dioxide and water, which then acts as a granulating liquid, potentially leading to an undesirable chain reaction. Hence, in such granulation, only a very small amount of water is initially added as the granulating liquid, and the effervescent reaction needs to be controlled by prompt drying of the granules. This drying can be performed in a subsequent pre-heated fluid bed drying or more conveniently in a single pot granulator using the aforementioned methods of vacuum, heated jacket, or microwaves [23].

In one example of this technology, TOPO granulation, an oscillating vacuum is applied intermittently during the granulation process in order to control the effervescent reaction and create only a surface modification of the citric acid particles. This controlled surface reaction of the acid with an alkaline carbonate forms a less reactive citrate layer of a few micrometers in thickness on the acid surface. Effervescent granules made with this technique are reportedly more stable and less moisture sensitive. Consequently, the final product made from these granules will be stable in storage while maintaining rapid reactivity when dissolved in water [24].

(For additional reading on Effervescent granulation, refer to Chapter 14 in this book.)

Alternatively, one patent describes a hot-melt extrusion process that can be used to granulate an effervescent formulation without the addition of water. This is possible using a hot-melt extrudable binder that can melt or soften under 150 °C, such as xylitol or polyethylene glycol. The choice of binder or binder combinations, and binder hydrophilicity or hydrophobicity, can be designed to modulate the rate of effervescence [25].

d) Foam Granulation

Foam granulation refers to the use of liquid binders in a foam form for wet granulation. This technique was first described for pharmaceutical wet granulation in a patent by Dow and later reported in a published industrial case study [26,27]. Foam granulation was developed to impart advantages in more efficient and homogenous dispersion of binder within the powder bed, avoiding overwetting, and also to reduce the drying time due to reduced use of solvent. Foam can reduce the "soak-to-spread" ratio resulting in the surface coating of powder with the liquid binder without extensive absorption. Less binder may be required for granulation. Tan et al. compared foam and drop nucleation ratios, demonstrating that foam dispersion provides better liquid distribution efficiency and uses less liquid binder to nucleate the same number of powder particles [28].

The foam granulation process requires specialized foaming equipment to generate the foam binder, but the delivery of the foam binder is done through a regular plastic tube, hence eliminating the need for nozzle-related optimization. The foam binder is made up of the common polymeric binders (e.g., HPMC and HPC) and surfactants as a foaming aid. Foam granulation application has been reported with high-shear granulators, and more recently with continuous twin screw granulators. Thompson et al. demonstrated the potential of foam granulation in a twin-screw extruder to granulate α-lactose monohydrate using methylcellulose as a binder. Comparing the new technology to a standard liquid injection process, the authors reported that foam granulation performed better in terms of process stability and granule size distribution, and the resultant granules had comparable strength and compressibility despite a lower binder usage [29].

The foam and powder bed interactions have been reported by several authors to describe the possible mechanisms for binder distribution and subsequent agglomeration. Koo et al. reported the different behaviors of the substrate powder-foam interaction, specifically focusing on foam drainage and half-life, which are relevant to nucleation and agglomeration during foam granulation. It was observed that the soluble substrate, lactose, resulted in destabilization of both HPMC and HPC foams, whereas the insoluble substrate, stearic acid, had little impact on the foam. This difference may impact binder distribution during foam granulation [30]. In the case of high drug load formulations, the drug represents the majority of the substrate to be granulated. Hence, the intrinsic mechanical properties of the drug particles will impact the consequent effects of wet granulation. In one example, foam granulation using HPC as a binder conferred enhanced plasticity for acetaminophen but the same was not observed for metformin [31].

Tan et al. proposed two mechanisms to explain the wetting and nucleation phenomena during a foam granulation process using high-shear granulator. The foam quality and powder flow pattern were two important factors leading to the predominance of either one of these mechanisms: foam drainage controlled localized wetting and nucleation, or a mechanical dispersion controlled wetting and nucleation [32].

e) Melt Granulation

Melt granulation also referred to as thermoplastic granulation is performed by replacing the typical granulating liquid with a meltable binder. The binder may be added in the solid-state and subsequently melted through frictional heat of the impeller movement, as well as heat from the jacketed granulator bowl [33]. Alternatively, the binder could be added in the molten state. In this technique, water addition may not be needed, and the drying step may be omitted. The use and choice of hydrophobic or hydrophilic meltable binders can impart additional functionality to modify the release and dissolution rate of drug actives.

Melt granulation may be performed in both low- and high-shear granulators. Most commonly, the vertical high-shear granulator and twin screw extruder are employed as they are both capable of precise and efficient product temperature control. Experiments studying the impact of both formulation and process variables have been extensively reported for the vertical high-shear granulator. Formulation variables investigated include the filler properties and their composition, the binder concentration, particle size, and binder viscosity [34–37]. Process variables studied include impeller speed and type, massing time, batch size, and product temperature [38–41]. End-point determination for melt granulation in a vertical high-shear granulator may also differ from conventional wet granulation due to the limited sensitivity of power consumption. A post-melt specific energy consumption method had been proposed as a more accurate process control tool [42]. Further studies reveal the complexity of this topic as the heating mechanism was also reported to influence the suitability of process control methods. Power consumption was found to be suitable for monitoring agglomerate growth under microwave-induced heating, while product temperature was a better indicator in conventional jacketed melt granulation. This was attributed to the disparities in heat acquisition rates and heating uniformities of the powders, as well as variation in baseline mixer power consumption between the two processes [43].

Previously, the relatively lower operating temperatures of jacketed high-shear granulators (50–90 °C) meant that only low-melting binders (e.g., waxes, polyethylene glycol, and lipids) could be utilized. However, the advent of twin-screw granulators allowed the usage of polymeric binders, which require a higher temperature to function in melt granulation. Batra et al. demonstrated the use of a twin-screw granulator for melt granulation at 130 °C and 180 °C for several HPC, HPMC, PVP, and methacrylate-based polymers. At binder amounts of 10% w/w, granules containing either metformin hydrochloride or acetaminophen were successfully produced and resulted in tablets of >2 MPa tensile strength [44]. The use of twin-screw granulator technology also has advantages in improving the dissolution of some poorly soluble drugs due to the fine dispersion of the drug in the microenvironment of the binder. This drug solubility improvement was reported by Melkebeke et al. using PEG as a binder in formulation with surfactants and maltodextrin as the filler [45]. On the other hand, using insoluble polymeric binders such as ethylcellulose can modify and retard the release of highly soluble drugs such as imatinib mesylate in a high dose tablet formulation [46]. The use of fluid bed granulators for melt granulation had also been reported to be a viable alternative to high-shear granulator equipment albeit with differences in granule size distribution and morphology owing to the different mechanisms of granule growth [47].

(For additional reading on Melt granulation refer to Chapter 19 in this book.)

f) Continuous Granulation

Continuous manufacturing can be defined as a process in which the input material(s) are continuously fed into and transformed within the process, and the processed output materials are continuously removed from the system (consisting of two or more unit operations) [48]. The advent of advanced technologies in processing and analytics, as well as the growing acceptance of major regulatory groups, has driven the pharmaceutical industry to seriously consider and implement continuous manufacturing. This emerging technology offers several benefits for the pharmaceutical industry, such as shorter processing time, reduced production steps, smaller footprint, ease of scale-up, real-time release, batch size flexibility, and greater real-time quality control (through Quality by Design and Process Analytical Technology).

Today, high-shear continuous granulation technology in pharmaceutical production is most commonly associated with the twin-screw granulator and this technology will be discussed in a separate chapter of this book. In this section, we describe other low- and high-shear continuous granulators available.

The rolling drum granulator is an example of a low-shear continuous granulation process. This granulator may be classified as a type of rotating shape granulator where particle agglomeration occurs via the collision of moistened powders during tumbling in a rolling cylindrical drum. Through this process, nucleation, growth by layering and/or coalescence, and consolidation can lead to the formation of granules. The drum of the granulator is installed in an inclined position to facilitate the gravitational movement of the material through the cylinder, and the ends may be open-ended or fitted with dam rings. Granulating liquid is added to the tumbling powder bed via nozzles or pipe systems, usually at or near the inlet end of the cylindrical drum. Scrappers are often installed to remove any material build-up on the drum wall. The main equipment parameters to consider during process development are the drum speed, the drum pitch angle, and drum length. Consequently, this impacts the hold-up volume and residence time of material in the granulator. The inclusion of baffles within the drum may also help to prevent segregation and to attain uniformity of the granulation more effectively [49].

Granules produced via the rolling drum granulator are generally coarse (2–20 mm), highly dense, and with a wide size distribution. For these reasons, and as the technology is also capable of very high throughput (up to 100 ton/h), the rolling drum granulator is more common in the fertilizer granulation and mineral processing industries [50].

Horizontal high-shear granulators can also be adapted to a high throughput continuous process requiring only three to six minutes for granulation with fill levels of 20–50% [51]. Similar to the batch equipment, rotating mixing elements in the form of specially designed blades can aid the fluidization of material and generate intense mixing of powder and liquid in the continuous granulator. In addition, the axial conveyance of the material from the inlet to the exit is facilitated by the mixing elements while maintaining an adequate back-mixing. Choppers may be installed to increase the turbulence in the mixing process, providing superior dispersion of agglomerates, primary particles, and fine particles. In some models, the mixing elements may differ in different sections along the length of the horizontal granulator (Figure 9.7). This is akin to the screw design in twin-screw granulators, and it can allow for different zones of conveyance, dispersing, and mixing for more sophisticated granulation requirements.

(For additional reading on continuous granulation refer to Chapter 13 in this book.)

9.3   GRANULATION OF THERAPEUTIC PROTEINS

The pharmaceutical industry is witnessing a paradigm shift from traditional small-molecule drugs to biological therapeutics. In 2016, 9 out of the top 10 global best-selling pharmaceutical products were biologics [52]. Biologics are therapeutic large molecules produced from biological sources

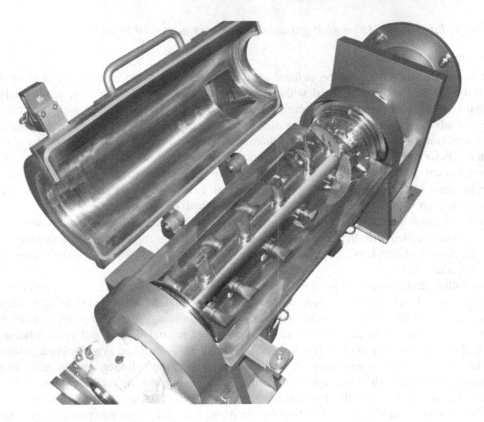

FIGURE 9.7   Lödige's Ring Layer Mixer CoriMix® Type CM 20 for Continuous Granulation.
Source: Courtesy of Gebrüder Lödige Maschinenbau GmbH.

and cover a broad range of products including recombinant proteins and their associated derivatives, vaccines, as well as cell-based and gene therapies. Of these, therapeutic proteins such as
monoclonal antibodies represent the most successful and commercialized category. The structural
complexity of therapeutic proteins confer the advantages of high potency and specificity; however,
its inherent lability presents formulation and bioavailability challenges to biopharmaceutical
scientists.

The oral bioavailability of therapeutic proteins is low due to physical and enzymatic degradation during gastrointestinal passage and low permeation across the mucosal barrier [53]. By
convention, therapeutic proteins are delivered via the parenteral route. It follows that parenteral
therapeutic protein products are preferably formulated as buffered solutions for injection unless
there are stability issues – in this case, the solution is freeze-dried and reconstituted before administration. Nevertheless, recent advances in the burgeoning field of protein therapeutics are
driving more complex biopharmaceutical formulation efforts to improve protein stability and
explore other non-invasive routes of administration. To this end, drying and granulation of therapeutic proteins into powders are gaining traction. The solid-state confers stability due to decreased molecular mobility of the protein and protection against pH, as well as mechanical and
interfacial stresses in solution [54]. Depending on the drying and granulation technique employed,
particle morphology and bulk properties of therapeutic protein powders can be engineered for
various pharmaceutical applications, such as pulmonary or nasal delivery, and of particular interest
– tableting or capsule-filling for oral dosage forms. These technologies will be discussed in the
following sections, with emphasis on the process stability of the therapeutic protein, which is a

critical challenge. This will be illustrated by formulation examples and their related pharmaceutical applications.

9.3.1 Protein Stability and Formulation Strategies

To understand the application of granulation technology to therapeutic proteins, first, we need to appreciate the structural complexity and lability of these large molecules, which are distinct from the classical small molecule drugs.

Proteins are chemically and structurally complex macromolecules with the flexibility to adopt a vast number of conformations, depending on environmental conditions. Nevertheless, the native configuration of a monoclonal antibody is essential for its therapeutic function. Deviations from this native three-dimensional structure are characterized as protein degradation, which can be effected by physical (e.g., unfolding, aggregation, and precipitation) and chemical mechanisms (e.g., fragmentation, oxidation, and deamidation) [54]. These instabilities culminate in negative consequences such as loss in efficacy and immunogenicity.

Monoclonal antibodies are highly susceptible to physical and chemical stresses, such as temperature, pH, shear/shaking, ionic strength, surface adsorption, and organic solvents, to name a few [55]. During processing and manufacture of the drug product, the monoclonal antibody can be exposed to any of these conditions with deleterious effects on its chemical and physical stability, more often than not, leading to protein aggregation and precipitation.

The stress conditions encountered by monoclonal antibodies during processing into solid dosage forms remain a significant challenge in biopharmaceutical development. Various formulation strategies had been investigated to stabilize monoclonal antibodies against stress-induced degradation. These can be broadly classified into six common categories, namely, buffering salts (citrate, phosphate); sugars (sucrose, glucose, lactose, trehalose); polyols (polyethylene glycol, mannitol, sorbitol); amino acids (arginine, glutamate, glycine, alanine, phenylalanine); polymers (cyclodextrins, dextran, inulin); and surfactants (polysorbate 20/80) [56].

The stabilizing effect of these agents is generally considered to be due to preferential exclusion, which reduces access to aggregation-promoting hydrophobic regions of the protein. In addition, polymers can inhibit protein-protein interactions via steric hindrance, while surfactants can reduce the impact of interfacial stress on proteins by preferentially locating to interfaces. During drying, stabilizers with functional hydroxyl groups, such as amino acids, sugars, and polyols, act as a water substitute to maintain native protein conformation via hydrogen bonding. High molecular weight carbohydrates or polymers also provide a rigid, solid glassy matrix that limits molecular mobility of the embedded protein, thus suppressing aggregation [55,56].

9.3.2 Slugging and Compaction of Freeze-Dried Powder

The race is on for pharmaceutical companies to deliver the first oral therapeutic protein product. This has seen the foray of biopharmaceuticals into conventional small-molecule process platforms, most notably powder processing and tableting.

Although freeze-drying is the mainstay technology and represents the gold standard for stabilization of therapeutic protein formulations with a long line of established commercial products [57], it produces low-density powders, which owing to their high porosity and dispersibility are more suited to be reconstituted for parenteral delivery or to be administered via inhalation. For the processing of dry powders into oral dosage forms, a granulation step is required to impart suitable powder properties to lyophilized powders, namely, flow and compressibility. Dry granulation methods such as slugging are typically employed to minimize the degradation of proteins when exposed to moisture.

A biotechnology company, VHsquared has developed minitablets containing a protease-resistant, anti-TNFα variable domain antibody, V565, currently in Phase 2 clinical trials, for targeted treatment of inflammatory diseases of the colon [58]. As described in the invention, the lyophilized therapeutic protein is slugged with mannitol and magnesium stearate, then blended and compressed into minitablets with MCC and croscarmellose sodium. Targeted release to the colon was effected by pH-sensitive enteric coatings [59]. In another example, infliximab was stabilized in a freeze-dried glassy matrix of inulin followed by dry granulation to produce powders of sufficient flowability. The infliximab sugar glass was then tableted with MCC, croscarmellose sodium, silica, and sodium stearyl fumarate [60]. Compaction forces were found to exert a detrimental effect on therapeutic protein recovery [61].

9.3.3 SPRAY DRYING

Spray drying is an established granulation technology commonly employed for small-molecule pharmaceuticals due to its high throughput, continuous process, low cost, and capability for particle engineering. Optimization of process parameters affords control over particle size and morphology, such as in protein encapsulation applications or for the production of dried powders with good processability. The concern of applying this technology for biopharmaceutical proteins is the high processing temperature involved, as well as shear- and interfacial stresses induced by atomization. Another limitation relates to the suboptimal yield of conventional spray dryers, which is prohibitive for high-value biopharmaceuticals.

Despite these challenges, there is an increasing number of studies demonstrating the successful application of spray drying for biopharmaceutical protein formulations. Two key process approaches for minimizing thermal degradation during the spray drying process are a reduction in spray drying temperature and a decrease in the residence time of the protein. Outlet temperatures are typically maintained below 100 °C with low liquid feed rates when spray drying thermolabile biopharmaceuticals. With suitable optimization of process parameters, preferably via a design-of-experiments approach, enhanced product recovery has been demonstrated even for bench-top spray drying equipment. Bowen et al. attributed high recovery rates of >95% spray-dried monoclonal antibody to longer residence time (hence the ability to produce larger particles), and use of a stainless steel construct that was found to be more compatible to their monoclonal antibody of interest, as compared to glass [62].

Formulation strategies using protein stabilizing excipients similar to those used during freeze-drying, such as sugars (sucrose, lactose, trehalose) and sugar alcohols (mannitol, sorbitol), are commonly employed in spray drying of biopharmaceutical proteins. In addition, surfactants in the formulation act to stabilize the therapeutic protein against interfacial stress-induced aggregation. Residual moisture content is critical – increasing evidence goes against the dogma that drier is better; instead, optimal water content is demonstrated to be beneficial for the long-term stability of dried biopharmaceutical proteins [63].

One of the first studies to demonstrate the feasibility of spray drying monoclonal antibody formulations was by Andya et al. [64]. The authors demonstrated that protein aggregation could be minimized during spray drying and storage by stabilization with mannitol, trehalose, or lactose. However, it was interesting to note that protein glycation with lactose was observed during storage. This phenomenon highlights the need for protein-excipient compatibility to reduce the risk of undesirable chemical reactions with negative implications on the bioactivity of the monoclonal antibody. Gikanga et al. reported the successful production of a spray-dried, high concentration monoclonal antibody formulations on pilot scale equipment at >95% yield. Formulations stabilized by arginine or trehalose demonstrated long-term stability for monoclonal antibody potency and viability [65].

(For additional reading on Spray drying refer to Chapter 6 in this book.)

9.3.4 ELECTROSPRAY

Coaxial electrospray, also known as coaxial electrohydrodynamic atomization, is an emerging technology developed in the past decade for the encapsulation of therapeutic agents, such as drugs, proteins, and gene therapy. Utilizing an electric field, two independent coaxial liquid jets are elongated by electrical shear stress to form a Taylor cone at the nozzle tip, before breaking up into multilayer droplets, which are accelerated by a ground electrode for collection [66]. This technique allows precise control in the fabrication of core-shell particle geometry, which is advantageous for the encapsulation and protection of labile compounds such as therapeutic proteins. By convention, emulsification methods are commonly employed for encapsulation of proteins in lipid vesicles because of its relatively gentle and non-toxic conditions. However, several limitations exist with emulsification, namely low encapsulation efficiencies for water-soluble actives, and non-uniform particle size distributions. The mechanical stress involved during homogenization was reported to induce protein degradation, resulting in a loss in bioactivity. Zhang et al. prepared Ranibizumab poly (lactic-co-glycolic) acid (PLGA) microparticles using a coaxial electrospray process followed by freeze-drying for intravitreal injection and sustained drug release. The encapsulation efficiency of 70% was reported, and more importantly, the bioactivity of ranibizumab was retained above 80% at electrospray voltages below 5 kV [67].

9.3.5 EXTRUSION-SPHERONIZATION

Extrusion-spheronization is a multi-step process for the production of multiparticulates in the form of spherical pellets typically of <1 mm in size. The process involves wet granulation of the API with a spheronization aid, most commonly MCC, to form a wet mass, which is then subject to extrusion, spheronization, and a final drying step. Although commonly used for the manufacture of multiparticulates containing small-molecule drugs, there are few reports of extrusion-spheronization processes to date, which involve therapeutic proteins. One foreseeable challenge is the wet granulation step whereby the protein is subjected to interfacial and shear stresses at high concentration.

Nevertheless, advantages abound for a multiparticulate system in the application of oral delivery of therapeutic proteins. Multiparticulate dosage forms are associated with low gastric residence time; moreover, they afford a more consistent release across different gastrointestinal physiologies. ImmuCell developed its proprietary technology for the extrusion-spheronization of pellets containing bovine antibodies for the targeted colonic treatment of *Clostridium difficile* infection. The pellet core comprises the active antibodies, MCC, and polyethylene glycol, which is coated with an enteric coating of Eudragit S100 [68]. Human clinical trials demonstrated the robust performance of these multiparticulates and compelling evidence of colon-targeting.

(For additional reading on Extrusion/Spheronization refer to Chapter 12 in this book.)

9.4 ARTIFICIAL INTELLIGENCE IN GRANULATION

Artificial intelligence (AI) is gaining increasing interest in pharmaceutical R&D and manufacturing because successful AI implementation will facilitate improved decision-making. This will translate into cost-saving, higher-quality products, and increased speed to market.

This chapter focuses on the data-based modeling paradigm as opposed to mechanistic approaches such as population balance and discreet element modeling. The data-based models are more robust and simpler to build, and thus are more cost-effective to implement. They consist of "Neural Network" programs capable of making advanced calculations and analysis on collected data in a manner similar to the human brain's thinking processes. AI functions as a machine learning system, which becomes smarter as it responds to more data.

In the granulation process, AI models are built to predict the effect of process parameters or material properties on the final granule properties or the endpoint of the process. The artificial neural network (ANN) and neuro-fuzzy logic systems are among the most commonly used AI algorithm for high-shear granulation process modeling. The ANN models rely on training data set to learn the relationships among the granulation inputs and outputs, while the testing data set assesses the generalization performance of the developed model. Neuro-fuzzy logic is a hybrid technology that combines the learning ability of the neural network and the fuzzy logic function for expressing concepts intuitively. Fuzzy logic is a decision-making approach based on all intermediate possibilities in between the absolute yes and no. As opposed to the classical logic used in computers, which allows only true or false (0 or 1), fuzzy logic allows a different level of possibilities in the input to achieve a definite output.

The following sections will highlight several case examples of the application of AI in high-shear granulation process modeling that will enable accurate process control and facilitate scale-up.

9.4.1 APPLICATION OF AI IN TWIN-SCREW GRANULATION

Shirazian et al. [69] used ANN to predict the particle size distribution of pure MCC granules obtained using twin-screw granulation. The ANN model consists of three layers, that is, input, hidden, and output. The input is defined by the liquid binder to solid (L/S) ratios, screw speeds, material throughputs, and screw configurations. The output or response parameters are particle size distribution (PSD), d10, d50, and d90. Hidden layers reside in-between input and output layers. The hidden layers determine the relationships between features of the input in order to produce an output through an activation function. From the 24 experimental runs conducted, training and validation of the network were performed using 16 and 8 runs, respectively. The most accurate simulation was obtained using two hidden layers containing two nodes per layer with non-linear activation function for both layers and three-fold cross-validation method. A correlation coefficient, $R^2 = 0.99$ was obtained between model predictions and experimental data. The ANN model was proposed as a tool for the implementation of model predictive control in the development of continuous manufacturing of pharmaceuticals.

AlAlaween et al. [70] developed a new framework based on a fuzzy logic system (FLS) to model the twin-screw granulation process on a formulation based on MCC and mannitol. The input parameters are the material type, screw configuration, screw speed, L/S ratio, and powder feed rate, and the output is granule PSD. The first step of fuzzy logic mapping involves the development of FLSs with different structures, each using the process data from 26 runs. The data were randomly divided into a training set (70%) and testing set (30%), which determines the complex input-output relationship and the generalization capabilities of the models, respectively. Various rule bases covering all areas in the space studied were obtained from the FLSs. The rules giving minimum root mean square errors between the training and testing sets were extracted. They were assessed to determine the ones with the greatest contribution to the system and subsequently reduced into a single rule base via the singular value decomposition-QR factorization (SVD-QR) approach. The reduced FLS was able to characterize the twin-screw granulation process mathematically through accurate prediction of granule size distribution, and linguistically through a set of simple IF-THEN rules. An R^2 improvement of 16% and 29% was demonstrated by the proposed FLS versus standard FLS and ANN, respectively.

9.4.2 APPLICATION OF AI IN THE BATCH HIGH-SHEAR GRANULATION PROCESS

Yu et al. [71] have developed ANN models to predict the granule mean particle size (MPS) and span for the high-shear granulation process for mixer scales of 32 L, 60 L and 1500 L. Input variables representing the raw material properties, equipment geometries, and operating conditions were classified into seven groups as follows: mixer scale, relative swept volume, total relative swept volume, theoretical liquid availability, liquid injection factor, viscosity stokes number and liquid temperature. For the purpose of network training, interpolation was the preferred approach to extend the database to compensate for insufficient data. The best algorithm to predict both the MPS and span was Bayesian regulation back-propagation, and the optimal network structure was 7–8–1 (seven, eight, and one node in input, hidden, and output layers, respectively). The theoretical liquid availability as reflected by L/S ratio and powder-specific surface area was identified as the most important input variable based on its highest mean impact value (MIV) computed via an importance analysis. The average absolute relative error, standard deviation, and correlation coefficient were 7.18%, 7.72%, and 0.9657, respectively, for MPS, and 5.76%, 5.88%, and 0.9759, respectively, for span. The ANN developed were concluded to be a reliable and robust tool for prediction of the granulation process over a wide range of formulation properties, operating conditions, and production scales.

AlAlaween et al. [72] have developed an integrated model for high-shear granulation of calcium carbonate with polyethylene glycol 1000 as a binder. The input variables are impeller speed, granulation time, L/S ratio and impeller shape, and output variables are granule particle size (d10, d50, d90), binder content, and porosity. A full factorial design leading to 108 granulation experiments in total were carried out. Random division of process data into training (5/6) and testing (1/6) set was found to be optimal for the model development (Figure 9.8). An integrated network that predicted the final output via two modeling phases was developed. In the first phase, a number of models with different structures were trained using the inputs (x_1, x_2, ... x_N) and the target outputs (y_T). Then, the predicted output (y_{P1}, y_{P2}, ... y_{PM}) from each model and the target outputs (y_T) were used to train another model resulting in the final predicted output in the second phase. Modeling in both the phases was performed using the radial basis function (RBF) network. Improvement of the model to address potential bias in the predicted outputs (y_P) was performed by characterizing error residuals using the Gaussian mixture model (GMM). Granule properties prediction was shown to fall within 95% confidence interval. Better model performance was observed for the prediction of PSD versus binder content and porosity. The latter granule properties had demonstrated higher measurement errors and heterogeneity even within the same size range.

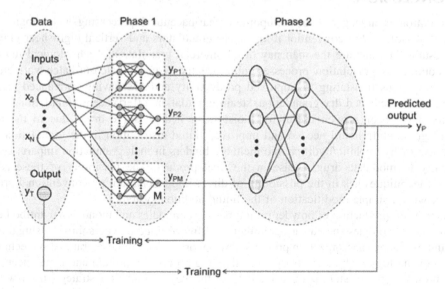

FIGURE 9.8 The Architecture of the Integrated Network Consisting of Two Modeling Phases ($x_N = N$ Number of Inputs, y_T = Target Output, M = Number of Models, y_{PM} = Predicted Output from Each Model, y_P = Final Pedicted Output).
Source: Adapted from AlAlaween et al. (2016).

The two-phase with multiple models approach worked in a complementary manner to model the complex input/output relationships (i.e., linear and nonlinear), leading to better acquisition of knowledge and hidden information for accurate predictions.

Landin [73] had reported an AI model based on the combination of neuro-fuzzy logic and gene expression programming (GEP) technologies for prediction of granulation endpoint in high-shear granulators of different scales as follows: 25 L, 65 L, 100 L, 600 L. This has enabled modeling for process scale-up. The 25 L, 200 L, and 600 L mixers were geometrically similar. The granule formulation consisted of 80% lactose, 18% maize starch, and 2% pregelatinized starch with a batch size of 0.3 kg/L in the mixers. The input variables were mixer volume, impeller diameter, impeller speed, percentage of liquid, wet mass density, and mean torque; and the output was impeller power. The neuro-fuzzy logic model was obtained using 41 datasets. Inputs were divided into submodels 1 and 2, with submodel 1 (impeller diameter, impeller speed, % liquid) being most influential on impeller power. The mixer volume was not found to be a critical input in the neuro-fuzzy logic model, leading to a mixer scale-independent model. GEP modeling was then performed using the chosen variables from neuro-fuzzy logic as inputs. Process data were randomly divided into three groups for training (33 datasets), error testing (3 datasets), and validation (5 datasets) of the GEP model. The GEP modeling has resulted in a transparent model consisting of a polynomial equation that accurately predicts the differential impeller power with $R^2 > 86.78\%$ for all mixer scales with similar or dissimilar geometries.

The predictive power of the data-based models arises from their ability to correlate complex and noisy relationships among input and output variables. The case examples presented in this section have highlighted the application of AI to enable process understanding and control and to facilitate scale-up of the high-shear granulation process. With increasing evidence and reports of successful process model implementation, AI will potentially be an essential part of the granulation process toolkit in the near future.

(For additional reading on Granulation process modelling refer to Chapter 23 in this book.)

9.5 CONCLUSIONS

Wet granulation is among the most important pharmaceutical processing technologies for the production of tablets. The conventional low-shear granulators and vertical high-shear granulators are well established and are the mainstay of commercial granulation. Technological innovations such as continuous granulation processes minimize the issue of batch-to-batch variability and reduce testing, thus translating to improved productivity and cost-saving. Advanced techniques such as moisture-activated dry granulation, steam granulation, effervescent granulation, and foam granulation have been proven useful for moisture or heat-sensitive drugs due to the minimal amount of granulating liquid needed and improved liquid distribution in the granulation powder bed. The use of hydrophilic/hydrophobic meltable binders in melt granulation imparts additional functionality to modulate drug release in the final product. The feasibility of these advanced granulation techniques lies in the possibility of direct implementation on conventional granulator equipment with a simple modification of the liquid addition system.

The successful production of powder prototypes for antibodies and monoclonal antibodies using conventional technologies such as dry granulation of freeze-dried powders through slugging, spray drying, and extrusion spheronization presents new opportunities for these granulation technologies. Advanced technology such as electrospray is showing promise in protein and gene encapsulation. Incorporation of protein stabilizing excipients is the key formulation strategy used with these processes. With the keen market interest to have biologic therapeutic agents as dried powders versus the conventional solution form for enhanced stability and convenience, granulation technologies are venturing into a new, challenging frontier.

The advances in computing power have allowed the application of artificial intelligence (AI) in the form of data-based process modeling on high-shear granulation processes, primarily through an artificial neural network and neuro-fuzzy logic system. The predictive power of the resultant process models has enabled more thorough process understanding and control, which will translate into reduced experimentation, increased speed, and reduced operation cost.

The continuous advancement of granulation technologies in terms of equipment design, processing techniques, formulation strategies, and process control will culminate in enhanced product quality and realization of solid dosage biologics in the near future.

REFERENCES

1. Shanmugam, Srinivasan. 2015. Granulation techniques and technologies: recent progresses. *BioImpacts: BI* 5 (1): 55.
2. Chirkot, Tom, and Cecil Propst. 2005. Low-shear granulation. In *Handbook of Pharmaceutical Granulation Technology*: CRC Press.
3. Cantor, Stuart L., Larry L. Augsburger, Stephen W. Hoag, and Armin Gerhardt. 2008. Pharmaceutical granulation processes, mechanism, and the use of binders. In *Pharmaceutical Dosage Forms-Tablets*, edited by Lary L. Augsburger, and Stephen W. Hoag: CRC Press.
4. Börner, Matthias, Marc Michaelis, Eva Siegmann, Charles Radeke, and Uwe Schmidt. 2016. Impact of impeller design on high-shear wet granulation. *Powder Technology* 295: 261–271.
5. Kardum, Jasna Prlić, Aleksandra Sander, and Darko Skansi. 2001. Comparison of convective, vacuum, and microwave drying chlorpropamide. *Drying Technology* 19 (1): 167–183.
6. McLoughlin, CM., WAM. McMinn, and TRA. Magee. 2000. Microwave drying of pharmaceutical powders. *Food and Bioproducts Processing* 78 (2): 90–96.
7. Loh, Z. H., C. V. Liew, C. C. Lee, and P. W. S. Heng. 2008. Microwave-assisted drying of pharmaceutical granules and its impact on drug stability. *International Journal of Pharmaceutics* 359 (1): 53–62.
8. Stahl, H. 2010. Comparing granulation methods. *GEA Pharma Systems*.
9. Ullah, I., R. Corrao, G. Wiley, and R. Lipper. 1987. Moisture activated dry granulation: a general process. *Pharm Technol* 11: 48–54.
10. Ullah, Ismat, Jennifer Wang, Shih-Ying Chang, Gary J. Wiley, Nemichand B. Jain, and San Kiang. 2009. Moisture-activated dry granulation – part I: A guide to excipient and equipment selection and formulation development. *Pharmaceutical Technology* 33 (11): 62–70.
11. Railkar, Aniruddha M., and Joseph B. Schwartz. 2000. Evaluation and comparison of a moist granulation technique to conventional methods. *Drug Development and Industrial Pharmacy* 26 (8): 885–889.
12. Takasaki, Hiroshi et al. 2019. Novel, lean and environment-friendly granulation method: Green fluidized bed granulation (GFBG). *International Journal of Pharmaceutics* 557: 18–25.
13. Takasaki, Hiroshi, Etsuo Yonemochi, Masanori Ito, Koichi Wada, and Katsuhide Terada. 2015. The importance of binder moisture content in Metformin HCL high-dose formulations prepared by moist aqueous granulation (MAG). *Results in Pharma Sciences* 5: 1–7.
14. Takasaki, Hiroshi, Etsuo Yonemochi, Masanori Ito, Koichi Wada, and Katsuhide Terada. 2016. The effect of water activity on granule characteristics and tablet properties produced by moisture activated dry granulation (MADG). *Powder Technology* 294: 113–118.
15. Takasaki, Hiroshi, Etsuo Yonemochi, Roman Messerschmid, Masanori Ito, Koichi Wada, and Katsuhide Terada. 2013. Importance of excipient wettability on tablet characteristics prepared by moisture activated dry granulation (MADG). *International Journal of Pharmaceutics* 456 (1): 58–64.
16. Christensen, L. H., H.E. Johansen, and T. Schaefer. 1994. Moisture-activated dry granulation in a high shear mixer. *Drug Development and Industrial Pharmacy* 20 (14): 2195–2213.
17. Moravkar, Kailas K., Tariq M. Ali, Jaywant N. Pawar, and Purnima D. Amin. 2017. Application of moisture activated dry granulation (MADG) process to develop high dose immediate release (IR) formulations. *Advanced Powder Technology* 28 (4): 1270–1280.
18. Hammer, Karl. 1984. Steam granulation apparatus and method (US4489504). U.S. Patent and Trademark Office.
19. Albertini, Beatrice, Nadia Passerini, M. L. González-Rodríguez, Cristina Cavallari, Maurizio Cini, and Lorenzo Rodriguez. 2008. Wet granulation as innovative and fast method to prepare controlled release granules based on an ion-exchange resin. *Journal of Pharmaceutical Sciences* 97 (3): 1313–1324.

20. Cavallari, C., B. Albertini, M. L. Gonzalez-Rodriguez, and L. Rodriguez. 2002. Improved dissolution behaviour of steam-granulated piroxicam. *Eur J Pharm Biopharm* 54 (1): 65–73.

21. Vialpando, Monica et al. 2013. Agglomeration of mesoporous silica by melt and steam granulation. Part I: a comparison between disordered and ordered mesoporous silica. *Journal of Pharmaceutical Sciences* 102 (11): 3966–3977.

22. Vialpando, Monica et al. 2013. Agglomeration of mesoporous silica by melt and steam granulation. Part II: screening of steam granulation process variables using a factorial design. *Journal of Pharmaceutical Sciences* 102 (11): 3978–3986.

23. Bertuzzi, Guia. 2016. Effervescent granulation. In *Handbook of Pharmaceutical Granulation Technology*, edited by Dilip M. Parikh: CRC Press.

24. Haac, D., Irmgard Gergely, and Christian Metz. 2012. The TOPO granulation technology used in manufacture of effervescent tablets. *TechnoPharm* 2 (3): 186–191.

25. Robinson, Joseph R., and James W. McGinity. 2000. Effervescent granules and methods for their preparation (US6071539). U.S. Patent and Trademark Office.

26. Keary, Colin M., and Paul J. Sheskey. 2004. Preliminary report of the discovery of a new pharmaceutical granulation process using foamed aqueous binders. *Drug Development and Industrial Pharmacy* 30 (8): 831–845.

27. Sheskey, Paul, and Colin Keary. 2004. Process for dispersing a fluid in solid particles (EP1438024B1). European Patent Office.

28. [] Tan, Melvin X. L., and Karen P. Hapgood. 2008. Wet granulation process via foams and drops. Paper read at American Institute of Chemical Engineers, Annual meeting, 2008.

29. Thompson, M. R., S. Weatherley, R. N. Pukadyil, and P. J. Sheskey. 2012. Foam granulation: new developments in pharmaceutical solid oral dosage forms using twin-screw extrusion machinery. *Drug Development and Industrial Pharmacy* 38 (7): 771–784.

30. Koo, Otilia M. Y., Jiangning Ji, and Jinjiang Li. 2012. Effect of powder substrate on foam drainage and collapse: Implications to foam granulation. *Journal of Pharmaceutical Sciences* 101 (4): 1385–1390.

31. Cantor, Stuart L., Sanjeev Kothari, and Otilia M. Y. Koo. 2009. Evaluation of the physical and mechanical properties of high drug load formulations: wet granulation vs. novel foam granulation. *Powder Technology* 195 (1): 15–24.

32. Tan, Melvin X. L., and Karen P. Hapgood. 2011. Foam granulation: binder dispersion and nucleation in mixer-granulators. *Chemical Engineering Research and Design* 89 (5): 526–536.

33. Voinovich, Dario, Mariarosa Moneghini, Beatrice Perissutti, and Erica Franceschinis. 2001. Melt pelletization in high shear mixer using a hydrophobic melt binder: influence of some apparatus and process variables. *European Journal of Pharmaceutics and Biopharmaceutics* 52 (3): 305–313.

34. Schæfer, Torben. 1996. Melt pelletization in a high shear mixer VI. Agglomeration of a cohesive powder. *International Journal of Pharmaceutics* 132 (1–2): 221–230.

35. Schæfer, Torben. 1996. Melt pelletization in a high shear mixer. X. Agglomeration of binary mixtures. *International Journal of Pharmaceutics* 139 (1–2): 149–159.

36. Schæfer, Torben, and Christina Mathiesen. 1996. Melt pelletization in a high shear mixer. IX. Effects of binder particle size. *International Journal of Pharmaceutics* 139 (1–2): 139–148.

37. Schæfer, Torben, and Christina Mathiesen. 1996. Melt pelletization in a high shear mixer. VIII. Effects of binder viscosity. *International Journal of Pharmaceutics* 139 (1–2): 125–138.

38. Schaefer, T., P. Holm, and H. G. Kristensen. 1990. Melt granulation in a laboratory scale high shear mixer. *Drug Development and Industrial Pharmacy* 16 (8): 1249–1277.

39. Schæfer, Torben, and Christina Mathiesen. 1996. Melt pelletization in a high shear mixer. VII. Effects of product temperature. *International Journal of Pharmaceutics* 134 (1–2): 105–117.

40. Schæfer, Torben, Birgitte Taagegaard, Lars Juul Thomsen, and H. Gjelstrup Kristensen. 1993. Melt pelletization in a high shear mixer. IV. Effects of process variables in a laboratory scale mixer. *European Journal of Pharmaceutical Sciences* 1 (3): 125–131.

41. Schæfer, Torben, Birgitte Taagegaard, Lars Juul Thomsen, and H. Gjelstrup Kristensen. 1993. Melt pelletization in a high shear mixer. V. Effects of apparatus variables. *European Journal of Pharmaceutical Sciences* 1 (3): 133–141.

42. Heng, Paul Wan Sia, Tin Wui Wong, Jian Jun Shu, and Lucy Sai Cheong Wan. 1999. A new method for the control of size of pellets in the melt pelletization process with a high shear mixer. *Chemical Pharmaceutical Bulletin* 47 (5): 633–638.

43. Liew, C. V., Z. H. Loh, P. W. S. Heng, and C. C. Lee. 2008. A study on microwave-induced melt granulation in a single pot high shear processor. *Pharmaceutical Development and Technology* 13 (5): 401–411.

44. Batra, Amol, Dipen Desai, and Abu T. M. Serajuddin. 2017. Investigating the use of polymeric binders in twin screw melt granulation process for improving compactibility of drugs. *Journal of Pharmaceutical Sciences* 106 (1): 140–150.

45. Van Melkebeke, Barbara, Brenda Vermeulen, Chris Vervaet, and Jean Paul Remon. 2006. Melt granulation using a twin-screw extruder: a case study. *International Journal of Pharmaceutics* 326 (1–2): 89–93.

46. Vasanthavada, Madhav et al. 2011. Application of melt granulation technology using twin-screw extruder in development of high-dose modified-release tablet formulation. *Journal of Pharmaceutical Sciences* 100 (5): 1923–1934.

47. Passerini, Nadia, Giacomo Calogerà, Beatrice Albertini, and Lorenzo Rodriguez. 2010. Melt granulation of pharmaceutical powders: a comparison of high-shear mixer and fluidised bed processes. *International Journal of Pharmaceutics* 391 (1–2): 177–186.

48. U.S. Food and Drug Administration. 2019. Quality considerations for continuous manufacturing – Guidance for industry (Draft guidance).

49. Behjani, Mohammadreza Alizadeh, Nejat Rahmanian, and Ali Hassanpour. 2017. An investigation on process of seeded granulation in a continuous drum granulator using DEM. *Advanced Powder Technology* 28 (10): 2456–2464.

50. Litster, Jim, and Bryan Ennis. 2004. Tumbling Granulation. In *The Science and Engineering of Granulation Processes*, edited by J. Litster, and B. Ennis: Springer Netherlands.

51. Gebrüder Lödige Maschinenbau GmbH. 2019. Continuous Ploughshare® - Mixer KM. Paderborn, Germany: Gebrüder Lödige Maschinenbau GmbH.

52. Lindsley, Craig W. 2017. New 2016 Data and Statistics for Global Pharmaceutical Products and Projections through 2017. ACS Publications.

53. Werle, Martin, Abdallah Makhlof, and Hirofumi Takeuchi. 2009. Oral protein delivery: a patent review of academic and industrial approaches. *Recent Patents on Drug Delivery & Formulation* 3 (2): 94–104.

54. Frokjaer, Sven, and Daniel E. Otzen. 2005. Protein drug stability: a formulation challenge. *Nature Reviews Drug Discovery* 4 (4): 298–306.

55. Wang, Wei. 2005. Protein aggregation and its inhibition in biopharmaceutics. *International Journal of Pharmaceutics* 289 (1-2): 1–30.

56. Emami, Fakhrossadat, Alireza Vatanara, Eun Ji Park, and Dong Hee Na. 2018. Drying technologies for the stability and bioavailability of biopharmaceuticals. *Pharmaceutics* 10 (3): 131.

57. Mensink, Maarten A., Henderik W. Frijlink, Kees van der Voort Maarschalk, and Wouter L. J. Hinrichs. 2017. How sugars protect proteins in the solid state and during drying (review): Mechanisms of stabilization in relation to stress conditions. *European Journal of Pharmaceutics and Biopharmaceutics* 114: 288–295.

58. Nurbhai, Suhail et al. 2019. Oral anti-tumour necrosis factor domain antibody V565 provides high intestinal concentrations, and reduces markers of inflammation in ulcerative colitis patients. *Scientific Reports* 9 (1): 1–12.

59. Crowe, Scott et al. 2019. Compositions (WO 2017/167997 Al). United States: VHSquared Limited.

60. Maurer, Jacoba M., Susan Hofman, Reinout C. A. Schellekens, et al. 2016. Development and potential application of an oral ColoPulse infliximab tablet with colon specific release: a feasibility study. *International Journal of Pharmaceutics* 505 (1–2): 175–186.

61. Gareb, Bahez et al. 2019. Towards the oral treatment of ileo-colonic inflammatory bowel disease with infliximab tablets: development and validation of the production process. *Pharmaceutics* 11 (9): 428.

62. Bowen, Mayumi, Robert Turok, and Yuh-Fun Maa. 2013. Spray drying of monoclonal antibodies: investigating powder-based biologic drug substance bulk storage. *Drying technology* 31 (13–14): 1441–1450.

63. Langford, Alex, Bakul Bhatnagar, Robert Walters, Serguei Tchessalov, and Satoshi Ohtake. 2018. Drying technologies for biopharmaceutical applications: Recent developments and future direction. *Drying Technology* 36 (6): 677–684.

64. Andya, James D. et al. 1999. The effect of formulation excipients on protein stability and aerosol performance of spray-dried powders of a recombinant humanized anti-IgE monoclonal antibody1. *Pharmaceutical Research* 16 (3): 350–358.

65. Gikanga, Benson, Robert Turok, Ada Hui, Mayumi Bowen, Oliver B Stauch, and Yuh-Fun Maa. 2015. Manufacturing of high-concentration monoclonal antibody formulations via spray drying—the road to manufacturing scale. *PDA Journal of Pharmaceutical Science and Technology* 69 (1): 59–73.

66. Zhang, Leilei, Jiwei Huang, Ting Si, and Ronald X. Xu. 2012. Coaxial electrospray of microparticles and nanoparticles for biomedical applications. *Expert Review of Medical Devices* 9 (6): 595–612.

67. Zhang, Leilei et al. 2015. Coaxial electrospray of ranibizumab-loaded microparticles for sustained release of anti-VEGF therapies. *PLOS One* 10 (8). doi:10.1371/journal.pone.0135608

68. Luck, Michael S., and Joseph H. Crabb. 2000. Colonic Delivery of Protein or Peptide Compositions. United States: ImmuCell Corporation.

69. Shirazian, Saeed, Manuel Kuhs, Shaza Darwish, Denise Croker, and Gavin M. Walker. 2017. Artificial neural network modelling of continuous wet granulation using a twin-screw extruder. *International Journal of Pharmaceutics* 521 (1–2): 102–109.

70. Wafa'H, AlAlaween, Bilal Khorsheed, Mahdi Mahfouf, Gavin K. Reynolds, and Agba D. Salman. 2020. An interpretable fuzzy logic based data-driven model for the twin screw granulation process. *Powder Technology* 364: 135–144.

71. Yu, Huiman, Jinsheng Fu, Leping Dang, Yuensin Cheong, Hongsing Tan, and Hongyuan Wei. 2015. Prediction of the particle size distribution parameters in a high shear granulation process using a key parameter definition combined artificial neural network model. *Industrial & Engineering Chemistry Research* 54 (43): 10825–10834.

72. Wafa'H, AlAlaween, Mahdi Mahfouf, and Agba D. Salman. 2016. Predictive modelling of the granulation process using a systems-engineering approach. *Powder Technology* 302: 265–274.

73. Landin, Mariana. 2017. Artificial intelligence tools for scaling up of high shear wet granulation process. *Journal of Pharmaceutical Sciences* 106 (1): 273–277.

10 Fluid Bed Processing

Dilip M. Parikh

CONTENTS

10.1   INTRODUCTION

The size enlargement of primary particles has been carried out in the pharmaceutical industry in a variety of ways. One of the most common unit operations used in the pharmaceutical industry is the fluid bed processing where the granules are produced in a single piece of equipment by spraying a binder solution onto a fluidized powder bed. This process is sometimes classified as the one-pot system because granulation and drying are carried out with the same equipment. The batch fluid bed granulation process is a well-established unit operation in the pharmaceutical industry; however, other process industries, such as food, nutraceutical, agrochemical, dyestuffs, and chemical, have adopted fluid bed granulation process to address particle agglomeration, dust containment, ease of material handling, and modifying particle properties to provide dispersibility or solubility to products, among other product enhancements.

Fluidization is the unit operation by which fine solids are transformed into a fluid-like state through contact with a gas. At certain gas velocities, the gas will support the particles, giving them freedom of mobility without entrainment. Such a fluidized bed resembles a vigorously boiling fluid, with solid particles undergoing extremely turbulent motion, which increases with gas velocity. The smooth fluidization of gas-solid particles is the result of an equilibrium between the hydrodynamic, gravitational, and interparticle forces.

Fluidization in a fluid bed process is critical for creating a homogeneous mixer of particles. Whether agglomerating, drying, or coating; fluidization at a proper level within the processor is required. Uneven fluidization will result in variation in the moisture content, particle size distribution, or un-granulated product resulting in poor content uniformity. Establishing the minimum fluidization velocity and controlling the bed by observing pressure drop across the bed and the filters will provide better control of the process.

The fluidization technique, as it is known today, began in 1942, with the work of the Standard Oil Company (now known as Exxon, in the United States) and M.W. Kellogg Company, to produce the first catalytic cracking plant on a commercial scale [1]. Fluid bed processing of pharmaceuticals was first reported by Wurster when he used the air suspension technique to coat tablets [2,3]. In 1960, he reported on granulating and drying a pharmaceutical granulation, suitable for the preparation of compressed tablets, using the air suspension technique. In 1964, Scott et al. [4] and Rankell et al. [5] reported on the theory and design considerations of the process using a fundamental engineering approach and employing mass and thermal energy balances. They expanded this application to the 30 kg capacity pilot plant model designed for both batch and continuous operation. Process variables, such as airflow rate, process air temperature, and liquid flow rate, were studied. Contini and Atasoy [6] later reported the processing details and advantages of the fluid bed process in one continuous step.

Wolf [7] discussed the essential construction features of the various fluid bed components, and Liske and Mobus [8] compared the fluidized bed and traditional granulation process. The overall results indicated that the material processed by the fluid bed granulator was finer, more free-flowing, and had homogeneous granules that, after compression, produced stronger and faster disintegration of tablets than the materials processed by conventional wet granulation. Reviews by Sherrington and Oliver [9], Pietch [10], and a series published on the topic of "fluidization in the pharmaceutical industry" [11–17] provide an in-depth background on the fundamental aspects of the fluidized bed and other granulation technologies. Earlier application of fluid bed was for efficiently drying of granulated or wet material. With the advent of newer technologies and drug delivery techniques, these units are now routinely used for granulation, particle coating by spraying binder, or polymer solution from the top, bottom, and tangential location to produce granules or modified release particles or pellets. Because of this versatility, these units are normally classified as multiprocessor fluid bed units.

The batch size increase using fluid bed granulation requires a good understanding of the equipment functionality, theoretical aspect of fluidization, excipient interactions, and, most of all, identification of the critical variables that affect the process of agglomeration.

This chapter will provide an essential understanding of the fluidization theory, and system description that makes up the fluid bed processor, and will discuss the critical variables associated with equipment, product, and the process. Since this process involves a large amount of air and fine powders and in some cases organic compounds as a binder solvent, understanding of safety precaution in installing and operating fluid bed equipment will be discussed as well.

10.2 FLUIDIZATION THEORY

The van der Waals forces have been established to be dominant during powder handling and fluidization, but the electrostatic forces also have a great influence on the behavior of the process. In the fluid bed process mixing effect is generally good for the particles between 50 and 200 μm. Fluidization behavior is a summation of various interactions and interparticle forces. When a packed bed of particles is subjected to a high upward flow of gas, the weight of particles is supported by the drag force exerted by the gas on the particles, and particles become fluidized. At low gas velocities, the bed of particles is practically packed, and the pressure drop is proportional to the superficial velocity. As the gas velocity is increased, a point is reached at which the bed behavior changes from fixed particles to suspended particles. The superficial velocity required to first suspend the bed particles is known as minimum fluidization velocity (U_{mf}). The minimum fluidization velocity sets the lower limit of possible operating velocities and the approximate pressure drop can be used to approximate pumping energy requirements. The flow required to maintain a complete homogeneous bed of solids in which coarse particles will not separate from the fluidized portion is very different from the minimum fluidization velocity. After the bed has been fluidized and the velocity of gas increased, the pressure drop across the bed stays constant, but the height of the bed continues to increase. When the rate of flow of gas increases, the pressure drop across the bed also increases until, at a certain rate of flow, the frictional drag on the particles equals the effective weight of the bed. These conditions and the velocity of gas corresponding to it are termed incipient fluidization and incipient velocity, respectively [18]. The relationship between the air velocity and the pressure drop is as shown in Figure 10.1 [19].

At the incipient point of fluidization, the pressure drop of the bed will be very close to the weight of the particles divided by the cross-sectional area of the bed (W/A). For the normal gas fluidized bed, the density of the gas is much less than the density of the solids and the balance of forces can be shown as

$$\Delta P_{mf} = \frac{W}{A}$$

where
where ΔP = pressure drop, ε_{mf} = minimum fluidization void fraction, A = cross-sectional area, W = weight of the particles, ρ_p = density of particles, and g/g_c = ratio of gravitational acceleration and gravitational conversion factor.

The fundamental phenomenon of fluidization was recently studied by the researchers [20] using the small-scale fluid bed unit. The purpose of the study was to compare experimental and computational minimum fluidizing velocities (U_{mf}) of pharmaceutical materials using the miniaturized fluid bed device. Using various materials, researchers found that the experimental method was more capable of describing the fluidizing behavior of pharmaceutical materials than the

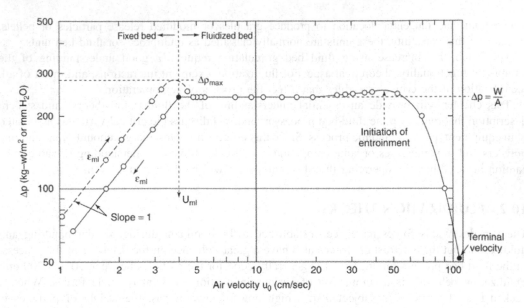

FIGURE 10.1   Relation Between Air Velocity and Pressure Drop.
Source: From Ref. [19].

computational approach. Computational models of fluidization are based on the behavior of various model particles. Computational models do not consider particle size and shape distributions, and cohesion and adhesion of pharmaceutical materials.

At gas flow rates above the point of minimum fluidization, a fluidized bed appears much like a vigorously boiling liquid; bubbles of gas rise rapidly and burst on the surface. The bubbles form very near the bottom of the bed, very close to the distributor plate, and as a result, the design of the distributor plate has a significant effect on fluidized bed characteristics. The bubbles contain a very small number of solids. Each bubble of gas in a wake contains a significant number of solids. As the bubble rises, it pulls up the wake with its solid behind it. As the velocity of the gas is increased further, the bed continues to expand, and its height increases with only a slight increase in the pressure drop. As the velocity of the gas is further increased, the bed continues to expand and its height increases, whereas the concentration of particles per unit volume of the bed decreases. At a certain velocity of the fluidizing medium, known as entrainment velocity, particles are carried over by the gas. This phenomenon is called entrainment. When the volumetric concentration of solid particles is uniform throughout the bed all the time, the fluidization is termed as the *particular*. When the concentration of solids is not uniform throughout the bed, and if the concentration keeps fluctuating with time, the fluidization is called *aggregative* fluidization. A *slugging bed* is a fluid bed in which the gas bubbles occupy entire cross-sections of the product container and divide the bed into layers. A *boiling bed* is a fluid bed in which the gas bubbles are approximately the same size as the solid particles. A *channeling bed* is a fluid bed in which the gas forms channels in the bed through which most of the air passes. A *spouting bed* is a fluid bed in which the gas forms a single opening through which some particles flow and fall on the outside.

The mechanisms by which air affects fluidization have been discussed by various researchers [12,13,21–23]. When the fluidizing velocity is greater than the incipient velocity, bubbles of air rise through the bed causing the mixing of particles. It is the gas passing through the bed in the form of bubbles that determines the degree of mixing. The extent of mixing appears to vary with the particle size. As the mean size of particles approaches zero, the mixing of particles less than 150 μm decreases. Different types of beds, described earlier, are formed depending upon the movement of bubbles through the bed. The pattern of movement of the gas phase in and out of bubbles depends on several factors, including minimum fluidization velocity and particle size. These movements affect heat transfer between air bubbles and particles. The air distributor at the bottom of the container has a controlling influence on the uniform distribution of gas, minimization of dead areas, and maximization of particle movement. The most common reason for mixing problems such as segregation in the fluid bed is the particle density differences. The main characteristic of the fluid bed is the relative velocity imparted to the particles, U_o, which is a strong function of the size of the particles and the gas velocity in the bed, and was shown to be given by

$$U_o \approx a\gamma^o = 18\frac{U_b a}{D_b}\delta^2$$

where a is the average particle size, γ^o is the interfacial energy, U_b is the bubble velocity, D_b is the bubble diameter, and δ is the dimensionless bubble spacing [24]. The first expression on the right-hand side of the equation applies to fluidized beds with no rotating parts where shear is induced by the motion of bubbles only. Recognizing the importance of particle size and density on the fluidization properties, Geldart found four fluidization modes described below (See Table 10.1 and Figure 10.2).

10.2.1 UNDERSTANDING THE PARTICLES

In 1973, Geldart classified powders into four groups by the solid and gas density difference and mean particle size and their fluidization properties at ambient conditions. The Geldart Classification of Powders is now used widely in all fields of powder technology. Understanding the nature of your product to be fluid bed processed is very critical. Geldart's classification of various particles is helpful and is provided in an abbreviated form in Table 10.1.

For any particle of known density ρ_p and mean particle size dp, the Geldart chart indicates the type of fluidization to be expected [1] (Figure 10.2).

The extent of segregation can be controlled in part by maintaining high fluidizing velocities and high bowl height to bowl diameter ratio. There are standard air velocities for various processes that can be used as guidelines. The standard velocities are based on the cross-sectional area at the bottom of the product container.

This is calculated by using the following formula for calculating the air velocity:

$$\text{Velocity (m/ sec)} = \text{air flow [cubic meter per hour (CMH)]} \div \text{area (square meters)} \times 3600$$

where airflow in CMH = airflow [cubic feet per minute (CFM)] × 1.696.

Standard air velocities are based on the application. Airflow velocities are normally 1.0–2.0 m/sec. For agglomeration, the air velocity required is normally five to six times the minimum fluidization velocity. Low air velocities, such as 0.8–1.4 m/sec are required for drying. The higher velocity is required during the early stages of drying because of the wet mass present in the bowl but is normally reduced when the product loses its moisture. The objective is to have good particle movement but to keep the material out of filters. Particle movement and quick-drying are important during the agglomeration process. An indication of good fluidization is a free downward flow of the granulation at the sight glass of the product container. However, improper fluidization can also be detected by monitoring the outlet air temperature. Every product has a unique constant rate of drying in which the bed temperature remains relatively constant for a significant length of time. Therefore, if the outlet temperature rises more rapidly than anticipated, it will indicate improper fluidization and the process may have to be stopped and manual or mechanical intervention may be required to assist the fluidization.

TABLE 10.1
Classification of Powders by Geldart

Group C Powders

- Cohesive powders
- They are difficult to fluidize, and channeling may occur
- Inter-particle forces greatly affect the fluidization behavior of these powders
- Mechanical powder compaction, before fluidization, greatly affects the fluidization behavior of the powder, even after the powder had been fully fluidized for a while
- Saturating the fluidization air with humidity reduces the formation of Agglomerates due to static charges and greatly improved the fluidization quality. The water molecules adsorbed on the particle surface presumably reduced the van der Waals forces
- $dp \sim 0{-}30\ \mu m$
- **Example: flour, cement**
  group C are difficult to fluidize

Group A Powders

- Size reduced by either using a wider particle size distribution or powders are easily Aeratable
- Characterized by a small Δp
- *Umb* is significantly larger than *Umf*
- Large bed expansion takes place before bubbling starts
- Gross circulation of powder even if only a few bubbles are present
- Large gas back mixing in the emulsion phase
- The rate at which gas is exchanged between the bubbles and the emulsion is high
- Bubble reducing the average particle diameter
- There is a maximum bubble size
- $\Delta p \sim 30{-}100\ \mu m$
- **Examples: milk flour**
  powders in group A exhibit dense phase expansion after minimum fluidization and before the commencement of bubbling

Group B Powders

- Bubbling
- $U_{mb}$and U_{mf} are almost identical
- Solids recirculation rates are smaller
- Less gas back mixing in the emulsion phase
- The rate at which gas is exchanged between bubbles and emulsion is smaller
- Bubbles size is almost independent of the mean particle diameter and
- the width of the particle size distribution
- No observable maximum bubble size
- $\Delta p \sim 100{-}1000\ \mu m$
- **Example: sand**
  group B bubble at the minimum fluidization velocity

Group D Powders

- Spoutable
- Either very large or very dense particles
- Bubbles coalesce rapidly and flow to a large size
- Bubbles rise more slowly than the rest of the gas percolating through the emulsion
- The dense phase has a low voidage
- $\Delta p \sim {>}1000\ mm$
- **Examples: Coffee beans, wheat, lead shot**
  in the group, D can form stable spouted beds.

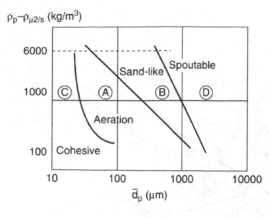

$\rho_p - \rho_{\mu 2/s}$ (kg/m³)

FIGURE 10.2   Geldart Classifications of Particles. *Source*: From Ref. [1].

10.3   SYSTEM DESCRIPTION

A fluid bed processor is a system of unit operations involving conditioning of process air, a system to direct it through the material to be processed and has the same air (usually laden with moisture) exit the unit void of the product. Figure 10.3 shows a typical fluid bed processor with all the components. These components and their utility for the granulation will be reviewed in this section.

At the downstream end of the fluid bed processor, an exhaust blower or a fan is situated to draw the air through the entire unit. This arrangement provides negative pressure in the fluid bed that is necessary to facilitate material loading, maintaining safe operation, preventing material escape, and carrying out the process under Good Manufacturing Practice guidelines, all of which will be discussed later in the chapter.

10.3.1   AIR HANDLING UNIT

A typical air preparation system includes sections for prefiltering incoming air, heating the air dehumidification, clean steam generating unit for rehumidification when needed, and final high-efficiency particulate air (HEPA) filter. Generally, outside air is used as the fluidizing medium in a fluid bed processor. For the air to be used for pharmaceutical products, it must be free of dust and contaminants. This is achieved by placing coarse dust filters (30–85%) in the air handling unit (AHU).

Through years of experience and dealing with various types of materials and various climate conditions, it is known that incoming air must be controlled very closely. As an example, it has been found that the humidity of the incoming air can greatly affect the quality of spray granulation, drying, or coating. Therefore, air preparation systems are now designed to better control the conditions of the incoming air. After the installation of the course prefilters, distinct heating or cooling sections are installed in the air handler depending upon the geographical location of the plant. In an extremely cold climate, where cooling coils (needed in summer months for maintaining uniform dew point) can freeze in winter, a preheating section is placed ahead of the cooling coils. A typical range for the air after pretreatment that one should aim at achieving is 15–30°C dry bulb and 3–5°C wet bulb. If the unit is located in a tropical or humid climate, the humidity removal section is employed first. The dehumidification of the air is extremely important where the outside air moisture varies over a wide range. In summer, in some parts of the world, when the outside humidity is high, dehumidification of the process air is required to maintain a specific dew point of the incoming air. On the other hand, during dry winter months, with low humidity in the incoming air, rehumidification may be necessary for some regions. A clean steam injector is used for

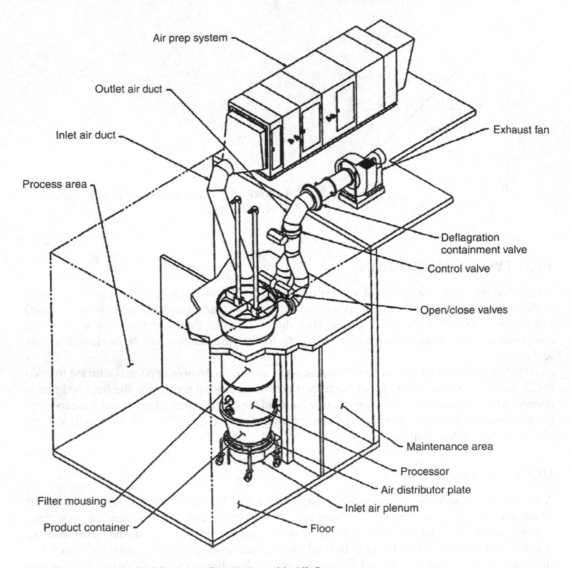

FIGURE 10.3 Fluid Bed Processor Installation with All Components.

rehumidifying the dry air. Generally, process air with a lower dew point has a higher affinity to entrain moisture reducing the processing time. When granulating extremely fine powders, an inlet air dew point of 15°C is beneficial to reduce static charges and facilitate uniform fluidization. In many processes, when preheating is required, a bypass loop can be used for preconditioning the air. This loop allows the required process temperature and humidity to be attained within the system ducts before the product is subjected to fluidization. After the conditioned air leaves the humidification/dehumidification section of the AHU, it is finally heated to the desired process air temperature and then passed through a HEPA filter of about 99.90–99.99% capacity. As the process air is treated and filtered, it is transported by the inlet duct into the lower plenum of the fluid bed unit.

10.3.2 PRODUCT CONTAINER AND AIR DISTRIBUTOR

With the air at the desired humidity and temperature, it is ready to be passed through the bed of solids. Figure 10.4a, 10.4b shows a typical product container with the air distributor. Another supplier offers single-air distributors where the open area can be changed by adjusting the slots underneath without using different air distributors mainly used for bottom spraying.

The air must be introduced evenly at the bottom of the product container through an inlet air plenum. Proper airflow in the inlet air plenum is critical to ensure that equal airflow velocities occur at every point on the air-distributor plate. If the air is not properly distributed before it reaches the bottom of the container, uneven fluidization can occur. To facilitate the even flow of powder in the product container, the conditioned air is brought in the plenum at various locations by certain manufacturers.

To properly fluidize and mix the material in the container, the correct choice of the container and air distributor must be made. The container volume should be chosen such that the container is filled to at least 35–40% of its total volume and no more than 90% of its total volume. The correct choice of the air distributor is important. These distributors are made of stainless steel and are available with a 2–30% open area. Typically, the distributor should be chosen so that the pressure drop across the product bed and air distributor is 200–300 mm of the water column. Most common air distributors are covered with a 60–325 mesh fine screen to retain the product in the container. This type of sandwiched construction (Figure 10.5a, b) has been used for the past 30 years in the fluid bed processors.

Keeping the screen and air distributors clean has been challenging. Partially to address the cleaning problems and partially to provide efficient processing, several manufacturers have introduced air distributors that eliminate the use of retaining screen. The overlap gill plat Figure 10.5b or air distributor with slotted angle (Figure 10.5a and adjustable air distributor (Figure 10.5c) are examples of newer designs available. The overlap gill plate was introduced in 1990 [25]. These new air distributors eliminate the need for a fine screen and perform dual functions as the efficient air distributor and product retainer. Other advantages claimed by the manufacturer are the ability to validate a clean in place (CIP) system, controlled fluidization, and directional flow of air to discharge the processed product from the container. Because there is no fine screen, these types of air distributors sometimes sift very fine particles through the screen, thus losing part of the batch in the

(a)   (b)

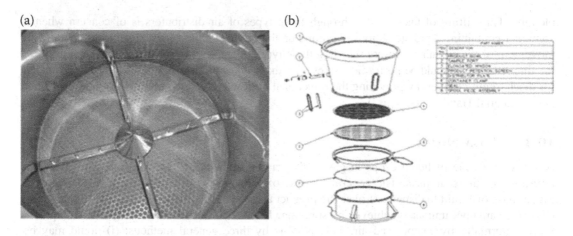

FIGURE 10.4   (a) and (b) Typical Air Distributors with Different Parts and Retaining Screens.

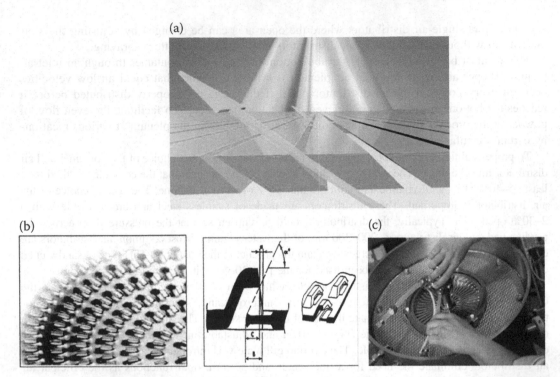

FIGURE 10.5 (a) Showing the Slotted Design Diskjet® Showing the Path of the Incoming Air (Source: Hüttlin (Syntegon), (b) Overlap Gill Plate Design (Source: GEA Pharma Systems), (c) Air Distributor with the Capability of Varying the Fluidization Velocity.
Source: Fluid Air accessed from the internet http://www.fluidair.com/fluid bed systems.htm#undefined 5.

plenum. This sifting of fine powder through these types of air distributors is of concern when a container containing a product is moved around on the production floor, losing some product due to movement of the container. Before selecting these types of single-plate air distributors, a sifting test for finer particles should be performed. However, these types of air distributors offer an advantage for discharging products by providing the directional airflow to the dried product from the container (see "Material Handling Options").

10.3.3 SPRAY NOZZLE

A spray is a zone of liquid drops in gas, and spraying is the act of breaking up a liquid into a multitude of these droplets. The general purpose of spraying is to increase the surface area of a given mass of liquid to disperse it over the product area. The primary concern is with the increase of surface area per unit mass achieved by spraying. The nozzle is an orifice through which liquid is forced, normally by compressed air. This is done by three general methods: (i) liquid may be sucked up by a pressure drop created over the nozzle cap, after which compressed air atomizes the liquid stream by disintegrating it with air jets, or (ii) the compressed air operates a piston arrangement that pushes the liquid through the orifice and then lets surface tension create a droplet, or (iii) impinge two pressure streams of liquid upon each other, and so form a highly dispersed, uniform spray.

The type of spray system is usually characterized by one of the four nozzle designs (Figure 10.6) [26].

1. Pressure nozzle: The fluid under pressure is broken up by its inherent instability and its impact on the atmosphere, on another jet, or on a fixed plate.

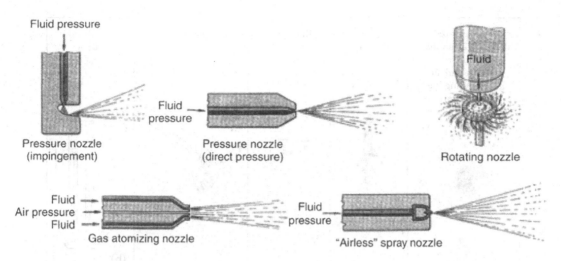

FIGURE 10.6 Types of Nozzles.
Source: From Ref. [26].

2. Rotating nozzle (rotary atomizer): Fluid is fed at low pressure to the center of a rapidly rotating disk and centrifugal force breaks up the fluid. These types of nozzles are used mainly in a spray drying application.

3. Airless spray nozzle: The fluid is separated into two streams that are brought back together at the nozzle orifice, whereupon impingement, they form drops.

4. Gas atomizing nozzle (two-fluid nozzle): The two-fluid (binary) nozzle where the binder solution (one fluid) is atomized by compressed air (second fluid) is the most commonly used nozzle for the fluid bed granulation (Figure 10.7b).

These nozzles are available as a single-port or multiport design. Generally, the single-port nozzles are adequate up to 100-kg batch, but for larger-size batches, multiport nozzles such as either three-port or six-port (Figure 10.7a) nozzle, are required. When these nozzles are air-atomized, the spray undergoes three distinct phases. In the first, the compressed air (gas) expands, essentially adiabatically, from the high pressure at the nozzle to that of the fluid bed chamber. The gas undergoes a Joule-Thomson effect, and its temperature falls. In the second, the liquid forms into discrete drops. During this atomization, the liquid's specific surface area usually increases 1000 times. In the third, the drops travel after being formed, until they become completely dry or impinge on the product particles. During this phase, the solvent evaporates, and the diameter of the drops decreases. The energy required to form a drop is the product of the surface tension and the new surface area. About 0.1 cal/g is needed to subdivide 1 g of water into 1 μm droplets. The air pressure required to atomize the binder liquid is set using a pressure regulator. The spray pattern and spray angle are adjusted by adjusting the air cap.

Optimum atomization is achieved by fine adjustment of the air cap and atomization air pressure measured at the nozzle. The binder solution is delivered to the nozzle port through a spray lance and tubing. The peristaltic or positive displacement pump is commonly used to pump the binder solution. The pneumatically controlled nozzle needle prevents the binder liquid from dripping when the liquid flow is stopped. Nozzle port openings of 0.8–2.8 mm in diameter are most common and are interchangeable.

The two-fluid nozzle in its simplified model is based on energy transmission as shown here:

Energy+Liquid→Two-Fluid Nozzle→Droplets+Heat

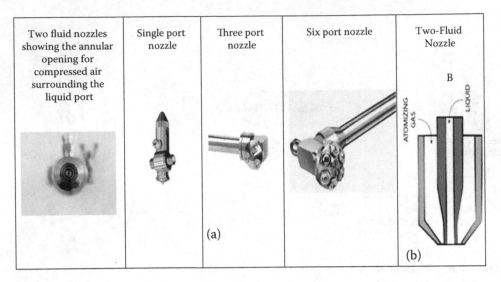

Two fluid nozzles showing the annular opening for compressed air surrounding the liquid port	Single port nozzle	Three port nozzle	Six port nozzle	Two-Fluid Nozzle

(a)

(b)

FIGURE 10.7   (a) Different Capacity Two Fluid Nozzles Used for Fluid Bed Granulation. (b) Schematic of the Binary (Two-Fluid) Nozzle.
Source: The Glatt Group.

The ratio of energy dissipation by heat and by the droplet-making process is difficult to measure. Masters [27] suggested that less than 0.5% of the applied energy is utilized in the liquid breakup. Virtually, the whole amount is imparted to the liquid and air as kinetic energy.

For top-spray granulation in a production size unit, nozzles placement may be required to be placed at various heights depending on the bed coverage required. To provide location flexibility for nozzle placement, some companies provide multiple ports to locate the nozzle.

Since nozzles are placed in the cloud of powder flowing in opposite direction to the flow of liquid from the nozzle, clogging of nozzles, or building up of product on nozzles or nozzle arm, poses problems. To overcome this, some companies have introduced the location of the nozzle in the product container (Figure 10.8), which offers nozzle arrangement above the air distributor in tangential position and allows for in-process inspection and reinsertion without the necessity to abort/pause the process. This installation is suitable for both, wet granulation and pellet layering. Alternatively the nozzle can be placed in the air distributor (Figure 10.9) spraying tangentially to the flow of powder. A similar approach with additional features is offered by GEA Pharma Systems with their Flex Stream™ system (Figure 10.10). Here the nozzle is placed on the side of the container, surrounded by passage through which a low-pressure process air, diverted from the lower plenum, enters around the nozzle and creates an area of spray pattern eliminating the possibility of overwetting of particles and keeping the nozzles clean [28]. The operational and capability of the FlexStream™ fluidized bed processor with swirling airflow were investigated using two DOE studies. It was established that the amount of binder solution affected the size, size distribution, flowability, and roundness of the granules, as well as the percentage of lumps produced. The amount of binder solution had a positive correlation with granule size and percentage of lumps but a negative correlation with size distribution and Hausner ratio. Binder solution spray rate also affected granule size positively while the distance between the spray nozzle and powder bed exerted a similar effect on the percentage of lumps. The authors also found that the percentage of fines was significantly affected by the inlet airflow rate. The distance between the spray nozzle and the powder bed showed a positive effect on the percentage of lumps produced.

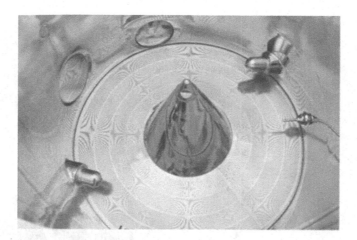

FIGURE 10.8 Three-Fluid Nozzle Position Just Above the Air Distributor for Granulation and Coating. *Source:* L.B. Bohle Maschinen + Verfahren GmbH.

This nozzle positioning approach away from the traditional top or bottom spray is the most significant change in the fluid bed technology. The effort here is to eliminate the different modules traditionally used for drying, granulating, or coating in the industry.

10.3.4 DISENGAGEMENT AREA AND PROCESS FILTERS

Once the air leaves the product bed, fine particles need to be separated from the air stream. Two zones are used in the fluid bed to separate particles from the airstream: the disengagement area and the exhaust filter. In the disengagement area, larger particles lose momentum and fall back into the bed. The velocity of the process air is highest at the center of the processor and approaches zero at the sidewalls. A process air filter system removes the particles from the exhaust air. The process air is filtered by using bags or cartridges. Bag filters are widely used there and are available as a single bag or with double-bag configuration, where one bag is mechanically shaking the particles while the other bag remains functional, thus facilitating uninterrupted fluidization. This alternate shaking of dual bags allows the process to be consistent from batch to batch. These filter bags are

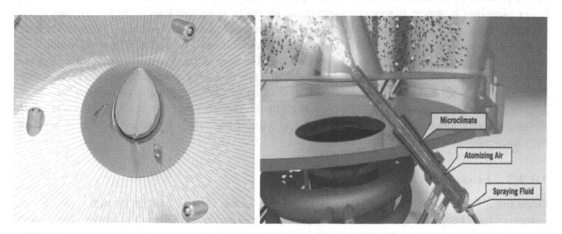

FIGURE 10.9 Three-Component Nozzle Position Within the Air Distributor for Granulation and Coating. *Source*: Hüttlin (Syntegon).

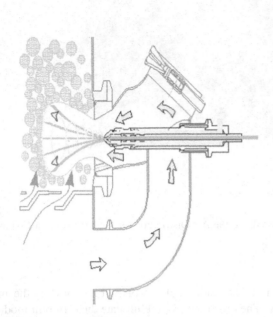
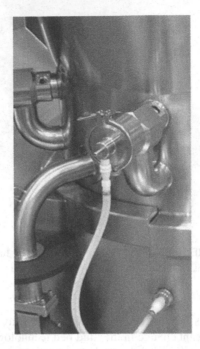

FIGURE 10.10   Nozzle Location in the Container of the FlexStream™ System.
Source: GEA Pharma System Wommelgem, Belgium.

constructed out of nylon, polyester, polypropylene, or polytetrafluoroethylene (PTFE) lined materials (Figure 10.11). To dissipate the potential static charges from the product particles, conductive fabrics are also available and are recommended. Cartridge filters lined with PTFE were introduced to the industry in the 1980s [29]. The standard filtration system normally contains a multiple cartridge filter system with an alternating blowback pulse arrangement allowing continuous product fluidization. A cleanable polyester 2-µm material is utilized for processing water-soluble and insoluble materials, which has an electrical conductivity for static-free operation. Recently, cartridges made of stainless steel suitable for the CIP system have been introduced [30]. Various suppliers of the process equipment have filter arrangements. The vertical filter cartridge claimed to provide better cleaning; however, it requires mechanical means to bring the filters down to replace them. Cartridge filters located at an angle do provide better access to take them out from the unit. They are equally effective. Figures 10.11 and 10.12 shows Commonly used process air filters for a fluid bed processor. The stainless steel cartridge filters are an expensive alternative to the cloth filter bags but provide the possibility of cleaning using an automated CIP system. For potent compound processing, these stainless steel cartridge filters with CIP system capability are normally recommended.

During the granulation or drying process, cloth filters with socks are mechanically shaken to dislodge any product adhered, while cartridge or cloth filters use a low-pressure compressed air blowback system to do the same.

10.3.5   EXHAUST BLOWER OR FAN

Once the air leaves the exhaust filters, it travels to the fan. The fan is on the outlet side of the system, which keeps the system at a lower pressure than the surrounding atmosphere. The airflow is controlled by a valve or damper installed just ahead or after the fan. Manufacturers of the fluid bed normally make the selection of the fan, based on the layout and the complexity of the system.

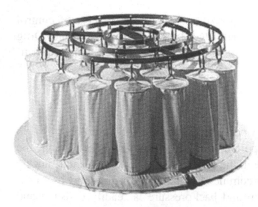

FIGURE 10.11 Conventional Cloth Filter Bag with Hanging Arrangements.
Source: Courtesy of the Freund-Vector Corporation. https://www.freund-vector.com/technology/fluid-bed-drying/.

Fan size is determined by calculating the pressure drop (ΔP) created by all the components that make up the fluid bed processor including the product at the highest design airflow volume.

10.3.6 Control System

A fluid bed granulation process can be controlled by pneumatic analog control devices, or state of the art, programmable logic controllers (PLCs), or computers. The electronic-based control system offers not only reproducible batches according to the recipe but also a complete record and printout of all the process conditions. Process-control technology has changed very rapidly, and it will

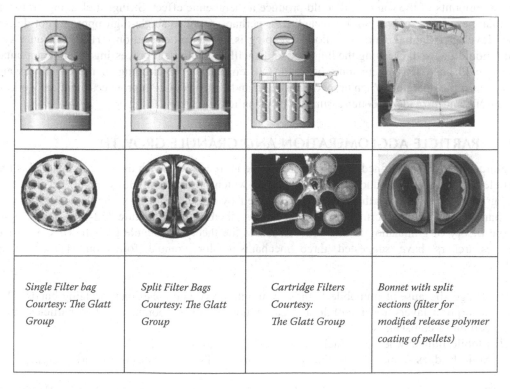

| Single Filter bag Courtesy: The Glatt Group | Split Filter Bags Courtesy: The Glatt Group | Cartridge Filters Courtesy: The Glatt Group | Bonnet with split sections (filter for modified release polymer coating of pellets) |

FIGURE 10.12 Commonly Used Process Air Filters for Fluid Bed Processor.
Source: Glatt Group.

continue to change as advances in computer technology take place, and as the cost of control systems fall. The CFR Part 11 requirements [31] mandated by the U.S. Food and Drug Administration (FDA) have created several approaches to assure these control systems are complying with the current regulation.

10.3.7 SOLUTION DELIVERY SYSTEM

The liquid delivery systems operate at low pressure. A peristaltic pump capable of delivering fluid at a controlled rate is desirable. The liquid is transported from the solution vessel through the tubing and atomized using a two-fluid (binary) nozzle in the fluid bed processor. In a multi-nozzle application for commercial processing, it is highly recommended that each nozzle port use a separate pump in case one of the nozzle port clogs up and backpressure is readily detected and remedial action is taken.

10.4 CLEANING FLUID BED PROCESSOR

The conventional method of cleaning fluidized bed equipment is by dismantling the piece of equipment and manually scrubbing or wiping the surfaces. This is not only time consuming but also difficult for larger equipment where the expansion chamber, filter housing, and dust collector areas cannot be easily accessed. It becomes even more challenging when the fluid bed is integrated with other process equipment. One of the challenges in fluid bed cleaning is the cleaning of filters. Generally, cloth filters are difficult to clean and assure the absence of previous products, hence companies dedicate the filters per product. During manufacturing solid dosage products, contamination/cross-contamination is a major concern, especially in high potency situations where minute amounts of the compound could produce a therapeutic effect. Stringent cleaning protocols are thus necessary, and testing for cleanliness, perhaps down to single-digit ppm or "not detectable" level, is essential. Normally, floor-sweeping is not permitted and only HEPA vacuum systems should be used. Cleaning the fluid bed and ancillary equipment processing potent compound, Clean In Place (CIP) system must be used. CIP eliminates the cleaning of the bag filters and exposure to the operator. When properly designed and validated, CIP reproduces identical working conditions and provides a better assurance of cleanliness.

10.5 PARTICLE AGGLOMERATION AND GRANULE GROWTH

Agglomeration can be defined as the size enlargement process, in which the starting material is fine particles and the final product is an aggregate in which primary particles can still be identified. The granules are held together with bonds formed by the binder used to agglomerate. Various mechanisms of granule formation have been described in the literature [32–34]. The chapter on the theory of granulation in this book discusses the theory of granule growth. To summarize, the researchers have suggested three mechanisms for granule formation. These are as follows:

1. Bridges because of immobile liquids form adhesional and cohesional bridging bonds. Thin adsorption layers are immobile and can contribute to the bonding of fine particles under certain circumstances.
2. Mobile liquids where interfacial and capillary forces are present.
3. Solid bridges formed due to the crystallization of dissolved substances during drying.

The type of bonds formed approaches through four transition states, described by Newitt and Conway-Jones [32] as (i) pendular, (ii) funicular, (iii) capillary, and (iv) droplet, which normally happens during spray drying.

Tardos et al. [35] investigated a comprehensive model of granulation. They developed a pendular bridge apparatus that can be used to test the bridge-forming characteristics of the binder and to determine binder penetration and spreading rates and the critical time of binder strengthening.

Iveson [36] worked to find a mathematical model for granule coalescence during granulation. He found that current models had one of the two limitations: either they only consider whether a bond formed on impact is strong enough to survive subsequent impacts or they fail to consider the possibility of bond rupture after formation at all. He developed a new model that considers both the effects of bond strengthening with time and the distribution of impact forces. He suggests that his models be combined with existing models that predict whether two granules stick initially on impact, and then be able to predict the probability of permanent coalescence.

Thermodynamics determines whether the wetting of the powder is favorable or not. Two aspects are essential, firstly the contact angle between particle and binder liquid and secondly the spreading of the liquid over powder particles.

In any wet granulation process, the surface energy of the starting, intermediate, or final products can be a key factor in understanding the processing operation and or the final product performance.

For a collision to be successful, two conditions must be met: (i) the particles must contact each other by a binder-wet region, and (ii) the viscous binder layer in this region must be able to dissipate the kinetic energy of the particles. Depending on the surface energy, a liquid binder droplet deposited on a smooth particle will either spread completely or form a film coating (total wetting case). As the efficiency of mixing and fluidization in a fluidized bed process is highly dependent on the nature and characteristics of the powder particles, the fluidized bed granulation process is inherently more sensitive to the properties of the starting materials than other commonly known techniques of wet granulation such as high shear granulation.

Agglomeration of hydrophilic particles results in a narrower granule size distribution than hydrophobic ones, most likely because granules above a certain critical size cannot be formed as the kinetic energy of granules during impact cannot be dissipated within the thin binder coating layer present on the particle surface. On the other hand, hydrophobic particles on which the binder droplets are more localized and thus thicker can grow to larger sizes. At the same time, due to lower fractional surface coverage of primary particles, a larger fraction of hydrophobic particles remains un-granulated.

Most of the fluid bed granulated products require an amount of wetting much less than the high shear granulation or spray dryer processed product.

In the fluid bed granulation process, the particles are suspended in the hot air stream and the atomized liquid is sprayed on it. The degree of bonding between these primary particles to form an agglomerated granule depends upon the binder used, physicochemical characteristics of the primary particles being agglomerated, and process parameters.

Schaefer et al. [38] and Smith and Nienow [39] have reported a description of the growth mechanisms in the fluid bed, where the bed particles are wetted by liquid droplets in the spray zone. Atomized liquid from the nozzle tends to spread over the particle surface, as long as there is an adequate wettability of the particle by the fluid [40]. Wet particles on impact form a liquid bridge and solidify as the agglomerate circulates throughout the remainder of the bed. Solid bridges then hold particles together. The strength of the binder determines whether these particles stay as agglomerates. These binding forces should be larger than the breakup forces and, in turn, depend on the size of the solid bridge. The breakup forces arise from the movement of the randomized particles colliding with each other and are related to the excess gas velocity and particle size.

If the binding forces are more than the breakup forces, either in the wet state or in the dry state, uncontrolled growth will proceed to an overwetted bed or production of excessive fines, respectively. If a more reasonable balance of forces is present, controlled agglomeration will occur, growth of which can be controlled. Maroglou and Nienow presented a granule growth mechanism in the fluid bed using model materials and a scanning electron microscope [41]. Iveson [37] and Goldschmidt [42] described the granule growth proportional to the collision frequency between the particles present in the granulator, and the fraction of successful collisions, that is., the fraction of collisions that lead to coalescing rather than rebound. For a collision to be successful, two conditions must be met: (i) the particles must contact each other by a binder wet region, and (ii) the viscous binder layer in this region must be able to dissipate the kinetic energy of the particles. Thielmann et al. [43] investigated the assumption that "better wetting means better granulation." Their experimental study concluded that the effect of surface properties resulted in having the hydrophilic particles resulting in smaller granules than hydrophobic ones and better wettability does not necessarily mean better granulation.

Figure 10.13 shows the various paths a liquid droplet can take and its consequences on the particle growth.

The mechanism of formation of a granule and subsequent growth primarily progresses through the following three stages:

1. Nucleation
2. Transition
3. Ball growth

Figure 10.14 shows the growth of the granule relative to the liquid added. At the beginning of the spraying stage, primary particles form nuclei and are held together by liquid bridges in a pendular state. The size of these nuclei depends upon the droplet size of the binder solution. As the liquid addition continues, more and more nuclei agglomerate and continue the transition from the pendular state to the capillary state.

The uniqueness of the fluid bed agglomeration process is how the liquid addition and drying (evaporation) steps are concurrently carried out. When the granulation liquid is sprayed into a fluidized bed, the primary particles are wetted and form together with the binder, relatively loose, and very porous agglomerates. Agglomeration between two particles will take place if the particles collide with each other and at least one of them is wet enough to form a liquid bridge. The sufficiently high moisture content of one colliding particle depends on the wetting and drying processes. Densification of these agglomerates is brought about solely by the capillary forces present in the liquid bridges. It is therefore important that the quantity of liquid sprayed into the bed should be relatively larger compared with that used in high-shear granulation. Although the wetting and nucleation step may be seen as a minor part of the granulation process it is nevertheless a vital part of the process, and spray rate conditions and particle flux in the spray zone have primary importance for the entire process and the resulting granule properties. Agglomerate can exist in several different spatial structures depending on the binder liquid saturation. It is the amount of liquid binder as well as the humidity conditions in the bed that determines the degree of saturation, which again determines the spatial structure of the final granule [44]. Drying a wet product in a fluid bed is a separate topic, but during the granulation process, it becomes an integral part of the process; hence, understanding fluid bed drying is important before we review the agglomeration process.

During agglomeration of amorphous powders and drying of amorphous granules in fluid beds, it remains difficult to provide a narrow particle size distribution and to avoid the generation of oversized particles. In fluid bed agglomeration, water or aqueous binder droplets are impacting on amorphous particle surfaces. The moisture is absorbed by the hydrophilic surface material generating a viscous solution. Particles impacting on this solution are adhering with a high probability due to effective energy dissipation by viscous forces and the generation of a 20 μm viscous bridge between the two particles. Thus, growth is often rather random and shear forces in the bed are not able to generate spherical particles by abrasion. Therefore, frequently random-shaped particles are obtained. If the liquid binder is finely atomized on the bed and the binder

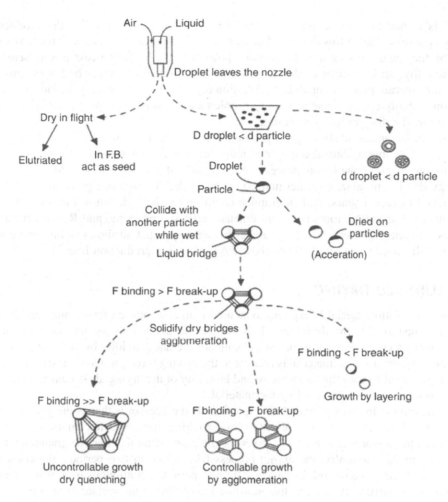

FIGURE 10.13 Mechanism of Granulation in a Fluid Bed.

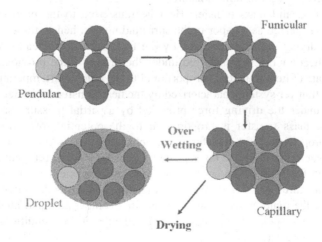

FIGURE 10.14 States of Liquid Saturation.

flow rate is rather low, more spherical particles are obtained. Generally, the produced agglomerates possess a rather low density. The size of agglomerates produced in fluid beds strongly depends on the shear forces within the moving powder bulk. As the process is very sensitive to its bed humidity, strict control of the condition of the fluidizing powder bed is of utmost importance for overall process reliability. Additionally, the use of binding liquids in this wet granulation technique may cause instability problems such as polymorphic transformations and degradation of the drug during processing.

Fluidized bed granulation shows great potential for continuous granulation. This stems from not only its consistent mixing but also the continuous and concurrent wetting and drying occurring throughout the entire granulation process. As a result of the US FDA's Process Analytical Technology (PAT) initiative, a greater understanding of the fluidized bed granulation process has been achieved in recent years. Although much attention has been drawn to the research and development of suitable PAT tools (e.g., viscometric, NIR spectroscopy, and Raman spectroscopy techniques) to control process conditions and characterize product attributes in-line, more work is required to fully implement and validate these PAT tools in a production line.

10.6 FLUID BED DRYING

When any moist solid material is exposed to an airstream at a constant temperature and humidity, moisture is transferred to the drying air. This transfer occurs as long as the material's moisture content is over its equilibrium moisture at the temperature and humidity of the drying air stream. The loss of moisture from the material is relative to the driving force for mass transfer. This driving force is proportional to both the temperature and humidity of the drying air stream and the internal resistance to mass transfer provided by the material.

One of the unique features of granulating in a fluid bed processor is that as the granulating fluid is added to the fluidized powders, constant drying is taking place with hot fluidization air.

A fluid bed processor is also used as a dryer for the granulation that may be granulated in a low or high-shear mixer. Normally, the drying process takes place in two periods, the constant rate period and the falling rate period. In the constant rate period, a continuous film of water exists at the surface of the particle. As long as this moisture is supplied to the surface at the same rate, it is removed from the surface through evaporation, the material dries at a constant rate. Once the drying process reduces the moisture content of the material to the critical moisture, surface moisture is no longer present and diffusion or capillary resistances within the material become significant. This causes the rate of moisture loss to be reduced and the total moisture decreases asymptotically toward the equilibrium moisture.

Drying involves heat and mass transfer. Heat is transferred to the product to evaporate the liquid, and mass is transferred as a vapor in the surrounding gas; hence, these two phenomena are interdependent. The drying rate is determined by the factors affecting heat and mass transfer.

In heat transfer, heat energy is transferred under the driving force provided by a temperature difference, and the rate of heat transfer is proportional to the potential (temperature) difference and the properties of the transfer system characterized by the heat-transfer coefficient. In the same way, mass is transferred under the driving force provided by a partial pressure or concentration difference. The rate of mass transfer is proportional to the potential (pressure or concentration) difference and the properties of the transfer system characterized by a mass-transfer coefficient.

The transfer of heat in the fluid bed takes place by convection. The removal of moisture from a product granulated in the fluid bed processor or other equipment essentially removes the added water called "free moisture" or solvent. This free moisture content is the amount of moisture that can be removed from the material by drying at a specified temperature and humidity. The amount of moisture that remains associated with the material under the drying conditions specified is called the equilibrium moisture content or EMC.

The evaporation rate of liquid film surrounding the granule being dried is related to the rate of heat transfer by the equation:

$$\frac{dw}{dt} = \frac{h \times A}{H} \times \delta T$$

where dw/dt is the mass transfer rate (drying rate), h is the heat transfer coefficient, A is the surface area, H is the latent heat of evaporation, and δT is the temperature difference between the air and the material surface.

Because fluid bed processing involves drying of a product in suspended hot air, the heat transfer is extremely rapid. In a properly fluidized processor, product temperature and the exhaust air temperatures should reach equilibrium. Improper air distribution, hence poor heat transfer in a fluidized bed, causes numerous problems such as caking, channeling, or sticking. The capacity of the air (gas) stream to absorb and carry away moisture determines the drying rate and establishes the duration of the drying cycle. Controlling this capacity is the key to controlling the drying process. The two elements essential to this control are inlet air temperature and airflow. The higher the temperature of the drying air, the greater is its vapor holding capacity. Since the temperature of the wet granules in a hot gas depends on the rate of evaporation, the key to analyzing the drying process is psychrometry [45–47].

Psychrometry is defined as the study of the relationships between the material and energy balances of water vapor-air mixture. Psychrometric charts (Figure 10.15) simplify the crucial calculations of how much heat must be added and how much moisture can be added to or removed from the air. The process of drying involves both heat and mass transfers. For drying to occur, there must be a concentration gradient, which must exist between the moist granule and the surrounding environment. As in heat transfer, the maximum rate of mass transfer that occurs during drying is proportional to the surface area, the turbulence of the drying air, the driving force between the solid and the air, and the drying rate. Because the heat of vaporization must be supplied to evaporate the moisture, the driving force for mass transfer is the same driving force required for heat transfer, which is the temperature difference between the air and the solid. Schaefer and Worts [48] have shown that the higher the temperature differences between incoming air and the product, the faster is the drying rate. Therefore, product temperature should be monitored closely to control the fluidized bed drying process.

In a batch fluidized bed dryer operated under a constant inlet air flow rate, the average moisture content of the particulates will pass through three distinct temperature phases (Figure 10.16). At the beginning of the drying process, the material heats up from the ambient temperature to approximately the wet-bulb temperature of the air in the dryer. This temperature is maintained until the granule moisture content is reduced to the critical level. At this point, the material holds no free surface water, and the temperature starts to rise further. The drying capacity of the air depends upon the relative humidity (RH) of the incoming air. At 100% RH, the air holds the maximum amount of water possible at a given temperature, but if the temperature of the air is raised, the RH drops and the air can hold more moisture. If air is saturated with water vapor at a given temperature, a drop-in temperature will force the air mass to relinquish some of its moisture through condensation. The temperature at which moisture condenses is the dew point temperature. Thus, the drying capacity of the air varies significantly during processing. By dehumidifying the air to a preset dew point, incoming air can be maintained at a constant drying capacity (dew point) and hence provide reproducible process times.

Julia ZH Gao et al. [50] studied the importance of inlet air velocity to dry product granulated in a high-shear granulator and dried in a fluid bed dryer. The manufacturing process involved granulating the dry components containing 63% water-insoluble, low-density drug in a high-shear granulator, milling the wet mass, and drying in a fluid bed dryer. The granules were dried at an

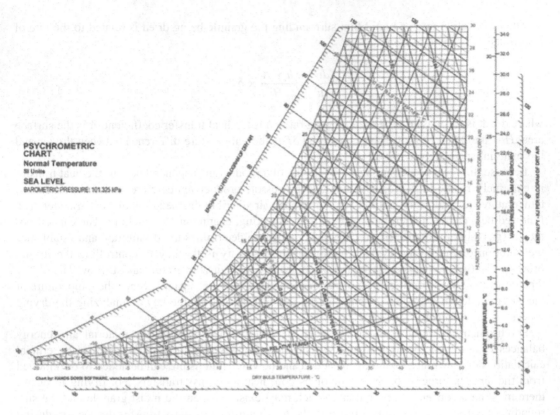

FIGURE 10.15   Psychrometric Chart.

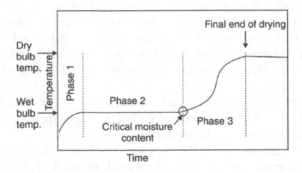

FIGURE 10.16   Product Temperature Changes During Drying.
Source: From Refs. [49,49A].

inlet air temperature of 60°C. Two different air velocities were examined for their effect on the drying uniformity of the product. The authors observed that the excessive velocity indicated by the rapid rise in the exhaust air temperature resulted in nonuniform drying of the product besides resulting in an inefficient process. Granules exhibit an intrinsic breakage propensity during drying, which is dependent on water content and the extent of stress exposed to the granules [51]. Water content and granule sizes are critical processes and quality parameters during the drying process. Nieuwmeyer et al. [52] expanded on the concept that the larger granules contain more water than smaller granules and developed a model to determine the water content of granule based on near-infrared (NIR) to monitor the drying process in a fluid bed. This model provided the median water content of granules and hence the drying endpoint. According to the authors, based on the amount of moisture in the granules, determined by the NIR technique, granule size determination can be made. This approach provides a faster way to determine the water content than the offline measurement more commonly employed.

The combination of granulating solvent and drying conditions could result in the conversion of some of the products to alternate crystalline forms during the drying process. To use NIR in fluid bed drying, knowing the basic properties of the drug substance being granulated is critical. Davis et al. [53] studied the drying of glycine and microcrystalline cellulose (MCC) (1:1) aqueous granulation in a fluid bed unit as well as in a tray dryer. Using the NIR, the researcher concluded that the slower drying techniques, such as tray drying, resulted in significantly less formation of α-glycine a polymorph. The drying rate determined the overall polymorph content. The faster the granulation was dried, the more rapid the increase in supersaturation concerning the metastable form and the greater the thermodynamic driving force for the nucleation and crystallization of the metastable form. The granulation rapidly dried by fluidized bed drying resulted in more crystallization of α-glycine than the granulations that were tray dried. Drying a high-shear wet granulated if not wet-milled could be very cohesive. In the case of cohesive materials in the fluid bed, the interparticle forces are considerable and they control the behavior of a bed. Thus, during the fluidization, the bed cracks into large portions, and the gas tends to flow into the gap between the fissures. Then, channeling occurs in the bed, and eventually, the gas-solid contact is very low, and heat and mass transfer operations are weakened. In such cases, a mechanical agitator as a part of the product container, for breaking up the cohesive granulation cake, is employed. The alternative is to pass the wet granulated product through a mill with four to eight mesh screen to break up the lumps.

10.7 GRANULATION PROCESS

As with any granulating system, with fluid bed granulation processing, the goal is to form agglomerated particles using binder bridges between the particles. To achieve a good granulation, particles must be uniformly mixed, and liquid bridges between the particles must be strong and easy to dry. Therefore, this system is sensitive to the particle movement of the product in the unit, the addition of the liquid binder, and the drying capacity of the air. The granulation process in the fluid bed requires a binary nozzle, a solution delivery system, and compressed air to atomize the liquid binder. Figure 10.17 shows the equipment setup for granulation using the fluid bed processor.

Thurn [54] in a 1970 thesis investigated details of the mixing, agglomerating, and drying operations, which take place in the fluid bed process. Results indicated that the mixing stage was particularly influenced by the airflow rate and air volume. It was suggested that the physical properties of the raw materials such as hydrophobicity might exert a strong influence upon the mixing stage. At the granulation stage, attention was paid to the nozzle and it was concluded that a binary design (two-fluid) nozzle gave a wide droplet size distribution yielding a homogeneous granule. The need for strong binders was recommended to aid granule formation and it was suggested that the wettability of the raw materials required attention. Several research papers have been published on the influence of raw material [37,48,53,55–68], binder type [5,8,47,53,62,64,69–78], binder concentration, and binder quantity [8,56,61,64,66,71,72,78–91]. Binder in the form of foam instead of liquid has been utilized by some pharmaceutical companies. Using foams of aqueous solutions of low molecular weight hypromellose polymers (E3PLV and E6PLV) or conventional solution for fluid bed granulation did not affect the physical properties of granules or tablets compressed from these granules. However, they found that because of foam, the granule formation is achieved more efficiently. It was further claimed that variables associated with nozzles were eliminated by using foam and that the water requirement was reduced along with shorter production time [91].

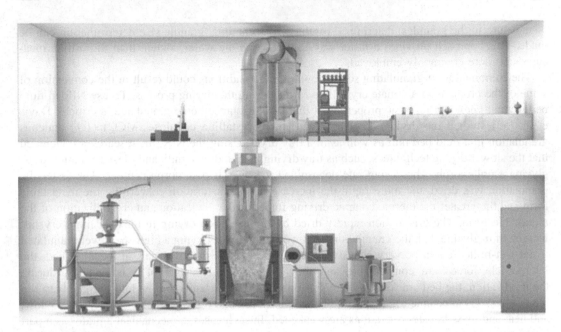

FIGURE 10.17 Typical Fluid Bed Processor Set Up Integrated with the Solution Delivery System and Discharge Through the Mill in the IBC.
Source: IMA, S.p.A. Italy.

10.8   VARIABLES IN GRANULATION

Factors affecting the fluid bed granulation process can be divided into three broad categories:

1. Formulation-related variables
2. Equipment-related variables
3. Process-related variables

10.8.1   FORMULATION-RELATED VARIABLES

Ideally, the particle properties desired in the starting material include a low particle density, a small particle size, a narrow particle size range, the particle shape approaching spherical, a lack of particle cohesiveness, and a lack of stickiness during the processing. Properties such as cohesiveness, static charge, particle size distribution, crystalline or amorphous nature, and wettability are some of the properties that have an impact on the properties of granules formed. The cohesiveness and static charges on particles present fluidization difficulty. The same difficulties were observed when the formulation contained hydrophobic material or a mixture of hydrophilic and hydrophobic materials. The influence of hydrophobicity of primary particles has been shown by Aulton and Banks [17], where they demonstrated that the mean particle size of the product was directly related to the wettability of the primary particles expressed as cos θ (where θ is the contact angle of the particles). It was also reported that as the hydrophobicity of the mix is increased, a decrease in granule growth is observed. Aulton, Banks, and Smith in a later publication showed that the addition of a surface-active agent such as sodium laurel sulfate improves fluidized bed granulation [92]. In a mixture containing hydrophobic and hydrophilic primary particles, granule growth of hydrophilic materials takes place selectively creating content uniformity problems. Formulating a controlled release granulation can be accomplished by using fluid bed granulation.

A controlled release matrix formulation of naproxen was successfully developed using fluid bed granulation [93].

The change in granulation when a new active pharmaceutical ingredient (API) is introduced, even the same material with a different lot number, can be caused by several factors. Surface free energy is considered as one of the material properties for a successful outcome of the granulation process [43].

10.8.1.1 Low-Dose Drug Content

Wan et al. [25] studied various methods of incorporating a low-dose drug such as chlorpheniramine maleate in lactose formulation with polyvinylpyrrolidone (PVP) as the granulating solution. They concluded that the randomized movement of particles in the fluid bed might cause segregation of the drug and that uniform drug distribution was best achieved by dissolving the drug in a granulating solution. The mixing efficiency of drug particles with the bulk material was found to increase in the proportion of the granulating liquid used to dissolve the drug. The optimum nozzle atomizing pressure was deemed to be important to avoid spray drying the drug particles or overwetting, which creates uneven drug distribution. Higashide et al. [94] studied the fluidized-bed granulation using 5-fluorouracil in the concentration of 0.3% in 1:1 mixture of starch and lactose. The hydroxypropyl cellulose (HPC) was used as the binder. The ratios of starch and lactose contained in the granules were measured gravimetrically. The researchers found that a bigger amount of the drug and starch was found in larger granules than in smaller granules. The results were attributed to the hydrophobicity of the 5-fluorouracil, starch, and the hydrophilicity of lactose.

10.8.1.2 Binder

A more general discussion on the types of binders used in the pharmaceutical granulations and their influence on the final granule properties can be studied in chapter 4 of this book. Different binders have different binding properties, and the concentration of individual binders may have to be changed to obtain similar binding of primary particles. Thus, the type of binder, binder content in the formulation, and concentration of the binder have a major influence on granule properties. These properties include friability, flow, bulk density, porosity, and size distribution.

Davies and Gloor [95,96] reported that the types of binders such as povidone, acacia, gelatin, and HPC all have different binding properties that affect the final granule properties mentioned earlier. Hontz [97] investigated MCC concentration, inlet air temperature, binder (PVP) concentration, and binder solution concentration effects on tablet properties. Binder and MCC concentrations were found to have a significant effect on tablet properties. Alkan et al. [98] studied binder (PVP) addition in solution and as a dry powder in the powder mix. They found a larger mean granule size when the dry binder was granulated with ethanol. However, when the binder was in solution the granules produced were less friable and more free-flowing. A similar finding was confirmed by other researchers [99,100]. Binder temperature affects the viscosity of the solution and, in turn, affects the droplet size. Increased temperature of the binder solution reduces the viscosity of the solution reducing the droplet size and hence producing a smaller mean granule size. Binder solution viscosity and concentration affect the droplet size of the binder. Polymers, starches, and high molecular weight PVP cause increased viscosity, which, in turn, creates larger droplet size and subsequently larger mean granule particle size [101].

Diluted binders are preferred because they facilitate finer atomization of the binder solution, provide the control of the particle size, reduce friability, and increase the bulk density even though the tackiness or binding strength may suffer [8,71–73,102].

Under conditions that optimal process parameters are selected, spreading of the binder over a substrate, binder-substrate adhesion, and binder cohesion are the main parameters that influence optimum granulation [103]. Planinsek et al. [104] investigated and concluded that the surface free energy of the formulation ingredients is important, and they found a good correlation between the spreading coefficient of binder over the substrate and the friability of the granules (Table 10.2).

TABLE 10.2

Heats of Vaporization for Commonly Used Solvents

Solvent	Solvent Boiling Point °C	Density (g/mL)	The Heat of Vaporization (kcal/g)
Methylene chloride	40.0	1.327	77
Acetone	56.2	0.790	123.5
Methanol	65.0	0.791	262.8
Ethanol	78.5	0.789	204.3
Isopropanol	82.4	0.786	175.0
Water	100.0	1.000	540.0

10.8.1.3 Binder Solvent

In most instances, water is used as a solvent. The selection of solvents such as aqueous or organic depends upon the solubility of the binder and the compatibility of the product being granulated. Generally organic solvents, because of their rapid vaporization from the process, produce smaller granules than the aqueous solution. Different solvents have different heats of vaporization as shown in Table 10.2. Incorporating a binder or mixture of binders of low melting point and incorporating it with the drug substance in the dry form can eliminate the requirement of solvent for the binder. The temperature of the incoming air is sufficient to melt the binder and form the granules. Seo et al. [105] studied fluid bed granulation using meltable polymers such as polyethylene glycol (PEG) 3000, or esters of PEG and glycerol (Gelucire 50/13). They showed that melt agglomeration by atomization of a melted binder in a fluid bed occurs by initial nucleation followed by coalescence between nuclei. The nuclei are formed by immersion of the solid particles in the binder droplets provided that the droplet size is larger than the size of the solid particles. The agglomerate growth rate is supposed to be practically independent of the droplet size if the binder viscosity is so low that the droplets can spread over the agglomerate surface. If the droplets are unable to spread because of high viscosity, the growth rate is supposed to be inversely proportional to the droplet size. These effects of droplet size are different from those seen in aqueous fluid bed granulation, probably because the aqueous process is affected by the evaporation of binder liquid.

10.8.2 EQUIPMENT-RELATED VARIABLES

10.8.2.1 Equipment Design

To fluidize and thus granulate and dry the product, a certain quantity of process air is required. The volume of the air required will vary based upon the amount of material that needs to be processed. The ratio of drying capacity of the process air and quantity of the product needs to be maintained constant throughout the scaling-up process. Most of the fluid bed units available are modular ones, where multiple processes, such as drying, granulating, bottom (Wurster) coating, rotary fluid bed granulating, or coating, can be carried out by changing the container specially designed for an individual process. The recent offerings by some manufacturers offer a single unit with nozzle configuration such that all of these processes can be carried out without changing the containers [106].

10.8.2.2 Air-Distributor Plate

The process of agglomeration and attrition because of random fluidization requires control of the particle during the granulation process. Optimization of the process requires control over fluidized particles. This is a complex phenomenon because of the prevailing fluidizing conditions and particle size distribution, which changes the process. As the conditioned air is introduced through the lower plenum of the batch fluid bed, the fluidizing velocity of a given volume of air determines how fluidization will be achieved.

Perforated air-distributor plates, described previously, provide an appropriate means of supplying air to the product. These plates are identified by their percentage of open area. Air-distributor plates that have 4 to 30 %open area are normally available. These interchangeable plates or plates with adjustable openings provide a range of loading capacities so that batches of various sizes can be produced efficiently and with uniform quality. To prevent channeling, an operator can select a plate with optimum lift properties. For example, a product with low bulk density requires low fluidizing velocity. A distributor plate having a small open area to give a large enough pressure drop may provide uniform fluidization of such a product without reaching entraining velocity and impinging the process filters. Alternatively, a product with higher bulk density can be fluidized and processed using a plate with a larger open area.

10.8.2.3   Fan (Blower) and Pressure Drop (ΔP)

The blower creates a flow of air through the fluid bed processor or a fan located downstream from the process chamber. This fan imparts motion and pressure to air using a paddle-wheel action. The moving air acquires a force or pressure component in its direction of motion because of its weight and inertia. This force is called velocity pressure and is measured in inches or millimeters of the water column. In operating duct systems, a second pressure that is independent of air velocity or movement is always present. Known as static pressure, it acts equally in all directions. In exhaust systems such as fluid bed processors, a negative static pressure exists on the inlet side of the fan. The total pressure is thus a combination of static and velocity pressures. Blower size is determined by calculating the pressure drop (ΔP) created by all the components of the fluid bed processing system. Proper selection of blower is essential in fluid bed design. A blower with appropriate ΔP will fluidize the process material adequately. However, a blower without enough ΔP will not allow proper fluidization of the product resulting in longer process time and improper granulation. A similar effect can be seen when a product with unusually high bulk density is processed in place of normal pharmaceutical materials, or an air-distributor plate offering high resistance because of its construction. This creates a pressure drop that the blower was not designed to handle. A properly sized blower or fan should develop sufficient ΔP so that the exhaust damper can be used in the 30-60% open position. Any additional components such as scrubbers, exhaust HEPA, police filters, catalytic thermal oxidizer, or overall length of the inlet or outlet duct and additional components in the AHU would require a larger blower/static pressure, which can be recommended by the supplier of the fluid bed processor.

10.8.2.4   Filters and Shaker/Blowback Cycle Mechanism

To retain entrained particles of process material, process filters are used. To maintain these filters from building up layers of fine process material, and causing higher pressure drop and thus improper fluidization, these filters are cleaned during the granulation process. When bag filters are used, mechanical means are used to clean them. This mechanical cleaning of the bag filters requires a cessation of airflow and thus the fluidization, during the filter cleaning process. In units with a single-bag house, this results in a momentary dead bed, where no fluidization takes place. This interruption in the process extends the processing time. To avoid process interruptions, a multi-shaking filter bag arrangement is desired, where the granulation process is continuous. Using bag filters with a blowback or using cartridge filters, where air under pressure is pulsed through the filters, the continuous filter cleaning process is achieved. Generally, filters should be cleaned frequently during the granulation step, to incorporate the fines in the granulation. This is possible if the cleaning frequency is high and the period between the filter cleanings is short. Rowley [107] reported the effect of the bag-shake/interval cycle. He discussed the possibility of improving particle size distribution by optimizing the shaking time and the corresponding interval between bag shakes.

Following general guidelines for filter cleaning frequency and duration are recommended.

Single-bag shaker unit: Frequency is 2–10 minutes between filter cleaning and 5-10 seconds for shaking. This may vary as the fine powders form granules and the frequency between the shakes or duration of shaking interval can be extended. In any case, the occurrence of the collapsed bed should be kept at a minimum in a single shaker unit.

Multiple-bag shaker unit: Since this is a continuous process, the frequency of shaking for each section is approximately 15–30 seconds between filter cleanings and about 5 seconds for shaking the filters. If a low-pressure blowback system is used for the bags, the frequency of cleaning is about 10–30 seconds.

Cartridge filters: These offer continuous processing and require a cleaning frequency of 10–30 seconds. The cleaning frequency and cleaning duration are now offered as an automated system where instead of having to base the cleaning frequency on time, the trigger point for filter cleaning is the buildup of a pressure drop across the filters. This automates the process and eliminates operator input.

10.8.2.5   Other Miscellaneous Equipment Factors

Granulator bowl geometry is considered to be a factor that may have an impact on the agglomeration process. The fluidization velocity must drop from the bottom to the top rim of the bowl by more than half to prevent smaller, lighter particles from being impinged into the filter creating segregation from heavier product components in the bowl. Generally, the conical shape of the container and expansion chamber are preferred where the ratio of the cross-sectional diameter of the distributor plate to the top of the vessel is 1:2. Most of the suppliers of these equipment offer units with a multiprocessor concept where a single unit can be used for drying, agglomerating, air-suspension coating, or rotary fluid bed processing by changing the processing container while the rest of the unit is common. This approach does eliminate the concerns about the geometry of the processor because of the way these units are constructed.

10.8.3   PROCESS-RELATED VARIABLES

The agglomeration process is a dynamic process where a droplet is created by a two-fluid nozzle and deposited on the randomly fluidized particle. The binder solvent evaporates leaving behind the binder. Before all of the solvent is evaporated other randomized particles form bonds on the wet site. This process is repeated numerous times to produce a desired agglomerated product. Several process variables control the agglomeration. Process variables most important to consider are listed as follows:

1. Process inlet air temperature
2. Atomization air pressure
3. Fluidization air velocity and volume
4. Liquid spray rate
5. Nozzle position and number of spray heads
6. Product and exhaust air temperature
7. Filter porosity and cleaning frequency
8. Bowl capacity

These process parameters are interdependent and can produce a desirable product if this interdependency is understood. Inlet process air temperature is determined by the choice of binder vehicle, whether aqueous or organic, and the heat sensitivity of the product being agglomerated. Generally, aqueous vehicles will enable the use of temperatures between 60°C and 100°C. On the other hand, organic vehicles will require the use of temperatures from 50°C to below room temperature. Higher temperatures will produce rapid evaporation of the binder solution and will produce smaller, friable granules. On the other hand, a lower temperature will produce larger, fluffy, and denser granules.

Figure 10.18 shows the relationship between the inlet and product air temperature, and outlet air humidity during the granulation process. The process of drying while applying spraying solution is a critical unit operation. This mass transfer step was previously discussed. The temperature, humidity, and volume of the process air determine the drying capacity. If the drying capacity of the air is fixed from one batch to the next, then the spray rate can also be fixed. If the drying capacity of the air is too high, the binder solution will tend to spray dry before it can effectively form bridges between the primary particles. If, on the other hand, the drying capacity of the air is too low, the bed moisture level will become too high and particle growth may become uncontrollable. This will result in unacceptable movement of the product bed.

As previously discussed, the appropriate process air volume, inlet air temperature, and binder spray rate are critical to achieving proper and consistent particle size distribution and granule characteristics. There are many ways to arrive at the proper operating parameters.

An excess of liquid feed, either over the whole bed or in a localized region, produces excessive and uncontrollable particle agglomeration and leads to a loss of fluidization, or what Nienow and Rowe [108] have called wet quenching.

Akio Miwa et al. [109] calculated the amount of water needed for the mixture of components before the fluid bed granulation. The range of an appropriate amount of water for each component in a model formulation was estimated with a refractive near infra-red (NIR) moisture sensor; using these values, the authors calculated the range of the suitable amount of water to add to the model formulation. The authors performed fluid bed granulation with NIR sensors and the calculated amount of water to conclude that the predictive method was able to calculate the amount of water needed for the granulation.

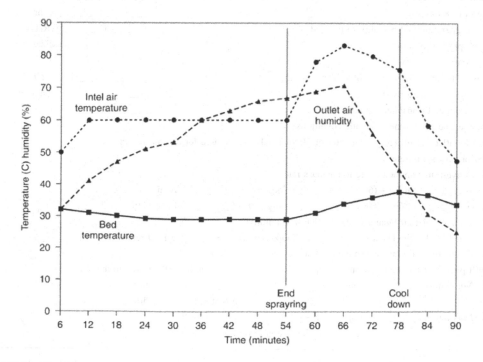

FIGURE 10.18   Temperature and Humidity Changes During the Granulation Process.

The following procedure was found by the authors to be one of the ways one can set the operating parameters when granulating with fluid bed processors.

1. Determine the proper volume of air to achieve adequate mixing and particle movement in the bowl. Avoid excessive volumetric airflow so as not to entrain the particles into the filters.
2. Choose an inlet air temperature that is high enough to negate weather effects (outside air humidity or inside room conditions). The air temperature should not be detrimental to the product being granulated. (*To achieve consistent process year-round, a dehumidification/ humidification system is necessary, which provides the process air with constant dew point and hence constant drying capacity.*)
3. Achieve a binder solution spray rate that will not spray dry and will not overwet the bed. This rate should also allow the nozzle to atomize the binder solution to the required droplet size.
4. As stated earlier, a typical air velocity used for spray granulation is from 1.0 to 2.0 m/sec. Table 10.3 is based on the psychrometric chart, which gives the first guess at determining the proper spray rate for a spray granulation process in a fluid bed processor (Table 10.3).

Variables in the fluid bed granulation process and their impact on the final granulation were summarized by Davies and Gloor [102], where they state that the physical properties of granulation are dependent on both the individual formulations and the various operational variables associated

---

TABLE 10.3
Calculation of Fluid Bed Spray Rate

Given Process data

Air volume range:

Minimum (1.2 m/sec)	_____m^3/hr
Maximum (1.8 m/sec)	_____m^3/hr
Inlet air temperature and humidity to be used:	_____°C_____ %RH
Solids in sprayed solution	_____% solids

From psychrometric chart

Air density at point where air volume is measured:	_____m^3/kg air
Inlet air absolute humidity (H):	_____g H_2O/kg air
Maximum outlet air absolute humidity (H):	_____g H_2O/kg air

(Follow the line of constant adiabatic conditions)

Use 100% outlet RH for spray granulator or 30–60% RH (as required for column coating)

Calculations for spray rate

Step 1. Convert air volumetric rate to air mass rate

Minimum _____m^3/hr ÷ (60 × _____m^3/kg air) = _____kg air/min

Maximum _____m^3/hr ÷ (60 × _____m^3/kg air) = _____kg air/min

Step 2. Subtract inlet air humidity from outlet air humidity:

_____(g H2O/kg air) H out – _____(g H2O/kg air) H in = _____g H_2O removed/kg air

Step 3. Calculate (minimum and maximum) spray rate of the solution:

This will provide a range of generally acceptable spray rates based on the airflow used in the unit

Step 1 (Minimum)_____ × step 2_____ ÷ [1 – (_____ % solids ÷100]

= _____spray rate g/min) at minimum air flow

Step 2 (Maximum)_____ × step 2 ÷ [1 – (_____ % solids ÷ 100]

= spray rate g/min) at minimum airflow

TABLE 10.4

Significant Variables and Their Impact on the Fluid Bed Granulation Process

Process Parameter	Impact on the Process	References
1. Inlet air temperature	Higher inlet temperature produces finer granules and lower temperature produces larger stronger granules.	76,85
2. Humidity	An increase in air humidity causes larger granule size, longer drying times.	38
3. Fluidizing airflow	Proper airflow should fluidize the bed without clogging the filters. Higher airflow will cause attrition and rapid evaporation, generating smaller granules and fines.	17, 20, 76
4. Nozzle and position	A binary nozzle produces the finest droplets and is preferred. The size of the orifice has an insignificant effect except when binder suspensions are to be sprayed. Optimum nozzle height should cover the bed surface. Too close to the bed will wet the bed faster producing larger granules, while too high a position will spray-dry the binder, create finer granules, and increase granulation time.	62
5. Atomization air volume and pressure	The liquid is atomized by the compressed air. This mass-to-liquid ratio must be kept constant to control the droplet size and hence the granule size. The higher liquid flow rate will produce a larger droplet and larger granule and the reverse will produce smaller granules. At a given pressure and an increase in orifice size will increase droplet size.	38, 62,87,91
6. Binder spray rate	Droplet size is affected by liquid flow rate, and binder viscosity, and atomizing air pressure and volume. The finer the droplet, the smaller the resulting average granules.	17. 60,68, 76 , 91,

with the process. The solution spray rate increase and subsequent increase in average granule size resulted in a less friable granulation, higher bulk density, and a better flow property for a lactose/corn starch granulation. Similar results were obtained by an enhanced binder solution, decreasing nozzle air pressure, or lowering the inlet air temperature during the granulation cycle. The position of the binary nozzle concerning the fluidized powders was also studied. It was concluded that by lowering the nozzle, binder efficiency is enhanced, resulting in an average granule size increase and a corresponding decrease in granule friability.

The significant process parameters and their effect on the granule properties are summarized in Table 10.4.

Maroglou [110] listed various parameters affecting the type and rate of growth in batch fluidized granulation (Table 10.4) and showed the influence of process parameters and the material parameters on the product.

10.9 FLUIDIZED HOT MELT GRANULATION (FHMG)

Melt granulation belongs to the group of hot-melt technologies, which represent an alternative to the classical solvent-mediated technological processes of agglomeration. Melt granulation is an emerging technique based on the use of binders that have a relatively low melting point (between 50°C and 80°) and act as a molten binding liquid. Combining low melting binders with powders and using the fluid bed hot air to melt the binders that effectively act as a liquid binder to form granules. The application of this approach can also produce solid dispersion of poorly soluble drugs to increase the solubility and bioavailability. The main advantage of hot-melt processes is the absence of solvents, which can be efficiently utilized in enhancing the chemical stability of moisture sensitive drugs and also improving their physical properties. Moreover, the drying phase is eliminated, which results in a more economical and environmentally friendly process. There are also some limitations to using melt granulation processes. Melt granulation or thermoplastic granulation is based on agglomeration carried out using a binder material, which is solid at room temperature and softens and melts at higher temperatures (i.e., 50–90°C). When melted, the action of the binder liquid is similar to that in a wet-granulation process. The binder is added either in a powder form to the starting material at ambient temperature, followed by heating the binder above its melting point (in situ granulation), or in a molten form, sprayed on the heated materials in fluid bed (spray-on granulation).

Kkeeca et al. [111] showed that melt granulation using hydrophilic binders is an effective method to improve the dissolution rate of poorly water-soluble drugs. The binder addition procedure was found to influence the dissolution profile obtained from granules produced in FHMG. The spray-on procedure resulted in a higher dissolution rate of carvedilol from the granules. FHMG has been proposed as an approach to taste masking of bitter drugs [112]. Waxy binders have been used in the preparation of conventional and sustained-release tablets [113], and more recently in the preparation of fast-release tablets [114]. Yanze et al. [115] reported the preparation of effervescent granules using PEG 6000 as a melt binder using fluidized bed melt granulation. The melt solidification technique for the preparation of sustained-release ibuprofen beads with cetyl alcohol has been studied in the laboratory [116].

Abbereger et al. [117], Seo et al. [118] Tan et al. [119] and Boerefijn et al. [120] investigated the effect of binder spray rate droplet size, particle size, bed temperature, atomization air pressure, and fluidization air velocity on the process performance, using polyethylene glycol as a model binder and glass ballotini and lactose as seeds. The results indicated that the melt flow rate and fluidization air velocity strongly affect how the agglomerates are formed and the resulting particle size.

Each phase of the granulation process must be controlled carefully to achieve process reproducibility. When binder liquid is sprayed into a fluidized bed, the primary particles are wetted and form together with the binder, relatively loose, and very porous agglomerates. Densification of these agglomerates is brought about almost solely by the capillary forces present in the liquid bridges. A portion of the liquid is immediately lost by evaporation; it is therefore important that the liquid binder sprayed into the bed should be relatively large in quantity compared with that used in the high- or low-shear granulation process. The particle size of the resulting granule can be controlled to some extent by adjusting the quantity of binder liquid and the rate at which it is fed, that is, the droplet size. The mechanical strength of the particles depends principally on the composition of the primary product being granulated and the type of the binder used. Aulton et al. [121] found that lower fluidizing air temperature, a dilute solution of binder fluid, and a greater spray rate produced better granulation for tableting.

10.10 PROCESS CONTROLS AND AUTOMATION

The agglomeration process is a batch process, and accurately repeatable control of all critical process parameters (CPPs) is necessary for a robust system. At the same time, it is a good example of a multivariate process in which effective and reliable process control tools are necessary to ensure end-product quality. The initial nucleation that takes place as the droplet hits the particle surfaces in the fluidized powder bed is characterized by a fast agglomerate growth rate. This phase is followed by a slower granule growth phase or a transition phase where the amount of nongranulated fines has substantially decreased [53]. In this transition region, the slower growth kinetics enables easier process control, and the process endpoint will most likely be found in this place. Earlier designs of the fluid

(a) (b)

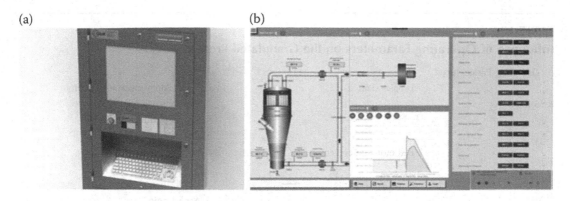

FIGURE 10.19 (a, b) PLC-Based Control Panel and Screen.
Source: The Glatt Group.

bed processor used pneumatic controls, which provided safe operation in hazardous areas but relied heavily on human actions to achieve repeatable product quality and accurate data acquisition. Current designs use PLCs and personal computers (PCs) to achieve sophisticated control and data acquisition. The operating conditions are controlled to satisfy parameters of multiple user-configured recipes and critical data is collected at selected time intervals for inclusion in an end-of-batch report. Security levels protect access to all user-configured data with passwords permitting access only to selected functions. With the appropriate security level not only are operating conditions configured but also the identification of each valid recipe and operator is entered. The identification is verified before any operator actions are permitted and are included with the end-of-run report. The use of computer-related hardware requires some additional validation, but with coordination between the control system provider and the end user, the validation of software can be managed. Figure 10.19a, b shows a PLC-based control panel with a typical operator screen.

The most important sensors for control of the drying process are inlet and exhaust air temperature and a sensor for airflow measurement, located in the air transport system. Other sensors for the spray agglomeration process are product bed temperature, atomization air pressure and volume, pressure drops (across the inlet filter, the product container with the product being processed, and outlet process air filter), inlet air humidity or dew point, process filter cleaning frequency and duration, spray rate for the binder solution, and total process time (Table 10.5).

All of these sensors provide constant feedback information to the computer. These electronic signals may then be stored in the computer's memory and then recalled as a batch report. With this ability to recall data analysis, greater insight can be gained into the process.

10.10.1 ADVANCES IN PROCESS CONTROL AND AUTOMATION

The degree of the instrumentation of pharmaceutical unit operations has increased. This instrumentation provides information on the state of the process and can be used for both process control and research. A central part of optimizing production is increasing the level of automation. Besides monitoring the process parameters, several approaches are being developed for measuring the moisture of the product to determine the endpoint of the process and consequently the in-process particle size analysis. Numbers of publications discuss on-line moisture measurement and process end-point determination using NIR.

10.10.1.1 Near-Infrared (NIR)

The non-destructive character of vibrational spectroscopy techniques, such as NIR, makes them novel tools for in-line quality assurance [122]. NIR has been widely used for the measurement of

TABLE 10.5

Influence of Operating Parameters on the Granulated Product

A. Operating Parameters

	Droplet size	NAR[a] Atomization air velocity
Rheology		Surface tension
		Nozzle position
		Nozzle type
	Bed moisture content	Solution type and feed rate
		Bed temperature
		Fluidization velocity
		Aspect ratio
		Nozzle position and atomization velocity
		Air distributor design
		Jet grinding
	Binder solution/suspension concentration	Bridge strength and size Rheology
B. Material Parameters		
	Binder solution/suspension concentration	Bridge Strength and size
		Rheology
	Type of Binder	Molecular length and weight
	Wettability	Particle-solvent interaction
		Surface tension
		Viscosity
	Material to be granulated	Average particle size
		Size distribution
		Shape and porosity
		Drying characteristics
		Density and density differences[b]

Notes
a   NAR is the ratio of air-to-liquid flow rates through the nozzle of a twin fluid atomizer expressed either in mass units or in volume units (air at STP).
b   Especially important relative to elutriation and segregation.

water in various applications [123]. NIR can be applied for both quantitative analyses of water and for determining the state of water in solid material. This gives a tool for understanding the physicochemical phenomena during the manufacture of pharmaceutical granulation. Accurate NIR in-line particle size analysis of moving granules is challenging because the scattering and absorptive properties of the granules vary. Also, since particle size data are not directly obtained using NIR techniques, pretreatment of spectra and chemometric modeling are needed.

The pharmacopeias have defined some characteristics of analysis with NIR [124,125]. Developing a functional automation system requires new measuring techniques; new in-line measuring devices are needed [126–130]. Solid-water interactions are one of the fundamental issues in pharmaceutical technology. The state of water in a solid material may be characterized using X-ray diffraction, microscopic methods, thermal analysis, vibrational spectroscopy, and nuclear magnetic resonance spectroscopy [131]. Traditionally, the control of fluidized bed granulation has based on indirect measurements. These control methods applied to utilize the properties of process air by Schaefer and Worts [48]. Frake et al. [132] demonstrated the use of NIR for in-line analysis of the moisture content in pellets of size 0.05–0.07 mm during spray granulation in the fluid bed processor. Rantanen et al. [133,134] described a similar approach for moisture content measurement using rationing of three to four selected wavelengths. He with his coworkers reported that the critical part of the in-line process was the sight glass for probe positioning that was continuously blown with heated air. They also reported spectra baselines caused by particle size and refractive properties of the in-line samples; they recurred to analyze several data pretreatments to eliminate these effects on their fixed wavelength setup. Solvents other than water have also been evaluated for real-time quantification. Nieuwmeyer et al. [52] determined the particle size and the drying endpoint of granules using NIR. Lipsanen et al. [135] evaluated the instrumentation system to determine the parameters expressing the changing conditions during the spraying phase of a fluid bed process using an inline spatial filtering technique (SFT) probe to the variations in properties of the product being processed. Vazquez recently provided a comprehensive review of FT-NIR application in measuring fluid bed drying end [136]. Rantanen et al. [137] used NIR to monitor the moisture as well as airflow. Using in-line multichannel NIR, the multivariate process data collected was analyzed using principal component analysis (PCA). The authors showed that a robust process control and measurement system combined with reliable historical data storage can be used for analyzing the fluid bed granulation process. PCA modeling proved a promising tool to handle multidimensional data that was collected and for the reduction of the dimensionality of process data. FT-NIR spectra gave useful information for understanding the phenomenon during granulation. Rantanen et al. [138] further studied the application of NIR for fluid bed process analysis. The authors used NIR to study moisture measurement combined with temperature and humidity measurements. By controlling the water during the fluid bed granulation, the granulation process was controlled. They concluded that the varying behavior of formulations during processing can be identified in a real-time mode. Thus, they found that NIR spectroscopy offered unique information on granule moisture content during all phases of granulation.

10.10.1.2   Other Approaches for Process Control

(a). Self-Organizing Maps

On-line process data is usually multidimensional, and it is difficult to study with traditional trends and scatter plots. Rantanen et al. [139] have suggested a new tool called "self-organizing maps" (SOM) for dimension reduction and process state monitoring. As a batch process, granulation traversed through several process states, which was visualized by SOM as a two-dimensional map. Besides, they demonstrated how the differences between granulation batches can be studied.

(b). At-Line Measurement

Laitinen et al. presented a paper at a recent conference [140] proposing an at-line optical technique to study particle size. Using a CCD camera with optics and illumination units with stabilized collimated light beams, the authors took two images of 36 granule samples by illuminating the samples alternatively. Two digital images with matrices of their grayscale values were obtained and the differences between the two matrices were calculated. This method provided a very rapid (1 min/sample) measurement of particle size with a very sample size (less than 0.5 g).

(c). Focused Beam Reflectance Measurement (FBRM)

This device uses a focused beam of laser light that scans in a circular path across a particle or particle structure passing in front of the window. Upon hitting the particle, light is scattered in all directions. Hu et al. [141] investigate granule growth in a fluidized bed granulation (FBG). The chord length distribution (CLD) measured by the FBRM was used to represent granule particle size distribution (PSD). The CLD evolution measured by the FBRM confirmed that the granule agglomeration was mainly dominated by the binder on the granule surface.

The light scattered back toward the probe is used to measure the chord length or the length between any two points on a particle. Such devices are supplied commercially and claim to be useful for monitoring on-line measurement of particle size in the fluid bed granulation process. A newly developed FBRM C35 utilizes a mechanical scraper to prevent the probe from fouling.

(d). Parsum Spatial Filtering Technique (SFT)

With the Parsum probe (Figure 10.20), laser light obscuration signal from individual particles can be translated into size information for analysis by the extended spatial filter as particles pass through an aperture on the probe tip. In wet granulation, probe fouling could be one of the most significant obstacles that hinder representative and accurate measurement. Pressurized air is used to disperse particles in the Parsum probe and minimize fouling, an extended spatial filter can convert light obscuration signals from individual particles into size information for analysis. Measurement range spans from 50 μm up to 6 mm at velocities up to 50 m/s. Particle size calculations are based on statistical evaluation of a specified quantity of individual particles. The chord length of an individual particle is measured, which is the link between two points on the perimeter of the measured particle's projection face. Huang et al. demonstrated that Parsum is a useful tool for in-line particle size characterization during fluid bed granulation for a formulation containing 40% (w/w) BCS class 4 compound granulated with 10% (w/w) aqueous solution of povidone (KollidonK25). All data generated by the Parsum probe during production can be utilized by the multivariate statistical methodology to study batch-to-batch variation and evaluate overall batch performance [142–144].

A process control strategy based on the real-time process and product measurement information was used to develop a feed-forward control strategy using spatial filter velocimetry (SFV) [145–151] and focused beam reflectance measurement (FBRM) [152,153] and moisture was used to determine the optimum drying temperature of the consecutive drying phase via real-time monitoring of process (i.e., spraying temperature and spray rate) and product (i.e. granule size distribution and moisture) parameters during spraying period. Besides this feed-forward strategy, a quantitative Partial Least Square (PLS) model for in-line moisture content prediction of the granulated end product was built using NIR data. Thus, combining SFV and moisture trajectories, real-time monitoring of the granulation and drying progress desired density requirement was accomplished [154].

(e). Artificial Neural Network

Neural networks have been used by scientists for optimizing formulations as an alternative to statistical analysis because of their simplicity for use and the potential to provide detailed information. The neural network builds a model of the data space that can be consulted to ask "what if" kinds of questions. Recently, there has been an interest in the industry for using artificial neural network (ANN) for process control. Similar to the human brain, an ANN predicts events or information based upon learned pattern recognition. ANNs are computer systems developed to mimic the operations of the human brain by mathematically modeling its neurophysiological structure (i.e., its nerve cells and the network of interconnections between them). In ANN, the nerve cells are replaced by computational units called neurons and the strengths of the interconnections are represented by weights [155]. This unique arrangement can simulate some of the neurological processing abilities of the brain such as learning and concluding

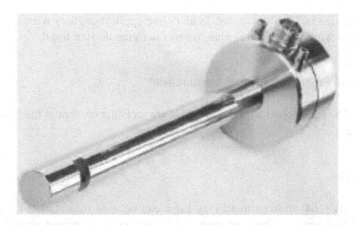

FIGURE 10.20 Parsum Probe.
Source: Malvern Instruments. https://www.malvernpanalytical.com/en/products/product-range/parsum-range.

experience [156]. Using the process control system, quality assurance results, or energy usage data, an ANN develops supervisory setpoints for the system. When ANN and process-control systems are used together, they form a production control system. Product control occurs when a system measures defined product attributes in real-time and use the knowledge to adjust the control system. While the process-control system runs the process (i.e., fans, motors, and heaters), the ANNs control the moisture level and consistency of the product. The fluidized-bed processor process-control system includes an operator interface, sensing elements, and final control elements. The inputs, in that case, are inlet air temperature, outlet air temperature, airflow rate, and energy consumption. Additional contributing factors are the fouling coefficient of the dryer bags, the quantity of a product in the processor, and the type of product with its unique characteristics. Watano et al. [157] described a practical method for moisture control in fluid bed granulation utilizing neural networks. Wet granulation of pharmaceutical powder was conducted using an agitation fluidized bed, and moisture content was continuously measured by the IR moisture sensor. A neural network system for moisture control was developed using moisture content and its changing rate as input variables, and the moisture control characteristics were investigated by the neural network system with backpropagation learning. Good response and stability without overshoot were achieved by adopting the developed systems. This system also maintained favorable stability under various operating conditions. Several researchers have published papers detailing the use of ANN for different applications [158–160]. Behzadi et al. [161] reported on the validation of a modified fluid bed granulator. Sucrose was granulated under different operating conditions and their effects on the size distribution, flow rate, repose angle, and tapped and bulk volumes of the granulation were measured. A generalized regression neural network (GRNN, a variation of radial basis function networks) was used to model the system. A good correlation was found between the predicted and experimental data. A review of the literature suggests a strong interest on the part of researchers in applying neural networks to the development of modified release oral solid dosage forms

(f). Three-Dimensional Particle Measurement

To address the issues with in-line measurement of particle size because probes and windows appearing prone to coating, Närvänen et al. [162] used a camera-described image analysis method to measure particle size in 3D and in color. In an online application, they were able to successfully retrieve images and were able to determine the median granule size trend.

(g). Triboelectric Probe for Moisture Measurement

Portoghese et al. [163] developed a method to measure moisture content in the fluid bed by using a triboelectric probe.

(h). Fuzzy Logic

Koerfer and Simutis [164] showed that fuzzy logic can be used for simulated real-time observations of fluidized bed agglomeration process and in general to eliminate several trials and error approach for the process. Watano and coworkers [165] have used fuzzy logic to control granulation processes in agitatating fluid bed. Additional information on process control for granulation processes can be obtained in Chapter 26 of this book.

10.11   PROCESS SCALE-UP

In fluid bed granulation, the spreading of the binder liquid droplets in the powder bed is much more crucial, because it is the phenomenon that controls most of the agglomeration. The process parameters are all interdependent, hence it is critical to obtain a stable regime by fully balancing the different input variables as you scale up the process. Scale transfer in fluid bed granulation involves similar equipment designs, parameters related to starting materials, input variables – such as spraying conditions, amount of solvent energy input, and efficiency – and processing time. More detailed engineering treatment can be seen in Chapter 24 of this book.

10.11.1   SCALE-UP AND EQUIPMENT DESIGN

The scale-up from the laboratory equipment to production size units is dependent on equipment design. The importance of scalability is well-understood and accepted by the manufacturers of fluid bed processors. Various sizes in their product line are logically designated and manufactured. The design and selection of the processor are very important for the laboratory and production unit. Because airflow is one of the components of the drying capacity of a fluid bed system, the ratio of air volume per kilogram or liter of the product is very critical to achieve linear scale-up. The other design feature is the cross-sectional area of the product container, and how it has been designed throughout the various sizes that a manufacturer supply. The relationship between various sizes of the process containers can be utilized to calculate the scale-up of binder spray rate, and if the cross-sectional area is designed linearly, then the spray rate scale-up can be linear. Nozzle position should always be such that it should cover the powder bed, and hence the location and the number of nozzle ports are an important consideration as you scale up.

10.11.2   SCALE-UP AND PROCESS FACTORS

The fluid bed agglomeration process is a combination of three steps, namely, dry mixing, spray agglomeration, and drying to the desired moisture level. The granule size is directly proportional to the bed humidity during granulation [47], and hence control of this humidity during scale-up is essential.

Gore et al. [166] studied the factors affecting the fluid bed process during scale-up. The authors found that processing factors that most affected granule characteristics were processing air temperature, the height of the spray nozzle from the bed, rate of binder addition, and the degree of atomization of the binder liquid.

The atomizing air pressure and the wetness of the bed are two of the most important elements of fluid bed granulation. A higher atomizing air pressure yields a finer droplet of binder solution. Therefore, granule growth (as described earlier in this section) is affected by the atomizing air pressure. A major factor, which must be considered during the scale-up of the fluid bed granulation process, is maintaining the same droplet size of the binder for assuring successful scale-up. Another study [167] confirmed the influence of spray nozzle setup parameters and drying capacity of the air. The study concluded that more attention should be to the easily overlooked nozzle atomizing air pressure and volume. When considering the atomizing air pressure, attention must be paid to ensure enough air is delivered to the nozzle tip. This can be assured by placing air pressure and volume measurement devices at the nozzle. The data also show that the drying capacity of the process air influences the final granulated particle size.

Jones [168] has suggested various process-related factors that should be considered during the scale-up of fluid bed processing. Because of the higher degree of attrition in the larger unit compared with the smaller unit, the bulk density of the granulation from the larger fluid bed is approximately 20% higher than the smaller unit. He also reemphasized the importance of keeping the bed moisture level below the critical moisture level to prevent the formation of larger agglomerates. Since the higher airflow along with the temperature (drying capacity) in a larger unit provides a higher evaporation rate, one must maintain the drying capacity in the larger unit such that the bed temperature is similar to the smaller unit bed temperature. This can be accomplished either by increased spray rate, increased air temperature, increased airflow, or by the combination of these variables to obtain suitable results. Since the ratio of bed depth to the air distributor increases with the size of the equipment, the fluidization air velocity is kept constant by increasing the air volume. In the past, the scale-up was carried out by selecting the best guess process parameters. The recent trend is to employ the factorial and modified factorial designs and search methods. These statistically designed experimental plans can generate mathematical relationships between the independent variables such as process factors and dependent variables such as product properties. This approach still requires an effective laboratory/pilot-scale development program and an understanding of the variables that affect the product properties.

In summary, when scaling up, the following processing conditions should be similar to the pilot-scale studies:

1. Fluidization velocity of the process air through the system
2. The ratio of granulation spray rate to drying capacity of fluidization air volume
3. The droplet size of the binder spray liquid

Each of these values must be calculated based on the results of the operation of the pilot size unit. Pilot size equipment studies should also be conducted in a wide range to determine the allowable operating range for the process.

Matharu and Patel [169] presented a scale-up case study where a low-dose multiple-strength product (0.5–5% w/w active) was sprayed granulated and scaled up from a pilot-scale fluid bed processor and scaled up to production size equipment. Their approach was based on matching air velocity between the two scales of operation. The impact of droplet size was determined by varying the independent parameters. Based on their study, the authors have suggested an equation, which takes into account material and equipment parameters. Rambali [170,171] scaled up the granulation process from small (5 kg) to medium (30 kg) to large (120 kg) to obtain a target geometric mean granule size of 400 μm. The scaling-up was based on the relative droplet size and the powder bed moisture content at the end of the spraying cycle. The authors found that the effect of the change in relative droplet size on the granule size was different for each fluid bed. They applied an experimental design on the small- and medium-scale unit, and regression models for the granule size were proposed to scale up the granulation process on the small to medium scale. Using only the relative droplet size, authors were able to scale up the process to the larger unit.

10.12 PROCESS TROUBLESHOOTING

In the life cycle of a product, troubleshooting is inevitable. Over the years, a raw material vendor may stop supplying an ingredient, requiring a replacement. A producer may change the manufacturing process, and while the new material may meet the specifications on their certificate of analysis, it may have an unexpected and adverse impact on your product or process. A material for exhaust air filters may be discontinued affecting process air volume performance. Finding a new fabric and identifying a test that will quantify its equivalence is certainly a challenge, and the list goes on. With all of this in mind, when does process troubleshooting start? When does a production batch fail? When do the finished product attributes begin to drift toward the failure limits? When did the process and equipment parameters begin to drift? Or does it start during formulation development? Process troubleshooting should be both proactive and reactive. A product that is formulated well and a process that has a broad operating window and is well characterized will be easier to troubleshoot once the inevitable occurs. The goal during the development process is this: for a well-designed product, the raw materials and process variables and their impact on critical quality attributes (CQA) are generally well understood. Applying statistics, via the design of experiments (DoE), will quantify the impact of the variables and the robustness of a product and its process. Continued use of DoE can confirm these findings during scale-up to pilot and production scale equipment, and this leads to the establishment of operating ranges that were derived experimentally rather than arbitrarily (e.g., applying operational qualification [OQ] limits).

10.12.1 METRICS: GRANULE PROPERTIES AND TABLETING

The variables in fluidized bed processing have an impact on granule properties such as particle size distribution and bulk (and tap) density, two metrics that are valuable tools in product and process understanding as well as in retrospective (or reactive) troubleshooting. These are likely to impact tablet attributes such as hardness, friability, disintegration, and possibly dissolution rate. Unfortunately, in too many instances, particle size distribution (both before and after any milling or sizing step) and bulk and tap densities are not routinely recorded as in-process parameters beyond the process validation activities. They may be taken under protocol up to that point, but to avoid the potential that a specification may eventually be required (possibly leading to granulation batch rejections on an arbitrary basis), these metrics are often eliminated from the batch records for routine production. This is unfortunate. If a production batch exhibits failures such as delamination of tablets or friability, the troubleshooter must work from the tablet press backward. Granulation machine parameters may give insight into the root cause and the properties of the granules themselves will likely help to confirm the findings. The fluid bed spray granulation process should take place slowly and deliberately, building granules to the desired size range by the precise control of CPPs. A subsequent milling step should not substantively alter the particle size distribution of the dried granulation. It should merely shift the small fraction (typically less than 5%) of oversized granules into the size range of the aggregate. It should also not be of an aggressive type of milling that may dramatically affect the performance of the granulation on a tablet press. By nature, fluid bed granules are porous and friable in comparison with those made using a high shear granulator. They do not need the force of a high shear mill to break the oversized agglomerates. A high shear mill may do a considerable amount of damage to the granules, causing an unnecessary number of fines, and this would almost certainly impact the tableting properties. A comparison of the particle size distributions taken before and after the milling step will expose the magnitude of the impact of the mill.

A poorly functioning spray nozzle will typically cause a combination of fines and coarse, dense granules. It does so as a consequence of nonuniformity of droplets – the majority is a fine mist, but there is likely to be a component of very large droplets (exceeding 50 μm) that form granules with nearly liquid centers and the resulting particle size distribution may be bimodal. The consequent dense granules will result in nonuniformity of moisture distribution because there is little interstitial porosity. Internal moisture cannot move to the surface for evaporation. The surfaces may dry and "case hardened" making it all the more likely that the moisture will become entrapped. In some cases, the wet granules will blind the screen during the final milling step, and in others, the mill will grind them finer and mask their existence. In either case, there is a strong possibility that their presence will have an adverse impact on tableting properties. It may seem that taking the moisture content of granules of various sizes would be an effective metric for identifying this problem. However, by the time the batch has been tableted, the moisture will be equilibrated in the remaining granulation and the disparity shadowed. If the problem is seen in a particular granulation batch, moistures should be taken as soon as the batch has finished. In a dried granulation, the high density of these granules may be revealed in the particle size distribution as a rogue peak, and bulk and tap density numbers for the aggregate will likely increase.

10.12.2 Proactive Troubleshooting – Design of Experiments

A comment often heard when discussing the formulation and product development is as follows: "DoE? We don't have the time or the resources to do it." A consequence is that all too often a product that is successful in the clinic is a menace on the manufacturing floor. When used effectively in small-scale batches, DoE is a learning tool – it helps identify and quantify CPPs. The selected-response variables may extend well beyond the CQAs, sometimes teaching one things one didn't expect. At the pilot scale, successful experimentation in a broadened domain establishes the operating limits for the CPPs. A machine's operating limits are too often selected either arbitrarily or simply reflect the OQ ranges identified during the equipment qualification stage of the installation. Unfortunately, these values are generated from the data taken from an empty machine, and this will almost certainly not reflect the behavior during batch processing. Finally, a limited number of early production-scale batches should confirm the results of the pilot-scale DoE.

Figure 10.21 shows the particle size distributions for a series of batches produced on a pilot scale (220 L) top spray fluidized bed granulator for a domain screening study.

There is a significant response within the selected domain for the parameters being evaluated. Isolating the results by process parameters, the responses can be seen individually in Figures 10.22–10.24. In Figure 10.22, it is apparent that inlet air temperature has a significant impact on the average particle size, with the peak shifting from 250 μm (60 mesh) for the high inlet temperature experiment to 420 μm (40 mesh) for the low value. What is notable is that the size distribution is very narrow – in each batch, more than 50% is retained on one screen. It also profoundly impacts the bulk density for the granulation – 0.43 g/cc and 0.52 g/cc, a 20+% difference. This commonly has a considerable influence on tableting properties, particularly on the potential for delamination and tablet friability (commonly seen with low-density granulations).

In Figure 10.23, it is also apparent that the spray rate has an impact, and in this case, the domain value selected as "high" was too high.

Resulting granulation was coarse; though after milling, it was reasonable in particle size distribution. However, it took a considerable amount of time for the sizing step, and the difference before and after milling was notable. As a consequence, the domain was adjusted and the high value for spray rate was lowered. This particular batch teaches a valuable lesson – a goal of DoE is to quantify the impact of process parameters on the selected response variables. To gain the most knowledge about the robustness of a product, it is prudent to operate within a broad domain, but this exposes the process to the potential that a batch may fail, diminishing the power of the DoE to an extent. For this reason, it is suggested that the first batch or two processed for

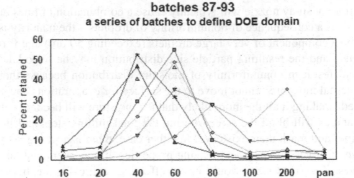

FIGURE 10.21   Particle Size Distribution for a Fluid Bed Spray Granulation DoE.
Source: The Glatt Group.

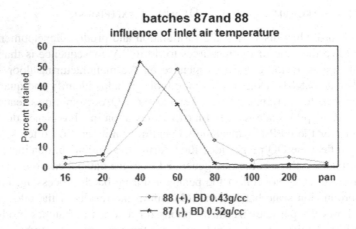

FIGURE 10.22   The Influence of Inlet Air Temperature on Particle Size and Bulk Density (High and Low Values).
Source: The Glatt Group.

the study are intentionally (not randomly) selected as the candidates that have the greatest propensity to fail – the extremes of the DoE. If a batch "fails" during processing, meaning that it cannot be produced successfully or dramatically impacts productivity or efficiency, the domain should be revisited. Complete randomization of a series of experiments may not be the best alternative because if a batch produced in the middle of the study is a disaster, some of the power of the study may be lost, or other batches may need to be added (e.g., edge points in a center composite design). As the figures demonstrate, there is a notable response for particle size distribution and bulk density within the tested domain. Interestingly, all batches tableted successfully – hardness, friability, disintegration, and dissolution all met specifications. The product and process are robust. What is also interesting is that the DoE revealed something unexpected – the response variables need not be limited to product considerations. A fluidized bed spray granulation process starts with raw materials that are small in particle size. The outlet air filter type must be selected with care to assure that the yield and potency of the finished product will be acceptable. Additionally, from a productivity perspective, it is best if multiple batches can be

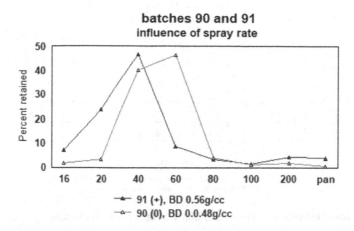

FIGURE 10.23 The Influence of Spray Rate on Particle Size and Bulk Density (Center Point and High Values).
Source: The Glatt Group.

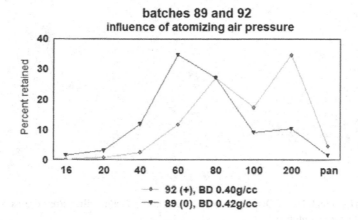

FIGURE 10.24 The Influence of Atomizing Air Pressure on Particle Size and Bulk Density (Center Point and High Values).
Source: The Glatt Group.

produced without the need for outlet air filter cleanings. The need to remove, replace, and clean an outlet filter after every batch is undesirable. Operators and the work area are exposed to the airborne product, and the time for the exchange impedes productivity and increases the chances of damage to the filter because of excess handling and washing. In this series of experiments, it was seen that outlet filter differential pressure was strongly related to the moisture of the product during the spray granulation process. Figure 10.26 shows the filter pressure response for the first few minutes of processing.

Batch "C" (Figure 10.25) shows a filter pressure peaking at 500 mm, and at this pressure, even for a short duration, there is a possibility of catastrophic failure (rupture or separation of the filter from its "D" ring). Partial or complete loss of the batch is a possibility and should be avoided if at all possible. A process air volume "ramp" of about 10 minutes (rising from a lower value initially to the desired high airflow rate for the duration) was employed to eliminate the problem at the front end of the process. However, batches produced with low in-process moistures during spraying resulted in filter pressure building to a high level later as the batch progressed, and this too is

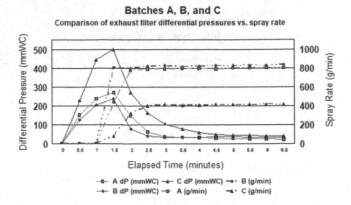

FIGURE 10.25   Filter Differential Pressure and Spray Rate for Various Batches.
Source: The Glatt Group.

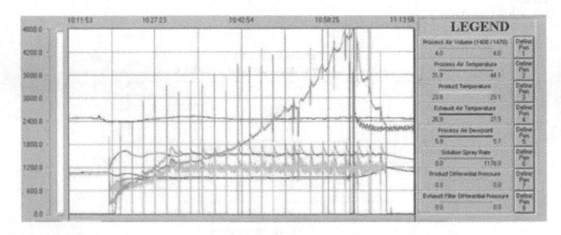

FIGURE 10.26   Historical Trend Display Showing Escalating Outlet Filter Pressure as a Consequence of lOw In-process Moisture Content.
Source: The Glatt Group.

undesirable. High spray rates kept the filter pressure low from beginning to end, and from a production perspective, this is far more attractive. Multiple batches can be produced, improving operating efficiency and keeping operator exposure to the API at a minimum. Tracings for filter differential pressure for dry and wetter batches are illustrated in Figures 10.26–10.27.

For commercialization, the scale-up (tech services) staff can select from a variety of process conditions. However, it is in the company's best interest to select a process that yields higher in-process moisture so that productivity is enhanced. Both the shorter process time and the opportunity to produce many batches between filter washings are strongly positive findings of the DoE study.

10.12.3   REACTIVE TROUBLE SHOOTING: ACQUIRED DATA AS A PROCESS TROUBLESHOOTING TOOL

A significant number of companies continue to record in-process data by hand (via the process operators). The typical recording interval depends on the total process time, but in general, it is once every 10–15 minutes. Although it is an accurate representation of the process when the

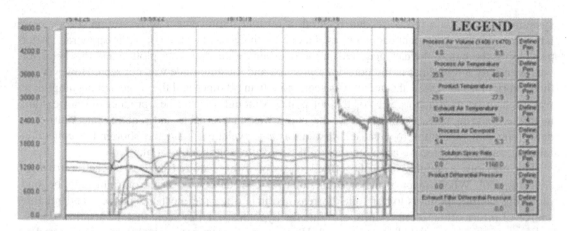

FIGURE 10.27 Historical Trend Display Showing Outlet Filter Pressure at a Low and Constant Value as a Consequence of Higher In-process Moisture Content.
Source: The Glatt Group.

operator recorded the readings, it is of very little use for retrospective troubleshooting. A fluid bed process is very dynamic and the "point in time" numbers do not reflect the intrinsic and rapid oscillation of parameters such as process air volume and product and filter differential pressure. Additionally, erratic variability in the spray rate, which would indicate a spray nozzle defect, would not be reflected at all in the handwritten data. Electronically acquired data is superior from the perspective that it is recorded more frequently. The typical recording interval is 30–60 seconds, and as such, the resolution is improved by a factor of 10× to 30×. It is also not subjective, as is the operator's collected data. The increased resolution affords the possibility that the root cause for the out of spec batch can be identified. Figure 10.28 shows a tracing for spray rate in which the erratic peaks and troughs are an indication of a defective spray nozzle. This type of behavior is a frequent reason for poor particle size distribution. A granulation produced under these conditions may exhibit a bimodal particle size distribution with the coarse fraction containing higher moisture content than the aggregate, as described earlier.

The benefit of historical data is illustrated in Figure 10.28, in which the data recording rate was 60 seconds.

However, some process variables, including spray rate, react much more quickly, and at this interval, much of the actual behavior is lost. By contrast, a historical trend utility in some control

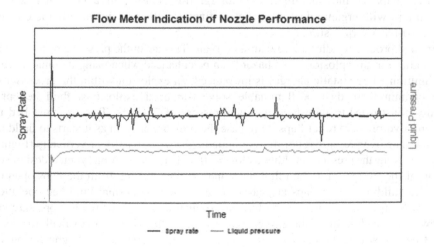

FIGURE 10.28 Tracing Showing Erratic Spray Nozzle Performance.
Source: The Glatt Group.

systems displays data in one-second interval, a 60-fold improvement in resolution. In a recent laboratory trial, a spray pump defect caused a one- to three-second surge or lag in spray rate. After processing the batch, the data acquired in the one-minute interval were plotted and this behavior was seen only a few times in the hour-long process, and the amplitude was not seen. However, on the historical trend screen, the defect was seen more than 30 times and the surge and lag amplitude was seen to be as much as 50% of the set point. Although the finished product did not exhibit negative consequences, the behavior of the pump was unacceptable and requires intervention to determine and repair the root cause. Resolution is "revelation," and the shorter the collection interval, the more effective acquired data will be as a troubleshooting tool.

The previous examples show the effectiveness of using acquired data as a reactive trouble-shooting tool. When minor or major excursions for CPP occur or a batch outright fails, beyond inquiring of the operators to sort out the reasons, it is often the most independent and reliable source of information. It can confirm or refute the hypothesis. It may seem that the acquired data is only as effective as a troubleshooting tool. However, it is extremely valuable for process under-standing and anticipating a problem before it becomes sufficiently serious that a batch or series of batches is lost. As such, the examination of the data for ALL batches is highly recommended.

10.12.4 Process Trouble Shooting Summary

Table 10.6 addresses "frequently asked questions" concerning process troubleshooting. For several issues, common root causes are listed. There are approaches to problem-solving proposed as well. In general, the fluidized bed spray granulation process yields CQA via a selection of process variables that methodically and intentionally produce the granulation. Some form of trouble-shooting is inevitable at some point during the life cycle of the product. However, a well-designed formulation and process, as well as granule metrics and instrumentation, should permit a sa-tisfactory resolution to the problems commonly encountered.

10.13 SAFETY IN FLUID BED

For an explosion to occur, three conditions must exist: an ignition source, a fuel, and oxygen. With an explosion, oxygen reacts with the fuel releasing heat and gases. If a dust explosion occurs in free space, a fireball of a considerable extent arises. If the dust explosion occurs in a closed container, then there is a sudden pressure rise that is mainly decided by the following factors: type of dust, size of the dust, dust/oxygen ratio, turbulence, precompression, tem-perature, the shape of the container, and an ignition source. In a container without pre-compression and with organic dust of sufficient fineness, the pressure inside the container can rise to over 10-bar overpressure.

The fluid bed process handles a large amount of air. This air in the presence of fine product dust poses a potential for an explosion. This hazard can be enhanced when using flammable solvents. If sufficient ignition energy (static charge) is introduced, an explosion within the processor can take place. To contain these dust or flammable solvent-induced explosions, fluid bed processors are normally constructed to withstand the overpressure of 2.0 bars. Two-bar fluid bed units are provided with overpressure relief flaps, to release the pressure as soon as it starts to build up inside the processor. The overpressure relief flaps mounted either horizontally or vertically (Figure 10.29) are designed to vent the pressure buildup as low as 0.06 bar. The two-bar vented design shows the propagation of the overpressure the relief flaps and the duct leading from the flaps open up to the outside of the building. These flaps are gasketed and sealed so normal fluid bed operation is not affected. It was an accepted practice to have a production unit with two-bar pressure shock in-tegrity; however, the cleaning of the gasket area around the flaps is always difficult to avoid having the product be exposed to the outside during as a result of overpressure, a suppression system is used to contain the possible overpressure front from leaving the unit. The suppression system

TABLE 10.6
Summary of Troubleshooting Process Challenges

Issue	The Most Likely Root Cause
1. Poor particle size distribution (coarse, wet granules mingled with acceptable granules and fines)	Spray nozzle performance
Proposed action	Before the processing of any batch, conduct a functional test of the spray nozzle to assure that it is performing correctly. Poor particle size control and nonuniform distribution of moisture is most commonly the fault of a defective spray nozzle. An effective spray nozzle cleaning/maintenance and testing program is essential. A functional check of the spray nozzle at the anticipated spray rate and atomizing air pressure/volume must be conducted after a major cleaning. Replacement of the nozzle head (port and air cap assembly) between batches is generally sufficient as a minor clean to assure proper performance. The reason for this is that the O-rings and sealing from which the defects originate are in the nozzle body itself. If this component is not disturbed between batches, it is highly unlikely that the nozzle will malfunction during a subsequent batch.
2. Lumps/large aggregates	Coalescence of granules – transition into ball growth
Proposed action	Transition into ball growth is typically seen in the latter stages of the spraying process. Ball growth is indicated by the presence of a considerable number of very large lumps comprising granules, not starting material. The resolution of the problem depends on discerning its onset. The progression of particle size growth is a powder to nuclei to uniform agglomerates. As granule size grows, there is less overall surface area to accumulate the spray liquid. The velocity and pattern density also decreases and there is a tendency for the material in proximity to the spray nozzle to be overwetted. The excess surface moisture results in the coalescence of granules and eventually ball growth. While this is not a common occurrence, it is undesirable and should be mitigated. This can be done either by an increase in fluidization air volume or a slight decrease in spray rate at the time the ball growth would usually begin. Because the resulting "balls" comprise porous agglomerates, they may dry reasonably well. However, their size typically leads to a slower moisture loss and consolidation at the base of the product container. As a consequence, they are not seen in the sample port and final moisture cannot include their contents. After milling, it is not uncommon for the final moisture content to be higher than that taken at the end of the drying process.
3. Nonuniform distribution of potent insoluble API	Particle size incompatibility – API and excipients
Proposed action	The root cause of the nonuniformity must be identified. A particle size distribution should be conducted, and the assay can be performed on the various fractions (generally up to 6 sieve sizes). Often the cause is a particle size incompatibility between the API and the granulation excipients, and this will be seen as super potency in one or more of the sieve fractions. The purpose of a binder is to immobilize the API in a matrix with the other materials. A relatively rigid granule structure at the end of drying and after milling is essential. Examination of the Certificate of Analysis for the API should reveal the particle size distribution, but

(Continued)

TABLE 10.6 (Continued)

Issue	The Most Likely Root Cause
	it says nothing of its shape. Needle-like materials are problematic in that a particle size distribution (using sieve analysis) is a 2D test for a 3D material. Scanning electron microscopy (SEM) will reveal particle shape and subjectively the size distribution. If the material is found to be the root cause, either an additional step to bring it into compatibility with the excipients will be needed (e.g., milling) or the specification to the vendor must be narrowed. If the API particle size is very small but the material is cohesive, small soft lumps of API likely remain in the finished granulation. In comparison to high-shear granulation, there is far less mechanical stress in the fluidized-bed process. If the API is added as a dry material to other excipients in the product container, it is suggested that it be co-milled with one of the excipients before its addition to the remaining materials. The shear of the pre-milling process would be sufficient for de-lumping and would give the mixing process a head start.
	It is common practice at the end of a spray granulation process to shake filter fines into the product container. If this layer is substantial and contains principally very fine material, it should be assayed for potency. If the material is found to be superpotent, the mechanicals for the filter system must be checked. In alternating shaking types of processors, often a gas-tight flap has lost its ability to seal completely and it must be repaired. A consequence is that there is still air flowing past it during shaking, therefore fines cannot be released from the stiffened filter fabric. This may be externally manifested by a comparatively high filter differential pressure from start to finish in the process. In cartridge filter systems, the effect is similar material adhering to the filter material cannot be released by the compressed air pulse while fluidization air continues through the cartridge. The release is only possible at the end of the batch when fluidization ceases. If this is an issue during process development and scale-up, irrespective of the type of filter shaking, it may be possible to mitigate by trying different types of filter materials. In any case, the problem should be addressed and solved before it is released to routine production.
4. Low potency of potent API	The poor initial distribution of API, demixing of API, preferential retention of API on machine surfaces (expansion chamber, outlet air filter)
Proposed action	Any residue in the machine tower should be assayed for potency and checked for particle size and distribution to ascertain if it is of primary size or wetted agglomerates. If the material is fine and dry, it may have demixed due to the electrostatic charge. This can potentially occur during vacuum charging, or during a product warm-up step before spraying if the temperature is high or the step exceeds 1–2 min. In both cases, the fluidization air is dry, and the environment is fertile for an electrostatic charge. If there is considerable residue and it is superpotent, the process can be adjusted such that fluidization forces the granular product into the upper reaches of the expansion chamber and the outlet air filter to "sand" the residue from these surfaces (during the middle and later stages of spraying). If the filter material that has been used to produce the product is no longer available, a replacement must be found. It should be noted that there is no standardized test for determining either porosity (the size of particle that can be retained) or permeability (quantity of airflow per unit time at a given pressure difference across the fabric). Essentially, one must rely on performance with the product for which it is intended to be used. A production batch (one or more)

TABLE 10.6 (Continued)

Issue	The Most Likely Root Cause
	must be earmarked as "experimental" and processed using the current recipe. If the filter differential pressure is lower, there is some risk that the yield will also be less. There is also the potential for the API to be lost if it is small in particle size. If this is the case, yet another type of fabric should be tested—the fabric should not dictate process conditions but must be selected to serve the product and process.
5. Poor process air temperature control at low process air volume settings	Operation of the machine at too close to the qualified lower limit for temperature and airflow
Proposed action	This is an unfortunate characteristic when the process starts at low air volume and temperature. The airflow sensor accuracy is diminished at low air flows, and the ability of an air handler to control a low temperature at low airflow is an extreme challenge and should be avoided if possible. A higher air volume is recommended even if it results in material being captured in the outlet air filter. If the filter system functions correctly, these fines will be returned regularly to be exposed to the spray liquid, ultimately becoming agglomerates. Evidence of this is a steady decay in filter differential pressure during spraying.
6. Bed stalling (*in regions of the product container*)	High in-process and end-spray moisture content.
Proposed action	Experimentation to determine the operating domain (design space) should identify an in-process moisture profile that reaches a failure limit. If this is done and in-process testing includes sampling for moisture, bed stalling would then be seen as a consequence of a breach of this moisture "threshold." A common cause for a sudden shift from success to failure in routine production is the calibration of the process air volume sensor. Many fluidized-bed spray granulations, particularly those with insoluble raw materials, have spraying conditions in which the air leaving the machine tower is saturated with moisture. The liquid spray rate slightly exceeds the drying capacity of the process air; therefore, the bed builds in moisture. Routine (quarterly or semiannual) machine calibration always includes the process air volume sensor, and of all of the instruments on a fluid bed processor, this is the most difficult to calibrate. Some companies conduct point checks in which the instrument and its transmitter are calibrated while disconnected. Others employ a loop check in which the testing instruments are installed in tandem with the sensor connected in the loop or a second instrument is used in the ductwork to independently confirm the accuracy of the machine-indicated value. In either case, if a change is made to the sensor, the user of the processor will not likely see the impact in any of the readings. For example, assume that calibration found the air volume sensor to be indicating a reading that is 5% higher than the actual. When it is corrected, the first batch-processed may be found to have in-process and end-spray moisture contents that are higher than usually seen. All of the operator interface terminal (OIT) indicated process parameters are the same as usual, but the batch outcome is different. The problem rests with the air volume sensor (its changed transmitter). If the process operates at saturation, the inlet and product temperature will not change – it represents the condition for each cubic meter or cubic foot of air entering and leaving the batch (at saturation). A sensor found to be off by 5% will mean that less water is being evaporated per unit time, therefore the bed is gaining moisture more quickly. If

(Continued)

TABLE 10.6 (Continued)

Issue	The Most Likely Root Cause
	moisture gain is sufficiently rapid, the ball growth or bed stalling threshold may be reached, and the batch will be at risk. It is strongly suggested that all calibration data, especially involving changes to any instrument be discussed with the equipment users so that the impact of these types of issues can be anticipated and are no "surprises."

Abbreviation·. API, active pharmaceutical ingredient.

consists of low-pressure sensors located within the processor. These sensors are designed to trigger a series of fire extinguishers (containing ammonium phosphate), as soon as a preset level (generally 0.1 bar) of pressure is set within the processor (Figure 10.30).

To contain any overpressure 10 or 12 bar units are available. They have a quick-acting valve, so when and if overpressure occurs in the unit, the quick-acting valve located in the inlet, as well as exhaust ducts, acts, and the pressure front is contained within the unit because the units are designed to withstand overpressure of up to 12 bar. Figure 10.31 shows the quick-acting valves and Figure 10.32 shows a 12-bar non-vented dome above the filter housing and a 2-bar vented area above the filter housing showing explosion relief panel.

With the introduction of potent and costly drug substances, the 2-bar design is being replaced with 10- or 12-bar designs Figure 10.31 shows the Ventex-ESI and quick-acting valves for passive control of the overpressure front. Figure 10.32 shows the 2- bar as well as a 12-bar unit. Most of the pharmaceutical dust explosions studied [172] show the overpressure reaching 9 bars with a K_{st} value (constant of explosion speed) of 200. An overpressure in a 10- or 12-bar unit is contained within the unit. A 10- to a 12-bar designed unit does not require any explosion relief panels or gaskets. This eliminates the concerns about the cleaning of the gaskets and flaps. Another advantage of a 10- to 12-bar unit is that, in case of explosion, the processor containing potent drug substance is contained inside the unit and the explosion does not pose an environmental problem as with the 2.0-bar unit. Figure 10.33 shows the overpressure valve in action.

The deflagration valve such as Ventex-ESI requires less maintenance than the active valve previously used in the industry. An explosion force (pressure wave) moving ahead of the flame front hurls the poppet forward to the valve seat providing an airtight seal. The poppet once seated is locked in by a mechanical shutoff device, which retains the seal until manually reset. The three basic

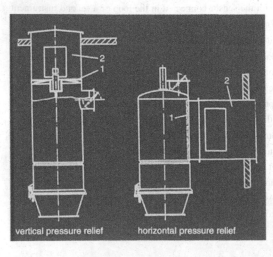

vertical pressure relief   horizontal pressure relief

FIGURE 10.29 A Two-Bar Unit Overpressure Relief Panels Showing Vertical Relief and a Side Relief.

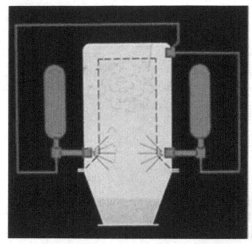

FIGURE 10.30 Overpressure Suppression System.

(a)

(b)

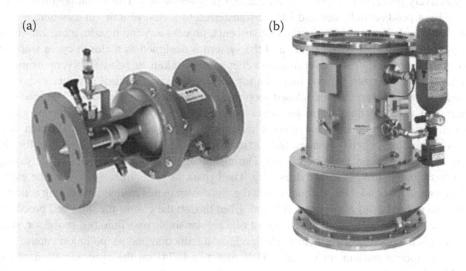

FIGURE 10.31 (a) Ventex SEI Valve (Deflagration Valve) and (b) Quick Action Stop Valve. *Source:* The Glatt group.

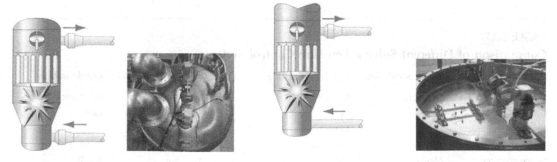

FIGURE 10.32 12-Bar Non-Vented Dome Above the Filter Housing and a 2-Bar Vented Area Above the Filter Housing Showing Explosion Relief Panels. *Source*: The Glatt Group.

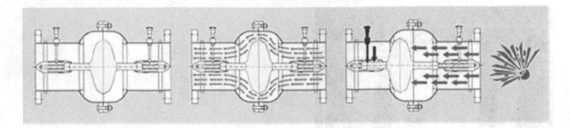

FIGURE 10.33 Explosion Protection Valve in Action.
Source: The Glatt Group.

versions of the standard mechanical Ventex valve are available with a set pressure of 1.5 psi and a maximum pressure of 150 psi. The Ventex-ESI valve closes by the explosion pressure wave, without external power for horizontal or vertical operation. Figure 10.33 shows how the Ventex valve closes. The pressure wave of an explosion pushes the closing device against a seal. When closed, the valve is locked and effectively prevents the spread of flames and pressure waves. The actual position of the valve is shown by a position indicator and can be transferred to a control unit via a switch.

In the case of granulation requiring flammable solvents, process air, and nozzle, atomization air is replaced by an inert gas such as nitrogen, and the system is designed as a closed cycle with the solvent recovery capability [173]. Several approaches can be taken to handle solvent from the process. Table 10.7 summarizes various methods for solvent emission control systems.

Kulling and Simon [18] reported the closed-loop system shown in Figure 10.34. The inert gas (generally nitrogen) used for fluidization circulates continuously. An adjustable volume of gas is diverted through the bypassed duct where solvent vapors are condensed, and solvent collected. The circulating gas passes through the heat exchanger to maintain the temperature necessary for the evaporation of the solvent from the product bed. During the agglomeration and subsequent drying process, the solvent load in the gas stream does vary. The bypass valve controls the flow of the gas to the heat exchanger and the condenser. By controlling the gas stream in this manner, the drying action is continued until the desired level of drying is reached. Even though the cost of the fluid bed processor with the solvent recovery is generally double the cost of a regular single pass fluid bed processor, such a system offers effective measures for both explosion hazard reduction and air pollution control.

In 1994, the European parliament issued ATEX directive [174] on the approximation of the laws of the Member States concerning equipment and protective systems intended for use in potentially explosive atmospheres. As of July 2006, organizations in the EU must follow the directives to protect employees from explosion risk in areas with explosive atmospheres. There are

TABLE 10.7

Comparison of Different Solvent Emission Control Systems

Considerations	Water Scrubbing	Catalytic Burning	Carbon Absorption	Condensation
System	Open cycle	Open cycle	Open cycle	Open cycle with N_2
Capital cost	High	Low	Moderate	Low
Energy requirement	High	Low		
Installation	External	External	External	Internal
Space required	Medium	High	Moderate	Small
Flexibility	Medium	Medium	Low	Good
Waste treatment	Required	CO_2/H_2O emission treatment	Required	Concentrated

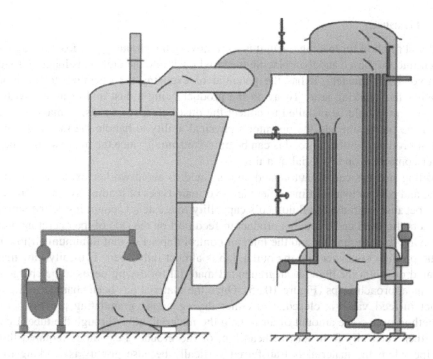

FIGURE 10.34 Schematic of a Closed-Loop Fluid Bed Processor with Solvent Recovery.

two ATEX directives (one for the manufacturer and one for the user of the equipment): The directive was updated in 2014.

The ATEX Directive 2014/34/EU covers equipment and protective systems intended for use in potentially explosive atmospheres. The directive defines the essential health and safety requirements and conformity assessment procedures, to be applied before products are placed on the EU market. It is aligned with the new legislative framework policy, and it is applicable from April 20, 2016, replacing the previous Directive 94/9/EC [175].

ATEX gets its name from the French title of the 2014/34/EU directive: Appareils destinés à être utilisés en ATmosphères EXplosibles.

Employers must classify areas where hazardous explosive atmospheres may occur into zones. The classification is given to a particular zone, and its size and location depend on the likelihood of an explosive atmosphere occurring and its persistence if it does. Areas classified into zones (0, 1, 2 for gas-vapor-mist and 20, 21, 22 for dust) must be protected from effective sources of ignition. Equipment and protective systems intended to be used in zoned areas must meet the requirements of the directive. Zones 0 and 20 require category 1 marked equipment; zones 1 and 21 required category 2 marked equipment; and zones 2 and 22 required category 3 marked equipment. Zones 0 and 20 are the zones with the highest risk of an explosive atmosphere being present. All manufacturers of fluid bed processors in Europe must comply with this directive.

Similar requirements for safety guidelines are implemented by the Occupational Safety and Health Administration (OSHA) in the United States.

10.14 MATERIAL HANDLING OPTIONS

The transfer of materials to and from the fluid bed processor is an important consideration. The loading and unloading of the processing bowl can be accomplished by manual mode or by automated methods.

10.14.1 LOADING

The traditional method for loading the unit is by removing the product bowl from the unit, charging the material into the bowl, and then placing the bowl back into the unit. This loading is simple and cost-effective. Unfortunately, it has the potential of exposing the operators to the product and contaminating the working area. To avoid the product being a dust and cleaning hazard, a dust collection system should be installed to collect the dust before it spreads. A manual process also depends on the batch size and the operator's physical ability to handle the material and the container full of product. Furthermore, this can be time-consuming since the material must be added to the product container, one material at a time.

The loading process can be automated and isolated to avoid worker exposure, minimize dust generation, and reduce loading time. There are two main types of loading systems. These systems are similar because both use the fluid bed's capability to create a vacuum inside the unit. Here the product enters the fluid bed through a product in-feed port on the side of the operating unit. This is done by having the fan running and the inlet air control flap set so that minimum airflow may pass through the product container and the outlet flap is almost fully open. Typically, raw materials to be granulated or when the high shear granulated material for drying needs to be charged into the fluid bed this approach helps (Figure 10.35). Once the material has been charged to the fluid bed, the product in-feed valve is closed, and either drying or the granulating process started. This transfer method uses some amount of air to help the material move through the tube. Loading can be done either vertically from an overhead bin, or the ground. Less air is required through the transfer pipe when the material is transferred vertically because gravity is working to help the process. Vertical transfer methods do require greater available height in the process area. Loading by this method has the advantages of limited operator exposure to the product and allows the product to be fluidized as it enters the processor. This method also reduces the loading time. The disadvantage of this type of system is the cleaning required between different products since a number of transfer sources have to be cleaned.

10.14.2 UNLOADING

As with loading, the standard method for unloading is by removing the product bowl from the unit. Once the bowl is removed, the operator may scoop the material from the bowl, which is the most time consuming and impractical method, because of its potential for exposure to the product. Alternatively, the product can be vacuum-transferred to a secondary container or unloaded by placing the product bowl into a bowl dumping device as shown in Figure 10.36a, b.

This hydraulic device is installed in the processing area. The mobile product container of the fluid bed processor is pushed under the cone of the bowl dumper and coupled together by engaging the toggle locks. Subsequently, the container is lifted hydraulically, pivoted around the lifting column, and rotated 180° for discharging. The use of the bowl dumping device or vacuum unloading device still requires that the product bowl be removed from the unit. There are contained and automated methods for unloading the product while the product bowl is still in the fluid bed processor. The product may either be unloaded out of the bottom of the product container or from the side. Until recently, the most common contained method is to unload the material from the bottom of the unit. This requires the ceiling height high enough to accommodate or the installation becomes a multistoried installation.

There are two types of bottom discharge options: gravity or pneumatic gravity discharge (Figure 10.37) allows for the collection of the product into the container, which is located below the lower plenum. If the overall ceiling height limitation prevents from having the discharge by gravity, the gravity/pneumatic transfer combination can be considered. The gravity discharge poses

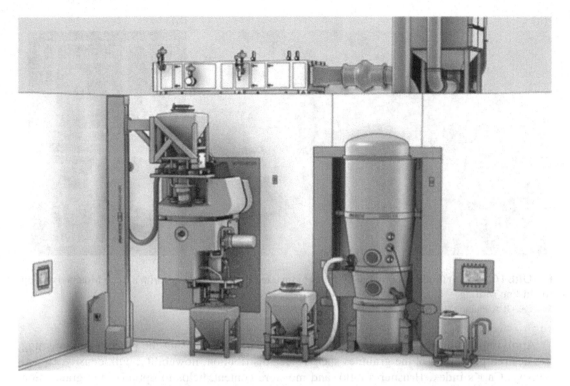

FIGURE 10.35 Ingredients from Integrated Bulk Container (IBC) Being Transferred to Fluid Bed.
Source: Courtesy IMA S.p.A, Italy.

cleaning problems since the process air and the product discharge follow the same path; assurance of cleanliness is always of prime concern.

The desire to limit the processing area and development of the overlap gill air distributor mentioned earlier in the chapter has prompted the consideration of the side discharge as an option. The product bowl is fitted with the discharge gate, as shown in Figure 10.38a, b.

Most of the product being free-flowing granules flows through the side discharge into a container. The remainder of the product is then discharged by manipulation of the airflow through the overlap gill air distributor. The discharged product can be pneumatically transported to an overhead bin if the dry milling of the granulation is desired. The contained system for unloading the product helps to isolate the operator from the product. The isolation feature also prevents the product from being contaminated from being exposed to the working environment. Material handling consideration must be thought of, early in the equipment procurement process. Fluid bed processing, whether used as an integral part of high-shear mixer/fluid bed dryer or as a granulating equipment option, production efficiency, and eventual automation, can be enhanced by considering these loading and unloading options.

10.15 OPTIMIZATION OF FLUID BED GRANULATION PROCESS

Fluid bed granulation is a multivariable process. Numerous parameters affect process optimization. The designed space approach to optimize the granulation process is used for some time in the industry. To establish a design space, a range of process parameter settings that have been demonstrated to provide the predetermined and defined end-product quality must be established. It is a multidimensional combination and interaction of input variables and process parameters, which can be varied within the design space but still provide assurance of quality [176].

(a)   (b)

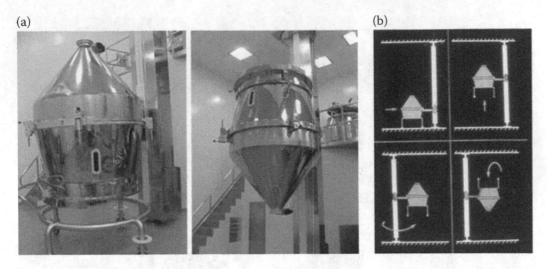

FIGURE 10.36   (a) Product Discharge System. (b) Inverted Product Container with a Cone Mounted on Top for In-line Milling.
Source: GEA Pharma System.

Applying and understanding the critical process parameters during the process and targeting the desired properties of the granules such as size distribution, flowability, bulk density, tapped density, Carr's index, Hausner's ratio, and moisture content, helps to optimize the granulation process. Type of diluent, binder concentration, the temperature during mixing, granulation, and drying, spray rate, and atomization pressure are some of the critical formulation and process parameters. Design space for process parameters such as atomization pressure and compression force and its influence on tablet characteristics can be evaluated [177]. A quality by design (QbD) strategy to optimize the fluid bed granulation was successfully implemented with process analytical tools by Lourenco et al. [178]. Variability of the excipients from batch to batch poses challenges to optimize the granulation process. Gavan et al. [179] demonstrated that the fluid bed granulation can be adapted through accurate control of critical process parameters (CPPs) to eliminate the variability brought by possible API or excipient changes. Therefore, assuring consistent end-product quality and maintaining its characteristics within the Quality Target Product Profile (QTPP) is possible with constant monitoring of the manufacturing process. The micro NIR spectrometer was successfully used as a robust PAT monitoring tool that offered a real-time overview of the moisture level and allowed the supervision and control of the granulation process. Merkuu et al. [180] examined the effect of process conditions, such as the inlet air temperature, atomizing air pressure, and the amount of binder solution in the fluidized bed granulation process. Huolong Liu et al. optimized the online granulation process by developing a multi-scale Three Stage Population Model (TSPBM) to describe the granule size distribution evolution of each stage of the top-spray fluidized bed granulation process. Based on the developed model, an online optimization strategy is proposed to improve the granule size distribution prediction of top-spray fluidized bed granulation, which utilized an improved differential evolution (DE) algorithm to solve the optimization problem [172]. Otsuka et al. investigated the most important variables in the process of manufacturing granules by applying the principal component analysis (PCA) method [181].

The authors performed PCA for Acetaminophen granulation against 13 physicochemical properties. As a result, the pressure transmission ratio, die wall force, and Carr's flowability index was found to be crucial variables for manufacturing tablets. The results were verified by multiple regression analysis and the optimized operational conditions produced the desired granules.

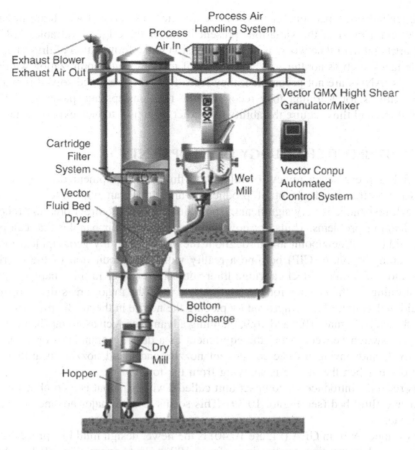

FIGURE 10.37 Loading and Unloading Setup with Bottom Discharge in an Integrated System.
Source: Courtesy of the Freund Vector Corporation.

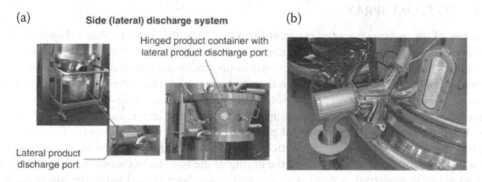

FIGURE 10.38 (a) Side Discharge Glatt. (b) Side Discharge.
Source: The Glatt Group (a); GEA Pharma Systems (b).

The procedure of principal component analysis (PCA) was published by Karl Pearson in 1901. PCA aims at reducing plenty of observed variables to a small number of latent variables. The latent variables are called factors or principal components. Principle component analysis is a method of reducing the dimensionality of a data set that contains a large number of interrelated variables while retaining the variation present in the data set. This is achieved by transforming to a new set of variables, called principal components, which are uncorrelated, and which are ordered so that the first few retain most of the variations present in all of the original variables [182]. The application of artificial neural networks is a new dimension in the formulation of drugs because of the unique advantages such as nonlinearity, the ability of modeling and optimization with a small set of experiments. ANNs are not programed, they learn from the presented solved problems. Using different algorithms for learning, they recognize the relationships and patterns within the data presented to them and thus acquire the ability to predict responses to new experimental conditions.

10.16   FLUID BED TECHNOLOGY DEVELOPMENTS

Parikh [183] has presented a review of all of the fluid bed equipment developments. Among various advances, the development of production units that can withstand more than 12-bar pressure shock resistance is very significant. These units do not require a pressure relief duct and associated cleaning problems. Units are now equipped with the air handler that can provide designated humidity and dew point air, throughout the year and at any geographical location. The fluid bed cleaning in place (CIP) became a reality with the introduction of the overlap gill air distributors and the stainless-steel cartridge filters described earlier in this chapter.

The positioning of the nozzles for granulation is one of the major areas that most of the suppliers of fluid bed systems have improved by placing the nozzle in the air distributors or tangential position as shown in Figures 10.8 and 10.9, claiming advantages such as no mechanical adjustment is necessary to switch between using the equipment as a dryer, a granulator or a coater, ease of nozzle removal, and having a three-component nozzle, and avoid nozzle "bearding" problems, which may occur when the nozzle is spraying from the top.

Glatt has recently introduced a compact unit called Twin Pro® that is a combination of a high-shear mixer and fluid bed (see Figure 10.39). This seems to be a major advance in an integrated system approach.

The Air Connect™ from GEA (Figure 10.40) is the newer design fluid bed processor for small-scale research and production applications (from 100 g up to more than 10 kg). Suitable for granulation, drying, and coating.

10.17   BOTTOM SPRAY

The coating of the particles is carried out most frequently using the Wurster column (Figure 10.41a, b). The Wurster process is the most popular method for coating particles. The Wurster-based coating process does not contain any fluid bed regions in the traditional sense, as it is a circulating fluid bed process. Four different regions within the equipment can be identified: the up-bed region, the expansion chamber, the down bed region, and the horizontal transport region. The coating process consists of three phases: the start-up phase, the coating phase, and the drying and cooling phase. During the coating phase, several processes take place simultaneously. They are as follows: the atomization of the coating solution or suspension, transport of the atomized droplets of the coating solution to the substrate, and the drying of the film. Even though particle coating with a bottom spray is preferred, a number of products have been coated using the top spray in the fluid bed. Recently, Ehlers and coworkers [184] coated ibuprofen powder particles with HPMC using a top spray without agglomerating powders.

Bottom spray coating (Figure 10.41a) is also used for agglomeration as well as particle coating as it was developed originally. As seen earlier in this chapter, by placing the nozzles tangentially, most of the manufacturers have improved the operational difficulties encountered when nozzle plugging required that the process be stopped to pull the nozzle during the coating process. By placement of nozzles tangentially, some manufacturers claim that separate modules to carry out agglomeration, coating, and drying will not be needed. Of the modification of the basic Wurster Technique, a column within column (HS collar) was introduced by Glatt to minimize

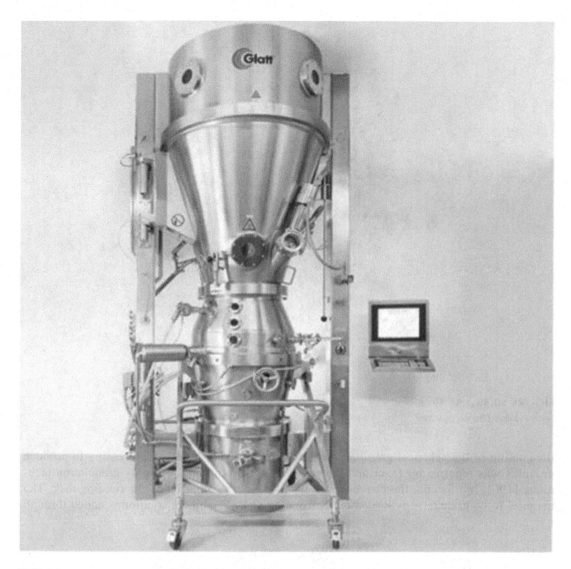

FIGURE 10.39 Twin Pro®- Combination of High Shear and a Fluid Bed All in One.
Source: The Glatt Group.

agglomeration during coating and enabling a higher spraying rate. Further modification of the Wurster was introduced by GEA Pharma systems as a coating as well as bottom spray granulating technique with an introduction of Precision Coater® as shown in Figure 10.41b.

Researchers have discussed the incorporation of microwaves in the laboratory fluid bed processor [185,186]. Fluid bed process using organic solvent requires inert gas such as nitrogen to replace the air used for fluidization as discussed earlier in the chapter. It is accompanied by the solvent recovery system.

10.18 ROTARY INSERTS

The other advance of significance is the development of a rotary fluid bed, for producing denser granulation. Modules were introduced by various manufacturers and the technology is discussed below. The 1972 patent [187] for the rotor technology was awarded for the equipment and coating of the granular material. The subsequent patents [188,189] were awarded for

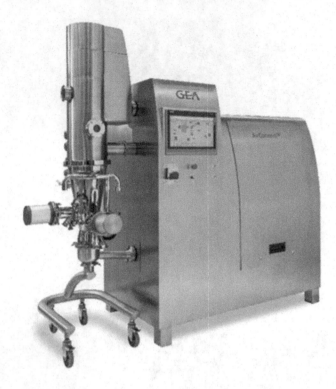

FIGURE 10.40   Air Connect.
Source: GEA Pharma Systems.

the coating of the spherical granules. An advantage of rotary fluid bed processing to produce granules was reported by Jager and Bauer over the conventional top spray granulation technique [190]. In this unit, the conventional air distributor is replaced by the rotating disk. The material to be granulated is loaded on the rotating disk. The binder solution is added through

(a)   (b)

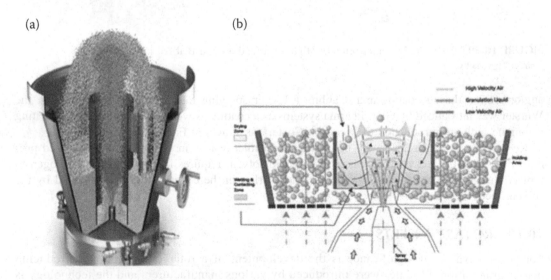

FIGURE 10.41   (a) Typical Wurster Coater. (b) Precision Coater®.
Source: IMA S.p.A. (a); GEA Pharma Systems (b).

the atomization nozzle located tangentially to the wall of the bowl. The centrifugal force creates a dense, helical doughnut-shaped pattern. This type of motion is caused by the three directional forces.

The vertical movement is caused by the gap or slit air around the rotating disk, the gravitational force folds back the material to the center, and the centrifugal force caused by the rotating disk pushes the material away from the center. The granulation produced in the rotary fluid bed processor shows less porosity compared with the conventionally agglomerated product in the fluid bed processor. (Figure 10.42a, b)

Türkoglu et al. produced theophylline granulation using a rotary fluid bed [191]. The formulation contained lactose, starch, and MCC along with theophylline. They reported that the granules produced were spherical and dense. Three different drug level formulations were evaluated. The authors concluded that a rotary fluid bed as a wet granulator has the potential to obtain a better drug content uniformity for tablets even at low API levels such as 1% in comparison with conventional fluidized beds. The use of the rotary fluid bed to produce spherical granules for a modified release application

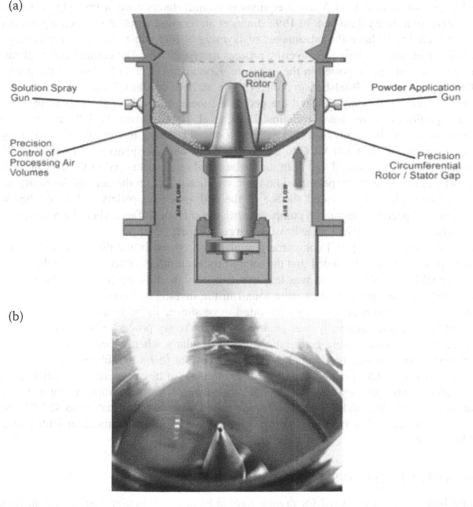

FIGURE 10.42 Rotary Fluid Bed Processing Modules. (a) GXR Rotor (Source: Freund-Vector Corp) (b) Rotor Module. (Source: The Glatt Group).

is reported by several authors. Rotary fluid bed technology was reviewed by Li et al. [192] and its usefulness was described to produce the pellets. The comparison of the rotary fluid bed processing with the multiple-step extrusion and spheronization was reported by Robinson et al. [193]. The authors manufactured acceptable immediate-release acetaminophen pellets using both of these techniques. The quality of the pellet produced improved as the minimum quantity of product was increased in the rotary fluid bed processor. The advantage of using a single unit such as a rotary fluid bed over multiple unit processes involving several pieces of equipment is as described.

The rotary fluid bed is used for producing a pellet by layering the active drug suspension or solution onto nonpareil cores and subsequently coating them with polymers to impart modified release properties [194]. Hileman et al. [195] reported the production of immediate spheres of a poorly water-soluble drug in a rotary fluid bed by layering the active drug suspension onto non-pareil cores. These immediate release spheres were then overcoated with an ethylcellulose/HPMC hydroalcoholic solution in the same unit eliminating the need for additional process and handling steps. Iyer et al. evaluated the layering of the aqueous solution of phenylpropanolamine hydro-chloride with different binders [196]. The layered beads were coated in the rotoprocessor and the Wurster Coater to compare the utility of rotoprocessor as a piece of equipment not only to produce pellets but to coat them as well. Various equipment manufacturers have promoted powder layering on the pellets, in a rotary fluid bed. In 1992, Jones et al. received a patent for such a process [197]. The process claims to have the advantages of layering a drug substance with a relatively small amount of liquid, thus making this layering process more efficient. The commercial application of this process has not been reported in the literature. Korakianiti et al. [198] studied the preparation of pellets using a rotary fluid bed granulator. The authors concluded that the rotor speed and amount of water significantly affected the geometric mean diameter of the pellets and they pro-posed an equation to show that correlation. Pišek et al. [199] studied the influence of rotational speed and surface of the rotating disk on pellets produced by using the rotary fluid bed. They used a mixture of pentoxifylline and MCC to produce pellets using a suspension of Eudragit® NE 30 D as a binder. The results showed that both the surface and rotational speed of the disk influence the shape, surface, and size of the pellets while there was less effect on the density, humidity content, and yield. They found the textured surface of the disk produced pellets with a rougher surface when rotational speed was increased compared with the smooth surface, where increased rotational speed produced more spherical pellets with a larger diameter.

Kristensen and Hansen [200] compared granulation prepared in the fluid bed with a top spray and rotary processor and concluded that the rotary processor offers better maneuverability in terms of the obtainable granule size and was less influenced by the flow properties of the starting ma-terials. Similar tablet characteristics were found in the investigated types of equipment. The ap-plicable range of liquid addition rates was found to be similar in the rotary processor and the top spray fluid bed module. Generally, wet granulation in the rotary processor was found to be a good alternative to conventional fluid bed granulation, particularly when cohesive powders with poor flow properties or formulations with low drug content are to be granulated by a fluidizing air technique. Kristensen [201] in another study of granulation of binary mixtures of MCC and either lactose, calcium phosphate, acetaminophen, or theophylline, in a 1:3 ratio, using a 50% (w/w) aqueous solution of PEG and water as the binder liquid, demonstrated that up to 42.5% w/w PEG can be incorporated and maybe an alternative process to the melt granulation with hydrophilic meltable binders.

10.19 INTEGRATED SYSTEMS

The fluid bed technology is used for drying, agglomerating, coating, and pelletization. However, the industry is using the fluid bed processor for drying, when there is a requirement for higher bulk density granulation, or a low concentration of hydrophobic drug formulation is required to be incorporated in a large quantity of excipients, companies prefer granulating the product in a high shear mixer and drying it in the fluid bed dryer. To facilitate these two separate operations, an integrated system is set up in several companies where the transfer of wet mass from high shear is passed through a mill before loading in the fluid bed. This approach is preferred because of several advantages such as minimizing material handling, less operator exposure to the product dust, space savings, and so on. It is normally economically beneficial if such a system is dedicated to a single product.

Figures 10.43 and 10.44 show a typical integrated system where containment is considered for controlling dust and cross-contamination. When these two-unit operations are integrated as a single unit, several points must be considered. Following is the list of some of the questions readers may want to consider:

1. Engineering layout and the footprint, ceiling height requirements.
2. How will the high shear mixer be loaded with powders by gravity, vacuum, or manually?
3. How will the binder solution be prepared and delivered to the mixer?
4. How will the granulation endpoint be determined and reproduced?
5. How will the discharge from the high shear mixer be accomplished?
6. Are the process parameters for granulation in high shear and fluid bed drying established and are reproducible, indicating a robust process?
7. How will the product be discharged from the fluid bed dryer? Does it require sizing and blending with the lubricants?
8. Is this system dedicated to a single product or multiple products?
9. How will this system be cleaned?
10. Will the control of a process be done individually for each unit or by an integrated control system?

For the potent compound processing requiring high-shear granulation and fluid bed drying, some companies have introduced a lab size unit with isolators and glove box. For a commercial scale, a contained unit is designed that minimize or eliminate the operator exposure to the potent compound. Such a system is costly and does require an enormous amount of time for process and cleaning validation.

In the case of APIs of lower toxicity, the major driving force in design is to prevent the possibility of product contact with the free environment. For APIs of high potency, the major concern in design is to protect the workforce from hazardous material. This has led to the use of barrier technology, downward laminar flow booths, and other containment technology. Innovative design solutions are required to provide practical answers to the problems of containment and cleanliness. APIs are becoming more and more potent, meanwhile, more than 50% of all NCE (New Chemical Entities) are classified as potent (Occupational Exposure Limit (OEL) <10 μg/m3). Furthermore, health and safety authorities all around the world are putting a greater focus on the protection of operators dealing with these substances. In response, suppliers of various hardware components have developed a huge variety of containment solutions, making it difficult to decide which is the best, even for experienced people.

A typical contained system with high shear granulation and fluid bed drying could be set up as follows: **Granulation**: integrated line comprising high shear mixer, integrated wet mill, wet product transfer line from the high shear mixer to fluid bed dryer, fluid bed processor, integrated dry mill and vacuum transfer system for dried granules from fluid bed processor to IBC. **Material handling**: IBCs with containment valve, Vibratory feeder and blending prism, disposable high containment interface like Hicoflex® which consists of two complementary and self-closing half couplings which seal off dust-tight and independently of each other, for discharging API from isolator and charging into high shear, IBC filling station at the discharge of fluid bed, post hoist, containment valve on a tablet press, IBC wash station, Wash In Place (WIP) drain frame.

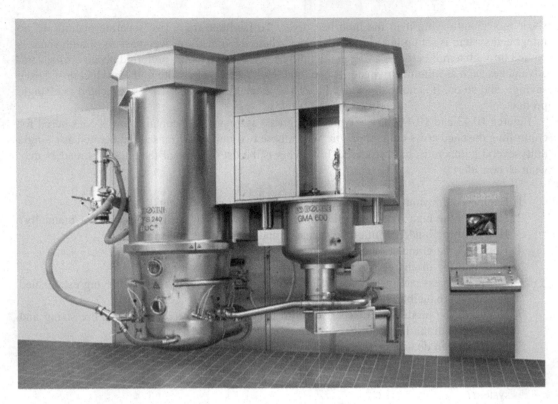

FIGURE 10.43   Integrated System Showing High Shear Mixer Next to the Fluid Bed Unit.
Source: L.B. Bohle Maschinen + Verfahren GmbH.

10.20   CONTINUOUS GRANULATION SYSTEMS

Continuous processing has long received support from the FDA, which has been interacting with the European Medicines Agency (EMA) and aligns well with the FDA's process analytical technology (PAT) and process validation guidance. The term "continuous" is applied to all production or manufacturing processes that run with a continuous flow. With that definition, continuous processing of solid dosage products in the pharmaceutical industry means starting the

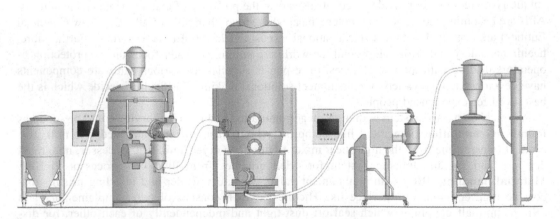

FIGURE 10.44   Integrated System with the In-line Mill at the Discharge of High Shear Mixer Feeding into a Fluid Bed with a Side Discharge into a Mill into an IBC via a Vacuum.
Source: Courtesy IMA S.p.A. Italy.

process from the synthesis of API to the final packaging of tablets or capsules 24/7 all year around. In the 1980s, Koblitz and Ehrhardt [202] reported on continuous wet granulation and drying. The article focused on continuous variable frequency fluid bed drying. Berkovitch in a Manufacturing Chemist article [203] quoted some researchers presenting these concepts in a symposium. Continuous processing of pharmaceuticals, including a process for solid oral dosage form manufacturing, was also discussed by Kawamura [204].

Drivers for continuous manufacturing in the pharmaceutical industry include the fact that New Chemical Entities (NCEs) are getting more potent/toxic. Small, dedicated suites are suitable to serve as "containments" for highly potent drugs. Investment costs for multi-product facilities for highly potent oral solid dosage products are exaggerated due to segregation measures. FDA initiative and the recent availability of compact integrated systems from equipment and software suppliers. Perceived operational and labor savings for high volume products.

Continuous granulation in fluid bed is more common where a large quantity of product is required. The current interest in continuous granulation focuses on a combination of high-shear/twin-screw extruders coupled with a continuous dryer. The following are some of the systems offered by the equipment suppliers.

Many unit operations are intrinsically continuous and are well understood. For all remaining unit operations, equipment is available. Experiences with continuous wet granulation have been positive. Opportunities to adopt a continuous process exist and should be built on a QbD approach, which will require more advanced control systems with simple and more complex PATs. It must be realized that not all products or processes will be manufactured with a continuous granulation approach. Every API will have to be evaluated for its capability to be a candidate for continuous granulation and a pertinent process will have to be developed for it.

A typical laboratory size continuous unit (Figure 10.45) consists of a 16 mm twin-screw granulator (TSG) and a truly continuous dryer with a throughput range from 0.1–2.5 kg/h. Preblended powders are fed via an integrated loss-in-weight feeder (Gericke) to the TSG, in which powder and liquid are delivered onto two co-rotating screws. Both components are continuously conveyed, mixed, and sheared to produce granules that leave the granulator into the continuous drying section.

LÖDIGE (Figure 10.46) offers a continuous granulation system in which a premixed mixture of composition is fed in the system and at a very high rotation speed the product is moved through the horizontal drum as a ring layer. Liquid addition is done by injectors or through the hollow shaft. The granulated product is then fed into a continuous fluid bed dryer with a varying fluidization velocity as the product is transferred through the dryer and further processed as required.

GEA Pharma Systems offers Consigma integrated granulation/ drying and tableting system (Figure 10.47). Based on the twin-screw wet granulation and the fluid bed drying, this integrated

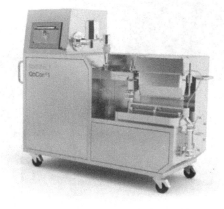

FIGURE 10.45   Qb Con 1 Laboratory-Scale Continuous Granulation and Drying System.
Source: L.B. Bohle Maschinen + Verfahren GmbH.

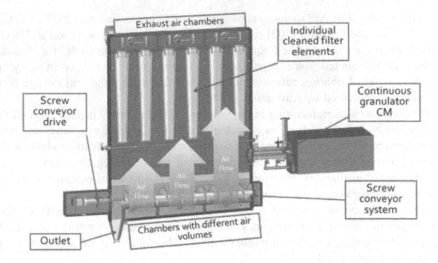

FIGURE 10.46 LÖDIGE Continuous Granulation and Drying System.
Source: LÖDIGE, Germany.

system is capable of producing between 0.5 and 200 kg of the product depending on the size of the system. In twin-screw continuous wet granulation, powdered solids, and binder pass through a twin-screw extruder, usually with co-rotating screws, resulting in a granulated product that is dried continuously, milled and blended, and compressed.

To avoid potential changes in the granulation density over time with twin-screw granulator resulting in bimodal particle size distribution and to avoid the particle segregation, Hüttlin (now Syntegon) has a newly developed continuous granulation platform called Xelum (Figure 10.48).

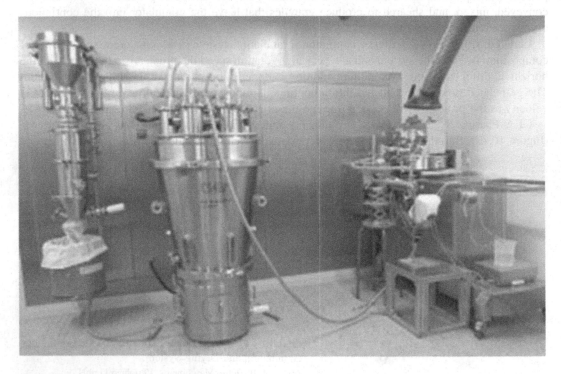

FIGURE 10.47 Consigma Continuous Granulation System.
Source: GEA Pharma Systems.

This platform doses active ingredients and excipients as discrete masses and not as continuous mass flow. The system doses mix and granulates individual packages, so-called X-keys, which continuously run through the process chain and are discharged successively as granules. Because of the soft sensors employed, the system does not require a steady-state operation.

Glatt offers a new Modular Continuous System (MODCOS) (Figure 10.49). MODCOS is a multipurpose platform designed for the continuous production of coated tablets from powder. The entire process chain, from the powder dosing of the active pharmaceutical ingredients (APIs) and excipients through wet granulation, drying, and tableting to tablet coating, is put together according to the customer's requirements.

Bohle offers a continuous granulation system called QbCon® 25 (Figure 10.50), which facilitates the continuous production of granulation and drying. The system can be integrated to produce tablets and coating.

As of this writing, US FDA has approved two products utilizing continuous manufacturing. However, having the process understanding and robust risk management program with continuous manufacturing will be the key to its successful implementation. This manufacturing approach must be seen as the platform for process development that is enhanced by continuous manufacturing.

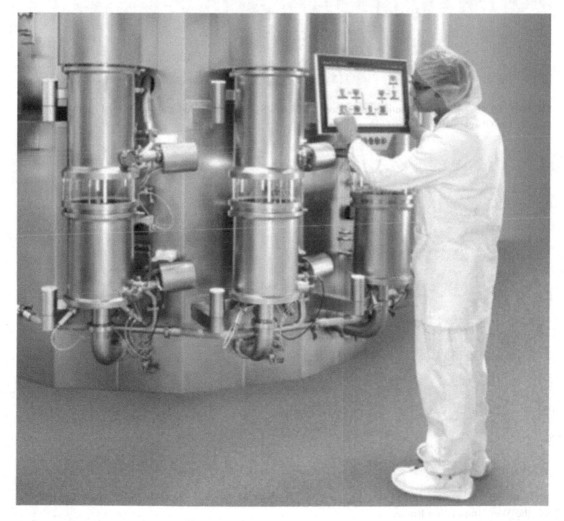

FIGURE 10.48 The Xelum Platform.
Source: Hüttlin (Syntegon) Germany.

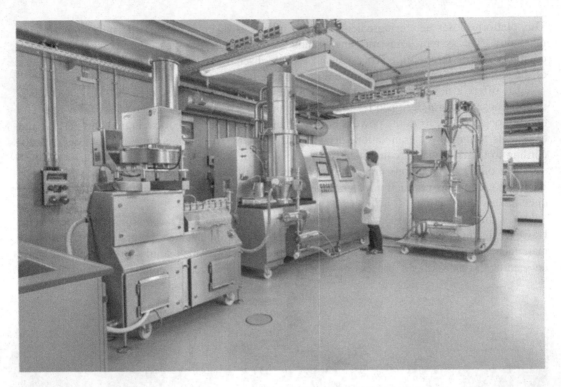

FIGURE 10.49   Modular Continuous System (MODCOS) with Fluid Bed and Ancillary Equipment.
Source: The Glatt Group.

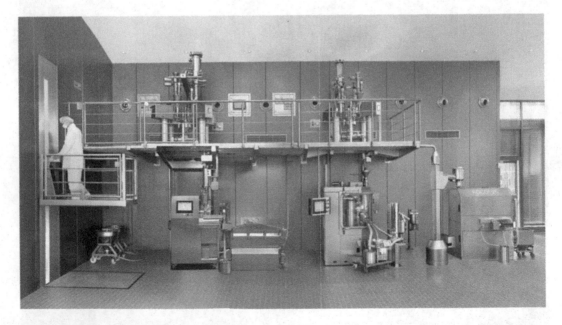

FIGURE 10.50   Continuous Manufacturing Systems (QbCon® 25 wet) - from Powder to the Coated Tablet via the Wet Granulation Route.
Source: L.B. Bohle Maschinen + Verfahren GmbH.

Continuous manufacturing provides renewed attention to PAT, process control, and on-line instrumentation. Implementation of continuous processing will be based on how manufacturers will overcome the challenges of compliance, process design, process control, and ultimately quality.

(A detailed treatment of continuous granulation is given in Chapter 13 of this book.)

10.21 CONCLUSION

The fluid bed dryer was used as an efficient way to dry a product because of the suspension of wet particles in the hot air stream. However, over the past 40 years of development in the pharmaceutical industry and the proliferation of the batch fluid bed processing technology in other industries such as food, polymer, and detergent have provided the opportunity to use the batch fluid bed processor for granulation, drying, particle coating, and pelletization. The advances in the fluid bed can be attributed to several factors. The needs of formulators, the requirements of the regulators, and technological innovations from the manufacturers of this technology are responsible for these advances. The result of these changes provided units that are paint-free, modular, and safer, in compliance with the cGMPs, and can perform various processes that were not thought of before.

The fluid bed process like other granulation technique requires understanding the importance of characterization of the raw materials, especially of a drug substance, the process equipment, limitations of the selected process, establishment of in-process control specifications, characterization of the finished product, and cleaning and process validation.

Over the past 20 years, process analytical technology has provided different approaches to understand this complicated unit operation. The interrelationship of process parameters is very critical as you establish the process parameters. We now have the modern computerized control panels and various on-line/in-line measurement options available for process control. If one reviews the history of innovation for this unit operation, the rate of equipment modification or improvement is relatively slow compared with the various process-control options being developed. The proper understanding of the process during the development stage will provide a robust process for the commercial application.

Acknowledgment: Some of the contents of this chapter were contributed by Mr. David Jones in the third edition of this book, who passed away in January 2016. His absence is sorely missed by the author and the pharmaceutical industry.

REFERENCES

1. Kunii, D., Levenspiel, O. Fluidization Engineering. New York: John Wiley & Sons Inc., 1968.
2. Wurster, D. E. Preparation of compressed tablet granulations by the air-suspension technique. II. J Am Pharm Assoc 1960; 49:82.
3. Wurster, D. E. Air-suspension technique of coating drug particles; a preliminary report. J Am Pharm Assoc (Sci Edi) 1959; 48(8):451–454.
4. Scott, M. W. et al. Continuous production of tablet granulation in Fluid Bed I. Theory and design considerations. J Pharm Sci 1964; 53(3):314–319.
5. Rankell, A. S. et al. Continuous production of tablet granulations in a fluidized bed. II. Operation and performance of equipment. Pharma Sci 1964; 53(3):320.
6. Contini, S., Atasoy, K. Fluid bed granulation, a modern economic method for tableting and encapsulation. Pharm Ind 1966; 28:144–146.
7. Wolf, G. Fluidized layer spray granulation. Drugs Made Germany 1968; 11:172–180.
8. Liske, T., Mobus, W. The manufacture and comparative aspects of fluidized layer spray granulation. Drugs Made Germany 1968; XI:182–189.
9. Sherrington, P. J, Oliver, R. Granulation monograph. In: Goldberg, AS Sr., ed. Powder Science and Technology. London: Heyden, 1981.
10. Pietch, W.B. Fluidization phenomena and fluidized bed technology. In: Fayed, ME, Otten, L, eds. Handbook of Powder Science and Technology. New York: Van Nostrand Reinhold, 1984.

11. Hersey, J. A. Fluidized bed technology – an overview. Int J Pharm Tech Prod Manuf 1981; 2(3):1–3.
12. Thiel, W. J., The theory of fluidization and application to the industrial processing of pharmaceutical products. Int J Pharm Tech Prod Manuf 1981; 2(5):5–8.
13. Thiel, W. J., Solids mixing in gas fluidized beds. Int J Pharm Tech Prod Manuf 1981; 2(9):9–12.
14. Littman, H., An overview of flow in fluidized beds. Pharm Technol 1985; 9(3):48.
15. Whitehead, A. B., Behavior of fluidized bed systems. Pharm Technol 1981; 2(13):13–18.
16. Story, M. J., Granulation and film coating in the fluidized bed. Pharm Technol 1981; 2(19):19–23.
17. Aulton, M. J., Banks, M. Fluidized bed granulation, factors influencing the quality of the product. Pharm Technol 1981; 2(24):19–27.
18. Kulling, W., Simon, E. L. Fluid bed technology applied to pharmaceuticals. Pharm Technol 1980; 4(1):79–83.
19. Gomezplata, A., Kugelman, A. M., Processing systems. In: Marchello, J. M., Gomezplata, A., eds. Gas-Solid Handling in the Process Industries. Chemical Processing and Engineering. Vol. 8. New York: Marcel Dekker Inc., 1976.
20. Räsänen, E., et al. The characterization of fluidized behavior using a novel multi-chamber microscale fluid bed. J Pharm Sci 2004; 93:780–791.
21. Davis, L., et al. Trans Inst Chem Eng 1966; 44T:293.
22. Gorrodnichev, V. I., et al. (English Translation). Pharm Chem J (USSR) 1974; 8:298.
23. Kirk-Othmer. Fluidization in Encyclopedia of Chemical Technology. Vol. 10, 3rd ed. New York: Wiley-Interscience, 1981:548–581.
24. Ennis, B. J., Tardos, G.I., Pfeffer, R. A micro-level-based characterization of granulation phenomena. Powder Technol 1991; 65:257–272.
25. Wan Lucy, S.C., Heng Paul, WS, Muhuri, G. Incorporation and distribution of a low dose drug in granules. Int J Pharm 1992; 88:159–163.
26. Long, G. E., Spraying theory and practice. Chem Eng 1978; PP73–PP77.
27. Masters, K. Spray Drying: An Introduction to Principles, Operational Practice, and Application. 2nd ed. New York: John Wiley & Sons Inc., 1976.
28. Heng, P. W. S., et al. Investigation on side-spray fluidized bed granulation with swirling airflow. AAPS PharmSciTech; 2013; 14(1):211–221.
29. Japanese Patent Application 61–259696, 1986.
30. Swiss Patent 0176/93, 1993, US Patent 5,444,892, 1995, European Patent number 0572356A1.
31. Guidance for Industry, Part 11, Electronic Records; Electronic Signatures – Scope and application. 2003.
32. Newitt, D. M., Conway-Jones, J. M., A contribution to the theory and practice of granulation. Int J Pharm Tech Prod Manuf 1958; 36:422.
33. Record, P. C., A review of pharmaceutical granulation technology. Int J Pharm Tech Prod Manuf 1980; 1:32.
34. Rumpf, H. The strength of granules and agglomerates. In: Krepper, W, ed. Agglomeration. New York: Interscience, 1962:379–418.
35. Tardos, GI, Khan, MI, Mort, PR. Critical parameters and limiting conditions in binder granulation of fine powders. Powder Technol 1997; 94:245–258.
36. Iveson, S. M., Granule coalescence modeling: including the effects of bond strengthening and distributed impact separation forces. Chem Eng Sci 2001; 56:2215–2220.
37. Thielmann, F., et al. The effect of primary particle surface energy on agglomeration rate in fluidized bed wet granulation. Powder Technol 181 (2008) 160–168
38. Schaefer, T., Worts, O. Control of fluidized bed granulation I effects of spray angle, nozzle height, and starting materials on granule size and size distribution. Arch Pharm Chem Sci Ed 1977; 5:51–60.
39. Smith, P. J., Nienow, AW. Particle growth mechanism in fluidized bed granulation. Chem Eng Sci 1983; 38(8):1223–1231, 1323–1240.
40. Aulton, M. E., Banks, M. Fluidized bed granulation-factors including the quality of the product. Int J Pharm Tech Prod Manuf 1981; 2(4):24–29.
41. Maroglou, A., Nienow, A. W. Fourth Symposium on Agglomeration. Toronto, Canada: Iron & Steel Society Inc., 1985:465–470.
42. Goldschmidt, M. J. V. Hydrodynamic modeling of fluidized bed spray granulation. Ph.D. Thesis, Twente University, Enschede, Netherlands, 2001.
43. Thielmann, F. et al. The effect of primary particle surface free energy on agglomeration rate in fluidized bed wet granulation. Powder Technol 2007; doi: 10.1016/j.powtec.2006.12.015.
44. Jain, K. Discrete characterization of cohesion in gas-solid flows. Master Thesis, School of Engineering, University of Pittsburgh, Pittsburgh, Pennsylvania, 2002.

45. McCabe, W. L., Smith, JC. Unit Operations of Chemical Engineering. New York, NY: McGraw-Hill, 1956.

46. Green Don, W., ed. Perry's Chemical Engineer's Handbook, Section 20. New York, NY: McGraw-Hill, Inc., 1984.

47. Rankell, R. S., Liberman, HA, Schiffman, RF. Drying in the Theory and Practice of Industrial Pharmacy. 3rd ed. Philadelphia: Lea & Feabiger, 1986.

48. Schaefer, T. Worts, O., Control of fluidized granulation III, effects of the inlet air temperature, and liquid flow rate on granule size and size distribution. Control of moisture content of granules in the drying phase. Arch Pharm Chem Sci Ed 1978; 6(1):1–13.

49. Parikh, D. M., Airflow in batch fluid-bed processing. Pharm Technol 1991; 15(3):100–110.

49A. Rowe, P. N., et al. Trans Inst Chem Eng 1965; 32T: 271.

50. Julia, Z. H., et al. Importance of inlet velocity in fluid bed drying of a granulation prepared in a high shear mixer. AAPS PharmSciTech, 2000; 1(4):1–4.

51. Nieuwmeyer, F. J. S., Vromans, H. Granule breakage during drying processes. Int J Pharm 2007; 329:81–87.

52. Nieuwmeyer, F. J. S., et al. Granule characterization during fluid bed drying by the development of a near-infrared method to determine water content and median granule size. Pharm Res 2007; 24(10):1854–1861.

53. Davis, T. D., et al. Modeling and monitoring of polymorphic transformations during the drying phase of wet granulation. Pharm Res 2004; 21(5):860–866.

54. Thurn, U. Mischen, Granulieren und Trocknen pharmazeutischer Grundstoffe in heterogenen Wirbelschichten (Mixing, granulating and dryingpharmaceutical Basic materials in heterogeneous fluidized beds) Dissertation no. 4511, Eidgenossischen Technischen, Hochschule, Zurich, 1970.

55. Liske, T., Mobus, W. The manufacture and comparative aspects of fluidized layer spray granulation. Drugs Made Germany 1968; 11(4):182–189.

56. Schaefer, T., Worts, O. Control of fluidized bed granulation V, factors affecting granule growth. Arch Pharm Chem Sci Ed 1978; 6:69–82.

57. Ormos, Z. Pataki, K. Hung, J., Indust Chem 1979; 7:89–103.

58. Ormos, Z. Pataki, K. Hung, J., Indust Chem 1979; 7:105–117.

59. Banks, M. Ph.D. Thesis,. C.N.A.A. Leicester Polytechnic, 1981.

60. Galmen, M. J. Greer, W. Fluid Technol Pharm Manuf International Conference, Paper 2, 1982.

61. Veillard, M et al. Int J Pharm Tech Prod Mfg 1982; 3(4):100–107.

62. Georgakopoulos, PP et al. The effects of using different grades of PVP and gelatin as binders in the fluidized bed granulation and tabletting of lactose. Pharmazie 1983; 38(4):240–243.

63. Jinot, J. C., et al. STP Pharma 1986; 2(13):126–131.

64. Shinoda, A., et al. Yakuzaigaku 1976; 36(2):83–88.

65. Aulton, M. E. et al. The wettability of powders during fluidized bed granulation. J Pharm Pharmacol 1977; 59P(suppl)

66. Schepky, G. Acta Pharm Technol 1978; 24(3):185–212.

67. Aulton, M. E., Banks, E. Proc Intl Conf Powder Technol Pharm Basel, Switzerland: Powder Advisory Center, 1979.

68. Kocova et al. Drugs Made Germany 1983; 26(4):205–211.

69. Davies, W. L., Gloor, WT. Batch production of pharmaceutical granulations in a fluidized bed. II Effects of various binders and their concentrations on granulations and compressed tablets. J Pharm Sci 1972; 61(4):618–622.

70. Rouiller, M., et al. Acta Pharm Technol 1975; 21(2):129–138.

71. Ormos, Z. Pataki, K., Stefko, B. Studies in granulation in a fluidized bed IX. Effects of concentration of various binders upon granule formation. Hung J Indust Chem 1979; 7:131–140.

72. Ormos, Z. Pataki, K. Stefko, B., Studies in granulation in a fluidized bed X. Effects of the relative amounts of various binders upon granule formation. Hung J Indust Chem 1979; 7:141–151.

73. Ormos, Z. Studies in granulation in a fluidized bed XI Approximate description of the particle size distribution. Hung J Indust Chem 1979; 7:153–163.

74. Ormos, Z. Studies in granulation in a fluidized bed XII, Bed expansion of fluidized heterodisperse granule masses. Hung J Indust Chem 1979; 7: 221–235.

75. Kocova El-Arini, S. Pharm Ind 1981; 43(7):674–679.

76. Jager, K. F., Bauer, KH. Acta Pharm Technol 1984; 30(1):85–92.

77. Nouh, A. T. I., Pharm Ind 1986; 48(6):670–673.

78. Bank, A., et al. Proc Conf Appl Phys Chem 1971; 2:687–692.

Pharmaceutical Granulation Technology

79. Davies, W. L, Gloor, W. T. Batch production of pharmaceutical granulations in a fluidized bed. III Binder dilution effects on granulation. J Pharm Sci 1973; 62(1):170–172.
80. Ormos, Z. Pataki, K. Csukas, B. Hung, J Indust Chem 1973; 1:307–328.
81. Ormos, Z., Pataki, K., Csukas, B. Hung, J Indust Chem 1973; 1:463–474.
82. Johnson, M. C. R. et al. Proceedings: Evaluation of small scale fluidiz ed bed granulation unit. J Pharm Pharmacol 1975; 2–80.
83. Schaefer, T., Worts, O. Control of fluidized bed granulation IV. Effects of binder solution and atomization on granule size and size distribution. Arch Pharm Chem Sci Ed 1978; 6:14–25.
84. Gorodnichev, V. I. et al. Pharm Chem J (USSR) 1980; 14(10):72–77.
85. Ceschel, G. C. et al. II Farmaco Ed Prat 1981; 36(6):281–293.
86. Rangnarsson, G., et al. Influence of granulating method on bulk properties and tabletability of high dose drugs. Int J Pharm 1982; 12:163–171.
87. Meshali, M., El-Banna, H. M., El-Sabbagh, H. Use of factorial design to evaluate granulations prepared in a fluidized bed. Pharmazie 1983; 38(5):323–325.
88. Hajdu, R., Ormos, Z. Hung, J Ind Chem 1983; 12:425–430.
89. Devay, A., et al. Acta Pharm Technol 1984; 30(3):239–242.
90. Alkan, M. H., Yuksel, A. Granulation in fluidized bed II-Effect of binder amount on the final granules. Drug Dev & Ind Pharm 1986; 12(10):1529–1543.
91. Sheskey, P., et al. Foam technology: the development of a novel technique for the delivery of aqueous binder systems in high shear and fluid-bed wet-granulation applications. Poster @ AAPS Annual Meeting, October 26–30, 2003.
92. Aulton, M. E. Fluid Technol Pharm Manuf International Conference, Paper 3, Powder Advisory Center, London, 1982.
93. Dahl, T. C, Bormeth, A. P. Naproxen controlled release matrix tablets: fluid bed granulation feasibility. Drug Dev Ind Pharm 1990; 16(4):581–590.
94. Higashide, F., et al. Dependence of drug content uniformity on particle sizes in fluidized bed granulation. Pharm Ind 1985; 47(11):1202–1205.
95. Davies, W. L, Gloor, WT Jr. Batch production of pharmaceutical granulation in fluidized bed II: effects of various binders and their concentrations on granulations and compressed tablets. J Pharm Sci 1972; 61:618.
96. Davies, W. L., Gloor, W. T. Jr. Batch production of pharmaceutical granulation in fluidized bed III: binder dilution effects on granulation. J Pharm Sci 1973; 62:170.
97. Hontz, J. Assessment of Selected Formulation and Processing Variables in Fluid Bed Granulation. Ph.D. Thesis, University of Maryland at Baltimore, 1987. Dissertation Abs Int 1987; (6):1655-B.
98. Alkan, H., et al. Doga Tu J Med Pharm 1987; 11(1):1–7.
99. Wan, L. S. C., Lim, K. S. Effect of polyvinylpyrrolidone solutions containing dissolved drug on a characteristics of lactose fluidized bed granules. STP Pharm 1988; 4(7):560–571.
100. Wan, L. S. C., Lim, K. S. Mode of action of polyvinylpyrrolidone as a binder on fluidized bed granulation of lactose and starch granules. STP Pharm 1989; 5(4):244–250.
101. Schaefer, T., Worts, O. Control of fluidized bed granulation II, estimation of droplet size of atomized binder solution. Arch Pharm Chem Sci Ed 1977; 5:178–193.
102. Davies, W. L., Gloor, W. T., Jr. Batch production of Pharmaceutical granulation in fluidized bed. I: Effects of process variables on physical properties of final granulation. J Pharm Sci 1971; 60(12):1869–1874.
103. Krycer, I., Pope, D. G., Hersey, J. A., An evaluation of tablet binding agents: Part 1: solution binder. Powder Technol 1983; 34:39–51.
104. Planinsek, O., et al. The utilization of surface free-energy parameters for the selection of a suitable binder in fluidized bed granulation. Int J Pharm 2000; 207:77–88.
105. Seo, A., Holm, P., Schaefer, T. Effects of droplet size and type of binder on the agglomerate growth mechanisms by melt agglomeration in a fluidized bed. Eur J Pharm Sci 2002; 16:95–105.
106. GEA Pharma. Flexstream Brochure and Web site. Available at: https://www.gea.com/en/products/dryers-particle-processing/fluid-beds/flexstream-fluid-bed-processor.jsp, and A Company Brochure and Web site. Available at: http://www.niro-pharma-systems.com.
107. Rowley, F. A., Effects of the bag shaking cycle on the particle size distribution of granulation. Pharm Technol 1989; 13(9):78–82.
108. Nienow, A. W., Rowe, P. N., Fluid bed granulation ll, Separation Process Services, Harwell, December 1975.

109. Miwa, A., et al. Prediction of a suitable amount of water in fluidized bed granulation of pharmaceutical formulations using corresponding values of components. Int J Pharma 2008; 352:202–208.

110. Maroglou, A., Nienow, A. W. Fluidized bed granulation technology and its application to tungsten carbide. Powder Metall 1986; 29(4):15–25.

111. Simon, Kukeca et al. Characterization of agglomerated carvedilol by hot-melt processes in a fluid bed and high shear granulator. Int J Pharm 2012; 430:4–85.

112. Kidokoro, M., Haramiishi, Y., Sagasaki, S., Yamamoto, Y., Application of fluidized hot-melt granulation (FHMG) for the preparation of granules for tableting. Drug Dev Ind Pharm 2002; 28:67–76.

113. Jones, D., Percel, P., Coating of multiparticulates using molten materials: Formulation and process consideration, in multiparticulate oral drug delivery. In: Ghebre-Sellassie, I., ed. Multiparticulate Oral Drug Delivery. 1st ed. New York: Marcel Dekker, 1994: 113–142.

114. Perissutti, B., Rubessa, F., Moneghini, M., Voinovich, D. Formulation design of carbamazepine fast-release tablets prepared by melt granulation technique. Int J Pharma 2003; 256:53–63.

115. Yanze, F., Duru, C, Jacob, M. A., process to produce effervescent tablets: fluidized bed dryer melt granulation. Drug Dev Ind Pharm 2000; 26:1167–1176.

116. Maheshwari, M., Ketkar, A., Chauhan, B., Patil, V., Paradkar, A., Preparation and characterization of ibuprofen–cetyl alcohol beads by melt solidification technique: effect of variables, Int J Pharma 2003; 261:57–67.

117. Abbereger, T., et al. The effect of droplet size and powder particle size on the mechanisms of nucleation and growth in fluid bed melt agglomeration. Int J Pharm 2002; 249:185–197.

118. Seo, A., et al. Effect of droplet size and type of binder on the agglomerate growth mechanisms by melt agglomeration in fluidised bed. J Pharm Sci 2002; 16:95–105.

119. Tan, H. S., et al. Kinetics of fluidised melt granulation I: The effect of process variables. Chem Eng Sci 2006 16;1586–1601.

120. Boerefijn, R., et al. Studies of fluid bed granulation in an industrial R & D context. Chem Eng Sci 2005; 60:3879–3890.

121. Aulton, M. E. et al. Mfg Chem Aerosol News 1978; 12:50–56.

122. Workman, J. Jr. A review of process near-infrared spectroscopy: 1980–1994. J Near Infrared Spectrosc 1993; 1:221–245.

123. Osborne, B. G., Fearn, T, Hindle, PH. Practical NIR Spectroscopy with Applications in Food and Beverage Industry Analysis. 2nd ed. Harlow, UK: Longman, 1993:227.

124. USP XXVII 2004.

125. European Pharmacopoeia. Near Infra-Red Spectrometry, 2004:59.

126. Callis, J., Illman, D, Kowalski, B. Process analytical chemistry. Anal Chem 1987; 59:624A–637A.

127. Beebe, K et al. Process analytical chemistry. Anal Chem 1993; 65:199R–216R.

128. Blaser, W et al. Process analytical chemistry. Anal Chem 1995; 67:47R–70R.

129. Hassel, D, Bowman, E. Process analytical chemistry for spectroscopists. Appl. Spectrosc 1998; 52:18A–29A.

130. Workman, J. Jr et al. Process analytical chemistry. Anal Chem 1999. 71:121R–180R.

131. Brittain, H. Methods for the characterization of polymorphs and solvates in polymorphism in pharmaceutical solids. In: Brittain, H, ed. Polymorphism Pharm Sol. Vol. 95, 1st ed. New York: Marcel Dekker Inc., 1999: 227–278.

132. Frake, P., et al. Process control and end-point determination of fluid bed granulation by application of near-infrared spectroscopy. Int J Pharm 1997; 151:75–80.

133. Rantanen, J., et al. Use of near-infrared reflectance method for measurement of moisture content during granulation. Pharm Dev Technol 2000; 5(2):209–217.

134. Rantanen, J., et al. On-line monitoring of moisture content in an instrumented fluidized bed granulator with multi-channel NIR moisture sensor. Powder Technol 1998; 99:163–170.

135. Lipsanen, T., et al. Particle size, moisture, and fluidization variations described by indirect in-line physical measurements of fluid bed granulation. AAPS PharmSciTech 2008; 9(4):1070–1077.

136. Vazquez R. E., Optimization of drying-end-points measurements for the automation of a fluidized-bed dryer using FT-NIR spectroscopy. Master of Science Thesis, University of Puerto Rico, 2004.

137. Rantanen, J., et al. Next-generation fluidized bed granulator automation. AAPS PharmSciTech 2000; 1(2):10.

138. Rantanen, J., et al. Process analysis of fluidized bed granulation. AAPS PharmSciTech 2001; 2(4):21.

139. Rantanen, J. T., et al. Visualization of fluid bed granulation with self-organizing maps. J Pharm Biomed Anal. 2001; 24(3):343–352.

140. Laitinen, N., et al. At-line particle size analysis with a novel optical technique during a fluidized-bed granulation process. Poster @AAPS Annual Meeting, 2002.

141. Hu, X. et al. Study growth kinetics in fluidized bed granulation with at-line FBRM. Int J Pharma 2008 Jan 22;347(1–2):54–61. Epub 2007 Jul 3.

142. Huang, J., et al. A., PAT approach to enhance process understanding of fluid bed granulation using in-line particle size characterization and multivariate analysis. J Pharm Innov 2010; 5:58–68 DOI: 10.1007/s12247-010-9079

143. Schmidt-Lehr, S., Moritz, H., Jürgens, K. C. Online control of particle size during fluidized bed granulation. Pharm Ind 2007; 69:478–484.

144. Petrak, D. Simultaneous measurement of particle size and particle velocity by the spatial filtering technique. Part Syst Char. 2002; 19:391–400.

145. Burggraeve, A., et al. Evaluation of in-line spatial filter velocimetry as PAT monitoring tool for particle growth during fluid bed granulation. Eur J Pharm Biopharm 2010; 76:138.

146. Burggraeve, A., et al. Batch statistical process control of a fluid bed granulation process using in-line spatial filter velocimetry. Eur J Pharm Sci 2011; 42:584.

147. Fischer, C., et al. Restoration of particle size distribution from fiber-optical in-line measurements in fluidized bed processes. Chem Eng Sci 2011; 66:2842–2852.

147A. Hartung, A., et al. Role of continuous moisture profile monitoring by in-line NIR spectroscopy during fluid bed granulation. Drug, Dev Ind Pharma 2011; 37:274–280.

148. Hauag, J., et al. A PAT approach to enhance process understanding of fluid bed granulation using in-line particle size characterization and multivariate analysis. J Pharma Innov 2010; 5:58–68.

148A. Närvänen, T. Particle size determination during fluid bed granulation-Challenges and ppportunities 19th Helsinki drug research. Eur J Pharm Sci, Helsinki, Finland 2008, 34:S12.

149. Närvänen, T., et al. Gaining fluid bed process understanding by in-line particle size analysis. J Pharm Sci 2009; 98:1110–1117.

149A. Närvänen, T. et al. Controlling granule size by granulation liquid feed pulsing. Int J Pharma 2009; 357:132–138.

150. Petrak, D., et al. In-line particle sizing for real-time process control by fiber-optical spatial filtering technique (SFT). Adv Powder Technol2011; 22:203–208.

151. Schmidt-Lehr, S., et al. Online-control of the particle size during fluid-bed granulation/evaluation of a novel laser probe for a better control of particle size in fluid-bed granulation. Pharm Ind 2007; 69:478–484.

152. Hu, X. H. et al. Study growth kinetics in fluidized bed granulation with at-line FBRM. Int J Pharma 2008; 347:54–61.

152A. Haug, J., et al. A PAT approach to improve process understanding of high shear wet granulation through in-line particle measurement using FBRM C35. I Pharm Sci 2010; 99:3205–3212.

153. Tok, A., et al. Monitoring granulation rate processes using three PAT tools in a pilot-scale fluidized bed. AAPS PharmSciTech 2008; 9:1083–1091.

154. Buurggraeve, A., et al. Development of fluid bed granulation process control strategy based on the real-time process and product measurements. Talanta, 100 293–302.

155. Jha, B. K., Tambe, S. S., Kulkarni, B. D. Estimating diffusion coefficients of a micellar system using an ANN. J Colloid Interface Sci 1995; 170:392–398.

156. Bourquin, J., et al. Basic concepts of ANN modeling in the application to pharmaceutical development. Pharm Dev Technol 1997; 2(2):95–109, 111–121.

157. Watano, S., Takashima, H, Miyanami, K. Control of moisture content in fluidized bed granulation by neural network. J Chem Eng 1997; 30(2):223–229.

158. Leane, M. M., Cumming, I, Corrigan, OI. The use of artificial neural networks for the selection of the most appropriate formulation and processing variables in order to predict the in vitro dissolution of sustained release minitabs. AAPS PharmSciTech 2003; 4(2):26.

159. Vandel, D., Davari, A., Famouri, P. Modeling of fluidized bed neural networks. Proceedings of 32nd IEEE SSST. Florida: FAMU-FSU Tallahassee, 2000.

160. Quantrille, T. E., Liu, Y. A. Artificial Intelligence in Chemical Engineering. San Diego: Academic Press, 1991.

161. Behzadi, S. S. et al. Validation of fluid bed granulation utilizing artificial neural network. Int J Pharma 2005; 291(1–2):139–148.

162. Närvänen, T. et al. A new rapid on-line imaging method to determine particle size distribution of granules. AAPS PharmSciTech 2008; 9(1):282–287.

163. Portoghese, F., Berruti, F., Briens, C. Continuous on-line measurement of solid moisture content during fluidized bed drying using Triboelectric probes. Powder Technol 2007; doi:10.1016/jPowtec2007.01.003.

164. Koerfer, R., Simutis, R. Advanced process control for fluidized bed agglomeration. Inf Technol Control 2008; 37(4):285–293.

165. Watano, S., Sato, Y., Miyanami, K. Control of granule growth in fluidized bed granulation by an image processing system. Chem Pharm Bull 1996; 44:1556–1560.

166. Gore, A. Y., McFarland, D. W., Batuyios, N. H. Fluid bed granulation: factors affecting the process in laboratory development and production scale-up. Pharm Technol 1985; 9(9):114.

167. Bonck, J. A. Spray granulation presented at the AIChE Annual Meeting, Orlando, Florida, USA, November 1993.

168. Jones, D. M. Factors to consider in fluid bed processing. Pharm Technol 1985; 9(4):50.

169. Matharu, A. S., Patel, MR. A new scale-up equation for fluid bed processing. Poster Presentation AAPS Annual Meeting, alt Lake City, UT, USA, 2003.

170. Rambali, B., Baert, L., Massart, D. L. Scaling up of the fluidized bed granulation process. Int J Pharma 2003; 252(1–2):197–206.

171. Simon, E. J. Fluid bed processing of bulk solids. Paper presented at the Third International Powder Technology and Bulk Solids Conference, PowTech, Harrogate, England, Heyden & Sons, 1975:63–73.

172. Huolong, Liu et al. Online optimization of a top-spray fluidized bed granulation process based on a three-stage population balance model. https://www.researchgate.net/publication/313559147 accessed Nov11 2019.

173. Kulling, W. Method and apparatus for removing a vaporized liquid from gas for use in a process based on the fluidized bed principle. US patent 4,145,818, March 27, 1979.

174. ATEX Directive 94/9/EC of the European Parliament and the council, March 23, 1994 and July 2006.

175. Guidelines to Directive 2014/34 EU (ATEX) /EU Guidelines, second edition 2017. https://osha.europa.eu/en/legislation/guidelines/guidelines-directive-201434-eu-atex.

176. US Food and Drug Administration. Food and drug administration announces new progress toward "21st Century" regulation of pharmaceutical manufacturing. 2003. http://www,fda.gov/cder/gmp/index.htm.

177. Djuriš J., et al. Design space approach in optimization of fluid bed granulation and tablets compression process. Sci World J Vol 2012. DOI:10.1100/2012/185085.

178. Lourenco V., et al. A Quality by Design study applied to an Industrial Pharmaceutical fluid bed granulation. Eur J Pharma Biopharmaceutics 2012; 81:438–447.

179. Gavn, A., et al. Fluidised bed granulation of two APIs: QbD approach and development of a NIR in-line monitoring method. Asian J Pharm Sci. DOI:10.1016/j.ajps.2019.03.003.

180. Merkku P., et al. Influence of granulation and compression process variables on flow rate of granules and on tablet properties, with special reference to weight variation. Int J Pharma 1994; 102:117–125.

181. Otsuka, T., et al. Application of principal component analysis enables to effectively find important physical variables for optimization of fluid bed granulation. Int J Pharma 2011; 409: 81–88.

182. Jolliffe, I. T. Principal Component Analysis. New York: Springer.

183. Parikh, DM. Fluid bed processing in the 1990s. Tabletting and granulation yearbook. Pharm Tech 1996; (suppl):40–47.

184. Ehlers, H., et al. Improving flow properties of ibuprofen by fluidized bed particle thin coating. Int J Pharma 2009; 368:165–170.

185. Doelling, M. K., et al. The development of a microwave fluid bed processor I: construction and qualification of a prototype laboratory unit. Pharm Res 1992; 9(11):1487–1492.

186. Doelling, M. K., Nash, RA. The development of a microwave fluid bed processor II: drying performance and physical characteristics of typical pharmaceutical granulations. Pharm Res 1992; 9(11):1493–1501.

187. Funakoshi, Y., et al. Process for coating granular materials. US Patent 3,671,296. June 20, 1977.

188. Funakoshi, Y., et al. Process for coating granular materials. US Patent 4,034,126. July 5, 1977.

189. Abe, E., Hirosue, H. Method and apparatus for continuously coating discrete particles in turning fluidized bed. US Patent 4,542,043. Sept 17, 1985.

190. Jager, K. F., Bauer, KH. Effect of material motion on agglomeration in the rotary fluidized -bed granulator. Drugs Made Germany 1982; 25:61–65.

191. Türkoglu, M., He, M., Sakr, A. Evaluation of rotary fluidized bed as a wet granulation equipment. Eur J Pharm Biopharm 1995; 41(6):388–394.

192. Li, S. P. et al. Recent advances in microencapsulation technology and equipment. Drug Dev Ind Pharm 1988; 14(2–3):353–376.

193. Robinson, R. L., Hollenbeck, G. Manufacture of spherical acetaminophen pellets: comparison of rotary processing with multiple-step extrusion and spheronization. Pharm Technol 1991; 15(5):48–56.
194. Parikh, D. M. Layering in rotary fluid bed a unique process for the production of spherical pellets for controlled release. Presented at Interphex-USA, New York, NY, 1991.
195. Hileman, G. A., Sarabia, R. E. Manufacture of immediate and controlled release spheres in a single unit using fluid bed otor insert. Presented at the Annual Meeting of the American Association of Pharmaceutical Scientists (AAPS), Poster PT 6167, San Antonio, Texas, USA, 1992.
196. Iyer, R. M., Augsburger, L. L., Parikh, D. M. Evaluation of drug layering and coating: effect of process mode and binder level. Drug Dev Ind Pharm 1993; 19(9):9891–9998.
197. U.S. patent 5, 132, and 142, 1992.
198. Korakianiti, E. S., et al. Optimization of the pelletization process in a fluid bed rotor granulator using experimental design. AAPS PharmSciTech 2000; 1(4):35.
199. Pišek, R., et al. Influence of rotational speed and surface of rotating disc on pellets produced by direct rotor pelletization. Pharm Ind 2000; 62:312–319.
200. Kristensen, J., Hansen, V. W. Wet granulation in rotary processor and fluid bed: comparison of granule and tablet properties. AAPS PharmSciTech 2006; 7:PPE1–PPE10.
201. Kristensen, J. Investigation of a 2-step agglomeration process performed in a rotary processor using PEG solutions as the primary binder liquid. AAPS PharmSciTech 2006; 7(4):89.
202. Koblitz, T., Ehrhardt, L. Continuous variable-frequency fluid bed drying of pharmaceutical granulations. Pharm Technol, March 1985.
203. Berkovitch, I. From batch to continuous pharmaceutical engineering. Manuf Chem, August 1986: 43–45.
204. Kawamura, K. Continuous processing of pharmaceuticals. In Swarbrick, J, Boyle, J, eds. Encyclopedia of Pharmaceutical Technology. 3rd Edition. New York: Marcel Dekker, 1990.

11 Single-Pot Processing

Griet Van Vaerenbergh and Harald Stahl

CONTENTS

11.1 INTRODUCTION

Single-pot processing was developed to provide a way to mix, granulate, dry and blend pharmaceutical granulations in a single device. Although any system that combines these processes into a single piece of equipment can be called a single-pot processor, this chapter only covers processors that comprise a high- or low-shear mixer granulator (similar to conventional granulators) outfitted with a variety of drying options. Fluid-bed processors, which also combine mixing, granulating, and drying processes into a single unit operation, are covered in another chapter in this book (Chapter 10).

When single-pot processing was initially introduced, high- or low-shear granulators were fitted with a vacuum system, combined with a heat-jacketed bowl, to provide a drying method in a single "pot." Today, processors are available that provide vacuum drying with microwaves or that percolate gas under low pressure into the vacuum chamber (processing bowl), or – in a more recent development – include fluid-bed drying into a high shear granulator [1]. Another very interesting improvement is the use of swinging processing bowls [2]. Since the design of the granulators at the

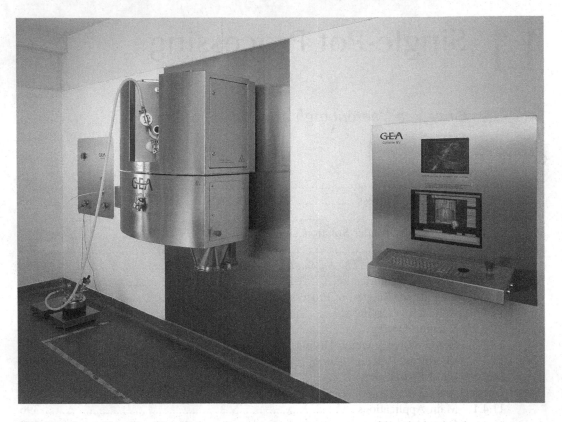

FIGURE 11.1 UltimaPro 75 microwave/vacuum single-pot processor with swinging bowl.
Source: Courtesy of GEA Group, Wommelgem, Belgium.

basis of single-pot processors varies from manufacturer to manufacturer, the same is valid for those machines (Figures 11.1–11.4).

Single-pot processors for the pharmaceutical industry have been available for years. They received renewed interest in the mid-1980s when microwaves were coupled with a vacuum to enhance the drying operation. Microwaves applied to drying pharmaceutical granulations became synonymous with single-pot processing and it was thought that this technology would eventually become the norm for granulation-based processing. Several major pharmaceutical companies purchased production-scale units following successful trials conducted at vendor pilot facilities. In the ensuing years, when the technology did not become as popular as expected, there were rumors that microwave systems could not be validated and suffered from excessive regulatory hurdles [3]. The reality is neither; single-pot technology has continued to evolve during the past decade. It has de-emphasized its association with microwave drying while continuing to demonstrate its appropriate role in granulation technology.

In a production setting, single-pot processing offers a number of advantages. By integrating granulating and drying capabilities into a single unit, capital investment in equipment and good manufacturing practice (GMP) floor space may be lower than other alternatives. The number of material handling steps is reduced and, consequently, the total processing time may be shorter while maintaining a high yield and keeping production support to a minimum. Environmental variables, such as humidity, are eliminated from the manufacturing process, which may offer benefits when processing moisture-sensitive formulations. Best practice is to outfit a single-pot processor with clean-in-place (CIP) systems, thereby enhancing operator safety by minimizing exposure to the product both during manufacturing and cleaning [4]. Requirements for solvent recovery systems are lower for single-pot processors compared with fluid-bed dryers. Single-pot

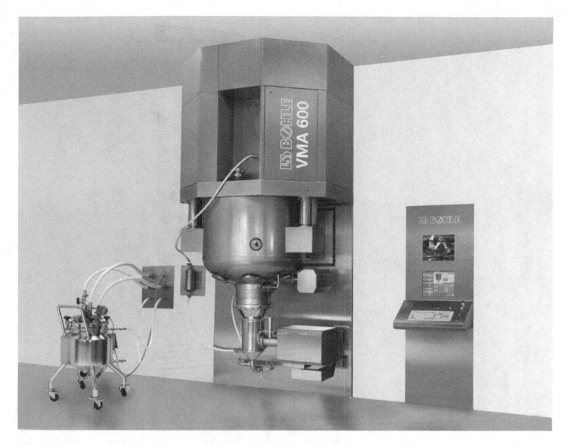

FIGURE 11.2 VMA600 microwave/vacuum single-pot processor.
Source: Courtesy of L.B. Bohle Group, Ennigerloh, Germany.

processors outfitted with vacuum are attractive for evaporating solvents that are explosive or for containing drug substances with low-exposure limits. Table 11.1 shows a summary of the main application areas of single-pot processors, which will be discussed in more detail later in the chapter.

The versatility and compactness of small-scale (3–25 L) single-pot processors also make the technology attractive for development and pilot laboratory facilities. Within the past decade, equipment manufacturers began to offer single-pot processors that can accommodate the batch sizes required during early development (0.3 g–10 kg). The processors can be used as mixer blenders for direct compression formulations or as mixer granulators to prepare wet granulations for fluid-bed drying. They can also be utilized as a single processing unit for all the steps required for granulation preparation. Some vendors offer the option of upgrading their small-scale processors. For example, a user can initially purchase a single-pot processor with vacuum drying capabilities and add a microwave drying system at a later date. Consequently, single-pot processors should be given strong consideration when equipping a development laboratory or pilot plant intended to offer a variety of pharmaceutical formulation processing options.

11.2 TYPICAL SINGLE-POT PROCESS

The steps and sequence of manufacturing pharmaceutical granulations using single-pot processing are the same as those that use alternative technologies, except that several of the stages are done in the same product chamber. The majority of production installations make use of its mixing,

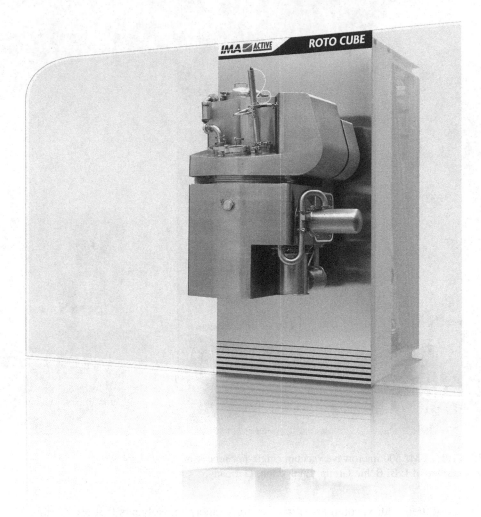

FIGURE 11.3 Rotocube single-pot granulator.
Source: Courtesy of IMA Group, Lucca, Italy.

granulating, and drying capabilities during the processing of a single batch. It's important to note the absence of a milling step between granulation and drying. Reducing the number of process steps has the advantage of a reduction in process time and operations, whereas the drawback is that there is no option to break up any lumps generated during granulation. Single-pot operations, therefore, require excellent control of the granulation process to prevent the formation of oversized material.

11.2.1 Dry Mixing

Powders are loaded into the single pot either manually (for development- and pilot-scale units) or by a conveying system (for production-scale units). Vacuum pump(s) used for the drying operation can also be used to charge the processor. Pneumatic and vacuum conveying systems, as well as

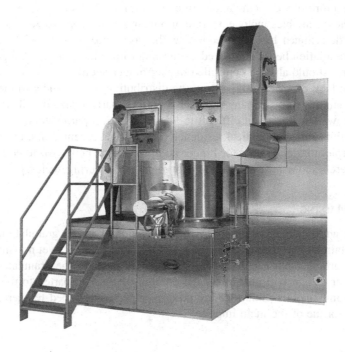

FIGURE 11.4 VAC 600 vacuum single-pot processor.
Source: Courtesy of Diosna, Osnabrück, Germany.

TABLE 11.1
Main Applications of Single-Pot Processors

1)	Expensive Products
2)	Short Campaigns (many different products)
3)	Highly potent (toxic) products
4)	Granulation with organic solvents
5)	Effervescent production

gravity feeding from an intermediate bulk container (IBC), contribute to minimizing operator exposure to the drug product. The powders are mixed in the dry state until the desired degree of uniformity is obtained. Depending on the geometry of the processing bowl and the efficiency of its mixing blades, optimal mixing for most processors generally occurs when the bowl is charged at 50–75% of capacity. Batch size, impeller speed, and mixing time are variables that affect the desired degree of blend homogeneity before the addition of the binder solution.

11.2.2 ADDITION OF BINDER SOLUTION

Once dry mixing is completed, the binder solution is added through a spray lance connected to a solvent delivery system (e.g., a pressure pot or peristaltic pump). For highly viscous binder solutions, it is advantageous to use the vacuum system of the processor to suck it into the processor.

Because the single-pot processor is operating as a granulator at this point, all variables considered during the manufacture of wet granulations in conventional high- or low-shear mixer granulators are applicable. Those variables include the rate of binder action, droplet size, and spray pattern (the latter two being determined by the selection of the spray nozzle and the distance between the nozzle tip and granulation bed). The speed of the main impeller and the chopper, as well as the jacket temperature, should also be controlled during binder addition.

Because of the lack of a wet milling step, the distribution of the binder in the powder bed is a critical aspect of single-pot processing to achieve optimal particle size distribution. When scaling up the process, however, it is often difficult to keep the critical parameters – such as droplet size and spray flux – the same for identical residence times [5]. In recent years, innovations related to introducing multiple nozzle systems for binder addition in production-sized equipment have been introduced to overcome the issue of the changing spray flux during scale-up.

11.2.3 Wet Massing

Following binder addition, additional energy may be required during granulation until the desired consistency is obtained. The speeds of the main impeller and chopper, wet massing time and jacket temperature are variables that can affect the physical attributes of the granulation. Like the bowl shape, the impeller design will also affect the amount of shear imparted to the granulation. The granulation endpoint may be controlled by process time, product bed temperature, energy consumption, or the torque of the main impeller.

11.2.4 Drying

After granulation, the material is dried using one of four approaches: (a) vacuum drying, (b) gas-assisted vacuum drying, (c) microwave vacuum drying or (d) fluid-bed drying. Details of each drying method are summarized in the "Drying Methods for Single-Pot Processors" section. The product bed is usually stirred at a low intensity during the drying process to facilitate solvent removal and promote uniform drying, as well as to prevent the caking of the granulation on the chamber walls. Agitation may be applied by slowly tilting the bowl or operating the impeller at a low speed – either continuously or intermittently – throughout the drying stage. Caution must be exercised to avoid granule breakdown during drying, which may result in unfavorable compression characteristics [6]. Variables for vacuum drying include the level of vacuum maintained in the bowl, the jacket temperature and the degree of agitation. In addition to the parameters listed for vacuum drying, gas-assisted vacuum drying must also consider the type of drying gas used and its rate of delivery. When microwave vacuum drying is used, all of the variables used for vacuum drying are applicable, as well as the level of microwave power used to dry the granulation. If the yield is of greater importance than process time, a viable option is to follow the product and wall temperatures very closely and only use the applied microwaves as the source of drying energy. This mode of operation minimizes the amount of material sticking to the walls; however, it prolongs the drying operation and reduced the overall throughput. This option is of special interest for the processing of highly expensive materials.

If required, cooling can be conducted after the drying operation. The heated water or steam in the bowl jacket, which supplied conductive heat during the drying process, can be replaced with a glycol-water solution to provide a contact surface as low as 10 °C. Another way to cool the granulation is by purging a cooling gas into the single pot while agitating the granulation bed.

11.2.5 Sizing and Lubrication

Once the granulation is dried, it is usually necessary to size it. This may be accomplished by discharging the material through an inline mill into a receiving vessel in which it can be blended with any remaining excipients (e.g., a lubricant or flavor). This process design maintains the containment benefits of the single-pot process. Alternatively, the remaining excipients may be added to the single-pot processor and blended with the granulation before discharging and milling. This approach requires that the lubricant be adequately distributed during milling and material transfer during compression.

11.3 DRYING METHODS FOR SINGLE-POT PROCESSORS

11.3.1 CONDUCTIVE DRYING

The bowls of single-pot processors are generally jacketed for temperature control, which minimizes condensation of the granulating solvent and assists with solvent evaporation during drying. As a result, conductive heating provided by the heat-jacketed lid and walls of the single pot contributes to the drying process. Its dependence on the transfer of heat through pharmaceutical powders, which are poor heat conductors, prevents its use as the sole mode of drying in single-pot processors. Equation (11.1) addresses the conductive drying component of solvent removal.

Heat transfer from the vessel walls to the granulation bed is governed by

$$Q = hS\Delta T \tag{11.1}$$

where
Q = the energy exchange
h = the exchange coefficient
S = the contact surface of the heated wall
ΔT = the temperature difference between the contact wall and the granulation.

The rate of drying can be facilitated either by increasing the contact area between the granulation and the vessel walls (which can be achieved by agitating the product or utilizing a tilting bowl) or by maximizing the temperature difference between the vessel walls and product (either through increasing the jacket temperature or maintaining the temperature of the product as low as possible during processing).

Equation (11.2) is a simple relation that may be of some value when scaling up processes using conductive heating [7].

$$\frac{t_b}{t_a} = \frac{(A/V)_a}{(A/V)_b} \tag{11.2}$$

where
t = drying time
A = heat transfer surface (m^2)
V = vessel working volume (m^3)
a = refers to pilot scale
b = refers to production scale.

This relation accounts for the ratio of the surface area of the jacketed bowl and the volume of the product requiring drying.

11.3.2 VACUUM DRYING

Single-pot processors using vacuum drying may be considered if the product must be dried at a low temperature (<40 °C), if solvent recovery is required or if the potential for explosion is high. A vacuum is maintained within the vessel, thereby lowering the temperature at which the granulating solvent evaporates. Because vapors are removed from the processing bowl, vacuum drying provides a convenient means of solvent recovery.

De Smet [8] has discussed the theory, advantages, and limitations of vacuum drying. Aqueous granulations require a large amount of energy during drying, which is generally supplied by the transfer of heat through conduction from the jacketed bowl to the product. The amount of energy required for water removal is dependent on the level of vacuum applied to the vessel and the osmotic pressure of dissolved substances. As additional material dissolves in the water, the osmotic pressure increases, and additional energy is necessary to drive off the water. Therefore, as the material becomes drier, the amount of energy necessary to evaporate the water increases and the rate of evaporation slows. Processing times in vacuum dryers are often long, owing to the limited contact of the granulation with the heat from the jacketed walls and the slow rate of evaporation of the solvent from the interior of the granules.

The drying rate of the vacuum component is dependent on the following relation:

$$V = ks\Delta P \tag{11.3}$$

where
    V = evaporation rate
    k = rate coefficient
    s = total surface of granules
    ΔP = the vapor pressure difference between the granules and the surrounding space.

The rate of drying can be facilitated by increasing the level of vacuum (decreasing the pressure within the bowl) to increase the differential between the granule and the bowl vapor pressure. Figure 11.5 is a typical drying curve for a vacuum drying process. When the moisture content of the granulation is high, the rate of drying is constant because solvent evaporation from the product surface occurs readily. As the level of moisture on the granule surface decreases, water must migrate from the interior of the granule before evaporation. As a result, the rate of evaporation progressively decreases.

During vacuum drying, several problems can arise. For example, granule damage may occur owing to excessive attrition as the bed is agitated during drying. Vacuum systems should contain adequate filtering or blowback to prevent the loss of granulation "fines" through the vacuum line, which may compromise the drug uniformity within the processed batch.

A condenser positioned between the processor and the vacuum pump should always be used, especially for granulations manufactured using organic solvents. The condensate must be sufficiently cooled to prevent it from being released into the atmosphere. Also, filters may become blocked owing to condensation forming on the filter or the entrapment of solid particles. The blockage of the filters reduces the level of vacuum that can be pulled on the bowl and puts the pump under excessive strain.

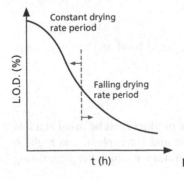

FIGURE 11.5 Typical vacuum drying curve.

11.3.3 Gas-Assisted Vacuum Drying

Accelerating the drying process in vacuum dryers is often limited by the characteristics of the product or equipment. Bowl temperature is generally defined by the physicochemical stability of the product, which can limit the use of higher temperatures to expedite drying. Increasing the contact area between the product and the vessel is difficult without significantly altering the design of the equipment. Excessive agitation of the product can lead to considerable granule attrition, which can result in poor granulation flow and compression properties.

Gas-assisted vacuum drying improves the efficiency of single-pot processors that use vacuum drying by continuously introducing a small stream of gas through the granulation to facilitate solvent removal. Drying continues at lower temperatures (compared with tray and fluid-bed drying), but at shorter processing times than vacuum drying alone and with the capability of reaching lower moisture contents.

The gas may be introduced into the unit through openings in the bottom of the vessel or through the mixing blades (Figure 11.6). Compressed air or nitrogen (mixed with or without air) are commonly used gases for these units. The rate of gas flow and the level of vacuum applied to the bowl can be adjusted for a specific product to optimize the drying conditions.

The introduction of gas into a vacuum chamber facilitates the drying process through several actions. The constant flow of gas through the product improves the transport of moisture from the product to the vacuum solvent recovery system [9]. Introducing gas into the bowl also increases the vapor pressure driving force [10]. The pressure gradient across the vessel is increased, resulting in a reduction in the rate at which water molecules recombine and increasing the net rate of evaporation. This causes the product temperature to be reduced, which increases the temperature differential between the granules and the bowl wall. The gas also reduces drying time by increasing the heat transfer coefficient from the bowl to the bed. In addition to improving the heat transport through the bed, the gas can reduce or eliminate product sticking to the sides of the vessel walls because it improves flow and dries the particle surfaces more quickly. As the vessel wall is the only notable source of drying energy, this technology is best used in case of

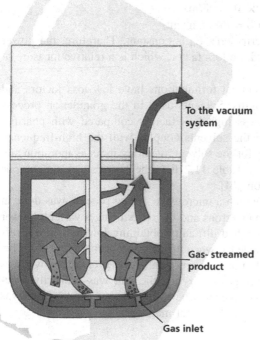

To the vacuum system

Gas- streamed product

Gas inlet

FIGURE 11.6   Gas-assisted vacuum drying principle. *Source*: Courtesy of GEA Group, Wommelgem, Belgium.

- small batch sizes (good surface-to-volume ratio)
- heat-insensitive materials (allows operation at a higher wall temperature)
- organic solvents (require only a fraction of the energy that water needs for evaporation). Additionally, the boiling temperature corresponding to the actual vacuum level is much lower for organic solvents than for water, generating a larger temperature difference between the product bed and the vessel.

11.3.4 MICROWAVE VACUUM DRYING

High-shear granulators with microwave vacuum drying capabilities provide the fastest drying rates in the single-pot processor family. Microwave drying is based on the absorption of electromagnetic radiation by dielectric materials, the theory of which has been extensively described [11–13]. Microwaves are a form of electromagnetic energy that are similar to radio waves, the frequencies of which fall between 300 and 3000 MHz (between radio and optical waves, see Figure 11.7). The two frequencies allocated for domestic, scientific, medical, and industrial purposes are 915 and 2450 MHz. Pharmaceutical processors generally use 2450 MHz because this frequency is more desirable when used in conjunction with a vacuum. Single-pot processors incorporating microwave drying are constructed of stainless steel because the metal is a common reflector of microwave energy and retains the energy within the processing chamber. Teflon is essentially inert to microwaves, making it a suitable material for components required in the processing bowl (e.g., the windows through which microwaves enter the processing bowl).

The energy absorption of materials exposed to microwaves is described by Eq. (11.4) [12,13].

$$P = 2\pi f V^2 E_o E_r \tan \delta \qquad (11.4)$$

where
  P = the power density of the material (W/m^3)
  f = frequency (Hz)
  V = voltage gradient (V/m)
  E_o = dielectric permittivity of free space (8.85 × 10^{-12} F/m)
  E_r = dielectric constant of the material and tan δ = loss tangent.

For a constant electric field strength, V, the term $2\pi f V^2 E_o$ is constant. Therefore, the power absorbed is proportional to the term $E_r \tan \delta$, called the loss factor, which is a relative measure of how easily a material absorbs microwave energy.

Various materials commonly used in pharmaceutical formulations have low loss factors and only absorb microwave energy at high field strengths. Solvents used in the granulation process (water, ethanol, isopropanol, etc.), however, possess high loss factors compared with pharmaceutical powders [12]. The dipolar component of the solvents couples with the high-frequency electromagnetic field to produce high heating rates for the solvent, resulting in its evaporation and subsequent removal from the processing chamber. Table 11.2 lists the loss factors for various components in a typical pharmaceutical granulation [14].

Lucisano and Moss [15] performed a study in which a microwave drying process was done in two different processors, one using fixed-output magnetrons and the other using a variable-power magnetron. The unit using fixed-output magnetrons had difficulty obtaining low moisture levels (<0.3%) because the E-field safety set point was exceeded when the moisture went below 1%. This problem did not occur for the unit using the variable-power magnetron because forward power was reduced as the E-field increased. During the late stages of drying, the unit was primarily functioning as a vacuum dryer, as the amount of microwave energy being introduced into the bowl was minimal. Nowadays, most microwave dryers use variable-output magnetrons.

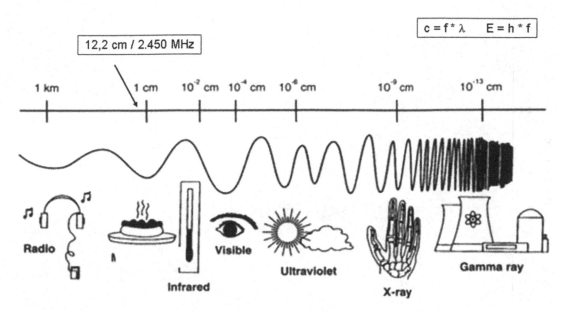

$$c = f * \lambda \qquad E = h * f$$

FIGURE 11.7 The electromagnetic spectrum.

The use of a vacuum during microwave drying lowers the temperature at which the solvent volatilizes, thereby limiting the temperature to which the material is exposed. For example, at a vacuum of 45 mbar, water-based granulations will dry at approximately 31 °C. Once most of the water is removed from the process, the temperature of the material will rise as components in the mixture with lower loss factors start to absorb the microwaves. If too much vacuum is applied to the system, there is a potential for granule breakdown owing to the excessive pressure between the core and surface of the granules. Microwaves are typically applied in a vacuum range of 30–100 mbar. Introducing microwaves into a less than 30 mbar vacuum risks ignition of the surrounding atmosphere, a condition known as "arcing."

Control of the drying process is achieved through the simultaneous measurement of product temperature, forward power, and reflected power. Figure 11.8 depicts the level of microwave forward power, microwave reflected power and product temperature at various times during the drying process. During the initial stage, the product temperature remains relatively constant as the free solvent is preferentially evaporated and the reflected power remains relatively low. The amount of vacuum applied to the bowl and, to a lesser extent, the bowl jacket temperature will affect the actual product

TABLE 11.2
Loss Factors for Typical Pharmaceutical Ingredients

Pharmaceutical Ingredient	Loss Factor at 20 °C
Lactose	0.02
Mannitol	0.06
Microcrystalline cellulose	0.15
Corn starch	0.41
Isopropanol	2.9
Water	6.1
Ethanol	8.6

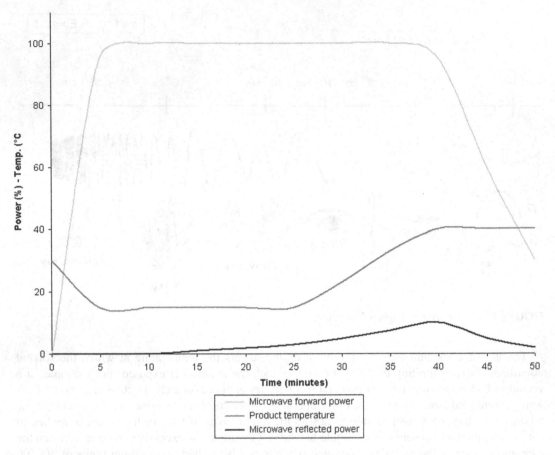

FIGURE 11.8   Relationship between microwave forward power, microwave reflected power, and product temperature during microwave vacuum drying.

temperature observed. As drying progresses at a constant rate of forward power, the amount of absorbed energy decreases as the material dries, thereby increasing the amount of free energy. As the free energy increases, a corresponding increase in the reflected power is also observed.

The rise in reflected power is accompanied by an increase in product temperature, which is simultaneously monitored while the magnetron output power is reduced. This is necessary because the loss factors for some pharmaceutical components are so small that very low moisture levels can be achieved before the temperature rises. For such materials, the reflected power can rise sharply once most of the solvent has evaporated, resulting in significant temperature gains.

The rise in temperature and reflected power signifies that the end of the drying process is approaching. Several factors, such as the loss factors of the formulation components, microwave power and the solvent retention properties of the solids, influence the point at which the previous relation will occur. For example, lactose has a low loss factor and shows a sharp rise in reflected power, followed by a slow temperature rise. Conversely, starch has a high loss factor and de-monstrates a fast temperature rise followed by a slow rise in reflected power.

One of the concerns often raised when considering microwave drying for pharmaceutical compounds is the stability of the product. However, experience has shown that the stability of pharmaceutical granulations dried by microwaves is comparable with that provided by alternative methods. Microwaves are nonionizing and do not possess the amount of energy required for the formation of free radicals or the liberation of bound-water conditions that foster product instability (Figure 11.7).

Since the introduction of microwave drying at the end of the 1980s, numerous new and supplemental drug applications that include the use of microwave vacuum drying of wet granulations have been approved by the US Food and Drug Administration (FDA). We are unaware of any instance in which the FDA required additional stability or analytical testing beyond that normally required for other methods of manufacture. Mandal [16], Moss [17], and others [18,19] have also published or presented data showing the comparability of the physicochemical characteristics of a granulation dried in microwave processors versus tray dryers and fluid-bed dryers.

When microwaves were first introduced, some authors [20] concluded that microwave drying could not be generally recommended because of the inability to control the microwaves after they enter the drying cavity and the risk of unacceptable thermal damage to active substances with high loss factors (high dielectric constants). The routine production of pharmaceutical products by several installations of single-pot processors using microwave vacuum drying indicates that their general concerns can be addressed by the proper selection of formulation components and process parameters.

Another aspect to consider when introducing microwaves into a single-pot processor is the safety of the operator (related to the potential leakage of microwave energy). Industrial microwave processors are expected to meet the guidelines for microwave leakage specified by the Center for Devices and Radiological Health within FDA and by the American National Standards Institute [21,22]. The guideline is 1 mW/cm^2 maximum exposure at a frequency of 2450 MHz at a distance of 5 cm from any surface of the microwave cavity before purchase and 5 mW/cm^2 at any such point during its lifetime. Survey meters for the detection of microwave leakage are relatively inexpensive and should be purchased by users of single-pot processors that incorporate microwave drying. The survey meters are calibrated before shipment and returned to the supplier for recalibration at periodic intervals. Their use should be incorporated in standard operating procedures for the equipment. Operator readings that exceed the guideline limit are often indicative of deteriorating seals around the lid cavity.

In addition to energy leakage standards, microwave processors are designed with safety interlocks to prevent accidental exposure. For example, the magnetrons can be activated only if the microwave cavity (bowl of the processor) is operating under vacuum, usually 30–100 mbar. If the vacuum falls outside this range, as in the unlikely event that an operator inadvertently tries to open the lid during microwave vacuum drying, the magnetrons are disabled. Vendors also incorporate additional safeguards to ensure that microwave power is disabled when access to the bowl is required.

Because of popular misconceptions about the use of microwave ovens (e.g., stainless steel should not be used in a microwave cavity) and electromagnetic radiation (all types cause biological effects), a training program should be instituted in any facility that uses microwave drying. This will demystify any unfounded concerns about the technology and foster a rational approach to a sound safety and maintenance program.

11.3.5 FLUID-BED DRYING

For more than 50 years, fluid-bed drying has been a standard drying process in the pharmaceutical industry. It is an excellent method for the controlled, gentle, and even drying of wet solids. The intensive heat/mass exchange of the fluidized bed product makes this method particularly effective and timesaving. With time, the design and performance of fluid-bed equipment have been significantly enhanced and the level of process understanding has improved. As this book contains a whole chapter on this technology (chapter 10), we will not go into detail here.

Recently, however, Glatt GmbH has fused high-shear technology with fluid-bed drying: the TwinPro*. After high-shear granulation is complete, the bottom of the granulator is slightly lowered, enabling fluidizing gas to enter the product. This thus allows gentle fluid-bed drying of the granulate without having to transfer it to another equipment, thus creating a single-pot processor [23].

11.4 APPLICATIONS

Because of the different technologies incorporated into a single-pot processor, it is capable of executing many different processes – apart from wet granulation and drying – and small modifications or additional options can extend the flexibility even further. This chapter discusses the main applications and some of the possible "special" processes that can take place in a single-pot processor. Although many of these processes are used in the pharmaceutical industry, scientific literature about them is rare. The main reason for this is that many of these processes were developed by the pharmaceutical industry as product-specific solutions. This does not imply, however, that these processes cannot be used more widely.

11.4.1 MAIN APPLICATIONS

11.4.1.1 Expensive Products

When producing expensive pharmaceutical products, the yield is one of the most important criteria to consider. Compared with the combination of a high-shear granulator and a fluid-bed dryer or even a fluid-bed spray granulator, a single pot has a much smaller surface area in contact with the product. Also, no fluidization with the associated risk of material sticking to the process filters happens. Should a processor equipped with microwaves be used, the microwave energy can be used to evaporate the granulation liquid while, at the same time, the wall temperature of the processor is kept close to that of the product, minimizing the amount of material that sticks to the processor wall. As a result, yields in excess of 99% can be realized.

11.4.1.2 Short Campaigns/Multiple Products

For multiproduct facilities with short campaigns, the changeover time between products and the exclusion of cross-contamination are two major factors to consider when selecting the production process. Both aspects are significantly influenced by the cleaning system provided on the equipment.

All single-pot processors on the market are equipped with a more or less extensive CIP system. Vendors have made a great effort to optimize their design and enable CIP procedures that can be validated [4]. The focus has been to eliminate any dead spots in the equipment where the cleaning water cannot reach and include cleaning spray balls in critical product contact areas, such as the product filter and discharge valve. Drying of the single-pot processor after the cleaning cycle to prepare the equipment for a subsequent batch can be done using the system's own vacuum drying system and jacketed bowl, making a separate drying unit redundant.

A nice case study of an evaluation of a CIP system on a pilot-scale single-pot processor is given in Ref. 4. In this study, it has been shown that a complete changeover from one product to the next can take place in less than two hours. Therefore, single-pot processors have a much shorter downtime compared with fluid-bed processors in terms of product changeover.

11.4.1.3 Highly Potent (Toxic) Products

One of the main drivers for the use of single-pot systems is the need to process potent substances such as hormones. Reasons for this are the small surface area in contact with the product (e.g., compared with a fluid bed), the tight execution of a single pot, the reduced risk of product entering the technical space (and thereby creating a risk for maintenance operators), the negative-pressure processing and the availability of a CIP system. As always, when dealing with potent substances, three main areas of concern exist, which are

- cleaning,
- loading and unloading the processor,
- sampling.

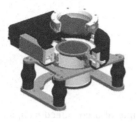
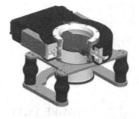
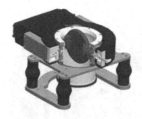

UNDOCKED AND CLOSED   DOCKED AND CLOSED   DOCKED AND OPEN

FIGURE 11.9   Functional principle of a split butterfly valve.
Source: Courtesy of GEA Group, Eastleigh, UK.

As already mentioned, modern single pots are equipped with CIP capabilities, eliminating the risk of exposure during the cleaning operation. For the loading and unloading of potent substances from and to up- and down-stream processes, split butterfly valves are commonly used. The functional principle of a split butterfly valve is shown in Figure 11.9.

Depending on their specification, split butterfly valves offer containment performances down to 20 ng/m^3 of airborne particles. To achieve the highest levels of containment, split valves can be fitted with dust extraction technology to remove any residual powders after the material transfer has occurred.

For small-scale batches or multiproduct facilities, there is a growing trend for single-use containment products, including single-use split valves and flexible bags with an integrated containment interface such as Hicoflex® (Figure 11.10). These single-use technologies can provide levels of containment that mirror those of traditional split butterfly valves. Additionally, as the Hicoflex® bags are transparent, operators can visibly check for full product transfer and can easily manipulate the bags to encourage product flow. Disposing of the bags eliminates the chance of cross-contamination and the need to validate container cleaning.

Although the use of process analytical technology (PAT) to eliminate sampling – as described in other chapters of this book – offers the most comprehensive approach when dealing with potent substances, it is also possible to sample in a contained manner. The BUCK® Sampler is based on the functional principle of split butterfly valves (Figure 11.11).

Hicoflex® functional description

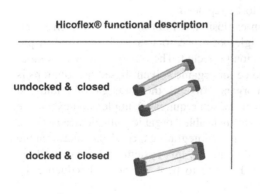

undocked & closed

docked & closed

docked & opened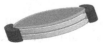

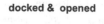

FIGURE 11.10   Functional principle of the Hicoflex® system.
Source: Courtesy of GEA Group, Eastleigh, UK.

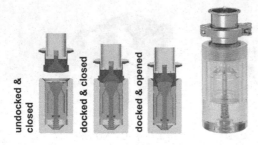

FIGURE 11.11   Principle of a contained sampler.
Source: Courtesy of GEA Group, Eastleigh, UK.

11.4.1.4   Organic Solvent Processing

Although there is a general trend in the pharmaceutical industry to replace organic solvents in granulation with water-based formulations, this is not possible for all products, because of their characteristics (e.g., instability of the active ingredient when in contact with water). The use of organic solvents in a granulation process poses specific challenges to the equipment, especially related to safety and environmental aspects.

The primary safety concern during the granulation and drying processes, especially when working with organic solvents, is the prevention of explosions. Bulk powder, dust clouds, and flammable vapors all have the potential to explode. Adequate grounding and ventilation during loading and discharging the vessel – and controlling the various processing conditions – can reduce the risk of explosion. In Europe, all equipment used in a potentially explosive atmosphere needs to be compliant with ATEX guidelines [24].

Two approaches are generally taken toward explosion protection in single-pot processors. One consists of removing oxygen from the processing chamber and replacing it with an inert gas (e.g. nitrogen) before any mixing takes place. The removal of oxygen reduces the risk of explosion by eliminating one of the necessary elements to create an explosion. Compared with a similar strategy of avoiding explosions in, for example, a fluid-bed processor, a single-pot processor will require minimal amounts of nitrogen. However, using nitrogen as a replacement gas also poses certain risks and requires some additional safety measures to be applied in the production and technical areas, such as oxygen sensors that warn the operators should the oxygen level in the room becomes too low (owing to potential leakage of the nitrogen gas from the supply lines or the equipment).

The other approach is to design the equipment to contain the explosion. Examples of 10–16 bar compatible high-shear granulators and single-pot processors are now readily available on the market. The downside of this approach is that – should an explosion take place – the equipment will most likely be severely damaged and will need to be replaced.

Apart from the measures taken to avoid or contain explosions within the processing chamber, the electrical, electronic, and mechanical parts of single-pot processors that will be used in potentially explosive atmospheres also need to be explosion protected. The other reason why single-pot processors are often the production method of choice for organic solvent-based granulations is environmental considerations. When granulating with organic solvents, the outlet gas of a fluid-bed dryer will contain some grams of organic solvents per m³, which requires a complex and expensive treatment system; in a single-pot system, only the (condensable) organic solvent needs to be treated. This can be handled cost-effectively and efficiently by integrating a condenser between the processor bowl and the vacuum pump. When installed correctly, this system will remove all organic vapors from the exhaust air, thereby avoiding the need to treat the air and reducing the amount of waste to be treated (only the recovered solvent).

11.4.1.5   Effervescent Production

The production of effervescent tablets is, first of all, a conventional oral solid dosage form manufacturing process, which has to accommodate some unusual features because of the special characteristics of the product. For example, adding a "normal" amount of water for granulation would initiate the effervescent reaction in the granulator and deplete the effervescent power of the formulation.

To granulate effervescent products, many different production techniques can be used, ranging from dry granulation methods and two-step granulation (granulating the acid and alkali phases separately) to one-step granulation using water or organic solvents. The process is discussed in detail in Chapter 14 of this book. For the one-step granulation methods, the use of a single-pot processor offers many benefits. Apart from the overall advantage of eliminating product transfer between a granulator and a dryer, a single-pot processor allows for easy solvent recovery by condensation (if organic solvents have been used as the granulation liquid), compared with the quite complex system for the exhaust gas treatment required for a fluid-bed dryer (see earlier in the chapter).

When water is used as a granulation liquid for effervescents, the eponymous reaction will start and cause a chain reaction. The critical point in such a process is to stop this reaction at the correct time by evaporating the water that has been created. In a single-pot processor, this can be very easily and accurately achieved by switching on the vacuum drying system (possibly supplemented with gas-assisted drying or microwave drying) [25,].

11.4.2 OTHER APPLICATIONS

11.4.2.1 Melt Granulation

Melt granulation is a process in which the binder solution of the standard wet granulation process is replaced with a meltable binder, such as a wax or PEG, which is generally added in solid form and melted during the process by adding the necessary energy. Chapter 19 of this book discusses various methods of producing melt granulation in detail.

The most common production technique for melt granulation uses extruders, but melt granulation in a high-shear mixer has also been extensively described in the literature. In this process, the necessary energy to melt the binder is provided either by the mixer arm (mainly in laboratory scale equipment) or by a heated jacket [26,27,28]. If the meltable binder used absorbs microwaves (e.g., PEG), using a single-pot processor equipped with microwave drying can present major time savings to the production process.

Providing the melting energy by the impeller or the heated jacket can be a very time-consuming process, especially in production-scale equipment. Microwaves are an instant source of energy that penetrates the product and can provide the energy faster and immediately where needed. In a comparison between the use of the heated jacket to melt the binder (PEG 3000) and the use of a heated jacket supplemented with microwaves, the latter method not only proved to be more than twice as fast but also reduced the granulation time threefold [29], although this information was contradicted in another study [30]. More investigations are warranted on this topic.

Another step when a single-pot processor can present a major advantage compared with the standard production techniques, and especially compared with using a high-shear mixer, is cooling. To achieve a stable "dry" granule from a melt granulation process, the product needs to be cooled to room temperature. In a high-shear mixer, the cooling process is done by circulating cold water or a glycol-water mixture in the bowl jacket. As the contact surface between the product and the jacket is limited, the cooling process generally takes a long time. If the process is done in a single-pot processor equipped with a gas-assisted vacuum drying system, this configuration can be used to pass cold air or even liquid nitrogen through the product to aid the cooling process and reduce the cooling time considerably. If liquid nitrogen is used, even a fivefold reduction of the cooling time is achievable [29].

11.4.2.2 Pellet Production

For the production of spheres or pellets, in most cases, an extrusion/spheronization process is used.

There are, however, many references in the literature detailing the production of pellets using a high-shear mixer, most of which concern melt pelletization [27–29,31–34]. Considering the previous discussion regarding melt granulation, a single-pot processor can, of course, also be used for this process for the same reasons. Also, for other pelletization processes that don't involve meltable binders, the use of a single-pot processor can be advantageous. Several references describe the use of a high-shear mixer for such processes [35,36]; yet, so far, none can be found that refer to single-pot processors. Nevertheless, a standard pellet formulation often contains microcrystalline cellulose, which needs a high water content to obtain a good granule/pellet quality. Drying the pellets is always a part of the production process. The advantage of a single-pot processor is that the whole process of pelletization and drying can be done in the same equipment, making product transfers redundant and thereby reducing the risk of product loss and contamination and enhancing both containment and operator safety.

To enhance the pelletization/spheronization process, many vendors of high-shear mixers/single-pot processors offer special mixing tools to produce pellet-like granules. Depending on the geometry of the equipment, this special mixing tool has either more (up to six) or less (two) mixing blades than a standard mixing tool, which generally has three mixing blades (Figure 11.12). All special pellet-mixing tools have, however, the same purpose: to simulate the product behavior in a spheronizer and enhance the spheronization process that occurs in the mixer.

11.4.2.3 Crystallization

Although a high-shear mixer/single-pot processor is mainly intended for powder processing, it is possible to do crystallization or recrystallization processes in this type of equipment as well. Starting from either a solution or a powder that has been dissolved in a suitable solvent, the speed of the drying process can be controlled to achieve the desired crystallization process. Using vacuum drying only, the drying process will be slow and gradual. Temperatures during this process will remain low, creating an environment for slow crystal growth. When microwaves are used, the process will be considerably faster and the temperature of the product will most likely be higher than under "pure" vacuum conditions. The crystals that result from such a crystallization process will have different characteristics than those derived from vacuum drying. When choosing the appropriate settings for the drying/evaporation process, crystals with specific properties can be obtained by combining vacuum and microwave drying.

The main advantage of doing a (re)crystallizing process in a single-pot processor is that the possibility exists to granulate the product at the same time by varying the mixer speed during the drying process. The resulting product will be suitable for tableting without the necessity of executing other processing steps (apart from lubrication).

11.5 SCALE-UP OF DRYING PROCESSES

Because the rate of solvent removal during vacuum drying is dependent on a favorable surface area/volume ratio, the drying time in a vacuum processor often increases substantially during scale-up – as described by Eq. (2). Microwave vacuum drying is relatively insensitive to the surface area/volume ratio and does not suffer the same inefficiency as vacuum drying during the transition from the pilot- to the production-scale. Pearlswig et al. [37] reported successfully scaling a microwave vacuum drying process for a moisture-sensitive formulation that required a drying endpoint of less than 0.2%. The drying time remained within a 30–45-minute range throughout the scale-up from 15 kg (Vactron 75) to 300 kg (Vactron 600), whereas the time for vacuum drying increased threefold. After additional scale-up to 600 kg in a Vactron 1200, the drying time rose slightly to a 50–55-minute range. Poska [18] also reported attaining equivalent drying times when scaling-up in Spectrum processors ranging from a bowl size of 65–300 L. Figure 11.10 compares typical drying curves for a lactose-starch granulation prepared in single-pot processors using vacuum drying, gas-assisted vacuum drying or microwave vacuum drying. Although

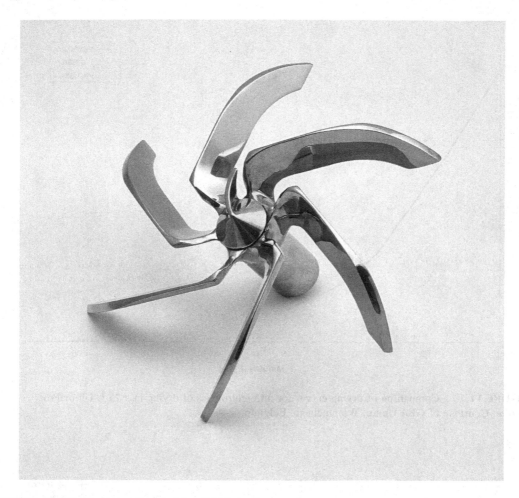

FIGURE 11.12 Example of a special pelletizing mixer arm.
Source: Courtesy of GEA Group, Wommelgem, Belgium.

not as rapid as microwave vacuum drying, gas-assisted vacuum drying can decrease the drying time by up to 50% compared with vacuum drying alone. As the wall of the vessel is the only source of drying energy in this example, the scale is of major importance for the drying time [38].

When performing feasibility trials on a development- or pilot-scale single-pot processor, it is important to be aware of the maximum energy input capacity of the corresponding production-scale processor. In Figures 11.13 and 11.14, the drying times for each drying method in pilot-scale and production-scale single-pot processors are shown. Although for processors equipped with microwaves, the drying time is relatively independent of the scale, a significant increase in drying time is observed for vacuum and gas-assisted vacuum drying processes.

11.6 REGULATORY CONSIDERATIONS

Single-pot processors combine established technologies into a single piece of equipment and, in general, deserve no special regulatory consideration when using them to develop a new product or to manufacture an approved one. Robin and colleagues [6] surveyed eight European regulatory agencies in 1992 to determine the implications of converting from fluid-bed drying to microwave vacuum drying within a single-pot processor. The majority of the agencies required only process validation data and three suggested limited stability data (up to six months of accelerated data).

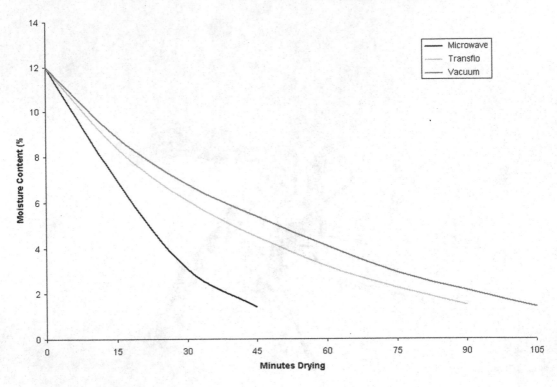

FIGURE 11.13   Comparison of drying curves for different modes of drying in a 75 L UltimaPro.
Source: Courtesy of GEA Group, Wommelgem, Belgium.

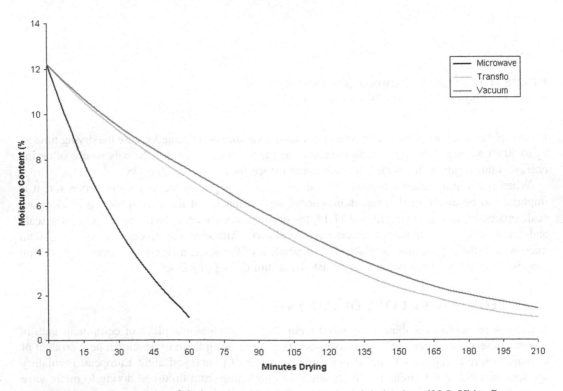

FIGURE 11.14   Comparison of drying curves for different modes of drying in a 600 L UltimaPro.
Source: Courtesy of GEA Group, Wommelgem, Belgium.

These requests were no different from those expected for similar types of manufacturing changes (e.g., changes in process or equipment).

Manufacturers considering converting to a single-pot process for an immediate release, oral solid dosage form (tablets, capsules, or similar) with an approved manufacturing process should consult their appropriate regulatory agencies governing the practices they use to manufacture their products. For drug products sold in the United States, manufacturers should refer to FDA's SUPAC IR Guidance document [39] that addresses scale-up and post-approval changes for marketed products. This document describes the levels of change that may be made in a manufacturing process and equipment. It outlines the chemistry, manufacturing and control (CMS) tests and documentation for each level of change, as well as the appropriate regulatory filing (Annual Report, Prior Approval Supplement or other).

Take, for example, a tablet formulation that's currently granulated using a high-shear granulator and dried in a tray dryer. The drug manufacturer wishes to replace this process with a single-pot processor that incorporates high-shear granulation and gas-assisted vacuum drying. This conversion would be viewed as a change in equipment to a different design and operating principles (defined as a Level 2 equipment change in the SUPAC IR Guidance document). Such a change requires the manufacturer to submit a Prior Approval Supplement, with up to three batches with three-month accelerated stability data (depending on the duration of commercial experience with the product). The submission would also require updated batch records, including the new equipment and the generation of multipoint dissolution profiles. The requirements for this conversion are, however, the same as those for swapping from a tray dryer to a fluid-bed drying process.

11.7 VALIDATION OF SINGLE-POT PROCESSORS

Because single-pot processors combine standard engineering approaches into a single processor, their validation should pose no special problems. Other sources adequately describe the validation of granulating and drying processes [40], although validating the microwave drying system and process control/monitoring of the drying endpoint deserve special mention.

For the operational qualification of microwave components, such as forward and reflected power, and arc detection, we suggest that customers contact the vendors because of the specialized nature of microwave systems. The cost associated with the calibration equipment is difficult to justify; microwave systems should operate reliably following proper set-up and qualification, and require no more periodic maintenance than other granulation approaches.

When microwave processors were first introduced, there was the expectation that E-field would be a reliable indicator of the drying endpoint. With experience, users found that the E-field tends to be too variable; most now view it as a safety feature that monitors the microwave field within the drying cavity. Most microwave dryers on the market today do not even include E-field monitoring anymore because of the associated validation difficulties.

Product temperature, time, cumulative forward power, and reflected power are proving to be more reliable indicators of the drying endpoint – with verification by some in-process control that directly measures the moisture content of a product sample. The industrial processes in operation today all use one of these approaches for endpoint determination. With the pharmaceutical industry moving toward the use of PAT; however, equipment vendors are also investigating the possibility of applying this concept to single-pot processors and thereby eliminating the necessity to take product samples.

11.8 PROCESS ANALYTICAL TECHNOLOGY

As PAT will be discussed extensively in other chapters of this book, the main focus of this chapter is to outline the areas of application of PAT in a single-pot processor. The goal of PAT is to gain better process understanding, resulting in optimized process control and, eventually, real-time product release by means of online monitoring and the measurement of critical quality attributes (CQAs). The product characteristics that are critical during single-pot processing are

- homogeneity of the active in the powder mixture,
- particle size distribution of the granules, which is significantly influenced by the distribution of liquid and binder, and
- moisture content of the product after drying.

Most single-pot processors are equipped with a number of "standard" measuring techniques that give an indication about these CQAs, such as product temperature and mixer torque or power, but these are not direct measurements on the CQAs themselves.

More advanced online measuring techniques can also be integrated to monitor and measure these characteristics. One of the most promising techniques to use in a single-pot processor is near infrared (NIR) spectroscopy, as it can be used during different stages of the single-pot process: during dry mixing, NIR is used to monitor blend homogeneity, whereas, during drying, the same probe—using a different analysis algorithm—can be used to monitor moisture content.

Other techniques have been reported for measuring granulate quality during the high-shear granulation process, such as power consumption, Raman spectroscopy, capacitance measurements, microwave measurements, imaging, focused beam reflectance measurements, spatial filter velocimetry, stress and vibration measurements, as well as acoustic emissions [41,42].

Some specific points of attention, when applying PAT measurements to single-pot processing, are as follows:

- The powders in a single-pot processor move at a high speed during the process; the chosen monitoring method should have the capability to meet this speed to make the necessary snapshots needed to show the changes taking place in the process
- During the wet granulation process, the product goes through different degrees of wetness; most products become sticky during one or more of these stages and this can obscure the optical sensors and lead to false measurements, so an inline cleanable system is advised
- Containment is often a reason to adopt single-pot processing; when applying NIR as a PAT measurement tool, it is good practice to take a baseline before every batch; as this is done by placing a white standard in front of the sensor, a problem may occur with containment unless a system is chosen that can take the white reference spectrum including the whole optical path without breaking containment.

To assist you with developing PAT techniques for single-pot processors, many equipment vendors now have application labs in which single-pot processors are equipped with PAT ports and tools and where specialists can assist.

11.9 CONTROL SYSTEMS AND DATA ACQUISITION SYSTEMS

Users of single-pot processors may use one or all of its processing features (mixing, granulating, drying, or others). The accompanying data acquisition system must collect, display, and record the relevant processing conditions and granulation behavior for each cycle. The degree of sophistication of the system may depend on the location in which the processor is used (Figure 11.15).

In a development setting, the sequence of cycles is often interrupted to collect samples for analysis, and the user is interested in capturing as much information as possible to help define a suitable processor for a particular formulation. In many cases, the control system for a

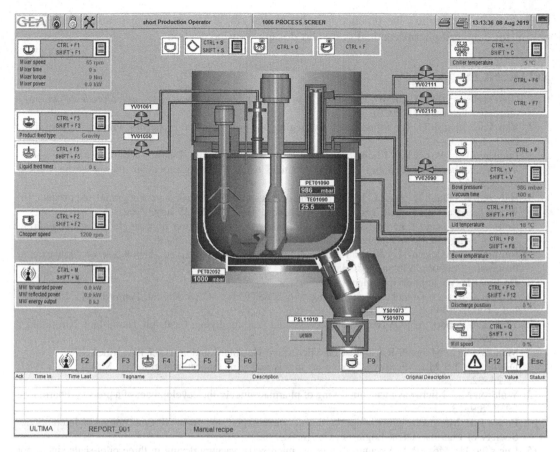

FIGURE 11.15 Screen of a typical control system for a single-pot processor.
Source: Courtesy of GEA Group Wommelgem, Belgium.

development environment can be limited to a manual control system. The data acquisition system, however, needs to be more sophisticated to be able to register all the relevant process data.

In production, the manufacturing sequence and process parameters are predefined and validated, and information needs are reduced to monitoring critical parameters. In these settings, an automatic control system with recipes to reduce operator intervention is indispensable. The data acquisition system may or may not be as sophisticated as the one used in development settings, depending on the batch record data requirements.

For troubleshooting and trend analysis, however, the information requirements of development and production converge, and data acquisition systems for single-pot processors should seek to address the needs of both types of users.

All data acquisition systems are considered to generate electronic records. If these electronic records are used as batch documentation, the acquisition system needs to be compliant with FDA 21 CFR part 11. Most vendors have addressed these issues by including password control, audit trails and point verification systems.

11.10 CONCLUSION

During the past 40 years since its introduction, single-pot processing has developed into a mature and generally accepted production technique. Even if, historically, the technology was used because of its specific advantages for effervescent production, potent compounds, organic solvents, or multiproduct facilities, the practice has shown that single-pot processing is also an attractive option for standard pharmaceutical oral solid dosage form production.

REFERENCES

1. Glatt website 2020. TwinPro® The fusion of two batch processes. www.glatt.com/en/products/twinpror/ (accessed February 21, 2020).
2. Van Vaerenbergh G. The influence of a swinging bowl on granulate properties. Pharm. Technol. Eur. 2001; 13(3):36–43.
3. Lucisano L.J., Poska R.P. Microwave technology-fad or the future. Pharm Technol 1990; 14:38–42.
4. Van Vaerenbergh G. Cleaning validation practices using a one-pot processor. Pharm Technol 2004; 16(2):26–34.
5. Hapgood K., Plank R., Zega J., Use of dimensionless spray flux to scale up a wet granulated product. In: World Congress on Particle Technology 4, Sydney, Australia, 21–25 July, 2002.
6. Robin P., Lucisano L.J., Pearlswig D.M. Rationale for the selection of a single pot manufacturing process using microwave/vacuum drying. Pharm Technol 1994; 18:28–36.
7. Bellini G., Pellegrini L. Non adiabatic drying. In: Goldberg E, ed. Handbook of Downstream Processing. London: Chapman & Hall, 1993.
8. De Smet P. Vacuum drying. Manuf Chem 1989; 37–39:37.
9. Technical Report. Granulation and drying with SYSTEM-VAGAS. Bristol, Pennsylvania, LB Bohle, Inc., 19007. 1996.
10. Technical Report. AEROVAC system, accelerated vacuum drying. Eastleigh, Hampshire, Niro-Fielder Ltd. 1993.
11. Metaxas A.C., Meredith R.J. Industrial Microwave Heating. London: Peter Peregrines, 1983.
12. Doyle C., Cliff M.J. Microwave drying for highly active pharmaceutical granules. Manuf Chem 1987; 78:23–32.
13. Waldron M.S. Microwave vacuum drying of pharmaceuticals: the development of a process. Pharm Eng 1988; 8:9–13.
14. Poska R.P. Microwave processing: the development experience revisited. Proceedings of International Society of Pharmaceutical Engineers Congress, 1992.
15. Lucisano U., Moss R.A. Vacuum drying vs. microwave-vacuum drying in three pilot-scale single pot processors using sodium acid pyrophosphate as the model granulation. AAPS Annual Meeting, San Antonio, Texas, 1992.
16. Mandal T.K. Evaluation of microwave drying for pharmaceutical granulations. Drug Dev Ind Pharm 1995; 21:1683–1688.
17. Moss R.A. Demonstration-microwave/vacuum drying of pharmaceuticals. AAPS Annual Meeting, Washington DC, 1991.
18. Poska R. Integrated mixing granulating and microwave drying: a development experience. Pharm Eng 1991; 11:9–13.
19. Van Scoik K. Microwave vacuum processing in the Vactron 300. AAPS Annual Meeting, Washington DC, November 1991.
20. Duschler G., Carius W., Bauer K.H. Single-step granulation method with microwaves: preliminary studies and pilot scale results. Drug Dev Ind Pharm 1995; 21:1599–1610.
21. U.S. Food and Drug Administration. Performance standards for microwave and radio frequency emitting products. 21 Code of Federal Regulations, Part 1030. General Services Administration, Washington, DC, April 1, 2008.
22. IEEE. IEEE standard for safety levels with respect to human exposure to electric, magnetic, and electromagnetic fields, 0 Hz to 300 GHz. In IEEE Std C95.1-2019 (Revision of IEEE Std C95.1-2005/ Incorporates IEEE Std C95.1-2019/Cor 1-2019): 1-312, 4 Oct. 2019.
23. Glatt 2018. Glatt combines high shear granulation with a fluid bed dryer. Manuf Chem. https://www. manufacturingchemist.com/news/article_page/Glatt_combines_high_shear_granulation_with_a_fluid_ bed_dryer/143958 (accessed February 21, 2020).
24. Eur-Lex. Directive 94/9/EC of the European Parliament and the Council of 23 March 1994 on the approximation of the laws of the member states concerning equipment and protective systems intended for use in potentially explosive atmospheres. https://eur-lex.europa.eu/legal-content/EN/ALL/?uri= celex:31994L0009 (accessed November 23, 2020).
25. Stahl H. Manufacturing effervescent tablets. Pharm Technol 2003; 15(4):25–28.

26. Schaefer T. Melt agglomeration with polyethylene glycols in high shear mixers. Thesis for doctoral degree in pharmacy. Copenhagen: The Royal Danish School of Pharmacy, 1996—.
27. Schaefer T., Holm P., Kristensen H.G. Melt pelletisation in a high shear mixer. I. Effects of process variables and binder. Acta Pharm Nord 1992; 4:133–140.
28. Schaefer T., Mathiesen C. Melt pelletisation in a high shear mixer. IX. Effects of binder particle size. Int J Pharm 1996; 139:139–148.
29. Van Vaerenbergh G. Melt granulation with polyethylene glycol in a one-pot processor. Internal document, GEA Pharma Systems, available upon request.
30. Loh Z.H., Sia B.Y., Heng P.W., Lee C.C., Liew, C.V. Evaluation of the physicochemical properties and compaction behavior of melt granules produced in microwave-induced and conventional melt granulation in a single pot high shear processor. AAPS PharmSciTech 2011; 12:1374.
31. Heng P.W., Wong T.W., Chan L.W. Influence of production variables on the sphericity of melt pellets. Chem Pharm Bull (Tokyo) 2000; 48:420–424.
32. Hamdani J., Moës A.J., Amighi K. Development and evaluation of prolonged release pellets obtained by the melt pelletization process. Int J Pharm 2002; 245:167–177.
33. Thies R., Kleinebudde P. Melt pelletisation of a hygroscopic drug in a high shear mixer. Part 1. Influence of process variables. Int J Pharm 1999; 188(2):131–143.
34. Voinovich D., Moneghini M., Perisutti B., Franceschinis E. Melt pelletization in high shear mixer using a hydrophobic melt binder: influence of some apparatus and process variables. Eur J Pharm Biopharm 2001; 52(3):305–313.
35. Vonk P., Guillaume C.P.F., Ramaker J.S., Vromans H., Kossena N.W.F. Growth mechanisms of high-shear pelletisation. Int J Pharm 1997; 157(1):93–102.
36. Ramaker J.S., Albada Jelgersma M., Vonk P., Kossen N.W.F. Scale-down of a high-shear pelletisation process: flow profile and growth kinetics. Int J Pharm 1998; 166(1):89–97.
37. Pearlswig D.M., Robin P., Lucisano L.J. Simulation modeling applied to the development of a single-pot process using microwave/vacuum drying. Pharm Technol 1994; 18:44–60.
38. Stahl H. Single pot systems for drying pharmaceutical granules. Pharm Technol Eur 2000; 12(5):23–34.
39. FDA. Immediate release solid oral dosage forms: scale-up and postapproval changes: chemistry, manufacturing, and controls; in vitro dissolution testing; in vivo bioequivalence documentation; guidance. Fed Reg 1995; 60:61638–61643.
40. Berry I.R., Nash R.A., eds. Pharmaceutical Process Validation. New York: Marcel Dekker, 1993.
41. Faure A., York P., Rowe R.C. Process control and scale-up of pharmaceutical wet granulation processes: a review. Eur J Pharm Biopharm. 2001;52(3):269–277.
42. Hansuld E.M., Briens L. A review of monitoring methods for pharmaceutical wet granulation. Int J Pharm. 2014;472(1–2):192–201.

12 Extrusion/Spheronization as a Granulation Technique

David F. Erkoboni

CONTENTS

12.1   INTRODUCTION

Extrusion/spheronization is a multi-step process capable of producing uniformly sized spherical particles. The shaped particles can have many uses within the framework of pharmaceutical drug delivery. This chapter will discuss the use of the process as a granulation method for use in producing free-flowing spherical granules. Its first [1] and third [2] editions were written by Erkoboni [1] and the second edition was written by Mehta, Rekhi, and Parikh [3].

The extrusion/spheronization process is widely utilized in the pharmaceutical industry. Its primary use is as a method of producing multi-particulates or multiple units for use in immediate or controlled-release applications. In immediate-release applications, multiple units in a dosage form can readily disperse throughout the gastrointestinal (GI) tract. They can also improve the dissolution of poorly soluble drugs, depending on excipient composition, as indicated by A. Dukieć-Ott et al. [4]. In controlled-release applications, the release is typically controlled through the application of a rate controlling membrane or coating, as demonstrated by T. Maejima et al. [5], or by the use of polymer diffusion or erosion type matrix, as shown by H. Kranz et al. [6] and K. A. Mehta et al. [7], respectively.

As pharmaceutical dosage units, pellets are defined as small, free-flowing, spherical or semi-spherical particles made up of fine powders or granules of bulk drugs and excipients by a variety of processes, extrusion-spheronization being one. The major advantage of extrusion/spheronization over other methods of producing drug-loaded spheres, pellets, or granules is the ability to incorporate high levels of active components without producing excessively large particles. This is critical to the production of pharmaceutically acceptable free-flowing spherical granules, as well as the pellets used for the more typical applications. Heilman et al. showed that pellets having a drug loading level of 80% can be produced reproducibly [8].

The process is more efficient than other techniques for producing spheres or pellets for controlled release dosage forms; however, it is more labor and time-intensive than the more common granulation techniques. Therefore, it should be considered as a granulating technique when the essential particle properties cannot be produced using more conventional techniques. Pharmaceutical development scientists have been able to use this processing method more easily and reliably due to advances made in equipment as well as an ever-expanding material and process understanding.

Extrusion/spheronization equipment engineering has made the equipment simpler to use. Formulation and process work conducted at academic institutions as well as in industry has progressed the understanding of the manufacturing process thus making it simpler to use. Pellets or spherical granular particles offer scientists a great deal of development flexibility. Chemically incompatible ingredients, for instance, can be incorporated into a single capsule using multiple pellet types, each containing one of the incompatible ingredients. Similarly, incompatible ingredients can be compressed into a tablet by coating spherical particles containing the ingredients with an immediate release barrier coat before blending them with other ingredients. Pellets of different release characteristics can be combined to achieve the desired release pattern of the active ingredients. Pellets or spherical granules are characterized by a low surface-area-to-volume ratio compared with powder or granules, which provides an excellent coating substrate.

Typically, pellets range in diameter between 0.25 and 1.5 mm. They are normally filled into hard gelatin capsules, or eventually compressed into tablets, which can disintegrate into individual pellets after oral administration. Granules produced by extrusion/spheronization can have a more narrow size distribution, higher density, and more spherical shape than granules produced using conventional techniques. These properties, when needed, can have significant advantages over more typical granule properties. They can also have undesirable effects if, for instance, the granules flow too well, or if the density is high enough to impede compression or cause segregation. These issues are discussed here.

Spheronization is a process invented by Nakahara in 1964. The patent describes a "Method and Apparatus for Making Spherical Granules" from wet powder mixtures [9]. The equipment described in the patent was commercialized by Fuji Denki Kogyo Co. under the trade name Marumerizer[®]. The process went widely unnoticed in the pharmaceutical industry until 1970 when two articles were published by employees of Eli Lilly and Co. Conine and Hadley described the steps involved in the process including (1) dry blending, (2) wet granulation, (3) extrusion, (4) spheronization, (5) drying, and (6) screening (optional) [10]. Reynolds went on to further describe the equipment and the mechanics of the process including the movement of the particles within the spheronizer [11]. Both publications cite desirable product attributes that can be achieved, including good flow, low dusting, uniform size distribution, low friability, high hardness, ease of coating, and reproducible packing. Additionally, the resulting pellets offer not only technological advantages, as mentioned before but also therapeutic advantages such as less irritation of the GI tract and a lowered risk of side effects due to dose dumping and reproducibility of the drug blood levels as demonstrated by K. A. Mehta et al. [12]. The interest in extrusion-spheronization has continued to grow from the time these articles were published through to today. Interest was initially driven by academia and the industry. Today the process has become a common approach to producing spheres and pellets for multi-particulate applications. The development of pellets for sprinkler type dosage forms are being developed for a pediatric population. The increased popularity in recent years is, in part, due to a growing understanding of the effects of process parameters and material characteristics. Vervaet et al. presented a thorough review of the various aspects of extrusion-spheronization [13].

Hot-melt extrusion (HME) and subsequent spheronization have gained academic and industrial attention with both sectors working to progress understanding of the critical formulation and process variables to control the process and produce a stable product. This process extension of extrusion-spheronization is being evaluated, and in some cases used, to solve some current issues, including solubilization of poorly soluble drugs. For pharmaceutical systems, this method has been used to prepare controlled release granules, readily deformable granules, effervescent granules, taste-masked granules, and granules-containing solid drug in polymer solutions or fine particle dispersion of drug facilitate solubilization. The bioavailability of the drug substance has been demonstrated to improve when it is dispersed at the molecular level using hot-melt extrusion. Several examples of melt-extruded molecular dispersions were presented by Breitenbach and Mägerlein [14].

Fully rounded spheres or pellets having similar properties for multi-particulate delivery systems can likewise be prepared, as demonstrated by C. R. Young et al. [15 and 16]. The advantage of HME is that it does not require the use of solvents or water and fewer processing steps are needed, making the process somewhat simpler, efficient, and continuous. The disadvantage of HME is that it may require greater understanding and typically employs high temperatures around and over 100 degrees centigrade as a requirement. Another possibility is the use of conventional extrusion after wet granulation with a low melting material, such as polyethylene glycol (PEG), incorporated. Once spheronized, the extrudate can be charged into a spheronizer with a jacketed bowl and spheronized with the jacket temperature at or above the melting point of the low melting material. This will soften or melt the low melting material, resulting in a more plastic mass, and allowing the forces during spheronization to round the particle. The resulting pellet can have immediate or sustained release depending on the low melting material used.

12.2 APPLICATIONS

There are many potential applications for spherical granules, including use in both immediate [4] and controlled release dosage forms [12]. S. Almeida-Prieto et al. discussed immediate and controlled release from pellets produced by extrusion/spheronization by adjusting the levels of various starches [17]. K. A. Mehta et al. showed that the use of polymer matrix systems prepared by extrusion spheronization could be used to achieve zero-order release with poorly soluble drugs [18]. R. Mallipeddi et al. demonstrated fine particle ethylcellulose could be used to produce well-formed spherical pellets containing water-soluble drugs [19]. The pellets or spherical particles resulted in immediate drug release. Granules such as these could be compressed into controlled release matrix tablets though, as shown by A. M. Agrawal et al. [20]. Effervescent dosage forms for rapid delivery can be prepared as well as taste-masked and chewable products. M. Repka et al. reviewed articles describing the use of hot melt extrusion to form effervescent granules as well as pelletization by spheronization [21]. P.C. Kayumba et al. discussed the taste-masking of pediatric dosage forms using coated pellets prepared by extrusion-spheronization [22].

Immediate and modified release of the poorly soluble drug can be achieved by preparing solid solutions, dispersing the drug in polymers, incorporating self-emulsifying systems, or solubility enhancers, such as emulsifiers, surfactants, and pH modifiers in the formulation. Hot-melt extrusion followed by warm temperature spheronization can be used to prepare rounded fine particles of solid dispersions or solid solutions, having a narrow size distribution [15]. Rapid cooling of the discharged pellets can help ensure the stability of the desired properties or state. This can be done by discharging into a bed of liquid nitrogen. The hot processing can be used to improve immediate release solubility as well as delay or sustain dissolution depending on the excipients used. This hot extrusion and spheronization process has advantages over using wet extrusion-spheronization to further process solid dispersions or solid solutions. Continued secondary wet processing of these materials can lead to an undesirable change in the properties or state of the dispersion or solution, resulting in a change in the target functionality. R. Jackowicz et al. compared dissolution from a powdered solid dispersion as compared to pellets, prepared using extrusion-spheronization from a similar physical mixture and solid dispersion. Dissolution from the powdered solid dispersion was faster and more complete than from the pellets [23].

M. Serratoni et al. demonstrated that the preparation of pellets containing drug dissolved in a self-emulsifying system results in improved dissolution. Further incorporation of a release controlling membrane can modulate the release [24]. I. Matsaridou et al. demonstrated the influence of surfactant hydrophobic-lipophobic balance (HLB) and oil/surfactant ratio on the properties of self-emulsifying pellets [25]. Bioadhesive granules or pellets can be formulated to enhance the absorption of drugs with a narrow absorption window. G.A. Awad et al. evaluated the use of bioadhesive pellets containing polyacrylic acids [26]. F.J.O. Varum et al. developed pellets for colonic delivery by coating bioadhesive pellets with an enteric coating [27].

Regardless of the application, the spherical granules can be filled into capsules or compressed into tablets. The applications or possible combinations are endless. Two or more actives can easily be combined in any ratio in the same dosage form. These combination products can contain actives that are incompatible or have varying release profiles. Immediate release and controlled release spheres or granules can be combined resulting in unique release profiles. Processed particles can be used as a method to limit drug migration. Physical characteristics of the active ingredients and excipients can be modified to improve physical properties and downstream processing. As an example, a low-density, finely divided active can be pelletized to increase density, improve flow, and limit dusting, as demonstrated by I.M. Jalal et al. [28]. Dense multi-particulates disperse evenly within the GI tract and can be used to prolong gastrointestinal transit times or improve tolerance of some compounds. The effect of density was investigated and discussed by M. Clarke et al. [29] and J.E. Devereus et al. [30]. Regardless of the application, care must be taken to achieve the required sphere or granule properties for the given application.

Pellets or spheres for controlled release coating applications likely have significantly different physical requirements than granules for compression. A product to be coated for controlled release should have a uniform size distribution, good sphericity, and surface characteristics as well as low friability. Once coated, the pellet should have the desired release characteristics. Additionally, if the coated pellets are to be compressed into tablets, they will require sufficient strength to withstand the forces of compression. Upon disintegration of the tablet, the individual spheres must retain their original release profile.

Physical properties such as flow, density, friability, porosity, and surface area are important for spherical granules intended for compression into tablets. The granules should have good deformation and bonding characteristics to form tablets with desirable physical properties. Drug release from the final dosage form must meet the target specification.

A product produced using extrusion-spheronization can range from barely shaped, irregular particles with physical properties similar to a conventional granulation to very spherical particles having properties that are drastically different. The targeted properties of the extruded and spheronized product should be determined by the requirements of the application. C.W. Woodruff et al. discussed the effect of process variables on the properties of particles produced by extrusion-spheronization [31]. Tableting characteristics can be modified by altering either (1) the composition of the spherical particles, as shown by J. P. Schwartz et al. [32], (2) the granulating fluid, as discussed by G. P. Millili et al. [33], (3) the physical characteristics as demonstrated by H. Santos et al. [34] and Salako et al. [35] or (4) the process conditions used to produce them as indicated by H.J. Malinowski et al. [36]. Compaction studies conducted on spheres similar to those used for controlled release applications show that the bonding and densification that occur during extrusion-spheronization can alter the deformation characteristics of some materials [33]. Microcrystalline cellulose (MCC), which deforms plastically in the dry powder state, exhibits elastic deformation followed by brittle fracture once spheronized after granulation with water [32]. The deformation characteristics, coupled with the larger size particles, result in reduced bonding sites and the production of weak compacts. A compaction profile of MCC and spheres prepared from MCC is shown in Figure 12.1.

The point is not to dwell on the properties required for each application, but rather to reinforce the fact that each application will have very specific requirements. One must first understand the

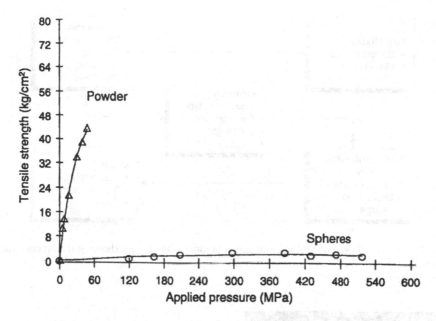

FIGURE 12.1 Compaction profiles of microcrystalline cellulose powder and spheres. *Source*: From Ref. [32].

properties required and then tailor the process to yield the desired effects. The effects of process and formulation variables are discussed here.

A review of the literature shows that most investigators have tried to understand small components of this process, isolated from other effects, focusing on the particular formulation or process parameters. It is valuable to have a detailed understanding of the main variables; however, this approach fails to take into consideration the high degree of interaction that exists between the variables. The use of statistical experimental design is a valuable tool to understand not only the main effects but also the interactions that can have a profound effect on the characteristics of the resulting particles. H.J. Malinowski et al. used a factorial design to determine the effect of spheronization process variables and evaluate granulations [36,37]. D.F. Erkoboni et al. determined the effect of process and formulation variables on sphere properties [38]. M. Chariot et al. used a factorial design to evaluate process variables [39] and K.K. Saripella et al. assessed the effect of formulation and process variable on the production of drug-loaded pellets [40]. Additionally, these techniques are extremely useful during product/process development or optimization to understand the effect of variables and control them to produce a product having the desired attributes [8].

After pointing out the benefits of design methodology in this application, it should be understood that, for simplicity, much of the discussion to follow will address the various topics individually. In reality, however, they truly cannot be isolated from one another. The remainder of this chapter will review and discuss the general process, the equipment types, and the effect of process and formulation variables on the properties of spherical granules.

12.3 GENERAL PROCESS DESCRIPTION

Extrusion-spheronization is a multi-step process typically requiring at least five units of operation with an optional sixth screening step. First, the materials are dry mixed (1) to achieve a homogeneous powder dispersion and then wet granulated and (2) to produce a sufficiently plastic wet mass. The wet mass is extruded (3) to form rod-shaped particles of a uniform diameter that are

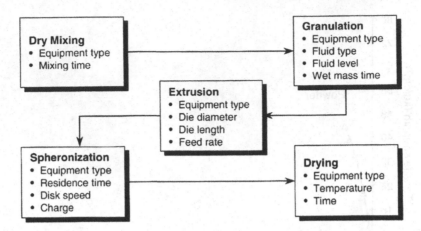

FIGURE 12.2 Process flow chart of the extrusion-spheronization process showing the process variables for each individual step.
Source: Ref. [41].

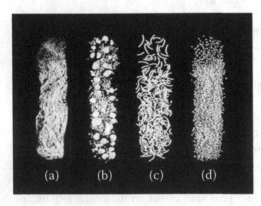

FIGURE 12.3 A product produced by the first four extrusion-spheronization process steps. (a) Powder from dry mixing (b) Granules from granulation (c) Extrudate from extrusion and (d) Spheres from spheronization.

charged into a spheronizer and rounded off (4) into spherical particles. The spherical particles are then dried (5) to achieve the desired moisture content and optionally screened (6) to achieve a targeted size distribution. In a modification to the process, hot-melt processing does not require a separate granulation step, as the granulation occurs during the hot extrusion. Additionally, cooling replaces the drying step.

The process flow diagram, shown in Figure 12.2, has been used by R.E. O'Conner et al. to show each of the process steps along with critical variables associated with them [41]. The end product from each of the steps is shown in Figure 12.3.

12.4   EQUIPMENT DESCRIPTION AND PROCESS PARAMETERS

12.4.1   DRY MIXING

During the first step, powders are dry mixed to achieve a uniform dispersion prior to wet granulation. It is generally carried out in the same mixer used for the granulation; however, if a continuous granulator (or hot-melt extruder) is used, a separate mixer may be required for the dry mix. This step is typically taken for granted because wet massing follows. The uniformity of the dry mix, however, can have a significant effect on the quality of the granulation and, in turn, the spherical particles produced. Uneven distribution of materials having wide differences in properties such as size and solubility can result in localized over-wetting, at least initially, during the granulation step. The more soluble and finely divided components can also dissolve and become part of the granulating fluid. The fluids, rich in soluble compounds, can either remain as overwet regions or, with continued wet massing, can be redistributed. J.E. Ojile et al. discuss the effect of drug distribution during wet massing on granule uniformity [42]. Sphere or granule uniformity (size and shape) is very much dependent on the uniform distribution and composition of the granulating fluid, which includes not only the solvent but any dissolved ingredients.

12.4.2 GRANULATION

The second step is granulation, during which a wet mass having the requisite plasticity or deformation characteristics is prepared. With a few exceptions, this step is similar to conventional granulation techniques used to produce products for compression. It is typically carried out in a batch-type mixer/granulator; however, any equipment capable of producing a wet mass, including the continuous type, can be used. Batch type processors include planetary mixers, vertical and horizontal high shear mixers, and sigma blade and ribbon mixers. An example of a continuous mixer is a continuous high shear twin screw mixer/extruder, which was studied by P. Kleinebudde et al. [43], C. Schmidt et al. [44] and A. Kumar et al. [45]. The high shear twin screw mixer/ extruders have mixer/feeders, which are capable of shearing and kneading the feed materials. Dry powders and fluids are fed in through separate ports and mixed by the action of the extruder blades and screws. The mixer/extruder can be configured to customize the amount of shear and energy used in the process by changing the configuration of the mixing blades. This can have an impact on the properties of the extrudate produced as demonstrated by N.O. Lindberg et al. [46]. As with the batch processors, it is critical to achieving a uniform level of fluid within the wet mass. The proper fluid/solids ratio is accomplished by maintaining a steady powder and fluid feed into the mixer/ extruder. Both are critical; however, the powder feed is the most problematic. Small variations in feed rates can cause significant shifts in the fluid content of the granulation and, therefore, the quality of the spherical particles produced.

The two major differences in the granulation step for extrusion/spheronization, as compared to typical granulations for compression, are the amount of granulating fluid required and the importance of achieving uniform dispersion of the fluid. The amount of fluid needed to achieve pellets or spheres of uniform size and sphericity, using extrusion-spheronization, is likely to be greater than that for a conventional high-shear granulation intended for tableting. The less size uniformity required for the application, the closer the fluid level should be to a conventional granulation. Instruments have been used to characterize the flow characteristics of granulations for use in extrusion-spheronization such as a ram extruder as used by Harrison et al. [47] and a torque rheometer as used by Landin et al. [48]. They are useful tools in quantifying the rheological effect of formulation and process variations in the granulation. The ram extruder has been used to characterize the flow of wet masses through a die as shown by Baert et al. [49]. Granulation flow has been divided into stages. They are (1) compression, where the materials are consolidated under slight pressure, (2) steady-state flow, where the pressure required to maintain flow is constant, and (3) forced flow, where an increase in force is required to maintain flow. The three stages are shown in the force versus displacement profile in Figure 12.4. The change from steady-state to forced flow is caused by the movement of fluid under pressure. Extrusion in a ram extruder is continuous, and this phenomenon is less likely to be seen in extruders that are discontinuous such as gravity-fed models. A diagram of a ram extruder is shown in Figure 12.5.

Regardless of the mixer used, one must remember that the downstream process steps of extrusion and spheronization are very dependent on the level of granulating fluid contained in the granulation and the quality of its dispersion. Over or under-wet granulations can cause an abundance of coarse or fine particles, respectively, while uneven wetting can cause a high degree of variation in particle size within the batch over the processing period. High-energy mixers such as

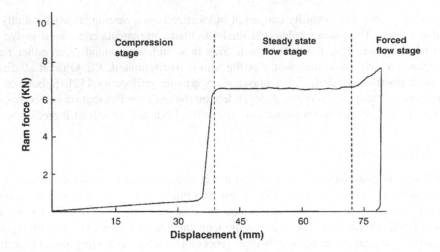

FIGURE 12.4 A force-displacement profile for a microcrystalline cellulose-lactose-water mixture showing the three stages of extrusion on a ram extruder: compression, steady-state flow, and forced flow (ram speed: 4 mm/sec; die diameter: 1.5 mm; L/R ratio: 12).
Source: From Ref. [50].

high-shear mixers and high-shear twin screw mixer/extruders can cause a significant rise in temperature within the wet mass. It may be necessary to use a jacket to guard against heat build-up. High temperatures can result in a greater than tolerable level of evaporation or an increase in the solubility of some of the solids as demonstrated by L. Baert et al. [49,51]. A reduction in a fluid

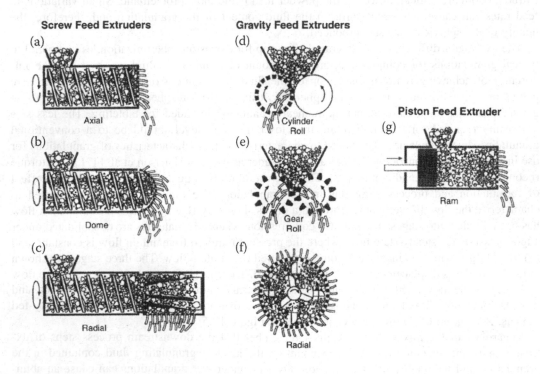

FIGURE 12.5 Schematic diagrams of extruder types used in extrusion-spheronization.

will reduce the plasticity of the granulation. This will likely cause a finer, more porous, less dense, less uniform, and less spherical granulation to be produced. The objective of downstream processing will determine if some of these effects are desirable or not. If the effects of less fluid are desirable, it is better to add less fluid, control the environmental conditions, and understand the effects of process variables, such as speed and time. If the effects of less fluid are undesirable, greater fluid and effective use of process variables to control the process are again necessary.

An increase in the solubility of the drug due to an increase in temperature will increase the weight ratio of granulating fluid to solids since the solute is then part of that fluid. C.C. Ku et al. demonstrated that the temperature of the granulating fluid had a significant effect on the size distribution of pellets or spherical granules produced [52]. The water or fluid solubility of the drug in the granulation plays a key role in determining the granulation endpoint for the extrusion/spheronization process. A highly soluble drug will dissolve in the granulation fluid, whereas a highly insoluble drug will have wetting problems during the granulation step and remain part of the solid during granulating and wet massing.

12.4.3 Extrusion

The third step is the extrusion step, which forms the wet mass into rod-shaped particles. The wet mass is forced through dies and shaped into small cylindrical particles having a uniform diameter. The extrudate particles break at similar lengths under their own weight. The extrudate must have enough plasticity to deform but not so much to adhere to other particles when collected or rolled in the spheronizer.

Extruders come in many varieties, but can generally be divided into three classes, based on their feed mechanism. They include those that rely on a screw, gravity, or a piston to feed the wet mass into the extrusion zone as described by R.C. Rowe [50]. Examples of extruders from each class are shown in Figure 12.5. Screw feed extruders include the (a) axial or end plate, (b) dome, and (c) radial type, while gravity feed extruders include (d) cylinder, (e) gear, and (f) radial types. The screw and gravity-fed types are used for development and manufacturing with the radial varieties being the most popular for pharmaceutical applications. The piston feed or ram extruder (g) is primarily used in research as an analytical tool.

Screw extruders have either one (single) or two (twin) augers that transport the wet mass from the feed area to the extrusion zone. During the transport process, the screws compress the wet mass removing most of the entrapped air. Studies have been conducted on the ram extruder to understand this compression or consolidation stage. They have shown that the apparent density of the wet mass plug before extrusion is approximately equal to the theoretical apparent particle density, indicating that nearly all of the voids were eliminated, as determined by P.J. Harrison et al. [53]. Twin-screw extruders generally have higher throughput than single screw models, while single screw extruders compress and increase the density of the extrudate more. Other features that can affect the density of the extrudate are the spacing of the turnings on the screw and the space between the end of the screw and the beginning of the die, as described by D.C. Hicks and H.L. Freese [54]. Turnings that are wide and regularly spaced minimize the amount of compression during material transport. Screws with closer or progressively closer spacing between the turnings will result in more compression and produce a denser extrudate. Space between the screw and the die results in a void into which material is deposited and compressed. The greater space, the more compression takes place before extrusion. As material builds up, pressure increases and causes the material to be forced, under hydraulic pressure, to flow through the die. When space between the screw and the die is at a minimum, extrusion takes place as material is compressed in the nip, between the extruder blade and the die.

The primary difference between the various types of screw extruders is in the extrusion zone. An axial or dome extruder transports and extrudes the wet mass in the same plane. Axial extruders force the wet mass through a flat, perforated endplate, typically prepared by drilling holes in a

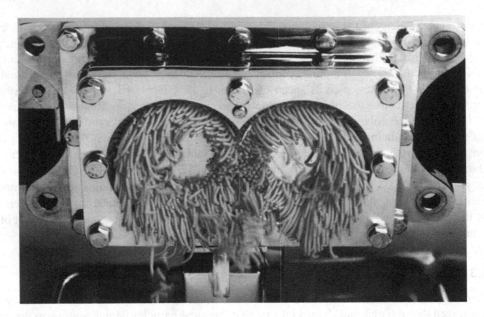

FIGURE 12.6   Twin screw axial extruder.
Source: Courtesy of LCI Corporation.

plate. The thickness of the plate can be more than four times the hole diameter, resulting in high die length to radius (L/R) ratios. A twin-screw axial endplate extruder is shown in Figure 12.6.

Dome extruders use a dome or half sphere-shaped screen as the die. The screen is prepared by stamping holes in metal stock having a similar thickness to the hole diameter. This results in a die L/R ratio of about 1:2; however, variations in screen thickness are possible resulting in a slightly higher or lower ratio. A dome extruder is shown in Figure 12.7.

Unlike axial and dome extruders, radial extruders extrude the wet mass perpendicular to the plane of transport. Material is transported to the extrusion zone where it is wiped against the screen

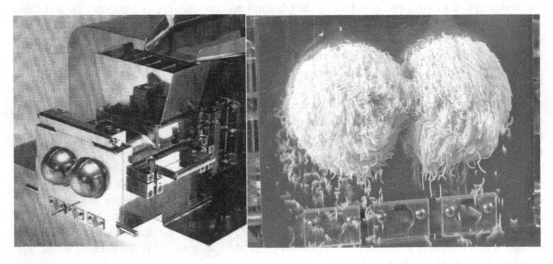

FIGURE 12.7   Dome extruder.
Source: Courtesy of LCI Corporation.

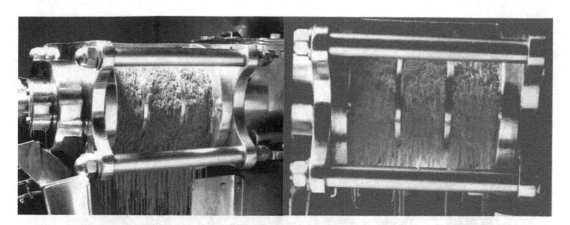

FIGURE 12.8 Side views of the extrusion zone of a radial extruder.
Source: Courtesy LCI Corporation.

die by an extrusion blade. The mass is forced through the die by pressure generated at the nip. A screw feed radial extruder is shown in Figure 12.8.

As with dome-type extruders, the die is a stamped screen. Due to the shorter die lengths and the increase in the number of holes or dies, dome and radial extruders have the advantage of higher throughput as compared to the axial type.

As with almost every extrusion-spheronization process step, heat build-up during extrusion is a significant concern. This is especially true of the screw fed extruders. Axial extruders generate heat due to their long die lengths. Radial extruders can have a significant heat differential over the width of the screen. Materials fed into the beginning or back of the extrusion zone will have the lowest temperature. However, as material moves to the end or front of the zone, the temperature increases due to the longer residence time of the material. Of the screw feed extruders, the dome type has the highest rate of throughput and is least likely to generate significant heat over an extended period, as it allows for uniform extrusion and shear over the extrusion screen. Since radial and dome extruders use stamped dies or screens, they are the most fragile and susceptible to damage due to high forces. Care must be taken to minimize the force required by formulation and fluid optimization, which will be discussed later in this chapter.

Gravity-fed extruders include cylinder, gear, and radial types. The cylinder and gear both belong to a broader class referred to as roll extruders. Both use two rollers to exert force on the wet mass and form an extrudate. The cylinder extruder has rollers in the form of cylinders, one solid and one hollow with drilled holes to form the dies. The wet mass is fed by gravity into the nip area between the two cylinders and forced through the dies into the hollow of the cylinder. Gear-type extruders have rollers in the form of hollow gears. The dies are holes drilled at the base of each tooth. The wet mass is forced through the holes and collected in the hollow of the gears as the teeth and the base areas mesh. The gears of a gear extruder are shown in Figure 12.9 to illustrate the teeth.

The last type of gravity feed extruder to be discussed is the radial type. Of the gravity-fed extruders, it is the most widely used. One or more arms rotate to stir the wet mass as it is fed by gravity. Rotating blades wipe the wet mass against the screen, creating localized forces sufficient to extrude at the nip. There is no compression prior to extrusion, which is the major difference between the gravity and screw feed radial extruders. A gravity-fed extruder is shown in Figure 12.10. Additionally, a schematic showing the extrusion zone and principle of operation is shown in Figure 12.11.

The primary extrusion process variables are the feed rate, die opening, and die length. The fluid content of the granulation is also very critical since the properties of the extrudate and resulting spheres are very dependent on the plasticity and cohesiveness of the wet mass. The process

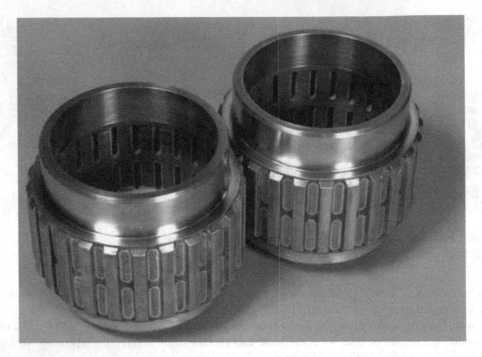

FIGURE 12.9   Gears of a gear-type extruder.
Source: Courtesy of AC Compacting Corporation.

(a)   (b)

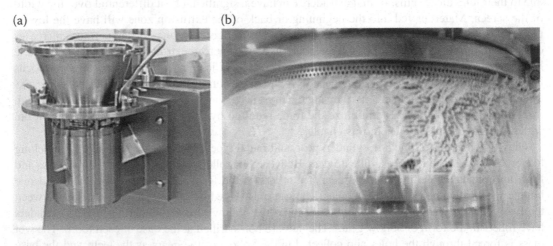

FIGURE 12.10   Gravity-fed rotary extruder; (a) front view and (b) close-up showing extrusion zone.
Source: Courtesy of GEA.

variables and fluid content have been the focus of many studies. P.J. Harrison et al. studied the flow of the wet mass as it is forced through a die [46,47,53,53,55,56]. They determined steady-state flow (described earlier and shown in Figure 12.4) was essential to produce smooth extrudate that results in uniformly sized spherical particles having good sphericity and surface characteristics. Materials and processes that did not result in a steady-state, a condition referred to as forced flow, produced extrudate having surface impairments. In moderate cases, the surface is rough, while in more severe cases, a phenomenon commonly referred to as shark-skinning occurs. Examples of the smooth extrudate and shark-skinned extrudate are shown in Figure 12.12. There continue to be differences of opinion regarding the value of smooth extrudate in the production of spherical

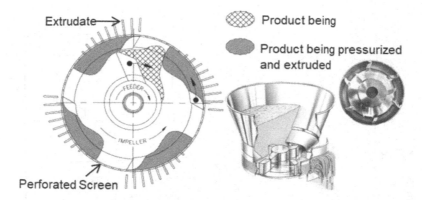

FIGURE 12.11   Gravity-fed rotary extruder; (left) Schematic of the extrusion zone and (right) Principle of operation of a gravity-fed extruder.
Source: Courtesy of GEA.

particles, commonly referred to as spheres, beads, and pellets, intended for use in multi-particulate drug delivery systems. Spherical granules intended for applications such as tablet or capsule granules as well as granules for filling into sachet type units do not require uniformity in size and therefore less care needs to be taken in the extrusion step.

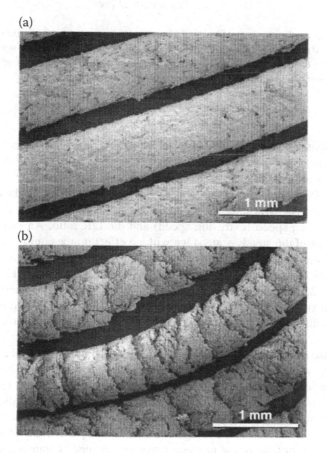

FIGURE 12.12   SEMs showing an example of (a) smooth extrudate and (b) extrudate having a surface impairment, or shark-skinning.

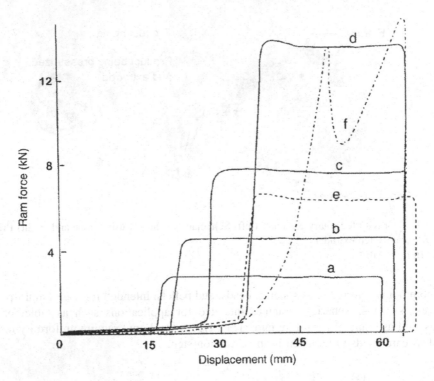

FIGURE 12.13 Force displacement profiles at various moisture contents of mixtures of microcrystalline cellulose and water: (a-d) microcrystalline cellulose-lactose-water (5:5:6); (e) lactose-water (8:2); (f) at a ram speed of 4 mm/sec, die diameter of 1.0, and a length/radius ratio of 12. Percentage of moisture content of microcrystalline cellulose-water mixture: a. 59.4; b, 51.1; d, 45.0.
Source: From Ref. [47].

Force displacement profiles of MCC and water at various ratios; MCC, lactose, and water at a 5:5:6 ratio; and lactose and water at an 8:2 ratio, developed by Harrison et al., are shown in Figure 12.13 [47]. Steady-state was possible with the MCC and MCC: lactose samples but not with lactose alone. As can be seen with the MCC samples, the duration of the compression stage was water-level dependent with no effect seen on the steady-state stage. Additional studies indicated the effect of ram speed (extrusion speed) and die L/R ratio. An increase in ram speed increased the duration of the steady-state stage with no effect on the compression stage. The L/R ratio did not affect either compression or steady-state. Wet mass composition, therefore, influenced the ability to achieve steady-state while the water level and ram speed influenced duration. Higher water levels decreased the force to produce steady-state flow but increased the duration. Faster ram speeds (extrusion rates) increased the duration of steady-state and increased the force. As discussed next, other investigators have reported the correlation between extrusion force and sphere quality.

Harrison et al. also indicated that a uniform lubricating layer at the die wall interface must occur to eliminate the slip-stick phenomenon responsible for forced flow [47]. The development of a lubricating layer was dependent on the length of the die (a minimum length required), wall shear stress, and upstream pressure loss. They represent the frictional forces at the die wall interface and the estimated pressure loss at zero die length in the barrel of the ram extruder. The method for deriving these values is described in the reference article. These parameters allow for a quantitative comparison between formulations and process; however, no specific values can be targeted since they vary with materials.

TABLE 12.1

Average Pore Diameter and Bulk Density of Extrudate Composed of DCP–Avicel PH-101–Water Mixture, Extruded Using Screens with a Different L/R ratio])

Composition DCP-Avicel-Water (w/w)	L/R Ratio of Screen	Average Pored Diameter (µm)	Bulk Density (g/mL)
150:380:470	4	0.982	1.132
150:400:450	4	0.992	1.211
150:380:470	2	1.249	0.949
150:400:450	2	1.292	0.947

Source: From Ref. [59].

Pinto et al. also showed that, at slow ram speeds, water moves toward the die wall interface and acts as a lubricant resulting in reduced extrusion forces [57]. At higher speeds, water is unable to move rapidly through the mass resulting in higher forces. They indicated the water content and its distribution are critical in determining the particle size and sphericity of the product. Lower water content and higher speed will reduce the size and sphericity of the particles. The extrusion speed and water content should be adjusted to achieve the desired effect. Other researchers have investigated the effect of die length using gravity feed radial extruder. Hellén et al. indicated the extrudate became smoother and more bound as the L/R ratio of the die was increased [58]. Vervaet et al. reported that a higher L/R ratio enables the use of lower water levels to achieve a more bound extrudate [59]. This also increased the range (drug loading and water level) over which quality spheres could be produced. They attributed the increased latitude and capability to increased densification and resulting well-bound extrudate. The average pore diameter and bulk density reported for extrudate prepared from various MCC:DCP:water ratios at two L/R ratios are shown in Table 12.1.

Baert et al. also indicated a similar increase in latitude when a cylinder extruder having an L/R ratio of 4 was compared to a twin-screw extruder having an L/R ratio of close to 1.8 [60]. Other studies have shown there is an optimal pressure range over which extrudate capable of yielding acceptable spheres can be produced. Shah et al. demonstrated the correlation between screen pressure yield and density [61]. A high yield of spheres within a targeted narrow size distribution was produced as long as the screen pressure was maintained within a given range. The relationship between yield and screen pressure is shown in Figure 12.14.

While many of the researchers have indicated a need for a more cohesive extrudate, few have expressed a need to remove all surface impairments. Some researchers have indicated that spheres having acceptable characteristics can be produced from extrudate having shark-skinning. O'Connor and Schwartz have found the presence of shark-skinning to be advantageous in facilitating the breakage of the extrudate during the spheronization step [62].

Experimental design studies conducted to concurrently investigate the effect of extrusion as well as other process and formulation variables have indicated the extrusion variables to be less significant than granulating fluid level or variables of the spheronization step. Hasznos et al. determined that extruder speed had little effect on the size distribution of the final product or moisture change during processing, as compared to the spheronization variables [63]. Hilemann et al. indicated that when water/MCC ratios are held constant, a change in screen size results in a significant change in the size distribution [64]. However, in a study where the water level was included as a variable, Erkoboni et al. showed the effect of screen size on size distribution to be small compared to the effect of a change in water level. A change in water level can shift the mean

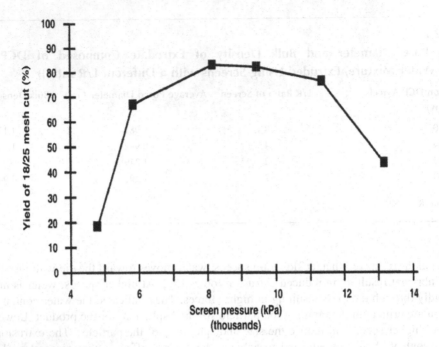

FIGURE 12.14 The effect of extruder screen pressure on the yield of particles within an acceptable distribution.
Source: From Ref. [61].

size and still result in an acceptable distribution [38]. This is in agreement with earlier work by I.M. Jalal et al. who also showed the mean particle size is typically smaller than the size of the screen itself due to shrinking during the drying step [28].

12.4.4 SPHERONIZATION

The fourth step in the extrusion-spheronization process is the spheronization step. It is carried out in a relatively simple piece of equipment. The working parts consist of a cylindrical bowl having fixed sidewalls with a rapidly rotating bottom plate or disk. The rounding of the extrudate into spheres is dependent on frictional forces. The forces are generated by the particle to particle and particle to equipment interaction. For this reason, the disk is generally machined to have a grooved surface, which increases the forces generated as particles move across its surface. Predominantly, disks having two general geometric patterns are produced, a cross-hatched pattern with the groves running at right angles to one another and a radial pattern with the groves running radially from the center. The two varieties are shown graphically in Figure 12.15 (a and b). Some studies have shown the rate of spheronization to be faster with the radial pattern; however, both plates will result in an acceptable product [50]. A third pattern that is available but not widely used is the striated edge pattern is shown in Figure 12.15 (c). Several researchers, including H. Michie et al. [64], have suggested it performs favorably compared to the others, but it has not been broadly adopted.

During the spheronization step, the extrudate is transformed from rod-shaped pellets into spherical particles. This transition occurs in various stages. Once charged into the spheronizer, the extrudate is drawn to the walls of the extruder due to centrifugal forces. From here what happens is very much dependent on the properties of the extrudate. Under ideal conditions, the extrudate breaks into smaller, more uniform pieces. Within a short period of time, the length of each piece is

(a)   (b)   (c)

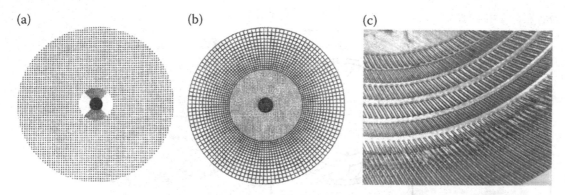

FIGURE 12.15 Spheronizer disks having three geometric patterns: (a) a cross-hatched pattern with the groves running at a right angle to one another, (b) a radial pattern with the groves running radially from the center, and (c) a striated edge pattern with a change in the groove size and space between groves at increasing plate diameters.
Source: Courtesy of GEA; adapted from Ref. [64].

approximately equal to the diameter, due to attrition and rapid movement of the bottom plate or disk. The differential in particle velocity as they move outward to the walls, begin to climb the walls, and fall back onto the rotating bed, along with the angular motion of the disk, results in a rope-like formation [11]. Figure 12.16 shows a graphic representation of the spheronizer charge movement and rope-like formation (a and b) as well as an empty spheronizer (c) and a running spheronizer showing the actual rope formation (d). This formation can be a critical indicator of the quality of the granulation or extrudate. The disk rotating without movement of the product indicates a severely over-wet condition. This condition is caused either by a granulation that was initially over wet or migration of water or a fluid ingredient to the surface of the extrudate during extrusion or spheronization.

The transformation from a cylinder-shaped extrudate to a sphere occurs in various stages. Three models have been proposed to describe the mechanism and are shown graphically in Figure 12.17. The model proposed by Rowe in 1985 describes a transition whereby the cylindrical particles (12.17-2a) are first rounded off into cylindrical particles with rounded edges (12.17-2b), then form dumbbell-shaped particles (12.17-2c), ellipsoids (12.17-2d) and finally spheres (12.17-2e) [50]. The second model proposed by Baert et al. in 1993 suggests that the initial cylindrical particles (12.17-1a) are deformed into a bent-rope-shaped particle (12.17-1b), then form a dumbbell with a twisted middle (12.17-1c). The twisting action eventually causes the dumbbell to break into two spherical particles with a flat side having a hollow cavity (12.17-1d). Continued action in the spheronizer causes the particles to round off into spheres (12.17-1e). When the sphere is fractured, a hollow particle is revealed [65]. The third model was proposed by Koestner et al. in 2010. It was described as a combination of a pelletization and an agglomeration mechanism. Cylindrical extrudate (12.17-3a) is rounded off into dumbbell-shaped rounded cylinders with fractured fines (12.17-3b). Particles combining with the fines through an agglomeration process with the particles rounding into an ellipsoid shape (12.17-3c). Continued motion in the spheronizer results in further rounding to form spheres (12.17-3d) [66]. The exact mechanism for a given formulation is likely composition dependent. If the extrudate is overwet, particle growth will occur resulting in broad size distribution. Under-wet extrudate will not have enough plasticity to further round off in the spheronizer resulting in the formation of dumbbells.

The scanning electron micrographs (SEMs) in Figure 12.18 show an example of round spheres produced from a sufficiently plastic mass and dumbbells from elastic extrudate that would not deform further.

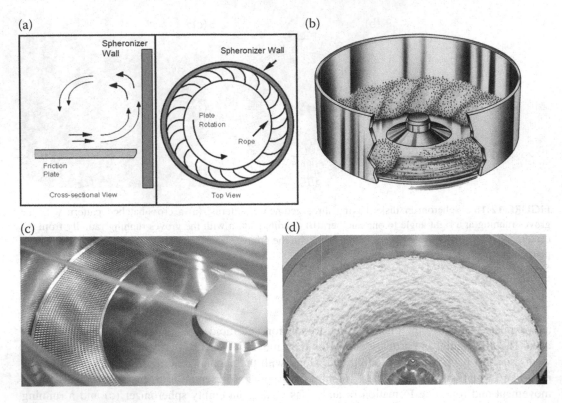

FIGURE 12.16 A graphic representation of (a) and (b) the characteristic rope-like formation in a spheronizer bowl during operation as well as (c) an empty spheronizer and (d) a running spheronizer.
Source: Courtesy GEA Pharma Systems.

Of the two process steps unique to extrusion/spheronization, the first, extrusion, is a continuous process while the second, spheronization, is a batch process. To make the process viable for commercial operations, two systems have been developed to enable the extruder to continuously feed material to the spheronizer(s). The first system is a semi-continuous shuttle system and the second is a cascade system. The shuttle system is typically used when uniform particles are required, such as for controlled release coating applications. The cascade system, however, can be used for applications where less size and shape uniformity are required, such as granulations intended for compression.

The shuttle system uses two spheronizers in parallel. It is designed to fill one spheronizer while the second is in the middle of its cycle, continue to collect extrudate in a shuttle receptacle while they are both full and operational, and fill the second after it empties and the first unit is in the middle of its cycle. The shuttle system operation is shown graphically in Figure 12.19. A picture of a spheronizing system having an extruder, a shuttle system to fill two spheronizers, and twin spheronizers is also shown in Figure 12.20.

The cascade operation uses one or more spheronizers that are modified to have the disks some distance below the discharge chute [54]. This results in a spheronization zone with a fixed volume. The product is continually fed from either the extruder or a previous spheronizer. As the charge volume grows from incoming material, some product is discharged by overflow into the discharge chute. The residence time is therefore dictated by the feed rate. A broader size and shape distribution are due to the percentage of material that does not reside in the spheronization zone for the intended period of time. The number of spheronizers placed in the sequence depends on the desired outcome. However, if only a slight rounding with minimal densification is required, one

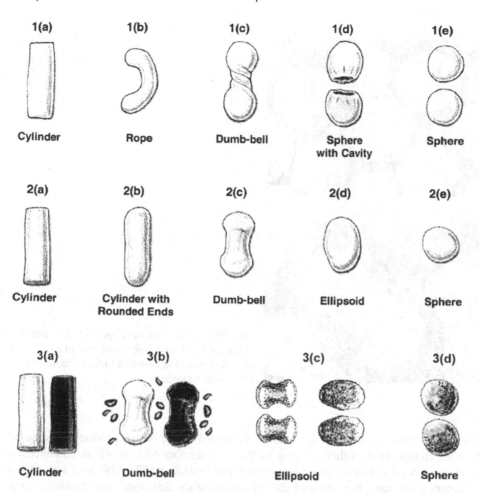

FIGURE 12.17 A graphic representation of the two models proposed to describe the mechanism of spheronization. The model proposed by Baert et al. [65] describes a transition from initial cylindrical particles (1a) into a bent rope (1b), dumbbell (1c), two spherical particles with a hollow cavity (1d), and spheres (1e). The model proposed by Rowe [50] describes a transition from cylindrical particles (2a) into cylindrical particles with rounded edges (2b), dumbbells (2c), ellipsoids (2d) and spheres (2e). (From Refs. [55] and [43]). The model proposed by Koester et al. [66] describes a transition from cylindrical particles (3a) into rounded cylindrical particles or dumbbells with fractured fines (3b), ellipsoids agglomerated with fines (3c) and spheres (3d).
Source: From Refs. [65], [50], and [66].

spheronizer with a short residence time will be sufficient. The cascade operation is shown graphically in Figure 12.21.

Variables in the spheronization step include spheronizer size, charge, disk speed, and residence time. Several studies have shown each of the variables has the potential to play a significant role in influencing the physical characteristics of the resulting product. Hasznos et al. showed that a higher disk speed and longer residence time increased the coarse fraction and mean diameter and decreased the fine fraction [63]. The faster speed and longer time also increased moisture loss during the process. Since the moisture loss can reduce the plasticity of the particle, it can have the same effect as an under-wet granulation. The particles may not round off into spheres and stay as deformed cylinders or dumbbells. Higher spheronizer charges reduced the moisture loss. They also suggested that an interaction between spheronizer speed and residence time indicated the total

(a)

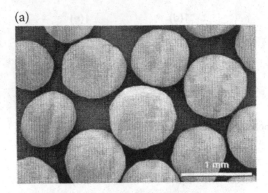

(b)

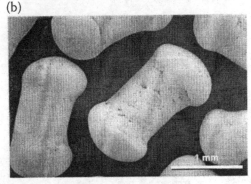

FIGURE 12.18 An example of (a) round spheres produced from a sufficiently plastic mass and (b) dumbbells that would not deform further produced from under wet elastic extrudate.

number of revolutions of the disk was critical. A change in one of the variables could be offset by an opposite change in the other, as long as the total number of revolutions remained constant. Hellén et al. showed similar moisture loss during spheronization [67]. Also, they indicated that the major factors influencing the shape of the spheres were the disk speed and residence time. High speed and a long time produced more spherical particles. Wan et al. indicated that a minimum disk speed and residence time were required to round the cylinder-shaped extrudate [68]. Furthermore, an increase in speed or time, up to a limit, increased the median diameter of the spheres while higher speeds and longer times caused a reduction in size. Short residence times at high disk speeds resulted in small but round particles.

Several investigators have reported the effect of disk speed and residence time on density. Woodruff and Neussle reported the variables do not affect the density of the spheres as compared to the density of the granulation and extrudate [31]. These results conflict with most of the other studies; however, they are likely due to the use of mineral oil in the formulation. Mineral oil can reduce the frictional forces at the die wall during extrusion and between particles and equipment surfaces during spheronization. Many investigators including Malinowski and Smith reported an increase in either disk speed or residence time increased density [37,38,67, and 69]. Mehta et al. studied the effect of spheronization time on the pellet hardness and drug release [7]. Pellet hardness increased with spheronization time for an initial period after which no increase was observed. The increase is likely due to the densification that occurs during the spheronization step. In another study, Mehta et al. showed the effect of spheronization time on the porosity parameters of the pellets [70]. A residence time of 2–10 minutes increased the number of pores and the total pore surface area and decreased the pore diameter. Beyond this time, for up to 20 minutes of spheronization time, the porosity was unchanged. O'Connor et al. indicated that the friability of placebo spheres decreased with increasing residence time while the mean particle diameter decreased [41].

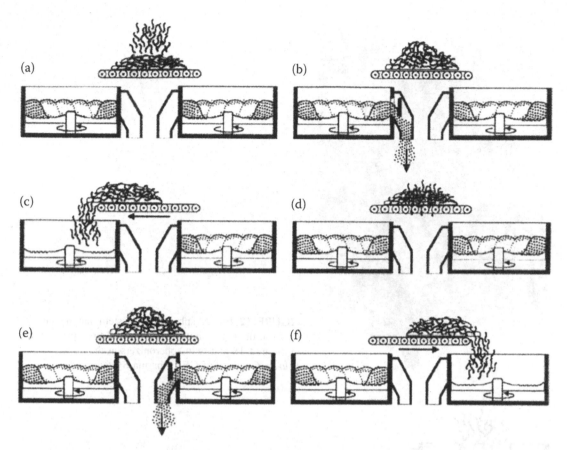

FIGURE 12.19 A graphic representation of a twin spheronizer shuttle system using two spheronizers in parallel and shuttle receptacle: (a) when both units are full the shuttle receptacle collects extrudate, (b) after one empties, (c) the shuttle box fills it, (d–f) the cycle repeats itself for the second unit.
Source: From Ref. [54].

12.4.5 DRYING

Drying is the final step in the process. This can be accomplished in any dryer that can be used for conventional type granulations, including tray dryers, column-type fluid beds, and deck-type vibratory fluid beds. Each of the drying techniques has advantages; however, the major differences are based on the rate of water removal. Tray drying is the slowest of the processes. Fluidized bed dryers result in a much more rapid drying rate because of the higher air volumes and the potential use of higher inlet temperatures. Column fluid beds are batch dryers, while the deck type dryers offer the advantage of a continuous process. Both have been used successfully in drying products produced by extrusion/spheronization. The drying process must be chosen based on the desired particle properties.

Pellets or granules to be dried in fluid bed equipment will have to withstand the fluidization process and resist attrition and maintain integrity. A more rapid rate in a fluid bed will likely minimize the effects of migration. This phenomenon can affect the number of particle properties. Tray drying is a slow process in a static bed. Because of this, it can offer the greatest opportunity for the drug to migrate toward the surface and recrystallize as indicated by A.M. Dyer et al. [71]. The increased active concentration at the surface of the particle can increase the rate of dissolution. This recrystallization, however, can cause a problem for applications requiring film coating since the smooth surfaces developed by the spheronization process would be damaged. Additionally, the

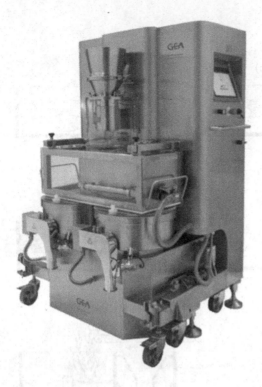

FIGURE 12.20 A spheronizer system having an extruder at the top, a shuttle system to fill two spheronizers in the middle, and twin spheronizers at the bottom. *Source*: Courtesy of GEA Pharma Systems.

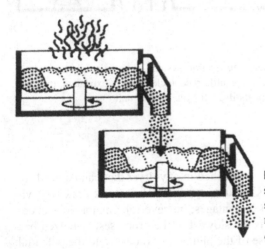

FIGURE 12.21 A graphic representation of a cascade spheronizer operation using two spheronizers. One of the spheronizers discharges into the second by overflow making the spheronization step continuous. *Source*: From Ref. [54].

crushing strength of tray dried particles will likely be greater than their fluid bed counterparts. The slow recrystallization in the static bed allows for crystal bridges to develop as the fluid is removed and the solute recrystallizes. The drying rate will also affect pellet or granule hardness. Slower rates will result in lower porosity and higher hardness.

12.5 FORMULATION VARIABLES

The composition of the wet mass is critical in determining the properties of the particles produced. This is clearly understood if we look at what material behaviors are required during each of the process steps. During the granulation step, a plastic mass is produced—a simple enough task if ended there. The materials must form a plastic mass, deform when extruded, and break off to form uniformly sized cylindrical particles. A minimal amount of granulating fluid should migrate to the surface during extrusion and the particles should stay discrete during collection. During spheronization, the particles must round off to form uniformly sized spheres. They must not dry out due to temperature or air volume or grow in size due to agglomeration. The fact is, a lot is asked from materials used in this process. This is especially true of formulations containing high percentages of active where low levels of excipients are used to impart the desired properties to the mass.

The importance of using sphere-forming excipients was noted early on. Conine and Hadley cited the necessity of using microcrystalline cellulose [10]. Reynolds went on to indicate the need for either adhesive or capillary type binders [11]. He cited cellulose gums, natural gums, and synthetic polymers as adhesives and microcrystalline cellulose, talc, and kaolin as capillary type binders. Since then much work has been conducted in an attempt to understand the significance of material properties. Some of the studies are discussed here.

O'Connor et al. studied the behavior of some common excipients in extrusion-spheronization [41]. The materials were studied as single components using water as the granulating fluid in an attempt to understand their application in the process. Of the materials tested, only the MCC or MCC with sodium carboxymethyl cellulose (Na-CMC) were capable of being processed. Others including dicalcium phosphate, lactose, starch, and modified starch did not process adequately, as single entities.

In an additional study, O'Connor et al. investigated the effect of varying drug, excipient, and excipient: drug ratios [62]. At low drug levels, they found the spheronizing excipient(s) played the most significant role in determining sphere properties. They found that, for low dose applications, MCC was the best excipient to use since it formed the most spherical particles. At moderate drug loading (50%), MCC as well as the two products consisting of MCC co-processed with Na-CMC (Avicel® RC-581 and Avicel® CL-611) resulted in acceptable spheres. At higher loading levels, however, the MCC did not yield acceptable spheres and the co-processed materials did. The spheres produced using Avicel® CL-611 were the most spherical. In addition, they found dissolution to be dependent on the type of excipient used and the solubility and concentration of the active. Spheres containing MCC remained intact and behaved as inert matrix systems, while those containing the co-processed products formed a gel plug in the dissolution basket and were described as water-swellable hydrogel matrix systems. The release profiles for spheres containing each of the excipients and theophylline in a 50:50 ratio are shown in Figure 12.22. Release profiles for spheres containing different drug loads are shown in Figure 12.23. An increase in drug load resulted in an increased release rate. Release profiles for spheres containing actives having different solubilities, including chlorpheniramine maleate, quinidine sulfate, theophylline, and hydrochlorothiazide, are shown in Figure 12.24. An increase in drug solubility resulted in an increased release rate.

L. Baert and J.P. Remon showed the effect of granulating fluid level on the release of drug from pellets [65]. Two model drugs were used, theophylline, which has a solubility of 1 g in 125 ml and sulfamethoxazole, which is practically insoluble. In each case, pellets were prepared using three granulating fluid levels. The dissolution rate was inversely proportional to the granulating fluid level with the higher levels resulting in slower release rates. See Figures 12.25 and 12.26.

Mehta et al. demonstrated the use of polymethacrylate polymers such as Eudragit L 100-55 and Eudragit S-100 in the development of controlled-release pellets [18,73] by extrusion-spheronization. The polymethacrylate polymers can be used as a pellet forming and release rate governing polymers for developing a controlled release drug delivery system without the use of MCC in the matrix. An eroding matrix capable of controlling the release of insoluble actives is formed.

Zhou et al. produced matrix pellets by combining microcrystalline waxes, pregelatinized starches, and hydrolyzed starches with model drugs, such as Ibuprofen and chloroquine phosphate [74]. They concluded the combination of microcrystalline waxes and pregelatinized starches or

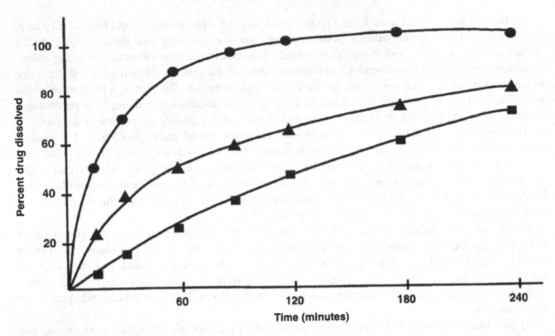

FIGURE 12.22 Dissolution profiles of spheres containing 50% theophylline in different Avicel® MCC types: ●Avicel® PH-101, ▲, Avicel® RC-581; ■, Avicel® CL-611.
Source: From Ref. [72].

maltodextrins is a flexible system for the production of matrix pellets, even with a high drug concentration. Additionally, they concluded that the drug release with such a system could be modeled by varying the type and the concentration of the wax and the starch. Tapia et al. described factors influencing the mechanism of release from sustained release matrix pellets, produced by the extrusion-spheronization process [75]. They demonstrated pellets that form a hydrogel during dissolution and sustain the release of the drug without a coating can be prepared.

Kleinebudde et al. concluded that during the extrusion process, the water content in the extrudate and pellet porosity was increased as the degree of polymerization of MCC and powder cellulose in the matrix were increased [76]. Millili and Schwartz demonstrated the effect of granulating with water and ethanol at various ratios. The physical properties of the spheres changed significantly as the ratio of the two fluids was varied. Spheres could not be formed with absolute ethanol but were possible with 5:95 water: ethanol. An increase in the water fraction resulted in a decrease in porosity, friability, dissolution, and compressibility and an increase in density. The porosity of spheres granulated with 95% ethanol was 54% while the water granulated product had a porosity of 14%. When greater than 30% of water was used, spheres remained intact throughout the dissolution test. As previously discussed, water granulated spheres were very difficult to compress while spheres granulated with 95% ethanol were significantly more compressible [33]. A tablet hardness versus compression forces profile is shown in Figure 12.27. Millili et al. proposed a bonding mechanism, referred to as autohesion, to explain the differences in the properties of spheres granulated with water and ethanol [77]. "Autohesion" is a term used to describe the strong bonds formed by the inter-diffusion of free polymer chain ends across particle-particle interfaces.

Using a ram extruder, Harrison et al. demonstrated that steady-state flow could not be achieved with lactose [47]. Additionally, they demonstrated the reduced sensitivity of MCC to small changes in moisture as determined by the force required to induce plug flow in a cylinder. Comparing MCC to a blend of MCC/lactose and 100% lactose, they found that, with lactose, small

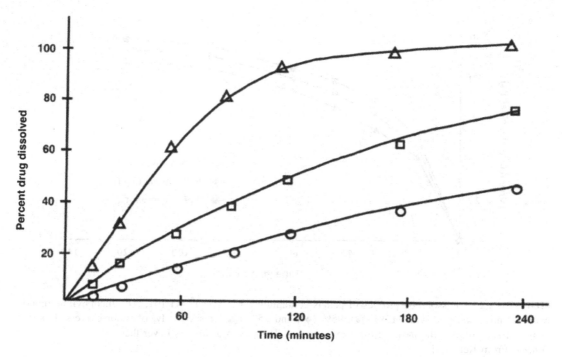

FIGURE 12.23 Dissolution profiles of spheres containing different concentrations of drug in Avicel® CL-611: ○, 10%; □, 59%; Δ, 80%.
Source: From Ref. [72].

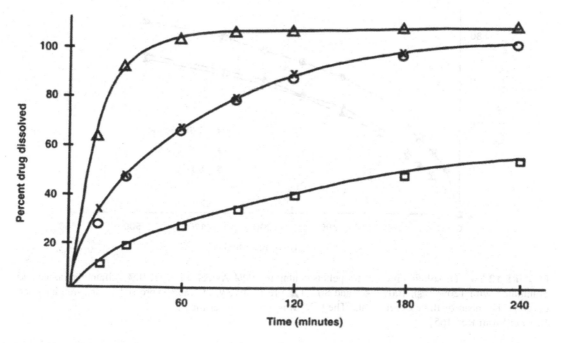

FIGURE 12.24 Dissolution profiles of spheres containing 10% drug in Avicel® PH 101: Δ, chlorphenarimine maleate; ○, quinidine sulfate, X, theophyline; □ hydrochlorothiazide.
Source: From Ref. [72].

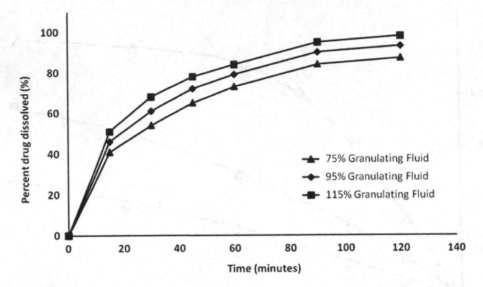

FIGURE 12.25   Dissolution profiles of pellets containing 80% Avicel® PH 101, 20% theophylline mono-hydrate and granulated with 115% (■), 95% (♦), and 75% (▲), respectively, of water expressed as dry weight. Each curve is the mean of three experiments. The C.V. was always lower than 2%.
Source: From Ref. [65].

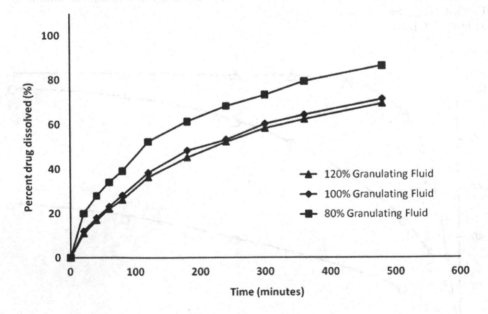

FIGURE 12.26   Dissolution profiles for pellets containing 90% Avicel® PH 101, 10% sulfamethoxazole and granulated with 120% (■), 100% (♦), and 80% (▲) respectively, of water expressed as dry weight. Each curve is the mean of three experiments. The C.V. was always lower than 2%.
Source: From Ref. [65].

changes in moisture caused large changes in force, while with MCC, larger changes in moisture were required to have similar effects on the force.

Baert et al. used mixtures of microcrystalline cellulose and co-excipients at various ratios to demonstrate the effect of solubility and the total fluid on extrusion forces [49]. They showed that if

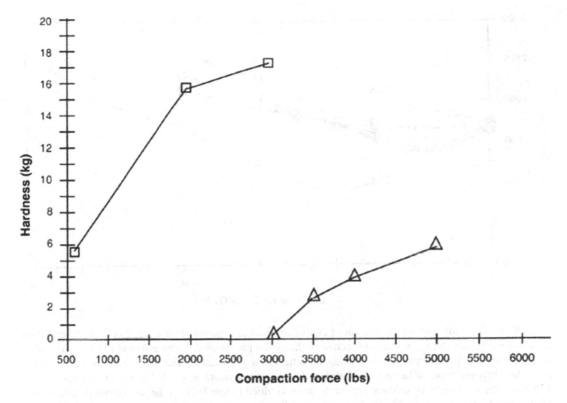

FIGURE 12.27 The effect of varying compression force on the hardness of compacted 16/30-mesh spheres of 10% theophylline-Avicel® PH101: Λ, spheres prepared by water; □, spheres prepared by 95% ethanol granulation.
Source: From Ref. [33].

the co-excipient was insoluble, such as dicalcium phosphate, the force required to extrude increased with increasing levels of co-excipient. When a soluble excipient such as lactose was used, the force required to extrude decreased with the addition of the initial amounts of lactose. After a certain level, however, the reduction in force stopped and began to increase. This was due to the initial solubilization of lactose and the resulting increase in the total fluid level. Once the fluid was saturated, the remaining lactose was not soluble and the force began to increase. The increase began at about 10% lactose level for α-lactose and 20% for β-lactose. This was due to the difference in solubility between the two materials. The effects of dicalcium phosphate and various lactose grades on the extrusion force is shown in Figure 12.28.

Funck et al. showed that low levels of common binders could be used to produce high drug-loaded spheres with microcrystalline cellulose [78]. Materials such as carbomer, sodium carboxymethylcellulose (Na-CMC), hydroxypropyl cellulose (HPC), hydroxypropylmethylcellulose (HPMC), povidone (PVP), and pregelatinized starch were used. All materials were capable of producing spheres of acceptable quality. Dissolution testing showed spheres containing HPC and HPMC remained intact during testing while spheres containing starch, PVP, and Na-CMC disintegrated. Lender and Kleinebudde reported that spheres produced with powdered cellulose had higher porosity and faster dissolution than those made using MCC [79]. Spheres could not be produced using only powdered cellulose and drug; a binder was required. The higher porosity of the spheres prepared from powdered cellulose may be beneficial for applications requiring compression. F. Podczeck showed that spheres could be produced using colloidal silica as the main excipient as long as a non-ionic surfactant was used in the granulating fluid. Pellets made from only colloidal silica and surfactant were very fragile but when an active or co-excipient was added, the strength was

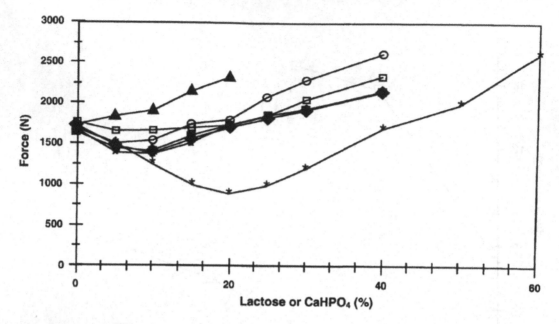

FIGURE 12.28 Influence of the amount of lactose or dicalcium phosphate dehydrates (% total weight) on the extrusion forces (N) for mixtures of lactose or dicalcium phosphate dehydrate-Avicel PH 101-water after granulation with a planetary mixer. Each endpoint is the mean of six values. The SD is lower than 3% for each point. Six different types of lactose were used: α- lactose monohydrate 80 mesh, □; α-Lactose monohydrate 200 mesh, ○; α-lactose monohydrate 325 mesh, ♦; spray-dried lactose DCL 11, ■; anhydrous β-lactose DCL 21, x; anhydrous α-Lactose DCL 30, *; one type of dicalcium phosphate dehydrate was used, ▲. *Source*: From Ref. [49].

improved and sufficient for downstream processing. Rapid disintegration and dissolution were notable characteristics with silica [80].

Feilden et al. showed that increasing the particle size of lactose resulted in forced flow and high extrusion forces, which then resulted in poor-quality extrudate and spheres having a wide size distribution [71]. This was attributed to the increased pore diameter of the mixture containing the coarse lactose, which allowed greater movement of water. Chien and Nuessle showed the use of a surfactant, such as sodium lauryl sulfate, reduced the migration of the drug to the surface of the sphere during drying by reducing the surface tension of the granulating fluid [72]. The reduction in surface tension also made it difficult to produce a cohesive extrudate in some cases.

Some miscellaneous observations include the following. Reynolds reported that excess extrudate friability can be overcome by incorporating more MCC, binder, or water in the granulation [11]. Erkoboni et al. indicated that sphere hardness was most affected by the level of MCC in the formulation and the level of granulating fluid used [38]. Hileman et al. showed that MCC had a narrower water range over which quality spheres could be made compared to MCC co-processed Na-CMC [69]. Hellén et al. showed that the surface characteristics were influenced by the water level with higher water levels giving smoother surfaces [67]. Mehta et al. showed that changing the concentrations of pellet forming and release rate controlling polymers in the matrix altered the dissolution kinetics of a poorly soluble drug [7].

12.6 COMPRESSION OF SPHERICAL GRANULES OR PELLETS

Pellets produced by extrusion-spheronization are typically used in controlled release applications. They are generally produced for filling into hard gelatin capsules or compression into a tablet dosage form without fracture or rupture of the pellet. The tablets are normally intended to disintegrate and the gelatin capsule shell to dissolve, releasing discrete, intact pellets into the gastrointestinal tract. The dosage forms are generally intended to deliver the active content through a modified release technique.

Spherical or somewhat rounded particles, however, can have other advantageous properties in the compression of tablets, filling of capsules, and production of other less common dosage forms such as sachets. Some of the granule properties that can be favorable to compression are improved flow, increase density, reduced friability, low dusting, taste-making, and stability. These properties were cited by a number of investigators, including J.W. Conine and H.R. Hadley [10], A.D. Reynolds [11], C.W. Woodruff, and N.O. Nuessle [31].

Care must be taken to tailor the formulation and process to maximize desirable qualities while minimizing any undesirable effects. As an example, the spherical pellets produced for controlled release or multi-particulate dosage forms are not suitable particles or granules for compression. They flow too freely, do not blend well with other compression aids such as lubricants, and, depending on their composition, likely require excessive force to fracture [10]. We have reviewed the factors affecting the properties of spherical multi-particulates produced by spheronization. Generally, the more spherical, denser particles are not preferred for compression. Physical properties conducive to compression can be produced by reducing the forces that cause consolidation. This includes optimizing variables such as the granulating fluid level, granulating fluid composition, wet mass mixing time, extrusion screen size, spheronizer disk speed, and residence time. Some of the factors are discussed ahead relative to compression.

Variations in material composition and the process can result in products having broad differences in physical properties. The first step in developing a pellet or granule using extrusion-spheronization should be building a reasonable understanding of the required particle properties. The formulation and process conditions used should be intended to achieve the target properties. Following the principles of the Quality by Design (QbD) initiative is an ideal way of accomplishing this goal. A quality target profile outlining critical quality attributes (CQA) of the intermediate granules as well as the final drug product should be created. Understanding the critical material attributes (CMA) and critical process parameters (CPP) required to achieve the CQA is necessary. Pharmaceutical Quality by Design is discussed in a review article by L. X. Yu et al. [73]. The use of statistical experimental design techniques is useful in both screenings to understanding the effect of materials and process variables as well as optimizing once the effects are understood. This type of approach is essential when using a technique such as extrusion/spheronization. The formulation variable and process parameters do not behave independently of one another.

Spherical granules or pellets have been shown to react differently to compaction and consolidation than powders of the same material. Think of the process pathway that transforms the powders to pellets as a continuum. The extremes represent properties that are not desirable. There are process conditions along the path that could result in a desirable product that meets the needs of the product being produced.

Wang et al. reported compression of lactose/MCC compositions at various ratios in both powder and pellet form [74]. Compacts made from the pellets had a different compaction and consolidation mechanism than the similar powders. The powders show an increase in tensile strength with increase MCC levels while compacts prepared from the pellets showed an opposite trend. Schwartz et al. [32] also demonstrated the compaction characteristics of MCC processed into spheres are significantly different than the original powder. The powder material forms hard compacts at low compression forces, while the spheres are not compressible and form soft compacts, even at high forces. They indicated that spheres prepared from MCC showed a high degree of visco-elasticity over the entire compression range. The inclusion of co-excipients, such as lactose and dicalcium phosphate, increases the compactability by decreasing the visco-elastic resistance or pressure range over which the spheres behave elastically. A reduction in visco-elastic resistance was seen with

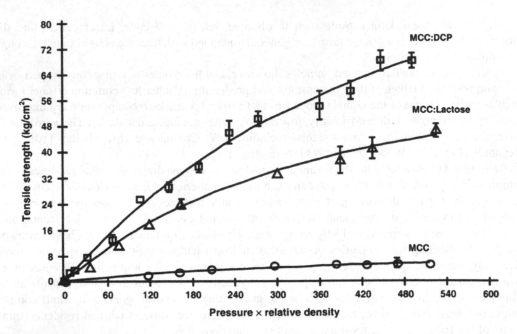

FIGURE 12.29 The effect of excipients on the compaction profile of spheres: compaction profiles of spheres containing 10% theophylline with either MCC, MCC-DCP, or MCC-lactose in a 22.5:67.5 ratio using the Leuenberger model.
Source: From Ref. [32].

spheres containing both lactose and dicalcium phosphate; however, dicalcium phosphate had a greater effect. Compaction profiles of spheres containing 10% theophylline with either MCC, MCC/dicalcium phosphate (DCP), or MCC/lactose in a 22.5/67.5 ratio are shown in Figure 12.29.

A similar phenomenon was reported by Maganti and Celik when pellets produced by rotor granulation were compressed [75]. They compared the compaction behavior of pellet formulations, mainly consisting of MCC, to that of the powders from which they were formed and also found significant differences. The powders examined were found to compact by plastic deformation and produced strong compacts, while the pellets exhibited elastic deformation and brittle fragmentation, resulting in compacts of lower tensile strength. This can be explained by the fact that the pellets, which are large and spherical in shape as compared to the small, irregular powder particles they are composed of, have a low surface to volume ratio, which might result in a decreased area of contact between the particles as they consolidate. Nicklasson et al. investigated the compression behavior of pellets consisting of MCC, with or without other excipients such as (PEG) and DCP [76]. Deformation of the aggregates was found to depend on three deformation characteristics, namely, the capacity for, the mode of and the resistance to deformation. High surface deformation refers to the great ability of the pellets to conform to the surface of the surrounding pellets. In pellets containing the soft component, the primary particles can reposition within the agglomerate and the ability to fill the intragranular pore space is increased. For pellets containing hard materials, the compaction stress may give local failure at pellet surfaces. Thus, the material properties of the primary particles constituting the pellets are important for the compression behavior of pellets. In several studies, various soft materials have been incorporated in pellets to modify their deformability and compatibility. N.O. Iloañusi and J.B. Schwartz investigated the effect of glyceryl behenate on the compaction of microcrystalline cellulose beads or pellets containing acetaminophen [77]. They found beads containing the waxy material required less force to form cohesive tablets. Salako et al. found that pellets containing theophylline and MCC were hard and less brittle than the ones containing glyceryl monostearate, which were soft pellets [78]. The soft pellets were found to fracture under low compression pressures and were able to form a coherent network of a deformable material in the tablets at higher pressures. The hard pellets were unable to form such a network at high pressures and were found to reduce more in volume without bond formation than soft pellets. F. Nicklasson and G. Alderborn studied the modulation of the tableting behavior of pellets through the incorporation of polyethylene glycol and found that these soft pellets had an increased propensity to deform and an altered mode of deformation compared to the relatively hard MCC pellets [79].

The size of the pellets can also have a bearing on their compression behavior. Small pellets are less affected than larger ones by the compaction process as shown by J.L. Haslam et al. [90] and B. Johansson et al. [91]. Smaller beads were significantly stronger, relative to their size, than larger ones, and larger pellets were much more readily deformed.

12.7 SUMMARY

Extrusion/spheronization is a versatile process capable of producing granules, pellets, or spheres having unique physical properties. Since it may be more labor and time-intensive than the more common granulation techniques, it should be considered as a granulating technique when the desired properties cannot be produced using more conventional techniques. Potential applications are many, including both immediate and controlled release. Regardless of the application, care must be taken to understand the desired properties and the formulation and process variables capable of achieving them. The principles of Quality by Design (QbD) are a useful tool in development and production. Understanding the critical quality attributes of the intermediate granules and the final product target properties is essential. An understanding of critical material attributes and process parameters will allow the granule and quality attributes of the product to be achieved.

The use of statistical experimental design for formulation and process development is strongly recommended due to the high degree of interactions between the variables. Lastly, new technologies such as hot-melt extrusion (HME) of continuous extrusion granulation with spheronization are gaining considerable interest in the pharmaceutical drug delivery arena for solving specific problems. Benefits include improved processing efficiency, enhanced taste masking, improved solubility for poorly soluble drugs, and improved drug bioavailability.

REFERENCES

1. D. Erkoboni, "Extrusion –Spheronization for Granulation" in Handbook of Pharmaceutical Granulation Technology, DM Parikh (Editor), Marcel Dekker, NY 1997.
2. D. Erkoboni, "Extrusion–Spheronization for Granulation" in Handbook of Pharmaceutical Granulation Technology, DM Parikh (Editor), Marcel Dekker, NY 2010.
3. K. A. Mehta, G. S. Rekhi, D. M. Parikh, "Extrusion–Spheronization for Granulation" in Handbook of Pharmaceutical Granulation Technology, D. M. Parikh (Editor), Marcel Dekker, NY 2005.
4. A. Dukieć-Ott, J. P. Remon, P. Forman, C. Vervaet, Immediate release of poorly soluble drug from starch-based pellets prepared via extrusion/spheronization, European J Pharm and Biopharm; 67: 715–724 (2007).
5. T. Maejima, J. W. McGinity, Influence of film additives on stabilizing drug release rates from pellets coated with acrylic, Polymers, Pharm Dev and Tech, 2(2), 211–221 (2001).
6. H. Kranz, K. Jürgens, M. Pinier, J. Siepmann, Drug release from MCC- and carrageenan-based pellets: experimental and theory, European J Pharm and Biopharm; 73: 302–309 (2009).
7. K. A. Mehta, M. S. Kislalioglu, W. Phuapradit, A. W. Malick, N. H. Shah, Effect of formulation and process variables on matrix erosion and drug, release from a multiunit erosion matrix of a poorly soluble drug, *Pharm Tech* February, 26–34, (2002).
8. G. A. Hileman, S. R. Goskonda, A. J. Spalitto, S. M. Upadrashta, Response surface optimization of high dose pellets by extrusion spheronization, Int. Journal of Pharmaceutics, 100: 71–79 (1993).
9. Nakahara, U. S. Patent 3,277,520 (October 1966).

10. J. W. Conine, H. R. Hadley, Preparation of small solid pharmaceutical spheres, *Drug and Cosm. Ind.*, 106: 38–41 (1970).

11. A. D. Reynolds, A new technique for the production of spherical particles, *Manuf. Chem. Aerosol News*, 41: 40–43 (1970).

12. K. A. Mehta, M. S. Kislalioglu, W. Phuapradit, A. W. Malick, J. Ke, N. H. Shah, In vivo release performance of nifedipine in dogs from a novel Eudragit, based multi-unit erosion matrix., *Drug Delivery Tech*, January/February, 2(2): 38–42 (2002).

13. C. Vervaet, L. Baert, J. P. Remon, Extrusion-spheronization: A literature review, *Int J. Pharm.*, 116: 131–146 (1995).

14. Breitenbach J. and Mägerlein M., Melt extruded molecular dispersions. *Pharmaceutical Extrusion Technology*, Ghebre-Sellassie (editor), Marcel Dekker Inc. NY (2003).

15. C. R. Young, J. J. Koleng and J. W. McGinity, Production of spherical pellets by a hot-melt extrusion and spheronization process, Int. J. Pharm., 242: 87–92 (2002).

16. C. R. Young, J. J. Koleng and J. W. McGinity, Properties of drug-containing spherical pellets produced by hot-melt extrusion and spheronization, J. Microencapsulation, 20 (5), 613–625 (2003).

17. S. Almeida-Prieto, C. I. de Sá Ferreira da Rocha, J. Blanco-Méndez, F. J. Otero-Espinar, Fast and controlled release of triamcinolone acetonide from extrusion-spheronization pellets based on mixtures of native starch with dextrin or waxy maize starch. Drug Dev. and Ind. Pharm., 33: 945–951 (2007).

18. K. A. Mehta, M. S. Kislalioglu, W. Phuapradit, A. W. Malick, NH Shah, Release performance of a poorly soluble drug from a novel Eudragit based multi-unit erosion matrix, *Int. J. of Pharm.*, 213: 7–12 (2001).

19. R. Mallipeddi, K. K. Saripella, S. H. Neau, Use of fine particle ethylcellulose as the diluent in the production of pellets by extrusion-spheronization, Saudi Pharmaceutical Journal, 22: 360–372 (2014).

20. A. M. Agrawal, S. H. Neau, P. L. Bonate, Wet granulation fine particle ethylcellulose tablets: effect of production variables and mathematical modeling of drug release, AAPS PharmSci, 5 (2): E13.

21. M. A. Repka, S. K. Battu, S. B. Upadhye, S. Thumma, M. M. Crowley, F. Zhang, C. Martin, J. W. McGinnity, Pharmaceutical applications of hot-melt extrusion: Part II, Drug Dev. and Ind. Phar., 33: 1043–1057 (2007).

22. P. C. Kayumba, N. Huyghebaert, C. Cordella, J. D. Ntawukuliryayo, C. Vervaet, J. R. Remon, Quinine sulfate pellets for flexible pediatric drug dosing: Formulation development and evaluation of taste-masking efficiency using the electronic tongue, Eur. J. pf Pharma and Biopharma., 66 (3):460–465 (2007).

23. R. Jackowicz, E. Nürnberg, B. Pieszek, B. Kluczykowska, A. Maciejeqska, Solid dispersion of keto-profen in pellets, Int. Journal of Pharmaceutics, 206: 12–21 (2000).

24. M. Serratoni, M. Newton, S. Booth, A. Clarke, Controlled drug release from pellets containing water-insoluble drugs dissolved in a self-emulsifying system, Eur. J. of Pharm. And Biopharm., 65: 94–98 (2007).

25. I. Matsaridou, P. Barmpalexis, A. Salis, I. Nikolakakis The influence of surfactant HLB and oil/sur-factant ratio on formulation and properties of delf-emulsifying pellets and microemulsion reconstitu-tion, AAPS PharmSciTech, 13(4):1319–1330 (2012).

26. G. A. Awad, C. A. Chartueau, P. Allain, J. C. Chaumeil, Formulation and evaluation of bioadhesive pellets containing different carbomers made by extrusion-spheronization, STP Pharma Sciences, 12: 157–162 (2002).

27. FJO Varum, F. Veiga, J. S. Sousa, A. W. Basit, Mucoadhesive platforms for targeted delivery to the colon, Int J of Pharm, 420: 11–19 (2011).

28. I. M. Jalal, H. J. Malinowski, W. E. Smith, Tablet granulations composed of spherical-shaped particles. J. Pharm Sci, 61: 1466–1468 (1972).

29. G. M. Clarke, J. M. Newton, M. B. Short, Comparative gastrointestinal transit of pellet systems of varying density, Int. J. of Pharm., 114: 1–11 (1995).

30. J. E. Devereus, J. M. Newton M. B. Short, The influence of density on the gastrointestinal transit of pellets, J. Pharm. Pharmacol., 42: 500–501 (1990).

31. C. W. Woodruff, N. O. Nuessle, Effect of processing variables on particles obtained by extrusion-spheronization, J. Pharm. Sci., 61: 787–790 (1972).

32. J. P. Schwartz, N. H. Nguyen, R. L. Schnaare, Compaction studies on beads: compression and con-solidation parameters, Drug Dev. and Ind. Pharm., 20: 3105–3129 (1994).

33. G. P. Millili, J. B. Schwartz, The strength of microcrystalline cellulose pellets: The effect of granulating with water/ethanol mixtures, Drug Dev. and Ind. Pharm., 16: 1411–1426 (1990).

34. H. Santos, F. Veiga, M. E. Pina, J. J. Sousa, Compaction, compression, and drug release properties of diclofenac sodium and ibuprofen pellets comprising xanthan gum as a sustained release agent, Int. J. of Pharm. 295: 15–27 (2005).

35. M. Salako, F. Podezeck, J. M. Newton, Investigations into the deformability and tensile strength of pellets, Int. J. of Pharm. 168: 49–57 (1998).

36. H. J. Malinowski, W. E. Smith, Effect of spheronization process variables on selected tablet properties, J. Pharm. Sci., 63: 285–288 (1974).

37. H. J. Malinowski, W. E. Smith, Use of factorial design to evaluate granulations prepared by spheronization, J. Pharm. Sci. 64: 1688–1692 (1975).

38. D. F. Erkoboni, S. A. Fiore, T. A. Wheatley, T. Davan, The effect of various process and formulation variables on the quality of spheres produced by extrusion/spheronization. Poster presentation, AAPS national meeting (1991).

39. M. Chariot, J. Francès, G. A. Lewis, D. Mathieu, R. Phan Tan Luu, HNE Stevens, A factorial approach to process variables of extrusion-spheronization of wet powder masses, Drug Dev. and Ind. Pharm., 13: 1639–1649 (1987).

40. K. K. Saripella, N. C. Loka, R. Mallipeddi, A. M. Rane, S. H. Neau, A quality by experimental design approach to assess the effect of formulation and process Variables on the Extrusion and Spheronization pf Drug-Loaded Pellets Containing Polyplasdone® XL-10, AAPS PharmSciTech, 17 (2): 368–379 (2016).

41. R. E. O'Connor, J. Holinez, J. B. Schwartz, Spheronization I: processing and evaluation of spheres prepared from commercially available excipients, Am. J. of Pharm., 156: 80–87 (1984).

42. J. E. Ojile, C. B. Macfarlane, A. B. Selkirk, Drug distribution during massing and its effect on dose uniformity in granules, Int. J. of Pharm., 10: 99–107 (1982).

43. P. Kleinebudde, H. Lindner, Experiments with a twin-screw extruder using a single-step granulation/extrusion process, Int. J. of Pharm., 94: 49–58 (1993).

44. C. Schmidt, P. Kleinebudde, Influence of the granulation step on pellets prepared by extrusion/spheronization, Chem. Pharm Bull., 47(3): 403–412 (1999).

45. A. Kumar *et al.*, Linking granulation performance with residence time and granulation distributions in twin-screw granulation: An experimental investigation, Eur. J. Pharm. Sci., 90: 25–37 (2016).

46. N. O. Lindberg, C. Tufvesson, P. Holm, L. Olbjer, Extrusion of an effervescent granulation with a twin-screw extruder, Baker Perkins MPF 50 D. Influence in intragranular porosity and liquid saturation, Drug Dev. and Ind. Pharm., 14: 1791–1798 (1988).

47. P. J. Harrison, J. M. Newton, R. C. Rowe, The characterization of wet powder masses suitable for extrusion/spheronization, J. Pharm. and Pharmacol. 37: 686–691 (1985).

48. M. Landín, R. C. Rowe, P. York, Characterization of wet powder masses with a mixer torque rheometer. 3. Nonlinear effects of shaft speed and sample weight, J. Pharm. Sci., 85: 557–560 (1995).

49. L. Baert, D. Fanara, P De Baets, J. P. Remon, Instrumentation of a gravity feed extruder and the influence of the composition of binary and tertiary mixtures on the extrusion forces, J. Pharm and Pharmacol., 43: 745–749 (1991).

50. R. C. Rowe, Spheronization: a novel pill-making process?, Pharm. Int., 6: 119–123 (1985).

51. L. Baert, J. P. Remon, P. Knight, J. M. Newton, A comparison between the extrusion forces and sphere quality of a gravity feed extruder and a ram extruder, Int. J. of Pharm. 86: 187–192 (1992).

52. C. C. Ku, Y. M. Joshi, J. S. Bergum, N. B. Jain, Bead manufacture by extrusion/spheronization: a statistical design for process optimization, Drug Dev. and Ind. Pharm., 19: 1505–1519 (1993).

53. P. J. Harrison, J. M. Newton, R. C. Rowe, The application of capillary rheometry to the extrusion of wet masses, J. of Pharm., 35: 235–242 (1987).

54. D. C. Hicks, H. L. Freese, "Extrusion and Spheronization Equipment" in *Pharmaceutical Pelletization Technology*, I. Ghebre-Sellassie (Editor), Marcel Dekker, New York, pp 71–100 (1989).

55. P. J. Harrison, J. M. Newton, R. C. Rowe, Flow defects in wet powder asses, J. Pharm. and Pharmacol., 37: 81–83 (1984).

56. P. J. Harrison, J. M. Newton, R. C. Rowe, Convergent flow analysis in the extrusion of wet powder masses, J. Pharm. and Pharmacol., 37: 81–83 (1984).

57. J. F. Pinto, G. Buckton, J. M. Newton, The influence of four selected processing and formulation factors on the production of spheres by extrusion and spheronization, Int. J. of Pharm., 83: 187–196 (1992).

58. L. Hellén, J. Ritala, P. Yliruusi, P., Merkku, E. Kristoffersson, Process variables of the radial screen extruder: I. Production capacity of the extruder and the properties of the extrudate, J. of Pharm. Tech. Int., 4: 50–60 (1992).

59. C. Vaervaet, L. Baert, P. A. Risha, J. P. Remon, The influence of the extrusion screen on pellet quality using an instrumented basket extruder, Int. J. of Pharm. 107: 29–39 (1994).

60. L. Baert, J. P. Remon, JAC Elbers, EMG Van Bommel, Comparison between a gravity feed extruder and a twin-screw extruder, Int. J. of Pharm., 99: 7–12 (1993).

61. R. Shah, M. Kabadi, D. G. Pope, L. L. Augsberger, Physico-mechanical characterization of the extrusion/spheronization process. Part I: Instrumentation of the extruder, Pharm. Res. 11: 355–360 (1994).

62. R. E. O'Connor, J. B. Schwartz, "Extrusion and spheronization technology" in Pharmaceutical Pelletization Technology, I. Ghebre-Sellassie (Editor), Maecel Dekker, New York, pp 187–216 (1989).

63. L. Hasznos, I. Langer, M. Gyarmathy, Some factors influencing pellet characteristics made by an extrusion/spheronization process, Part I.: Effects on size characteristics and moisture content decrease of pellets, Drug Dev. and Ind. Pharm. 18: 409–437 (1992).

64. H. Michie, F. Podczeck, J. M. Newton, The influence of plate design on the properties of pellets produced by extrusion spheronization, Int. J. of Pharm., 434: 175–182 (2012).

65. L. Baert, J. Remon, Influence of amount of granulating liquid on the drug release rate from pellets made by extrusion spheronization, Int. J. of Pharm., 95: 135–141 (1993).

66. M. Koester, M. Thommes, New insights into the pelletization mechanism by extrusion/spheronization, AAPS PharmSciTech, 11(4): 1549–1551 (2010).

67. L. Hellén, J. Yliruusi, P. Merkku, E. Kristoffersson, Process variables of instant granulator and spheronizer: I. physical properties of granules, extrudate, and pellets, Int. J. of Pharm., 96: 197–204 (1993).

68. LSC Wan, PWS Heng, C. V. Liew, Spheronization conditions on spheroid shape and size, Int. J. of Pharm., 96: 59–65 (1993).

69. G. A. Hileman, S. R. Goskonda, A. J. Spalitto, S. M. Upadrashta, A factorial approach to high dose product development by an extrusion/spheronization process, Drug Dev. and Ind. Pharm. 19: 483–491 (1993).

70. K. A. Mehta, M. S. Kislalioglu, W. Phuapradit, A. W. Malick, N. H. Shah, Effect of formulation and process variables on porosity parameters and release rates from a multi-unit erosion matrix of a poorly soluble drug, J. Con. Rel 63: 201–211 (2000).

71. A. M. Dyer, K. A. Khan, M. E. Aulton, Effect of the drying method on the mechanical and drug release properties of pellets prepared by extrusion, Drug Dev. and Ind. Pharm., 20: 3045–3068 (1994).

72. R. E. O'Connor, J. B. Schwartz, Spheronization II: drug release from drug-diluent mixtures, Drug Dev. and Ind. Pharm., 11: 1837–1857 (1985).

73. K. A. Mehta, M. S. Kislalioglu, W. Phuapradit, A. W. Malick, N. H. Shah, Multi-unit controlled release systems of nifedipine and nifedipine: Pluronic F-68 solid dispersions: Characterization of release mechanisms., Drug. Dev. Ind. Pharm., 28(3), 275–285 (2002).

74. F. Zhou, C. Vervaet, J. P. Remon, Matrix pellets based on the combination of waxes, starches and maltodextrins, Int. J. Pharm. 133: 155–160 (1996).

75. C. Tapia, G. Buckton, J. M. Newton, Factors influencing the mechanism of release from sustained release matrix pellets, produced by extrusion/spheronization, Int. J. Pharm., 92: 211–218 (1993).

76. P. Kleinebudde, M. Jumaa, F El Saleh, Influence of degree of polymerization on the behavior of cellulose during homogenization and extrusion/spheronization, AAPS PharmSci, 2(18): (2000). https://doi.org/10.1208/ps020321.

77. G. P. Millili, R. J. Wigent, J. B. Schwartz, Autohesion in pharmaceutical solids, Drug Dev. and Ind. Pharm., 16: 2383–2407 (1990).

78. JAB Funck, J. B. Schwartz, W. J. Reilly, E. S. Ghali, Binder effectiveness for beads with high drug levels, Drug Dev. Ind. Pharm., 17: 1143–1156 (1991).

79. H. Linder, P. Kleinebudde, Use of powdered cellulose for the production of pellets by extrusion/spheronization, J Pharm. and Pharmacol., 46: 2–7 (1994).

80. F. Podczeck, A novel aid for the preparation of pellets by extrusion spheronization, Pharm. Tech. Eur., 20(12): 26–31 (2008).

81. K. E. Fielden, J. M. Newton, R. C. Rowe, The influence of lactose particle size on the spheronization of extrudate processed by a ram extruder, Int. J. of Pharm., 81: 205–224 (1992).

82. T. Y. Chien, N. O. Nuessle, Factors influencing migration during Spheronization, *Pharm. Technol.*, 4: 44–48 (1985).

83. L. X. Yu et al., Understanding pharmaceutical quality by design, AAPS Journal, 16(4): 771–783 (2014).

84. C. Wang, G. Zhang, N. H. Shah, M. H. Infeld, A. W. Malick, J. W. McGinity, Compaction properties of spheronized binary granular mixtures, Drug Dev. Ind. Pharm., 21: 753–779 (1995).

85. L. Maganti, M. Celik, Compaction studies on pellets I. Uncoated pellets, Int. J. of Pharm., 95: 29–42 (1993).

86. F. Nicklasson, Compression mechanics of pharmaceutical aggregates- studies on the tableting of spheronized aggregates with varying composition and porosity, PhD Thesis, Uppsala University, Sweden, 2000.

87. N. O. Iloañusi, J. B. Schwartz, The effect of wax on compaction of microcrystalline cellulose beads made by extrusion and Spheronization, Drug Dev. Ind. Pharm., 24: 37–44, (1998).

88. M. Salako, F. Podczeck, J. M. Newton, Investigations into the deformability and tensile strength of pellets, Int. J. Pharm. 168: 49–57, (1998)

89. F. Nicklasson, G. Alderborn, Modulation of the tableting behavior of microcrystalline cellulose pellets by the incorporation of polyethylene glycol, Eur. J. Pharm. Sci., 9: 57–65 (1999).

90. J. L. Haslam, A. E. Forbes, G. S. Rork, T. L. Ripkin, D. A. Slade, D. Khossravi, Tableting of controlled release multiparticulates, the effect of millisphere size and protective overcoating, Int. J. Pharm.,173: 233–242 (1998).

91. B. Johansson, F. Nicklasson, G. Alderborn, Effect of pellet size on the degree of deformation and densification during compression and on compactability of microcrystalline cellulose pellets, Int. J. Pharm. 163: 35–48 (1998).

13 Continuous Granulation

Chris Vervaet, Thomas De Beer, and Valérie Vanhoorne

CONTENTS

13.1 INTRODUCTION: CONTINUOUS PROCESSING OF SOLID DOSAGE FORMS

For decades, the manufacturing of solid dosage forms in the pharmaceutical industry has been synonymous with batch processing, using a series of unit operations to modulate the properties of the material being processed. According to the Food and Drug Administration (FDA) definition, batch manufacturing uses "a specific quantity of a drug or other material that is intended to have uniform character and quality, within specified limits, and is produced according to a single manufacturing order during the same cycle of manufacture". When the predetermined endpoint of the batch process is reached, the unit operation is finished, and only then product quality is assessed, via off-line analysis in quality control labs using a wide array of (often destructive) analytical tools. During off-line analysis, the processing cycle is stopped and the in-process materials are stored in the manufacturing plant until it is assured that product quality meets the predefined quality parameters. If these quality standards are not met, the entire batch is either rejected or reprocessed.

In contrast, a continuous manufacturing process relies on the "one in, one out" principle, as new materials are continuously added to the process and finished products are continuously removed at the same rate to ensure a constant material volume in the process chamber. The basic difference between batch-wise and continuous manufacturing is illustrated in Figure 13.1. The quality during continuous production is assured by incorporating at-line, on-line, or in-line process analytical technology (PAT) measurements into the process stream, which allow continuous monitoring of critical process parameters as well as continuous inspection of quality attributes of raw materials, intermediates, and end product. When the monitored parameters remain within the acceptable ranges defined during the development phase, the outcome of the process is guaranteed. Any deviation from the predefined range can be rapidly corrected by real-time adjustment of process parameters via a feedback or feedforward control system. Since continuous processing does not rely on off-line measurement to determine if the material quality is within the predefined

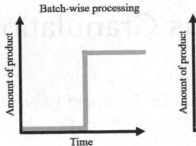
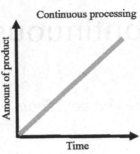

FIGURE 13.1 Schematic Illustration of the Basic Difference between Batch-Wise (Left) and Continuous (Right) Manufacturing. During Batch-Wise Manufacturing, Materials are Charged at the Start of the Process and Discharged When the Predetermined Endpoint is Reached, While Continuous Manufacturing Materials are Continuously Charged and Discharged at the Same Rate.

specifications, there is no need to interrupt the manufacturing process to make critical decisions about product quality, thus reducing cycle time and space required for material storage.

The pharmaceutical industry has been slow to adopt the concept of continuous processing, although its value has already been proven in other industries (polymer, food, dairy, electronics, automobile, and petrochemical), which have implemented fully continuous production processes for many years [1–3]. In these industries, the drivers for the shift toward continuous processing were not limited to the reduced costs, the ease of automation, and the short response time to growth when higher output is required, but also the higher yield, additional process knowledge gained, and improved product quality (due to the multiple in-process analyzers built into a continuous manufacturing line) were essential features that stimulated the implementation of continuous processing.

Although batch processes are often characterized by limited process control (possibly resulting in a batch rejection or reprocessing), high labor costs (due to the multiple manual interventions during processing), high production costs, excessive inventories, and scale-up issues, this mode of processing prevailed within the pharmaceutical industry as it has been hesitant to move from batch processing toward continuous processing for several reasons.

Historically, innovation within the pharmaceutical industry has been mainly through the introduction of new drugs and to a lesser extent via novel drug delivery platforms. Because of the high value of the manufactured goods and the associated high profit margins, there was no driver for innovation in conventional pharmaceutical manufacturing processes of solid dosage forms, even when one was aware that the manufacturing process was run suboptimally. However, faced with greater pressure to reduce costs (e.g., due to the competition from generics or the small drug pipeline) and based on the opportunities offered by continuous processing toward process control (to reduce process variability), the incentives are currently present to introduce continuous processing within the pharmaceutical production plant, and companies are implementing this concept in their strategies. Stringent regulatory constraints within the pharmaceutical industry were initially perceived as another barrier, as they allowed little room for change and significantly contributed to the aversion to bring new manufacturing technologies to the attention of the regulators (to avoid delaying regulatory approval).

However, the current emphasis on quality-by-design and PAT initiatives by the regulatory authorities has lowered this hurdle [4–7]. By its very nature, continuous processing with automated and real-time in-process monitoring and control fits perfectly within these concepts. The PAT framework for Innovative Pharmaceutical Manufacturing and Quality Assurance describes a regulatory framework, which stimulates the development and implementation of new efficient tools during pharmaceutical development, manufacturing, and quality assurance while maintaining or improving the current level of product quality assurance [4]. On the basis of the concept that quality cannot be tested into the product but must be built in by design, the PAT and quality-by-design initiatives aim to introduce new technologies into the pharmaceutical manufacturing process to better respond to the changing marketplace, and continuous processing is an integral part of this strategy to move toward a risk- and science-based approach for pharmaceutical processing as "facilitating continuous processing to improve efficiency and manage variability, using small-scale equipment," has been identified in the PAT initiative as a way to improve quality, safety, and efficiency [4,5]. Based on these regulatory initiatives, pharmaceutical manufacturers should be encouraged to exploit the benefits of continuous processing.

Another regulatory-related issue when introducing continuous processing is that the conventional method to identify a batch is not applicable anymore for continuous processes. However, the FDA batch definition can also accommodate continuous processes as "batch" within the definition does not refer to the mode of manufacturing, but to a quantity of material having uniform character and quality (within specified limits). Hence, several options for batch definition during continuous processes are applicable, for example, amount of material manufactured within a specified production interval or corresponding to a specific amount of raw material processed. Meanwhile, regulatory authorities such as the Food and Drug Administration (FDA), European Medicine Agency (EMA), and Pharmaceuticals and Medical Devices Agency (PMDA) stated that there are no regulatory hurdles toward the implementation of continuous manufacturing and encourage its adoption to pursue ameliorated product quality [8]. Furthermore, a new guideline (due 2021) by the International Conference on Harmonization aims at clarification and harmonization of international regulatory requirements applicable to continuous manufacturing, and the FDA published a draft guidance for industry providing insight into the FDA's opinion on quality considerations for continuous manufacturing [9,10]. Currently, four pharmaceutical companies were granted approval by the American, European, or Japanese regulatory authorities for at least one continuously manufactured drug product [11].

The importance of continuous manufacturing will certainly increase over the coming years, and it is certain to make an impact on the manufacturing of solid dosage forms as there are many advantages associated with this mode of manufacturing, which are all related to important economic (cost and time) and quality drivers for change:

- Increased quality control, which improves product uniformity, reduces the amount of rejected or reprocessed material, and increases process efficiency and productivity.
- Less scale-up issues: increasing the production capacity does not require larger equipment (with a development, optimization, and validation phase at each scale), but only an extension of process time on the same equipment using the same process settings, providing enormous flexibility and eliminating material and technology transfer. Given that a continuous process mainly operates under steady-state conditions, the product of a given quality can be produced for any length of time.
- More flexibility: time, and not the size of the equipment, determines the total material output, hence the demand for the product can dictate how many hours the system will operate.
- Smaller production footprint: smaller equipment, fewer good-manufacturing-practice areas, and quality control and assurance labs (as a result of integrated process monitoring), and reduced warehouse space (due to the elimination of storage of intermediates in between unit operations).
- Lower cost: less labor (less personnel assigned to quality control and quality assurance, fewer manual interventions), less waste (improved product quality and less material rejection), shorter development times (fewer process steps, fewer bioequivalence studies), less utilities and resources for heating, ventilation and air conditioning.
- More efficient use of equipment: equipment is only profitable when in operation and the overall equipment effectiveness (i.e., the percentage of time the equipment is making product compared with the maximum) during batch processing within the pharmaceutical industry is too low (typically 30%, with 74% being considered a "good" pharmaceutical process) [12].

- Real-time release based on real-time production records via in-process monitoring (rather than final product testing following batch manufacture).
- Less product at risk provided a sufficient level of plug flow is maintained and that accurate and continuous in-process monitoring with feedback systems is in place (hence the importance of PAT to allow adjustment of the variables to maintain the critical quality attribute (CQAs) of the product within the target levels).
- Ease of automation (reducing labor costs, operator interventions, and human errors, possibility to run the light-off process).
- Enclosed process (no material transfer needed as the different unit operations are directly linked, providing containment for toxic and highly potent drugs).

13.2 CONTINUOUS GRANULATION

A shift toward continuous processing in the pharmaceutical industry is not as extreme as it may sound since several pharmaceutical unit operations are inherently continuous (e.g., roller compaction, tablet compression, hot-melt extrusion, spray drying, packaging, milling), that is, they have a constant flow of material in and out of the equipment. However, they are typically run to process a fixed amount of material (i.e., a batch process), but the capability is present to rapidly change toward the continuous production concept. Continuous tablet manufacturing via dry granulation can, for example, be achieved by combining blending, roller compaction, milling, and tableting into a continuous manufacturing cycle.

However, the challenge for the pharmaceutical industry is to modify the inherently batch processes (e.g., wet granulation, drying, coating) into continuous techniques to fully benefit from the advantages associated with continuous processing in systems that rely on these unit operations. As wet granulation is the most applied popular method to improve material properties (e.g., flow properties, homogeneity, compressibility) via an agglomeration procedure, development of a continuous granulation step was required to introduce a fully continuous production line of solid dosage forms as conventional fluid-bed and high-shear granulators operate in batch-wise mode [13].

Although the amount of material processed can be increased by prolonging the process run time, this does not entirely eliminate the need of having continuous granulators of different sizes as each continuous granulator has a maximum throughput capacity, and for certain applications, this might result in a very long process time to be economically feasible. Faced with this problem, the company can either run the process on two parallel continuous production lines with limited capacity or use a single continuous granulation system having larger dimensions. However, as the dynamic range of a continuous granulator is larger compared with a batch granulator, fewer equipment sizes are required, and in addition, to process the same amount of material, the overall size of a continuous processor is smaller compared with batch granulators.

A critical aspect of a continuous granulation technique is the product homogeneity at start-up and shut-down. Whereas material loss during batch processing only occurs during material transfer between different unit operations, the yield of a continuous process is mainly determined by the time required to reach steady-state conditions within the granulation chamber and by the end-of-batch material holdup in the granulator. As these factors are independent of the amount of material processed, they have less of an impact when larger quantities are processed (i.e., during commercial manufacturing) compared with processing a smaller material volume during the development phase. Following the start-up phase, in-process controls and feedback loops must ensure that the output parameters remain within the predefined intervals to maintain steady-state conditions in response to variations in, for example, raw materials.

Another challenge is to obtain a uniform material residence time in the continuous granulator. This essentially requires a plug flow of the material in the granulator to minimize the effects of a residence time distribution on product quality. In contrast, all materials processed via a batch-wise unit operation

TABLE 13.1
Overview of the Various Continuous Granulation
Techniques Available for Processing of Pharmaceuticals

Mechanical granulation
- High-shear granulation (ring layer granulation)
- Twin-screw granulation
- Roller compaction

Fluidized-bed granulation

Spray drying

Spray congealing

have, by the very nature of the process, the same residence time. Whereas plug flow moves the material directly from feed zone toward the discharge zone (resulting in a well-defined residence time for all materials), incoming material is mixed with material already present in the granulation chamber when back mixing occurs (i.e., material retention time is less controlled and variable).

Different continuous granulation techniques available are listed in Table 13.1. Although roller compaction, spray congealing, and spray drying (possibly linked to a continuous fluid bed or with a fluid bed integrated at the bottom of the spray drying chamber to increase granule size and flow properties [14]) can also be used for the continuous production of granules, these applications are not discussed in this chapter as these agglomeration techniques are reviewed in detail in other chapters of this handbook. This chapter covers continuous fluid-bed drying, twin-screw granulation, and ring layer granulation and focuses on the critical process parameters affecting the granule quality. Additionally, the integration of continuous wet granulation in continuous manufacturing lines is discussed. Over recent years, twin-screw granulation has emerged as preferred continuous wet granulation technique for improvement of the flowability, homogeneity, and compressibility of materials which is reflected in the numerous scientific studies available.

13.3 CONTINUOUS FLUID-BED GRANULATORS

Conventional batch fluid-bed systems have been adapted for continuous processing, the main modifications being a continuous powder inlet valve and a continuous classifying device to limit the outlet from the granulation chamber to only agglomerated materials. The latter is based on an air separator, which retains undersized particles in the granulation chamber, whereas larger agglomerates are not withheld by the upward airflow and are removed from the granulation process based on their mass (Figure 13.2). The velocity of the upward airflow is controlling the particle size of the granulated material. As it is essential to maintain steady-state conditions during processing, strict control of the powder feed system is required as a new particle has to be added to the process chamber for every particle removed from the system. If the input and output rates are not matched, either the material will accumulate in the granulation chamber or the process will run out of particles; however, even before these extremes occur, the powder/liquid ratio will change, thus affecting the agglomerate growth rate and granule characteristics. This design provides limited control over material residence time as the first-in/first-out principle of material flow in the granulation chamber cannot be guaranteed. Another disadvantage is that all processes (mixing, granulation, and drying) take place at the same time inside a single chamber; hence, dry and wet granules can interact with each other.

In contrast, the different phases of a granulation process are spatially separated in a horizontal fluid bed (Figure 13.3) as different functional zones (product feed zone, product mixing and

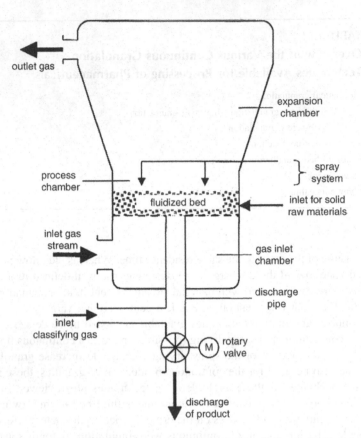

FIGURE 13.2 Continuous Fluid-Bed Granulator. The Granule Size is Controlled by an Upward Airflow, Which Retains Undersized Particles in the Granulation Chamber. (Reprinted with permission from M. Jacob, *Granulation equipment* (In: Handbook of Powder Technology, A.D. Salman, M.J. Hounslow, J.P.K. Seville, eds., 2007), 417–476).

preheating zone, spraying zone, drying zone, cooling zone, and discharge zone, which are not necessarily mechanically separated from each other) can be identified based on the flow rate, temperature, and relative humidity of the fluidizing/drying air and on the presence of top- or bottom-spray nozzles. This allows sequential mixing, heating, agglomeration, and drying as the product passes through the longitudinal granulation chamber. The movement of material from the feed zone toward the discharge zone of the horizontal fluid bed can be controlled via a specific air distribution plate (gill-shaped openings), via vibration of the granulation chamber, or using a sloped powder bed (as fluidized particles have a liquid-like flow behavior) to guarantee directional transport of the powder, without segregation of the powder particles. Despite the efficient air-driven material transport in the horizontal fluid-bed dryers, they are characterized by broad residence time distributions (e.g., up to 60 minutes at a throughput of 60 kg/h) [15]. However, for traceability and minimization of diverted non-compliant material in case of disturbances, plug flow is preferred for control of continuous granulation processes. Additionally, continuous horizontal fluid-bed dryers require a large amount of material at start-up as the equipment is filled with raw material similar to batch processing, and only after this material has been granulated, the process switches to the continuous mode by introducing the material via an inlet valve and discharging granules via an outlet valve. Thus, horizontal fluid beds are not favored for pharmaceutical continuous production.

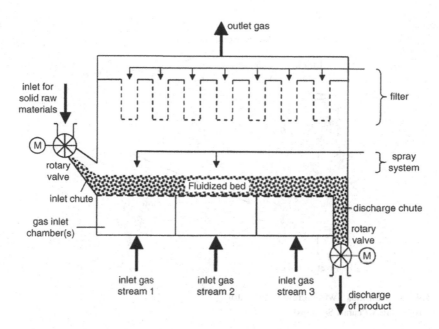

outlet gas

inlet for solid raw materials

filter

rotary valve

spray system

inlet chute

Fluidized bed

discharge chute

gas inlet chamber(s)

rotary valve

inlet gas stream 1

inlet gas stream 2

inlet gas stream 3

discharge of product

FIGURE 13.3 Continuous Horizontal Fluid-Bed Granulator. (Reprinted with permission from M. Jacob, *Granulation equipment* (In: Handbook of Powder Technology, A.D. Salman, M.J. Hounslow, J.P.K. Seville, eds., 2007), 417–476.).

13.4 TWIN-SCREW GRANULATION

Twin-screw granulation is the most applied continuous wet granulation technique. It was first described by Keleb et al. who successfully produced lactose granules by removing the die of a co-rotating intermeshing twin-screw extruder and through the addition of distilled water or an aqueous polyvinylpyrrolidone solution as granulation liquid to the extruder [16]. Removal of the die drastically reduced the pressure build-up at the barrel end and avoided compression of the granules, yielding medium-density granules [16]. Along the length of the screws, different process steps take place, that is, mixing, granulation, conveying, and discharging. The confined space (typically 0.1–0.5 mm) between screws and barrel ensures intense mixing and efficient granulation within a short and controllable time period. The screws can typically be configured modularly and consist of conveying elements, kneading elements, or specific shaping elements (e.g., comb mixing elements, size control elements). Figures 13.4 and 13.5 depict a continuous twin-screw granulator and a typical twin-screw configuration consisting of two blocks of each six kneading elements at a stagger angle of 60°, respectively.

Residence time distributions vary roughly between 2 to 20 seconds, depending on the process settings and screw configuration, whereas the residence time distributions during batch-wise granulation are in the order of tens of minutes [17–20]. The short residence time during twin-screw granulation ensures that steady-state conditions are quickly reached, and in combination with a minimal product holdup, this allows processing at a small scale (e.g., during drug product development phases) with limited material loss using the same equipment as for commercial manufacturing. The stability and repeatability of the process were evaluated by Vercruysse et al., by monitoring of critical granule and tablet quality attributes, and process descriptors (e.g., torque, temperature barrel jacket) during three five-hour runs, granulating a commercial formulation [21]. Although a stabilization period was observed for the process descriptors, the quality of the granules and tablets produced during this period was not affected. Additionally, the process proved highly repeatable [21].

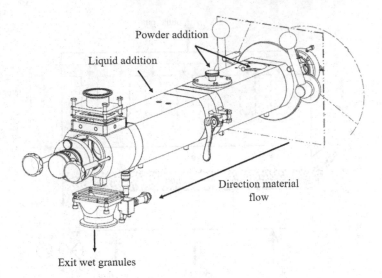

Powder addition

Liquid addition

Direction material
flow

Exit wet granules

FIGURE 13.4 Continuous Twin-Screw Granulator.
(*Source*: Copyright: GEA Pharma Systems).

Keleb et al. compared granulation via twin-screw granulation and high-shear granulation [22]. Formulations with high paracetamol or cimetidine content could be processed via twin-screw granulation, whereas conventional high-shear granulation required an additional binder. Twin-screw granulation proved a robust process toward raw material variability as lactose particle size (90–450 mesh) and morphology only had a minor influence on granule and tablet properties, whereas granulation in a high-shear mixer was more affected by these variables. Further, the paracetamol and cimetidine granules prepared via twin-screw granulation had a higher process yield and lower friability compared with high-shear processing. Furthermore, Lee et al. compared the quality of microcrystalline cellulose (MCC) granules produced via twin-screw granulation and high-shear granulation [23]. Scanning electron microscopy (SEM) images showed that, in contrast to the spherical and smooth granules produced via high-shear granulation, granules produced via twin-screw granulation exhibited an irregular shape and rough surface. Flat edges likely induced

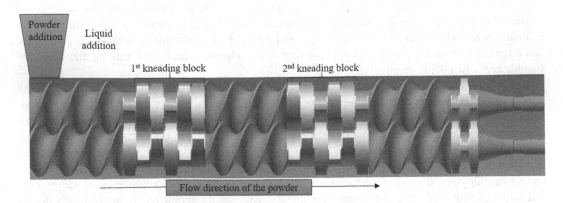

Powder
addition

Liquid
addition

1st kneading block   2nd kneading block

Flow direction of the powder

FIGURE 13.5 Typical Screw Configuration Used During Twin-Screw Granulation, Consisting of Conveying Elements and Two Blocks of Each Six Kneading Elements at a Forward Stagger Angle of 60°. (Reprinted from A. Kumar et al., "Linking granulation performance with residence time and granulation liquid distributions in twin-screw granulation: An experimental investigation." *European Journal of Pharmaceutical Sciences* 90 (2016): 25–37, with permission from Elsevier).

by kneading elements were identified in the twin-screw granulated granules. Additionally, uniaxial bulk confined compression tests disclosed that the continuously produced granules were three to four times weaker than the granules produced via high-shear granulation which was attributed to the higher porosity of the former as shown via mercury porosimetry and X-ray tomography.

Compared with high-shear granulation and fluid-bed granulation, less water was required to efficiently agglomerate a placebo lactose formulation with or without a binder via twin-screw granulation [16,22–24]. Additionally, Lee et al. reported that the liquid-to-solid (L/S) ratio operating window yielding acceptable granules is wider for twin-screw granulation compared to high-shear mixing [23].

In recent years, the twin-screw granulation process was intensively studied, improving our understanding of the granulation mechanism and the interplay between process parameters, material attributes, and final granule (and tablet) quality. Altogether, twin-screw granulation is currently the most promising continuous technique to replace batch-wise granulation techniques.

13.4.1 CRITICAL PROCESS PARAMETERS

Acknowledging the potential of twin-screw granulation, numerous researchers investigated the impact of screw design, formulation, and process variables on the granule quality. However, as these studies were performed on granulators varying in scale and geometry, on diverse formulations, and in the different process parameter ranges, conclusions are sometimes contradictory and/ or restricted to specific experimental regions. Key process variables that must be considered to optimize granule quality are the screw configuration, liquid-to-solid (L/S) ratio, screw speed, temperature, and powder feed rate.

Research unanimously points at the L/S ratio as the most influential process parameter affecting the granule quality which is inherent to the wet granulation principle. Adding more water favors liquid and solid bonds' formation, resulting in larger, denser, and stronger particles [17,24–30,32].

Reports on the effect of screw speed and throughput separately are contradictory at times. Most studies described a limited or no effect of screw speed on the granule size distribution [26,28,33,34], while others found a negative [23,30] or positive correlation [28,32] between screw speed and granule size distribution. Similarly, some studies reported on larger granules produced at higher powder feed rates [27,33,35], while others reported the opposite or no effect [26,34,36]. Although this could be attributed to formulation-dependent effects, this is probably also due to the exploration of different experimental regions covering different degrees of barrel fill level. The barrel fill level is the ratio of wet mass volume to the total available volume in the barrel and is determined by the barrel and screw dimensions, screw speed, and powder feed rate. While the actual fill level is rarely determined, the specific feed load (SFL) and powder feed number (PFN) can be used as surrogate descriptors (Eqs. 13.1 and 13.2) [28,37,38]. Whereas SFL only relies on the screw speed and powder feed rate, PFN also takes material properties into account which enables comparison between different materials

$$\text{SFL} = \frac{\text{powder feed rate}}{\text{screw speed}} \tag{13.1}$$

$$\text{PFN} = \frac{\text{powder feed rate}}{\text{powder bulk density} * \text{screw speed} * \text{free barrel volume}} \tag{13.2}$$

Lute et al. investigated the influence of L/S ratio and barrel fill level, estimated by the SFL and PFN, on the residence time distribution and quality of MCC and lactose granules [28]. The mean residence time decreased with increasing fill levels as a result of more pressure-driven flow. Whereas the granule size of the lactose formulation was not affected by different fill levels, the median granule size of MCC granules decreased at higher fill levels [28]. For MCC, at identical SFL, PFN values were higher compared to lactose. This signifies that due to differences in material properties, the barrel fill level was higher for MCC than lactose at identical screw speed and powder feed rate, which resulted in higher shear forces breaking the MCC granules. Further, in contrast to MCC, lactose is well-soluble which favors bridge formation between particles and the creation of stronger particles less affected by the fill level. Finally, as lactose dissolves during granulation, a stickier mass was created in the granulator, resulting in longer mean residence times for granulation of lactose compared to MCC making the latter more sensitive to fill level changes [28].

Djuric et al. compared granulation of lactose and dicalcium phosphate (DCP) on two granu-lators with similar screw configurations but differing in free barrel volume and screw diameter [33]. Increasing the powder feed rate (and thus also the barrel fill level) generally yielded larger granule size distributions [33]. This is in contrast to the study of Lute et al [28]. However, Djuric et al. also reported that the observed effect was much more pronounced using the granulator barrel with a lower free volume [33]. Thus, it is recommended to take formulation properties and free barrel volume into account, either by calculating the actual fill level or the PFN as a surrogate descriptor, for a fair evaluation of the effect of process parameters affecting the fill level. In contrast to the conflicting reports on the effect of powder feed rate on particle size, most studies reported stronger and denser granules at higher powder feed rates, which was attributed to enhanced densification in the function of the fill level [26,33,35].

The effect of barrel temperature is not often studied in the literature. Nevertheless, granulation of well-soluble formulations at higher temperatures favored granule formation, allowing more material to solubilize during the short processing time. This, in turn, created more solid bonds upon crystallization of dissolved material, yielding larger and stronger granules [27,29,34].

13.4.2 SCREW CONFIGURATION

Combining different screw elements, endless screw designs can be configured. However, screw configurations generally consist of one or two kneading zones separated by conveying elements and a conveying zone at the screw end. Van Melkebeke et al. demonstrated that conveying ele-ments after a kneading zone eliminated oversized granules, thereby increasing the yield [39]. In contrast to the kneading zone, conveying elements are partially filled with the filling degree depending on the applied process parameters.

Conveying elements with different pitch lengths are available. Djuric and Kleinebudde demonstrated that conveying elements with smaller pitch lengths exhibited a detrimental effect on the process yield, increasing both the fines and oversized granule fractions as the smaller volumes between the screw flights resulted in uneven material distribution between the flight chambers and limited interaction with material in other chambers [40]. Similarly, Liu et al. reported that con-veying elements with a larger pitch length after a kneading zone increased the fraction of medium-sized granules [41].

Kneading elements induce shear forces on the wetted mass which results in intense liquid-powder mixing and squeezing of granulation liquid to the granule surface. They vary in thickness and can be positioned at stagger angles of 30, 60, and 90° in forward or backward direction. Increasing the forward stagger angle, especially up to 90°, results in longer mean residence times and more plug flow behavior which is reflected in higher torque values and formation of larger, denser, and stronger granules, although this effect is also dependent on the screw filling degree [19,39,42]. Positioning the kneading elements backward induces even more restriction with the transport of material relying on pressure-driven flow. However, such configurations are not often used as they result in dense lumps, flake-like granule shapes, and/or blockage, especially when a high number of kneading elements are used [40,43]. Inclusion of more kneading elements in the screw configuration generally prolongs the mean residence time and restricts axial mixing but favors liquid-powder mixing, resulting in larger, denser, and stronger granules [18,19,24,24,34,40]. Overall, kneading zones consisting of four to eight kneading elements at a forward stagger angle of

60° are most commonly used. A commonly used screw configuration including two kneading zones of each six kneading elements at a forward stagger angle of 60° is shown in Figure 13.5.

Further, other screw element designs were evaluated, including tooth mixing elements, comb mixing elements, screw mixing elements, and size control elements, to maximize the granule fractions suitable for downstream processing ([24,35,42,44]). Although their use is not widely applied, some of these elements show the potential to limit the fines and oversized fractions of the granules.

Comb mixing elements (also referred to as distributive mixing elements) consist of an angular-cutted ring positioned perpendicular to the screw axis and an annular ring [44]. Depending on the angle of the cuts, forward material movement is promoted or hindered. This design was adopted from extrusion processes and is hypothesized to provide distributive mixing [42,44]. Slightly different designs are available [35,42]. Sayin et al. performed a dedicated study on the comb mixing elements including three screw mixing elements in a screw configuration further consisting of conveying elements [44]. The comb mixing elements were positioned at the screw end, either next to each other or separated by a small conveying zone, and the direction of the annular ring was facing the upstream screw elements or directed toward the screw end [44]. Compared to screws exclusively consisting of conveying elements, all screw configurations with comb mixing elements resulted in narrower granule size distributions with fewer fines and oversized granules. However, when the annular ring of the elements was facing the screw end, monomodal granule size distributions were obtained at lower L/S ratios. Inclusion of the comb mixing elements with annular ring toward the screw end also proved beneficial compared to more conventional screw configurations with a kneading zone consisting of seven kneading elements at an angle of 30° backward and 90° or 60° forward as the screw configurations with comb mixing elements yielded spherical granules with a monomodal size distribution [42,44]. Despite their capacity to narrow granule size distributions, it should be noted that in contrast to the conventional kneading and conveying elements, the comb mixing elements are not self-cleaning which could limit their implementation in pharmaceutical processes [44].

Vercruysse et al. found that replacing a length corresponding to two L/D or four L/D conveying elements by screw mixing elements (Figure 13.6, left) at the screw end significantly reduced the oversized granule fraction while no additional fines were created, which indicated these elements induced breakage and layering [24]. Additionally, positioning these screw mixing elements at the screw end resulted in lower and more stable torque values [24]. The screw mixing elements have some transport capacity as the geometry of screw mixing elements resembles conveying elements, but their flight tip design induces more backflow and distributive material mixing [24]. The design of the screw mixing elements was optimized making them self-cleaning by introducing several planes in the channel depth between the screw flights. Similarly to the effect of the screw mixing elements, the resulting size control elements (Figure 13.6, right) reduced the fraction of oversized granules without creation of fines [29].

When granulating controlled release formulations containing 20% (w/w) hydroxypropylmethylcellulose (HPMC), Thompson et al. reported on the formation of twisted noodle-shaped granules unsuitable for downstream processing originating from the screw flights of conveying elements positioned after a non-conveying zone [45]. It was hypothesized that the creation of a liquid-rich granule surface in the kneading zone in combination with a highly viscous wet mass typical of HPMC as a controlled release excipient resulted in the twisted noodle-shaped granules [45]. Formation of such granules could only be avoided by positioning either kneading elements or comb mixing elements at the screw end [45]. In contrast, Vanhoorne et al., processing controlled release formulations containing up to 40% (w/w) HPMC using screw configurations with conveying elements at the screw end, reported the formation of granules similar in shape to immediate release granules [46,47]. Even when processing an identical formulation and using a similar screw configuration as that by Thompson et al., Vanhoorne et al. only found twisted noodle-shaped granules at excessive L/S ratios. Therefore, it was concluded that the granulator design (e.g., smaller clearance between granulator screws and barrel in the study of Thompson et al.) and formulation

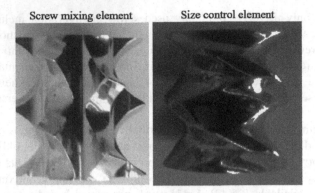

FIGURE 13.6   Screw Mixing Element (Left) and Size Control Element (Right). (Reprinted from C. Portier et al., "Continuous twin screw granulation: Influence of process and formulation variables on granule quality attributes of model formulations." *International Journal of Pharmaceutics* 576, 25 (2020): 118981, with permission of Elsevier).

characteristics (particularly high water absorption capacity of MCC) were likely to take part in the formation of aberrantly shaped controlled release granules [47].

13.4.3   Granulation Mechanism

Most studies merely linked equipment, process, and formulation settings to the quality of granules collected at the granulator exit, without studying the different phenomena occurring spatially along the screw length. To elucidate the twin-screw granulation mechanism, granules can be collected from different screw compartments via screw pullouts or granules corresponding to different screw compartments can be produced using a modified granulation barrel allowing rearrangement of the screw elements to obtain granules from the desired compartment [41,43,48,49]. The latter approach offers the possibility to collect much larger amounts of granules allowing more extensive granule characterization and was applied by Verstraeten et al. in a particularly thorough study investigating the effect of screw speed, throughput, and L/S ratio on the granule size and shape, and on the distribution of liquid, active pharmaceutical ingredient (API) and porosity over different size fractions of two formulations with different hydrophobicity [49]. Two screw configurations with either one or two kneading blocks, consisting of six kneading elements at a stagger angle of 60° and two thin kneading elements at the screw end, were used. The granulation mechanism derived from these experiments is schematically presented in Figure 13.7.

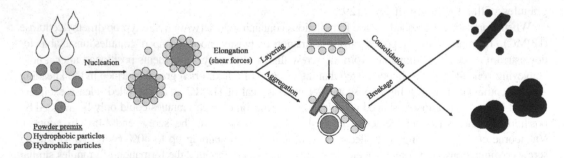

FIGURE 13.7   Schematic Visualization of the Twin-screw Granulation Mechanism as Presented by Verstraeten et al. (Reprinted from M. Verstraeten et al., "In-depth experimental analysis of pharmaceutical twin-screw wet granulation in view of detailed process understanding." *International Journal of Pharmaceutics* 529, 1–2 (2017): 678–693, with permission of Elsevier).

In the first screw compartment consisting of conveying elements, granulation liquid was added to the powder blend resulting in immersion nucleation with the formation of wetted, porous, and oversized granules next to primary particles. Uneven API and liquid distribution over the different granule size fractions were observed as hydrophobic particles were layered on top of nuclei of hydrophilic particles which were preferentially nucleated. This effect is most pronounced at low L/S ratios as under these conditions hydrophobic particles remain mainly unwetted and consequently ungranulated.

Next, loose granules were densified and elongated as the wet mass is pushed through the small gap between the kneading elements and the barrel wall, thereby squeezing the liquid toward the granule surface. Such liquid-rich granule surface favored further layering and aggregation of particles. At low L/S ratios, brittle granules were created which were mainly subject to breakage. Especially for hydrophilic formulations processed at a low L/S ratio, this resulted in a heterogeneous distribution of water over the granule size fractions, indicating the need for a second kneading zone for successful granulation. In contrast, applying high L/S ratios yielded plastic granules which were predominantly consolidated in the kneading department, resulting in homogeneous liquid distribution and unimodal size distribution. These granules were further consolidated in the second kneading zone, shifting the granule size distributions slightly to smaller particles. The two thin kneading elements at the screw end did not affect the granule size at low L/S ratios, while they induced breakage of oversized granules at high L/S ratios.

In contrast to the narrow and unimodal granule size distributions obtained after batch-wise granulation, several authors reported on the bimodal granule size distributions after twin-screw granulation [17,23,24,26,26,28,30,44]. These granule size distributions typically evolve toward narrower unimodal size distributions at higher L/S ratios, giving rise to the hypothesis that this was due to uneven liquid distribution over the granule fractions at low L/S ratios [17,20,43,44]. However, using a screw configuration with two kneading zones, Verstraeten et al. demonstrated that the granulation liquid was homogeneously distributed over the granules at the granulator outlet, independently of the applied L/S ratio. Nevertheless, granulation at low L/S ratios yielded bimodal granule size distributions, consisting of smaller spherical and larger elongated granules, whereas narrow unimodal granule size distributions were obtained at higher L/S ratios. Therefore, Verstraeten et al. concluded that the bimodal granule size distribution often observed after twin-screw granulation at relatively low L/S ratios was not linked to uneven liquid distribution over the granules (as earlier hypothesized) but due to the limited availability of liquid at the granule surface which hinders aggregation [49].

Narrow monomodal granule size distributions are generally preferred to minimize the risk of segregation during downstream processing and to ensure uniform drying of the wet granules. Although oversized granules could be eliminated by milling the dried granules, it should be noted that the creation of fines is an undesirable side-effect of milling [24].

13.4.4 Heat-Assisted Twin-Screw Granulation

During conventional twin-screw granulation, water is typically used as a solvent to establish particle bonding. Optionally, binders can be added either in the granulation liquid or in the powder blend to favor granulation. Continuous melt granulation using a twin-screw granulator is also possible via the inclusion of a thermoplastic binder in the powder blend instead of the addition of granulation liquid and application of higher barrel temperatures. Applying melt granulation, the subsequent drying step typical of wet granulation processes is eliminated.

Recently, heat-assisted twin-screw dry granulation was introduced [50–52]. In this case, granulation was exclusively induced by moderate heating at temperatures below the glass transition temperature or melting temperature of the ingredients, as no water was added to the process. Unlike conventional twin-screw granulation, the heat-assisted granulation process is not susceptible to moisture-induced degradation while it is also expected to be less prone to heat-induced degradation than twin-screw melt granulation. Additionally, in contrast to melt granulation which relies upon heating above the glass transition temperature or melting temperature of the ingredients, no molecular level mixing is anticipated. However, while Kallakunta et al. and Ye et al. indeed observed no loss of crystallinity after heat-assisted twin-screw granulation of a controlled release formulation, Ye et al. did detect interactions between the API and polymers [50,52]. Currently, only the aforementioned studies are available on heat-assisted twin-screw granulation. Its potential as a generically applicable continuous dry granulation technique is currently unclear. Kallakunta et al. reported that the plasticity and compactability of polymers and APIs included in the formulation influence successful granulation, while Ye et al. indicated that inclusion of a lubricant was necessary to limit friction and prevent equipment abrasion during processing [50,52].

13.5 RING LAYER GRANULATION

A continuous ring layer granulator consists of a cylindrical process chamber including a rotary impeller with configurable blades and one or multiple nozzles for granulation liquid addition (Figure 13.8). Due to the high rotation speed of the impeller (up to 4000 rpm), centrifugal forces dominate over gravimetric forces, resulting in a forward-moving concentric annular layer of product in the process chamber. Granules are formed by the intimate mixing of liquid and powder induced by the impeller [20,53]. At lower impeller speed and without liquid addition, the equipment can also be used for mechanical mixing of powders as at such conditions a free-falling movement or fluidization of the powder particles is obtained.

Up to now limited academic studies investigated the ring layer granulation process [20,53,54]. Järvinen et al. compared the quality of granules produced via ring layer granulation and batch-wise granulation processes (high-shear granulation and fluid-bed granulation), whereas Meng et al. dedicated one study to the determination of the critical process parameters affecting granule and tablet quality and compared the quality of granules produced via ring layer granulation and

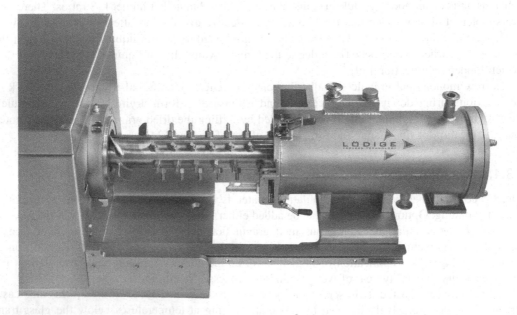

FIGURE 13.8 Continuous Ring Layer Granulator (Corimix® by Lödige Process Technology). (*Source*: Copyright: Lödige Process Technology, Paderborn, Germany).

twin-screw granulation in another study [20,53]. Meng et al. identified impeller speed and L/S ratio as critical process parameters, whereas throughput exhibited a limited impact on the granule quality [20,53]. However, it should be noted that only a fraction (10–20 kg/h) of the operational throughput region (maximal throughput 80 kg/h) of the ring layer granulator was investigated which does not exclude throughput as a critical process parameter. Increasing the L/S ratio and impeller speed during ring layer granulation yielded larger, denser, stronger, and more spherical granules with excellent flowability. The effect of the L/S ratio is in accordance with its effect in other wet granulation processes, that is, favoring granule growth and consolidation. The impact of applying a higher impeller speed on the granule quality was attributed to the more frequent interparticle collisions resulting in more granulation liquid squeezed to the granule surface and consequently more consolidation of the granules.

In contrast to the granules produced via twin-screw granulation, narrow granule size distributions and spherical granules were obtained after ring layer granulation which was attributed to higher shear forces and more frequent collisions during the latter process [20,53]. Despite the higher mechanical input during ring layer granulation, the porosity of granules produced during ring layer and twin-screw granulation was similar and higher than typically encountered after batch-wise high-shear granulation. This was attributed to the short residence time during both processes which limited consolidation. The residence time distributions during twin-screw granulation and ring layer granulation were narrow and in the same order of magnitude (<12 seconds), making them ideally suited for continuous manufacturing from a traceability point of view. Comparing the quality of granules produced via twin-screw granulation and ring layer granulation, it should be noted that the screw configuration (consisting of conveying elements and comb mixing elements) was kept constant during twin-screw granulation, although it is a highly influential variable [20]. Järvinen et al. reported that the granules produced via ring layer granulation resembled those produced via batch-wise high-shear granulation, whereas granules produced via batch-wise fluid-bed granulation were more porous [54].

13.6 DOWNSTREAM PROCESSING AND INTEGRATED MANUFACTURING LINES

In recent years, several equipment manufacturers (e.g., Glatt, L.B. Bohle Maschinen + Verfahren, GEA Pharma Systems, Lödige Process Technology) designed integrated continuous lines for the production of tablets via continuous wet granulation. Such lines typically consist of a dosing station with loss-in-weight feeders, a continuous blender for mixing the API with excipients, a twin-screw (or ring layer) granulator, (semi-)continuous dryer, mill, feeder, and blender for the external phase, and finally a rotary tablet press. An example of an integrated continuous line including a twin-screw granulator is shown in Figure 13.9.

Similarly to the short residence times during twin-screw or ring layer granulation, residence times in the subsequent unit operations are preferably short as well. Up to now only fluid-bed drying after twin-screw granulation is described in academic literature [55–57]. As broad residence times are inherent to continuous fluid-bed drying, semi-continuous segmented fluid-bed dryers were designed to ensure a certain degree of plug flow during fluid-bed drying. Granules are continuously fed into a specific cell of such a segmented fluid-bed dryer for a set time (i.e., filling time) after which the next cell is filled while drying of granules in the previous cells is continued. Thus, next to the airflow and air temperature, the cell filling time can be varied. This principle is demonstrated in Figure 13.10 for a segmented dryer with six cells.

Truly continuous dryers are also commercially available, but to date, none of these systems were evaluated in academic literature. Whereas Freund Vector developed a continuous spiral dryer based on the use of a high-speed airflow, L.B. Bohle Maschinen + Verfahren and Lödige Process Technology made adaptations to the horizontal fluid-bed drying process to ensure plug flow. The

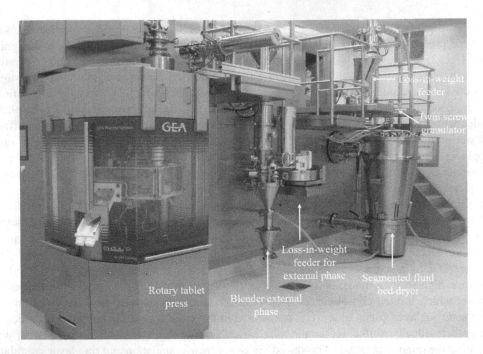

FIGURE 13.9 Integrated Line (ConsiGma^{TM} by GEA Pharma Systems) for Continuous Manufacturing of Tablets Consisting of a Loss-in-Weight Feeder, Twin-Screw Granulator, Segmented Fluid-Bed Dryer, Mill, Loss-in-Weight Feeder, and Blender for External Phase, and a Rotary Tablet Press.
(*Source*: Copyright: GEA Pharma Systems).

continuous dryer of L.B. Bohle Maschinen + Verfahren was integrated after a twin-screw granulator. In this dryer concept, wet granules fall on a perforated vibrating particle transport grid through which conditioned air gently fluidizes the granules (Figure 13.11) [58]. Conveying speed and airflow are independent variables which, next to the airflow temperature, allow steering of the drying process. This continuous fluid-bed dryer design offers short and narrow residence time distributions ideally suited for drying after continuous wet granulation [58]. In the continuous fluid-bed dryer of Lödige Process Technology, a screw is integrated for the forced conveyance which, according to the manufacturer, results in narrow residence time distributions ("Commercial Information by Lödige Process Technology"). This drying process is commercially available linked to a ring layer granulator.

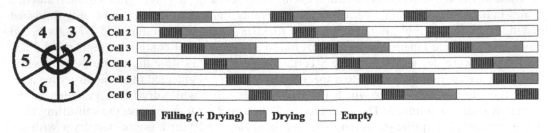

FIGURE 13.10 Operating Principle of a Segmented Fluid-Bed Dryer Comprising Six Cells. (Reprinted from F. De Leersnyder et al., "Breakage and drying behavior of granules in a continuous fluid-bed dryer: Influence of process parameters and wet granule transfer." *European Journal of Pharmaceutical Sciences* 115 (2018): 223–232, with permission of Elsevier).

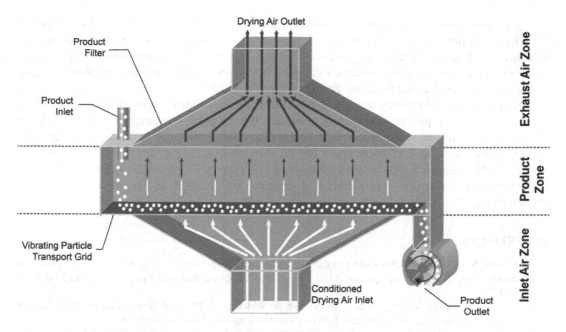

FIGURE 13.11   Operating Principle of the Truly Continuous Fluid-Bed Dryer of L.B. Bohle Maschinen + Verfahren (part of the QbCon® system) Which Ensures Narrow Residence Time Distributions Through Mild Vibration and Fluidization of Particles on the Transport Grid.
(*Source*: Copyright: L.B. Bohle Maschinen + Verfahren GmbH, Ennigerloh, Germany).

Addressing the need for short and controllable drying of granules, Schmidt et al. evaluated the potential of in-barrel-drying, where a part of the granulator barrel is heated to temperatures of 205–215°C, to eliminate the drying step after twin-screw granulation [59]. Complete drying while adding sufficient water for effective granulation proved challenging given the short residence time in the granulator but was achieved for the studied formulation. Although the principle of in-barrel-drying is attractive, its generic applicability and impact on product degradation require further study.

TABLE 13.2

Overview of Granule CQAs and Associated PAT Technology for Their Monitoring and Control (Reprinted from Vanhoorne and Vervaet, "Recent progress in continuous manufacturing of oral solid dosage forms" International Journal of Pharmaceutics 579 (2020): 119194, with permission of Elsevier)

Granule CQA	PAT Technology	References
Granule size distribution	NIR spectroscopy	[60–62]
	Particle size analyzers	[61]
Granule moisture content	NIR spectroscopy	[56,62–65]
Content uniformity	NIR spectroscopy	[62]
	Raman spectroscopy	[37]
Solid state	NIR spectroscopy	[56,60]
	Raman spectroscopy	[56,60]

Up to now, only a few studies were performed on fully integrated continuous lines. Whereas Stauffer et al. pointed at the importance of such studies to reveal interactions between unit operations, De Leersnyder et al. highlighted that the impact of the transportation mode of wet granules (pneumatic vs. gravimetric) on the granule size distribution of dried granules was more influential compared to the fluid-bed drying parameters [55,57].

Along with the availability of mature manufacturing technology, successful implementation of PAT probes for process monitoring promoted the adoption of continuous processing for the manufacturing of oral solid dosage forms. Table 13.2 presents an overview of granule CQAs and associated PAT techniques for their monitoring and control. Interestingly, near infrared (NIR) spectroscopy allows to monitor all granule CQAs, although this might not be achievable for every formulation and depends on the NIR sensitivity of the studied formulation.

REFERENCES

1. Plumb, K. "Continuous Processing in the Pharmaceutical Industry: Changing the Mind Set." *Chemical Engineering Research and Design* 2005; 83 (6):730–738. https://doi.org/https://doi.org/10.1205/cherd. 04359.
2. Rockoff, J. "Drug Making Breaks Away from Its Old Ways." *The Wall Street Journal* 2015. https://www.wsj.com/articles/drug-making-breaks-away-from-its-old-ways-1423444049.
3. Van Arnum, P. "Continuous Processing: Moving with or against the Manufacturing Flow." *Pharmaceutical Technology* 2008; 32 (9):55–58.
4. Food and Drug Administration. "Guidance for Industry. PAT – A Framework for Innovative Pharmaceutical Development, Manufacturing and Quality Assurance." U.S. Department of Health and Human Services. 2004. https://www.fda.gov/media/71012/download.
5. International Conference on Harmonisation. 2009. "Q8(R2)." https://www.ema.europa.eu/en/documents/scientific-guideline/international-conference-harmonisation-technical-requirements-registration-pharmaceuticals-human-use_en-11.pdf.
6. Lee, S. L., TF O'Connor, X. Yang et al. "Modernizing Pharmaceutical Manufacturing: From Batch to Continuous Production." *Journal of Pharmaceutical Innovation* 2015; 10 (3):191–199. https://doi.org/10.1007/s12247-015-9215-8.
7. Yu, L. X., G. Amidon, M. A. Khan et al. "Understanding Pharmaceutical Quality by Design." *The AAPS Journal* 2014; 16 (4): 771–783. https://doi.org/10.1208/s12248-014-9598-3.
8. Nasr, M., M. Krumme, Y. Matsuda et al. "Regulatory Perspectives on Continuous Pharmaceutical Manufacturing: Moving From Theory to Practice" *Journal of Pharmaceutical Sciences* 2017; 106 (11): 3199–3206. https://doi.org/https://doi.org/10.1016/j.xphs.2017.06.015.
9. Food and Drug Administration. "Quality Considerations for Continuous Manufacturing - Guidance for Industry - Draft Guidance." 2019. https://www.fda.gov/media/121314/download. Accessed April 27th 2020.
10. ICH. 2018. "ICH Q13: Continuous Manufacturing of Drug Substances and Drug Products - Final Concept Paper.". https://database.ich.org/sites/default/files/Q13_EWG_Concept_ Paper.pdf.
11. Vanhoorne, V., and C. Vervaet. "Recent Progress in Continuous Manufacturing of Oral Solid Dosage Forms." *International Journal of Pharmaceutics* 2020; 579:119194.
12. Vervaet, C., and J. P. Remon. "Continuous Granulation in the Pharmaceutical Industry." *Chemical Engineering Science* 2005; 60 (14): 3949–3957. https://doi.org/10.1016/j.ces.2005.02.028.
13. Leane, M., K. Pitt, G. K. Reynolds et al. "Manufacturing Classification System in the Real World: Factors Influencing Manufacturing Process Choices for Filed Commercial Oral Solid Dosage Formulations, Case Studies from Industry and Considerations for Continuous Processing,". *Pharmaceutical Development and Technology* 2018; 23:964–977.
14. Masters, K. "Process Stages and Spray Drying Systems." In: Keith Masters edited by, *Spray Drying in Practice*. Spray Dry Consult International, 2002:39–96.
15. Gotthardt, S., A. Knoch, and G. Lee. "Continuous Wet Granulation Using Fluidized-Bed Techniques I. Examination of Powder Mixing Kinetics and Preliminary Granulation Experiments." *European Journal of Pharmaceutics and Biopharmaceutics* 1999; 48 (3): 189–197. https://doi.org/https://doi.org/10.1016/S0939-6411(99)00050-8.
16. Keleb, E. I., A. Vermeire, C. Vervaet, and J. P. Remon. "Twin Screw Granulation as a Simple and

Efficient Tool for Continuous Wet Granulation." *International Journal of Pharmaceutics* 2004a; 273 (1): 183–194. https://doi.org/https://doi.org/10.1016/j.ijpharm.2004.01.001.

17. E. l. Hagrasy, A. S., J. R. Hennenkamp, M. D. Burke, J. J. Cartwright, and J. D. Litster. "Twin Screw Wet Granulation: Influence of Formulation Parameters on Granule Properties and Growth Behavior." *Powder Technology* 2013; 238: 108–115. https://doi.org/https://doi.org/10.1016/j.powtec.2012.04.035.

18. Kumar, A., M. Alakarjula, V. Vanhoorne et al. "Linking Granulation Performance with Residence Time and Granulation Liquid Distributions in Twin-Screw Granulation: An Experimental Investigation." *European Journal of Pharmaceutical Sciences* 2016; 90: 25–37. https://doi.org/https://doi.org/10.1016/j.ejps.2015.12.021.

19. Kumar, A., J. Vercruysse, M. Toiviainen et al. "Mixing and Transport during Pharmaceutical Twin-Screw Wet Granulation: Experimental Analysis via Chemical Imaging." *European Journal of Pharmaceutics and Biopharmaceutics* 2014; 87 (2):279–289. https://doi.org/https://doi.org/10.1016/j.ejpb.2014.04.004.

20. Meng, W., L. Kotamarthy, S. Panikar et al. "Statistical Analysis and Comparison of a Continuous High Shear Granulator with a Twin Screw Granulator: Effect of Process Parameters on Critical Granule Attributes and Granulation Mechanisms." *International Journal of Pharmaceutics* 2016; 513 (1): 357–375. https://doi.org/https://doi.org/10.1016/j.ijpharm.2016.09.041.

21. Vercruysse, J., U. Delaet, I. Van Assche et al. "Stability and Repeatability of a Continuous Twin Screw Granulation and Drying System." *European Journal of Pharmaceutics and Biopharmaceutics* 2013; 85 (3, Part B): 1031–1038. https://doi.org/https://doi.org/10.1016/j.ejpb.2013.05.002.

22. Keleb, E. I., A. Vermeire, C. Vervaet, and J. P. Remon. "Extrusion Granulation and High Shear Granulation of Different Grades of Lactose and Highly Dosed Drugs: A Comparative Study." *Drug Development and Industrial Pharmacy* 2004; 30 (6): 679–691. https://doi.org/10.1081/DDC-120039338.

23. Lee, K. T., A. Ingram, and N. A. Rowson. 2013. "Comparison of Granule Properties Produced Using Twin Screw Extruder and High Shear Mixer: A Step towards Understanding the Mechanism of Twin Screw Wet Granulation." *Powder Technology* 238: 91–98. https://doi.org/https://doi.org/10.1016/j.powtec.2012.05.031.

24. Vercruysse, J., A. Burggraeve, M. Fonteyne et al. "Impact of Screw Configuration on the Particle Size Distribution of Granules Produced by Twin Screw Granulation." *International Journal of Pharmaceutics* 2015; 479 (1):171–180. https://doi.org/https://doi.org/10.1016/j.ijpharm.2014.12.071.

25. Dhenge, R. M., J. J. Cartwright, M. J. Hounslow, and A. D. Salman. "Twin Screw Wet Granulation: Effects of Properties of Granulation Liquid." *Powder Technology* 2012; 229: 126–136. https://doi.org/https://doi.org/10.1016/j.powtec.2012.06.019.

26. Dhenge, R. M., R. S. Fyles, J. J. Cartwright, D. G. Doughty, M. J. Hounslow, and A. D. Salman. "Twin Screw Wet Granulation: Granule Properties." *Chemical Engineering Journal* 2010; 164 (2): 322–329. https://doi.org/https://doi.org/10.1016/j.cej.2010.05.023.

27. Fonteyne, M., A. Correia, S. De Plecker et al. "Impact of Microcrystalline Cellulose Material Attributes: A Case Study on Continuous Twin Screw Granulation." *International Journal of Pharmaceutics* 2015; 478 (2): 705–717. https://doi.org/https://doi.org/10.1016/j.ijpharm.2014.11.070.

28. Lute, S., R. Dhenge, and A. Salman. "Twin Screw Granulation: An Investigation of the Effect of Barrel Fill Level." *Pharmaceutics* 2018; 10 (2): 67. https://doi.org/10.3390/pharmaceutics10020067.

29. Portier, C., K. Pandelaere, U. Delaet et al. "Continuous Twin Screw Granulation: Influence of Process and Formulation Variables on Granule Quality Attributes of Model Formulations." *International Journal of Pharmaceutics* 2020a; 576:118981. https://doi.org/https://doi.org/10.1016/j.ijpharm.2019.118981.

30. Tu, W. D., A. Ingram, and J. Seville. "Regime Map Development for Continuous Twin Screw Granulation." *Chemical Engineering Science* 2013; 87: 315–326. https://doi.org/https://doi.org/10.1016/j.ces.2012.08.015.

31. United States government. "Code of Federal Regulations 21. (210.3) - Definitions." https://www.govinfo.gov/content/pkg/CFR-2012-title21-vol4/pdf/CFR-2012-title21-vol4-sec210-3.pdf. Accessed online April 27th 2020.

32. Vanhoorne, V., B. Bekaert, E. Peeters, T. De Beer, J. P. Remon, and C. Vervaet. . "Improved Tabletability after a Polymorphic Transition of Delta-Mannitol during Twin Screw Granulation." *International Journal of Pharmaceutics* 2016b; 506 (1): 13–24. https://doi.org/https://doi.org/10.1016/j.ijpharm.2016.04.025.

33. Djuric, D., B. Van Melkebeke, P. Kleinebudde, J. P. Remon, and C. Vervaet. "Comparison of Two Twin-Screw Extruders for Continuous Granulation." *European Journal of Pharmaceutics and Biopharmaceutics* 2009; 71 (1): 155–160. https://doi.org/https://doi.org/10.1016/j.ejpb.2008.06.033.

34. Vercruysse, J., D. Córdoba Díaz, E. Peeters et al. "Continuous Twin Screw Granulation: Influence of Process Variables on Granule and Tablet Quality." *European Journal of Pharmaceutics and Biopharmaceutics* 2012; 82 (1): 205–211. https://doi.org/https://doi.org/10.1016/j.ejpb.2012.05.010.

35. Djuric, D., and P. Kleinebudde. "Continuous Granulation with a Twin-Screw Extruder: Impact of Material Throughput." *Pharmaceutical Development and Technology* 2010; 15 (5): 518–525. https://doi.org/10.3109/10837450903397578.

36. Dhenge, R. M., K. Washino, J. J. Cartwright, M. J. Hounslow, and A. D. Salman. "Twin Screw Granulation Using Conveying Screws: Effects of Viscosity of Granulation Liquids and Flow of Powders." *Powder Technology* 2013; 238: 77–90. https://doi.org/https://doi.org/10.1016/j.powtec.2012.05.045.

37. Harting, J., and P. Kleinebudde. "Optimisation of an In-Line Raman Spectroscopic Method for Continuous API Quantification during Twin-Screw Wet Granulation and Its Application for Process Characterisation." *European Journal of Pharmaceutics and Biopharmaceutics* 2019; 137:77–85. https://doi.org/10.1016/j.ejpb.2019.02.015

38. Portier, C., K. Pandelaere, U. Delaet et al. "Continuous Twin Screw Granulation: A Complex Interplay between Formulation Properties, Process Settings and Screw Design." *International Journal of Pharmaceutics* 2020b; 576:119004. https://doi.org/https://doi.org/10.1016/j.ijpharm.2019.119004.

39. Van Melkebeke, B., C. Vervaet, and J. P. Remon. "Validation of a Continuous Granulation Process Using a Twin-Screw Extruder." *International Journal of Pharmaceutics* 2008; 356 (1):224–230. https://doi.org/https://doi.org/10.1016/j.ijpharm.2008.01.012.

40. Djuric, D., and P. Kleinebudde. "Impact of Screw Elements on Continuous Granulation with a Twin-Screw Extruder." *Journal of Pharmaceutical Sciences* 2008; 97 (11): 4934–4942. https://doi.org/https://doi.org/10.1002/jps.21339.

41. Liu, Y., M. R. Thompson, and K. P. O'Donnell. "Function of Upstream and Downstream Conveying Elements in Wet Granulation Processes within a Twin Screw Extruder." *Powder Technology* 2015; 284: 551–559. https://doi.org/https://doi.org/10.1016/j.powtec.2015.07.011.

42. Thompson, M. R., and J. Sun. "Wet Granulation in a Twin-Screw Extruder: Implications of Screw Design." *Journal of Pharmaceutical Sciences* 2010; 99 (4):2090–2103. https://doi.org/https://doi.org/10.1002/jps.21973.

43. E. l. Hagrasy, A. S., and J. D. Litster. "Granulation Rate Processes in the Kneading Elements of a Twin Screw Granulator." *AIChE Journal* 2013; 59 (11): 4100–4115. https://doi.org/10.1002/aic.14180.

44. Sayin, R., A. S. E. l. Hagrasy, and J. D. Litster. "Distributive Mixing Elements: Towards Improved Granule Attributes from a Twin Screw Granulation Process." *Chemical Engineering Science* 2015; 125: 165–175. https://doi.org/https://doi.org/10.1016/j.ces.2014.06.040.

45. Thompson, M. R., and K. P. O'Donnell. "'Rolling' Phenomenon in Twin Screw Granulation with Controlled-Release Excipients." *Drug Development and Industrial Pharmacy* 2015; 41 (3): 482–492. https://doi.org/10.3109/03639045.2013.879723.

46. Vanhoorne, V., L. Janssens, J. Vercruysse, T. De Beer, J. P. Remon, and C. Vervaet. "Continuous Twin Screw Granulation of Controlled Release Formulations with Various HPMC Grades." *International Journal of Pharmaceutics* 2016c; 511 (2): 1048–1057. https://doi.org/https://doi.org/10.1016/j.ijpharm.2016.08.020.

47. Vanhoorne, V., B. Vanbillemont, J. Vercruysse et al. "Development of a Controlled Release Formulation by Continuous Twin Screw Granulation: Influence of Process and Formulation Parameters." *International Journal of Pharmaceutics* 2016a; 505 (1): 61–68. https://doi.org/https://doi.org/10.1016/j.ijpharm.2016.03.058.

48. Li, H., M. R. Thompson, and K. P. O'Donnell. "Understanding Wet Granulation in the Kneading Block of Twin Screw Extruders." *Chemical Engineering Science* 2014; 113: 11–21. https://doi.org/https://doi.org/10.1016/j.ces.2014.03.007.

49. Verstraeten, M., D. Van Hauwermeiren, K. Lee et al. "In-Depth Experimental Analysis of Pharmaceutical Twin-Screw Wet Granulation in View of Detailed Process Understanding." *International Journal of Pharmaceutics* 2017; 529 (1): 678–693. https://doi.org/https://doi.org/10.1016/j.ijpharm.2017.07.045.

50. Kallakunta, V. R., H. Patil, R. Tiwari et al. "Exploratory Studies in Heat-Assisted Continuous Twin-Screw Dry Granulation: A Novel Alternative Technique to Conventional Dry Granulation." *International Journal of Pharmaceutics* 2019; 555:380–393. https://doi.org/10.1016/j.ijpharm.2018.11.045

51. Liu, Y., M. R. Thompson, K. P. O'Donnell, and S. Ali. "Heat Assisted Twin Screw Dry Granulation." *AIChE Journal* 2017; 63 (11): 4748–4760. https://doi.org/10.1002/aic.15820.

52. Ye, X., V. Kallakunta, D. W. Kim et al. "Effects of Processing on a Sustained Release Formulation Prepared by Twin-Screw Dry Granulation." *Journal of Pharmaceutical Sciences* 2019; 108:2895–2904. https://doi.org/10.1016/j.xphs.2019.04.004

53. Meng, W., J. Dvořák, R. Kumar et al. "Continuous High-Shear Granulation: Mechanistic Understanding of the Influence of Process Parameters on Critical Quality Attributes via Elucidating the Internal Physical and Chemical Microstructure." *Advanced Powder Technology* 2019b; 30 (9): 1765–1781. https://doi.org/https://doi.org/10.1016/j.apt.2019.04.028.

54. Järvinen, M. A., M. Paavola, S. Poutiainen et al. "Comparison of a Continuous Ring Layer Wet Granulation Process with Batch High Shear and Fluidized Bed Granulation Processes." *Powder Technology* 2015; 275: 113–120. https://doi.org/https://doi.org/10.1016/j.powtec.2015.01.071.

55. De Leersnyder, F., V. Vanhoorne, H. Bekaert et al. "Breakage and Drying Behaviour of Granules in a Continuous Fluid Bed Dryer: Influence of Process Parameters and Wet Granule Transfer." *European Journal of Pharmaceutical Sciences* 2018; 115: 223–232. https://doi.org/https://doi.org/10.1016/j.ejps.2018.01.037.

56. Fonteyne, M., D. Gildemyn, E. Peeters et al. "Moisture and Drug Solid-State Monitoring during a Continuous Drying Process Using Empirical and Mass Balance Models." *European Journal of Pharmaceutics and Biopharmaceutics* 2014b; 87 (3): 616–628. https://doi.org/https://doi.org/10.1016/j.ejpb.2014.02.015.

57. Stauffer, F., V. Vanhoorne, G. Pilcer et al. "Managing API Raw Material Variability in a Continuous Manufacturing Line – Prediction of Process Robustness." *International Journal of Pharmaceutics* 2019; 569:118525. https://doi.org/https://doi.org/10.1016/j.ijpharm.2019.118525.

58. Meier, R., D. Emanuele, and P. Harbaum. "Important Elements in Continuous Granule Drying Processes - Experiences from Lab and Production Scale." *Technopharm* 2020; 10 (2): 92–101.

59. Schmidt, A., H. de Waard, P. Kleinebudde, and M. Krumme. "Continuous Single-Step Wet Granulation with Integrated in-Barrel-Drying." *Pharmaceutical Research* 2018; 35 (8):167. https://doi.org/10.1007/s11095-018-2451-0.

60. Fonteyne, M., J. Vercruysse, D. Córdoba Díaz, et al. "Real-Time Assessment of Critical Quality Attributes of a Continuous Granulation Process." *Pharmaceutical Development and Technology* 2013; 18 (1): 85–97. https://doi.org/10.3109/10837450.2011.627869.

61. Meng, W., A. D. Román-Ospino, S. S. Panikar et al. "Advanced Process Design and Understanding of Continuous Twin-Screw Granulation via Implementation of in-Line Process Analytical Technologies." *Advanced Powder Technology* 2019a. https://doi.org/10.1016/j.apt.2019.01.017.

62. Pauli, V., Y. Roggo, P. Kleinebudde, and M. Krumme. "Real-Time Monitoring of Particle Size Distribution in a Continuous Granulation and Drying Process by near Infrared Spectroscopy." *European Journal of Pharmaceutics and Biopharmaceutics* 2019. https://doi.org/10.1016/j.ejpb.2019.05.007.

63. Chablani, L., M. K. Taylor, A. Mehrotra, P. Rameas, and W. C. Stagner. "Inline Real-Time Near-Infrared Granule Moisture Measurements of a Continuous Granulation–Drying–Milling Process." *AAPS PharmSciTech* 2011; 12 (4): 1050–1055. https://doi.org/10.1208/s12249-011-9669-z.

64. Continuous drying with a defined retention time distribution. Commercial Information by Lödige. https://www.loedige.de/en/machines/continuous-fluid-bed-dryer-granucon/. Accessed April 27th 2020.

65. Fonteyne, M., J. Arruabarrena, J. de Beer et al. "NIR Spectroscopic Method for the In-Line Moisture Assessment during Drying in a Six-Segmented Fluid Bed Dryer of a Continuous Tablet Production Line: Validation of Quantifying Abilities and Uncertainty Assessment." *Journal of Pharmaceutical and Biomedical Analysis* 2014a; 100: 21–27. https://doi.org/https://doi.org/10.1016/j.jpba.2014.07.012.

Section III

Product-Oriented Granulations

14 Effervescent Granulation

Guia Bertuzzi

CONTENTS

14.1 INTRODUCTION

Effervescence has proved its utility as an oral delivery system in the pharmaceutical and dietary industries for decades. In Europe and the United States of America, effervescent granules and tablets are widespread, and their use is growing in other countries [1]. Effervescent granulation is an important step of "fizzy" dosage forms' production that most of the time cannot be avoided to achieve the desired characteristics of the effervescent tablets. It is a critical step because it can affect the stability of the final dosage forms. The first effervescent preparations were described over two centuries ago, in the official compendia, in powder forms to use as cathartic salts. Later, in 1815, a patent describes "a combination of neutral salt or powder which possesses all the properties of the medicinal spring of Seidlitz in Germany, under the name of Seidlitz Powders," containing sodium potassium tartrate, sodium bicarbonate, and tartaric acid, in the proportions 3:1:1, respectively [2]. Effervescent granules and tablets have become more and more popular as dosage forms because they are promptly soluble, easy to take, and ensure quick therapeutic action.

The effervescent forms are defined within Pharmacopeias as "those granules or tablets to be dissolved in water before administration to patients." They are used to administer water-soluble active ingredients, especially when the large dosage is required. A typical effervescent drug for oral administration can take more than 2 g of the active ingredient in tablets that can weigh up to 5 g with a diameter of 25 mm or in sachets in case a larger dosage is required. Effervescent tablets or granules are uncoated and generally contain acidic substances and carbonate or bicarbonate that react rapidly to release carbon dioxide once dissolved in water. The disintegration of the tablets usually occurs within two minutes or even less, because of the evolution of bubbles of carbon dioxide. The effervescent form is in fact widely proposed for pain relief and anti-inflammatory therapies. In certain cases, they can shorten significantly drug absorption rate in the body as compared with traditional tablets, resulting in a quicker therapeutic effect [3].

Effervescent dosage forms also enhance patient compliance. They are easier to administer, particularly helpful to patients, like children, who are not able to swallow capsules or tablets. A pleasant taste, because of carbonation, helps to mask the bad taste of certain drugs. This could also help to avoid the gastric side effect of certain drugs [4]. They are easy to use and appeal to consumers for color and fizzy appearance more than traditional dosage forms. For example, a study shows that patient compliance has increased when the chloroquine phosphate was administered as an effervescent tablet because of the faster response onset than uncoated tablets [5]. Effervescent drugs also have other advantages over conventional pharmaceutical forms. They substitute liquid forms when the active ingredient has a little stability in the water as they are administered only by prior dissolving of the tablet in water. Active ingredients that are not stable in liquid form are most of the time more stable in effervescent form.

Disadvantages of such solid dosage forms are more related to production technology even if processing methods and equipment are the same as the conventional ones. In general, product requirements are similar to conventional granules, namely particle size distribution and shape, along with content uniformity of the active ingredient, to produce satisfactory free-flowing granules capable of tableting using a high-speed rotary tablet press. However, it is also necessary to focus attention on some aspects of the manufacturing procedure, including compression and packaging because effervescent dosage forms are challenging for their stability and consequently critical to make. The pharmaceutical industry faces many issues, especially in the preparation of effervescent tablets, as it is certainly the application for which the choice of the process technology is at least as important as the formulation design.

14.2   THE EFFERVESCENT REACTION

Effervescence is the evolution of gas bubbles from a liquid, as a result of a chemical reaction. The most common reaction for pharmaceutical oral solid dosage forms is the autocatalytic acid–base reaction between sodium bicarbonate and citric acid.

$$3NaHCO_3(aq)[252g(3\ mol)] + H_3C_6H_5O_7(aq)[192g(1\ mol)]$$
$$\Rightarrow 3H_2O(aq)[54g(3\ mol)] + 3CO_2[132g(3\ mol)] + 3Na_3C_6H_5O_7(aq)[258g(1\ mol)]$$

This reaction starts in presence of water, even with a very small amount, as a catalyzing agent, and because water is one of the reaction products, it will accelerate and will be very difficult to stop. For this reason, the whole manufacturing, packaging, and storage of effervescent products have to be planned by minimizing the contact with water.

Considering the stoichiometric ratios in the reaction, it is quite easy to understand the reason why effervescent doses are so large.

Recently, some effervescent systems have been prepared to act as penetration enhancers for drug absorption, not only in oral forms but also in some topical products, such as skin or vaginal applications. In these cases, the reaction takes place directly after administration, in the mouth because of saliva [6], on the wounds because of blood serum [7], or when formulated in a suppository to treat vaginal infections, the effervescence is provoked by the moisture of the vaginal mucosa [8] to adjust the pH [9].

There are other forms, the effervescence of which is based on a different reaction upon carbon dioxide formation. Effervescence in these cases is due to reactants that evolve hydrogen peroxide and oxygen, which are safe for human use even if they are not suitable for oral administration but can be employed in preparations for external use such as antibacterial for dental plate cleaning [10].

14.3 FORMULATION

The criteria to choose the raw materials for effervescent products are similar to those for conventional granules and tablets, since in either case, good flowability, compressibility, and compactability are the targets to achieve. The intrinsic characteristics of effervescent forms bring some considerations that will limit the choice of raw materials, including the selection of active ingredients. The moisture content of the raw material is a very significant aspect because it affects the compressibility and stability of the tablets. To avoid premature effervescent reaction during the process or once the granules or tablets are packed, raw materials with very low moisture content have to be used. Since an effervescent form is required to dissolve within two minutes or less in a glass of water (about 100 mL), raw materials' solubility and rate of solubility are other significant aspects. The active ingredient must be either soluble, water-dispersible, or at least solubilized by salt formation during the dissolution in the glass of water. The rest of the excipients, such as additives like sweeteners, coloring agents, and flavors, also have to be water-soluble.

For all these considerations, the list of the excipients for this dosage form has not changed much for many years. However, the physical properties of these raw materials have recently improved to smooth critical aspects in manufacturing and ensure consistent high quality. Many different grades for each material are commercially available, including some pre-formulated grades, which allow in some cases to skip the granulation process since they are specifically designed for direct compression [11]. Formulators should choose the excipient grade based on the characteristics of the active ingredient, dosage, release profile, and process technology available. Therefore, the ultimate use of the effervescent granules or tablets mainly affects the choice of raw materials.

To design an effervescent formula, it is necessary to consider the stoichiometric ratios in the reaction and the carbon dioxide solubility in water, which is 90 mg/100 mL of water (in Standard Temperature and Pressure conditions, which is defined to be 273 K (0 degrees Celsius) and 1 atm pressure (or 105 Pa)). The suggested ratio between acid and alkaline components is about 0.6, but sometimes it might be required to increase the acid source to get a pleasant taste. In fact, the alkaline–acid ratio controls both the effervescence capacity and the taste of the solution to administer. When the solubility of the active ingredient is not pH-dependent, the alkaline–acid ratio can be optionally selected. This ratio can also be determined according to the pH that is required for dissolving the active ingredient. In fact, when the active solubility increases at the acid side, the pH of the solution is lowered by adding an excess of the acidic agent. Conversely, an excess of alkaline sources must be added when the active ingredient is more soluble at higher pH [12]. However, another approach that can be used to increase the active ingredient solubility is to increase the volume of carbon dioxide to be generated by increasing the alkaline component in the formulation.

As far as other excipients, such as diluents or binders, are concerned, there is very little space for the formulator to play with, because of the large dimension of the tablet due to the effervescent system. Additional binders for effervescent dosage form cannot enhance compressibility, because the tablet has a larger size in the first place and to not limit the prompt dissolution rate when put in the glass with water.

In the latest development in effervescent forms, some formulations have been designed to control the rate of effervescence, to obtain a rapid, intermediate, or slow rate. The rate control is related to the ratio of the acid–alkaline components, but the chemical properties of the effervescent excipients or their combinations can influence it, especially when a slow rate of effervescence is required [13].

14.4 RAW MATERIALS

The ingredients of effervescent dosage forms require having low moisture content and to be easily soluble. Because of the nature of the effervescence reaction, additional excipients are sparingly used as the alkaline and acid ingredients are also the fillers to get a tablet bulk. They are, indeed, in such a large amount that tablets are much larger than the conventional ones. In case it would be necessary to add a filler, sodium bicarbonate is widely selected because of its lower cost and because it does not influence the final pH of the solution and increases the effervescence effect. Sodium chloride and sodium sulfate are other possible fillers; they are high-density crystalline powders that are very compatible with the other ingredients.

Additives are added in small amounts to make the tablets more attractive for users. Flavors, colors, and sweeteners are used as usual in all the formulations.

14.4.1 Acid Materials

Necessary acidity for effervescence can be provided by three main sources: food acids, acid anhydrides, and acid salts. Food acids, citric acid, tartaric acid, and ascorbic acid are the most commonly used because these have a nice taste and are odorless, not expensive, and easy to handle.

14.4.1.1 Citric Acid

Citric acid is the more often used acidic ingredient because of its good solubility and pleasant taste. It is mainly commercially available in powder and is either colorless or in white crystals. The particle size grades are coarse, medium, fine, and powder (only anhydrous). It is very soluble in water and soluble in ethanol [14]. It can be used as a monohydrate or anhydrate, depending on the selected equipment technology and process conditions. Anhydrous citric acid is less hygroscopic than the monohydrate [15]. However, caking of the anhydrous ingredient may occur upon prolonged storage at humidity greater than 70%. Citric acid monohydrate is used in the preparation of effervescent granules, while the anhydrous form is widely used in the preparation of effervescent tablets; the monohydrate melts at 100°C and releases the water of hydration at 75°C. For this reason, it can be used as a binder source in hot-melt granulation.

14.4.1.2 Tartaric Acid

It is very soluble in water and very hygroscopic, more than citric acid. In the effervescence reaction with sodium bicarbonate, it behaves like citric acid in producing an evident effervescence. It must be used in a higher amount to get the proper stoichiometric proportions, being a diprotic acid, while citric is a triprotic acid. In terms of compressibility, it is also comparable to citric acid [16].

14.4.1.3 Ascorbic Acid

It is white in crystalline form and light yellow in fine powder. It is not hygroscopic, and this may be helpful in production because it is easier to handle. It is freely soluble in water (1 g in about 3 mL) and absolute ethanol [17]. If exposed to light, it gradually gets dark. Its behavior in the effervescent reaction with sodium bicarbonate is comparable to the other acids (citric and tartaric) in terms of the release rate of carbon dioxide.

14.4.1.4 Acid Anhydrides

Anhydrides of food acids are a potential acid source as they are precursors of the corresponding acid by hydrolyzation in water. The effervescent effect is strong and sustained by the continuous production of acid in the solution. Water has to be avoided for the whole process when anhydrides are part of a formulation; otherwise, they would be hydrolyzed into the corresponding acid before its use [18].

14.4.1.5 Acid Salts

Sodium dihydrogen phosphate, amino acid hydrochlorides, acid citrate salts, etc. are acid salts that are used in effervescent formulation since they are water-soluble and react quickly with alkaline sources. In combination with another of the above-mentioned acids, they work as a pH buffering agent during drug administration, thus promoting active ingredient absorption while mitigating possible undesired side effects for the stomach [19].

14.4.1.6 Other Less Frequent Sources of Acid

Fumaric and nicotinic acid, which are not hygroscopic, have lower water solubility than that of the others.

Malic acid is highly hygroscopic and soluble but has less acid strength than the tartaric or citric acids. It is sometimes preferred for its smooth and light taste.

Acetylsalicylic acid, though active ingredient, which is very commonly administered in effervescent preparations, is used in combination with other acid sources for its low water solubility.

Adipic acid is not used as an acid source because of its low water solubility but can be found in effervescent formulas as a lubricant. It has given good results as a lubricant for effervescent calcium carbonate tablets [20].

14.4.2 Sources of Carbon Dioxide

Carbonate salts are the most popular source for effervescence; bicarbonate forms are more reactive than carbonates, providing a stronger effervescence effect.

14.4.2.1 Sodium Bicarbonate

It is the major source of carbon dioxide in effervescent forms, which is able to provide a yield of 52% of carbon dioxide. It is commercially available in many different grades according to particle size, from free-flowing uniform granule to fine powder, which is odorless and slightly alkaline in taste. When heated to about 50°C, sodium bicarbonate begins to dissociate into carbon dioxide, sodium carbonate, and water. On heating to 250–300°C, for a short time, sodium bicarbonate is completely converted into anhydrous sodium carbonate. However, the process is both time- and temperature-dependent, with 90% conversion completed within 75 minutes at 93°C [21]. Being a nonelastic material, it has very low compressibility, but this issue is overcome when produced by spray-drying technique. Directly compressible grades are now also available with some additives such as polyvinylpyrrolidone (PVP) or silicone oil [22].

14.4.2.2 Sodium Carbonate

It is commercially available in three different forms, all very soluble in water: anhydrous, monohydrate, and decahydrate. It is more resistant to the effervescent reaction, and in some formulations, it can be used as a stabilizing agent in an amount not exceeding 10% of the batch size since it absorbs moisture preferentially, preventing the effervescent reaction to start. Of course, the anhydrous form is preferred for this purpose [12]. A particular grade of modified sodium bicarbonate is available whose surface is coated with a carbonate layer to increase bicarbonate stability so as to be suitable for direct compression [23,24].

14.4.2.3 Potassium Bicarbonate and Potassium Carbonate

They are lesser soluble than the corresponding sodium salts and are more expensive. They can partially substitute the sodium salts when a reduced amount of sodium ion is required [25].

14.4.2.4 Calcium Carbonate

Precipitated calcium carbonate occurs as fine, white odorless, and tasteless powder or crystals. Its water solubility is very poor and is not soluble in ethanol or isopropanol. It is a high-density powder that is not suitable for direct compression. It is normally used as a drug in effervescent tablets for patients who suffer from calcium shortage. It can also be used as an alkaline source because it provides stability to the effervescent system [26].

14.4.2.5   Sodium Glycine Carbonate

Sodium glycine carbonate provides a light effervescence reaction but brings rapid disintegration of the tablets, so it is often applied in the preparation of fast dissolving sublingual tablets. It is much more compressible than the other alkaline compounds, and it has been found suitable for direct compression [27].

14.4.3   BINDERS

In general the use of a binder is usually necessary to provide the tablet the proper hardness to handle them. In effervescent formulations use of binder is limited by the fact that any binder, even if water-soluble, tends to retard the tablet disintegration and take some moisture into the tablets. Therefore, the amount of binder in a given formula will be a compromise between desired granule strength and desired disintegration time.

As will be described in the section "Wet Granulation," water itself is an effective binder for effervescent granules when granulated with all the components together. A small amount of water, finely distributed on the powder bed, acts as a binder by partially dissolving the raw materials and preparing them for agglomeration. Other solvents, for example, ethanol and isopropanol, can be used as a granulating liquid to dissolve dry binders. The binder choice in wet granulation is also related to the method of production and, consequently, the amount of granulating liquid. In fact, when both the alkaline and acidic components are granulated together with water, it would not make sense to put a binder in the formulation because the small amount of water will never activate it due to being not enough for dissolving it.

The most popular binder for effervescent tablets is polyvinylpyrrolidone (PVP) due to its strong binding power at low concentration in the formula, effective from 2%. PVP K25 and K30 are preferred for their good water solubility and do not retard the drug dissolution rate, thus matching the final purpose of effervescent tablets. They are used in water, alcohol, and hydroalcoholic solutions [12] and can also be used for dry granulation. Binders normally used for dry granulation, such as lactose, mannitol, and dextrose, are almost inappropriate because they would be effective only in a larger amount than that allowed by effervescent formulations.

14.4.4   LUBRICANTS

Tableting is a critical step of effervescent production, and selecting the lubricant is one of the most important issues because of the chemical–physical nature of the lubricants. As most of the lubricants have low water solubility, they tend to inhibit the tablet disintegration, which, as already said, must be very rapid in case of effervescent tablets. The effervescent tablets – mainly for marketing reasons – are often required to provide a clear transparent solution, that is, without any insoluble "film" formation on the water surface or any residue left. When selecting a lubricant, proper attention must be given to its solubility in water, along with its compatibility with the active ingredient therapeutic action.

Many different lubricants have been tested to establish the most appropriate condition for effervescent tablets, including the opportunity to carry out external lubrication of the granules directly in the dies of the tablet press [28].

Lubricant substances, known as suitable for effervescent manufacturing, are sodium benzoate, sodium acetate, L-leucine, and carbowax 4000. Combinations of lubricants have also become a possibility. Literature reports calcium and potassium sorbates and micronized polyethylene glycol (PEG) with calcium ascorbate or trisodium citrate [29]. Spray-dried L-leucine and PEG 6000 are also considered as a successful mix [30]. Other lesser soluble lubricants are still however used in formulating effervescent tablets. In any case for good lubrication, a balance should be found between compression efficiency and water solubility. Magnesium stearate is commercially available in combination with sodium lauryl sulfate, a surfactant agent that helps in dispersion [31].

14.4.5 ADDITIVES

In order to improve the taste and appearance of effervescent preparations, some additives are also put in little quantity in the formulas. Water-soluble flavors like lemon, orange, and other fruit essences are particularly suitable to achieve the organoleptic requirements. They are usually about 0.5%–3.0% of the final dose. Most of the time flavors are combined with sweeteners like sorbitol, sucrose, aspartame, stevia, and saccharin sodium. Coloring agents can include all the dies soluble and suitable for food such as the FD&C ones, and all the natural coloring substances amount to about 0.1%–3.5% of the dose. In addition, surfactants or antifoaming agents can be used to improve the performance of the effervescent preparation at the time of use.

14.5 MANUFACTURING OF EFFERVESCENT FORMS

Manufacturing conditions are crucially important even for the stability of the products once they are packed. Almost all the raw materials used for effervescent manufacturing are highly hygroscopic, so moisture absorption from the environment air must be prevented to avoid the effervescent reaction to start prior to use and ensure reliable shelf life.

The whole production process, dispensing and sieving of the raw materials, granulation, blending of other ingredients (if required), lubricant addition, compression, and packaging, can be carried out within a completely closed and integrated handling system. Materials' handling utilizing intermediate bulk containers and their blender also allows reducing product transfers and limiting exposure as shown in Figure 14.1.

In case open handling and pneumatic transfer systems are used, it is highly recommended to maintain the airflow in the manufacturing area at the minimum level of moisture content [32]. Recommended working conditions throughout the plant are relative humidity (RH) below 20% and uniform constant temperature at 21°C. However, it is known that 25% of RH at controlled room temperature (25°C) is enough to prevent the granules or tablets from sticking to the machines and from capturing moisture from the environment [33].

Granulation of effervescent products is most of the time executed in batch mode and can significantly influence the characteristics of the final forms, granules primarily, or tablets as well. The lubrication of granules, compression, and packaging of both granules and tablets should also be carefully addressed.

The challenge in compressing effervescent granules is given by many factors. Tablets need to have large dimensions because most of their contents consist of the effervescent parts, which typically have low compressibility themselves. These raw materials occupy the majority of space in the dosage formula so there is little opportunity for other excipients to contribute to compression improvement. Another challenge of compression can also be due to limitations in types and quantity of lubricants to use. Lubricants, if not well balanced, could affect negatively the dissolution time, the taste, and the appearance of the ready-to-use potion. For all these reasons, the compression phase has to be carried out carefully and requires using pre-compression and high compression force. To overcome lubrication issues within the formula, sometimes the tablet press can be equipped for carrying out external lubrication of the granules. Antiadherent or lubricant ingredients are sprayed from ancillary dosing equipment (Figure 14.2), directly into the dies of the tablet press, just before filling phase, so as to prevent sticking of granules on dies and punches [34]. This technique is widely used in the nutraceutical industry; it allows using less material than that used in intrinsic lubrication, improving the tensile strength of tablets and at the same time reducing the tablet ejection force. An alternative technique to achieve better tablets, not described in the literature but sometimes used in practice that helps to increase the hardness of effervescent tablets,

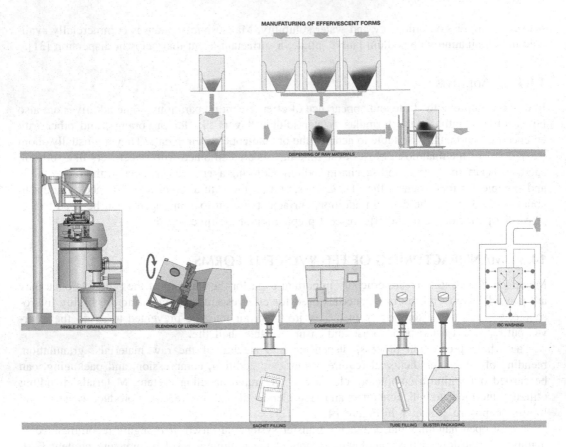

FIGURE 14.1 Typical process flow diagram for effervescent forms.
Source: From IMA S.p.A., Bologna, Italy.

consists of compressing the granules while still slightly wet. Later, tablets are dried and brought to achieve the right moisture for their stability by a step in static ventilated oven or fluid bed.

Packaging for both, granules and tablets, must be operated, as already mentioned, in strictly controlling humidity environment and by selecting a kind of packaging that provides a suitable moisture barrier. The critical aspects of the packaging of effervescent drugs are obviously related to the stability of either tablets or granules. The main objective is to protect them, as much as possible, first during packaging operations, later, once they are packed, to preserve them for reasonable shelf life and ensure stability long after the pack is open. In the old times, packaging for effervescent preparations consisted of wrapping the acid and alkaline components separately, to avoid the premature effervescent reaction until use. All the effervescent drugs can be nowadays packed in individual dose units, in airtight containers made of protective aluminum foil or plastic laminates. Tablets can also be packed by stacking them one by one into plastic or metal tubes, which have almost the same diameter as that of the tablets, so as to minimize the air which remains in contact with the tablets. The tubes must be resealed every time, after taking out each tablet. Tablets can also either be wrapped in an aluminum foil before tube filling or put naked into tubes containing silica gel at the internal side of the cap. These are given as the best solutions for achieving long-term stability [35]. For tablets that are packed in aluminum strips or blisters, it is essential that the packaging machine has a fine control on the temperature of the welding unit, so as to obtain an accurate sealing but avoid overheating that could provoke the release of residual water from the tablets that could start effervescence reaction later [36].

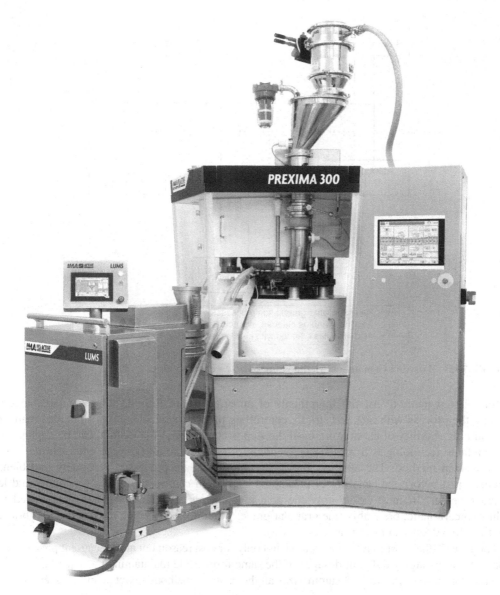

FIGURE 14.2   LUMS, dosing equipment for external lubricant addition in a tablet press.
Source: From IMA S.p.A., Bologna, Italy.

14.6   GRANULATION METHODS

The 1911 edition of British Pharmacopoeia reported a detailed description of the manufacturing procedure [37].

> *"Effervescent granules consist of an effervescing basis of citric and tartaric acids and sodium bicarbonate, with or without sugar, and other ingredients. The ingredients are thoroughly mixed, placed in a suitable vessel, heated between 95° and 105°. When the mixture has, by careful manipulation, assumed a uniformly plastic condition, it is passed through a sieve of suitable mesh to produce granules of the required size. The granules are dried at a temperature not exceeding 55° and should be stored in well-closed containers."*

Only a few aspects have substantially changed in modern methods since then.

Two main methods can be executed with various granulation technology:

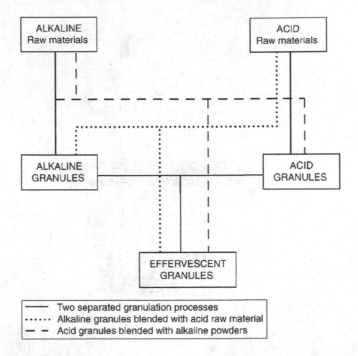

FIGURE 14.3   Possible Granulation Methods for Effervescent Granules.

Single-step method: All the ingredients of an effervescent formula are granulated together, running the process with care and strictly controlling process parameters, in a contained manner to maintain the stability of the mixture until the step is completed. This method can be applied to all the available technologies from the dry blending of powders to all types of granulation.

Multi-step method: The alkaline and acid components are processed separately and blended together, just before the tableting or packaging step. Both can be granulated separately and later mixed together. In most cases, only the acid components are granulated and then mixed with sodium bicarbonate, preferably fine granular grade. Other additives, such as flavors and lubricants, can then be added and mixed later on.

The latter is the most convenient method, not only for cost reason but also because it provides more flexibility in managing different dosages of the same form while maintaining the same batch size for the granulation step. Figure 14.3 summarizes all the possible methods to obtain effervescent granules.

14.6.1   Granulation Technologies

14.6.1.1   Dry Blending of Powders

The dry blending of powders would be the ideal process for effervescent tablet manufacturing, but it is limited to ingredients with proper compressibility that are able to ensure a homogeneous mixture with no risk of segregation. It is recommended when the active ingredient cannot be wet granulated because it is unstable in the presence of water or contains some water of crystallization that could be difficult to manage during granulation. It is a quick and simple way of manufacturing in bin tumblers, ribbon, twin-cone, and V-type blenders and suitable for continuous mixers but requires the right selection of raw materials, possibly already available in granular form.

14.6.1.2   Dry Granulation

Dry granulation usually performed by roller compaction of pre-blended bulk is an appropriate technology for its simplicity since effervescent drug stability is preserved by no use of water [38].

It takes low operational costs, facilitates process containment, and allows high product throughput. Dry granulation is suitable for continuous manufacturing and offers the opportunity to recycle back materials in case the proper particle size distribution is not achieved. Operations and required space are relatively less and consequently room air conditioning is reduced too. On the other hand, not all the excipient grades are suitable for such technology. In some cases, the use of more sophisticated pre-treated raw materials with favorable properties for this technology may not be convenient even considering all the potential above-described advantages.

14.6.1.3   Wet Granulation

Wet granulation is still the preferred method for making effervescent granules despite the criticality of higher risk to affect the stability of the final form.

Also in case of effervescent drugs, wet granulation assures homogeneous granules with consistent content uniformity that are suitable for sachet filling or, in case of compression, capable to provide uniform tablets in terms of either weight, thickness, or hardness.

As previously explained, granulation process in the multi-step method (granulation of separate acid or alkaline ingredients) is most convenient since it is a regular granulation process that often runs with a water-based binder and does not require to use explosion-proof equipment. It is also quite usual to granulate only one of the effervescent sources and adds the other one in powder during the final blending. While in the case of the single-step method (all the ingredients granulated together), it is essential to handle the process with great care because the granulating liquid might interact with the powders initiating the effervescent reaction.

14.6.1.4   Wet Granulation According to Single-Step Method

The peculiar process that distinguishes effervescent granulation consists of processing all the components of the formulation according to a single-step method, where the challenge is to stabilize the moisture-sensitive components in the air still preserving their rapid reactivity in the water of the final form.

The single-step method applied to wet granulation provides effervescent granules directly by granulating the acid and the alkaline materials with nonreactive or reactive liquids with reference to the effervescence reaction.

It is possible to use either water only as a binder, thus controlling the effervescent reaction, or nonreactive liquids, like absolute ethanol or isopropanol, but in this case, it is necessary to use a binder to get the agglomeration of the particles of the raw material.

A very small amount of water, usually not more than 1% of the batch size, can be finely sprayed onto the solid mass bulk to initiate the effervescent reaction. Some carbon dioxide is released, and some water too, which acts as the binder as well. It takes a few minutes (approximately 5–10) to obtain wet granules. As the rate of effervescent reaction rapidly increases after its start, an immediate drying of the granules is necessary to control and stop the effervescent reaction. This works well for a single-pot processor (high-shear mixer with vacuum dryer) [39] or fluid-bed granulator avoiding transferring wet granules from the granulator to the dryer. Single-pot processing especially is very suitable for controlling the effervescence reaction by vacuum. With the single-pot processor, it is in fact possible to suddenly switch on the drying phase by creating a vacuum and heating the process bowl, just after the granulation phase when wet granules are well massed. The vacuum is created in a few seconds, which immediately provokes the decrease of the water boiling point down to about 20°C. At the same time, the process bowl is heated up to provide more energy for water evaporation. In a few seconds, the free water released on the surface of the granules is removed and the effervescent reaction stops. The application of microwaves, combined with a vacuum inside the bowl of the high-shear granulator, can also be used to stop the effervescent reaction and dry the effervescent granules [40].

Drying effervescent granules under vacuum takes a shorter time than drying conventional granules granulated with water because the water to be removed is in a very small amount. However, drying still remains a critical step since it is hard to remove even the smallest quantity of water from hydrophilic or hygroscopic materials (Figure 14.4). The water evaporation rate from

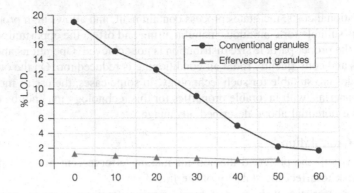

FIGURE 14.4   Drying rate of effervescent granules, compared with conventional granules in a single-pot processor.
Source: From IMA Active Laboratory Archive, IMA S.p.A, IMA ACTIVE Division, Bologna, Italy.

effervescent granules becomes lower toward the end of the drying phase because more energy is required to remove the inner water tightly bonded to the particles. Consequently, the drying time increases scaling up from pilot single-pot processor to industrial scales (Figure 14.5).

14.6.1.4.1 Case Study

An example of effervescent aspirin produced in a single-pot processor Roto Cube 600 equipped with vacuum and tilting bowl (Figure 14.6).

The formulation consists of:

Anhydrous citric acid 116.6 kg
Sodium bicarbonate   154.2 kg
Sodium carbonate   39.2 kg
Acetylsalicylic acid   50 kg

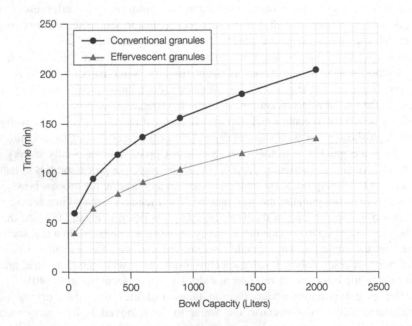

FIGURE 14.5   Drying Time Scale Up for Single-Pot Processing.
Source: From IMA Active Laboratory Archive, IMA S.p.A, IMA ACTIVE Division, Bologna, Italy.

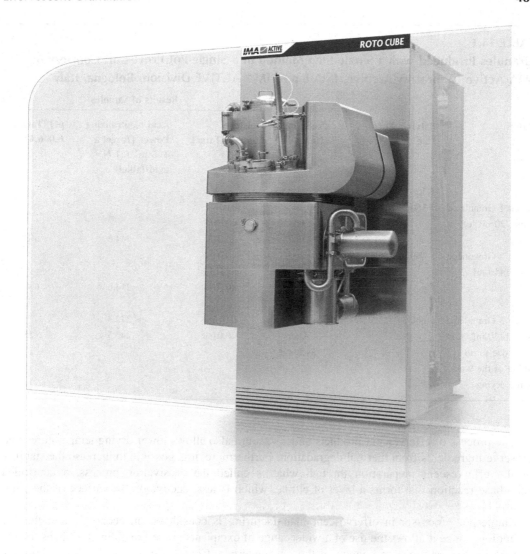

FIGURE 14.6 "Roto Cube" Single-Pot Processor for High-Shear Granulation and Vacuum Drying. *Source*: From IMA S.p.A., Bologna, Italy.

The effervescent bulk is granulated first, with very small amounts of water (2–4 mL/kg) sprayed in very fine droplets. The acetylsalicylic acid is added later, in the final blending, after granulation is completed.

The results of the three batches are reported in Table 14.1.

The whole batch time is reasonably quick, and batch 3 has lower yield due to some product sticking onto the bowl walls. In batch 3, drying was performed keeping the single-pot bowl static, instead of using the tilting bowl, a typical functionality available for a sing-pot processor that enhances drying, moving gently the bulk while drying.

TABLE 14.1

Granules Produced with a Single-Step Method in a Single-Pot Processor. Courtesy of IMA Active Laboratory Archive, IMA S.p.A, IMA ACTIVE Division, Bologna, Italy

Batch	Batch Size	Yield		Sampling Time	Results of Samples		
					Moisture Content (Target ≤ 0.1%)	Acid Neutralizing Power (Target ≥ 185 mL 0.1 N acid/tablet)	pH (Target 6.0–6.4)
	kg	kg	%	min			
Batch 1 Granulated with 720 mL of water	360	352.2	97.80	30	0.048%		
				60	<0.01%		
				90	<0.01%	244.6	6.1
Batch 2 Granulated with 1440 mL	360	336.4	93.44	30	<0.01%		
				60	<0.015%		
				After discharge	<0.01%	244.6	6.4
Batch 3 Granulated with 1440 mL*Low yield due to no tilting of the bowl while drying	360	323.5	89.86*	60	0.075%	229.8	
				After discharge	<0.01%	245.5	6.25

The process of effervescent products under vacuum also allows lower drying temperatures that preserve ingredients from thermal degradation. Furthermore, it is possible to increase the stability of the effervescent preparation through what is called the passivation process, a controlled acid–base reaction that forms a layer of citrate, which is less reactive on the surface of the citric acid [41].

Single-pot processor in effervescent manufacturing is considered an economic and flexible technology since it allows the use of a wider range of excipients grades, avoiding problems related to particle size or moisture content of the raw materials. Granules produced by this technology appear fine, but their flow properties are however good for tableting properties [42].

Within the overall advantages of single-pot technology, it is important to consider that water-based granulation with vacuum drying has also reduced running cost since it avoids the use of explosion-proof equipment and does not consume a huge quantity of process air that requires expensive pre-treatment of filtration and dehumidification as typically needed by the fluid-bed technology.

However, fluid-bed dryers are widely used to make effervescent granulation especially when granules are designated to sachets' filling. In fluid-bed granulation, the water or binder solution is sprayed from the top over the effervescent mixture while it is suspended in a flow of warm, dry air. The humidity and temperature of the air are key parameters for either granulation or drying which occurs in practice at the same time so as to control the effervescence reaction.

All the components of an effervescent mixture can be granulated together in a single-step method in a conventional fluid-bed granulator dryer. Granulation occurs when water is sprayed on the fluidized bed, initiating the effervescent reaction. The reaction stops when water is not sprayed anymore and the drying phase is continued with warm dry air [43] until the final moisture content is reached. Subsequent patent applications show how to make effervescent granules, using the fluid-bed rotor granulator, a version with tangential spray, and polyvinylpyrrolidone (PVP) as binder dissolved in alcohol instead of water. A clever process is to layer alternatively the acid materials with alkaline ones while still using the rotary fluid-bed system [44]. The process consists of two or three subsequent steps to produce effervescent spheres by layering the acid components over alkaline spheres or vice versa. Binding liquid still is a hydroalcoholic solution of PVP. The first step is the granulation of alkaline components in the rotary fluid bed. In the second step, the granulating solution is sprayed in combination with the acidic powders, which deposit on the alkaline spheres creating an external acid layer separated by a neutral layer of the binder. As agglomeration is completed, the drying phase with hot air starts without any interruptions. In literature, we find that apomorphine effervescent can also be made by the multi-layering technique in a fluid [45].

As seen in the last example, it is sometimes preferable to granulate with a hydroalcoholic solution to initiate a lighter effervescence to keep the reaction under better control during the process. The use of alcohol is indispensable in case a binder, like PVP, is included in the formulation. In fact, the required water amount to dissolve PVP, to obtain the binding solution, would be too much, and it would not be possible to manage the effervescent reaction. To work with organic solvents, it is a must to install fully explosion-proof equipment possibly with an accessory solvent's recovery utility that will limit the emission of vapors in the atmosphere.

14.6.1.5 Hot-Melt Process

Hot melt is an alternative process, which is discussed in detail in another chapter of this book, which is suitable for the single-step method in making effervescent granules. Hot-melt granulation can be carried out in a single-pot processor with the capability to heat up the process bowl when the mixture is formulated with a relatively low melting binder, PEG 4000, and cetyl alcohol, for instance [46]. Another dry, simple, and rapid type of process includes applying melt granulation in an air-forced oven to a mixture of anhydrous citric acid and sodium bicarbonate added to PEG 6000 [47]. A similar process is applied to a fluid-bed spray granulator where low melting point binders are PEGs or polyoxyethylene glycols [48]. Hot-melt extrusion deserves attention due to the growing interest in continuous manufacturing.

The formulations for this technology must contain a hot-melt extrudable binder and can be processed with either single or multiple step methods. Preferred binders are the PEGs with a molecular weight in the range of 1000 to 8000, but some other polymers are investigated. Binder percentage varies according to the formulation in a range of 20% to 40% of the total weight, and the required melting temperature is less than 150°C. Selection of the temperature range can be critical because the degradation of the active ingredient as well as decomposition of the effervescent components may occur. This range is usually from about 50°C to about 120°C. It is possible to adjust the temperature and rate of extrusion to control the effervescence rate of the final dosage form [49]. Another patent [50] for hot-melt extrusion with twin-screw processor concerns porous effervescent granules formed from a blend comprising an acid and a base obtained with an *in situ* granulating agent, which is a portion of the acid ingredient that melts during granulation.

14.7 CONCLUSION

Three effervescent granulation technologies summarized in Figure 14.7 were evaluated: dry granulation, wet granulation, and hot-melt granulation. The choice of the proper granulation technology is related to either the therapeutic purpose of the granules, production needs, or facilities design. All these aspects should be considered during formulation and selecting the raw materials with appropriate physical characteristics such as particle size, density, flowability, compressibility, and moisture content.

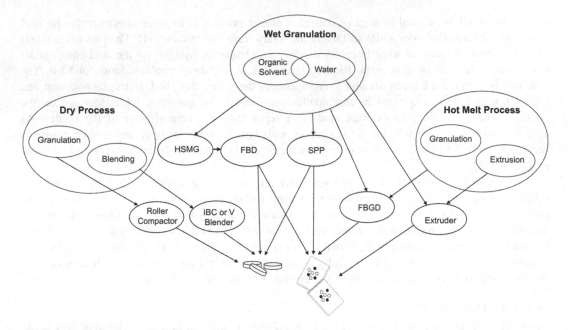

FIGURE 14.7   Map of Granulation Technologies for Effervescent Solid Forms.

REFERENCES

1. GME. Effervescent products market size, trends & analysis - forecasts to 2026. January 25, 2020. Available at https://www.globalmarketestimates.com.
2. Homan P. Seidlitz — the morning-after powder. The Pharmaceutical Journal 2001; 267(7179):911–936.
3. Moeller PL, et al. Time to onset of analgesia and analgesic efficacy of effervescent acetaminophen 1000 mg compared to tablet acetaminophen 1000 mg in postoperative dental pain: a single-dose, double-blind, randomized, placebo-controlled study. Journal of Clinical Pharmacology 2000; 40(4):370–378.
4. İpci K, et al. Effervescent tablets: a safe and practical delivery system for drug administration. ENT Updates 2016; 6:46–50.
5. Yanze MF, et al. Rapid therapeutic response onset of a new pharmaceutical form of chloroquine phosphate 300mg: effervescent tablets. Tropical Medicine & International Health 2001; 6(3):196.
6. Pather SI, et al. Sublingual buccal effervescent. US Patent US2011/0212034 A1 2011.
7. Rapp M. Fibrin-based glue granulate and corresponding production method. WO Patent WO/2000/ 038752 2000.
8. Sánchez MT, Ruiz MA, Castán H, Morales ME. A novel double-layer mucoadhesive tablet containing probiotic strain for vaginal administration: design, development, and technological evaluation. European Journal of Pharmaceutical Sciences 2018; 112:63–70.
9. 王世锋. Metronidazole, clotrimazole, and chlorhexidine vaginal effervescent tablet and preparation method. CN Patent CN101406463B 2012.
10. 苏桂珍 史鲁秋 李华山. Effervescent tablet for false teeth as well as preparation method and application of effervescent tablet. CN Patent CN102552054B 2013.
11. Popescu C, Zhou L, Nienow C, Lefevre Ph. Ascorbic acid stability in effervescent tablets formulated with direct compressible maltitol. AAPS Annual Meeting, San Diego, CA, 2014.
12. Merrifield DR, Laurence P, Doughty G. Pharmaceutical formulations. US Patent US6,077,536 2000.
13. Patel SG, Siddaiah M. Formulation and evaluation of effervescent tablets: a review. Journal of Drug Delivery & Therapeutics JDDT 2018; 8(6):296–303.
14. Rowe RC, Sheskey PJ, Quinn ME. Handbook of Pharmaceutical Excipients 6th Edition, Royal Pharmaceutical Society of Great Britain, London, UK. 2009:181–183.
15. Gothoskar AV, Kshirsagar S. A review of patents on effervescent granules. Pharmaceutical Reviews 2004.
16. Rowe RC, Sheskey PJ, Quinn ME. Handbook of Pharmaceutical Excipients 6th Edition, Royal Pharmaceutical Society of Great Britain, London, UK. 2009:731–732.

17. Rowe RC, Sheskey PJ, Quinn ME. Handbook of Pharmaceutical Excipients 6th Edition, Royal Pharmaceutical Society of Great Britain, London, UK. 2009:43–46.
18. Repta AJ, Higuchi T. Synthesis, isolation, and some chemistry of citric acid anhydride. Journal of Pharmaceutical Sciences 1969; 58:1110–1113.
19. Bilgic M, et al. Effervescent formulations comprising second-generation cephalosporin. WO Patent WO2011/093833 A2 2011.
20. Hoss Carr G. Adipic acid as a tableting lubricant. Us Patent US3,584,099 1971. Available at https://patentimages.storage.googleapis.com/49/80/96/3d3dfbf6cab564/US3506756.pdf.
21. Chemical Book. 2017. Sodium bicarbonate Available at: https://www.chemicalbook.com/product-chemicalpropertiescb7492884_en.htm.
22. Saleh SI, Boymond C, Stamm A. Preparation of direct compressible effervescent components: spray-dried sodium bicarbonate. International Journal of Pharmaceutics 1988; 45(1–2):19–26.
23. Mohapatra A, Parikh RK, Gohel MC. Formulation, development, and evaluation of patient-friendly dosage forms of metformin, Part-III: soluble effervescent tablets. Asian Journal of Pharmaceutics 2008;177–181.
24. Effer Soda® Technical Sheet. Available at https://www.spipharma.com/en/products/functional-excipients/effer-soda/.
25. Duvall RN, Gold G. Effervescent analgesic antacids composition having reduced sodium content. EP Patent EP0377906 A2 1993.
26. Tritthart W, Piskernig MA, Kölb G. Effervescent formulations. US Patent US 6,242,002 B1 2001.
27. Chiesi P, et al. Pharmaceutical compositions containing an effervescent acid-base couple. US Patent US 6,284,272 2001.
28. Alexander TA. Lubricant for use in tableting. US Patent US 5,843,477 1998.
29. Daher LJ. Lubricant for use in tableting Bayer Corporation, USA. US Patent US 5,922,351 1999.
30. Rotthaeuser B, Kraus G, Schmidt PC. Optimization of an effervescent tablet formulation using a central composite design optimization of an effervescent tablet formulation containing spray-dried l-leucine and polyethylene glycol 6000 as lubricants using a central composite design. European Journal of Pharmaceutics and Biopharmaceutics 1998; 46(1):85–94.
31. Rudnic EM, Schwartz JD. Oral solid dosage forms. The Science and Practice of Pharmacy 21st Edition, In: Remington JP, Beringer P. Lippincott Williams & Wilkins, eds. Philadelphia, PA, USA 2006:891–893.
32. Armandou J-P, Mattha AG. Establishment of a geographical and chronological map for relative humidity (R.H.) in an effervescent tablets manufacturing and storage building. Pharmaceutica Acta Helvetiae 1982; 57:287–289.
33. Mohrle R. Effervescent tablets. In: Lieberman HA, Lachman L, eds. Pharmaceutical Solid Dosage Forms. Vol 1. Marcel Dekker, Inc., New York 1980:225–258.
34. Daher LJ. Lubricant. US Patent US 5,922,351 13 1999.
35. Özer YA, et al. Evaluation of the stability of commercial effervescent ascorbic acid tablets by factorial design. STP Pharma Science 1993; 3(4):313–317.
36. Yadav AV, Yeole PG, Gaud RS, Gokhale SB. Text Book of Pharmaceutics. Pragati Books Pvt. Ltd., India 2016:208.
37. Pharmaceutical Society of Great Britain. The British Pharmaceutical Codex: An Imperial Dispensatory for the Use of Medical Practitioners and Pharmacists. Pharmaceutical Society of Great Britain, London, UK 1923:1265–1266.
38. Antonio MW. Roller compaction as a method for effervescent tablet preparation. Purdue University, ProQuest Dissertations Publishing, Indiana, USA 1997: 9953744. Available at https://search.proquest.com/docview/304400896.
39. Manufacturing Chemist. Choosing effective granulation strategies for effervescent formulations. January 30, 2019. Available at https://www.manufacturingchemist.com/news/article_page/Choosing_effective_granulation_strategies_for_effervescent_formulations/150405.
40. Stahl H. Drying of pharmaceutical granules in single pot systems. Die Pharmazeutische Industrie, 1999; 61(7):656–661.
41. Koeberle M. Granulation technologies for effervescent products. Tablets & Capsules Solid Dose Digest. March 12, 2018. Available at https://www.tabletscapsules.com/enews_tc/2018/issues/tcnews_03_12_18expert.html.
42. Pearlswig DM. Simulation modeling applied to the single pot processing of effervescent tablets, Master's Thesis, North Caroline State University, Raleigh, North Carolina, 1995.

43. Coletta V, Kennon L. New preparative technique for effervescent products. Journal of Pharmaceutical Sciences 1964; 53 (12):1524–1525.

44. Aiache J-M, et al. Effervescent microsphere and method for making them. US Patent US 6,210,711 B1 2001.

45. Larsen F. Effervescent formulation comprising apomorphine. WO Patent WO 2004/026309 A1 2004.

46. Diyya ASM, Thomas NV. Formulation and evaluation of metronidazole effervescent granules. IJPSR 2018; 9(6):2525–2529.

47. Yanze FM, Duru C, Jacob M. Process to manufacture effervescent tablets: air forced oven melt granulation. Die Pharmazie 2000; 55(12):919–924.

48. Yanze FM, Duru C, Jacob M. A process to produce effervescent tablets: fluidized bed dryer melt granulation. Drug Development and Industrial Pharmacy 2000; 26(11):1167–1176.

49. Robinson JR, McGinity JW. Effervescent granules and methods for their preparation. US Patent US 6,649,186 B1 2003.

50. Padmanabhan B, et al. Effervescent composition and method for making it. WO Patent WO2016042372AI 2016.

15 Granulation of Plant Products and Nutraceuticals

Dilip M. Parikh

CONTENTS

15.1 INTRODUCTION

For centuries, food has been used for the prevention and treatment of disease as well as botanicals and herbal formulations that contribute to the daily diet of macro- and micronutrients intake. Nutraceuticals and dietary supplements have been interchangeability used to describe products made from plants, animals, or minerals which may show therapeutic activity. Ancient texts of India and China contain exhaustive depictions of the use of a variety of plant-derived medications. In India, Ayurveda medicine recognized the beneficial influence of food and plant consumption and intake on human health. Since millennia, the primary focus of the Ayurveda has been the establishment of the healthy condition and removal of the disease condition. Nutraceuticals made from the plants are the food components made from herbal or botanical raw materials, which are used for preventing or treating different types of acute and chronic maladies. Also known as functional foods and phytochemicals, nutraceuticals are the bioactive chemical and natural compounds that have the medicinal properties to treat and cure several disorders.

The term "nutraceutical" was coined from "nutrition" and "pharmaceutical" in 1989 by Stephen DeFelice, MD [1]. According to DeFelice, nutraceutical can be defined as, "a food (or part of a food) that provides medical or health benefits, including the prevention and/or treatment of a disease." However, the term nutraceutical as commonly used in marketing has no regulatory definition [2]. However, "The Dietary Supplement Health and Education Act" (DSHEA) in the United States formally defined "dietary supplement" using several criteria [3] as follows:

A dietary supplement

- *is a product (other than tobacco) that is intended to supplement the diet that bears or contains one or more of the following dietary ingredients: a vitamin, a mineral, an herb or other botanical, an amino acid, a dietary substance for use by man to supplement the diet by increasing the total daily intake, or a concentrate, metabolite, constituent, extract, or combinations of these ingredients.*
- *is intended for ingestion in pill, capsule, tablet, or liquid form*
- *is not represented for use as a conventional food or as the sole item of a meal or diet.*
- *is labeled as a "dietary supplement."*
- *It does not claim any specific ailment treatment*
- *a dietary substance for use by a person to supplement the diet by increasing the total dietary intake; or a concentrate, metabolite, constituent, extract, or combination of any ingredient*

Thus, nutraceuticals (as per the proposed definition) differ from dietary supplements in the following aspects:

- *Nutraceuticals must not only supplement the diet but should also aid in the prevention and/or treatment of disease and/or disorder*
- *Nutraceuticals are represented for use as a conventional food or as the sole item of meal or diet.*
- *The dietary supplement product does not include.*
- *"(i) an article that is approved as a new drug under section 505, certified as an antibiotic under section 507, or licensed as a biologic under section 351 of the Public Health Service Act (42 U.S.C. 262), or*
- *"(ii) an article authorized for investigation as a new drug, antibiotic, or biological for which substantial clinical investigations have been instituted and for which the existence of such investigations has been made public.*

The nutraceuticals have many therapeutic benefits and are especially relevant as antifatigue or for preventing or delaying several age-related diseases, that is, arthritis, cancer, metabolic and cardiovascular diseases, Alzheimer's, Huntington's disease, osteoporosis, cataracts, brain disorders, etc. [4]. The therapeutic potential of herbal drugs depends on its form, whether parts of a plant, simple extracts, or isolated active constituents. Herbal medicine is now globally accepted as a valid alternative system of therapy in the form of pharmaceuticals, functional foods, etc., a trend recognized and advocated by the World Health Organization (WHO). The US Pharmacopeia has established guidelines for standardization, tests, assays, and other specifications for the dietary supplements [5]. Various studies around the world, especially in Europe, have been initiated to develop scientific evidence-based rational herbal therapies.

Ayurveda has recommended several drugs from indigenous plant sources for the treatment of asthma and allergic disorder, and has been successful in controlling these diseases as well. Some herbal drugs which are mainly used in the treatment of asthma are *Albezzia Lebbeck, Euphorbia Hirta, Adhatoda Vasica,* and *Allium Capa. Madhavi lata (Hiptage benghalensis),* native to India and the Philippines, is a vine-like plant that is often cultivated in the tropics for its attractive and fragrant flowers. It is used medicinally in India. Its bark, leaves, and flowers are aromatic, bitter, acrid, astringent, vulnerary, expectorant, cardiotonic, anti-inflammatory, and insecticidal.

In the last decades, the number of research papers and debate about the potential use of nutraceuticals and food supplements has grown exponentially [4A]. Examples of nutraceuticals widely used nowadays are the polyvitamins, omega-3 fatty acids, carotenoids, and polyphenols (anthocyanins, proanthocyanidins, flavanones, isoflavones, and ellagic acid). Another category of nutraceuticals that are quickly growing in the past two decades is the "Probiotics." The oral delivery of probiotics is hampered by the low instability of the bacteria in the Gastro Intestinal Tract and consequent loss of viability under the effect of high acidity and bile salt concentrations. The problem of oral delivery of the nutraceuticals at an acceptable bioavailability has been tackled by formulators with various degrees of success. For probiotics delivery, the bacteria could be immobilized into a polymer matrix, which is a kind of enteric system that remains intact in the stomach but degrades and dissolves in the intestine. The advent of nanotechnology for pharmaceutical applications has opened a new avenue for stability, solubility, and/or permeability enhancement of problematic nutraceuticals [6–9].

Recent regulatory relaxation in most of the countries for Cannabis has sparked interest in the nutraceutical industry. Cannabis (also known as marijuana) is the most frequently used illicit (in some countries) psychoactive substance in the world. Cannabis does have therapeutic properties for certain indications. These therapeutic applications pertain only to certain cannabinoids and their synthetic derivatives. There are over 480 natural components found within the Cannabis sativa plant, of which 66 have been classified as "cannabinoids" chemicals unique to the plant. Cannabidiol (CBD) is probably the most abundant cannabinoid, contributing up to 40% of cannabis resin.

15.2   NUTRACEUTICAL MARKET

A major factor contributing to the growth of the global herbal medicine market is the increasing demand for natural medicines, thus increasing research funding for herbal medicines. Multiple applications of herbal medicines are expected to enhance market growth. According to the National Center for Biotechnology Information, in 2015, the World Health Organization (WHO) reported that around 70% to 80% of people globally rely on herbal sources for their treatment. It was reported by the American Botanical Council, in September 2017, that in 2016 the sale of herbal supplements increased by 7.7% in the United States. The Global Herbal Medicine Market is expected to register a Compound Annual Growth Rate (CAGR) of 5.88% to reach USD 1,29,689.3 million until 2023. The global herbal medicine market, based on region, is divided into the Americas, Europe, Asia-Pacific, and the Middle East and Africa. Americas are estimated to account for the third-largest market share during the forecast period. This is due to the growing use of herbal medicines in the United States. According to the National Center for Biotechnology Information, in 2017, it was reported that herbal supplements were majorly used for conditions such as cancer (43.1%), stroke (48.7%), and arthritis (43%) in the United States. The herbal medicine market in the Middle East and Africa is expected to observe a slow growth due to less awareness and in-depth knowledge about herbal drugs in this region [10]. Europe is expected to hold the largest share and estimated to be the fastest-growing region, of the global herbal medicine market, because of extensive R&D for herbal medicine, increasing funding for research on medicinal plants and growing preference for herbal drugs in the European region. Asia-Pacific is expected to account for the second-largest market share during the forecast period. The factors responsible for market growth in this region are the adoption of traditional medicines by pharmaceutical companies, researchers, and policymakers.

15.3   REGULATORY LANDSCAPE AROUND THE WORLD

For the regulation of dietary supplements, there is no global consensus on how the category of products known variously as dietary supplements, natural health products (NHPs), complementary medicines, or food supplements in different countries is defined. For example, a product is considered to be a dietary supplement and regulated as a food in the United States, whereas in another jurisdiction, it may be considered either a food supplement or a therapeutic good (complementary medicine) or a therapeutic good (a prescription medicine) or potentially even a controlled substance. In the United States, these products are not allowed to claim any medical benefits but are available without a prescription. Nutrient content claims are regulated by the Food and Drug Administration (FDA) under the Nutrition Labeling and Education Act (NLEA) [11]. The FDA has provided a guidance document to distinguish between structure/function claims and disease claims [12].

In Canada, these products are called Natural Health Products (NHP), regulated under the Canadian Food and Drugs Act. Recent changes in regulating NHPs consist of the following five major components: 1. a three-class system of NHPs based on risk, 2. requirements and pathways for licensing NHPs, 3. site licensing modifications, 4. quality guidance redevelopment for NHPs, and 5. compliance transition over time [13].

Most of the world treats dietary supplements like a prescription drug. In Latin America, Asia, and Europe, dietary supplements must show the efficacy, and manufacturers must meet quality standards with that of the manufacturing of prescription drugs.

In the European Union (EU), nutraceuticals, and functional foods have no specific legal status.

However, most of these products are covered by legislation on food supplements, fortified foods, and dietetic foods and to the extent that health claims are made by the European Union (EU) legislation covering nutrition and health claims. Article 6 of Regulation 178/2002 also firmly establishes scientific risk analysis as the basis of the decision-making process in matters of food law in the EU. All foods making nutrition or health claims are subject to specific legislation since 2006 (Regulation 1924/2006). The system put in place is based on the pre-marketing approval of all claims [14,15]. The use of botanicals for therapeutic or preventive purposes in medicinal products has been harmonized in the EU by the Traditional Herbal Medicinal Product Directive (THMPD 2004/24) [16].

Two important areas not yet harmonized in the EU for food supplements include:

* Maximum levels of vitamins and minerals used in food supplements
* The use of ingredients other than vitamins and minerals (including botanicals) for nutritional/physiological purposes, where these ingredients are not regarded as novel foods.

If medicinal claims are made based on "traditional use" as defined in Directive 2004/24/EC [16A], or the herb is considered medicinal by function, the product may be categorized as a "Traditional Herbal Medicinal Product (THMP)," provided the time-related criteria are met. These time-related criteria are 30 years of usage overall, of which 15 years are in the EU [17].

(*with the recent exit of the United Kingdom from the EU, UK regulations regarding Neutraceuticals are not clear, whether UK will continue to follow the same regulations as the EU until authorities come up with the new regulations is not clear at this writing*).

In Japan, regulatory authorities approve these products by categorizing products based on their composition and the functionality claims after the supporting evidence is submitted for approval.

Germany has the most rigorous set of regulations, and this is reflected in the way nutraceuticals are dispensed to the consumers, through pharmacies only, except for herbal products with German names.

In Australia, medicinal products containing ingredients such as herbs, vitamins, minerals, nutritional supplements, and homeopathic and certain aromatherapy preparations are referred to as "complementary medicines" and are regulated as medicines under the Therapeutic Goods Act, 1989.

The Russian system for controlling the circulation of food supplements is largely harmonized with those in Europe and the United States, including indications for use of such products, except biologically active food supplements, which have stricter regulations [18].

In India, the responsibility of framing and regulating standards for nutraceuticals rests with the Food Safety and Standards Authority of India (FSSAI) as outlined in the Food Safety Act, 2006, and updated in 2011. This authority will be in charge of categories like functional foods, nutraceuticals, dietetic products, and other similar products [19–22].

Chinese health food industry has grown dramatically in the past two decades and become the second-largest health foods/dietary supplements market in the world. Chinese FDA (SFDA) has similar regulations and the requirements to prove the claims of included ingredients [23,24].

15.4 MANUFACTURE OF NUTRACEUTICALS

Various types of nutraceuticals typically manufactured are as follows:

- Nutraceuticals ground, dried, powdered, and either mixed or decoction extracted and further processed from plant materials
- Nutraceuticals extracted or purified from plants
- Foods that have added active ingredients other than vitamins or minerals and have been scientifically demonstrated to provide health benefits beyond their basic nutritional functions.
- Nutraceuticals produced, extracted, or purified from marine sources
- Nutraceuticals that are produced, extracted, or purified from animals and micro-organisms

15.4.1 PREPARATION OF EXTRACT

According to the World Health Organization (WHO), nearly 20,000 medicinal plants exist in 91 countries including 12 mega biodiversity countries. The premier steps to utilize the biologically active compound from plant resources are extraction, pharmacological screening, isolation and characterization of bioactive compounds, toxicological evaluation, and clinical evaluation. The formulation of herbal medicines is challenging particularly when using fresh plants for robust tablet forms due to the inherent poor tableting properties of most herbal or powdered plant parts. Because of the compression difficulties and the low bulk density, herbal products are formulated as capsules. Extraction, on the other hand, offers standardization of the extracted and concentrated tincture, thereby diminishing the variability of the dry mass and its properties in the tincture. For plants with active constituents, the most common practice is to extract the active compound(s) with the extraction process. The basic process includes steps, such as pre-washing, drying of plant materials, freeze-drying, or grinding, to obtain a homogenous sample and extract with the solvent system. Proper actions must be taken to assure that potential active constituents are not lost, distorted, or destroyed during the preparation of the extract from plant samples. The selection of the solvent system largely depends on the specific nature of the bioactive compound that is targeted. The extraction of hydrophilic compounds uses polar solvents such as methanol, ethanol, or ethyl-acetate. As the target compounds may be non-polar to polar and thermally labile, the suitability of the methods of extraction must be considered. For extraction of more lipophilic compounds, dichloromethane or a mixture of dichloromethane/methanol in the ratio of 1:1 is used. In some instances, extraction with hexane is used to remove chlorophyll [25]. There are various methods, such as sonification, heating under reflux, and soxhlet extraction, where compounds have a limited solubility in the solvent being used. Besides, plant extracts are also prepared by maceration or percolation of fresh green plants or dried powdered plant material in water and/or organic solvent systems. The other modern extraction techniques include solid-phase micro-extraction, supercritical-fluid extraction, pressurized-liquid extraction, microwave-assisted extraction, solid-phase extraction, and surfactant-mediated techniques, which possess certain advantages. Conventional organic solvent extraction techniques face issues of safety, involving more labor, and are time-consuming [26,27]. Often referred to as subcritical water extraction, "Pressurized Hot Water Extraction" (PHWE) is an efficient and greener method for the extraction of bioactive compounds from plant materials [28]. The main parameters which influence its extraction efficiency are namely the temperature, extraction time, flow rates, and addition of modifiers/additives. The extraction of certain compounds is dependent on pressurized water with different applied temperature. Thus, the stability and reduced solubilities of certain compounds at elevated temperatures are critical. Researchers reported the use of PHWE with methanol as an auxiliary solvent, *Bidens pilosa* plant. The temperature was an important factor to effectively extract pharmacologically relevant metabolites *dicaffeoylquinic acid (diCQA)* and *chicoric acid (CA),* which are known to possess anti-HIV properties, and their analogs from *B. pilos,* thus showing that the extraction efficiency of PHWE can be greatly enhanced by introducing an auxiliary solvent [29].

15.4.2 DOSAGE FORM MANUFACTURING CHALLENGES

15.4.2.1 Sourcing and Standardization

Plant materials are chemically and naturally variable. Herbal drugs are usually mixtures of many constituents. The active principle(s) is (are), in most cases, unknown. The source and quality of the raw material are variable. One of the major constraints in using plants in pharmaceutical discovery is the lack of reproducibility of activity for over 40% of plant extracts. Reproducibility is the major problem, as the activities detected during screening often do not repeat when plants are re-sampled and re-extracted. This problem is largely due to differences in the biochemical profiles of plants harvested at different times and locations, differences in variety, and variation in the methods used for extraction and biological activity determination. Furthermore, the activity and efficacy of plant extracts/medicines often result from additive or synergistic interaction effects of the components. Therefore, a strategy should be used to evaluate the qualitative and quantitative variations in the content of bioactive phytochemicals of plant material. Standardization, optimization, and full control of growing conditions could result in the cost-effective and quality-controlled production of many herbal medicines.

15.4.2.2 Physicochemical Properties of Powdered Plants and Herbal Parts

Particle shape and size distribution are particular concerns for flow while formulating a dosage form. Botanical powders, particularly barks and roots, are notorious for needle-like fibers. The best way to minimize the presence of fibers is to mill the powder to a very fine particle size before blending. Besides, low bulk density and variable particle sizes pose an additional challenge. These typically inhibit flow and ultimately cause problems. Poor flow may result in great difficulty in processing the material, especially on high-speed tableting or encapsulation equipment, leading to problems with fill weight variation and content uniformity. Other issues that pose challenges in flow, particularly with botanicals, are moisture absorption, oiliness, waxy consistency, and static electricity. Hygroscopicity may contribute to poor flow as well as adversely influence both physical and chemical stability. All of these factors inhibit flow by causing the product to become clumpy, gritty, or sticky. The most common solution is to add a glidant. Glidants have an extremely small particle size (140 to 400 mesh) and work by coating the surface of larger particles to reduce friction, absorb excess moisture, and enhance flow. Examples of glidants are silicon dioxide, calcium silicate, and talc among others. Density differences in these ingredients can be addressed by granulating these plant products. Minerals in the formulation taste bad. They also tend to react with vitamins and other nutrients, especially in the presence of heat and moisture. There are serious bioavailability, solubility, and tolerability issues to be addressed, and sometimes, addressing one set of concerns exacerbates another set. A formulator must take all these technical and nutritional factors into account to develop the most efficacious product possible. Some of the technologies used to overcome challenges posed by mineral fortification and to improve bioavailability include microencapsulation, taste-masking, stabilization with other carriers (hydrolyzed proteins or polysaccharides), chelation, micropulverization, and liposome applications. Mineral chelates [30] and effervescent mineral–vitamin formulation soluble in water are also growing in popularity [31]. The largest issue with trace minerals is homogeneity. If you consider that the recommended use rates for all of these nutrients are measured in micrograms, it becomes a challenge to get that small amount blended across a typical batch so that a label claim can be guaranteed.

15.4.2.3 Microbiological Issues

The raw materials, pharmaceutical ingredients, and active ingredients used in the manufacture of nutritional and dietary articles may range from chemically synthesized vitamins to plant extracts and animal byproducts. Microbiological process control, control of the bioburden of raw materials, and control of the manufacturing process to minimize cross-contamination are necessary to guarantee acceptable microbial quality in the final dosage forms. Raw materials, excipients, and active substances as components of nutrition and dietary supplements can be a primary source of microbiological contamination. To assure minimum microbiological challenges, incoming raw material, its bioburden, and its proportionate quantity used in the formulation should be determined. Specifications should be developed, and sampling plans and test procedures should be employed to guarantee the desired microbiological attributes of these materials. From a microbiological perspective, the development of the formulation of nutritional or dietary supplements includes an evaluation of raw materials and their suppliers and the contribution made to the products by each ingredient and the manufacturing processes [16A; see Table 15.1].

15.4.2.4 Quality Challenges

Botanical extracts and blends present particular challenges for detecting misidentification and contamination. The presence of adulterants and contaminants of both biological and chemical nature

---

TABLE 15.1

Microbiological Attributes of Non-Sterile Nutritional and Dietary Supplements [16A]

Botanical Preparation	Definition
Chopped or powderedbotanicals	Hand-picked portions of the botanical (e.g., leaves, flowers, roots, tubers, etc.) that are air-dried, chopped, flaked, sectioned,ground, or pulverized to the consistency of a powder.
Botanical extracts	Extracts are solid or semisolid preparations of a botanical that are prepared by percolation, filtration, and concentration by evaporation of the percolate. The extracting material may by alcoholic, alkaline, acid hydro-alcoholic, or aqueous. Typically, an extract is 4 to 10 times as strong as the original botanical. The extracts may be semisolids or dry powders termed powdered extracts.
Tinctures	Tinctures are solutions of botanical substances in alcohol obtained by extraction of the powdered, flaked, or sectioned botanical.
Infusions	Infusions are solutions of botanical principles obtained by soaking the powdered botanical in hot or cold water for a specified time and straining. Typically, infusions are 5% in strength.
Decoctions	Decoctions are solutions of botanicals prepared by boiling the material in water for at least 15 minutes and straining. Typically, decoctions are 5% in strength.
Fluid extracts	A fluid extract is an alcoholic liquid extract made by the percolation of a botanical so that 1 mL of the fluid extract represents 1 g of the botanical.
Botanicals to be treated with boiling water before use	Dried botanicals to which boiling water is added immediately before consumption.

in supplements is also challenging. Zhang et al. classified quality issues of herbal medicine into two categories: external and internal. External issues are contamination (e.g., toxic metals, pesticide residues, microbes, adulteration, and misidentification), and internal factors are the complexity and non-uniformity of the ingredients in herbal medicines [32]. Analytically, the identification of plant constituents is of a particular challenge. Even when easily identified whole plants or plant parts are used, unless the chain of custody is tight, and the exact manufacturing process is known and well-characterized, the quality of extracts and blends such as those found in many botanical products is difficult to determine. Analytical methods and reference standards are lacking for many of the thousands of different bioactive ingredients in dietary supplements. The availability of analytical procedures is difficult to develop for some of the plant extracts. Analytical techniques for a mixture of plants/herbs in supplements are further complicated because the active compound(s) is often unknown. The DSHEA does not set a framework for quality except to state that manufacturers are prohibited from introducing products posing "significant or unreasonable risk" into interstate commerce; must get pre-market approval from FDA for "New Dietary Ingredients;" must follow labeling regulations (accuracy, label disclaimers, or notification of claims); and must have substantiation that claims are truthful and not misleading [33]. The safety of dietary supplements depends largely on dose. The possibilities of excessive intake of nutrients from dietary supplements are greater where supplements are available over the counter and where several food items are fortified with vitamins and minerals.

The presence of adulterants and contaminants of both biological and chemical nature in supplements is also challenging. Certain categories of supplements, such as athletic performance, sexual performance, and weight loss products, are particularly prone to the deliberate "spiking" with unlabeled extraneous or synthetic substances to confuse analytical techniques and even occasionally the addition of active synthetic drugs. Purity is a special problem for individuals with inborn errors of metabolism for specific nutrients such as vitamin B-6 or choline who require reliable, high-quality sources of the nutrient [34].

15.5 FORMULATION AND PROCESSING

Herbs and plant products for herbal therapies are usually prepared by grinding or steeping the parts of a plant that are believed to contain medicinal properties. The ground plant matter is called the "macerate." The macerate is soaked in a liquid referred to as the "menstruum" to extract the active ingredients. Herbal infusions are prepared by treating the herb with water or alcohol or mixtures of the two; a coarsely ground drug boiled in water for a definite period is known as a decoction, and tinctures are solutions of the active principles of the drug in alcohol and water. This extraction process leads to the production of the herbal preparations in the form of fresh juice, hot and cold infusions, decoctions, tinctures, pastes, and powders referred to as "pulverata." The resulting therapies come in several forms, including oral tablets, capsules, gel caps, extracts, and infusions. Solid or powdered extracts are prepared by evaporation of the solvents used in the process of extraction of the raw material. Herbal extracts, including *b-sitosterols* (found in Saw Palmetto berry), *Cernilton* (pollen extract), and *Pygeum Africum* (African plum), have been clinically evaluated for use in the treatment of benign prostatic Hyperplasia [35]. Kumadoh et al. prepared *Enterica* dosage form, from *Enterica* herbal decoction which consisted of a combination of plant materials obtained from 12 plants and mixing decoction with absorbents like starch, kaolin, light magnesium carbonate, and bentonite to produce dried granules. Resulting granules were encapsulated [36]. To produce dosage forms, several problems not applicable to synthetic drugs influence the quality of herbal drugs and pose processing problems. To manufacture solid dosage forms from these plant materials or minerals, vitamins, and other nutritional ingredients, different granulation processes that are described in this book can be used. Following a few examples will illustrate how various formulation strategies and process technologies can be used to process dietary supplements and plant-based products.

15.5.1 DIRECT COMPRESSION

Depending upon the quantity and physical properties of the ingredient, a direct compression process can be utilized to produce tablets or capsules. Generally, the dietary supplement contains more than one plant or mineral ingredient, and direct compression may not be feasible. A number of plant extracts are spray-dried, further processed by using direct compression and dry compaction such as slugging or roller compaction, or wet granulated in high-shear mixers. The direct compression method was used for the preparation of nutraceutical tablets containing clove [37]. The fast-dissolving tablets were prepared with a mixture of powdered cloves and crospovidone as a super disintegrant and magnesium stearate and talc by direct compression.

In one case study, the herbal product consisted of spray-dried Teng tea powdered extract at a concentration of 14%. The active ingredient could not be processed by wet granulation because it became very sticky when exposed to water. To avoid a solvent granulation process, a formulation for direct compression was developed with Teng tea extract, as well as with ginseng extract using Starch 1500 along with other excipients. Colorcon has listed several case studies where the formula contained a mixture of 22.5% spray-dried extract (SDE) and 67.5% crude herb powder, which left only 10% of the formulation for excipients. However, by using Starch 1500, the formulation met the criteria for disintegration and hardness [38].

Brahmbhatt et al. collected fresh leaves of *Hiptage Benghalensis,* dried, and ground to a fine powder. The extract was obtained from the powder, concentrated, and used with other excipients to make tablets with a direct compression tablet. Wet granulation was also performed using the same extract along with polyvinylpyrrolidone (PVP) K 30 and starch which showed the best results upon evaluation compared to direct compression [39]. Because of hygroscopicity, of a spray-dried extract of *Maytenus ilicifolia,* wet granulation could not be carried out. The extract was blended with other ingredients and slugged, milled, and processed as follows:

The spray-dried extract from M. ilicifolia was blended in a Turbula mixer with other excipients of magnesium stearate. Slugs were produced at a compression force of 22.0 ± 1.0 kN using flat-faced tooling 17 mm in diameter on a single-punch tablet press. The slugs were crushed in a dry granulator to obtain granules with a particle size of < 2.00 mm. The resulting material was passed through an oscillating granulator using a 1.0-mm sieve. The granulate fraction between 250 and 1000 μm was chosen for tablet optimization [40].

15.5.2 SPRAY DRYING

Spray-dried extracts (SDEs) often have a small particle size and consequently poor flow, which may result in variation in weight and poor content uniformity within tablets. Spray-dried extracts (SDEs) from medicinal plants are often used as active components in solid dosage forms because of their better stability. However, these products generally present deficient rheological properties, inadequate compressibility, and high sensitivity to atmospheric moisture, resulting in difficult direct compression, as medicinal plants are often used as active components in solid dosage forms because of their better stability [41]. Particle size can be enlarged by granulation to increase the flow rate. *Phyllanthus niruri* is a medicinal plant widely distributed and used in folk medicine to treat kidney stone ailments and viral hepatitis. Pharmacological experiments confirm its therapeutic efficacy and safety. Daniel Guajardo-Flores et al. spray-dried black bean extract powders and used it in different formulations for the production of nutraceutical capsules with reduced batch-to-batch weight variability. Factorial designs were used to find an adequate maltodextrin–extract ratio for the spray-drying process to produce black bean extract powders. They were also able to show retention of flavonoids and saponins from black bean extract powder, which decreases with the increase of maltodextrin concentration in the spray-drying feed [42].

15.5.3 FLUID-BED GRANULATION

Herb *"Xuchunchongji"* consists of 17 different medicinal herbs. It is difficult to dry the extract from the plant due to its viscous nature. To dry the extract, researchers sprayed the extract on substrate containing 1:2 ratio of dextrin and sucrose, producing the desired granules in a fluid-bed granulator [43]. Bennelli et al. reported the feasibility of fluidized beds for seed agglomeration of rosemary (*Rosmarinus officinalis*) extract compositions and attempted to form a product with adequate physicochemical properties. Lipid- and carbohydrate-based compositions with different viscosities were top sprayed onto fluidized beds of cassava flour or sugar pellets as seed particles [43A].

15.5.4 ROLLER COMPACTION

Roller compaction of a milled botanical (*Baphicacanthus cusia*) with and without a binder, poly-vinylpyrrolidone (PVP), was conducted. Larger-sized and less friable granules were obtained with decreasing roller speed. The addition of PVP affected the flowability and binding capacity of the herbal powder blend, which influenced the size and friability of the granules. The co-milling of PVP with the herbal powder enhanced the flow of the blends and the effectiveness of the binder, which contributed favorably to the roller-compacted product [44]. Aloe vera gel is the colorless gel contained in the inner parts of the fresh leaves. Chemical analysis has revealed that this clear gel contains amino acids, minerals, vitamins, enzymes, proteins, polysaccharides, and biological stimulators. Fast-dissolving tablets of the nutraceutical, freeze-dried Aloe vera gel were prepared by the dry granulation method utilizing the factorial design. The results of multiple regression analysis revealed that to obtain a fast-dissolving tablet of the Aloe vera gel, an optimum concentration of mannitol and a higher content of microcrystalline cellulose should be used [45]. Spray-dried extract of *Maytenus ilicifolia*, widely used in Brazil, as anti-inflammatory, analgesic, and anti-ulcerogenic, was dry granulated using roller compaction process. The compressional behavior of spray-dried extract and granules made from roller compaction was characterized by Heckel plots. The tablet properties of powders, granules, and formulations containing high extract doses were compared [46].

15.5.5 WET GRANULATION

A number of these ingredients are hygroscopic and thus may require non-aqueous granulation or are roller compacted to produce dense-enough granules for compression or encapsulation. *Rauwolfia serpentine* powder is soft in nature, is poor in die filling, and deforms by initial frag-mentation. Patra et al. [47] compared the granulating roots of *Rauwolfia serpentine* with starch paste and compared resultant granulation with a direct compression blend. The compression results from both granulations showed that wet granulated product had better flow property, compressi-bility, and compactibility compared to direct compression formulations. *Phyllanthus niruri* spray-dried extract (SDE) often has a small particle size and consequently poor flow. Because of its water solubility and unknown stability of the major active substance, this extract was granulated with Eudragit E in acetone to make granulation, which provided free-flowing granules with lower moisture sorption behavior than original extract. The mechanical properties of the tablets were found to be dependent on the Eudragit E proportion within the granules and the compression force; therefore, a higher proportion of Eudragit E with a smaller compression force resulted in a better release of the SDE from the tablets [48]. A patent describes similar granulation of a Chinese herb extract, which was granulated with excipients and dried [49]. There are multiple specific chemical entities classed as phytosterols, including but not limited to *beta-sitosterol, campesterol*, and *stigmasterol*. Typical phytosterol could contain a single or mixture of these sterols. Because of its hydrophobic waxy nature, it is difficult to mill, resulting in clogged mill screen, and it does not flow after micronization. The low bulk density and waxy nature causes compression problems. As such granulation of these sticky sterols with silicon dioxide before processing and granulating with PVP in a high-shear mixer and fluid-bed drier was reported [50]. Granola is an aggregated baked food product often eaten as a breakfast cereal containing natural ingredients such as oats, nuts, and honey. It generally displays a high degree of friability. Pathare et al. [51] studied the effect of binder spray rate and nozzle air pressure on the granule size and texture properties of granola breakfast cereal prepared by fluidized bed granulation. The industrial production of granola is typically undertaken by employing a mixer granulator (e.g., a large bowl with impeller) or in a high-shear mixer granulator as described by Bas et al. [52]. A review of the attributes of granola breakfast cereal produced by wet granulation was reported by Pathare et al. [53].

Chewable tablets of *Amalaki* from *Emblica Officinalis Gaertn* family were prepared by granulating with a non-aqueous solution of 10% PVP in ethanol, and after drying, extra granular excipients were added and compressed [54].

15.5.6 NANOTECHNOLOGY

The advent of nanotechnology for pharmaceutical applications has opened a new avenue for stability, solubility, and/or permeability enhancement of problematic nutraceuticals. In this context, nanometric systems in the absence or presence of carriers have been attempted. In absence of a carrier, nanonization of the bioactive nutraceutical overcomes its "grease ball" nature and improves its wettability and dissolution rate. In the presence of a carrier, several nanocarriers such as nanocapsules, micelles, and nanoparticles can be used. However, biocompatibility and biodegradability-related issues are crucial. Biodegradable FDA approved polymers, for example, polyesters, are favored by formulators to develop nutraceutical-loaded nanoparticles.

15.5.7 CANNABIS AND CANNABIDIOL (CBD) PROCESSING

Cannabis has been consumed in one form or another for thousands of years, but it wasn't until 1964 that a team led by the Israeli researcher Raphael Mechoulam identified Tetrahydrocannabinol (THC) as the molecule that had psychoactive results. American neurologist Russo and Mechoulam in 2010, at a conference, presented a paper called "Taming THC," which compiled more than 400 studies that strengthened the case for the role terpenes played in the variable effects of Cannabis. Despite lingering prohibitions in 17 states, legal cannabis is already an $8 billion industry in the United States [55, 56]. Cannabis does have therapeutic properties for certain indications. These therapeutic applications pertain only to certain cannabinoids and their synthetic derivatives. There are over 480 natural components found within the Cannabis sativa plant, of which 66 have been classified as "cannabinoids," chemicals unique to the plant. The most well known and researched of these, delta-9-tetrahydrocannabinol (Δ9-THC), is the substance primarily responsible for the psychoactive effects of cannabis. Three classes of cannabinoids, the Cannabigerol (CBG), Cannabichromene (CBC), and Cannabidiol (CBD), are not known to have any such psychological effect. Tetrahydrocannabinol (THC), Cannabinol (CBN), cannabidiol (CBDL), and some other cannabinoids, on the other hand, are known to be psychologically active to varying degrees. Cannabidiol (CBD) is probably the most abundant cannabinoid, contributing up to 40% of cannabis resin. Synthetic cannabinoids (SCs) emerged in the 1970s when researchers were first exploring the endocannabinoid system and attempting to develop new treatments for cancer pain. Since 2008, more than 160 SCs have been identified in various products, 24 of which appeared in 2015 [57]. A patent describing the alternative solution for the administration of cannabis was reported providing an oral, buccal, or sublingual preparation such that single doses of one of THC or CBD or both are delivered between 1 and 30 mg per single dose. Other objects of the invention include methods of making the oral sublingual or buccal preparations for treating diseases and other medical conditions and also for recreational purposes [58]. Another patent describes the manufacturing of granules of cannabinoid for oral dosage administration. The inventors developed granules made of lactose particles held together by a binding component comprising a cannabinoid and a lipophilic matrix containing at least 80% wt. of sucrose monoester of a C8-C18 fatty acid [59].

15.6 STORAGE AND STABILITY

Plant products contain a variety of biologically active compounds, and some of these include iso-flavones, flavonoids, carotenoids, bioactive peptides, and vitamins. Proper storage is important from harvesting to final manufacturing of the plant/herbal products. Low-temperature storage is always recommended for phytochemicals. Chang et al. concluded that the phenolic stability of hawthorn (*Crataegus pinnatifida* var. *major*) was affected by the storage temperature [60]. Dry powders are stored for a long time before being used in the dosage form manufacturing, and the producer needs to understand, without testing before use, that the intended "dose" of the plant product may not be what ends up in the dosage form. For example, *ginsenoside* in ginseng preparation was found to vary dose from 0% to a high of 9% [61–62].

Kopleman and Augsburger studied the challenges analyzing the active principle and determined the challenges of processing the popular herbal product St. John's Wort (*Hypericum perforatum*). The authors concluded that storage of the botanical product should be kept at a minimal temperature, and care should be taken to avoid not only oxygen and light but humidity as well. They further concluded that chemical extraction of the crude material, as well as further processing, may significantly influence the physical and chemical characteristics of the powdered commercial extract. Therefore, the supplement manufacturer needs to perform a complete physicomechanical and chemical characterization when extracts are purchased from multiple suppliers [63].

15.7 GMP AND NUTRACEUTICALS

Adulteration and contamination of herbal medicines appear to be common in countries that have lenient controls in regulating their purity. Adulteration in Asian medicines mostly results from the misidentification of plants. The US FDA and other investigators have also reported the presence of prescription drugs, including glyburide, sildenafil, colchicines, adrenal steroids, alprazolam, etc., in products claiming to contain only natural ingredients [64]. On June 25, 2007, the US FDA issued the final rules for the nutraceutical/dietary supplement industry Good Manufacturing Practice (GMPs) for the nutraceutical industry. This is the big change for the industry in the United States where these nutraceutical products were classified up until now under the "food" category and were not subject to the same level of CGMP requirements, which has now changed. This will require manufacturers to conduct a gap analysis. Whether the issue is cross-contamination or product consistency, the challenge remains the same, to balance procedural and engineering changes to manage risk and cost effectively. The DSHEA gave the FDA the express responsibility to regulate the manufacturing processes of dietary supplements, and the FDA issued its first proposed rule in 2003 [65]. In June 2007, it issued its final rule [66] which requires all dietary supplement manufacturers to ensure by June 2010 that production of dietary supplements complies with *current* good manufacturing practices, and these are manufactured with "controls that result in a consistent product free of contamination, with accurate labeling" [67]. Besides, the industry is now required to report to the FDA "all serious dietary supplement related adverse events."

15.7.1 KEY REQUIREMENTS OF THE FINAL RULE

The CGMPs apply to all domestic and foreign companies that manufacture, package, label, or hold dietary supplements, including those involved with the activities of testing, quality control, packaging, and labeling, and distribute them in the United States (referred to herein as "companies").

Each company involved in manufacturing, packaging, labeling, or holding dietary supplements is responsible for only those CGMPs that relate to its activities. The Final Rule is limited to only those involved with dietary supplements – it does not extend to entities that manufacture, package, label, or hold only dietary ingredients, or to persons engaged only in activities associated with the harvesting, 67storage, or distribution of raw agricultural commodities that will be incorporated into dietary supplements by other persons. Additionally, the Final Rule does not apply to retail establishments holding dietary supplements only for purposes of direct retail sale to individual consumers, although this exception does not include a retailer's warehouse or another storage facility, nor does it extend to warehouses or storage facilities that sell directly to individual consumers. In 2010, FDA released Current Good Manufacturing Practice in Manufacturing, Packaging, Labeling, or Holding Operations for Dietary Supplements; Small Entity Compliance Guide [68].

15.8 CONCLUSION

Plant materials are used throughout the developed and developing world as home remedies, in over-the-counter drug products, and as raw material for the pharmaceutical industry, and they represent a substantial proportion of the global drug market. Therefore, it is essential to establish internationally recognized guidelines for assessing their quality. The possibility of herb–drug interactions is important, but "under-research" is an issue. The World Health Assembly in resolutions WHA31.33 (1978), WHA40.33 (1987), WHA42.43 (1989), and WHA56.31 (2003) has emphasized the need to ensure the quality of medicinal plant products by using modern control techniques and applying suitable standards [69–72] The toxicity benchmarks for herbal drugs depend on purity, herbs containing toxic substances, bioavailability, and reported adverse effects. The selection of the manufacturing process to produce a solid dosage form requires understanding the process most suitable for the intended product and intimate knowledge of analytical techniques to determine the active moiety and its potency. Granulating plant products and nutraceuticals require their appropriate physicochemical characteristics, before embarking on the chosen technique. Sometimes the capsule formulation could be forgiving compared to the tablet formulation. The incorporation of various ingredients increases the complexity of formulating and stability of the final dosage forms. Herbal medicines can act through a variety of mechanisms to alter the pharmacokinetic profile of concomitantly administered drugs. Numerous examples exist of drug and herbal interactions. These effects may potentiate or antagonize drug absorption or metabolism, the patient's metabolism, or cause unwanted side reactions.

REFERENCES

1. Brower V Nutraceuticals: poised for a healthy slice of the healthcare market? Nat Biotechnol 1998;16: 728–731.
2. Zeisel SH Regulation of "Nutraceuticals." Science 1999;285: 185–186.
3. Food and Drug Administration. Dietary Supplement Health and Education Act of 1994. USFDA 1994.
4. Gonzalez-Sarrias A, Larrosa M, Garcia-Conesa MT, Tomas-Barberan FA, Espin JC Nutraceuticals for older people: facts, fictions, and gaps in knowledge. Maturitas 2013;75: 313–334.
4A. Yeung AWK, Mocan A, Atanasov AG Let food be thy medicine and medicine be thy food: a bibliometric analysis of the most cited papers focusing on nutraceuticals and functional foods. Food Chem 2018;269: 455–465.
5. Dietary Supplements and Herbal Medicine United States Pharmacopeia 2019. https://www.usp.org/products/dietary-supplements-compendium.
6. Espin JC, Garcia-Conesa MT, Tomas-Barberan FA Nutraceuticals: facts and fiction. Phytochem 2007;68: 2986–3008.

7. Yallapu MM, Jaggi M, Chauhan SC Curcumin nanomedicine: a road to cancer therapeutics. Curr Pharm Des 2013;19: 1994–2010.
8. Yallapu MM, Jaggi M, Chauhan SC Curcumin nanoformulations: a future nanomedicine for cancer. Drug Discov Today 212;17: 71–80.
9. Yallapu MM, Jaggi M, Chauhan SC Scope of nanotechnology in ovarian cancer therapeutics. J Ovarian Res 2010;3:19.
10. Herbal medicine market research report - global forecast till 2023. July 2019. Available at info@marketresearchfuture.com.
11. Federal Food, Drug, and Cosmetic Act US FDA. Nutrition Labeling and Education Act of 1990 1990.
12. FDA Guidance for industry: structure-function claims small entity compliance guide. 2002. Available at http://www.fda.gov/Food/GuidanceComplianceRegulatoryInformation/GuidanceDocuments/DietarySupplements/ucm103340.htm.
13. Health Canada A new approach to natural health products. 2012. Available at http://www.hc-sc.gc.ca/dhp-mps/prodnatur/nhp-new-nouvelle-psn-eng.php.
14. EAS Strategic Advice How to apply the nutrition and health claims regulation. 2010. Available at http://www.eas.eu.
15. Food Supplements Europe The application of the Nutrition and Health Claims Regulation 1924/2006. Guidance for food operators. 2013.
16. Directive 2004/24/EC of the European Parliament and of the Council of 31 March 2004 amending, as regards traditional herbal medicinal products, Directive 2001/83/ EC on the Community code relating to medicinal products for human use. 30/04/ 2004. Official Journal of the European Union: L136/85.
16A. USP 31 <2023> Microbiological attributes of non-sterile nutritional and dietary supplements USP29–NF24 Page 3087 Pharmacopeial Forum: Volume No. 30(5) Page 1818].
17. Directive 2004/24/EC of the European Parliament and of the Council of 31st March 2004 amending, as regards traditional herbal medicinal products, Directive 2001/83/ EC on the Community code relating to medicinal products for human use Official Journal L 136, 30/04/2004, p. 0085-0907.
17A. Therapeutic Goods Act-USA government 1989 https://www.legislation.gov.au/Series/C2004A03952
18. Tutelyan V, Sukhanov B Biologically active food supplements: modern approaches to quality and safety assurance. Vopr Pitaniya 2008;77(4): 4–15.
19. India. Food Safety and Standards Act 2006. 2006 http://www.commonlii.org/in/legis/num_act/fsasa2006234/.
20. India together: legislative brief. 2006 Available at: http://www.indiatogether.org/2006/feb/lawsfoodsafe/htmal/hilite.
21. FICCI study on implementation of Food Safety and Standard Act 2006: an industry perspective. 2011 Available at http://www.indiaenvironmentportal.org.in/Files/food_safety_study.pdf.
22. Food Standards and Safety Authority of India The food safety and standards regulations. 2011. Available at http://fssai.gov.in/GazettedNotifications.aspx.
23. SFDA Critical points for the technical evaluation of health food re-registration (SFDA permission division notification No 390, 2010; issued September 26, 2010). 2010. Available at http://www.sfda.gov.cn/WS01/CL0055/54296.html.
24. SFDA Critical points on technical evaluation of health foods (SFDA Permission Division Notification No 210, 2011; issued May 28, 2011). 2011.
25. Cosa P, Vlietinck AJ, Berghe DV, Maes L Anti-infective potential of natural products: How to develop a stronger in vitro 'proof-of-concept'. J Ethnopharmacol 2006;106: 290–302.
26. Lee J, Scagel CF Chicoric acid: chemistry, distribution, and production. Front Chem 2013;1: 40–41.
27. Teo CC, Tan SN, Yong J, Hew CS, Ong ES Pressurized hot water extraction (PHWE). J Chromatogr A 2010;1217: 2484–2494.
28. Asl AH, Khajenoori M Subcritical water extraction. In: Nakajima H (ed). Mass transfer—advances in sustainable energy and environment-oriented numerical modeling. InTech, Rijeka, 2013: 459–487.
29. Gbashi S, et al. The effect of temperature and methanol-water mixture on pressurized hot water extraction (PHWE) of anti-HIV analogs from Bidens Pilosa. Chem Cent J 2016;10: 37.
30. Ashmead SD, Pedersen M. US Patent 6,426,424 B1, Composition and method for preparing granular amino acid chelates and complexes, July 30, 2002.
31. DeWayne Ashmead H, Petersen RV, US patent 4,725,427, Effervescent vitamin-mineral granule preparation, February 16, 1988.
32. Zhang J, Wider B, Shang H, Li X, Ernst E Quality of herbal medicines: challenges and solutions. Complement Ther Med 2012;20: 100–106.

33. FDA Dietary Supplement Health and Education Act of 1994 (United States Public Law 103–417; 103rd Cong., 25 October 1994). Food and Drug Administration, Department of Health and Human Services, Washington, DC.

34. Dwyer J Dietary supplements: regulatory challenges and research resources. Nutrients 2018;10(1): 41.

35. Braeckman J The extract of Serenoa repens in the treatment of benign prostatic hyperplasia: a multi-center open study. Curr Ther Res 1994;55: 776–785.

36. Kumadoh D, et al. Development of oral capsules from Enterica herbal decoction-a traditional remedy for typhoid fever in Ghana. J App Pharma Sci 2015;(04): 083–088.

37. Tiwari RK Formulation development of fast dissolving tablet of clove - the best nutraceutical analgesic tablet. Asian Food Sci J 2018;1(3): 1–7.

38. Starch 1500® Partially Pregelatinized Maize Starch. From Colorcon website (https://www.color con. com/products-formulation/all-products/excipients/tablets/starch-1500).

39. Brahmbhatt T, et al. Development and evaluation of various herbal formulations for anti-asthmatic plant extract. IJPRBS 2012;1(3): 317–327.

40. Soares LAL, Ortega GG, Petrovick PR, Schmidt PC Optimization of tablets containing a high dose of spray-dried plant extract: a technical note. AAPS PharmSciTech 2005;6(3): E367–E371.

41. Broadhead J, Rouan SKE, Rhodes CT The spray-drying of pharmaceuticals. Drug Dev Ind Pharm 1992;18:1169Y1206.

42. Guajardo-Flores D, et al. Influence of excipients and spray drying on the physical and chemical properties of nutraceutical capsules containing phytochemicals from black bean extract. Molecules 2015;20: 21626–21635.

43. Cui F, Liu G, Yang M, Zhuang D, Pang X Studies on direct granulation of compound herbal extracts using fluidized-bed granulator. Proceedings of the SCEJ Symposium on Fluidization 2001. Available at http://sciencelinks.jp/j-east/article/200215/000020021502A0153136.php.

43A. Bennelli L, et al. Fluid bed drying and agglomeration of phytopharmaceutical compositions. Powder Technol 2015;273: 145–153.

44. Heng PWS, Chan LW, Liew CV, Chee SN, Soh JLP, Ooi SM Roller compaction of crude plant material: influence of process variables, polyvinylpyrrolidone, and co-milling. Pharm Dev Technol 2004;9: 135–144.

45. Madan J, Sharma AK, Singh R Fast dissolving tablets of aloe vera gel. Trop J Pharm Res 2009;8(1): 63–70.

46. Soares LAL, Ortega GG, Petrovick PR, Schmidt PC Dry granulation and compression of spray-dried plant extracts. AAPS PharmSciTech 2005;6(3): E359–E366.

47. Patra CN, Pandit HK, Singh SP, Devi MV Applicability and comparative evaluation of wet granulation and direct compression technology to rauwolfia serpentina root powder: a technical note. AAPS PharmSciTech 2008;9: 1.

48. de Souza TP, Martínez-Pacheco R, Gómez-Amoza JL, Petrovick PR Eudragit E as excipient for production of granules and tablets from Phyllanthus niruri L spray-dried extract. AAPS PharmSciTech 2007;8(2): 34.

49. Sung-I T. USPTO Application #: 20080233215, Excipient and an improved method for manufacturing extracted, evaporated, granulated botanical herb product. 2007.

50. Bubnis W, et al. World patent WO2007038596 A2, Phytosterol nutritional supplement, 2007.

51. Pathare PB, Bas N, Fitzpatrick JJ, Cronin K, Byrne EP Production of granola breakfast cereal by fluidized bed granulation. Food Bioprod Process 2012;90: 549– 545.

52. Bas N, Pathare PB, Catak M, Fitzpatrick JJ, Cronin K, Byrne EP Mathematical modeling of granola breakage during pipe pneumatic conveying. Powder Technol 2011;2061–2): 170–176.

53. Pathare PB, Byrne EP Application of wet granulation processes for granola breakfast cereal production. Food Eng Rev 2011;3: 189–.

54. Santhosh SB, et al. Development of chewable tablet from *Dugdhamalakyandi Yoga*: an Ayurveda preparation. Anc Sci Life 2012;32(1): 34–37.

55. Greenberg G Cannabis scientists are chasing a perfect High, New York Times Magazine, April 1, 2020.

56. Lafaye G, et al. Cannabis, cannabinoids, and health. Dialogues Clin Neurosci 2017;19(3): 309–316.

57. Mills B, Yepes A, Nugent K Synthetic cannabinoids. Am J Med Sci 2015;350(1): 59–62.

58. Sekura RD, Moore RM, Larabee TM, US Patent US20160058866A1, Alternative solutions for the administration of cannabis-derived botanical products.

59. de Vries JA, et al., US Patent US20150132400A1, Granulate containing cannabinoid, a method for its manufacture and oral dosage unit comprising such granulate.

60. Chang Q, Zuo Z, Chow MSS, Ho WKK Effect of storage temperature on phenolics stability in hawthorn (Crataegus pinnatifida var. major) fruits and a hawthorn drink. Food Chem 2006;98(3): 426–430.
61. Anonymous Herbal roulette. Consumer Rep 1995;60(11): 698–705.
62. Cui J, et al. What do commercial ginseng preparation contain? Lancet 1994;344: 134.
63. Kopleman SH, Augsburger LL. Selected physical and chemical properties of commercial Hy pericum perforatum extracts relevant for formulated product quality and performance. AAPS PharmSci 2001; 3(4): 26.
64. Ernst EJ Intern Med Adulteration of Chinese herbal medicines with synthetic drugs: A systematic review. J Intern Med 2002; 252: 107–113.
65. CFSAN FDA issues dietary supplements final rule. 2007.
66. FDA Final rules: current good manufacturing practice in manufacturing, packaging, labeling, or holding operations for dietary supplements. Federal Register. 2007.
67. U.S. Food and Drug Administration FDA issues dietary supplements final rule. Press release. 2007. Available at http://www.fda.gov/bbs/topics/NEWS/2007/NEW01657.html.
68. US FDA-Dietary Supplements Guidance Documents & Regulatory Information 2010. https://www.fda.gov/regulatory-information/search-fda-guidance-documents/small-entity-compliance-guide-current-good-manufacturing-practice-manufacturing-packaging-labeling, December 2010.
69. WHO Basic Tests for Drugs, Pharmaceutical Substances, Medicinal Plant Materials, and Dosage Forms. World Health Organization, Geneva, 1998.
70. WHO Bulletin of the World Health Organization. Regulatory Situation of Herbal Medicines. A Worldwide Review. World Health Organization, Geneva, 1998.
71. WHO Regulatory Situation of Herbal Medicines: A Worldwide Review. World Health Organization, Geneva, 1998.
72. WHO69 WHO fifty-sixth world health assembly, WHA56.31, 2003.

16 Granulation Approaches for Modified-Release Products

Neelima Phadnis and Sree Nadkarni

CONTENTS

16.1 INTRODUCTION

For this chapter, "Modified Release (MR)" is an umbrella term that will be used for describing granulations and/or drug products with a variety of drug release patterns after administration, ex., sustained-release, controlled-release, pulsatile-release, and delayed-release products. Examples of some drug release patterns are shown in Figure 16.1.

An easily recognizable commercial MR formulation is Ambien CR™, where the benefits of extending the sleep-inducing effects of the active drug are readily apparent. The underlying basis for changing the release pattern of a drug from its dosage form (post-administration) is to influence the drug's concentration in the biological system and therefore modulate its therapeutic effects in a beneficial manner. Some other benefits of modifying the drug release pattern through dosage form modification are:

- Improvement of patient compliance
- Reduction in the dosing frequency
- Reduction in fluctuations (peaks and troughs) of drug plasma concentrations, in order to reduce concentration-related side-effects or improve effectiveness

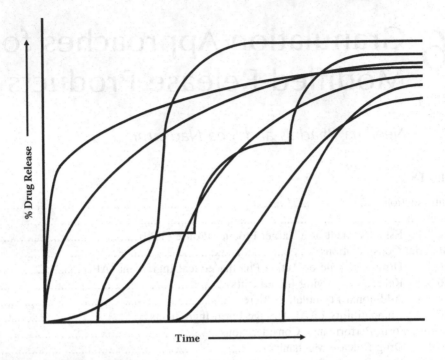

FIGURE 16.1   Drug release patterns as a function of time.

- Controlling the site of drug delivery in the gastrointestinal tract.

Traditionally, MR dosage forms were introduced to the market after the successful commercial launch of a conventional dosage form that demonstrated a safe and efficacious profile within the established therapeutic window (Chapter 22). This Product LifeCycle Management strategy was no doubt a combination of an organization's need to capitalize on the intellectual property window of commercial opportunity and deference to the complex technical nature of developing MR products.

More recently, MR is increasingly being considered earlier in the drug development cycle:

- As a potential avenue to progress a shrinking pool of viable molecules, rather than going back to the molecular drawing board.
- To accommodate market drivers that promote a user-friendly dosing regimen.

16.2 SCOPE

Dosage forms can be classified in several ways:

- Site of administration – oral, intranasal, transdermal, colonic, etc.
- Dosage form appearance – tablets, capsules, patch, an osmotic pump, etc.
- By technology platform – hot-melt extrusion, 3D printing, electrostatic deposition films, rapid release, etc.

Technically, rapid release granulations/dosage forms require modulation of drug release profiles to achieve rapid onset of release for quick onset of therapeutic action and may also get categorized as modified-release preparations. But given the scope of the topic, rapid release formulations are addressed under various related themes in Chapters 14, 18, and 19.

Modifying the release pattern of a drug involves leveraging elements that are already used in conventional dosage form development. Accordingly, material and process related aspects (including scale-up and regulations) for designing and manufacturing granulated MR dosage forms have significant overlap with topics covered in other chapters of this book. The subject matter in this chapter will, therefore, complement information covered elsewhere, offer items for consideration in designing a robust granulated MR product, and highlight applications with select case studies.

The reader is referred to additional literature [1,2] for coverage of non-granulated MR drug delivery systems.

To prepare a sound MR dosage form development strategy, it is important to first establish a comprehensive, well-defined target product profile (TPP). The TPP will thus form the basis for material considerations and dosage form performance considerations. These topics are elaborated below.

16.2.1 ESTABLISHMENT OF A TARGET PRODUCT PROFILE (TPP)

A successful granulated MR (GMR) dosage form development begins with a well-defined TPP. This TPP should include the objective of the exercise and may include one or more of the previously outlined benefits of MR dosing. A well-defined TPP will provide a clear perspective on the clinical and market requirements for a successful drug. It should include aspects such as:

- Therapeutically effective dose range
- Dosing frequency, i.e., twice a day versus once a day
- Target release profile, i.e., constant, zero-order release, or pulsatile release, including minimum and maximum therapeutically effective and safe plasma levels
- Dosage form considerations, i.e., tablet or a capsule, tablet size, shape, etc.

Establishment of a desirable TPP outline could start as early as the physico-chemical profiling of the drug substance as material supply and informational database evolves [3]. Generating this drug molecule specific TPP helps in managing expectations – on whether a granulated MR dosage form is realistic [4] – and in the framing of a GMR dosage form development strategy.

Limited drug supply, time, and investment in an interesting molecule may make generation of an MR TPP unrealistic, especially at an exploratory stage of the drug discovery development program. If this situation was to arise and an organization wish to keep its MR options open, a nanoparticles approach may be adopted. Nanoparticles are one unique platform that can bridge the gap between discovery supportive efforts and future MR dosage form development programs [5].

16.3 MATERIAL CONSIDERATIONS

16.3.1 DRUG MOLECULE OR ACTIVE PHARMACEUTICAL INGREDIENT (API)

Not all drug molecules are amenable to being formulated into a granulated MR dosage form, and an MR feasibility assessment is needed at the outset of the program. Once a TPP is established, MR feasibility can be carried out at any stage of development of a compound for which an MR dosage form is being considered. A fairly comprehensive assessment exercise for a drug molecule destined for MR dosage form development is outlined by Thombre [4] and is presented as a flowchart representation in Figure 16.2.

Taking the drug physicochemical, biopharmaceutical, and pharmacokinetic-metabolic properties into account and available technology, the end product of the assessment is a recommendation for an MR dosage form development strategy (Figure 16.2).

In the above assessment, two molecular characteristics are important

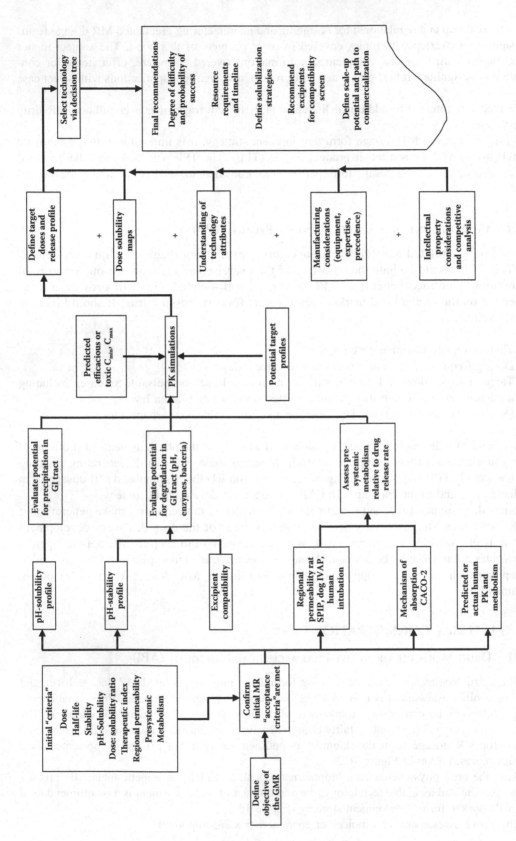

FIGURE 16.2 Modified release feasibility assessment flow chart. Reprinted from ref. 4 with permission from Elsevier. Abbreviations: MR: modified release; GI: gastrointestinal; IVAP: intestinal vascular access port; PK: pharmacokinetics; SPIP: single-pass intestinal perfusion.

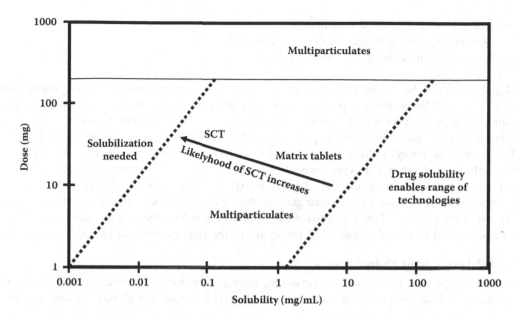

FIGURE 16.3 Example of a dose-solubility map to guide controlled release technology selection. Reprinted from Ref. 4 with permission from Elsevier. Abbreviation: SCT: swellable core technology.

- The API's Biopharmaceutical Classification System (BCS) categorization: it is useful in defining the bioavailability and route of administration. As illustrated in Chapter 22, a drug has to first exist as a dissolved moiety in the fluids at the site of absorption and pass through a biological barrier in order to reach the site of action. These two steps are governed by two defined characteristics of a molecule – its solubility and permeability. The BCS framework for the categorization of drugs was developed [6] a few years ago in recognition of the importance of these characteristics.
- The dose-solubility ratio: it is useful in MR technology selection

A number of GMR processes are available for supporting the above-identified dosage forms. GMR examples are highlighted in the section covering case studies.

In addition to the intrinsic API characteristics discussed above, a judicious selection of the API solid-state could also become an important exercise in MR dosage form development. An interesting strategy is presented by Chzranowski [7–9], whereby a salt form that is poorly soluble or practically insoluble in water in the pH range of 1.3 to 6.8 or 7.4 is chosen for incorporation into an MR dosage form.

16.3.2 Release-Modifying Ingredient(s)

The second most important ingredient in a GMR formulation is the ingredient or a combination of ingredients that enables modification of the drug release pattern. The two main classes of release modifiers are polymers and long-chain hydrocarbons.

16.3.2.1 Polymers

Not surprisingly, many of the polymers used for modulating drug release are high viscosity grades of polymers that are used as binders, at low aqueous concentrations, and are described in Chapter 4. When selecting a polymer for its functional utility, the following characteristics are closely examined [10]:

- Reproducibility of physical properties
- Non-interference with the drug's therapeutic action
- Chemical compatibility with the drug

MR polymers can be further classified according to their origin (synthetic, semisynthetic, and natural), pH-solubility profile (pH-independent or pH-dependent), or by their hydrophilic or lipophilic nature. Examples of polymers commonly used in MR formulations are:

Hydroxypropyl methylcellulose (hypromellose, HPMC), hydroxypropyl cellulose, hydroxyethyl cellulose, hydroxypropyl methylcellulose phthalate (HPMCP), Poly(2-hydroxy ethyl methacrylate), Poly(methyl methacrylate, Poly(vinyl alcohol), Poly(acrylic acid), Polyacrylamide, Poly(ethylene-co-vinyl acetate), Poly(methacrylic acid), Polylactides (PLA), Polyglycolides (PGA), Poly(lactide-co-glycolides) (PLGA), chitosan, chitin, guar gum, xanthan gum, alginic acid, alginates, and carrageenan.

Incorporation of the polymer or a mixture of polymers into the dosage form is determined by the physicochemical and biopharmaceutical properties of the drug as well as process requirements.

16.3.2.2 Long-Chain Hydrocarbons

Many waxes and fats provide modification of drug release due to their inherent hydrophobic/lipophilic characteristics. Examples included carnauba wax, glyceryl behenate, and glyceryl palmitostearate.

16.3.3 Additional Formulation Ingredients

Other materials for inclusion in the GMR are more specific to the selected granulation platform and are covered in the chapters dealing with specific processes ex. wet granulation and roller compaction.

16.3.4 Compatibility of All Dosage Form Ingredients

Adequate care must be taken to demonstrate a lack of negative interactions between dosage form components as outlined in Chapter 3. This feature of dosage form development is not unique to MR dosage forms and must be executed before launching into a viable GMR dosage form development program [11].

16.4 DOSAGE FORM PERFORMANCE CONSIDERATIONS

By definition, MR dosage forms are differentiated from conventional dosage forms by their distinctive drug release pattern. Knowledge of the following listed dosage form characteristics is useful in the design and production of MR dosage units with reproducible drug release patterns.

16.4.1 Drug Release Mechanism

Manner of drug release from granules (Figure 16.4) is typically either by diffusion, swelling, erosion, and dissolution, or a combination of the various mechanisms. Mechanistic understanding allows the scientists' insights into designing a formulation that can best accommodate the TPP.

This release mechanism is also dictated by the polymer characteristic and the stimulus it experiences in the release medium. Examples of the impact of formulation ingredients or environmental conditions on release modulating properties of hydrogels are provided in Table 16.1.

16.4.2 Drug Release Pattern and Predictability

Movement of drug molecules within and out of a dosage form is a mass transport phenomenon. Starting with the simplest diffusive flux equation also known as Fick's first law [12] that relates the amount of material flowing through a unit cross-section:

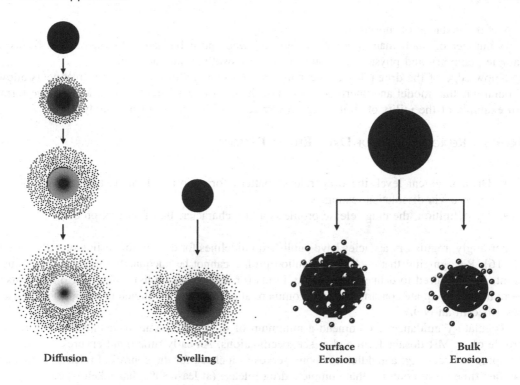

FIGURE 16.4 Schematic view of drug release mechanisms from granules.

$$J = -D(dC/dx)$$

Where
  J is the diffusional flux
  D is the diffusion coefficient or diffusivity
  C is the concentration, and

TABLE 16.1
Formulation Ingredients or Environmental Conditions that Modulate the Release of Drug from Hydrogels

Stimulus	Hydrogel Forming Polymer	Mechanism Causing Changes in Swelling, that in Turn Lead to the Release of Drug
pH	Acidic or basic	Change in pH
Ionic strength	Ionic	Change in ionic strength-change in concentration of ions
Chemical species	Electron accepting groups	Electron donating compounds-formation of a charge-transfer complex
Thermal	Thermoresponsive ex. Poly(N-isopropyl acrylamide)	Change in temperature-change in polymer-polymer and water polymer-interactions
Electrical	Polyelectrolyte	Applied electric field-membrane charging-electrophoresis of charged drug
Ultrasound irradiation	Ethylene-vinyl alcohol	Ultrasound irradiation-temperature increase

x is the distance of movement

A number of mathematical equations are reviewed and published in literature [13,14], taking sample geometry and physical phenomena, such as swelling, into account.

Knowledge of the drug release mechanism and availability of mathematical treatments allows simulations that model and interpret kinetics of the drug release process from MR dosage forms. An example of the utility of simulating drug release is illustrated in Case Study 5.

16.4.3 REPRODUCIBILITY OF DRUG RELEASE PATTERN

* On a practical level, the drug release pattern for a dosage form is typically established *in vitro* via dissolution testing.
* By definition, the drug release profile is a key characteristic of an MR product.

Accordingly, regulatory agencies have published guidelines for dissolution testing of MR products [15,16]. Recognizing that an MR dissolution profile cannot be adequately described by a single point, it is required to define acceptability limits (or set specifications) at multiple time points to demonstrate adequate conformance of a commercial product to that studied in a clinical setting and described in an NDA.

Regulatory guidances recommend a minimum of three time points to define the drug release profile of an MR dosage form and to set specifications. An early time point ensures that no dose dumping is occurring, a middle time point serves as a check for the control of release profile, and the last time point confirms that complete drug release (at least 80%) has taken place.

In order to establish specifications per regulatory agency guidelines, particular attention needs to be given to the dissolution method developed. An example of how various dissolution parameters may affect drug release is briefly covered in Case Study 5.

Two additional items relating to dissolution testing of MR products are:

1. *In vitro–in vivo correlation (IVIVC)*
   When a predictive mathematical model is able to describe a relationship between an *in vitro* property of a dosage form, ex., drug dissolution profile, and an *in vivo* response, ex., drug's extent of absorption, then an *in vitro–in vivo* relationship (IVIVR) is said to exist. IVIVR forms the basis for the determination of an IVIVC. The main objective of developing and evaluating an IVIVC is to establish the dissolution test as a surrogate for human bioequivalence studies, which in turn may reduce the number of bioavailability/bioequivalence studies performed during the initial development and approval process as well as with certain scale-up and post-approval changes. Additional details pertaining to bioequivalence are covered in Chapter 22. An example of an IVIVC for a commercial product is depicted in Figure 16.8 as part of the discussion in Case Study 3.
2. *Dose Dumping – Food Effects*
   As part of the effort to ensure and establish the unique drug release pattern of an MR product, the relationship between food and alcohol effects on the drug dissolution pattern must also be demonstrated. This topic is of particular concern for drugs with a narrow therapeutic window because the complete dose may be more rapidly released from the dosage form than intended, creating a potential safety risk for the study subjects or the ultimate consumer of the MR product.

Utility of *in vitro* dissolution testing for exploring this issue was recently highlighted [17,18].

16.5 TYPES OF MR GRANULATIONS AND CASE STUDIES

Granulated MR dosage forms may be classified as follows:

1. Matrix type
Depending on the physicochemical properties of the drug and the MR polymer(s), various granulation techniques can be employed. They include :
- Conventional (high shear or fluid bed) wet granulated tablets with hydrophilic or hydrophobic polymer (barrier coated or uncoated)
- Specialized granulation techniques, such as rotor granulation, extrusion–spheronization, melt granulation (using a high shear mixer), hot-melt extrusion, etc.
- Dry granulated (roller-compacted) tablets

2. Multiparticulates
- Granules in capsules
  o Non-spherical
  o Spherical

- Barrier-coated (spherical) granules

Chapters 9, 10, 11, and 12 cover specific process-related details for the production of granules classified above. Accordingly, processing effects on drug release patterns and decision making specific to GMR are highlighted in the form of case studies below.

16.5.1 CASE STUDY 1

In many cases, the move to MR is part of Product Lifecycle Management, and a conventional tablet dosage form is available as a starting point for formulation. From a manufacturing perspective, this strategy is advantageous because of the familiarity in handling the materials and known dosage form characteristics.

In this example [19] of how an "immediate release" (IR) wet granulated caplet formulation can be transformed to a controlled- or modified-release wet granulated formulation, Dow scientists took a model system containing Naproxen sodium as the model drug and successfully demonstrated the IR to MR transformation using Methocel K4MP as the drug release-retarding polymer (Table 16.2).

The change in the drug release pattern (Figures 16.5a and 16.5b; IR and MR) is evident for tablets compressed with granulation batches made at the laboratory scale (10 L), pilot scale (150 L), and with commercial-scale equipment (600 L).

TABLE 16.2
Composition of Foamed Binder Formulations

	Ingredient	Immediate Release Model Formulation		Modified Release Formulation	
		mg	(approx %)	mg	(approx %)
1	Naproxen sodium, USP	220	44.0	100	20.0
2	Methocel K4MP, USP	0	0.0	150	30.0
3	Methocel E5PLV, USP (7% solution)	8.72	2.0	8.81	1.0
4	Microcrystalline cellulose, NF	100	20	75	15
5	Fast Flo lactose-316, NF	152.5	30.5	167.5	33.5
6	Croscarmellose sodium	15	3.0	0	0.0
7	Magnesium stearate, NF	2.5	0.5	2.5	0.5

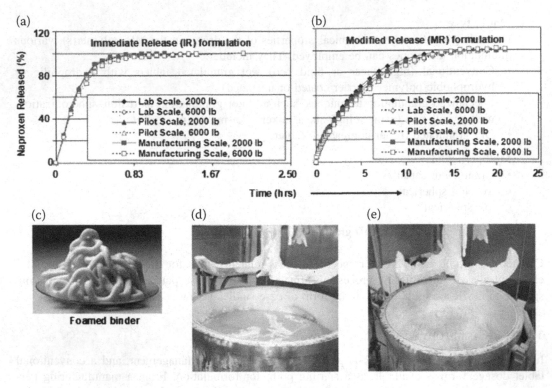

FIGURE 16.5 Foamed binder granulation. (a) dissolution of naproxen from IR tablets, (b) dissolution of naproxen from MR tablets, (c) foamed binder, (d) 600 L Gral containing 38.3 L of foamed binder on top of 135 kg of MR formulation powders (before wet massing step), (e) 600 L Gral after wet massing step during the batch process. Reprinted from Ref. 19 with permission from Dow.

Another interesting key process improvement covered in this publication is the use of a foamed binder solution that had a consistency of shaving cream (Figure 16.5c). Foamed binder solution use eliminates the need for piping, nozzles, and studies for demonstrating the effect of binder addition on granulation characteristics. This is a relatively new technology introduced by Dow in the last few years [20,21] and enables direct addition of the foam to the dry ingredients into the granulator, as shown in Figure 16.5d.

In conclusion, foam binder technology enables a relatively easy transformation of an IR to MR formulation and reduces the complexity of the scale-up process.

Over the last decade, foam binder granulation usage has gone up. However, caution is needed in readily adopting this process option for a high drug load (>80%) granulation that is subsequently compressed into tablets. Cantor et al [22] have showcased such an effort, by evaluating granules containing acetaminophen (APAP), metformin, and aspirin. These three model drugs were selected because of their intrinsic brittle, viscoelastic, and ductile properties, respectively. Various granules and compact properties were reported in the article. Foam granulation appeared to enhance the plasticity of granulated brittle material APAP and showed a mixed deformation effect on granulated ductile material, Aspirin. Surprisingly, foam granulation did not enhance the plasticity for granulated viscoelastic Metformin. This phenomenon was attributed to binder surface coverage. While modification of drug release is not claimed in this publication, a need for understanding the intrinsic mechanical property of a drug is highlighted.

Foam binder granulations are also generated using another process – twin-screw extrusion [23–25].

Twin-screw extrusion is becoming increasingly attractive because of its adaptability for continuous granulation manufacture and is the topic for Case Study 2.

16.5.2   CASE STUDY 2

Tan et al [26] studied the manufacture of modified-release verapamil tablets at 60% drug loading using a direct-molding melt granulation process with the twin-screw extruder. The influence of four factors – hydrophilic polymer type (Hypromellose HPMC K4M, Polyethylene oxide Polyox 1 M), hydrophobic polymer type (Glyceryl behenate Compritol®ATO 888, Glyceryl palmitostea-rate Precirol®ATO 5), a ratio of hydrophobic: hydrophilic polymer (30:10, 35:5), and process (direct molding, milling, and tableting of extrudates) – was investigated.

A sharp endothermic peak is detected in differential scanning calorimetry (DSC) profiles across all formulations post granulation, corresponding to the melting point of crystalline verapamil. Furthermore, powder X-ray diffraction patterns for all formulations corresponded to crystalline verapamil diffraction pattern, confirming that all formulations remain thermally stable post granulation.

Dissolution profiles of the formulations were measured following the USP method for ver-apamil hydrochloride extended-release tablets, using USP Apparatus II with a stirring speed of 50 rpm at $37 \pm 0.5°C$. Samples were collected automatically at 2, 3.5, 5, 8, 12, and 18 hours.

Statistical analysis of the dissolution profile at 12 hours showed that the type of hydrophilic binder (p = 0.005) and process (p = 0.005) were the significant main factors in determining the release profile (Figure 16.6).

HPMC K4M-based formulations demonstrated a faster release rate as compared to PEO 1 M-based formulations. In general, tablets compressed from milled extrudate exhibited faster release than directly molded tablets. The process had a statistically significant two-way interaction with the type of hydrophilic binder (p = 0.028) (Figure 16.7). The combination of hydrophilic binder type and the ratio of hydrophobic: hydrophilic binder in the formulation also had statistically significant two-way interactions (p = 0.033).

The results of this study demonstrated that direct-molded verapamil extended-release tablets can be manufactured by the hot-melt process using a twin-screw extruder. The dissolution release

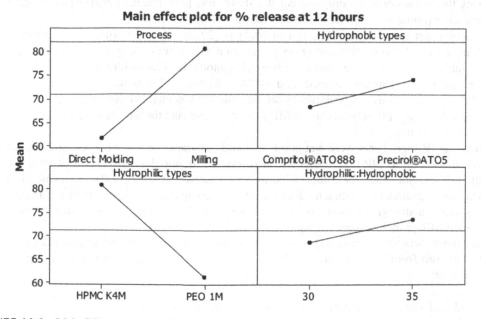

FIGURE 16.6   Main Effects plot for all formulations. Reproduced in part with permission from Ref. 26.

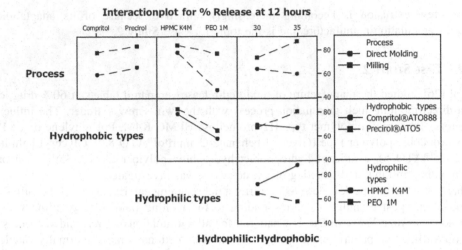

FIGURE 16.7 Interaction plot for all formulations. Reproduced in part with permission from Ref. 26.

profile of verapamil can be modulated by the type of hydrophilic polymer and to a lesser degree by the ratio of hydrophilic to hydrophobic polymers.

16.5.3 CASE STUDY 3

For some compounds with a short half-life, it is useful to maintain the clinical efficacy of the drug by prolonging the effective plasma level with additional drug release, once the target plasma concentration is achieved with a standard immediate-release formulation. Typically, this type of desired drug release pattern is achieved by a dosage form that is composed of two parts – an immediate release part and a modified-release part. A specific example is Zolpidem® extended-release or MR, which is a two-layer, biphasic tablet: One layer releasing approximately 60% of the dose immediately, and the second layer releasing the remainder of the drug content at a slower rate [27]. The drug release pattern and plasma concentration profile for Zolpidem® MR are shown in Figure 16.8 [28].

In a two-part publication, Ohmori and Makino [29,30] illustrate some of the challenges in developing an MR formulation, using dry granulation as one option to generate an MR matrix in a bilayer tablet. The model drug used was Phenylpropanolamine Hydrochloride (PPA). A target drug release profile was initially defined, and HPMC (Metolose 2280) was chosen as the release-modulating agent. Based on preliminary studies, the PPA content in the immediate release layer was pegged at 5 mg, PPA content in the MR layer at 20 mg, and the weight of each caplet layer was finalized at 200 mg.

Since the IR ingredients were wet granulated and the granule median particle size was 214 µm, wet granulation of the MR ingredients was also considered, initially. However, wet granulated MR granulation was not suited for compression using the bilayer tablet press. To overcome this hurdle and yet have a granulation with a median particle size comparable to that of the IR granules, roller compaction - a dry granulation process was adopted. The median particle size of the roller-compacted MR granulation was 225 µm.

Keeping in perspective the number of compression events, the drug release-modulating polymer would undergo from blending of ingredients to finished bilayer tablet, the following parameters were studied:

- order of filling granulation into the bilayer tablet press (Figure 16.9)
- roller compaction pressure of the MR granules

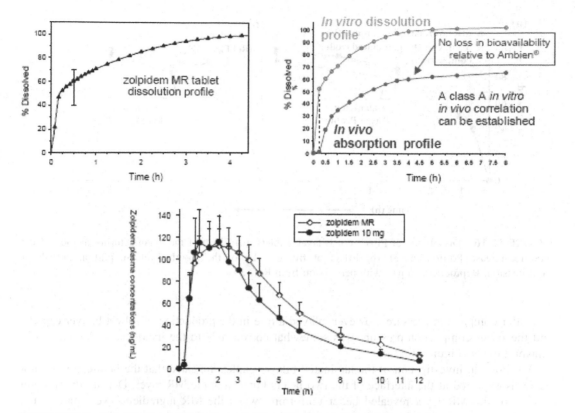

FIGURE 16.8 Zolpidem® modified-release (MR) tablets. Reproduced from Ref. 23.

order of filling granulation into the bilayer tablet press was not found to impact the drug release profile (Figure 16.10). This effect was attributed to the ability of HPMC to hydrate rapidly before the shape factor could additionally influence drug dissolution.

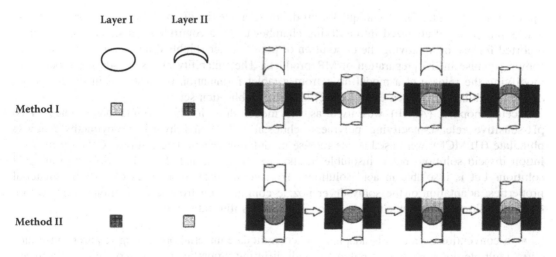

FIGURE 16.9 Schematic representation of bilayer compression. (▦) immediate release portion and (▨) modified-release portion. Reproduced in part with permission from Ref. 29.

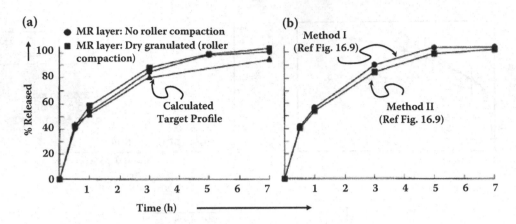

FIGURE 16.10 Dissolution of PPA from Bilayer Tablets. (a) Effect of the manufacturing method of the modified-release Portion (n = 6). (b) Effect of filling order of the modified-release portion in Bilayer Compression. Reproduced in part with permission from Ref. 29.

Roller compaction pressure, however, played a role in the production of robust bilayer caplets, and the roller compaction pressure was somewhat correlatable to the incidence of lamination in bilayer caplets (Figure 16.11a).

A follow-up investigation of the laminated bilayer caplets revealed that the lamination did not occur as expected at the interface of the two layers but within the MR layer. Density distribution studies of the MR layer revealed better uniformity when the MR ingredients were part of the second convexo-concave layer, as compared to the convexo-convex first layer. Images from one technique (CT scan) used to study the density distribution in tablets are shown in Figure 16.11b.

In conclusion, robust bilayer caplets with a target PPA release profile were produced when the wet granulated IR layer was compressed into the tablet press first, followed by a blend (0 kN roller compaction pressure) of the MR ingredients. While dry granulation was a good alternative to wet granulation, in this instance, granulation of the MR component did not result in a robust end product.

16.4.4 CASE STUDY 4

Spray drying (Chapter 5), a technique for producing granules by drying of a solution or suspension that is pumped and atomized into a drying chamber under a controlled gas stream, was initially reported for use in improving the dissolution of poorly water-soluble drugs. More recently, it has shown promise in the preparation of MR products. The suitability of a spray-drying process for modifying the release of a model drug from a tablet formulation is illustrated in the following example published by Chen et al. [31,32] as a two-publication set.

Acetaminophen (APAP) was used as the model drug in the formulations studied. Two pH-sensitive release-modifying polymers, chitosan (CHT) and hydroxypropylmethylcellulose phthalate (HPMCP), were used as the release modulating agents. Interestingly, CHT forms a solution in acid solutions but is insoluble in alkaline solutions, and HPMCP dissolves in alkaline solutions but is insoluble in acid solutions. To accommodate these types of differing material properties, adaptation of the spray dryer nozzle configuration from a conventional version to a 4-fluid version was attempted. This set of publications illustrated how

- a conventional process is adapted, to accommodate material processing requirements, and
- multiple combinations of polymers with differing properties may be combined in a meaningful manner for manufacturing an MR product having a drug release profile of choice

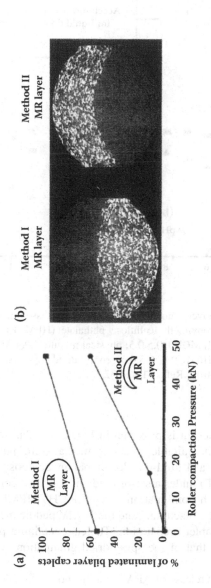

FIGURE 16.11 Bilayer caplets. (a) relationship between manufacturing method and percentage of laminated caplets. (b) CT of caplet cross-section in which the calcium from dibasic calcium phosphate present in the MR layer is seen as white spots. Reproduced in part with permission from ref. 30.

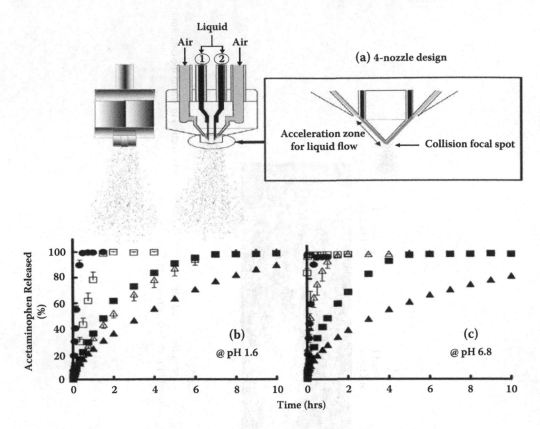

FIGURE 16.12 (a) Schematic of novel 4-nozzle design (b) & (c) dissolution profiles of Acetaminophen (APAP)–Chitosan (CHT)–hydroxypropylmethylcellulose phthalate (HPMCP) systems. symbol key: (●) APAP spray dried (■) APAP:CHT:HPMCP 1:0.5:0.5; physical mixture (▲) APAP:CHT:HPMCP 1:2.5:2.5; physical mixture (□) APAP:CHT:HPMCP 1:0.5:0.5; spray dried (△) APAP:CHT:HPMCP 1:2.5:2.5. Reproduced in part with permission from Refs. 31 and 32.

A diagram of the newer nozzle design is provided in Figure 16.12a. Solutions containing APAP and each polymer solubilized in suitable aqueous media were pumped separately through the two liquid-feed channels of a 4-fluid-nozzle, to obtain composite particles containing all 3 materials (APAP:CHT: HPMCP) under a set of predefined drying conditions. Tablets of spray-dried composite particles for each combination of APAP:CHT:HPMCP were obtained using a Carver press type "universal testing machine," and the JPXIV paddle method was used to generate APAP release profiles for each tablet preparation. Tablets containing physical mixtures of the 3 ingredients in the same ratios as that of the spray-dried granulations were also compressed and subjected to dissolution tests.

Figures 16.12b and 12c show the release of APAP as a function of time for tablets manufactured with various spray-dried granulations and physical mixtures of APAP, CHT, and HPMCP, in acid and alkaline media, respectively. From these dissolution profiles, it can be concluded that APAP release is influenced by the presence of pH-sensitive polymers. While a physical mixture of the drug and polymers demonstrate some slowing down of the drug release rate, especially in the acidic dissolution medium, a marked and somewhat pH-insensitive product is obtained in the case of spray-dried granules. Based on tablet dissolution profiles in the two media, superiority of the spray-drying technique as an MR granulation process versus a simple physical mixture for tablet production, is readily apparent.

To get a better understanding of how the process affected the processed material at a molecular level, physical characterization of the spray-dried granules and physical mixtures of the three ingredients by DSC, FTIR, and XRD were also undertaken. Studies revealed that APAP existed as a solid dispersion only in spray-dried granules and the carbonyl group in APAP hydrogen bonds with the amino group in CHT.

In conclusion, spray drying is a viable technique for the production of GMR dosage forms. Spray drying as a processing method for the production of MR granulations has also been studied for modification of drug delivery to the lung and in dosage forms for antibodies [33,34].

16.4.5   CASE STUDY 5

In a series of five related papers, Fukui et al. [35–39] provide an interesting example of comparing and contrasting the performance of granules obtained from three multiparticulate spherical GMR process methods for their drug release pattern. Phenylpropanolamine hydrochloride (PPA) at a 500 mg dose was used as the model drug, and ethylcellulose (EC) was chosen as the drug release-retarding agent. Capsules of drug-containing matrix granules prepared by the extrusion–spheronization process (Chapter 12) were compared with those prepared by a layering process in a rotor granulator (Chapter 11) or a fluid bed rotor granulator (chapter 10).

Starting with a simpler system, an understanding of the drug release process was first attempted, which then provided the ability to evaluate three different granulation techniques and identification of one MR granulation process that was most expedient from a commercial manufacturing perspective.

In the first part of the study, two grades of EC (#10 and #100) were used to generate granules by the extrusion–spheronization process. Because release of drug into the dissolution medium is influenced by shape, this granulation process ensured the production of a matrix granule possessing the simplest geometry – a sphere. A spherical geometry then enabled modeling of the drug release process. In this instance, two equations were deemed necessary for describing the entire drug release curve, as a function of time. They are:

1. Higuchi's square-root equation: for the initial part of the curve
   $m_t = k_H(t)^{1/2}$, where
   m_t is the amount of PPA released
   k_H is the apparent release rate constant, and
   t is the release time
2. The cube-root equation: for the later part of the curve
   $(1-m_t)^{1/3} = K_{App}(t)$, where
   m_t is the amount of PPA released
   K_{App} is the apparent release rate constant, and
   t is the release time

Granules containing EC#10 gave a better agreement between the theoretical and experimental data, and thus EC#10 was chosen as the drug release-modulating agent for further studies.

In the second part of the study, effect of EC#10 content and ethanol (EtOH; component of binder solution) content on drug release was studied in recognition of the fact that the composition of the binder solution influences granule properties. Upon physical examination of the granules, increasing EtOH and/or EC content in the binder solution facilitated formation of a smoother matrix structure. EtOH concentrations at and above 85% in the binder solution resulted in granules that exhibited a fairly constant value for the transition point at which PPA release changed from the square-root profile to the cube-root profile.

The dissolution method was challenged next in the third part of the series of experiments. Four parameters were evaluated for their potential influence on *in vitro* drug release. They were:

- volume of the buffer solution
- pH of the buffer solution
- paddle rotation speed, and
- dosage strength

The data suggested that the analytical method was appropriate for the intended purpose, and except for pH of the buffer solution, the other parameters had a lesser impact on the drug release profile.

The above-described studies now set the stage for comparison of PPA release from three granulations which differed mainly in the granulation process. The three granulation processes and corresponding drug release patterns of the resulting granules, reported in the fourth and fifth parts of the experimental series, are summarized in Figure 16.13.

While there were slight differences in the dissolution curves (Figure 16.14a) for capsules containing granules from the standard wet granulation process (designated Capsule A; matrix granules) and the rotor granulator (designated Capsule B; EC layered coating granules), their *in vivo* plasma concentration curves (Figure 16.14b) were comparable. Capsule A granules showed higher variability in the correlation curve of *in vitro* PPA release to *in vivo* PPA plasma concentration; therefore, authors concluded that Capsule B granulation was the more robust formulation.

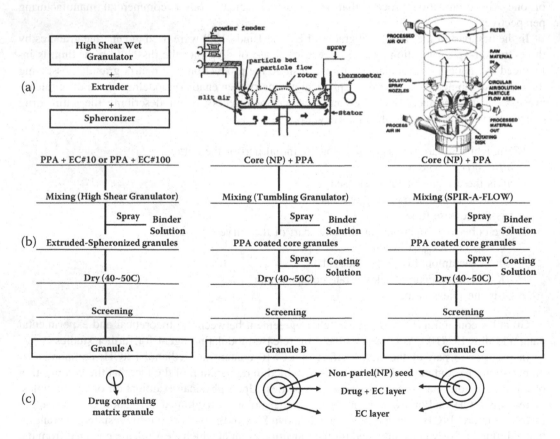

FIGURE 16.13 Summary of the three MR granulation methods used to prepare PPA granules. Schematic representation of (a) equipment, (b) process, and (c) granule: drawings not to scale. Reproduced in part with permission from refs. 38–41.

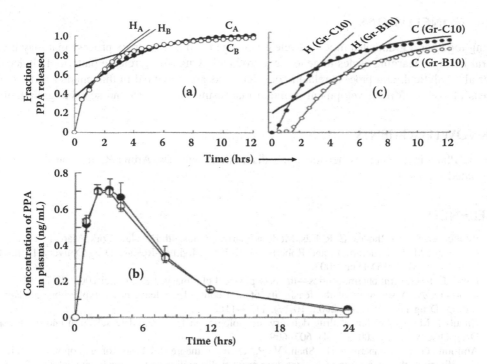

FIGURE 16.14 (a) Release and simulation curves (●) capsule A (○) capsule B. H_A Simulation using the square-root time law equation for capsule A. H_B Simulation using the square-root time law equation for capsule B. C_A Simulation using the cube-root time law equation for capsule A. C_B simulation using the square-root time law equation for capsule B.
(b) Concentration of PPA in the blood of beagle dogs: (●) capsule A and (○) capsule B.
(c) Release and simulation curves: (○) capsule B* and (●) capsule C. $H_{(Gr-C10)}$ simulation using the square-root time law equation for capsule C. $H_{(Gr-B10)}$ Simulation using the square-root time law equation for capsule B*. $C_{(Gr-C10)}$ Simulation using the cube-root time law equation for capsule C. $C_{(Gr-B10)}$ Simulation using the square-root time law equation for capsule B*. Note: capsule B and B* granulations only differ in the thickness of the EC coat. Reproduced in part with permission from Refs. 38 and 39.

Since EC layer coated granules performed better *in vivo* as compared to matrix granules, the fifth part of the experimental series examined the effects of two EC layer coating processes, i.e., rotor granulation and fluid bed rotor granulation (Spir-A-Flow) on the release of PPA. The PPA release profiles of EC layered granules varying in EC content between 6% and 10% for both processes were examined.

In contrast to the matrix granules, EC layered granules obtained by both processes exhibited a lag time in PPA release (Figure 16.14c). The lag time increased with EC content; therefore, this lag time was hypothesized to be an indicator of surface coverage by EC.

Matching simulation curves generated with previously developed mathematical model(s) to the PPA release profile curves of the newly prepared granules showed excellent agreement. This match enabled plotting the relationship between the apparent release rate constants (K_H and K_{app}) as a function of EC coating percentage. At the highest EC coating level (10%), K_H and K_{app} values for granules produced by either rotor granulation or fluid bed rotor granulation were similar. Since the fluid bed rotor granulation process did not result in a granulation with superior properties to those produced by simple rotor granulation, a change in process was not deemed necessary.

In conclusion, the rotor granulation process was identified as the most convenient GMR process for manufacturing an MR dosage form for the selected model drug.

16.5 CONCLUSIONS

Piecing together a granulated modified-release dosage form is a complex process that may involve several iterative learning cycles to generate a product having a drug release pattern of choice. Key material, analytical, and process-related considerations are presented in this chapter as tools for a successful dosage form development program that results in a robust and scalable granulation.

ACKNOWLEDGMENTS

Neelima Phadnis appreciates her unending discussions with Dr. Aruna Railkar on drug delivery and related topics.

REFERENCES

1. Banker, G. S. and Rhodes, C. R. Eds. Modern Pharmaceutics. 4th Ed. New York: Marcel Dekker, 2002.
2. Rathbone, M. J., Hadgraft, J., and Roberts, M. S. Eds. Modified-Release Drug Delivery Technology. New York: Marcel Dekker, 2003.
3. Fiese, E. F. General pharmaceutics—the new physical pharmacy. J Pharm Sci 2003, 92(7), 1331–1342.
4. Thombre, A. Assessment of the feasibility of oral controlled release in an exploratory development setting. Drug Discov Today 2005, 10(17), 1159–1166.
5. Chaubal, M. Application of drug delivery technologies in lead candidate selection and optimization. Drug Discov Today 2004, 9(14), 603–609.
6. Amidon, G. L., Lennernas, H., Shah, V. P., et al. A theoretical basis for a biopharmaceutic drug classification: the correlation of in vitro drug product dissolution and in vivo bioavailability. Pharm Res 1995, 12, 413–420.
7. Chzranowski, F. Preformulation considerations for controlled release dosage forms. Part I. Selecting candidates. AAPS PharmSciTech 2008, 9(2), 635–638.
8. Chzranowski, F. Preformulation considerations for controlled release dosage forms. Part II. Selected candidate support. AAPS PharmSciTech 2008, 9(2), 639–645.
9. Chzranowski, F. Preformulation considerations for controlled release dosage forms. Part III. Candidate form selection using numerical weighting and scoring. AAPS PharmSciTech 2008, 9(2), 646–650.
10. Rios, M. Polymers for controlled release formulation follows function. Pharm Tech 2005, 29(6).
11. Serajuddin, A. T. M., Thakur, A. B., Ghoshal, R. N., et al. Selection of solid dosage form composition through drug-excipient compatibility testing. J Pharm Sci 2000, 88(7), 696–704.
12. Diffusion and Dissolution. In Martin, A. N., Bustamante, P., and Chun, A. H. C. Eds. Physical Pharmacy. 4th Ed. PA: Lea & Febiger, 1993: 325.
13. Kanjickal, D. G., Lopina, S. T. Modeling of drug release from polymeric delivery systems-a review. Crit Rev Ther Drug Carrier Syst 2004, 21(5), 345–386.
14. Arifin, D. Y., Lee, L. Y., Wang, C. H. Mathematical modeling and simulation of drug release from microspheres: implications to drug delivery systems. Adv Drug Deliv Rev 2006, 58(12–13), 1274–1325.
15. FDA SUPAC-MR: modified release solid oral dosage forms scale-up and postapproval changes: chemistry, manufacturing, and controls; in vitro dissolution testing and in vivo bioequivalence documentation. 1997. Available at http://www.fda.gov/Cder/guidance/1214fnl.pdf.
16. Eudralex. Quality of Modified Release Products A) Oral Solid Dosage Forms B) Transdermal Dosage Forms Section I (Quality) CPMP/QWP/ 604/96], 3. 1999. http://www.emea.europa.eu/pdfs/human/qwp/060496en.pdf.
17. Chandaroy, P., Jiang, X., Lee, C., et al. In vitro alcohol-induced dose-dumping dissolution studies of generic modified-release oral drug products. AAPS J 2008, 10(S2).
18. Fadda, H. M., Sousa, L. L., Basit, A. W. Alcohol induced dose-dumping of modified release budesonide formulations in vitro. AAPS Journal 2008, 10(S2).
19. http://www.dow.com/PublishedLiterature/dh_0062/0901b803800629e6.pdf? (accessed April 2009).
20. Keary, C. M., Sheskey, P. J. Preliminary report of the discovery of a new pharmaceutical granulation process using foamed aqueous binders. Drug Dev Ind Pharm 2004, 30(8), 831–845.
21. Ji, J., Nunes, C. J., Bindra, D. S. Selection of binder addition technique in a high-shear wet granulation process: impact of formulation wettability. AAPS Journal 2008, 10(S2).

22. Cantor, S. L., Kothari, S., Koo, OMY. Evaluation of the physical and mechanical properties of high drug load formulations: wet granulation vs. novel foam granulation. Powder Technol 2009, 195, 15–24.

23. Thompson, M. R., Weatherley, S., Pukadyil, R. N., Sheskey, P. J. Foam granulation: new developments in pharmaceutical solid oral dosage forms using twin screw extrusion machinery. Drug Dev Ind Pharma 2012, 38(7), 771–784.

24. Rocca, K. E., Weatherley, S., Sheskey, P. J., Thompson, M. R. Influence of filler selection on twin screw foam granulation. Drug Dev Ind Pharma 2015, 41(1), 35–42.

25. Thompson, M. R., O'Donnell, K. P. "Rolling" phenomenon in twin screw granulation with controlled-release excipients. Drug Dev Ind Pharma 2015, 41(3), 482–492.

26. Tan, D. C. T., Chin, W. W. L., Tan, E. H., Hong, S., Gu, W., Gokhale R. Effect of binders on the release rates of direct molded verapamil tablets using twin-screw extruder in melt granulation. Int J Pharm 2014, 463, 89–97.

27. Doghramji, P. P. Insomnia: zolpidem extended-release for the treatment of sleep induction and sleep maintenance symptoms. MedGenMed 2007, 9(1), 11.

28. http://en.sanofi-aventis.com/binaries/03-06-10_GoldmanSachs_EN_tcm28-19683.pdf (accessed April 2009).

29. Ohmori, S., Makino, T. Sustained-release phenylpropanolamine hydrochloride bilayer caplets containing the hydroxypropyl methylcellulose 2208 matrix. I. Formulation and dissolution characteristics. Chem Pharm Bull 2000, 48(5), 673–677.

30. Ohmori, S., Makino, T. Sustained-release phenylpropanolamine hydrochloride bilayer caplets containing the hydroxypropyl methylcellulose 2208 matrix. II. Effects of filling order in bilayer compression and manufacturing method of the prolonged-release layer on compactibility of bilayer caplets. Chem Pharm Bull 2000, 48(5), 678–682.

31. Chen, R., Okamoto, H., Danjo, K. Particle design using a 4-fluid-nozzle spray-drying technique for sustained release of acetaminophen. Chem Pharm Bull 2006, 54(7), 948–953.

32. Chen, R., Takahashi, H., Okamoto, H., et al. Particle design of three-component system for sustained release using a 4-fluid nozzle spray-drying technique. Chem Pharm Bull 2006, 54(11), 1486–1490.

33. Seville, P. C., Li, H. Y., Learoyd, T. P. Spray-dried powders for pulmonary drug delivery. Crit Rev Ther Drug Carrier Syst 2007, 24(4), 307–360.

34. Kaye, R. S., Purewal, T. S., Alpar, H. O. Simultaneously manufactured nano-in-micro (SIMANIM) particles for dry-powder modified-release delivery of antibodies. J Pharm Sci 2009, 98(11), 4055–4068.

35. Fukui, A., Fujii, R., Yonezawa, Y., Sunada, H. Analysis of the release process of phenylpropanolamine hydrochloride from ethyl cellulose matrix granules. Chem Pharm Bull 2002, 50(11), 1439–1442.

36. Fukui, A., Fujii, R., Yonezawa, Y., et al. Analysis of the release process of phenylpropanolamine hydrochloride from ethyl cellulose matrix granules II. Effects of the binder solution on the release process. Chem Pharm Bull 2004, 52(3), 298–302.

37. Fukui, A., Fujii, R., Yonezawa, Y., et al. Analysis of the release process of phenylpropanolamine hydrochloride from ethyl cellulose matrix granules III. Effects of the dissolution condition on the release process. Chem Pharm Bull 2006, 54(8), 1091–1096.

38. Fukui, A., Fujii, R., Yonezawa, Y., et al. Analysis of the release process of phenylpropanolamine hydrochloride from ethyl cellulose matrix granules IV. Evaluation of the controlled release properties for *in vivo* and *in vitro* release systems. Chem Pharm Bull 2007, 55(11), 1569–1573.

39. Fukui, A., Fujii, R., Yonezawa, Y., Sunada, H. Analysis of the release process of phenylpropanolamine hydrochloride from ethyl cellulose matrix granules V. Release properties of ethyl cellulose layered matrix granules. Chem Pharm Bull 2008, 56(4), 525–529.

40. Maejima, T., Ohsawa, T., Kobayashi, M., et al. Factors effecting spherical granulation of drugs by tumbling granulation method. Chem Pharm Bull 1992, 40(2), 488–492.

41. Freund-Vector technical brochure. June 2009. Available at http://www.vectorcorporation.com/.

17 Granulation of Poorly Water-Soluble Drugs

Albert W. Brzeczko, Firas El Saleh, and Hibreniguss Terefe

CONTENTS

17.1   INTRODUCTION

Over the past several decades, advances in drug discovery techniques have been significant in identifying new and novel therapeutics agents in the pharmaceutical industry. Receptor mapping and molecular modeling coupled with high-throughput screening have revealed a plethora of drug candidates for numerous disease states. Because of the nature and the location of many of these receptors in a lipophilic membrane, drug candidates having the best molecular configuration and fitting into these receptors may, by design, be poorly water-soluble. It is estimated that 90% of new chemical entities in drug development are characterized as poorly water-soluble with a potential market impact projected at $145 billion [1]. Crestor® (rosuvastatin calcium), Nexium® (esomeprazole magnesium), and Sovaldi® (sofosbuvir) are drugs with significant therapeutic impact, which are classified as poorly water-soluble. This rise of more poorly water-soluble drug candidates in development presents a challenge to formulators of pharmaceutical oral solid dosage forms to improve the drug's bioavailability while maintaining product stability, both physically and chemically, as well as providing a robust commercial process.

From a historical perspective, the classification of drug solubility has been graded according to pharmacopoeial standards for solubility [2]. Ranging from freely water-soluble to water-insoluble, drug solubility is determined from its equilibrium solubility in water. In addition to categorization based on equilibrium solubility, a bioclassification system (BCS) has been created that categorizes a drug based not only on solubility but also on its permeability [3]. The BSC classes for solubility and permeability are given in Figure 17.1.

Initially designed as criteria for waiver of bioequivalence testing based on *in vitro* testing for immediate release, highly soluble, and highly permeable drugs (BCS 1) [4], the BCS has been a very valuable tool for determining formulation and processing strategies in the development of oral drug products. Consideration in the BCS solubility criteria is given to drug dose as well as to the

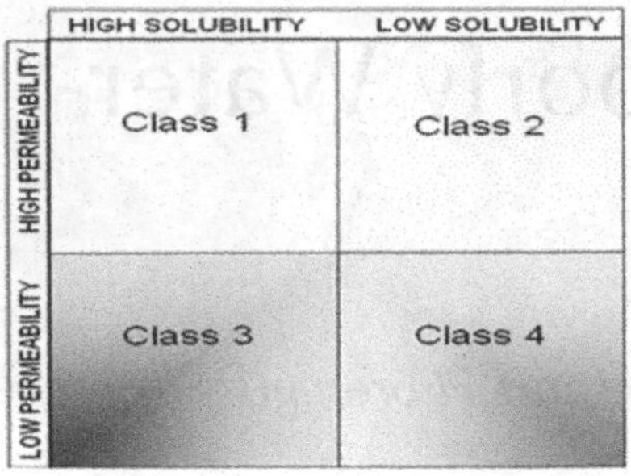

	HIGH SOLUBILITY	LOW SOLUBILITY
HIGH PERMEABILITY	Class 1	Class 2
LOW PERMEABILITY	Class 3	Class 4

FIGURE 17.1   BSC Classes for solubility and permeability.

pH solubility profile of a drug. Therefore, two drugs may be categorized as sparingly soluble, but drug A has a highest therapeutic dose of 1 mg and drug B has the highest dose of 100 mg; under the BCS guidance, drug A may meet the highly soluble criteria (either class 1 or 3), whereas drug B would be considered poorly soluble (class 2 or 4). For this chapter, granulation and formulation techniques will be primarily discussed for drugs considered as BCS class 2 and class 4.

As many chapters in this text reinforce, granulation techniques are important tools to aid in solving oral solid dosage development problems. Improving content uniformity, increasing tablet compressibility, enhancing powder flow, and, to some extent, improving dissolution rates and bioavailability are application examples in traditional granulation techniques. However, in perspective to a growing class of highly poorly water-soluble drugs, traditional practices may be somewhat limited to improve solubility and bioavailability. It is well documented that the use of surfactants in tablet formulations can improve dissolution rates of poorly soluble drugs [5]. However, as the limits of drug solubility move to lower solubilities ($\leq 10\,\mu g/mL$), traditional granulation techniques and outcomes yield to newer granulation techniques to effect a change to highly lipophilic and highly crystalline drugs to produce drug products with enhanced solubility and bioavailability. Spray drying, which had long been relegated to pharmaceutical excipients' production, has more recently emerged as a useful granulation technique in the manufacture of poorly water-soluble drug products [6]. In addition to reporting the emerging use of spray drying in pulmonary drug delivery and therapeutic proteins, Parikh notes the growing interest in producing amorphous solid dispersion (ASD) drug products through solvent-based spray drying. The face of dry-granulation techniques is also changing, wherein conventional compaction processing is yielding to thermal dry-granulation processing such as hot-melt extrusion (HME) and spray congealing (spray freezing). These thermal processes are employed to intimately mix polymers in a molten state [temperature at or above melting temperature (T_m) or glass transition temperate (T_g)] with poorly water-soluble drugs. The resulting solid solutions or solid dispersions have been reported to improve drug solubility and bioavailability when compared with physical mixtures of drug and polymers [7].

The focus of this chapter will be to highlight the role that granulation technology plays in improving the solubility of poorly water-soluble drugs, particularly around drug particle size reduction and nanoparticle technology, drug complexation, and solid drug dispersion.

Increasing drug solubility through particle size reduction has been a mainstay of the pharmaceutical industry. The Noyes–Whitney equation shows a direct relationship between the rate of dissolution and the surface area of the solid [8].

$$\frac{dW}{dt} = \frac{DA(C_s - C)}{L} \tag{17.1}$$

where $\frac{dW}{dt}$ is the rate of dissolution, A is the surface area of the solid, C is the concentration of the solid in the bulk dissolution medium, C_s is the concentration of the solid in the diffusion layer surrounding the solid, D is the diffusion coefficient, and L is the diffusion layer thickness.

Micronization techniques to decrease particle size and hence impart an increase in specific surface area of the drug include simple comminution processing such as jet milling and ball milling to produce drug particles of a size approaching 1 μm. Drugs, such as griseofulvin and spironolactone, have been shown to have improved dissolution rate and bioavailability when particle size reduction is employed [9,10]. However, with the discovery of more highly insoluble drugs, conventional milling techniques are limited. Newer nanoparticle drug delivery technologies employing specialized milling techniques and supercritical fluids (SCF) have been very effective to reduce drug particle size approaching 100 nm [11]. This significant increase in the surface area greatly increases the dissolution rate and potentially enhanced bioavailability. However, as drug particle sizes begin to approach oligomolecular units, the increase in particle surface energy results in spontaneous aggregation (Oswald's ripening), which must be controlled through formulation and/or process. Surface stabilization is typically achieved with the adsorption of a stabilizing agent to the nanocrystal particles.

Increased interest in drug complexation and solid dispersion technologies has emerged recently. Both require the intervention of hydrophilic excipients to increase the solubility of poorly water-soluble drugs. Cyclodextrins (CDs) and their derivatives have been central to this complexation research. CDs are unique cyclic oligosaccharides, wherein the hydrophobic nature of the interior ring surface promotes complexation with hydrophobic drugs. This often leads to a substantial increase in solubility for drug/CD complexes [12]. Unlike ordered complexes, solid dispersions represent molecular or near-molecular mixtures of drugs and hydrophilic excipients, which can result in a variety of states such as eutectic, solid solution, and glass suspension among others. Because the poorly soluble drug is evenly dispersed in a hydrophilic matrix, enhanced solubility is seen with techniques that produce solid dispersions [13]. Overall, granulation techniques used in the formation of stable and bioavailable drug nanoparticles, complexes, and solid dispersions have been established and have been proven commercially. A list of several commercially available drug products for each technology is given in Table 17.1 (additional products are included later in the chapter).

17.2 PARTICLE REDUCTION AND NANOPARTICLES

Particle size reduction has been widely used by the pharmaceutical industry to improve the dissolution rate of poorly water-soluble drugs. Conventional methods for reducing drug particle size such as hammer and jet milling are well established and, therefore, present economical, safe, and effective

TABLE 17.1

Several Commercial Products Using Solubility/bioavailability-Enhancing Technology

Technology	Drug	Product
Nanoparticle	Sirolimus	Rapamune®
Nanoparticle	Aprepitant	Emend®
Nanoparticle	Fenofibrate	Tricor®
α-Cyclodextrin	Limaprost	Opalmon®
α-Cyclodextrin	Alprostadil	Prostavasin®
Solid dispersion	Itraconazole	Sporanox®
Solid dispersion	Etravirine	Intelence®

pathways for the commercialization of products. However, certain limitations are inherent when conventional size reduction technologies are used. Drugs that are shear- and/or temperature-sensitive may be susceptible to degradation in comminution processing. Since comminution relies on particle fracture for size reduction, drugs with low-melting temperatures, or having thermoplastic characteristics may be difficult if not impossible to process by conventional milling. Reduced temperature milling such as cryomilling may be beneficial to aid in the size reduction of low-melting-temperature drugs. However, the most impactful of conventional milling is its limitation to improve drug dissolution rate as drugs approach water insolubility (<10 µg/mL). Nanoparticle as a drug delivery technique is well established for pharmaceuticals [14] and presents an improvement to conventional milling to enhance dissolution and bioavailability of poorly water-soluble drugs.

Nanoparticles are materials that are less than or equal to 1 µm in one dimension, and more specifically, a nanocrystal is a single crystalline in nature. In colloidal chemistry, nanoparticles are further limited to 100 nm or less; however, in the pharmaceutical area, nanoparticles can range in size from approximately 10 nm to 100 nm. Nanoparticle delivery systems are reported for oral, parenteral, and pulmonary drug delivery. Junghanns and Müller [15] report not only an increase in dissolution rate by surface area enlargement but also an increase in saturation solubility related to the dissolution pressure increase associated with nanoparticles. Optimal drug nanoparticles with the highest increase in saturation solubility have a 20- to 50-nm particle size and would be amorphous. Stabilization of the nanoparticle amorphous drug is required to confer adequate product shelf life.

17.3 NANOPARTICLES FOR POORLY WATER-SOLUBLE DRUGS

Nanoparticles for pharmaceutical applications are produced by two basic methods, comminution or a "top-down" method and precipitation or a "bottom-up" method. Within the comminution method are two primary particle size reduction techniques, bead milling and homogenization. The NanoCrystal® technology for nanoparticle formation is based on the bead milling process. Bead mills are favorable because they are less expensive, relatively simple to use, available at a small R&D scale, and readily scalable for commercialization. Milling media (beads), the dispersion medium, drugs, and other formulation aids (stabilizers) are charged into the milling chamber. Wet milling is essential to achieve smaller nanoparticle sizes when compared with dry bead milling processing. The dispersion medium would ideally be a non-solvent for the drug. For poorly soluble drugs, water often serves as the dispersion medium. Surfactants and stabilizers are essential in the production of nanoparticles by nanosuspensions. The choice of surfactant is dependent on the affinity of the surfactant for the drug surface and the physical nature of the interaction (i.e., steric or electrostatic). Generally, steric stabilization on nanoparticles is preferred. In some cases, a combination of low- and high-hydrophilic-lipophilic balance surfactants may be warranted. Milling media are available in a variety of materials, but to minimize contamination, yttria zirconium beads offer nearly contamination-free grinding [16]. The extent of bead erosion depends on milling material, suspension concentration, drug hardness, and milling time. Impact and shearing forces between the milling media and the suspended drug particles are responsible for particle reduction. Smaller milling media with a higher number of contact points are preferred to produce smaller nanoparticles. As a general rule, the size of the milling media is 1000 times the size of the desired nanoparticle size. Plug flow, where particles move at a uniform velocity in the mill, is preferred to achieve a consistent and reproducible grind and residence time. Milling times can be highly variable and are largely dependent on drug hardness, dispersion media, milling energy, surfactant and level used, temperature, and type and size of milling media. The wet suspension from bead mill processing can be dried for oral solid dosage manufacturing or the suspension can be used for delivery as a drug suspension.

In addition to wet bead milling, homogenization presents an additional technique for top-down nanoparticle formation. Within homogenization techniques, there are two processes reported for nanoparticle formation by disintegration, jet stream, and piston-gap homogenizations. Jet stream homogenizer produces nanoparticles through a collision of two fluid streams under high pressure, where particle collision and shear and cavitation forces lead to the disintegration of the drug particle. Microfluidizer can generate pressures up to 275 MPa and jet velocities of the colliding streams approaching 500 m/sec. As with wet bead milling, nanoparticle stabilization facilitated by a surfactant is required. Disadvantages of jet stream homogenizers as a particle disintegrator are its limitation on the minimum size and the high number of cycles required to achieve a homogeneous size distribution [17]. Panagiotou and Fisher compared jet stream homogenizer by disintegration and precipitation processes via microchannel reactors (MCR). They showed that the precipitation process was more efficient at achieving a smaller nanoparticle size for carbamazepine with a narrower particle size distribution (median particle size 304 nm vs. 604 nm by disintegration). The precipitation technique was performed in a single cycle, whereas 25 cycles were used for the disintegration technique.

Nanoparticle formation by piston-gap homogenizers was introduced by Müller et al. [18]. In this technology, a poorly soluble drug is dispersed in water and, by the force of a piston generating pressure up to 4000 bar, is passed through a narrow gap to affect particle reduction. Surfactants are required to facilitate size reduction and stabilize nanoparticles from ripening effects. Gap distances range from 5 to 25 μm and are dependent on the suspension viscosity. High-shear forces and turbulent flow play a role in particle reduction; however, cavitation forces are reported to have the greatest effect [19]. From Bernoulli's law, the cross-sectional volume flow in a closed system is constant. When the liquid is in the homogenizer gap, a significant increase in dynamic pressure and a decrease in static pressure occur. The liquid starts boiling at room temperature, rapidly forming bubbles. After leaving the homogenizer gap, bubbles rapidly collapse and implode under atmospheric pressure. This cavitation process generates great energy in drug size reduction.

Nanoparticles produced by precipitation (or "bottom-up" processing), as the name suggests, involve a controlled build of the drug particle from a solution. In this technique, the drug is dissolved in a solvent, and the drug solution is added in a controlled manner to a drug antisolvent under high agitation. The drug precipitates rapidly and in a controlled manner in the presence of the antisolvent by generating a large number of nucleation sites and limiting the subsequent growth. Bottom-up processing has an advantage to top-down processing in that particle formation can be done with heterogeneous materials to form cocrystals or coprecipitates, which may further enhance the solubility of the poorly soluble drug compared with the homogeneous drug nanoparticles. Crystal size is controlled by thermodynamic principles, transport phenomena, and reaction kinetics. The key to this process is the presence of homogeneous nanoscale regions throughout the crystallization volume. The process can be as simple as using a static mixer for nanoparticle precipitation. However, results obtained in the R&D lab may not readily scale to larger containers where hydrodynamics, vessel volume to the surface, and turbulence are not readily reproduced. Alternatively, a jet stream homogenization technology using MCR has been reported to replicate the single confined impinging jet reactor scale experience by stacking multiple jet impinging reactor units to achieve the desired production rate [17]. In this process, a drug solution is jet impinged into an antisolvent for the drug. Carbamazepine crystals, manufactured by the jet impinging process, were 150 to 300 nm wide and 2 to 5 μm in length, whereas drug particles by conventional mixing were 1 to 2 μm wide and less than 20 μm in length. Zhou et al. [20] showed that danazol nanoparticles made in the MCR process significantly increased specific surface area (14.32 vs. 0.66 m^2/g) and a dissolution rate in five minutes from 35% to 100% when compared with danazol particles "as received" [20].

Supercritical fluid (SCF) technology in pharmaceutical nanoparticles has gained great interest [21]. Carbon dioxide is the primary supercritical fluid used in this technology because it can be processed in mild operating conditions, both temperature and pressure, is chemically inert and non-flammable, and has minimal to low environmental impact compared with organic solvents. Solvent properties of supercritical CO_2 are mostly representative of non-polar solvents, but these properties can vary depending on the temperature and pressure conditions of the fluid. When organic solvents are used in processing, the miscibility of CO_2 with most organic solvents typically results in low residual solvent content, avoiding additional downstream processing. Vemavarapu et al. [22] reviewed the various supercritical fluid techniques used in particle formation, of which most use an antisolvent approach because of low drug solubility in supercritical CO_2. Two popular supercritical processes are supercritical antisolvent recrystallization (SAS) and the rapid expansion of super-critical solutions (RESS). SAS processing requires the drug to be solubilized into a solvent that is sprayed into SCF. The drug should be insoluble in the SCF and the organic solvent, miscible in SCF. As the SCF diffuses into the drug–solvent droplets, the miscible solvent expands with the SCF, and precipitation of the drug particles occurs. In a batch SAS process, the drug solution is sprayed into a vessel containing the SCF, whereas, in a continuous SAS process, the drug solution and SCF are introduced into the vessel concurrently. SAS process has greater flexibility in con-trolling particle growth through solvent(s) selection and by controlling the solvent extraction conditions of SFC. However, high residual solvent levels can result in particle agglomeration or crystal growth. Chattopadhyay and Gupta have reported an improvement in the SAS process to obtain smaller nanoparticles with narrower distribution [23]. Supercritical antisolvent precipitation with enhanced mass transfer utilizes an ultrasonic field to enhance mass transfer between the drug solution and SCF and prevents agglomeration due to increased mixing. Griseofulvin nanoparticles of 130 nm were obtained at 180 W energy input.

For supercritical processing, where the drug is soluble in the SCF, RESS processing is favored. These drugs tend to be highly lipophilic with low molecular weight (MW). RESS involves dissolving a drug or a drug–polymer mixture in SCF and spraying the SCF solution into a lower-pressure vessel. The rapid expansion by the solution reduces the density of the SCF and super-saturates the drug or a drug–polymer mix in the lower-pressure solution, resulting in precipitation of pure drug or drug–polymer particles with reduced size and narrow size distribution. Limitations of the RESS process are that few drugs are soluble in commonly used SFC and process throughput rates for precipitates are slow.

A fairly recent technology that is considered to apply to poorly water-soluble drugs that lack adequate volatile organic solvent solubility and/or are thermally labile is Microprecipitation (MBP) technology [24]. In this technology, a crystalline drug substance and an ionic polymer are dis-solved in polar solvents such as dimethylacetamide, dimethylformamide, and dimethylsulfoxide and slowly added into a large volume of antisolvent (cold acidified water) to induce controlled precipitation. The organic solvent is then removed by extraction and the material containing water dried by the forced-air oven or fluid-bed drying. Heat and moisture during final drying may promote crystallization.

17.4 COMPLEXATION

17.4.1 Background

While the techniques of micro/nanosizing and formation of solid dispersions/solutions are mainly beneficial for enhancing the solubility and the dissolution rate of drugs with a strong crystal lattice (so-called "brick dust" active pharmaceutical ingredients [APIs]), complexation techniques can be beneficial in increasing the solubility of hydrophobic drugs (so-called "grease ball " drugs) [25].

Complexation is well known in organic and inorganic chemistry. Complexes are entities comprising two or more molecules (or ions) that are bound to each other with non-covalent bonds, that is, only with physical forces such as hydrogen bonds or van der Waals bonds [26].

Such complexation reactions are an equilibrium between the free components and the complex as in the following equation:

$$mA + nB \Leftrightarrow A_m B_n \tag{17.2}$$

This reaction has an equilibrium constant that can be calculated as follows:

$$K_{mn} = \frac{[A_m B_n]}{A^m \cdot B^n} \tag{17.3}$$

where m and n are the number of the molecules of compounds, A and B (respectively), involved in the complexation, $A_m B_n$ is the formed complex, and K_{mn} is the stability constant of this complex. The higher this constant, the more likely the reaction is to form the complex. Conversely, when it is low, the substances involved in the complexation exist more in the free form than in the complex form.

Cyclodextrin (CDs) are the most pharmaceutically relevant substances that have been used to increase the solubility of drugs through the formation of so-called inclusion complexes. They can also form other types of complexes, so-called non-inclusion complexes or complex aggregates [27], similar in their structures to micelles. Native (non-substituted) CDs were first isolated and characterized in 1911 by Schardinger who identified α- and β-dextrins [28]. These two substances contain 6 or 7 α $(1 \rightarrow 4)$-linked D-glucopyranose subunits (Figure 17.2), and nowadays, they are called α- and β-CD. γ-CD, with eight glucopyranose subunits, was discovered in 1935 [29]. These are the native CDs used so far in pharmacy. In later stages, native CDs with more than eight glucose units were discovered [30], but they have not been used in pharmaceutical applications so far. CDs have different functionalities. They are used in pharmaceuticals mainly for drug stabilization, increasing drug solubility, preventing drug–drug or drug–excipient interactions, and taste masking. We are mainly interested in the solubility-increasing features in this chapter. A listing of pharmaceutical products using CD technologies is given in Table 17.2.

Cyclodextrins are crystalline, non-hygroscopic, cyclic oligosaccharides derived from starch. They have a shape of a hollow truncated cone, rather closer to a cylinder or also described as a toroid, with a rigid structure and a central cavity that can accommodate another molecule, the size of which varies according to the cyclodextrin type [3].

The upper, wider "rim" of the molecule is constituted of secondary hydroxyls (positions C2 and C3), and the narrower rim consists of primary hydroxyls (position C6). The "walls" or "cavity" are rather hydrophobic, enabling them to accommodate a hydrophobic guest, while the hydroxyls at the rims are hydrophilic and interact with water, hence the solubilization effect. Due to the formation of a perfectly rigid structure in the β-CD molecule, the secondary hydroxyls form intimate hydrogen

TABLE 17.2
List of CD-Based Products

Product	Manufacturer	API	Cyclodextrin	Dosage Form
BRIVIACT	UCB	Brivaracetam	BCD	Tablet
MAVENCLAD 10 mg tablets	Merck Serono	Cladribine	HPBCD	Tablet
Y+	Bayer	Drospirenone/ethinyl estradiol/ levomefolate calcium	BCD	Tablet
Gilenya	Novartis	Fingolimod HCl	HPBCD	Capsule
IVABRADINE SYNTHON 2.5MG FILM-COATED TABLETS	Synthon	Ivabradine	BCD	Tablet
Pramipexol STADA 0,7 mg Tabletten	STADA	Pramipexole dihydrochloride	BCD	Tablet
Perindopril HEXAL plus Indapamid 4 mg/1,25 mg Tabletten	Hexal/Sandoz	Prindopril erbumine/indapamide	BCD/HPBCD	Tablet

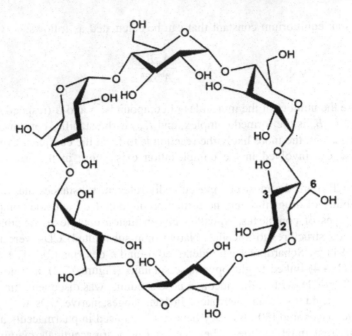

FIGURE 17.2 Structure of α-cyclodextrin, showing the positions for the primary hydroxyl at C6 and the secondary hydroxyls at C2 and C3.

bonds within the molecule and between the β-CD molecules, rendering their interaction with water very limited. β-CD has, therefore, a relatively low water solubility (18.5 g/L, at room temperature), whereas the structures of α- and γ-CD are less rigid and have a higher ability to interact with water, leading to higher solubility in water (145 and 232 g/L, respectively) [31]. The substitution of the hydroxyls within the CD molecule with various substituents often leads to increasing the solubility in water by disrupting the internal hydrogen bonding. 2-Hydroxypropyl betadex (2-HP β-CD), for instance, has a solubility in water up to 750 g/L [32]. In pharmaceutical applications, methyl

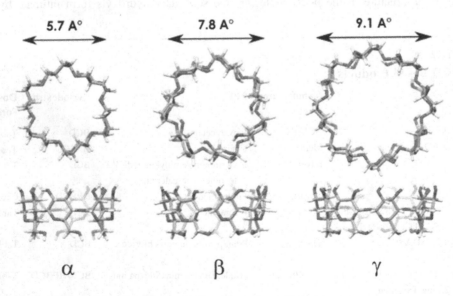

FIGURE 17.3 Three-dimensional structures of α-, β-, and γ-cyclodextrin.

(dimethyl, randomly methylated), 2-hydroxypropyl, and sulfobutyl-ether derivatives of β-CD and 2-hydroxypropyl γ-CD are used. Some of these derivatives are crystalline (methylated CDs), and some others are amorphous (hydroxyproxylated CDs) [33]. Complexes made from amorphous CDs are often amorphous. The following types can be found in pharmacopeias: Alfadex (α-CD), betadex (β-CD), and 2-hydroxypropyl betadex (2-HP β-CD), which are in both the European Pharmacopoeia and the United States Pharmacopoeia, while γ-cyclodextrin and sulfobutylether betadex (SBE-β-CD) are only listed in the United States Pharmacopoeia.

17.4.2 SELECTION OF SUITABLE CYCLODEXTRIN AND DETERMINATION OF STOICHIOMETRY

It is important to determine which cyclodextrin forms a complex or, more precisely, which kind of complex it forms with the studied API. Since α-, β-, and γ-CDs have internal cavities of increasing diameter and, therefore, volume, one of them would often be more suitable to be a host to a drug molecule than the others. This depends mainly on the shape and size of the drug molecule and how it fits into the cavity of the CD, as well as the ability to build hydrogen bonds and their hydrophobicity. As a simple rule of thumb for small-molecule APIs, an α-CD cavity is most suitable as a host for drugs with straight aliphatic chains, whereas β-CD is more suitable for simple aromatic ring structures and γ-CD is more suitable for larger structures consisting of several rings, such as steroids. This could best be explained as depicted in Figure 17.4. In most cases, only one type of CD would form a complex of a certain guest, considerably more stable than that with other types of CD.

Since this complexation concerns the complexation of a certain number of CD molecules with a certain number of API molecules, this has an impact on the overall drug load in the formulation. As an approximate example, since native CDs have a molecular weight (MW) of about 1000 Da, while many small-molecule drugs have an MW around 400 Da, a 1:1 complex (molar ratio CD:API) is approximately a 2.5:1 weight/weight ratio, that is, a drug loading of about 28.6% in the complex. If this is to be formulated into a tablet while adding other excipients, the drug load would drop below 25%. Since many tablets have a weight below 1000 mg, the maximum possible drug load would be around 250 mg. Another constraint is only for native β-CD and the fact that World Health Organization/Food and Agriculture Organization joint comity [34] set a maximum recommended daily intake of 5 mg/kg body weight per day. This constraint was reconfirmed by the European Food Safety Authority [35]. This means that for a person of 70 kg weight, not more than 350 mg β-CD should be ingested, and thus about 140 mg daily dose of the complexed drug, according to the example above.

Phase-solubility diagrams are an important tool for selecting the most suitable CDs for solubilizing the studied API. This test is conducted by preparing solutions of increasing concentrations of each tested cyclodextrin and adding a quantity of a drug that considerably surpasses its saturation concentration in water. The solutions are stirred or shaken in bottles for 48 hours and then filtered. The concentration of the dissolved drug (in Mol/L) is measured and plotted against

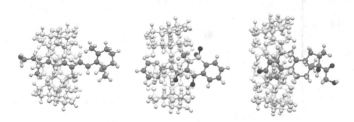

FIGURE 17.4 Assumed exemplary structures of complexes of α alpha-cyclodextrin-cyclodextrin with retinol (left), β beta-cyclodextrin-cyclodextrin with piroxicam (middle), and γ gamma-cyclodextrin-cyclodextrin with dexamethasone (right).

the concentration of cyclodextrin solution (also in Mol/L). The resulting curve would have one of the different shapes indicating a specific type of interaction between the drug and the tested cyclodextrin. More details about this can be found in a review by Brewster and Loftsson [36].

As already mentioned, cyclodextrins play the role of a host (CD) and the drug to be complexed, the guest (G), to form a so-called inclusion complex (CD·G). One or more cyclodextrin molecules would form a complex with one or more drug molecules. In the case of a 1:1 (molar ratio) complex, Eq. (3) could be written as follows:

$$K_c = \frac{[CD \cdot G]}{[CD] \cdot [G]} \tag{17.4}$$

The stability constant and stoichiometry can be determined using the method of continuous variations, also known as Job Plots [37,38], and monitoring band shifts with different analytical methods such as nuclear magnetic resonance and circular dichroism spectroscopy [38]. Also, the phase-solubility diagrams [38,39] isotherms are often used for the same purpose. For this, Eq. (4) could be rewritten as Eq. (5) [36] and used to calculate the K_c for 1:1 complexes based on the slope and intercept (D_0) of a regression line passing through the linear part of the phase-solubility diagram, in which both axes are expressed as Mol/L:

$$K_c = \frac{slope}{D_0 \cdot (1 - slope)} \tag{17.5}$$

The different methods of calculating K_c often lead to different results [40].

An example for calculating K_c using the phase-solubility diagram method and Eq. (4) can be seen in Figure 17.5.

The usual procedure for determining the CD type with the best solubility enhancement of the drug starts by making phase-solubility diagrams of the tested drug in various CDs and then choosing the most suitable one for the drug and application. An example is provided by Abdoh et al. [42]. They made solubility phase diagrams of diclofenac sodium in α-, β-, γ-, and hydroxypropyl (HP) β-CD in pH 2.8 and 6.5. The slope of the solubility curves of diclofenac sodium was highest with γ-CD, followed by HP β-CD, β-CD, and finally α-CD. Note that 1:1 complexes were formed for all types of CDs and in both pHs, with the exception of γ-CD at pH 5.8, where the diclofenac sodium formed a 2:1 diclo:γ-CD complex.

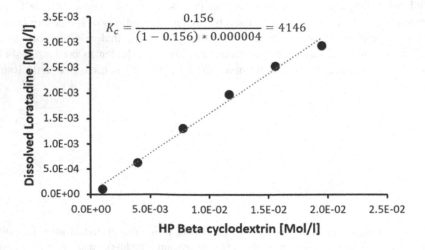

FIGURE 17.5   Solubility isotherm of loratadine in hpbcd solutions [41] with example K_c calculation.

Once the optimal CD and appropriate stoichiometry for the investigated drug have been established, a complex of the drug and this CD can be made using different methods. The classical method for preparing cyclodextrin complexes is in the liquid phase, usually by heating an aqueous solution of a CD, adding the drug in the suitable stoichiometric proportion [43,44], and then stirring the solution for several hours. The duration of the stirring is to be determined empirically. The solution is then cooled down slowly in a controlled way to obtain the complex in a crystalline form. The crystals are separated, rinsed, and dried. In a similar way, the drug is dissolved in an organic solvent mixture and added gradually to an aqueous solution of a CD, and the mixture is stirred for a certain time and resulting crystals are separated. This is feasible if the CD used is crystalline, like the native CDs. Such a method requires reactors for the preparation of a large quantity of the complex. This usually is not available in classical pharmaceutical production facilities. It is also important to note here that the used solvent should not disrupt the formation of the complex by competition [45].

17.4.3 COMPLEX PREPARATION METHODS

The most relevant methods of a complex preparation used in the context of this chapter are:

17.4.3.1 Spray-Drying and Fluid-Bed Granulation

In this process, the solution/suspension of the complex can be dried as is via spray drying [46–48], to obtain a dry powder. Similar results can be achieved using fluid-bed granulation by spraying the complex solution or suspension on a neutral carrier, for example, spraying a carvedilol–HP β-CD solution on lactose [49], or by using fluid-bed coating to spray piroxicam–HP β-CD on non-pareil beads [50]. Since the efficiency of the complexation can be enhanced by using polymers such as polyvinylpyrrolidone (PVP) [51,52], PEG-PVCL-PVAc, or hydroxypropyl methylcellulose (HPMC) [53,54], it would be very beneficial to use them in the preparation of granules or pellets using fluid-bed granulation or coating.

17.4.3.2 Kneading Process in High-Shear Mixer

The kneading process in a high-shear mixer is very similar to a wet granulation process, as only higher amounts of water or solvent–water mixtures are used. It is also most effective with cyclodextrins that have a low water solubility, that is, mainly BCD. The required amount of CD is kneaded or mixed with the amount of water needed to obtain a water content of about 15% to 20% of the final mass in a kneader or in a high-shear mixer. The API is then added as a mass of powder or in a pre-dissolved form in an appropriate organic solvent to the kneaded form of CD; the kneading process is continued until the complexation is complete [55]. The completion of the complexation can be often determined by a strong increase of power consumption of the motor and by a change in the appearance of the kneaded mass. Hutin et al. [56] investigated such a process and the factors influencing it. Water was added dropwise until the endpoint of complexation had been detected via torque measurements. The kneaded mass, once the complexation was complete, was dried in a tray dryer or a fluid-bed dryer. The temperature used in drying should be optimized as high temperatures might break the complex. Drying the complexes at a product temperature of 50°C should be suitable for most complexes.

17.4.3.3 Twin-Screw Kneading and Extrusion

Since the two main factors driving the complexation are the presence of water and mechanical shear, twin-screw kneading/extrusion is an excellent way to control such complexion process since both the amount of water used and the shear applied can be controlled. These factors can be controlled by changing process parameters such as water pump speed (in case of aqueous kneading), screw rotation speed, and screw configuration. Screw configuration can be used to control mechanical shear and residence time by selecting screw components that offer more shear and lead to higher retention of the material in the barrel, like kneading blocks, or reducing the shear and reducing the residence time by using simple conveying elements [57]. In case additional heat energy input is favorable for the complexation reaction, the barrel can be heated or cooled. If the end of the twin-screw extruder barrel is open without a die, the process is called twin-screw kneading. If a terminal die plate is mounted, the process becomes extrusion. By adding a die plate to the end of the barrel, the shear would be further increased, which could be beneficial for the complex formation. However, it could lead to some limitations by quickly reaching the maximum torque of the motor and, thus, bringing the process to a halt.

According to Fukuda et al. [58], hot-melt extrusion of ketoprofen with SBE-β-CD led to a significantly higher dissolution rate than with native β-CD or ketoprofen alone. Yoshii et al. [59] investigated the impact of kneading energy on the effectiveness of complexation and concluded that the fraction of limonene complexed increased sharply with the increase of torque. One way to further process the kneaded mass is to extrude it as a first step, and then apply spheronization to obtain disintegrating pellets [60]. The pellets can then be compressed into tablets. Yano et al. [61] prepared complexes of indomethacin and HPBCD using wet granulation and melt extrusion. In both cases, the dissolution rate of the drug was strongly increased compared to a physical mixture. The drug was completely amorphous, in the case of melt extrusion, or partially amorphous with wet extrusion. Malaquias et al. [62] investigated combining fluconazole with BCD or HPBCD and a thermoplastic polymer (HPC and HPMC) using a hot-melt extrusion process to modulate the drug release and also obtain taste masking of the API. This kind of process can also be used in modern continuous manufacturing lines. Thiry et al. [63] studied the effect of extruding a class II API, itraconazole, with high logP and very low water solubility, using a hot-melt extrusion process containing different β-CD and various derivatives as well as a thermoplastic polymer (Soluplus®). The formulation containing HP β-CD and randomly methylated β-CD achieved the highest drug release rate, considerably faster than the release from a formulation containing the drug and the polymer alone. Since such a process depends on the melt rheology of the materials used, the melt rheology was measured using a parallel plate melt rheometer.

17.4.3.4   Cogrinding

As already mentioned, mechanical energy input, that is, mechanical shear plays an important role in the formation of CD complexes. This was already discussed for the kneading process. However, if the drug is sensitive to water, dry processes such as comilling, cogrinding, or general mecanochemical processes would be a good alternative for the formation of CD complexes. Additionally, since there is no water added, dry processes do not require the removal of water at the end of the process, leading to energy and time savings. CD and drug in appropriate molar proportions are either firstly blended or directly inserted into a mill, like a vibrational ball mill [27,64–66] or a roll mill [67], and then the milling process is started. The variation of milling duration and milling speed/frequency can have an impact on the quality of the resulting complex and the solubility and dissolution rate of the complexed drugs [64].

17.5   SOLID DISPERSIONS

In the 1960s, coprecipitates as a formulation approach for poorly soluble drugs were reported in several publications. These systems primarily contained an intimate mixture of a drug and a water-soluble component by coprecipitation from a common solvent via the solvent evaporation process. The water-soluble component was typically a polymer such as PVP or a low molecular weight compound such as urea [68]. In 1971, Chiou and Riegelmann defined solid dispersions as "a dispersion of one or more active ingredients in an inert carrier at the solid-state, prepared by melting, solvent or melt-solvent method" and introduced a classification system of solid dispersions based on the possible physical states of the active ingredient and the carrier [69]. The concept of "Solid Dispersion" evolved when in 1991 Sekiguchi and Obi reported how to produce dispersions of poorly soluble drugs in a water-soluble carrier by forming eutectic mixtures with the aim to improve oral absorption [70].

Solid dispersion is one of the most important approaches employed in pharmaceutical product development to increase drug solubility and dissolution without a chemical modification of drug compounds. Compared with other conventional approaches, solid dispersion can reduce the size of drug particles to a much smaller level, even down to molecular dimension, and stabilize those physically modified compounds from agglomeration, crystallization, and phase separation through the understanding of the interaction between the drug compound and the carrier.

The term amorphous solid dispersion (ASD) refers to the dispersion of one or more active ingredients in a carrier matrix to enhance oral bioavailability. Depending on drug absorption behavior, the carrier can be a water-soluble polymer such as polyethylene glycol (PEG), polyvinylpyrrolidone (PVP), polyvinylpyrrolidone/vinyl acetate copolymers (PVP/VA), and hypromellose (HPMC) for poorly water-soluble active to enhance solubility, an insoluble polymer such as ethylcellulose (EC), or polymers with pH-dependent solubility such as hydroxypropyl methylcellulose phthalate (HPMCP), hydroxypropylmethylcellulose acetate succinate (HPMCAS), polyacrylates, and polymethacrylates (Eudragit) for modified release dosage forms. For poorly water-soluble compounds, ASD improves drug dissolution rate and solubility through size reduction, improved wettability, and amorphous transformation, resulting in enhanced bioavailability.

In the last decade or so, ASDs are gaining popularity and several products have been approved. Table 17.3 shows examples of ASD-based products [71–73].

17.5.1 Structures of Solid Dispersion

Having insight into the structures of solid dispersions is critical to clearly understand their dissolution characteristics. Irrespective of the method of preparation, solid dispersions can be described in two broad classes based on the magnitude of dispersion, oligomolecular level, or molecular level (Figure 17.6) [74].

Solid dispersions are classified as:

1. *Eutectic Mixtures:* A typical eutectic mixture is a mixture of two components (A and B) that melt at a single temperature lower than the melting points of the principal components. The two components (A and B) are completely miscible at the liquid (molten) state and form liquid solutions while they exhibit limited miscibility in the solid state. At a specific composition, the two components (A and B) crystallize simultaneously at a specific temperature forming a true eutectic mixture that has a microstructure different from the microstructure of either of the components (A or B). A molten mixture of the two components (A and B) at a composition different from the eutectic mixture, with one component crystallizing first resulting in one pure solid component and liquid solution. A true eutectic mixture is formed only at a specific composition of A and B (Fig. 17.7). One must bear in mind that unless the composition is exactly at the eutectic point, the dispersion will contain a mixture of the dispersion and one separated phase of the component in excess of eutectic composition. Differential scanning calorimetry (DSC) studies are often used to characterize eutectic mixtures in light of melting points. Eutectic mixtures of poorly soluble drugs and water-soluble carriers have been reported to enhance dissolution rates of poorly soluble APIs.
2. *Solid Solutions:* Solid solutions are formed when a solute (drug) is non-stoichiometrically mixed into the crystal lattice of a solvent (crystalline carrier) [75]. Solid solutions are further categorized as *continuous* and *discontinuous solid solutions* based on the miscibility and molecular size of the components. In *continuous solid solutions,* the components are miscible in all proportions, which occurs when the bonding strength between the solute and solvent molecules is greater than that of the individual components [76]. In *discontinuous*

TABLE 17.3

List of ASD-Based Products

Product Name	Drug Substance	Application Holder Company	ASD Method of Manufacturing	Polymer Used	Year of Approval
Cesamet	Nabilone	MYLAN SPECIALTY LP		PVP	1985
Isoptin	Verapamil	ABBVIE INC	Spray drying		1987
Sporanox	Itraconazole	JANSSEN PHARMACEUTICALS INC	Spray coating	HPMC	1992
Prograf	Tacrolimos	ASTELLAS PHARMA US INC	Spray drying	HPMC	1994
Rezulin	Troglitazone	PFIZER PHARMACEUTICALS LTD	HME	PVP	1997
Afeditab	Nifedipine	Elan	Spray drying	PVP	2010
Kaletra	Lopinavir/Ritonavir	ABBVIE INC	HME	PVP/PVA	2005
Intelence	Etarvine	JANSSEN R&D LLC	Spray drying	HPMC	2008
Zortress	Everolimus	JANSSEN R&D LLC	Spray drying	HPMC	2010
Norvir	Ritonavir	ABBVIE INC	HME	PVPVA	2010
Onmel	Itraconazole	SEBELA IRELAND LTD	HME	HPMC	2010
Afinitor	Everolimus	NOVARTIS PHARMACEUTICALS CORP	Spray drying	HPMC	2010
Incivek	Telaprevir	VERTEX PHARMACEUTICALS INC	Spray drying	HPMCAS	2011
Zelboraf	Vemurafenib	HOFFMANN LA ROCHE INC	Microprecipitation	HPMCAS	2011
Noxafil	Posaconazole	MERCK SHARP AND DOHME CORP	HME	HPMCAS	2013
Belsomra	Suvorexant	MERCK SHARP AND DOHME CORP	HME	PVPVA	2014
Viekira XR	Dasabuvir sodium, Ombitasvir, Paritaprevir, Ritonavir	ABBVIE INC	HME	PVP	2016
Venclexta	Venetoclax	ABBVIE INC	HME	PVPVA	2016
Kalydeco	Ivacaftor	VERTEX PHARMACEUTICALS INC	Spray drying	HPMCAS	2019

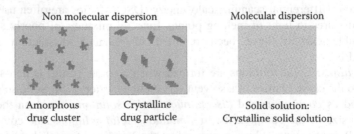

FIGURE 17.6 Solid dispersion at a non-molecular and molecular level.

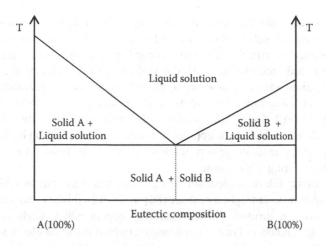

FIGURE 17.7 Phase diagram for a eutectic system [76].

solid solutions, solid solubility exists only at specific compositions of the mixture rather than over the entire compositional range [77]. Each component is completely miscible with the other component in specific compositional regions (α and β). The solubilization of one component in the other is temperature-dependent (Figure 17.8).

3. *Glass Solutions:* In glass solutions, the carrier is amorphous and the solute is molecularly dispersed in the amorphous carrier. It is a homogeneous single-phase system (characterized by a single T_g) in which the drug molecule is dissolved in a glassy solvent. Glass solutions are comparable to liquid solutions as the drug's particle size is reduced to its absolute minimum – the molecular dimension [78]. Unlike crystalline dispersion, the active is present as an amorphous form in glass solution, which further improves drug solubility by removing the lattice energy associated with the crystalline structure, according to Yalkowsky's general solubility equation:

$$\log S_w = 0.5 - \log K_{ow} - 0.001(MP - 25) \tag{17.6}$$

where S_w is aqueous solubility, K_{ow} is partition coefficient (octanol/water), and MP is the melting point of the drug [79].

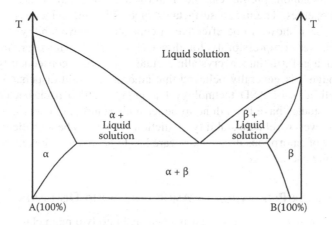

FIGURE 17.8 Typical phase diagram of solid solution [76].

Glass solutions may only be thermodynamically stable at low concentrations. Though it is generally believed that solid solutions could potentially improve drug dissolution, they are usually supersaturated with the intent to achieve higher drug loads; hence, they are prone to recrystallization and precipitation during dissolution. Recrystallization may be retarded by kinetic stabilization. Phase separation is the first step before recrystallization. For phase separation to occur, a certain degree of molecular mobility within the system will be required which may be slowed downed by storing solid solutions below the glass transition temperature (T_g). Careful selection of appropriate polymers that result in higher T_g and including antinucleating components in the formulation would also be helpful to limit recrystallization and precipitation during dissolution.

4. *Glass Suspensions:* Glass suspension is a homogeneous system in which the amorphous drug is suspended in an amorphous carrier [80]. If the miscibility of an amorphous drug in an amorphous carrier is limited, phase separation occurs which leads to the formation of amorphous drug-rich and polymer-rich domains (which could be characterized by two T_gs). Formulations that provide glass solutions at low drug loading may also transition to a glass suspension at higher concentrations. Because the drug is still in an amorphous form, it shows increased dissolution behavior compared to the crystalline form; however, it has a higher likelihood of recrystallization.

Though DSC and X-ray diffraction (XRD) studies are frequently conducted to provide interpretations to the properties of amorphous solid dispersions, the detection of ASD structure is not as simple as one may imagine. Questions still remain as to whether the active is dispersed at a molecular level to form a glass solution or is present as a separated amorphous phase, even though drug crystalline fusion energy is not detected in thermal analysis such as DSC. Great progress has been made by the work of Zografi et al. as well as others in the past few decades to better understand the basis of amorphous systems [81–84]. Compared to the crystalline counterpart, ASD are likely to improve the drug solubility and dissolution rate up to several hundred orders of magnitudes [85].

Vasconcelos et al. classified solid dispersions based on the composition and complexity of their formulations (Fig. 17.9) [86]. First-generation solid dispersions were prepared using crystalline carriers such as urea and sugar, which were the first carriers to be employed in solid dispersion. Second-generation solid dispersions include amorphous carriers which are usually polymers. These polymers include synthetic polymers such as povidone (PVP), polyethylene glycols (PEG), and polymethacrylate as well as cellulosic polymers such as hydroxypropyl methylcellulose (HPMC), ethylcellulose (EC), and hydroxypropyl cellulose (HPC). In third generation, it has been recently shown that the dissolution profile can be improved if the carrier has surface activity or self-emulsifying properties. The use of surfactants such as inulin, Gelucire 44/14, and Poloxamer 407 as carriers has been shown to be effective in enhancing bioavailability.

ASDs provide better compressibility for direct compression. However, most ASDs are not stable and tend to transform into a crystalline state over time, consequently losing solubility improvement. Though it is generally believed that amorphous solid dispersion can improve drug solubility, the application of ASD technology has greatly settled back because of the stability concern. Extensive studies have been done to better understand the factors governing amorphous stability recently; however, reliable stability prediction remains to be a challenge. Due to the very high hygroscopicity of amorphous drugs, extra care has to be taken to prevent moisture absorption during manufacturing and storage.

17.5.2 METHODS FOR PREPARATION OF AMORPHOUS SOLID DISPERSIONS

ASD manufacturing technologies are primarily classified into two main classes, solvent-based and non-solvent. Solvent-based technologies include spray drying, spray coating, coprecipitation, freeze-drying, electrospinning, supercritical fluid-based technologies, and microprecipitation. Non-solvent technologies include milling, ultrasonic-assisted compaction, melt granulation, melt extrusion, generally known as HME, and Kinetisol [87].

17.5.2.1 Hot-Melt Method

The hot-melt method to prepare solid dispersion was first demonstrated by Sekiguchi and Obi [70]. They produced an eutectic mixture consisting of sulfathiazole and a water-soluble inert carrier, urea. The active ingredient and the carrier were mixed and heated at a temperature above their melting points until all the components completely melted. The homogenous hot melt was quenched in an ice bath and then milled to reduce the particle size. Though cooling may introduce supersaturation, because of the fast solidification rate, the dispersed active ingredient was trapped within the carrier matrix without phase separation.

Hot-melt extrusion is a significant step forward for the commercial application of the hot-melt method. Hot-melt extrusion is a very common process in the plastics and polymer industry; however, it did not find application in the pharma industry until recently. The plastics industry utilizes single- or twin-screw extruders. In the pharma industry, the twin-screw extruder has gained acceptance due to its inherent design and operational characteristics [88]. A typical twin-screw extruder consists of:

1. An extruder drive motor,
2. A gear box that controls the direction and speed of the screw rotation,
3. Modular barrels with heating and cooling devices to control the barrel temperature and with flexible powder and liquid feed ports, and
4. A twin-screw shaft with modular screw elements configured in a fashion to achieve specific unit operations, and a die (Figure 17.10).

It is an excellently engineered, highly flexible, and controllable equipment. Understanding the process parameters and their impact on the material being processed and, as a result, on the critical quality attributes of the product is key to the successful development and manufacturing of a drug product.

Basic unit operations that take place in a melt extrusion process include feeding, melting and plasticization, melt conveying, mixing, venting/degassing, and pumping. A melt extrusion process can be flexibly designed to accommodate specific unit operations in a specific arrangement in order to manufacture a product with the desired product attributes. In the design of the process, it is imperative to understand the property of the material to be processed and the interactive impact of formulation parameters and process parameters on the quality attributes of the product.

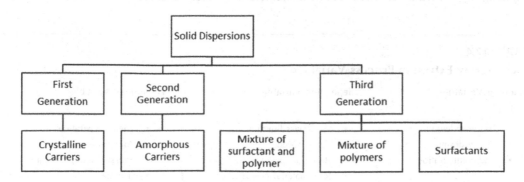

FIGURE 17.9 Classification of solid dispersions [86].

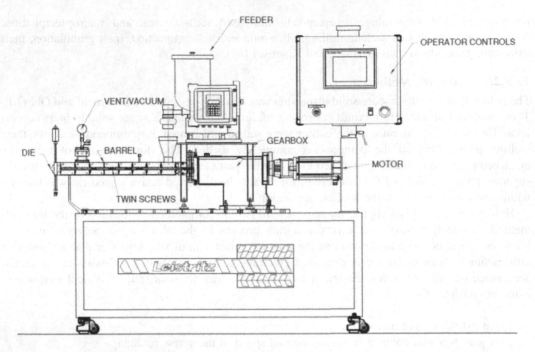

FIGURE 17.10 Scheme of a twin-screw extruder (leistritz, usa).

Twin-screw extrusion process parameters and variables can be classified into machine variables, independent process variables, and dependent variables [89,90] as shown in Table 17.4.

Hot-melt extrusion (HME) is currently one of the cutting-edge solubility enhancement manufacturing technologies that pharmaceutical development scientists consider when formulating poorly soluble drug substances to manufacture ASD-based products. In 1991, Ghebre-Sellassie introduced the use of HME process into the industry to enhance the solubility of troglitazone, a very poorly soluble drug that was approved by the Food and Drug Administration in 1997 [1].

Once HME was introduced for ASD manufacturing, many companies successfully utilized the process and got approval for commercial use. It is expected that many more ASD-based products made by HME would be approved in the coming years. The versatility of the twin-screw extrusion process would allow the use of more complex solubility enhancement formulations, and being a continuous process, its amenability to process analytical technology (PAT) would make it more desired for drug manufacturers as well as drug regulatory bodies [91].

As an illustration, the following unpublished case study provides insight into the successful application of HME as an efficient ASD manufacturing process to enhance the bioavailability of a

TABLE 17.4
Twin Screw Extrusion Process Variables

Machine Variables	Independent Variables	Dependent Variable
• Extruder length	• Feed/mass flow rate	• Melt temperature
• Screw design	• Screw speed	• Melt pressure
• Die configuration	• Barrel temperature	• Pressure along the barrel
	• Raw material properties	• Torque

poorly soluble drug as compared to a commercial product that was prepared by a solvent-based ASD manufacturing process [92]. The drug substance was a BCS Class IV molecule having an aqueous solubility of less than 1 µg/mL. An ASD of the drug substance was prepared in a PVP-based formulation. The formulation components were carefully mixed to obtain a uniform free-flowing pre-extrusion blend. The blend was melt-extruded at controlled processing conditions and pelletized to the appropriate size. The pellets were then filled into a capsule and stored in induction-sealed HDPE bottles with desiccant. A 12-human subject crossover biostudy against a marketed reference product consisting of spray-coated pellets was conducted in a fasted and fed state. The plasma concentration of the parent substance and the active metabolite were measured. As a result, the HME and the reference product AUC_∞ (ng/mL × h) were in fasted states 6704 and 4621, respectively, and in fed states 8074 and 3657, respectively. The HME capsules had a total exposure of 1.5- to 2.2-fold, which could potentially reduce the dose by 50%.

A less commonly used hot-melt method is spray congealing. In a general sense, spray congealing is quite similar to spray drying and also consists of an atomizer, cooling chamber, cyclone recovery, and separation unit [93]. A hot-molten slurry is formed by the melting of active ingredients and the thermoplastic polymer and then sprayed out of the atomizer to form droplets. These droplets are quickly solidified by the heat sink provided by cooled process airflow inside the cooling chamber. The cooled free-flowing particles are collected by cyclone recovery. As with spray drying, spray congealing usually yields particles of similar size and shape. However, properties such as density, moisture, and friability are most often independent of the process because, unlike spray drying, no mass transfer is involved in the solidifying of the droplets. Spray congealing also yields very fine particles and may enhance the drug dissolution rate by increasing specific surface area.

Novel technology in the manufacture of amorphous solid dispersion is KinetiSol®, a fusion-based process that utilizes frictional and shear energies to rapidly transition drug and polymer blend into a molten state. KinetiSol® rapidly and thoroughly mixes the active ingredient with its carrier on a molecular level to achieve a single-phase ASD system. The processing time is less than 20 seconds, and elevated temperatures are observed for typically less than 5 seconds before discharge and cooling. It is claimed that the process is applicable to a high melting point (>225°C) drug substances [94].

17.5.2.2   Solvent Evaporation Method

The solvent evaporation method provides another common way to prepare solid dispersions comprising of the active ingredient(s) and carrier(s). The active ingredient is forced into intimate contact with the carrier by dissolving them together in a common solvent(s). The homogeneous solution is then converted into a solid state by removing the solvent quickly. An important prerequisite for the application of the solvent evaporation method is that both the active ingredient and the carrier are sufficiently soluble or dispersible in the common solvent. Spray-drying technology is the most frequently used process to prepare solid dispersion on a continuous basis. Figure 17.11 shows the unit operations involved in a common spraying process.

The success of spray-drying technology attributes to its ability to not only remove the solvent rapidly, but also control the properties of the powder products: particle size, distribution, shape, uniformity, bulk density, and even particle configuration [95]. Coffee, detergent, milk, and excipient industry are excellent examples of spray-drying technology industry applications. The capability of rapid solvent removal also makes this technology a good fit for the preparation of ASD. In the spray-drying process, rapid solvent evaporation rapidly "freezes" the actives into the glass matrix and prevents the conversion from an amorphous state to a crystalline state. The spray-drying process consists of the following steps: (i) formation of a solution containing the active and the carrier; (ii) the solution is then atomized into fine droplets; (iii) the droplet is exposed to a heated gas media for drying; and (iv) the dry free-flowing powder is collected. However, the

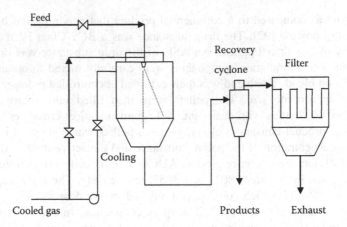

FIGURE 17.11 Main components of a typical spray drier [93].

particle formation process may not be as simple as one can imagine. Figure 17.12 presents the mechanism of particle formation in spray drying.

Many aspects of the particle formation process in spray drying are controlled by the relationship between surface recession and diffusion of the solutes. Radial demixing of components may occur during the drying process because of different diffusion rates of the components [96,97]. For drug/polymer solid dispersion system, a polymer-rich outer layer will be structured outside the solid dispersion particles because of the much less diffusion rate of polymer compared with drug molecules and could result in a delay of the onset of drug release. Although the radial demixing effect is not desired in most situations of solid dispersions, it does lead to the successful design of structured microparticles with functional layers, which can be used to further modify drug release behavior.

Powder density of spray-dried ASD can vary considerably and is typically a function of the level of solids in the spray-drying solution and the nature of the matrix polymer. During the rapid solvent evaporation at the droplet surface, a continuous polymer film forms trapping excess solvent which can result in ballooning at the particle surface leading to low bulk density particles with complete drying. By comparison, melt extrusion powders tend to have higher bulk density when compared to spray-dried powders.

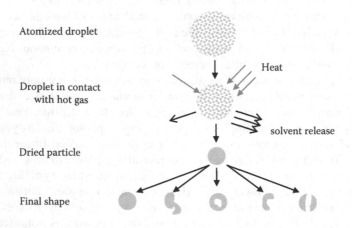

FIGURE 17.12 Mechanism of particle formation during spray drying [93].

17.5.3 CARRIERS

17.5.3.1 Polyethylene Glycol

PEGs are polymers of ethylene oxide, with an MW falling in the range of 200 to 300,000. As the MW increases, so does the viscosity. At MW up to 600, PEGs are liquid; in the range of 800 to 1500, they are semi-solid; from 2000 to 6000, they are waxy, and those with MW of 20,000 and above change to hard, brittle crystals at room temperature. Their solubility in water is generally good, but the dissolution rate decreases with increasing MW. The melting point of PEG is in a range of 37°C to 65°C and decreases as MW decreases [98].

The relatively low-melting points are advantageous for the manufacture of solid dispersion using the hot-melt extrusion method, especially for those heat-sensitive compounds. PEGs with MW of 1500 to 20,000 are usually employed in the manufacture of solid dispersion because in this MW range, the water solubility is still relatively high and the melting point is also high enough to produce pharmaceutical acceptable solids.

PEG 8000 was used to form a eutectic mixture with fenofibrate [99]. The study showed the eutectic composition by generating a phase diagram using hot-stage microscopy (HSM) and DSC. The *in vitro* dissolution study proved the improved solubility and dissolution rates of the eutectics solid dispersion compared with the pure drug. The dissolution rates and solubility were also found to increase as the PEG composition increased in the eutectics mixture. PEG is also used to prepare amorphous solid dispersion. A class IV drug, ritonavir, was selected to prepare amorphous solid dispersion with PEG 8000 [100]. The *in vitro* evaluation showed five-fold increases in solubility compared with a physical mixture of the same formulation. The bioavailability in beagle dogs showed a maximum of a 22-fold increase in AUC_{0-24hr} over the physical mixture. The importance of the PEG MW to the performance of the eutectic solid dispersion was illustrated in a study of five poorly water-soluble compounds formulated as eutectics with PEG 3350, PEG 8000, and PEG 20000 [101]. The study showed that the influence of PEG MW on dissolution performance is dictated by the drug--carrier interactions. Compounds with specific interaction with the carrier will have higher eutectic composition and faster dissolution than with lower MW PEG. The drug/carrier ratio apparently is another main influence on the performance of solid dispersion. If the percentage of the drug is too high, it will exceed the eutectic composition and form a separated crystalline region.

In general, PEG is an ideal carrier to form eutectic solid dispersion. However, its application in forming ASD is limited because of amorphous drug stability. Compared with other polymer carriers, the chain length of the PEG is still very short and incapable of amorphous stabilization, especially at high drug loading. Another limitation of PEG lies in the subsequent formulation into an acceptable solid dosage form. Solid dispersion in low MW PEG is often too soft and presents challenges to manufacture a tablet dosage form. For tablet formulations, the use of polyethylene oxides (higher MW) may be more appropriate.

17.5.3.2 Polyvinylpyrrolidone and Polyvinylpyrrolidone-Polyvinyl Acetate Copolymer

Polymerization of vinylpyrrolidone leads to PVP of MW ranging from 2500 to 3,000,000. The MW of PVP is specified by the K value, which is calculated using Fikentscher's equation (102).

PVP is an amorphous polymer with relatively high glass transition temperature, for example, glass transition temperature for PVP K30 has T_g of 163°C [98]. For this reason, PVP has limited application for the preparation of solid dispersion using hot-melt extrusion. The glass transition temperature also increases as MW increases. Because of their good solubility in a wide variety of organic solvents, they are particularly suitable for the preparation of solid dispersion using the solvent method. PVPs are also freely soluble in water, and their aqueous solubility decreases as the MW increases. The very good solubility can improve the wettability of the dispersed compound in many cases and offers improved dissolution rates.

The chain length of the PVP has a very significant influence on the dissolution rate of the dispersed compound from the solid dispersion. As the chain length increases, the aqueous solubility of PVP decreases, and the viscosity increases at a given concentration. Studies with coprecipitates of chloramphenicol and PVP revealed that the dissolution of chloramphenicol was reduced when high MW PVP was used as a carrier [103]. Similarly, the slower dissolution of indomethacin from PVP K90 compared with PVP K12 was attributed to the higher viscosity generated by PVP K90 in the diffusion boundary layer adjacent to the dissolving surface of the dispersion [104]. The dissolution rates of sulfathiazole and phenytoin were also found reduced as high MW PVPs were used as dispersion agent [105,106].

The drug/PVP ratio is another very important factor governing the drug release rate. It is not difficult to understand that the decrease of drug load leads to a higher dissolution rate of the dispersed compound because of the improvement of fineness of dispersion, for example, the dissolution rate of albendazole was found to decrease as formulated with less amount of PVP [107]. However, this is not always the case. In the case of the piroxicam/PVP solid dispersion system, the release rate increased as the drug/PVP ratio increased from 1:6 up to 1:4, after which the release fell again [108]. The XRD studies revealed that only the dispersion at 1:4 drug/PVP ratio was amorphous, all other formulations were either crystalline or semi-crystalline. The 1:4 ratio proved to be the optimal solid dispersion formula for the piroxicam/PVP K30 system.

It is well recognized that PVP facilitates the preparation of ASD. Simvastatin and PVP were prepared by the spray-drying process [109]. Initial characterizations of combined IR, DSC, and XRPD analysis confirmed the presence of amorphous simvastatin dispersed in PVP. The dissolution studies showed that the amorphous solid dispersion presented significant increases in both dissolution rate and saturation solubility over their dry blend. The *in vivo* evaluation in rats also justified the improvement in the therapeutic efficacy of the ASD over the crystalline counterpart.

The biggest challenge of the ASD in practice is their physical stability. The amorphous drug is not physically stable and tends to transform into crystalline counterpart, which does not have the dissolution and solubility advantages as the amorphous drug presents. PVP is not only well known as a solubilizer in solid dispersion, it is also widely recognized as a very effective amorphous stabilizer. Studies on celecoxib–PVP–meglumine ternary system suggested that PVP functions more as stabilizers and meglumine functions more like solubility enhancers in their amorphous solid dispersion [110]. The dissolution rate and saturation solubility of nilvadipine were found substantially decreased compared with the initial dissolution test of nilvadipine ASD [111]. The amorphous form physical stability of nilvadipine was improved by the use of nilvadipine/PVP/microcrystalline cellulose ternary solid dispersion system.

Polyvinylpyrrolidone/vinyl acetate (PVP/VA) are vinylpyrrolidone-based copolymers with about 40% vinylpyrrolidone being replaced by vinyl acetate. Compared with PVP, PVP/VA is less water-soluble and also has a lower glass transition temperature at the same MW. The use of PVP/VA as a solid dispersion carrier has been shown to lead to enormous increases in drug releases as well as amorphous stability. Poorly water-soluble drugs including indomethacin, lacidipine, nifedipine, and tolbutamide were dispersed into PVP and PVP/VA using hot-melt extrusion method [112]. The studies showed that the formation of glass solution depends on the temperature of melt extrusion. Physical stability difference was also observed between these solid dispersion systems because of the magnitude of hydrogen bonding between the drug and carrier.

17.5.3.3 Soluplus®

Soluplus®, a polyethylene glycol, polyvinyl acetate, and polyvinylcaprolactam-based graft copolymer (PVAc-PVCap-PEG), is a new amorphous amphiphilic polymer that can act as a solubilizer by forming micelles in solution. Its glass transition temperature (T_g) is 70°C and is specifically designed for ASD manufacturing with HME without the need to include a plasticizer. Another advantage of Soluplus® is the low hygroscopicity of the polymer, which will help stabilize the dispersion during storage. Soluplus® could successfully enhance the solubility of carbamaze-pine ([113].

17.5.3.4 Cellulose Derivatives

Celluloses are naturally occurring polysaccharides that are ubiquitous in the plant kingdom. They consist of high MW unbranched chains, in which the saccharide units are linked by b-1–4-glycoside bonds. By appropriate alkylation, the cellulose can be derivatized to form methylcellulose (MC), hydroxypropyl cellulose (HPC), hydroxypropyl methylcellulose (HPMC), and many other semi-synthetic types of cellulose. A further possibility for derivatization is the esterification of the cellulose to form compounds such as hydroxypropyl methylcellulose phthalate (HPMCP) and hypromellose acetate succinate (HPMCAS).

Both HPC and HPMC exhibit good solubility in a range of solvents including cold water. The average MW of the HPCs ranges from 37,000 to 1,150,000. Studies with flurbiprofen showed that the dissolution rate was improved as low MW HPC was used in the solid dispersion [114]. HPMCs have an average MW in a range from 10,000 to 1,500,000, and their glass transition temperatures are as high as 170°C to 180°C. Studies with tacrolimus compared the dissolution profiles of solid dispersions having HPMC, PVP, and PEG as a carriers [115]. Significant increases in dissolution rates were confirmed for the solid dispersions formulated with all these polymers. However, severe precipitation was observed for PVP- and PEG-based solid dispersions due to supersaturation. Though all three polymers were shown equally effective in dissolution rate improvement, their capabilities for maintaining supersaturation were significantly different and the rank order was HPMC > PVP > PEG. Studies with albendazole, a poorly water-soluble compound, showed that the release rate and bioavailability could be improved through the preparation of solid dispersion in HPMC [116]. Other drugs that exhibit faster release from solid dispersion in HPMC include poorly soluble weak acids nilvadipine and benidipine [117,118].

HPMCPs are cellulose esters, often used as enteric coatings but also investigated in ASD development. Their average MW ranges from 20,000 to 2,000,000. Depending on their grades, they dissolve at pH 5 (HP50) or pH 5.5 (HP55). Griseofulvin was transformed into the amorphous state by dispersing in HPMCP using the evaporation method [119] and exhibited a significant increase in dissolution rate. Using a spray-drying technique to form a solid dispersion in HP55, the dissolution rate of the antifungal drug MFB-1041 could be increased by a factor of 12.5 as compared with that of the micronized drug. Furthermore, the oral bioavailability in beagle dogs was almost 17 times better following the administration of the drug in solid dispersion form [120]. In the studies of poorly water-soluble drug HO-221, it was shown that the dispersion in HPMCP presented the equal release of the drug as the dispersion in pH-independent polymers, PVP and PVP/VA, at pH 6.5 buffer solution [121]. However, the oral bioavailability study in beagle dogs exhibited 30% to 60% absorption for solid dispersion in PVP/VA, whereas it was completely (100%) absorbed for solid dispersion with HPMCP. It was concluded that the incomplete absorption was due to the precipitation of the drug following rapid dissolution and formation of a supersaturated solution in the gastric fluid.

17.5.3.5 Polyacrylates and Polymethacrylates

Polyacrylates and polymethacrylates are glassy materials that are produced by the polymerization of acrylic and methacrylic acid, and derivatives of these polymers such as esters amides and nitriles. They are primarily used in oral capsule and tablet formations as film-coating agents and are commonly known by the trade name of Eudragit®. Eudragit E is often used to improve drug release since it is soluble in gastric fluid below pH 5 and swells at high pH, while Eudragit L and S are water-insoluble and used as desired to avoid release in the stomach. Eudragit L is more permeable than Eudragit S grade, and films of varying permeability can be obtained by mixing the two types together. Their capability of forming a water-insoluble film coat finds most of their pharmaceutical applications in the formation of the sustained-release formulation. Eudragit L has been successfully used to increase the dissolution of griseofulvin and spironolactone at a pH value of 6.8 [119].

17.5.3.6 Surfactants

The release behavior of many poor water-soluble compounds, especially those with very high lipophilicity, can be further improved through the incorporation of a surface-active agent in the solid dispersion. The most frequently used surfactants include polysorbate, sodium lauryl sulfate (SLS), and polyethylene-propylene glycol copolymer (poloxamer). Surface-active agents improve drug release mainly through increasing drug substance wettability and the solubilization effect. It is generally believed that there are two ways that the surfactant provides a solubilization effect to a poorly water-soluble compound. First, the hydrophobic and hydrophilic blocks of the surfactant tend to form structures well known as micelles in an aqueous solution, where drug compounds can be solubilized inside the hydrophobic core of the micelles. Second, the surfactant can also interact with the polymer carrier to form a structure known as aggregate, which can solubilize guest molecules inside the hydrophobic core, for instance, PVP was discovered to form aggregate as the presence of sodium lauryl sulfate in the solution [122,123]. Owing to their potential toxicity, surfactants are usually used carefully in a very small quantity, and they are always used in combination with other carriers. Surfactants may also exert a direct influence on drug absorption through alerting drug transport across the membrane [124]. Using hot-melt extrusion, Tween 80 and SLS were dispersed with API in three different polymers, PVP, PVP/VA, and HPMC. The study showed that significant dissolution rate increases by the surfactant as compared with the solid dispersions without surfactant [125].

REFERENCES

1. Terefe H. The origins of HME as a solubility enhancement manufacturing technology. Am Pharm Rev 2017;5:82–85.
2. United States Pharmacopeia and National Formulary (USP28-NF23) Supplement 1 Paperback – April 1, 2005. USP28/NF23, p. 9., 2005.
3. Amidon G. L., Lennernas H., Shah V. P., et al. A theoretical basis for a biopharmaceutic drug classification: the correlation of in vitro drug product dissolution and in vivo bioavailability. Pharm Res 1995;12:413–420.
4. Center for Drug Evaluation and Research, Waiver of in vivo bioavailability and bioequivalence studies for immediate release solid oral dosage forms based on a biopharmaceutic classification system. FDA, Rockville, USA 2017.
5. Heng P. W. S., Wan L. S. C., Ang T. S. H. Role of surfactants on drug release from tablets. Drug Dev Ind Pharm 2007;16(6):783–789.
6. Parikh D. Advances in spray drying technology: new applications for a proven process. Am Pharm Rev 2008;11(1):34–41.
7. Zheng X., Yang R., Tang X., et al. Part II: bioavailability in beagle dogs of nimodipine prepared by hot melt extrusion. Drug Dev Ind Pharm 2007;33(7):783–789.
8. Noyes AA, Wikipedia, 1897 Available at: http://en.wikipedia.org/wiki/Arthur_Amos_Noyes.
9. Yamamoto K., Nakano M., Arita T., et al. Dissolution rate and bioavailability of griseofulvin from ground mixture with microcrystalline cellulose. J Pharmakin Pharmadyn 1974;2(6):487–493.
10. McInnes G. T., Ashbury M. J., Ramsay L. E., et al. Effect of micronization on the bioavailability and pharmacologic activity of spironolactone. J Clin Pharmacol 1982;22(8–9):410–417.
11. Merisko-Liversidge E. M., Liversidge G. G. Drug nanoparticles: formulating poorly water soluble drugs. Tox Path 2008;36(1):43–48.
12. Soliman O. A. E., Kimura K., Hirayama F., et al. Amorphous spironolactone-hydroxypropylated cyclodextrin complexes with superior dissolution and oral bioavailability. Int J Pharm 1997;149 (1):73–83.
13. Kumar N., Jain A., Singh C., et al. Development, characterization and solubility of solid dispersions of terbinafine hydrochloride by solvent evaporation method. Asian J Pharm 2008;2(3):154–158.

14. Douglas S. J., Davis S. S., Illum L. Nanoparticles in drug delivery. Crit Rev Ther Drug Carrier Syst 1987;3:233–261.

15. Junghanns J. A. H., Müller R. H. Nanocrystal technology, drug delivery, and clinical applications. Int J Nanomed 2008;3(3):295–310.

16. PharmTech.com. The challenges of manufacturing nanoparticles through media milling. PharmTech.com 2008. Available at: http://pharmtech.findpharma.com/pharmtech/Article/The-Challenges-of-Manufacturing-Nanoparticles-thro/ArticleStandard/Article/detail/529752.

17. Panagiotou T., Fisher R. J. Form nanoparticles via controlled crystallization. Chem Engineer Prog 2008;104(10):33–39.

18. Müller R. H., Peters K., Becker R., et al. Nanoparticles – a novel formulation for the IV administration of poorly water soluble drugs. In. 1st World Meeting of the International Meeting on Pharmaceutics, Biopharmaceutics and Pharmaceutical Technology, Budapest, Hungary. 1995.

19. Müller R. H., Jacobs C., Kayser O. Nanosuspensions as particulate drug in therapy: rationale for development and what we can expect for the future. Adv Drug Deliv Rev 2001;471:3–19.

20. Zhou H., Wang J., Wang Q., et al. Controlled liquid antisolvent precipitation of hydrophobic pharmaceutical nanoparticles in a microchannel reactor. Ind Eng Chem Res 2007;46(24):8229–8235.

21. York P. Strategies for particle design using super critical fluid technologies. Pharm Sci Technol Today 1999;2:430–440.

22. Vemavarapu C., Mollan M., Lodaya M., et al. Design and process aspects of laboratory scale SCF particle formation systems. Int J Pharm 2005;292:1–16.

23. Chattopadhyay P., Gupta R. Production of griseofulvin using supercritical CO_2 antisolvent with enhanced mass transfer. Int J Pharm 2001;228(1–2):19–31.

24. Shah N., Sandhu H., Phuapradit W., et al. Development of novel microprecipitated bulk powder (MBR) technology for manufacturing stable amorphous formulations of poorly soluble drugs. Int J Pharm 2012;438(1–2):50–53.

25. Tuomela A., Saarinen J., Strachan C. J., et al. Production, applications and in vivo fate of drug nanocrystals. J Drug Deliv Sci Technol 2016;34:21–31.

26. Connors K. A. The stability of cyclodextrin complexes in solution. Chem Rev 1997;97(5):1325–1357.

27. Loftsson T., Másson M., Brewster M. E. Self-association of cyclodextrins and cyclodextrin complexes. J Pharm Sci 2004;39(5):1091–1099.

28. Schardinger F. Bildung kristallisierter polysaccharide (dextrine) aus stärkekleister durch microben. Centralbl Bakteriol Parasitenkd Abt. II 1911;29(1–3):188–197.

29. Freudenberg K., Meyer-Delius M. Über die Schardinger - Dextrine aus Stärke. Berichte der deutschen chemischen Gesellschaft (A and B Series). 1938;71(8):1596–1600.

30. French D., Pulley A. O., Effenberger J. A., et al. Studies on the Schardinger dextrins: XII. The molecular size and structure of the δ-, ε-, ζ-, and η-dextrins. Arch Biochem Biophys 1965;111(1):153–160.

31. Escotet-Espinoza M. S., Moghtadernejad S., Oka S., et al. Effect of material properties on the residence time distribution (RTD) characterization of powder blending unit operations. Part II of II: Application of models. Powder Technol 2019;344:525–544.

32. Blouquin P., Reginault P. Patent WO02056881. Fournier Tablets. 2002.

33. Szejtli J. Utilization of cyclodextrins in industrial products and processes. J Mater Chem 1997;7(4):575–587.

34. WHO. Evaluation of Certain Food Additives and Contaminants: Forty-Fourth Report of the Joint FAO/WHO Expert Committee on Food Additives. WHO, Geneva 1995.

35. EFSA Panel on Food Additives and Nutrient Sources added to Food (ANS), Mortensen A., Aguilar F., et al. Re-evaluation of β-cyclodextrin (E 459) as a food additive. EFSA J 2016;14(12):e04628.

36. Brewster M. E., Loftsson T. Cyclodextrins as pharmaceutical solubilizers. Adv Drug Deliv Rev 2007;59(7):645–666.

37. Barbosa J. S., Nolasco M. M., Ribeiro-Claro P., et al. Preformulation studies of the γ-cyclodextrin and montelukast inclusion compound prepared by comilling. J Pharm Sci 2019;108(5):1837–1847.

38. Mura P. Analytical techniques for characterization of cyclodextrin complexes in aqueous solution: a review. J Pharm Biomed Anal 2014;101:238–250.

39. Higuchi T., Connors K. A. Phase-solubility techniques. In: Reilley C., editor. Advances in Analytical Chemistry and Instrumentation. Interscience, New York 1965. p. 117–212.

40. Cirri M., Maestrelli F., Orlandini S., et al. Determination of stability constant values of flurbiprofen-cyclodextrin complexes using different techniques. J Pharm Biomed Anal 2005;37(5):995–1002.

41. El-Saleh M. C., Stoyanov E. The use of cyclodextrins in preparing a paediatric oral liquid dosage form

of Loratadine In. 10th World Meeting on Pharmaceutics, Biopharmaceutics and Pharmaceutical Technology. Glasgow, UK: APV; 2016. p. 60.

42. Abdoh A. A., Zughul M. B., Davies J. E. D., et al. Inclusion complexation of diclofenac with natural and modified cyclodextrins explored through phase solubility, 1H-NMR and molecular modeling studies. J Incl Phenom Macrocycl Chem 2007;57(1):503–510.

43. Braga S. S., Gonçalves I. S., Herdtweck E., et al. Solid state inclusion compound of S-ibuprofen in β-cyclodextrin: structure and characterisation. New J Chem 2003;27(3):597–601.

44. Caira M. R., Dodds D. R. Inclusion of nonopiate analgesic drugs in cyclodextrins. II. X-ray structure of a 1: 1 β-cyclodextrin - acetaminophen complex. J Incl Phenom Macrocyc Chem 2000;38(1):75–84.

45. Garcia-Rio L., Herves P., Leis J. R., et al. Evidence for complexes of different stoichiometries between organic solvents and cyclodextrins. Org Biomol Chem 2006;4(6):1038–1048.

46. Salustio P. J., Feio G., Figueirinhas J. L., et al. The influence of the preparation methods on the inclusion of model drugs in a beta-cyclodextrin cavity. Eur J Pharm Biopharm 2009;71(2):377–386.

47. Miletic T., Kyriakos K., Graovac A., et al. Spray-dried voriconazole-cyclodextrin complexes: solubility, dissolution rate and chemical stability. Carbohydr Polym 2013;98(1):122–131.

48. Mihajlovic T., Kachrimanis K., Graovac A., et al. Improvement of aripiprazole solubility by complexation with (2-hydroxy)propyl-beta-cyclodextrin using spray drying technique. AAPS PharmSciTech 2012;13(2):623–631.

49. Alonso E. C., Riccomini K., Silva L. A., et al. Development of carvedilol-cyclodextrin inclusion complexes using fluid-bed granulation: a novel solid-state complexation alternative with technological advantages. J Pharm Pharmacol 2016;68(10):1299–1309.

50. Zhang X., Wu D., Lai J., et al. Piroxicam/2-hydroxypropyl-beta-cyclodextrin inclusion complex prepared by a new fluid-bed coating technique. J Pharm Sci 2009;98(2):665–675.

51. Sule A., Szente L., Csempesz F. Enhancement of drug solubility in supramolecular and colloidal systems. J Pharm Sci 2009;98(2):484–494.

52. Vieira A. C. C., Ferreira Fontes D. A., Chaves L. L., et al. Multicomponent systems with cyclodextrins and hydrophilic polymers for the delivery of Efavirenz. Carbohyd Polym 2015;130:133–140.

53. Medarevic D., Kachrimanis K., Djuric Z., et al. Influence of hydrophilic polymers on the complexation of carbamazepine with hydroxypropyl-beta-cyclodextrin. Eur J Pharm Sci 2015;78:273–285.

54. Jug M., Becirevic-Lacan M. Multicomponent complexes of piroxicam with cyclodextrins and hydroxypropyl methylcellulose. Drug Dev Ind Pharm 2004;30(10):1051–1060.

55. Gil A., Chamayou A., Leverd E., et al. Evolution of the interaction of a new chemical entity, eflucimibe, with γ-cyclodextrin during kneading process. Eur J Pharm Sci 2004;23(2):123–129.

56. Hutin S., Chamayou A., Avan J. L., et al. Analysis of a kneading process to evaluate drug substance-cyclodextrin complexation. Pharm Tech 2004;28(10):112–124.

57. Meier R., Thommes M., Rasenack N., et al. Granule size distributions after twin-screw granulation – Do not forget the feeding systems. Eur J Pharm Biopharm 2016;106:59–69.

58. Fukuda M., Miller D. A., Peppas N. A., et al. Influence of sulfobutyl ether β-cyclodextrin (Captisol®) on the dissolution properties of a poorly soluble drug from extrudates prepared by hot-melt extrusion. Int J Pharm 2008;350(1–2):188–196.

59. Yoshii H., Furuta T., Okita E., et al. The increased effect of kneading on the formation of inclusion complexes between d-limonene and b-cyclodextrin at low water content. Biosci Biotechnol Biochem 1998;62(3):464–468.

60. Gazzaniga A., Sangalli M. E., Bruni G., et al. The use of β-cyclodextrin as a pelletization agent in the extrusion/ spheronization process. Drug Dev Ind Pharm 1998;24(9):869–873.

61. Yano H., Kleinebudde P. Improvement of dissolution behavior for poorly water-soluble drug by application of cyclodextrin in extrusion process: comparison between melt extrusion and wet extrusion. AAPS PharmSciTech 2010;11(2):885–893.

62. Malaquias L. F. B., Sa-Barreto L. C. L., Freire D. O., et al. Taste masking and rheology improvement of drug complexed with beta-cyclodextrin and hydroxypropyl-beta-cyclodextrin by hot-melt extrusion. Carbohydr Polym 2018;185:19–26.

63. Thiry J., Krier F., Ratwatte S., et al. Hot-melt extrusion as a continuous manufacturing process to form ternary cyclodextrin inclusion complexes. Eur J Pharm Sci 2017;96:590–597.

64. Borba P. A. A., Pinotti M., Andrade G. R. S., et al. The effect of mechanical grinding on the formation, crystalline changes and dissolution behaviour of the inclusion complex of telmisartan and β-cyclodextrins. Carbohydr Polym 2015;133:373–383.

65. Braga S. S., El-Saleh F., Oliveira C. L., et al. Co-amorphisation of simvastatin and β-cyclodextrin. In.

World Meeting on Pharmaceutics, Biopharmaceutics and Pharmaceutical Technology. Glasgow: APV; 2016.

66. Mura P., Bettinetti G. P., Cirri M., et al. Solid-state characterization and dissolution properties of naproxen-arginine-hydroxypropyl-beta-cyclodextrin ternary system. Eur J Pharm Biopharm 2005;59(1):99–106.

67. Kong R., Zhu X., Meteleva E. S., et al. Physicochemical characteristics of the complexes of simvastatin and atorvastatin calcium with hydroxypropyl-β-cyclodextrin produced by mechanochemical activation. J Drug Deliv Sci Technol 2018;46:436–445.

68. Bates T. R. Dissolution characteristics of reserpine-polyvinylpyrrolidone co-precipitates. J Pharm Pharmacol 1969;21:710–712.

69. Chiou W. L., Riegelman S. Pharmaceutical applications of solid dispersion systems. J Pharm Sci 1971;60(9):1281–1302.

70. Sekiguchi K., Obi N. Studies on absorption of eutectic mixture sulfathiazole and that of ordinary sulfathiazole in man. Chem Pharm Bull 1961;9:866–872.

71. Baghel S., Cathcart H., O'Reilly N. J. Polymeric amorphous solid dispersions: a review of amorphization, crystallization, stabilization, solid-state characterization, and aqueous solubilization of biopharmaceutical classification system class ii drugs. J Pharm Sci 2016;105(9):2527–2544.

72. US Food and Drug Administration, Approved Drug Products with Therapeutic Equivalence Evaluations, Orange Book, Rockville, USA. Available at: www.accessdata.fda.gov/scripts/cder/ob/index.cfm.

73. Zhang J., Han R., Chen W., et.al. Analysis of the literature and patents on solid dispersions from 1980 to 2015. Molecules 2018;23:1697.

74. Craig D. Q. M. The mechanisms of drug release from solid dispersions in water-soluble polymers. Int J Pharm 2002;231:131–144.

75. Moore M. D., Wildfong P. L. D., Aqueous solubility enhancement through engineering of binary solid composites: pharmaceutical application. J Pharm Innov 2009;4(1):36–49.

76. Leuner C. Improving drug solubility for oral delivery using solid dispersions. Eur J Pharm Biopharm 2000;50:47–60.

77. Bhatnagar P., Dhote V., Mahajan S. C., et al. Solid dispersion in pharmaceutical drug development: from basics to clinical applications. Curr Drug Deliv 2014;11:155–171.

78. Goldberg A. H., Gibaldi M., Kanig J. L. Increasing dissolution rates and gastrointestinal absorption of drug via solid solutions and eutectic mixtures. I. Theoretic consideration and discussion of the literature. J Pharm Sci 1965;55:482–487.

79. Yalkowsky S. Aqueous Solubility: Methods of Estimation for Organic Compounds. Marcel Dekker Inc, UK 1991.

80. Sakari M., Brown T., Chen X., et al. Enhanced drug dissolution using evaporative precipitation into aqueous solutions. Int J Pharm 2002;243:17–31.

81. Hancock B. C., Shamblin S. L., Zografi G. Molecular mobility of amorphous pharmaceutical solids below their glass transition temperature. Pharm Res 1995;12:799–806.

82. Taylor L., Zografi G. Spectroscopic characterization of interactions between PVP and indomethacin in amorphous molecular dispersions. Pharm Res 1997;14:1691–1698.

83. Matsumoto T., Zografi G. Physical properties of solid molecular dispersions of indomethacin with poly (vinylpyrrolidone) and poly(vinylepyrrolidone-co-vinyl-acetate) in relation to indomethacin crystallization. Pharm Res 1999;16:1722–1728.

84. Guo Y., Byrn S. R., Zografi G. Effects of lyophilization on the physical characteristics and chemical stability of amorphous quinapril hydrochloride. Pharm Res 2000;17:930–935.

85. Blagden N., Matas M., Gavan P. T., et al. Crystal engineering of active pharmaceutical ingredients to improve solubility and dissolution rates. Adv Drug Deliv Rev 2007;59:617–630.

86. Vasconcelos T., Sarmento B., Costa P. Solid dispersions as strategy to improve oral bioavailability of poor water soluble drugs. Drug Discov Today 2007;12(23–24):1068–1075.

87. Shah N., Sandhu H., Choi D. S., et al. Amorphous Solid Dispersions: Theory and Practice. Springer, Switzerland AG 2014.

88. Breitenbach J., Grabowski S., Rosenberg J. Extrusion von polymer wirkstoff-gemischen zur herstellung von areneiformen. Spekt d wissenschaft 1995;11:18–20.

89. Ghebre-Sellassie I., Martin C., Zhang F., et al. Pharmaceutical Extrusion Technology. 2nd ed. CRC Press, Florida 2018.

90. Giles H. F., Wagner J. R., Mount E. M. Extrusion – The definitive processing guide and handbook. Willam Andrew Inc., New York 2005.

91. Terefe H., Ghebre-Sellassie I. Comparative assessment of spray drying and hot melt extrusion as manufacturing processes for amorphous solid dispersions - part I: historical perspective. Am Pharm Rev 2019;22:6.

92. Terefe H. ExxPharma Therapeutics LLC, Unpublished study.

93. Killeen M. J. The process of spray drying and spray congealing. Pharm Eng 1993;14:57–64.

94. DiNunzio J. C., Brough C., Miller D. A., et al. Application of KinetiSol® dispersing for the production of plasticizer free amorphous solid dispersions. Eur J Pharm Sci 2010;40:179–187.

95. Mujumdar A. S., Filkova I. Drying '91. Elsevier Science Publishers, Amsterdam 1991. p. 55–73.

96. Vehring R., Foss W. R., Lechuga-Ballesteros D. Particle formation in spray drying. J Aerosol Sci 2007;38:728–746.

97. Chow A. H., Tong H. H. Y., Chattopadhyay P., et al. Particle engineering for pulmonary drug delivery. Pharm Res 2007;24:411–437.

98. Rowe R. C., Sheskey P. J., Weller P. J. Handbook of Pharmaceutical Excipients. 4th ed. Pharmaceutical Press, London and Chicago 2003.

99. Law D., Wang W., Schmitt E. A., et al. Properties of rapidly dissolving eutectic mixtures of poly (ethylene glycol) and fenofibrate: the eutectic microstructure. J Pharm Sci 2002;92:505–515.

100. Law D., Wang W., Schimitt E. A., et al. Ritonavir-PEG 8000 amorphous solid dispersions: in vitro and in vivo evaluation. J Pharm Sci 2003;93:563–570.

101. Vippagunta S. R., Wang Z., Horhung S., et al. Factors affecting the formation of eutectic solid dispersions and their dissolution behavior. J Pharm Sci 2006;94:294–304.

102. Robinson B. V., Sullivan F. M., Borzelleca J. F., et al. PVP: A Critical Review of the Kinetics and Toxicology of Polyvinylpyrrolidone (Povidone). Lewis Publishers Inc., Boca Raton 1990.p. 11–14.

103. Kassem A. A., Zaki S. A., Mursi N. M., et al. Chloramphenicol solid dispersion system I. Pharm Ind 1979;41:390–393.

104. Hilton J. E., Summers M. P. The effect of wetting agents on the dissolution of indomethacin solid dispersion systems. Int J Pharm 1986;31:157–164.

105. Simonelli A. P., Metha S. C., Higuchi W. I. Dissolution rates of high energy polyvinylpyrrolidone (PVP)-sulfathiazole coprecipitates. J Pharm Sci 1969;58:538–549.

106. Jachowicz R. Dissolution rates of partially water-soluble drugs from solid dispersion systems. II. Phenytoin Int J Pharm 1987;35:7–12.

107. Torrado S., Torrado J. J., Cadorniga R. Preparation, dissolution and characterization of albendazole solid dispersions. Int J Pharm 1996;140:247–250.

108. Tantishaiyakul V., Kaewnopparat N., Ingkatawornwong S. Properties of solid dispersions of piroxicam in polyvinylpyrrolidone K-30. Int J Pharm 1996;140:59–66.

109. Ambike A. A., Mahadik K. R., Paradkar A. Spray-dried amorphous solid dispersions of simvastatin, a low T_g drug: in vitro and in vivo evaluation. Pharm Res 2005;22:990–998.

110. Gupta P., Bansal A. K. Molecular interactions in celecoxib-PVP-meglumine amorphous system. J Pharm Pharmacol 2004;57:303–310.

111. Hirasawa N., Ishise S., Miyata H., et al. An attempt to stabilize nilvadipine solid dispersion by the use of ternary systems. Drug Dev Ind Pharm 2003;29:997–1004.

112. Kondo N., Iwao T., Hirai K., et al. Improved oral absorption of enteric coprecipitates of poorly water soluble drug. J Pharm Sci 1994;83:566–570.

113. Hu V. C. Y., Tajber L., Erxleben A., et al. Amorphous solid dispersions of sulfonamide/Soluplus® and sulfonamide/PVP prepared by ball milling. AAPS PharmSciTech 2013;14(1):464–474.

114. Yuasa H., Ozeki T., Takahashi H., et al. Application of the solid dispersion method to the controlled release of medicine. 6. Release mechanism of a slightly water soluble medicine and interaction between flurbiprofen and hydroxypropyl cellulose in solid dispersion. Chem Pharm Bull 1994;42:354–358.

115. Yamashita K., Nakate T., Okimoto K., et al. Establishment of new preparation method for solid dispersion formulation of tacrolimus. Int J Pharm 2003;267:79–91.

116. Kohri N., Yamayoshi Y., Xin H., et al. Improving the oral bioavailability of albendazole in rabbits by the solid dispersion techniques. J Pharm Pharmacol 1999;51:159–164.

117. Okimoto K., Miyake M., Ibuki R., et al. Dissolution mechanism and rate of solid dispersion particles of nilvadipine with hydroxypropylmethylcellulose. Int J Pharm 1997;159:85–93.

118. Suzuki M., Miyamoto N., Masada T., et al. Solid dispersions of benidipine hydrochloride. 1. Preparations using different solvent systems and dissolution properties. Chem Pharm Bull 1996;44:364–371.

119. Hasegawa A., Kawamura R., Nakagawa H., et al. Physical properties of solid dispersions of poorly water soluble drugs with enteric coating agents. Chem Pharm Bull 1985;33:354–358.

120. Kai T., Akiyama Y., Nomura S., et al. Oral absorption improvement of poorly soluble drug using solid dispersion technique. Chem Pharm Bull 1996;44:567–571.
121. Foster A., Hempenstall J., Tades T. Characterization of glass solutions of poorly water soluble drugs produced by melt extrusion with hydrophilic amorphous polymers. J Pharm Pharmacol 2000;53:303–315.
122. Nagarajan R. Solubilization of "guest" molecules into polymeric aggregates. Polym Adv Technol 2001;12:23–43.
123. Lange V. H. Wechselwirkung zwischen natriumalkylsulfaten und polyvinylpyrrolidone in wassrigen losungen. Kolloid-Z uZ Polymers 1971;243:101–109.
124. Malmsten M. Surfactants and Polymers in Drug Delivery. Marcel Dekker, Inc., New York 2002.
125. Ghebremeskel A. N., Vemavarapu C., Lodaya M. Use of surfactants as plasticizers in preparing solid dispersions of poorly soluble API: selection of polymer-surfactant combinations using solubility parameters and testing the processability. Int J Pharm 2007;328:119–129.

18 Granulation and Production Approaches of Orally Disintegrating Tablets

Tansel Comoglu and Fatemeh Bahadori

CONTENTS

18.1   DESCRIPTIONS OF ORALLY DISINTEGRATING DOSAGE FORMS

Orally disintegrating dosage forms or orally disintegrating tablets (ODT) are solid dosage forms that are able to dissolve or disintegrate in the oral cavity quickly by saliva without the need for water administration [1]. European Pharmacopoeia has used the term orodispersible tablet for tablets that disperse inside the mouth readily and within three minutes before swallowing [2]. The United States Food and Drug Administration (FDA) defined ODT as "a solid dosage form containing a medicinal substance or active ingredient which disintegrates rapidly usually within a matter of seconds when placed upon the tongue" [3]. Other literature has used terms such as fast disintegrating tablets (FDT), orodispersible tablets (ODT), oral dispersible system (ODS), rapidly disintegrating tablets (RDT), mouth dissolving tablets (MDT), and orally fast disintegrating tablets (OFDT).

ODTs provide the benefits of liquid and solid dosage forms together with additional special advantages. As a solid form, the stable, accurate, and unit dose of ODTs comes with small packing size which is easily handled by patients even during travels with no access to water. As a dosage form with high adsorption in mouth, pharynx, esophagus, and gastrointestinal epithelium, the bioavailability of ODTs competes with that of liquid forms that provide a fast and higher rate of action. As additional benefits, ODTs avoid hepatic metabolism by presenting pre-gastric adsorption which increases the bioavailability of drug molecules. Furthermore, they are easily administered in pediatric, geriatric, mentally retarded, and psychiatric patients and especially in patients with dysphagia, nausea, vomiting, or motion sickness [1,4].

ODTs have been formulated for many categories of drugs in which rapid absorption and fast increase in the peak plasma concentration are desired. This requires the fast entrance of saliva to the tablet matrix to achieve rapid disintegration. Thus, maximizing the porous structure of the tablet and incorporation of hydrophilic excipients with the appropriate disintegrating agents are the main approaches in the preparation of ODTs [5].

Variation in the metabolism of the drug molecule upon formulating in ODT is the most important factor that needs to be considered for the molecules as their oral dosage forms are already available. Since ODTs may face different degrees of pre-gastric absorption, they could not be counted as the bioequivalence to the similar conventional dosage forms. Drug safety and toxicity must be deliberated for the possible toxic metabolites generated by the first pass effect and/or for substantial fractions of the drug with possible absorption in the oral cavity [6].

18.2   DESIRED PROPERTIES OF ODTS

An ODT must be designed to have some criteria to have therapeutic efficacy and reliability. An ideal ODT

- Should be dispersible in the mouth usually within seconds with no need for water and without leaving any residue.
- Should be absorbed in the oral mucosa.
- The active material should be loaded insufficient amount.
- Should not have bad taste and smell and should deliver a satisfying feel.
- Should be compatible with existing taste-masking technologies.
- Should be robust to environmental circumstances.
- The manufacturing operations should be adaptable to the existing fabrication process.
- Should be compatible with the conventional packaging process with minimum risk of fragility [7–9].

18.3 THE NEED FOR THE DEVELOPMENT OF ORALLY DISINTEGRATING TABLETS (ODTS) AND THEIR DESIRED PROPERTIES

Different kinds of dosage forms have been formulated such as tablets, capsules, suspensions, and injections in the pharmaceutical area. In recent years, there have been increased requirements for more patient-friendly and compliant pharmaceutical formulations. Therefore, the requirements for developing new technologies in the pharmaceutical area are increasing every year. Considering these requirements, ODTs have been developed by the pharmaceutical industry [5,10–12]. They are new types of dosage forms that mediate the advantages of both solid and liquid types of drug formulations such as ease of use and stability. Requirements for ODTs have been explained here below, in terms of factors related to patients, efficacy, and manufacturing factors [13].

18.3.1 PATIENT FACTORS

ODTs are especially convenient for individuals who have problems in swallowing conventional solid dosage form. These include the following:

- Pediatric and geriatric populations who have a complication in swallowing of conventional oral dosage forms. ODTs are convenient for children and elderly patients as well as the individuals who would like to take their medication, anytime and anywhere, without water.
- The usage of conventional solid pharmaceutical forms can cause vomiting to patients who are under radiation therapy for cancer.
- ODTs are suitable dosage forms during the journey for patients with permanent nausea.
- Antipsychotic drug molecules can be more easily applied to schizophrenic patients by ODT formulations than traditional pharmaceutical forms [14,15].
- The safety profile of the dosage form is improved due to a decrease in the risk of choking or suffocation [16].
- ODT leaves a pleasant taste in the mouth; hence patients' attitudes toward medication may change [17].

18.3.2 EFFECTIVENESS FACTOR

Faster onset of action, high drug loading, and increased bioavailability are the main properties of ODT formulations. The disintegration of active material in the oral cavity provides pre-gastric absorption from many ODT formulations. In this way, the required therapeutic response begins quickly, and an increase in bioavailability can be achieved. In addition, because the active material which is formulated as ODTs does not undergo the first-pass metabolism, it can be also said that the bioavailability of the active substance directly increases [18].

18.3.3 MANUFACTURING FACTORS

Developing current technologies is critical to surviving in the pharmaceutical industry. A new patient-convenient drug formulation such as ODTs allows manufacturers to develop dosage forms. Moreover, enhanced patient compliance provided by ODTs leads to an increase in their production in the pharmaceutical industry [5]. ODTs can be adapted with the equipment and packaging devices available in the pharmaceutical industry at affordable costs. Packaging expenses are also important. No specific packaging is required in ODTs as they can be packaged in push-through blisters [19].

Some ODT formulations which are available in the pharmaceutical market have been shown in Table 18.1.

TABLE 18.1
Some ODT Formulations Which Are Available in the Pharmaceutical Market [5,14]

Manufacturing Technology	Active Ingredient	Brand Name	Category	Advantages
Zydis°	Loratadine	Claritin	Antihistaminic	Very fast disintegration
Orasolv°	Mirtazapine	Remeron	Antidepressant	Effervescent disintegration
Zydis°	Olanzapine	Zyprexa	Antipsychotic	Very fast disintegration
Zydis°	Ondansetron	Zofran ODT	Antiemetic	Very fast disintegration
Zydis°	Risperidone	Risperdal	Antipsychotic	Very fast disintegration
Zydis°	Rizatriptan	Maxalt	Antimigraine	Very fast disintegration
Flash Dose°	Tramadol	Ultram	Analgesic	Effectively taste masking
Dura Solv°	Zolmitriptan	Zomig	Antimigraine	Easy to formulate low dose of active ingredient

18.4   TECHNOLOGIES USED IN THE PRODUCTION OF ODTS

Many technologies are commonly used in preparing ODTs. Some of them have been shortly explained in the following.

18.4.1   COMPACTION METHODS

Various compaction methods such as dry granulation, direct compression, and wet granulation are used in the formulation of ODTs. The following technologies are based on the compaction mechanism.

18.4.1.1   Direct Compression Method

In cases where the right disintegrant/superdisintegrant and polyol-based excipients are available, some therapeutic agents could directly be compressed as ODTs with acceptable qualities. The direct compression method is cost-effective but the easiest manufacturing method for ODTs. The schematic view of the direct compression method was shown in Figure 18.1. The

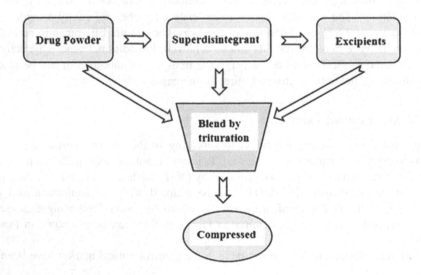

FIGURE 18.1   Schematic figure of the direct compression process.

disintegration of the ODTs can be prepared by direct compression that depends on the single or combined effects of disintegrants. Further information about superdisintegrants is given under the related title of this chapter [1]. Superdisintegrants increase the rate of disintegration and hence the dissolution. The presence of other formulation ingredients such as water-soluble excipients and effervescent agents further hastens the process of disintegration. For the success of ODTs, the tablet has to have a quick-dissolving property which is achieved by using superdisintegrants. The commonly used superdisintegrants have been shown in Table 18.3.

18.4.1.2   Wet Granulation

The ODTs can be manufactured through wet granulation by using plastic granules. If the used plastic material is polymeric, then it is necessary to prevent the growth of a viscous layer at the surface of ODT [20].

One technique to prepare these tablets is to mix the plastic material (e.g., spray-dried mannitol) with water penetration enhancers (e.g., maltodextrin) at specific ratios and compress them at low pressure. Consequently, the plastic deformation of the materials forms adjacent contact among the particles required for providing bonds between them. In this method, the plastic granules are divided by water, which causes an obstruct formation of a second layer on the ODT. Plastic granules keep the porous form after compression which results in fast disintegration because of a fast absorption of saliva from the ODTs. The wet granulation process has been shown schematically in Figure 18.2 [15].

Ghareeb and Mohammedways have prepared meclizine hydrochloride ODTs by using the wet granulation method. In this study, sodium starch glycolate, crospovidone, microcrystalline cellulose (MCC), and croscarmellose sodium at different ratios have been used as superdisintegrant. On the other hand, ammonium carbonate and camphor have also incorporated in ODTs as a subliming agent. Dissolution study results showed that the release of meclizine hydrochloride from ODTs prepared by wet granulation method and conventional tablet showed 100% and 49.32% drug release respectively at 15 minutes, which consequently indicates that enhancement of drug release

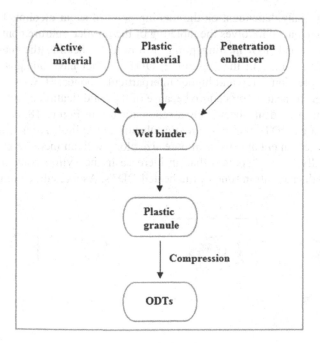

FIGURE 18.2   Schematic figure of the wet granulation process.

has been obtained by ODTs [21]. Sheshala et al. have prepared ondansetron ODTs with diverse superdisintegrants by wet granulation method. They have evaluated the ODTs both in *in vitro* and *in vivo* studies. *In vitro* disintegration time for all ODTs is reported between 5.8 and 33.0 seconds. The selected formulation with 15% Polyplasdone XL has released more than 90% of active material within five minutes [22].

Spray drying may also be classified as another wet granulation method for ODTs. In this method, all ingredients are integrated by hydrolyzed and non-hydrolyzed gelatins as supporting agents, sodium starch glycolate as a disintegrating agent, and mannitol as a bulking agent. The most important characteristic property of ODTs which are prepared with spray drying is the rapid dissolution time (<20 seconds) when contacted with water [11].

Nair et al. have developed a spray-drying form of risperidone nanosuspension using quality by design method. Nanosuspension of risperidone has been prepared by the antisolvent precipitation method using Poloxamer as a stabilizer. Spray-dried powder has been characterized not only by bulk properties but also formulated as an ODT. The prepared ODT was evaluated with *in vitro* characterization studies like disintegration time and dissolution studies. According to the results, ODTs formulated with spray-dried nanosuspension showed higher dissolution than marketed ODT formulation which may be due to the enhancement in solubility of risperidone during spray drying of nanosuspension [23].

18.4.1.3 Dry Granulation

In this method, high-density earth alkali metal salts and water-soluble carbohydrates are often reported to be unsuitable because of their rapid disintegration and the flavor they leave in the mouth. Low-density alkaline earth metal salts are also difficult to compress as a tablet. Because the content uniformity of these salts is insufficient, low-density alkaline earth metal salts or water-soluble carbohydrates are precompressed, and then the granules obtained are compressed into ODTs [24].

18.4.2 PHASE TRANSITION METHOD (CRYSTALLINE TRANSITION PROCESS)

This method is principally dependent on the melting point of sugar alcohols like xylitol, sorbitol, and mannitol. This technique involves the tableting of the powder mixture containing two different sugar alcohols of low and high melting points followed by heating the mass at a temperature between their melting points. In the beginning, ODTs do not have adequate hardness property because of low compression force and higher interparticular bonds. However, the hardness of the ODTs increases after the heating procedure because of the solidification of used sugar alcohols [1]. The phase transition method has been shown schematically in Figure 18.3.

Kuno et al. prepared ODTs that contained erythritol and xylitol. After heating both materials at 93 °C for 15 minutes, an enhancement in pore size along with an increase in tablet hardness was recorded. Additionally, it was reported that an increase in the xylitol content causes an increase in the hardness and disintegration time of the heated ODTs. As a result, a composition of low and

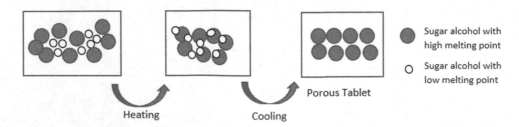

FIGURE 18.3 Schematic figure of the phase transition method.

high melting point sugar alcohols, as well as a phase transition event in the preparing procedure, is crucial to prepare ODTs without any specific device [25].

18.4.3 SUBLIMATION

Rapid disintegration property can be obtained by formulating into a porous mass by incorporating solid substances that volatilize fast like camphor, menthol, ammonium bicarbonate, thymol, and urea. In the sublimation method, ODTs are compressed by using tablet components, and after compression, the volatile substance is vaporized by pressure with the application of heat, and while the volatile substance leaves the mass, a porous structure is formed. Compressed tablets containing mannitol and camphor have been prepared by the sublimation technique. The tablets dissolve within 10–20 seconds and exhibit sufficient mechanical strength for practical use [26]. The most important advantage of this method is that the volatilization of these materials eliminates the complicated process associated with the lyophilization process [1].

Elbary et al. have prepared meloxicam ODTs using the sublimation method. They have used menthol, camphor, and thymol as volatile substances at various concentrations. According to the results of this study, meloxicam ODTs with fast disintegration time and drug release with enhanced hardness properties are successfully formulated by employing the sublimation technique [27].

Sutradhar et al. also formulated ODTs of domperidone using the sublimation method also. They used camphor as a volatilizing agent and Kollidon and Guar Gum as superdisintegrants. This study indicates that a proper balance should be provided between polymers and the disintegrating material formulated with a volatilizing material [28].

The sublimation method has been schematically shown in Figure 18.4.

18.4.4 LYOPHILIZATION (FREEZE DRYING)

Lyophilization is one of the key methods of creating acceptable and effective ODTs. Lyophilization process, or freeze drying, consists of freezing the aqueous complex followed by sublimation of solid water to the vapor phase under vacuum. A very porous material remains from this process with traces of water, which provides complete control of disintegration or dispersion of the solid dosage form. In the case of ODT, lyophilization can be applied, since it results in obtaining a palatable material that can disperse very fast, leaving a pleasant feel in the mouth. This method is very convenient for thermo-sensitive drug molecules. In such cases, the drug molecule is physically entrapped in the aqueous matrix, lyophilization of which gives a fluffy material, feasible for fast disintegration [29]. The lyophilization technique provides high porosity and specific surface area and gets dissolve quickly in the oral cavity providing high bioavailability. Mainly disadvantages of the lyophilization process are high cost, fragility, and time-consuming procedure [26].

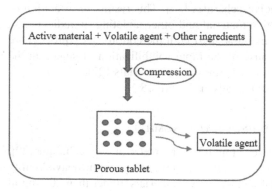

FIGURE 18.4 Schematic figure of the sublimation method.

Liew et al. have investigated the effect of starch and polymer types on the ODT which was prepared with lyophilized dapoxetine. Three polymers (HPMC, Carbopol 934, and Eudragit® EPO) and starch have been used as matrix materials in ODTs. The polymeric dispersion has been placed into a mold and kept at −20 °C for four hours before being freeze dried for 12 hours. According to the results, an increase in HPMC and Carbopol 934 concentrations, tablets gave higher hardness and longer disintegration time values. In contrast, it was reported that it was unable to form ODTs with adequate hardness at different concentrations with Eudragit®EPO [30].

Shoukri et al. have developed lyophilized ODTs in order to enhance the dissolution and absorption properties of nimesulide. Results show that lyophilized ODTs were disintegrated within several seconds, and they showed a faster dissolution rate than nimesulide simple powder drug [31].

Lai et al. have prepared different nanocrystal ODTs by lyophilization method using poloxamer 188 as a stabilizer to enhance the dissolution rate and solubility of piroxicam. According to the results of the study, ODTs have provided an enhanced piroxicam dissolution rate because of the nanosized drug particles [32].

18.4.5 MOLDING

ODTs can be prepared by the molding method easily. The molding method may be divided into two categories: compression molding and heat molding. Compression molding involves the wetting of powder mass, using hydroalcoholic solvents, which is then compressed as a tablet. The solvent is allowed to evaporate. Taste property of the drug is prepared by spray freezing the molten mixture of hydrogenated sodium carbonate and lecithin, with an active material-based tablet mass. In the heat molding process for the preparation of ODTs, molten tablet mass containing a dispersed drug and/or dissolved active material is used [26].

In the heat molding process, molten mass containing a dispersed drug or dissolved active material is used for the preparation of ODTs. In this method, suspension of the active material with water-soluble sugars such as lactose, sucrose, or sorbitol is prepared and then poured into blisters. The dispersion is then distributed into molds at room temperature to form a jelly and dehydrated at approximately 30 °C [1].

Modi and Pralhad have studied valdecoxib ODTs using this method. The drug has to be kneaded with polyvinyl pyrrolidone and compressed into a tablet. The dissolution studies of the prepared ODTs were then compared with that of the commercial products of valdecoxib. According to experimental results, the molding technique can be successfully used for improving dissolution properties of valdecoxib in ODT formulation [33].

18.4.6 COTTON CANDY PROCESS

This method benefits continuous flash melting and spinning procedure to produce a string of crystalline structures by producing a pattern of polysaccharides [34]. This results in formation of the candy floss matrix, which is blended with active material and other tableting ingredients and afterward compressed into ODTs [1]. The ODTs manufactured with the cotton candy process are highly porous and provide pleasant taste feel because of the rapid solubilization of sugars in the presence of water. But this process is not suitable for thermo-labile materials [29].

The cotton candy process has been shown schematically in Figure 18.5.

18.4.7 MELT GRANULATION (NANOCRYSTAL TECHNOLOGY/NANOMELT)

This process involves materials of which particle size is minimized by wet grinding technique [29]. The advantage of this method is that it is suitable for water-insoluble drugs with bioavailability problems. With the help of this process, ODTs that include active materials higher than 200 mg in

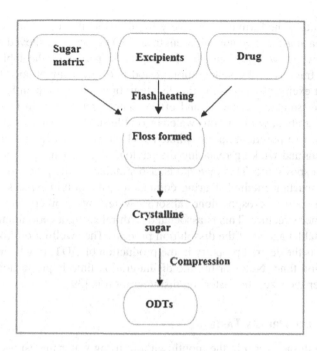

FIGURE 18.5 Schematic figure of the cotton candy process.

each ODT can be produced, and this method can be utilized without water or organic solvents as there is no drying step [26].

Hari et al. have prepared and evaluated of drotaverine hydrochloride ODTs by melt granulation method. Drug–polymer melt granules have been manufactured by using either compritol or precirol using distinct drug–polymer ratios of 1:7, 1:5, 1:2, and 1:1. According to taste evaluation results, the drug–polymer ratios 1:7 with compritol and (1:5) with precirol have been optimized. The granules have been prepared with an optimized drug–polymer ratio, and they have been evaluated. All the prepared drotaverine HCl ODTs that contain mannitol and melt granulated mixture have been characterized on the basis of orally disintegrating tablet criteria like taste and dissolution. Among these studies, ODTs prepared with croscarmellose sodium with mannitol as diluent gave complete drug release in 60 minutes with acceptable taste and mouth feel. Hence, ODT formulations prepared with croscarmellose sodium and mannitol by using this method show suitable ODT properties [35].

Sree et al. prepared ODTs of Levocetirizine by melt granulation technology. When the formulations have been tested for tablet weight variation, friability, wetting time, disintegration time, and *in vitro* drug release, all tablets have shown sufficient mechanic properties. Additionally, ODTs containing crospovidone have provided sufficient *in vitro* disintegration time and drug release [36].

18.5 CHALLENGES IN PREPARATION OF ODTS

ODT formulations consist of excipients including disintegrants, diluents, lubricants, and in some cases swelling agents, sweeteners, and flavoring agents. A combination of these materials generally is associated with the below-mentioned problems [37].

18.5.1 DISINTEGRATION PERIOD AND FRAGILITY

The priority in presenting an ODT dosage form is to provide fast disintegration at the oral cavity which is obtained by the occupation of a highly porous matrix in formulating the drug molecule.

The porous matrix causes the formation of a very fragile tablet that could smash during packing or transportation. Increasing the mechanical strength of ODTs can be achieved by using excipients with less porosity, which will prolong the disintegration period of the tablet. Thus, achieving balance in terms of fragility and disintegration period is of great importance [38].

Superdisintegrant excipients determine the disintegration and consequently the dissolution time of ODT. Other water-soluble excipients and effervescent agents used in ODT formulation help the process of disintegration, while fibrous water-insoluble structures such as crospovidone provide mechanical strength. Crospovidone, a crosslinked PVP derivative, acts through various mechanisms such as swelling and wicking releasing the payload drug. Disintegration is achieved by the strain recovery of crospovidone. This material is also suitable for the production of ODT using the wet granulation compaction method. During compaction, the polymer faces some deformations. Upon contact with saliva, crospovidone absorbs water by capillary forces which provide reassembly of polymer structure. This is associated with releasing a certain amount of energy that is able to break the tablet and start the dissolution process. The swelling of crospovidone does not cause gelling which is the desired property in the production of ODT, in which gelation causes the delay of disintegration time. Noteworthy, the disintegration time is proportional to the crospovidone size. The larger the size, the faster the disintegration is [39].

18.5.2 MASKING THE DRUG'S TASTE

The application of a dosage form in the mouth without using water intensifies the bad taste of the drug molecule. Successful masking of the bitter taste of the drug must be achieved to accomplish patient compliance. Flavors and sweeteners are the main excipients used in this order. Flavor oils, fruit essences, and aromatic oils are the most commonly used flavoring agents. Sweeteners, on the other hand, play multiple roles in ODT formulations. Sugar-based sweeteners are hydrophilic materials with bulking property and provide fast disintegrating while masking the drug taste. Artificial sweeteners like aspartame and sugars derivatives, and bulking agents like dextrose, fructose, isomalt, lactilol, maltitol, maltose, mannitol, sorbitol, starch hydrolysate, polydextrose, and xylitol are applied for these purposes.

18.5.3 FORMATION OF EUTECTIC MIXTURES

An eutectic system is a combination of different materials that freeze (also melt or solidify) in a temperature lower than either of its components. Water-soluble drug molecules form eutectic systems with the excipients, thus the freezing process remains incomplete during the lyophilization process. This results in the collapse of the system upon drying because of missing the backbone excipient system during the sublimation. In such cases, the employment of materials such as mannitol, which is capable of forming matrixes and inducing crystallinity, can help to increase the rigidity of matrix along with masking the taste of drugs [40]. According to some literature [41], the maximum dose for a hydrophilic drug molecule in an ODT formulation is 60 mg, while this amount is defined as 400 mg for the hydrophobic drugs because it has been evidenced that hydrophobic molecules could also create aggregates upon sublimation due to the high molecular weight.

18.5.4 SIZE OF TABLET AND AMOUNT OF DRUG

According to the United States Pharmacopeia, the dose of each ODT should not exceed 500 mg. Thus, the problem is associated with the preparation of ODT that originates from the low capacity of each unit of the dosage form for carrying a certain dosage of the drug molecule.

Similarly, the size of the dosage form needs to be around 8 mm, and it is required for the active ingredient to be carried within this mass area. As mentioned above, the limit for uploading hydrophobic drug molecules to ODT is 400 mg, and this amount decreases to 60 mg for the hydrophilic molecules.

A recent method consisting of melting drug molecules to nano size and granulation by adsorption of stabilizers on their surface has been used to enhance the capacity of ODT in carrying active ingredient molecules up to 200 mg per unit [42].

18.5.5 Safe Packing

A dosage form such as ODT, designated to be disintegrated in saliva, will also be sensitive to the moisture and physical conditions. Almost all ODT are hygroscopic and are not stable at normal temperature and humidity. This calls for custom-designed packing, so the pre-formulation studies on ODT are associated with the design and evaluation of the specialized packages at the very early stages of formulation development [43].

18.6 FORMULATION APPROACHES TO INDUCE FAST DISINTEGRATION IN ODTS USING GRANULATION METHODS

The excipients used to form ODTs are a diluent, a disintegrant or superdisintegrant, a lubricant, and in some cases a permeabilizing agent, a sweetener, and a flavoring agent [26].

The ratios of these excipients in a wide range are given in Table 18.2.

18.6.1 Disintegrants and Binders

Two main components of ODTs are disintegrants and binders. Many excipients play both roles in the preparation of these dosage forms. The order of their addition during the formulation process depends on the strategy and the purpose of formulation preparation. While the direct blending of excipients is a simple approach for incorporating the disintegrants and binders, granulation, a more complicated process, results in obtaining improved properties in ODT dosage forms. In wet granulation, binders are used as granulation liquid, while during the melt granulation, they are used in molten form. Spray coating of binder (such as mannitol) with a disintegrant (such as crospovidone) results in obtaining granules with enhanced surfaces in each of which fine disintegrant particles cover the mannitol particles, which not only provides fast disintegration due to the enhanced surface of formulation but also forms hard compacts due to an increase in the contact surface of particles [44].

One of the first reports on the preparation of ODTs which was published by Watanabe et al. used crystalline cellulose (as a binder) and low substituted hydroxypropyl cellulose (L-HPC, as disintegrant) [45]. Cellulose was used as a binder in the early 1990s, while further studies led the researchers to use bi-functional excipients with the binding-disintegrating property. This approach caused a shift from cellulose-based materials (primarily crystalline cellulose) toward

TABLE 18.2

The Percentages of Excipients Used in the Preparation of ODTs [26]

Excipient Category	Ratio (%)
Superdisintegrant	1–15
Binder	5–10
Lubricant	0–10
Diluent	0–85

sugar/polyol-based excipients. Watanabe et al. [45] used crystalline cellulose as binder, filler, and a provider for the tablet hardness, while L-HPC was used as a disintegrant. The advantages of cellulose in providing mechanical strength initiated the employment of cellulose derivatives in ODT preparation. Microcrystalline cellulose (MCC), which shows considerable compaction properties, is now the most widely used excipient due to swelling without gelation and capillary properties along with high dilution potential. The unique plastic deformation property of MCC originating from hydrogen bonds of neighboring particles makes this excipient very suitable for the fabrication process, especially tablet formation via compressing method. However, the mouth feel of this material mainly depends on its particle size. MCC as an insoluble particle in water (saliva) negatively affects the mouth feeling; however, further studies resulted in the successful development of spherical MCC particles with sizes reduced to 7 μm and consequently solved unpleasant mouth feeling-related problems [46]. The poor flow properties of MCC have been improved using α-lactose monohydrate which is a sugar/polyol-based excipient [47].

Sugar/polyol-based excipients provide numerous advantages including superior mouth feel, sweetening, and favorable property as fillers. The most famous polyol is mannitol. The advantages of using mannitol in the preparation of ODT dosage forms are

- the cooling sensation in mouth due to the negative heat of mannitol
- creamy mouth feel during the disintegration process
- sweet taste despite the low sugar content
- the lack of hygroscopic properties [48].

Not all sugar alcohol/polyols are as suitable as mannitol for successful ODT preparation. Lactose, xylitol, sorbitol, erythritol, and maltodextrin have also been used in this process; however, along with some advantages, none of them is a complete substitution for mannitol, due to high hygroscopic properties. Thus, other sugar alcohol/polyols are incorporated with mannitol during the granulation/compression procedures, especially to improve the hardness of ODT dosage forms. The compacts obtained under pressure using mannitol are poorly strong due to its fragmentation during compaction method, unlike other sugars such as lactose, sorbitol, or xylitol which produce stronger compacts upon fragmentation.

In some cases, Superpolystate©, PEG-6-stearate has been used in wet granulation and melt granulation process as a waxy binder (or as a super polystate) [49] to enhance the physical strength and the disintegration property of ODTs. This excipient has an hydrophilic lipophilic balance value around 9 which provides water diffusion and fast disintegration, while its physical property delivers stiffness to the ODT formulation [50]. For this purpose, an emulsion prepared from PEG-6-stearate is used as a granulating liquid in wet granulation, while in the melt granulation process, its molten form is used [50].

Finally, it has been evidenced that the ratio of the binder:disintegrant determines the period of disintegration, that is, while the ratio of MCC/L-HPC is in the range of 8:2 to 9:1, the ODT shows the fastest disintegration period [51].

Recently feasibility of excipients from the natural sources has attracted the attention of researches for ODT preparations. Agar powders and amino acids are the two main categories in this regard. Saccharides, the disintegrants with natural sources, can induce swelling without gelation. Similar to MCC, a decrease in particle size by grinding results in obtaining much faster disintegration periods. Amino acids such as proline, serine, L-lysine HCl, L-alanine, glycine, and L-tyrosine with high wettability property have been used as disintegration enhancers mainly in lyophilization and direct compression methods [52,53]. The penetration of water into the tablet produces a separation force between the hydrophilic and hydrophobic forces [53] disintegrating ODT. Thus, the ratio of non-polar (dispersion) to the polar component determines the surface energy and hence the disintegration period of an ODT. This could be achieved by tuning the ratio of hydrophobic/ hydrophilic amino acids incorporated in ODT formulation.

18.6.2 SUPERDISINTEGRANTS

This category of excipients is added to ODT dosage forms to achieve fast oral dispersion associated with a pleasant feeling in the mouth. The disintegration process generally starts with swelling, hydration, and changes in the volume of disintegrant material or by the production of disruptive changes in the tablet structure such as producing gases. The most famous disintegrants are sodium starch glyconate, crospovidone, alginic acid, calcium silicate and, croscarmellose. Other examples of superdisintegrants are listed in Table 18.3. Ideally, superdisintegrants enhance the compressibility and compatibility of a tablet without making any change in the mechanical strength of tablets even at the high drug doses [42].

Disintegrants are useful and necessary in the granulation process because they are intra-granularly very active and also effective in low concentrations with compatibility to both hydrophilic and hydrophobic drug molecules.

Natural superdisintegrants are superior to the synthetic ones due to their safe toxic profile and lower costs. Gums and mucilage are the best examples for this class of excipients which are abundantly available around the world. They are capable of swelling up to 5 times their original volume which consequently results in fast and effective disintegration of tablets. They also are more acceptable by the

TABLE 18.3
Disintegrants, Some Examples, and Related Comments [20,42]

Superdisintegrants	Example	Mechanism of Action	Special Comment
Crosscarmellose*	Crosslinked cellulose	Swells 4–8 folds in < 10 seconds.	Swells in two dimensions.
Ac-Di-Sol*		Swelling and wicking both.	Direct compression or granulation
Nymce ZSX*			Starch free
Primellose*			
Solutab*			
Vivasol*L-HPC			
Crosspovidone Crosspovidon M* Kollidon* Polyplasdone*	Crosslinked PVP	Swells very little and returns to original size after compression but acts by capillary action	Water-insoluble and spongy in nature so get porous tablet
Acrylic acid derivatives		Wicking	
Effervescence Substances (Citric acid, Tartaric acid)		Effervescent effect	Evolution of CO_2 after contact with water
Sodium starch glycolate Explotab* Primogel*	Crosslinked starch	Swells 7–12 folds in < 30 seconds	Swells in three dimensions and high levels serve as sustain release matrix
Alginic acid NF Satialgine*	Crosslinked alginic acid	Rapid swelling in aqueous medium or wicking action	Promote disintegration in both dry or wet granulation
Soy polysaccharides Emcosoy*	Natural super disintegrant	-	Does not contain any starch or sugar. Used in nutritional products
HPC (LH-11)		Swelling and wicking	Disintegration time max. 90 seconds
Calcium silicate		Wicking action	Highly porous, Optimum concentration is b/w 20 and 40%

patients and the public [54]. Some examples of natural superdisintegrants are *Plantago ovata, Cassia fistula, Hibiscus rosa sinensis,* Locust bean gum, Chitin and Chitosan, *Aloe vera,* Guar gum, Gum karaya, Agar, Fenugreek seed mucilage, Soy polysaccharide, Gellan gum, *Lepidium sativum* mucilage, *Aegle marmelos* gum, dehydrated banana powder, *Cassia tora,* and *Ocimum basilicum.*

18.6.3 TASTE MASKING USING DRY GRANULATION IN ODT DEVELOPMENT

The ODTs disintegrate in the oral cavity and release the active ingredients, which generally are unpalatable on the taste buds; thus, the taste-masking process is of great importance in the production of ODT dosage forms. The taste-masking technologies and agents currently used could be listed as coating, granulation, sweeteners, microencapsulation, taste suppressants, potentiators, solid dispersions, ion exchange resins, viscosity enhancers, complex formation, pH modifiers, and adsorbates.

Taste masking using granulation consists of granulation of drugs, using a granulation agent, and its coating using a taste-masking polymer. Granulation technologies for taste masking are further discussed in Table 18.4.

18.6.4 CHALLENGES IN SELECTION OF ODT DRUG CANDIDATES

There are several considerations regarding selecting the drug molecule for formulating as an ODT. These considerations could be classified into two groups, the drug molecules which are ideal for ODT dosage forms and the ones in which certain warnings must be deliberated.

Drug molecules ideal for ODT dosage forms are as follows [38]:

1. The drugs that have toxic metabolites after first pass effect or gastric degradation.
2. The molecules which are able to diffuse through upper gastrointestinal system (GIS) (log P > 1, or preferable > 2) or the ones that can penetrate oral mucosa.

Some of the promising drug candidates for developing ODTs are listed in Table 18.5.

Drug molecules that are not good candidates for ODT dosage forms are as follows:

1. The drugs which show significantly different pharmacokinetic behavior compared with the commercial dosage form after oral adsorption.
2. The drugs that initiate a new derivative in the oral cavity or in the pre-gastric segment of GIS.
3. ODT dosage forms must be very carefully administered to the patients who take anticholinergic medications.
4. Patients with Sjogren's syndrome or dryness of the mouth due to decreased saliva production.
5. Drugs with short half-life which need frequent dosing with bitter taste whose taste masking cannot be achieved or which require controlled or sustained release

18.7 CHARACTERIZATION OF ODTS PREPARED BY GRANULATION TECHNOLOGY

18.7.1 WETTING TIME

This implies the disintegration period. The faster the wetting, the shorter is the disintegration time. The ODT is placed in a petri dish containing 6 mL of water and two times folded paper tissue, and the time period for complete wetting is measured. This period is directly proportional to the contact angle [5].

TABLE 18.4

Some Granulation Technologies Used in Taste Masking of Bitter Drug Molecules; Revised Table from [55]

Granulating Agent(s)	Drug(s)	Percentage of Excipients	Granulation Method	Ref.
Sugar alcohol	Calcium containing compounds (e.g., CaCO3)	Concentration of sugar alcohol from about 5% to about 40% w/w	Melt granulation with sugar alcohol as the binding agent	[56]
Hydroxypropyl cellulose, hydroxypropyl methylcellulose, croscarmellose, and sodium alginic acid	Erythromycin	Drug: polymer ratio of 2.5:1 to 50:1	Drug molecule and, optionally, Tween 80 were added to the dispersion of granulating agents after which they were coated on microcrystalline cellulose beads in a fluid-bed processor.	[57]
Cyclodextrin	Dextromethorphan	Drug:polymer ratio of between 0.9:1 and 1:25	Mixing of drug with cyclodextrin followed by granulation; without complexation	[58]
pH-dependent polymer (e.g., Eudragit E-100) and sugar, solid support to coat drug–polymer mixture	Alprazolam	Drug–polymer mixture is 0.1 to 300% w/w relative to the weight of the solid support	Alprazolam-containing layer material, e.g., the combination of the alprazolam and the first taste-masking material, is used as a granulation binder. The resulting granulate is then coated with overcoating layers directly or first is coated with alprazolam-containing layers before the application of overcoating layers.	[59]
A neutral methacrylic acid ester copolymer and a binder	Norfloxacin	The polymer comprises 1 to 40% w/w of drug	Wet granulation. An aqueous dispersion of the neutral methacrylic acid ester copolymer along with a binder is added to the powdered drug, mixed with other excipients such as glidants and antiadhesives, and the resulting mixture is blended to form granules.	[60]

Further examples are found in the comprehensive review by Ayenew et al. [55].

TABLE 18.5

Some of the Promising Drug Candidates for ODTs; Published with Permission from [1]

Category of the Active Ingredient	Examples of the Active Ingredient
Antibacterials	Ciprofloxacin, tetracycline, erythromycin, rifampicin, penicillin, doxycycline, nalidixic acid, trimethoprim, sulphacetamide, sulphadiazine
Anthelmintics	Albendazole, mebendazole, thiabendazole, livermectin, praziquantel, pyrantel embonate, dichlorophen
Antidepressants	Trimipramine maleate, nortriptyline HCl, trazodone HCl, amoxapine, mianserin HCl
Antidiabetics	Glibenclamide, glipizide, tolbutamide, tolazamide, gliclazide, chlorpropamide
Analgesics/anti-inflammatory agents	Diclofenac sodium, ibuprofen, ketoprofen, mefenamic acid, naproxen, oxyphenbutazone, indomethacin, piroxicam, phenylbutazone
Antihypertensives	Amlodipine, carvedilol, diltiazem, felodipine, minoxidil, nifedipine, prazosin HCl, nimodipine, terazosin HCl
Antiarrhythmics	Disopyramide, quinidine sulphate, amiodarone HCl
Antihistamines	Acrivastine, cetrizine, cinnarizine, loratadine, fexofenadine, triprolidine
Anxiolytics, sedatives and hypnotics	Alprazolam, diazepam, clozapine, amylobarbitone, lorazepam, haloperidol, nitrazepam, midazolam phenobarbitone, thioridazine, oxazepam
Diuretics	Acetazolamide, clorthiazide, amiloride, furosemide, spironolactone, bumetanide, ethacrynic acid
Gastro-intestinal agents	Cimetidine, ranitidine HCl, famotidine, domperidone, omeprazole, ondansetron HCl, granisetron HCl
Corticosteroids	Betamethasone, beclomethasone, hydrocortisone, prednisone, prednisolone, methylprednisolone
Antiprotozoals	Metronidazole, tinidazole, omidazole, benznidazole

18.7.2 DISINTEGRATION TEST

It is obvious that the disintegration period for ODTs is much shorter than other oral dosage forms, and the related test needs to be done without water by saliva in conditions mimicking oral cavity; thus, the regular dissolution apparatus has been modified by several research groups to determine this very short time period. Bi et al. [47] have developed a new method for this regard in which the tablet in a sinker is placed in a container containing 900 mL of water at 37 °C, right below the water surface, and rotated by a paddle at 100 rpm. The disintegration time is measured when the tablet is completely disintegrated and passed through the screen of the sinker. It is possible to use a texture analyzer instrument in this order. In such a case, a flat-ended cylindrical probe is used to penetrate through the ODT immersed in water by applying a very small force. The distance traveled by the probe upon the disintegration of the tablet is measured and reported as the disintegration profile of the tablet as a function of time by the software of the instrument [61].

18.7.3 DISSOLUTION TEST

It has been reported that USP 2 paddle apparatus [62] is the most convenient instrument for the measurement of the dissolution time of ODTs. The preferred paddle speed is 50 rpm. Although dissolution condition listed in pharmacopeia monographs for the active ingredient is a good point to start the dissolution studies, other conditions such as 0.1 M HCl and buffer (pH 4.5 and 6.8) should be considered to evaluate the dissolution of ODT in the oral cavity [5].

18.7.4 MOISTURE UPTAKE STUDIES

Moisture uptake test is important to evaluate the stability of the final product containing several hygroscopic excipients. For this purpose, tablets are kept in a desiccator over calcium chloride at 37 °C for 24 hours. The tablets are weighted and exposed to 75% relative humidity for two weeks. The increase in weight of the tablet is compared to one tablet prepared without disintegrants at the end of this period [5].

18.8 FUTURE PROSPECTS

Along with numerous advantages of ODTs mentioned in this chapter, this dosage form is a good strategy to manage the life cycle of the pharmaceutical product and to elongate the patent period of an existing product. The strong market and demand of patients who need a convenient dosage anywhere at any time without water are expanding the target population of ODTs day by day [42]. Protein- and peptide-based therapeutics which degrade in GIS due to the acidic conditions and enzymatic reactions are the best candidates for the preparation of the next generation of disintegrating tablets. Other challenges on the way of these dosage form include the development of compatible methods for the production of ODTs using currently available industrial instruments and improving their physical strength and taste-masking capacities [38].

REFERENCES

1. Badgujar, Bhatu, and Atish Mundada. 2011. "The technologies used for developing orally disintegrating tablets: a review." *Acta Pharmaceutica* 61 (2):117–139.
2. European Pharmacopoeia Commission. 2013. "European Pharmacopoeia 8.0, Volume I." *Strasbourg: European Directorate for the Quality of Medicines of European Council* 242.
3. Food and Drug Administration. 2008. "Guidance for industry: orally disintegrating tablets." Center for Drug Evaluation and Research (CDER), Maryland, USA.
4. Aguilar, Johnny Edward, Encarna García Montoya, Pilar Pérez Lozano, Josep M Suñe Negre, Montserrat Miñarro Carmona, and José Ramón Ticó Grau. 2013. "New sedem-odt expert system: an expert system for formulation of orodispersible tablets obtained by direct compression." *Formulation Tools for Pharmaceutical Development* 137–154.
5. Hirani, Jaysukh J, Dhaval A Rathod, and Kantilal R Vadalia. 2009. "Orally disintegrating tablets: a review." *Tropical Journal of Pharmaceutical Research* 8 (2).
6. DeRoche, C. C. 2005. "Consumer preference for orally disintegrating tablets over conventional forms of medication: Evolving methodology for medication intake in dysphagia. Lecture presented at the 12th Annual Meeting of the Dysphagia Research Society, San Francisco, CA, 2–4 Oct. 2003." *Dysphagia* 20 (1):77–86.
7. Comoglu, Tansel, and Emine Dilek Ozyilmaz. 2019b. "Orally disintegrating tablets and orally disintegrating mini-tablets – novel dosage forms for pediatric use." *Pharmaceutical Development and Technology* 24 (7):902–914. doi: 10.1080/10837450.2019.1615090.
8. Awasthi, Rajendra, Gaurav Sharma, Kamal Dua, and Giriraj T Kulkarni. 2013. "Fast disintegrating drug delivery systems: a review with special emphasis on fast disintegrating tablets." *Journal of Chronotherapy and Drug Delivery* 4 (1):15–30.
9. Bharawaj, Sudhir, Vinay Jain, Shailesh Sharma, R. C. Jat, and Suman Jain. 2010. "Orally disintegrating tablets: a review." *Drug Invention Today* 2 (1).
10. Comoglu, T, O Inal, A Kargili, and B Pehlivanoglu. 2017. "Formulation, in vitro and in vivo evaluation of taste-masked rasagiline orally fast disintegrating tablets." *Pharmacy and Pharmaceutical Sciences* 6 (1):27–38.
11. Comoglu, Tansel, and Burcu Unal. 2015. "Preparation and evaluation of an orally fast disintegrating tablet formulation containing a hydrophobic drug." *Pharmaceutical Development and Technology* 20 (1):60–64.
12. Şenel, Sevda, and Tansel Comoglu. 2018. Orally disintegrating tablets, fast-dissolving, buccal and sublingual formulations. Taylor & Francis, London, U.K.

13. Bircan, Yağmur, and Tansel Çomoğlu. 2012. "Formulation technologies of orally fast disintegrating tablets." *Marmara Pharmaceutical Journal* 16 (2):77–81.

14. Comoglu, Tansel, and Emine Dilek Ozyilmaz. 2019a. "Orally disintegrating tablets and orally disintegrating mini-tablets–novel dosage forms for pediatric use." *Pharmaceutical Development and Technology* 24 (7):902–914.

15. Velmurugan, S, and Sundar Vinushitha. 2010. "Oral disintegrating tablets: an overview." *International Journal of Chemical and Pharmaceutical Sciences* 1 (2):1–12.

16. Indurwade, N H, and K.R. Biyani. 2000. "Evaluation of comparative and combined depressive effect of Brahmi, Shankhpushpi and Jatamansi in mice." *Indian Journal of Medical Sciences* 54 (8):339–341.

17. Allen Jr, V Loyd, Bingnan Wang, and John D Davies. 1997. Method of making a rapidly dissolving tablet. Google Patents.

18. Gupta, A, A K Mishra, V Gupta, P Bansal, R Singh, and A K Singh. 2010. "Recent trends of fast dissolving tablet-an overview of formulation technology." *International Journal of Pharmaceutical & Biological Archives* 1 (1):1–10.

19. Kuchekar, B S, A C Badhan, and H S Mahajan. 2003. " Mouth dissolving tablets: a novel drug delivery system." *Pharma Times* 35:7–9.

20. Brniak, Witold, Renata Jachowicz, and Przemyslaw Pelka. 2015. "The practical approach to the evaluation of methods used to determine the disintegration time of orally disintegrating tablets (ODTs)." *Saudi Pharmaceutical Journal* 23 (4):437–443.

21. Ghareeb, Mowafaq M, and Twana M Mohammedways. 2012. "Development and evaluation of orodispersible tablets of meclizine hydrochloride." *International Journal of Pharmaceutical Sciences and Research* 3 (12):5101.

22. Sheshala, Ravi, Nurzalina Khan, Mallikarjun Chitneni, and Yusrida Darwis. 2011. "Formulation and in vivo evaluation of ondansetron orally disintegrating tablets using different superdisintegrants." *Archives of Pharmacal Research* 34 (11):1945–1956.

23. Nair, Anu, Dignesh Khunt, and Manju Misra. 2019. "Application of quality by design for optimization of spray drying process used in drying of risperidone nanosuspension." *Powder Technology* 342:156–165.

24. Chowdary Kpr, K Ravi Shankar, and B Suchitra. 2014. "Recent research on orodispersible tablets–A review." *International Research Journal of Pharmaceutical and Applied Sciences* 4 (1):64–73.

25. Kuno, Yoshio, Masazumi Kojima, Shuichi Ando, and Hiroaki Nakagami. 2005. "Evaluation of rapidly disintegrating tablets manufactured by phase transition of sugar alcohols." *Journal of Controlled Release* 105 (1–2):16–22.

26. Hannan, P A, J A Khan, A Khan, and S Safiullah. 2016. "Oral dispersible system: a new approach in drug delivery system." *Indian Journal of Pharmaceutical Sciences* 78 (1):2.

27. Abd Elbary Ahmed, Adel A Ali, and Heba M Aboud. 2012. "Enhanced dissolution of meloxicam from orodispersible tablets prepared by different methods." *Bulletin of Faculty of Pharmacy, Cairo University* 50 (2):89–97.

28. Sutradhar, Kumar B, Dewan T Akhter, and Riaz Uddin. 2012. "Formulation and evaluation of taste-masked oral dispersible tablets of domperidone using sublimation method." *International Journal of Pharmacy and Pharmaceutical Sciences* 4 (2):727–732.

29. Pandey, Parijat, and Mandeep Dahiya. 2016. "Oral disintegrating tablets: a review." *International Journal of Pharma Research & Review* 5 (1):50–62.

30. Liew, Kai Bin, and Kok Khiang Peh. 2015. "Investigation on the effect of polymer and starch on the tablet properties of lyophilized orally disintegrating tablet." *Archives of Pharmacal Research* 1–10.

31. Shoukri, Raguia Ali, Iman Saad Ahmed, and Rehab N Shamma. 2009. "In vitro and in vivo evaluation of nimesulide lyophilized orally disintegrating tablets." *European Journal of Pharmaceutics and Biopharmaceutics* 73 (1):162–171.

32. Lai, Francesco, Elena Pini, Francesco Corrias, Jacopo Perricci, Maria Manconi, Anna Maria Fadda, and Chiara Sinico. 2014. "Formulation strategy and evaluation of nanocrystal piroxicam orally disintegrating tablets manufacturing by freeze-drying." *International Journal of Pharmaceutics* 467 (1–2):27–33.

33. Modi, Aftab, and Pralhad Tayade. 2006. "Enhancement of dissolution profile by solid dispersion (kneading) technique." *AAPS PharmSciTech* 7 (3):E87.

34. Asthana, Abhay, Swati Aggarwal, and Gayti Asthana. 2013. "Oral dispersible tablets: novel technology and development." *International Journal of Pharmaceutical Sciences Review and Research* 20 (1):193–199.

35. Hari, Kuralla, Saripilli Rajeswari, and V K Ramanamurthy. 2018. "Preparation and evaluation of orally disintegrating tablets of drotaverine hydrochloride using the sublimation technique." *International Journal of Pharmacy and Pharmaceutical Sciences* 10:85–95.

36. Sree, G P B, S N Siva, M Swetha, V R M Gupta, N Devanna, and S Madiha. 2013. "Formulation and evaluation of orodispersible tablets of levocetirizine by melt granulation technology." *Der Pharmacia Lettre* 5:107–115.

37. Nagar, Priyanka, Kusum Singh, Iti Chauhan, Madhu Verma, Mohd Yasir, Azad Khan, Rajat Sharma, and Nandini Gupta. 2011. "Orally disintegrating tablets: formulation, preparation techniques and evaluation." *Journal of Applied Pharmaceutical Science* 1 (04):35–45.

38. Roy, Anupam. 2016. "Orodispersible tablets: a review." *Asian Journal of Pharmaceutical and Clinical Research* 9 (1):19–26.

39. Hiremath, Praveen, Kalyan Nuguru, and Vivek Agrahari. 2019. "Material attributes and their impact on wet granulation process performance." In *Handbook of Pharmaceutical Wet Granulation*, 263–315. Elsevier, Cambridge, MA, USA.

40. Manivannan, Rangasamy. 2009. "Oral disintegrating tablets: a future compaction." *Drug Invention Today* 1 (1):61–65.

41. Amipara, Lalji Vajubhai, and M M Gupta. 2013. "Oral disintegrating tablet of antihypertensive drug." *Journal of Drug Delivery and Therapeutics* 3 (1).

42. Beri, Chiman, and Isha Sacher. 2013. "Development of fast disintegration tablets as oral drug delivery system-A review." *Indian Journal of Pharmaceutical and Biological Research* 1:3.

43. Kumar, Erande, and Joshi Bhagyashree. 2013. "Mouth dissolving tablets–A comprehensive review." *International Journal of Pharma Research & Review* 2 (7):25–41.

44. Okuda, Y, Y Irisawa, K Okimoto, T Osawa, and S Yamashita. 2009. "A new formulation for orally disintegrating tablets using a suspension spray-coating method." *International Journal of Pharmaceutics* 382 (1–2):80–87.

45. Watanabe, Yoshiteru, Keiichi Koizumi, Yoshiko Zama, Miyuki Kiriyama, Yoshiaki Matsumoto, and Mitsuo Matsumoto. 1995. "New compressed tablet rapidly disintegrating in saliva in the mouth using crystalline cellulose and a disintegrant." *Biological and Pharmaceutical Bulletin* 18 (9):1308–1310.

46. Ishikawa, Tatsuya, Baku Mukai, Shuji Shiraishi, Naoki Utoguchi, Makiko Fuji, Mitsuo Matsumoto, and Yoshiteru Watanabe. 2001. "Preparation of rapidly disintegrating tablet using new types of micro-crystalline cellulose (PH-M series) and low substituted-hydroxypropylcellulose or spherical sugar granules by direct compression method." *Chemical and Pharmaceutical Bulletin* 49 (2):134–139.

47. Bi, Y X, H Sunada, Y Yonezawa, and K Danjo. 1999. "Evaluation of rapidly disintegrating tablets prepared by a direct compression method." *Drug Development and Industrial Pharmacy* 25 (5):571–581.

48. Al-khattawi, Ali, and Afzal R Mohammed. 2013. "Compressed orally disintegrating tablets: excipients evolution and formulation strategies." *Expert Opinion on Drug Delivery* 10 (5):651–663.

49. Yang, Dong, Rajesh Kulkarni, Robert J Behme, and Pramila N Kotiyan. 2007. "Effect of the melt granulation technique on the dissolution characteristics of griseofulvin." *International Journal of Pharmaceutics* 329 (1–2):72–80.

50. Abdelbary, G, P Prinderre, C Eouani, J Joachim, J P Reynier, and Ph Piccerelle. 2004. "The preparation of orally disintegrating tablets using a hydrophilic waxy binder." *International Journal of Pharmaceutics* 278 (2):423–433.

51. Bi, Yunxia, Hisakazu Sunada, Yorinobu Yonezawa, Kazumi Danjo, Akinobu Otsuka, and Kotaro Iida. 1996. "Preparation and evaluation of a compressed tablet rapidly disintegrating in the oral cavity." *Chemical and Oharmaceutical Bulletin* 44 (11):2121–2127.

52. AlHusban, Farhan, Amr ElShaer, Jiteen Kansara, Alan Smith, Liam Grover, Yvonne Perrie, and Afzal Mohammed. 2010. "Investigation of formulation and process of lyophilised orally disintegrating tablet (ODT) using novel amino acid combination." *Pharmaceutics* 2 (1):1–17.

53. Fukami, Jinichi, Asuka Ozawa, Yasuo Yoshihashi, Etsuo Yonemochi, and Katsuhide Terada. 2005. "Development of fast disintegrating compressed tablets using amino acid as disintegration accelerator: evaluation of wetting and disintegration of tablet on the basis of surface free energy." *Chemical and Pharmaceutical Bulletin* 53 (12):1536–1539.

54. Pahwa, Rakesh, Shwetakshi Sharma, Abhinav Singh Rana, Anshul Garg, and Inderbir Singh. 2016. "Emergence of natural superdisintegrants in the development of orally disintegrating tablets." *Indo American Journal of Pharmaceutical Sciences* 3 (8):777–787.

55. Ayenew, Zelalem, Vibha Puri, Lokesh Kumar, and Arvind K Bansal. 2009. "Trends in pharmaceutical taste-masking technologies: a patent review." *Recent Patents on Drug Delivery & Formulation* 3 (1):26–39.

56. Bertelsen, Poul Egon, Peder Mohr Olsen, Carsten Martini Nielsen, and Magnus Wilhelm Tolleshaug. 2014. Melt granulation of a composition containing a calcium-containing compound. Google Patents.
57. Dabre, Rahul, Vishnubhotla Nagaprasad, and Rajiv Malik. 2007. Taste masked compositions of erythromycin a and derivatives thereof. Google Patents.
58. Stroppolo, Federico, Franco Ciccarello, Rita Milani, and Lorenzo Bellorini. 2004. Oral pharmaceutical compositions containing cyclodextrins as taste-masking agent. Google Patents.
59. Habib, Walid, and Derek Moe. 2006. Taste masking system for alprazolam. Google Patents.
60. Mukherji, Gour, Sandhya Goel, and Vinod Kumar Arora. 2003. Taste masked compositions. Google Patents.
61. El-Arini, Silvia Kocova, and Sophie-Dorothée Clas. 2002. "Evaluation of disintegration testing of different fast dissolving tablets using the texture analyzer." *Pharmaceutical Development and Technology* 7 (3):361–371.
62. Klancke, James. 2003. "Dissolution testing of orally disintegrating tablets." *Dissolution Technologies* 10 (2):6–9.

19 Melt Granulation

Shana Van de Steene, Valérie Vanhoorne, Chris Vervaet, and Thomas De Beer

CONTENTS

19.1 INTRODUCTION

Prior to tableting, granulation is a particle enlargement step that is often required in pharmaceutical manufacturing to facilitate the processing of raw materials into solid oral dosage forms to improve processability, compactability, flowability, and content uniformity of powder blends. Traditionally, the agglomeration process is performed via wet granulation whereby adding a solvent (often water), binding between powder particles, is initiated, which is followed by a drying step for consolidation [1,2]. Next to wet granulation, dry granulation is a second often used technique which has gained more interest over the past years and which requires no solvent for granulation; hence, no drying step has to be performed [3]. Roller compaction is a relatively simple dry granulation process that not only enables a significant increase in the bulk density of the material but also has a few drawbacks. A lot of fines and dust are formed during roller compaction, and this technique reduces the compaction properties of the powder particles [4]. Hence, processing via wet or dry granulation requires specific material properties (e.g., for wet granulation, the materials cannot be heat- or moisture-sensitive) and additional processing steps before obtaining the end product (e.g., drying for wet granulation and milling for dry granulation). A mutual drawback of both techniques is that the drug load in the formulation is limited which can be problematic for high-dose formulations [5,6].

With this in mind, melt (or thermoplastic) granulation is an interesting alternative technique to perform agglomeration due to its multiple advantages. Melt granulation can offer a solution to challenging formulations and is able to counter several of the disadvantages of wet and dry granulation. This technique uses a meltable binder which is solid at ambient temperature, establishes liquid bridges between particles when the binder melts in a heated powder bed to initiate agglomeration [i.e., moisture-sensitive active pharmaceutical ingredients (APIs) can be processed], and forms solid bridges to consolidate the agglomerates when reducing the temperature of the powder bed. The binder also remains in the formulation as a constituent which eliminates the drying step required for wet granulation to evaporate the granulation liquid [7–9]. The lack of drying in melt granulation also results in higher granule density and reduced porosity which is advantageous for the compactability [10]. Furthermore, the possibility to develop high-dose formulations with up to 95% of active pharmaceutical ingredient (API), the ability to modulate release kinetics of the API using different binders, and the relatively low processing temperatures can be added to the extensive list of advantages of melt granulation. An overview of the binders used for melt granulation is provided in Table 19.1 [3,8,9]. Batch-wise melt granulation offers the advantage that all unit operations can be performed in the same equipment which is not the case for wet granulation. As mixing, agglomerating, and forming of solid bridges are performed in a single-pot process, the risk of material loss due to transfers between different unit operations is minimized. A disadvantage that should be taken into account for melt granulation is the risk of thermal degradation of the API. However, by choosing a specific melt granulation technique (e.g., twin-screw melt granulation) in combination with a binder with a low melting temperature, the residence time of the API in the process can be minimized to avoid the risk of thermal degradation.

Although melt granulation offers several advantages compared to wet granulation, it is only since the 1990s that intensive studies have been conducted on high-shear melt granulation as the first batch-wise manufacturing process to perform melt granulation. Research on fluidized bed melt granulation increased in the early 2000s, and in the past decade, the pharmaceutical industry gained more and more interest in continuous (twin-screw) melt granulation [1,11]. This is reflected in the examples of commercialized products manufactured via melt granulation in Table 19.2.

The binder for melt granulation can be incorporated into the melt agglomeration process via two techniques: the melt-in method and spray-on or pour-on method. In the former method, the binder is blended with the active pharmaceutical ingredient (API) in solid form as powder or flakes, and the entire blend is heated to soften or liquify the binder to initiate particle agglomeration. In the latter method, the binder is melted separately before it is added to the API/excipient blend. The binders that are used in melt granulation can be polymers or waxes, and these typically have a relatively low melting point in the range of 50–90°C. Binders with a melting point below 50°C are

TABLE 19.1
List of Commonly Used Binders for Melt Granulation

Lipophilic Binders	Hydrophilic Binders
Beeswax	Polyethylene glycol (3000–20000)
Carnauba wax	Polyethylene oxide
Microcrystalline wax	Ethylene oxide–propylene oxide
Paraffin wax	Gelucire 50/13
Cetostearyl alcohol	Gelucire 44/14
Stearic acid	Polyvinylpyrrolidone
Palmitic acid	Polyvinyl acetate/polyvinylpyrrolidone
Glyceryl tripalmitate	Polyvinyl alcohol–polyethylene glycol copolymer and polyvinyl alcohol
Glyceryl tristearate	Hydroxypropyl cellulose (HPC)
Glyceryl palmitostearate	Hydroxypropyl methylcellulose
Glyceryl behenate	Hydroxypropyl methylcellulose acetate succinate (HPMC-AS)
Glyceryl monostearate	Acrylate-based copolymers (Eudragit E PO, Eudragit L100-55)
Hydrogenated soybean oil	
Hydrogenated castor oil	

TABLE 19.2
Overview of Commercialized Melt Granulation Products [12–14]

Name	Drug	Company	Process	Reason
Eucreas®	Metformin HCl/vildagliptin	Novartis	Twin-screw melt granulation	Moisture-sensitive
Certican®	Everolimus	Novartis	Fluid-bed melt granulation	Poor solubility
LCP-Tacro®	Tacrolimus	Lifecycle Pharma	Tumbling melt granulation	Poor solubility
Fenoglide®	Fenofibrate	Veloxis	Fluid-bed melt granulation	Poor solubility
Zithromax®	Azithromycin	Pfizer	Spray congealing	Taste masking

rarely used to avoid softening during downstream processing or storage. The binder preferably has a melting point below 90°C to keep the processing temperatures as low as possible to minimize the risk of thermal degradation. The binders can have very divergent properties which will result in different release profiles. Hydrophilic binders can be used for immediate release formulations, while hydrophobic binders allow developing sustained-release formulations. Using a mixture of hydrophilic and hydrophobic binders, the desired release profile can be achieved [1,3,8,15,16]. If a formulation is developed for sustained release, the structural integrity of the sustained-release matrices should also be maintained after oral administration to avoid dose-dumping.

Three different phases can be identified during a melt granulation process and are comparable to wet granulation: nucleation, coalescence, and the combined phenomena of attrition and breakage. Two granulation mechanisms are identified for melt granulation, distribution and immersion mechanisms which are illustrated in Figure 19.1. Both mechanisms can occur simultaneously, but which mechanism will occur preferentially depends on the various formulation and process parameters, for example, the particle size ratio of the API and binder. The distribution mechanism is promoted when the binder droplet size is smaller than the powder particles of the drug, while immersion dominates when the binder droplet size exceeds the particle size of the drug. In the distribution mechanism, the molten binder liquid is distributed on the surface of the primary particles, and nuclei (held together via liquid bridges) are formed via coalescence of primary particles. Agglomerate growth further occurs via coalescence of nuclei provided that liquid saturation is sufficient. In the case of immersion, nuclei are formed when the initial solid particles become immersed in the surface of a molten binder particle/droplet [1].

Next to binders, other excipients can be added to a formulation processed via melt granulation to enhance the bioavailability, stability, or processability of the drug in a solid oral dosage form.

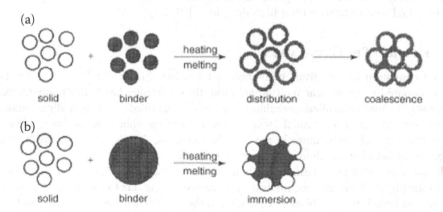

FIGURE 19.1 Agglomerate Formation Mechanism in Melt Agglomeration. (A) Distribution Mechanism and (B) Immersion Mechanism [17].

Plasticizers, anti-oxidants, disintegrants, surfactants, and lubricants are examples of excipients that can be added to the melt granulation process. To make a selection of an appropriate excipient, it has to fulfill the same requirements as set for the API: it should also be able to withstand the heat that is generated during the granulation process to guarantee the stability of the formulation [3,8].

19.2 BATCH MELT GRANULATION

19.2.1 HIGH-SHEAR GRANULATION

The equipment for high-shear melt granulation consists of a mixing bowl with a heated jacket and an impeller and a chopper as mixing elements inside the bowl. The main process settings for high-shear granulation that can be varied during high-shear melt granulation are the impeller speed and the jacket temperature. The melt granulation process can be divided into four different phases: mixing, heating, kneading, and cooling. The function of the impeller is to blend the powder and to distribute the binder homogeneously, while the chopper enables the breaking up of large agglomerates [18]. Both methods of binder addition mentioned in the introduction of this chapter can be applied for high-shear melt granulation: the melt-in and the spray-on/pour-on methods which are discussed in detail in the introduction. The main advantages of this technique are the production of high-density granules and the possibility to process highly viscous binders. The heat to melt the binder originates from the heating jacket via conductive heat transfer, while heat is also generated by the frictional forces of the impeller. The jacket temperature is ideally chosen slightly below the melting point of the binder during the heating and kneading phase, while it will be set at a much lower temperature during the mixing (i.e., to maintain a solid mass) and cooling (i.e., to solidify the binder) phase. The impeller speed is also increased during the heating and kneading phase which will generate more frictional forces and increase the product temperature to obtain granules with uniform quality attributes. Due to the design of the equipment, the contact surface between product and the heated jacket is limited, possibly resulting in an uneven heat exposure of the material which could lead to inhomogeneous binder distribution and uncontrolled non-uniform granule growth [8,17].

The high-shear mixer and the influence of process parameters were extensively investigated for melt granulation by the group of Schaefer and Kristensen in the first decade of this century. The endpoint of agglomeration in a high-shear mixer can be determined by measuring the power consumption of the impeller [19]. Schæfer et al. also showed that the distribution mechanism is promoted if the binder has a small particle size, low viscosity, and a high impeller speed [17,20]. During the past decade, substantially more research was performed on the impact of formulation parameters during high-shear melt granulation, but mainly for sustained- and controlled-release formulations and formulations with a high drug load [21–24].

19.2.2 FLUIDIZED BED GRANULATION

Fluid-bed granulation differs from high-shear granulation due to the low-shear forces in this process. Compared to high-shear melt granulation, this technique has better temperature control, and therefore, a more controlled granulation process is obtained. In a high-shear mixer, heat is originating not only from the heated jacket but also from the shear forces. Since these are negligible for the material temperature in the fluid bed process, the energy input can be completely controlled by monitoring the fluidization air temperature.

For fluidized bed melt granulation, both binder addition methods can be used. The binder can be blended in the physical mixture and melts during the processing due to the hot air that is circulating in the fluidized bed. When the binder is blended in the powder as coarse particles and the *in situ/* melt-in method is applied, the immersion mechanism is promoted with subsequent layering. If the binder is added as fine particles, the distribution mechanism will be the dominating nucleation mechanism followed by coalescence. The influence of the binder particle size can be seen in Figure 19.2 [7,11,19,26,27]. The binder particle size, binder content, binder viscosity, and granulation time appear to be the most influencing factors that determine granule size and shape for the *in situ* fluid-bed melt granulation technique (Figure 19.3). Smaller binder particles or a higher binder content will lead to a higher yield fraction. When large binder particles are combined with a low binder concentration, a low yield is obtained which is linked to a larger fraction of un-granulated powder particles when immersion and layering are the dominant agglomeration mechanism and the amount of binder in the formulation is insufficient. The granulation time is also identified as an influencing factor, and a longer granulation time results in larger granules, but the granule growth rate is dependent on the binder concentration [10,11,26].

The second method is the spray-on or pour-on method where the binder is continuously sprayed via a bottom- or top-spray nozzle until sufficient binder is added to achieve granulation. When the binder is sprayed onto a powder bed containing solid particles larger than the binder droplets, nucleation via the distribution mechanism mainly takes place followed by coalescence. Immersion is the dominant mechanism if the solid particles are smaller compared to the binder droplet size. Distribution results in a more open agglomerate structure, while immersion yields a denser structure. It can also be stated that a larger binder droplet size, as well as a higher viscosity, will result in larger granules [25,27]. This effect on granule size mainly takes place at low processing temperatures due to the high binder viscosity and the solidification of the binder. If higher processing temperatures are used, the droplet size and binder viscosity have a negligible influence on the final agglomerate size. The granulation process is also significantly affected by the binder spray rate, fluid-bed temperature, and atomizing air pressure, indicating that the spray nozzle conditions control the granule formation mechanism [28–30].

For the spray-on method, the granulation mechanism can be divided into different events. At first, the solid particles capture the binder droplets which is followed by the wetting of the particle. If a single particle is wetted, either the particle can collide with another particle to initiate agglomeration via liquid bridges or the binder solidifies before any collision occurs. Aggregation or coalescence continues until the binder solidifies or until the liquid bridges break. After solidification, breakage of these solid bridges is still possible which results in the generation of smaller granules [31]. The granule growth can be controlled easily for the melt-in method compared to the spray-on method as the coalescence of wetted particles is more likely in the spray-on method. Consequently, rapid granule growth can be initiated due to the higher frequency of coalescence of the wetted particles.

19.2.3 MELT PELLETIZATION

Spherical beads or pellets are formed via this melt process, yielding particles with a diameter between 0.5 and 2 mm, a lower porosity, and higher sphericity compared to other melt granulation techniques [32]. Melt pelletization can be performed in a high-shear or fluid-bed granulator by applying higher shearing forces and/or longer massing times [19]. A rotary processor (i.e., a fluid-bed granulator which is equipped with a rotational friction plate, Figure 19.4) is the most often used equipment to perform melt pelletization. The bottom plate in the granulator can have various textures to vary the shear forces on the material. Similar to a high-shear mixer, torque measurements of the rotational plate and the energy consumption can be monitored and used as a tool to determine the endpoint of spheronization, next to measuring the product temperature.

The melt pelletization process can be divided into a pre- and post-melting phase. During the latter phase, the temperature of the material exceeds the melting point of the binder to allow the binder to form liquid bridges between the solid particles. Furthermore, during this phase, the process parameters are set to ensure a smooth surface, lower porosity, and high sphericity of the granules [33,34].

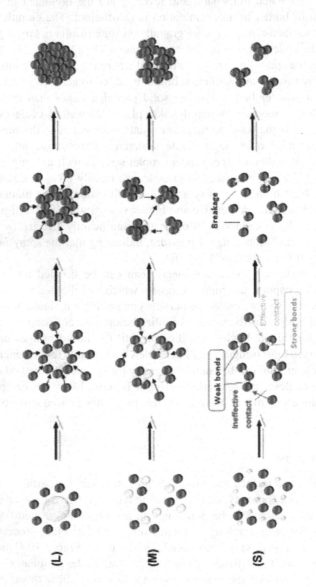

FIGURE 19.2 Proposed Agglomerate Growth Mechanisms During Fluidized Bed Melt Granulation in the Function of the Particle Size of the Binders. (L) Binder Size = 710–1000 μm; (M) Binder Size = 125–250 μm; (S) Binder Size = 45–90 μm [25].

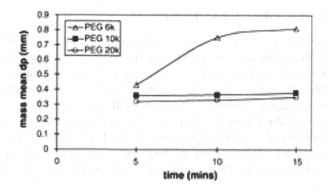

FIGURE 19.3 Effect of Granulation Time and Binder Viscosity on Mean Particle Diameter During Fluidized Bed Melt Granulation. (Formulation: Lactose/PEG 90/10 (w/w); Air Speed = 1.0 ms^{-1}, Granulation Temperature = 80°C, Initial Lactose Size = 54 μm) [10].

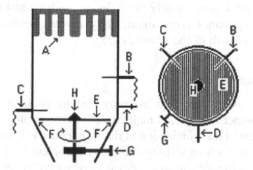

FIGURE 19.4 Schematic Drawing of the Rotary Processor (Left: Side View; Right: Top View): (A) Exhaust; (B) Upper Product Temperature Sensor; (C) Lower Product Temperature Sensor; (D) Sample Thief; (E) Friction Plate; (F) Air Gap; (G) Friction Plate Elevator; and (H) Cone [19].)

19.2.4 Tumbling Melt Granulation

Tumbling melt granulation is a technique where meltable and non-meltable material adheres to core beads using a centrifugal fluidizing granulator. This technique is less frequently used and studied compared to previously mentioned techniques in this chapter but is applied in some cases to formulate poorly soluble drugs as can be seen in Table 19.2. This is performed by adding a mixture of binder and particles to the heated beads in the centrifugal granulator. During granulation,

the processing temperature of the bed is set at least 5°C above the melting point of the binder in the formulation. The surface of the beads is gradually compacted and smoothened while maintaining the temperature and tumbling of the bed. When the granulation process is finished, the granules are cooled at room temperature. Preferably, the core beads have a narrow size distribution and a smooth surface to ensure the formation of a uniform layer which is especially important for sustained, controlled, or enteric formulations. Granulation temperature, particle size, and concentration of the raw materials should be optimized to achieve granules with good quality attributes [35,36]. Next to the former properties, the viscosity of the binder also influences the efficiency of the granulation process. A high viscosity binder hinders the distribution of the binder on the surface of the beads which results in fewer powder particles adhering to the beads and a more irregular surface of the beads [37].

19.3 CONTINUOUS MELT GRANULATION

Nowadays, the pharmaceutical industry is more and more interested in innovative manu-facturing techniques that allow continuous manufacturing to improve process efficiency. A few of the main drivers to make a switch from batch-wise to continuous melt granulation are the uniform heat transfer onto the powder bed with better control of the product temperature and more uniform granule quality attributes, the easy scale-up from development to industrial production capacity (only the production time must be extended), and the short residence time. While the material residence time for high-shear or fluid-bed melt granulation is also in the order of (tens of) minutes, the exposure of heat can – for some continuous techniques – be limited for only a few seconds. This significantly reduces the risk of thermal degradation of the API or excipients.

In batch-wise melt granulation, it is challenging to determine the endpoint of the process and to control the temperature of the product. For example, using a high-shear mixer, the product tem-perature is influenced by the heating of the jacket of the mixing bowl and by frictional forces during granulation. As product temperature in the mixing bowl as high as 100°C was recorded when the jacket temperature was set at only 50°C due to the frictional forces and the insufficient cooling capacity of the equipment, this can significantly increase the risk of thermal degradation of the API and uncontrolled growth of the granules [38].

19.3.1 SPRAY CONGEALING

During spray congealing, also referred to as spray chilling or spray cooling, a liquid melt is atomized in a cooling chamber. This liquid melt consists of the molten binder in which the API is dispersed or dissolved. Next to the atomization of the melt, cold gas is introduced into this chamber in the same direction as the melt to solidify the molten droplets [39] (Figure 19.5). Spray con-gealing can be compared as the solvent-free equivalent of spray-drying similar to high-shear melt granulation being the solvent-free equivalent of high-shear wet granulation [40].

Various molten carriers can be used for spray congealing which allows different applications of these microparticles. Immediate as well as controlled release particles can be developed for oral administration, and topical and parenteral applications depending on the binder used for the manufacturing of the microparticles. Spray-congealed particles can enhance the dissolution of poorly soluble drugs or microencapsulate liquids into solids [41]. While particles resulting from spray-drying typically result in hollow, low-density particles due to the evaporation of the solvent, the lack of an evaporation step during spray congealing results in dense spherical particles [39].

Microparticles produced via spray congealing are generally smaller than 500 µm, as the molten carrier in which the API is dissolved or dispersed is atomized into the cooling chamber [42]. As the process temperature in this chamber is below the melting point of the carrier, the small droplets congeal in contact with the cool airflow, forming solid spherical particles [41,43–45]. Next to the processing of small molecules, spray congealing also allows to incorporate large molecules, for example, proteins, in lipid microparticles [41,46].

For atomization, ultrasonic atomizers or wide pneumatic nozzles are used. The latter enables the formation of spherical and non-aggregated microparticles with high encapsulation efficiency. A disadvantage of spray congealing is the quite long exposure time to elevated temperatures (i.e., in the bulk reservoir of the molten liquid before atomization) with possible thermal degradation of APIs (e.g., protein conformational instability). After atomization in the congealing chamber, the droplets are rapidly cooled, but this fast cooling of the melt can enable a polymorphic transition which endangers the stability of the microparticles. Another major limitation of this technique is the drug load of the formulation that can be processed with spray congealing. If the drug load exceeds 25–30%, the viscosity of the melt is too high which prevents the atomization of the molten mass.

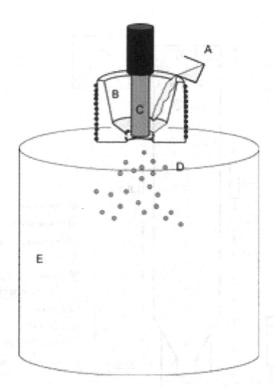

FIGURE 19.5 Schematic Representation (Not in Scale) of an (Ultrasonic) Spray Congealing Process: (A) Drug + Molten Carrier, (B) Temperature-Controlled Reservoir, (C) Atomizer, (D) Molten Droplets, and (E) Cooling Chamber [40].

However, in some cases, drug loads up to 50% could be achieved using a specific nozzle design. Preferably, the viscosity of the melt is lower than 500 mPas to obtain efficient atomization [39,47].

19.3.2 PRILLING

A second continuous melt granulation technique is prilling [48]. Prilling can be considered as a type of spray congealing where particles larger than 500 μm are formed, and both techniques are applied to produce solid lipid-based formulations to enhance the bioavailability or modify the drug release using lipophilic matrix materials (e.g., triglycerides, waxes, and fatty acids) [49,50]. A homogeneous liquid phase, consisting of API dissolved or dispersed in a molten lipid matrix, is pumped through a (vibrating) nozzle, and the resulting droplets solidify during their fall in the cooling chamber [48]. A schematic overview of the prilling technique is presented in Figure 19.6. Applications of this new and innovative manufacturing technique in the pharmaceutical industry are currently very limited due to the lack of knowledge. However, it allows to efficiently sustain the release rate of highly water-soluble APIs incorporated in a hydrophobic matrix [52,53].

Prilling requires no additional downstream processing steps and yields spherical particles with excellent flow properties and narrow size distribution (Figure 19.7). These quality attributes facilitate the filling of prills in capsules or sachets to produce multiparticulate formulations. These formulations provide flexibility to modify the dose or to combine prills with different drugs, matrices, or drug loads in one capsule or sachet, without changing the formulation or prilling process. The drug can be dissolved or dispersed in a lipophilic matrix where the choice of lipid and additives can modify the drug release. For example, pore formers or emulsifiers can be added to enhance the dissolution of the drug from the matrix [49].

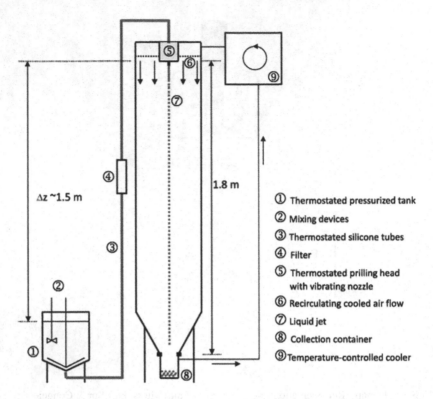

Δz ~1.5 m

1.8 m

① Thermostated pressurized tank
② Mixing devices
③ Thermostated silicone tubes
④ Filter
⑤ Thermostated prilling head
   with vibrating nozzle
⑥ Recirculating cooled air flow
⑦ Liquid jet
⑧ Collection container
⑨ Temperature-controlled cooler

FIGURE 19.6   Schematic Configuration of the Prilling Process (Not at Scale) [51].

A major disadvantage of this technique is the limited drug load (20–50%) that can be incorporated due to viscosity issues. The viscosity is limited to ensure homogenous droplet formation and to avoid blocking of the nozzle. This process also requires high prilling towers to ensure sufficient solidification of the prills which increases the cost of the process. In addition, relatively low throughput is obtained for this technique, but this can be countered by the use of multiple nozzles for droplet formation [48].

The critical process parameters are the homogeneity of the solubilized or dispersed mixture, the processing temperature, the viscosity of the formulation, and the cooling capacity to ensure rapid and uniform solidification of the droplets during prilling. If the mixture is not homogeneous, the drug concentration varies per droplet and viscosity fluctuations influence the droplet formation rate and uniformity. Generally, the processing temperature is 10°C above the melting temperature of the lipids present in the formulation, and a viscosity limit of 500 mPas is applied [39,51].

19.3.3 MELT EXTRUSION

Melt extrusion is typically performed with a single- or twin-screw extruder, using a co- or counter-rotating setup for the latter. During melt extrusion, a heated barrel ensures that the binder in the formulation melts or softens to initiate interactions between the particles. The screws ensure that the material is pumped through the die to yield an end product with a uniform shape (defined by the dimensions of the die) and high density. To transform these extrudates into small discrete agglomerates (i.e., granules), milling is needed as a downstream processing step. Melt extrusion can also produce other types of solid dosage forms (e.g., tablets, films, co-extruded formulations), but this is not within the scope of this chapter. For more information on these applications of melt extrusion, the reader is referred to the following papers [54–58].

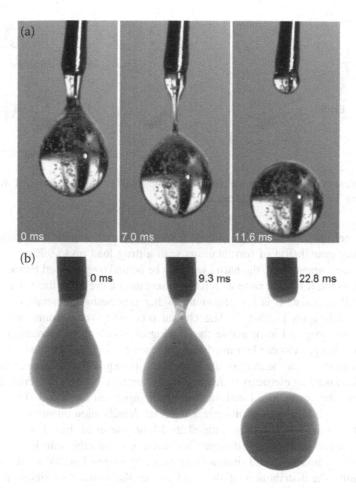

FIGURE 19.7 Spherical Droplet Formation at the Nozzle of (A) a Transparent 30% Metoprolol Tartrate in Behenic Acid Solution and (B) an opaque 10% Metformin in Behenic Acid Suspension in the Function of Time [52].

19.3.4 TWIN-SCREW MELT GRANULATION

A twin-screw extruder can be used to directly manufacture granules (in contrast to the melt extrusion process) provided that the densification of the formulation at the end of the extruder barrel is limited. Hence, this process is run without a die plate, allowing to discharge the material with minimal densification. The first granulation application with a twin-screw extruder was already described in 1988 for the production of an effervescent formulation of paracetamol [59]. In a twin-screw melt granulation process, the material is transported along the barrel using fully modular screws which consist of conveying, kneading, and optionally screw-mixing elements. The kneading elements, located in one or multiple kneading zones which can vary in location, number of kneading elements, and staggering angle between adjacent kneading elements, are essential to initiate interactions between solid particles and binder and form the agglomerates. Screw-mixing elements, which are typically placed at the end of the screw shafts, reduce the size of large lumps to yield a narrower granule size distribution [1,60]. The granule size distribution can also be modified after granulation by including a milling step in the process [61,62]. The screw config-uration can be optimized depending on the formulation properties and the required granule quality

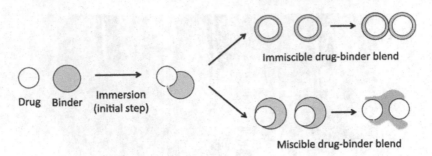

FIGURE 19.8 Visualization of Granule Growth Mechanism for a Miscible and Immiscible Binder Formulation During Twin-Screw Melt Granulation [1].

attributes for further downstream processing [1,63,64]. Twin-screw melt granulation is an efficient technique allowing granulation of formulations with a drug load up to 90%.

In twin-screw melt granulation, the barrel wall can be heated over a broad temperature range, even up to 200°C. But as the residence time within the granulation barrel is in the order of a few seconds, the risk of thermal degradation is less, allowing higher processing temperature compared to other melt granulation techniques [1,65–67]. The chosen processing temperature has to be below the melting point of the drug and at or above the melting or softening temperature of the binder. For some formulations, the process can be run adiabatically when – in case of a binder with a low melting or softening temperature – no heating of the barrel wall is required as sufficient shear and heat are generated from the kneading elements to achieve agglomeration. Next to the screw configuration and barrel temperature, the screw speed and material throughput can be varied. These two parameters determine the barrel fill level which influences material densification during processing [3,62,68].

Two granulation mechanisms were defined by Monteyne et al. based on the interactions between drug and binder, identifying different mechanisms in miscible and immiscible drug/binder blends. In case of a miscible blend, interactions (e.g., hydrogen bonds) occur between drug and binder which limits the distribution of the binder over the powder particles. In case of an immiscible blend, there is no interaction between drug and binder and therefore the distribution of the binder will be more homogenous. These mechanisms are schematically illustrated in Figure 19.8. Depending on the granulation mechanism, other process and formulation parameters are identified that have an influence on the granule properties. For a miscible system, the powder feed rate and consequently the barrel filling degree strongly affect the granule properties, whereas for an immiscible system, the binder concentration is influencing the granule properties [1,64].

19.4 FORMULATION AND PROCESS SELECTION FOR MELT GRANULATION

In order to select a formulation or a process for an API, it is important to gain knowledge about the physicochemical properties of the API and excipients and to determine the desired properties of the end product in terms of flowability, drug load, and drug release profile. Before developing a melt granulation process for an API, a formulation should be defined. The desired drug release profile has to be kept in mind when the binder is chosen. For a sustained-release formulation, hydrophobic binders like waxes, stearic acid, and glyceryl behenate can be selected, while immediate release profiles can be obtained using hydrophilic binders like polyethylene glycols, HPC, or HPMC (Table 19.1). The drug release can be even more controlled using multiple binders and optionally other excipients to enhance or delay the drug release as investigated by Monteyne et al. for a formulation with stearic acid and PEO [63,64,69].

In addition to the drug release profile, the miscibility of the API and the binder must be taken into account. If the formulation is miscible, interactions like hydrogen bonding can take place between API and excipients. These can influence the glass transition temperature of the binder due

TABLE 19.3

Overview of Granule Quality Attributes Obtained Depending on the Used Production Technique (– for Low Value Of Quality Attribute; + for High Value of Quality Attribute)

	Fluid-Bed Granulation	High-Shear Granulation	Tumbling Melt Granulation	Melt Pelletization	Spray Congealing	Prilling	Melt Extrusion	Twin-Screw Granulation
Density	–	+	+	+	+	+	+	–
Porosity	+	–	–	–	–	–	–	+
Compressibility	+	–	–	–	–	–	–	+
Sphericity	–	+	‡	+	+	‡	+	–
Drug load	+	+	–	–	–	–	+	‡
Residence time	+	+	+	–	+	+	–	–

to a plasticizing effect. Furthermore, it can affect the rheological properties of the binder or inhibit the distribution of the binder over the powder particles. In contrast, in an immiscible system, the binder can easily distribute over the powder particles once the binder is molten. The miscibility of all ingredients can be predicted by calculating the three-dimensional Hansen solubility parameters or it can be determined via differential scanning calorimetry (DSC) or spectroscopic analysis [9,64,70–73].

Next to the formulation, a process for melt granulation has to be selected. At first, a batch-wise or continuous process mode must be selected. Selection of the granule quality attributes which are required for efficient downstream processing (e.g., improved flowability or dissolution rate) is also critical. In Table 19.3, an overview of the obtained quality attributes per melt granulation technique is presented in order to facilitate the selection of a specific melt granulation technique [69,74].

REFERENCES

1. Monteyne, Tinne, Jochem Vancoillie, Jean Paul Remon, Chris Vervaet, and Thomas De Beer. 2016. Continuous Melt Granulation: Influence of Process and Formulation Parameters upon Granule and Tablet Properties. European Journal of Pharmaceutics and Biopharmaceutics 107. Elsevier B.V.: 249–262. doi:10.1016/j.ejpb.2016.07.021.
2. Patil, Hemlata, Roshan V. Tiwari, Sampada B. Upadhye, Ronald S. Vladyka, and Michael A. Repka. 2015. Formulation and Development of PH-Independent/Dependent Sustained Release Matrix Tablets of Ondansetron HCl by a Continuous Twin-Screw Melt Granulation Process. International Journal of Pharmaceutics 496 (1). Elsevier B.V.: 33–41. doi:10.1016/j.ijpharm.2015.04.009.
3. Batra, Amol, Dipen Desai, and Abu T. M. Serajuddin. 2017. Investigating the Use of Polymeric Binders in Twin Screw Melt Granulation Process for Improving Compactibility of Drugs. Journal of Pharmaceutical Sciences 106 (1): 140–150. doi:10.1016/j.xphs.2016.07.014.
4. Bacher, C., P. M. Olsen, P. Bertelsen, and J. M. Sonnergaard. 2008. Compressibility and Compactibility of Granules Produced by Wet and Dry Granulation. International Journal of Pharmaceutics 358 (1–2). Elsevier: 69–74. doi:10.1016/j.ijpharm.2008.02.013.
5. Dalziel, Gena, Ewa Nauka, Feng Zhang, Sanjeev Kothari, and Minli Xie. 2013. Assessment of Granulation Technologies for an API with Poor Physical Properties. Drug Development and Industrial Pharmacy 39 (7): 985–995. doi:10.3109/03639045.2012.687744.
6. Meeus, Liesbeth. 2011. Direct Compression versus Granulation. Pharmaceutical Technology Europe 23 (3).
7. Korteby, Yasmine, Yassine Mahdi, Kamel Daoud, and Géza Regdon. 2019. A Novel Insight into Fluid Bed Melt Granulation: Temperature Mapping for the Determination of Granule Formation with the in-Situ and Spray-on Techniques. European Journal of Pharmaceutical Sciences 127 (January). Elsevier: 351–362. doi:10.1016/J.EJPS.2018.09.003.
8. Lakshman, Jay P., James Kowalski, Madhav Vasanthavada, Wei Qin Tong, Yatindra M. Joshi, and Abu T. M. Serajuddin. 2011. Application of Melt Granulation Technology to Enhance Tabletting Properties of Poorly Compactible High-Dose Drugs. Journal of Pharmaceutical Sciences 100 (4): 1553–1565. doi:10.1002/jps.22369.
9. Mu, B., and M. R. Thompson. 2012. Examining the Mechanics of Granulation with a Hot Melt Binder in a Twin-Screw Extruder. Chemical Engineering Science 81: 46–56. doi:10.1016/j.ces.2012.06.057.
10. Walker, G. M., G. Andrews, and D. Jones. 2006. Effect of Process Parameters on the Melt Granulation of Pharmaceutical Powders. Powder Technology 165 (3): 161–166. doi:10.1016/j.powtec.2006.03.024.
11. Mašić, Ivana, Ilija Ilić, Rok Dreu, Svetlana Ibrić, Jelena Parojčić, and Zorica Đurić. 2012. An Investigation into the Effect of Formulation Variables and Process Parameters on Characteristics of Granules Obtained by in Situ Fluidized Hot Melt Granulation. International Journal of Pharmaceutics 423 (2). Elsevier: 202–212. doi:10.1016/J.IJPHARM.2011.12.013.
12. Monteyne, Tinne. 2016. Development of Formulation and Process Knowledge for Continuous Twin-Screw Melt Granulation. Ghent University.
13. Newman, Ann, Gregory Knipp, and George Zografi. 2012. Assessing the Performance of Amorphous Solid Dispersions. Journal of Pharmaceutical Sciences 101 (4): 1355–1377. doi:10.1002/jps.23031.
14. Watts, Robert O. Williams III, Alan B. Miller, Dave A. 2012. Formulating Poorly Water Soluble Drugs. Springer, New York. doi: 10.1007/978-1-4614-1144-4.
15. Monteyne, Tinne, Peter Adriaensens, Davinia Brouckaert, Jean Paul Remon, Chris Vervaet, and

Thomas De Beer. 2016. Stearic Acid and High Molecular Weight PEO as Matrix for the Highly Water Soluble Metoprolol Tartrate in Continuous Twin-Screw Melt Granulation. International Journal of Pharmaceutics 512 (1). Elsevier B.V.: 158–167. doi:10.1016/j.ijpharm.2016.07.035.

16. Tan, David Cheng Thiam, William Wei Lim Chin, En Hui Tan, Shiqi Hong, Wei Gu, and Rajeev Gokhale. 2014. Effect of Binders on the Release Rates of Direct Molded Verapamil Tablets Using Twin-Screw Extruder in Melt Granulation. International Journal of Pharmaceutics 463 (1). Elsevier: 89–97. doi:10.1016/J.IJPHARM.2013.12.053.

17. Schæfer, Torben. 2001. Growth Mechanisms in Melt Agglomeration in High Shear Mixers. Powder Technology 117 (1–2). Elsevier: 68–82. doi:10.1016/S0032-5910(01)00315-1.

18. Osborne, James D., Robert P. J. Sochon, James J. Cartwright, David G. Doughty, Michael J. Hounslow, and Agba D. Salman. 2011. Binder Addition Methods and Binder Distribution in High Shear and Fluidised Bed Granulation. Chemical Engineering Research and Design 89 (5). Elsevier: 553–559. doi:10.1016/j.cherd.2010.08.006.

19. Vilhelmsen, Thomas, Jakob Kristensen, and Torben Schæfer. 2004. Melt Pelletization with Polyethylene Glycol in a Rotary Processor. International Journal of Pharmaceutics 275 (1–2). Elsevier: 141–153. doi:10.1016/J.IJPHARM.2004.01.027.

20. Eliasen, Helle, Torben Schæfer, and H. Gjelstrup Kristensen. 1998. Effects of Binder Rheology on Melt Agglomeration in a High Shear Mixer. International Journal of Pharmaceutics 176 (1): 73–83. doi:10.1016/S0378-5173(98)00306-8.

21. Aoki, Hajime, Yasunori Iwao, Midori Mizoguchi, Shuji Noguchi, and Shigeru Itai. 2015. Clarithromycin Highly-Loaded Gastro-Floating Fine Granules Prepared by High-Shear Melt Granulation Can Enhance the Efficacy of Helicobacter Pylori Eradication. European Journal of Pharmaceutics and Biopharmaceutics 92 (May). Elsevier: 22–27. doi:10.1016/j.ejpb.2015.02.012.

22. Aoki, Hajime, Yasunori Iwao, Takeaki Uchimoto, Shuji Noguchi, Ryusuke Kajihara, Kana Takahashi, Masayuki Ishida, Yasuko Terada, Yoshio Suzuki, and Shigeru Itai. 2015. Fine Granules Showing Sustained Drug Release Prepared by High-Shear Melt Granulation Using Triglycerin Full Behenate and Milled Microcrystalline Cellulose. International Journal of Pharmaceutics 478 (2). Elsevier: 530–539. doi:10.1016/j.ijpharm.2014.11.058.

23. Ochoa, L., M. Igartua, R. M. Hernández, A. R. Gascón, M. A. Solinis, and J. L. Pedraz. 2011. Novel Extended-Release Formulation of Lovastatin by One-Step Melt Granulation: In Vitro and in Vivo Evaluation. European Journal of Pharmaceutics and Biopharmaceutics 77 (2). Elsevier: 306–312. doi:10.1016/j.ejpb.2010.11.024.

24. Shiino, Kai, Yasunori Iwao, Yukari Fujinami, and Shigeru Itai. 2012. Preparation and Evaluation of Granules with PH-Dependent Release by Melt Granulation. International Journal of Pharmaceutics 431 (1–2). Elsevier: 70–77. doi:10.1016/j.ijpharm.2012.04.031.

25. Zhai, H., S. Li, D. S. Jones, G. M. Walker, and G. P. Andrews. 2010. The Effect of the Binder Size and Viscosity on Agglomerate Growth in Fluidised Hot Melt Granulation. Chemical Engineering Journal 164 (2–3). Elsevier: 275–284. doi:10.1016/J.CEJ.2010.08.056.

26. Aleksić, Ivana, Jelena Đuriš, Ilija Ilić, Svetlana Ibrić, Jelena Parojčić, and Stanko Srčič. 2014. In Silico Modeling of in Situ Fluidized Bed Melt Granulation. International Journal of Pharmaceutics 466 (1–2). Elsevier: 21–30. doi:10.1016/J.IJPHARM.2014.02.045.

27. Zhai, H., S. Li, G. Andrews, D. Jones, S. Bell, and G. Walker. 2009. Nucleation and Growth in Fluidised Hot Melt Granulation. Powder Technology 189 (2). Elsevier B.V.: 230–237. doi:10.1016/j.powtec.2008.04.021.

28. Abberger, Thomas, Anette Seo, and Torben Schæfer. 2002. The Effect of Droplet Size and Powder Particle Size on the Mechanisms of Nucleation and Growth in Fluid Bed Melt Agglomeration. International Journal of Pharmaceutics 249 (1–2): 185–197. doi:10.1016/S0378-5173(02)00530-6.

29. Borini, G. B., T. C. Andrade, and Luis A. P. Freitas. 2009. Hot Melt Granulation of Coarse Pharmaceutical Powders in a Spouted Bed. Powder Technology 189 (3). Elsevier: 520–527. doi:10.1016/J.POWTEC.2008.08.004.

30. Seo, Anette, Per Holm, and Torben Schafer. 2002. Effects of Droplet Size and Type of Binder on the Agglomerate Growth Mechanisms by Melt Agglomeration in a Fluidised Bed. European Journal of Pharmaceutical Sciences 16 (3): 95–105. doi:10.1016/S0928-0987(02)00086-6.

31. Tan, H. S., A. D. Salman, and M. J. Hounslow. 2006. Kinetics of Fluidised Bed Melt Granulation I: The Effect of Process Variables. Chemical Engineering Science 61 (5). Pergamon: 1585–1601. doi:10.1016/J.CES.2005.09.012.

32. Kondo, Keita, Aya Kato, and Toshiyuki Niwa. 2015. Development of a Novel Pelletization Technique through an Extremely High-Shear Process Using a Mechanical Powder Processor to Produce High-

Dose Small Core Granules Suitable for Film Coating. International Journal of Pharmaceutics. Volume 483, Issues 1–2, Pages 101-109 doi: 10.1016/j.ijpharm.2015.02.026.

33. Heng, Paul Wan Sia, Tin Wui Wong, and Lai Wah Chan. 2000. Influence of Production Variables on the Sphericity of Melt Pellets. Chemical and Pharmaceutical Bulletin. Volume 48, Issue 3, Pages 420-424 doi:10.1248/cpb.48.420.

34. Schæfer, Torben, Birgitte Taagegaard, Lars Juul Thomsen, and H. Gjelstrup Kristensen. 1993. Melt Pelletization in a High Shear Mixer. IV. Effects of Process Variables in a Laboratory Scale Mixer. European Journal of Pharmaceutical Sciences 1 (3): 125–131. doi:10.1016/0928-0987(93)90002-R.

35. Maejima, Toru, Masashi Kubo, Takashi Osawa, Kingo Nakajima, and Masao Kobayashi. 1998. Application of Tumbling Melt Granulation (TMG) Method to Prepare Controlled-Release Fine Granules. Chemical & Pharmaceutical Bulletin 46 (3). Pharmaceutical Society of Japan: 534–536. doi:10.1248/cpb.46.534.

36. Maejima, Toru, Takashi Osawa, Kingo Nakajima, and Masao Kobayashi. 1997b. Preparation of Spherical Beads without Any Use of Solvents by a Novel Tumbling Melt Granulation (TMG) Method. Chemical & Pharmaceutical Bulletin 45 (3). Pharmaceutical Society of Japan: 518–524. doi:10.1248/cpb.45.518.

37. Maejima, Toru, Takashi Osawa, Kingo Nakajima, and Masao Kobayashi. 1997a. Effects of Species of Non-Meltable and Meltable Materials and Their Physical Properties on Granulatability in Tumbling Melt Granulation Method. Chemical & Pharmaceutical Bulletin 45 (11). Pharmaceutical Society of Japan: 1833–1839. doi:10.1248/cpb.45.1833.

38. Schæfer, Torben, and Christina Mathiesen. 1996. Melt Pelletization in a High Shear Mixer. VII. Effects of Product Temperature. International Journal of Pharmaceutics 134 (1–2). Elsevier: 105–117. doi:10.1016/0378-5173(95)04455-8.

39. Cordeiro, Paula, Márcio Temtem, and Conrad Winters. n.d. Spray Congealing: Applications in the Pharmaceutical Industry. Chimica Oggi 31 (5): 69–72.

40. Passerini, Nadia, Beatrice Albertini, Beatrice Perissutti, and Lorenzo Rodriguez. 2006. Evaluation of Melt Granulation and Ultrasonic Spray Congealing as Techniques to Enhance the Dissolution of Praziquantel. International Journal of Pharmaceutics 318 (1–2). Elsevier: 92–102. doi:10.1016/J.IJPHARM.2006.03.028.

41. Sabatino, Marcello Di, Beatrice Albertini, Vicky L. Kett, and Nadia Passerini. 2012. Spray Congealed Lipid Microparticles with High Protein Loading: Preparation and Solid State Characterisation. European Journal of Pharmaceutical Sciences 46 (5): 346–356. doi:10.1016/j.ejps.2012.02.021.

42. Passerini, Nadia, Beatrice Perissutti, Mariarosa Moneghini, Dario Voinovich, Beatrice Albertini, Cristina Cavallari, and Lorenzo Rodriguez. 2002. Characterization of Carbamazepine–Gelucire 50/13 Microparticles Prepared by a Spray-Congealing Process Using Ultrasounds. Journal of Pharmaceutical Sciences 91 (3). John Wiley and Sons Inc.: 699–707. doi:10.1002/jps.10085.

43. Albertini, Beatrice, Matteo Mezzena, Nadia Passerini, Lorenzo Rodriguez, and Santo Scalia. 2009. Evaluation of Spray Congealing as Technique for the Preparation of Highly Loaded Solid Lipid Microparticles Containing the Sunscreen Agent, Avobenzone. Journal of Pharmaceutical Sciences 98 (8). John Wiley and Sons Inc.: 2759–2769. doi:10.1002/jps.21636.

44. Morselli Ribeiro, Marilene D. M., Daniel Barrera Arellano, and Carlos R. Ferreira Grosso. 2012. The Effect of Adding Oleic Acid in the Production of Stearic Acid Lipid Microparticles with a Hydrophilic Core by a Spray-Cooling Process. Food Research International 47 (1). Elsevier: 38–44. doi:10.1016/J.FOODRES.2012.01.007.

45. Passerini, Nadia, Sheng Qi, Beatrice Albertini, Mario Grassi, Lorenzo Rodriguez, and Duncan Q. M. Craig. 2010. Solid Lipid Microparticles Produced by Spray Congealing: Influence of the Atomizer on Microparticle Characteristics and Mathematical Modeling of the Drug Release. Journal of Pharmaceutical Sciences 99 (2). John Wiley and Sons Inc.: 916–931. doi:10.1002/jps.21854.

46. Maschke, Angelika, Christian Becker, Daniela Eyrich, Josef Kiermaier, Torsten Blunk, and Achim Göpferich. 2007. Development of a Spray Congealing Process for the Preparation of Insulin-Loaded Lipid Microparticles and Characterization Thereof. European Journal of Pharmaceutics and Biopharmaceutics 65 (2). Elsevier: 175–187. doi:10.1016/J.EJPB.2006.08.008.

47. Li, Luk Chiu, Lihua Zhu, Jing-Feng Song, Jone-Shin Deng, Rubi Bandopadhyay, and Dale E Wurster. 2005. Effect of Solid State Transition on the Physical Stability of Suspensions Containing Bupivacaine Lipid Microparticles. Pharmaceutical Development and Technology 10 (2). Taylor & Francis: 309–318. doi:10.1081/PDT-54475.

48. Vervaeck, A., L. Saerens, B. G. De Geest, T. De Beer, R. Carleer, P. Adriaensens, J. P. Remon, and C. Vervaet. 2013. Prilling of Fatty Acids as a Continuous Process for the Development of Controlled Release Multiparticulate Dosage Forms. European Journal of Pharmaceutics and Biopharmaceutics 85 (3 PART A). Elsevier B.V.: 587–596. doi:10.1016/j.ejpb.2013.02.003.

49. Coninck, E. De, V. Vanhoorne, M. Boone, G. Van Assche, B. G. De Geest, T. De Beer, and C. Vervaet.

2020. Prilling of API/Fatty Acid Suspensions: Screening of Additives for Drug Release Modification. International Journal of Pharmaceutics 576 (February). Elsevier B.V.: 119022. doi:10.1016/j.ijpharm. 2020.119022.

50. Vervaeck, A., T. Monteyne, F. Siepmann, M. N. Boone, L. Van Hoorebeke, T. De Beer, J. Siepmann, J. P. Remon, and C. Vervaet. 2015. Fatty Acids for Controlled Release Applications: A Comparison between Prilling and Solid Lipid Extrusion as Manufacturing Techniques. European Journal of Pharmaceutics and Biopharmaceutics 97 (November). Elsevier: 173–184. doi:10.1016/j.ejpb.2015.09.011.

51. Séquier, F., V. Faivre, G. Daste, M. Renouard, and S. Lesieur. 2014. Critical Parameters Involved in Producing Microspheres by Prilling of Molten Lipids: From Theoretical Prediction of Particle Size to Practice. European Journal of Pharmaceutics and Biopharmaceutics 87 (3). Elsevier: 530–540. doi:10. 1016/j.ejpb.2014.03.005.

52. Coninck, E. De, V. Vanhoorne, A. Elmahdy, M. Boone, G. Van Assche, D. Markl, B. G. De Geest, T. De Beer, and C. Vervaet. 2019. Prilling of API/Fatty Acid Suspensions: Processability and Characterisation. International Journal of Pharmaceutics 572 (December). Elsevier B.V.: 118756. doi:10.1016/j.ijpharm.2019.118756.

53. Pivette, Perrine, Vincent Faivre, Lucia Mancini, Claire Gueutin, Georges Daste, Michel Ollivon, and Sylviane Lesieur. 2012. Controlled Release of a Highly Hydrophilic API from Lipid Microspheres Obtained by Prilling: Analysis of Drug and Water Diffusion Processes with X-Ray-Based Methods. Journal of Controlled Release 158 (3). Elsevier: 393–402. doi:10.1016/j.jconrel.2011.11.027.

54. Crowley, Michael M., Feng Zhang, Michael A. Repka, Sridhar Thumma, Sampada B. Upadhye, Sunil Kumar Battu, James W. McGinity, and Charles Martin. 2007. Pharmaceutical Applications of Hot-Melt Extrusion: Part I. Drug Development and Industrial Pharmacy 33 (9): 909–926. doi:10.1080/ 03639040701498759.

55. Lowinger, Michael B., Yongchao Su, Xingyu Lu, Robert O. Williams, and Feng Zhang. 2019. Can Drug Release Rate from Implants Be Tailored Using Poly(Urethane) Mixtures? International Journal of Pharmaceutics 557 (February). Elsevier: 390–401. doi:10.1016/J.IJPHARM.2018.11.067.

56. Repka, Michael A., Sunil Kumar Battu, Sampada B. Upadhye, Sridhar Thumma, Michael M. Crowley, Feng Zhang, Charles Martin, and James W. McGinity. 2007. Pharmaceutical Applications of Hot-Melt Extrusion: Part II. Drug Development and Industrial Pharmacy 33 (10). Taylor & Francis: 1043–1057. doi:10.1080/03639040701525627.

57. Repka, Michael A., Soumyajit Majumdar, Sunil Kumar Battu, Ramesh Srirangam, and Sampada B. Upadhye. 2008. Applications of Hot-Melt Extrusion for Drug Delivery. Expert Opinion on Drug Delivery 5 (12). Taylor & Francis: 1357–1376. doi:10.1517/17425240802583421.

58. Verstraete, G., P. Mertens, W. Grymonpré, P. J. Van Bockstal, T. De Beer, M. N. Boone, L. Van Hoorebeke, J. P. Remon, and C. Vervaet. 2016. A Comparative Study between Melt Granulation/ Compression and Hot Melt Extrusion/Injection Molding for the Manufacturing of Oral Sustained Release Thermoplastic Polyurethane Matrices. International Journal of Pharmaceutics 513 (1-2): 602–611. doi:10.1016/j.ijpharm.2016.09.072.

59. Lindberg, N.-O., C. Tufvesson, P. Holm, and L. Olbjer. 1988. Extrusion of an Effervescent Granulation with a Twin Screw Extruder, Baker Perkins MPF 50 D. Influence on Intragranular Porosity and Liquid Saturation. Drug Development and Industrial Pharmacy 14 (13). Taylor & Francis: 1791–1798. doi:10. 3109/03639048809151987.

60. Vercruysse, J., A. Burggraeve, M. Fonteyne, P. Cappuyns, U. Delaet, I. Van Assche, T. De Beer, J. P. Remon, and C. Vervaet. 2015. Impact of Screw Configuration on the Particle Size Distribution of Granules Produced by Twin Screw Granulation. International Journal of Pharmaceutics 479 (1). doi:10.1016/j.ijpharm.2014.12.071.

61. Kittikunakorn, Nada, J. Joseph Koleng, Tony Listro, Changquan Calvin Sun, and Feng Zhang. 2019. Effects of Thermal Binders on Chemical Stabilities and Tabletability of Gabapentin Granules Prepared by Twin-Screw Melt Granulation. International Journal of Pharmaceutics 559: 37–47. doi:10.1016/j. ijpharm.2019.01.014.

62. Kittikunakorn, Nada, Changquan Calvin Sun, and Feng Zhang. 2019. Effect of Screw Profile and Processing Conditions on Physical Transformation and Chemical Degradation of Gabapentin during Twin-Screw Melt Granulation. European Journal of Pharmaceutical Sciences 131: 243–253. doi:10. 1016/j.ejps.2019.02.024.

63. Melkebeke, Barbara Van, Brenda Vermeulen, Chris Vervaet, and Jean Paul Remon. 2006. Melt Granulation Using a Twin-Screw Extruder: A Case Study. International Journal of Pharmaceutics 326 (1–2). Elsevier: 89–93. doi:10.1016/J.IJPHARM.2006.07.005.

64. Monteyne, Tinne, Liza Heeze, Séverine Thérèse F. C. Mortier, Klaus Oldörp, Ingmar Nopens, Jean Paul Remon, Chris Vervaet, and Thomas De Beer. 2016. The Use of Rheology to Elucidate the Granulation

Mechanisms of a Miscible and Immiscible System during Continuous Twin-Screw Melt Granulation. International Journal of Pharmaceutics 510 (1). Elsevier B.V.: 271–284. doi:10.1016/j.ijpharm.2016.06.055.

65. Dhenge, Ranjit M., James J. Cartwright, Michael J. Hounslow, and Agba D. Salman. 2012. Twin Screw Granulation: Steps in Granule Growth. International Journal of Pharmaceutics 438 (1-2): 20–32. doi:10.1016/j.ijpharm.2012.08.049.

66. Keleb, E. I., A. Vermeire, C. Vervaet, and J. P. Remon. 2004. Twin Screw Granulation as a Simple and Efficient Tool for Continuous Wet Granulation. International Journal of Pharmaceutics 273 (1-2): 183–194. doi:10.1016/j.ijpharm.2004.01.001.

67. Weatherley, Sharleen, Bo Mu, Michael R. Thompson, Paul J. Sheskey, and Kevin P. O'Donnell. 2013. Hot-Melt Granulation in a Twin Screw Extruder: Effects of Processing on Formulations with Caffeine and Ibuprofen. Journal of Pharmaceutical Sciences 102 (12): 4330–4336. doi:10.1002/jps.23739.

68. Hagrasy, A. S. El, and J. D. Litster. 2013. Granulation Rate Processes in the Kneading Elements of a Twin Screw Granulator. AIChE Journal 59 (11): 4100–4115. doi:10.1002/aic.14180.

69. Shanmugam, Srinivasan. 2015. Granulation Techniques and Technologies: Recent Progresses. BioImpacts: BI 5 (1). Tabriz University of Medical Sciences: 55–63. doi:10.15171/bi.2015.04.

70. Greenhalgh, David J., Adrian C. Williams, Peter Timmins, and Peter York. 1999. Solubility Parameters as Predictors of Miscibility in Solid Dispersions. Journal of Pharmaceutical Sciences 88 (11). American Chemical Society: 1182–1190. doi:10.1021/js9900856.

71. Grymonpré, W., G. Verstraete, V. Vanhoorne, J.P. Remon, T. De Beer, and C. Vervaet. 2018. Downstream Processing from Melt Granulation towards Tablets: In-Depth Analysis of a Continuous Twin-Screw Melt Granulation Process Using Polymeric Binders. European Journal of Pharmaceutics and Biopharmaceutics 124 (March). Elsevier: 43–54. doi:10.1016/J.EJPB.2017.12.005.

72. Kidokoro, Motonori, Navnit H. Shah, A. Waseem Malick, Martin H. Infeld, and James W. McGinity. 2001. Properties of Tablets Containing Granulations of Ibuprofen and an Acrylic Copolymer Prepared by Thermal Processes. Pharmaceutical Development and Technology 6 (2). Taylor & Francis: 263–275. doi:10.1081/PDT-100002203.

73. Vasanthavada, Madhav, Yanfeng Wang, Thomas Haefele, Jay P. Lakshman, Manisha Mone, Weiqin Tong, Yatindra M. Joshi, and Abu T. Abu. 2011. Application of Melt Granulation Technology Using Twin-Screw Extruder in Development of High-Dose Modified-Release Tablet Formulation. Journal of Pharmaceutical Sciences 100 (5): 1923–1934. doi:10.1002/jps.22411.

74. Srivastava, Saurabh, and Garima Mishra. 2010. Fluid Bed Technology: Overview and Parameters for Process Selection. International Journal of Pharmaceutical Sciences and Drug Research 2 (4): 236–246.

Section IV

Characterization and Scale-UP

20 Sizing of Granulation

Gurvinder Singh Rekhi and Richard Sidwell

CONTENTS

20.1   INTRODUCTION

Tablets are the most frequently administered solid oral dosage forms in contemporary practice. Tablets consist of a mixture of powders or granules that are compacted in the die of a tablet press. Even though the popularity of directly compressible materials has increased, many powders are granulated to overcome the difficulties in obtaining an acceptable tablet dosage form and meeting the product specifications. The most challenging task in a tableting process is to achieve a constant volume of homogenous mixture to flow into the tablet die cavity. Unfortunately, most powder materials do not have inherently good flow properties. This, in turn, demands to change the physical characteristics of the powder or improving the design of the tablet press [1]. Therefore, granulation becomes an integral part of a pharmaceutical process that attempts to improve powder-flow characteristics.

The granule properties play a pivotal role in the final performance of a tablet; for example, granule size can affect the flowability and drying rate kinetics of wet granulations. The effect of granule size and size distribution on final blend properties and tablet characteristics is dependent upon formulation ingredients and their concentration as well as the type of granulating equipment and processing conditions employed. Therefore, granulation and sizing of granulation become critical unit operations in the manufacture of oral dosage forms [2,3]. To some extent, the same requirements are necessary in capsule manufacturing, especially when the drug is bulky or has poor flow properties, or in high-speed capsule-filling machines, where limited compaction occurs.

Few materials used in the manufacture of pharmaceutical solid oral dosage forms exist in the optimum size and must be reduced in size at some stage during commercial manufacturing. The advantages of sizing of granules in tablet formulation development are as follows:

1. Mixing and blending of pharmaceutical ingredients are easier and more uniform if the ingredients are of approximately the same size and distribution.
2. Improving color distribution. Milling may reduce the tendency for mottling and hence improve the uniformity of color from batch to batch.
3. Wet milling produces uniformly sized wet granules, which promotes uniform and efficient drying.
4. Improving uniformity of dosage units by virtue of uniformity of particle-size distribution and reduction in the segregation of the mix.
5. Enhancing flow properties reduces weight variation and improves content uniformity.
6. Increasing surface area because of particle-size reduction may enhance the dissolution rate, and thereby, the drug's bioavailability.
7. Reducing dust reduces workers' exposure.

Size reduction alone is not a panacea for all tableting problems. There are some disadvantages to size reduction that may affect the final characteristics of a dosage form, such as degradation of the drug or a change in the polymorphic form as a result of the excessive heat generated, or increase in surface energies leading to agglomeration. Hence, in optimizing the manufacture of pharmaceutical dosage forms, it is important not only to characterize the formulation ingredients but also to study their effect on the manufacturing process (i.e., whether a granulation should be milled and to what extent based on the final product specifications).

The objective of this chapter is to focus on the sizing of granulation after drying in a wet granulation process. Furthermore, the process of wet milling for obtaining uniformly sized granules for uniform drying will also be addressed. A full discussion of the theories of comminution or equipment description is beyond the scope of this chapter. Details of various types of equipment used in the size-reduction process, their merits and demerits, and variables affecting the size-reduction process, scale-up factors, and relevant case studies to be considered in the development and optimization of tablet and capsule manufacture will be addressed.

20.2   THEORY OF COMMINUTION OR SIZE REDUCTION

Comminution, or size reduction, is the mechanical process of reducing the size of particles or aggregates. There is, as yet, only a basic understanding of the mechanism and quantitative aspects of milling [4,5]. The reduction of particle size through fracture requires the application of mechanical stress to the material to be crushed or ground. Materials respond to this stress by yielding, with consequent generation of strain. In the case of a brittle material, a complete rebound occurs on release of applied stress to the yield point, at which fracture would occur. In contrast, plastic material would neither rebound nor fracture. The vast majority of pharmaceutical solids lie somewhere between these extremes and thus possess both plastic and brittle properties.

The energy expended by comminution ultimately appears as surface energy associated with newly created particle surfaces, internal free energy associated with lattice changes, and heat. For any particle, there is the minimum energy required that will fracture it; however, conditions are so haphazard that many particles receive impacts that are insufficient for fracture and are eventually fractured by the excessively forceful impact. As a result, most efficient mills use <1% to 2% of the energy input to fracture particles and to create new surfaces. The rest of the energy is dissipated in the form of heat from the plastic deformation of the particles that are not fractured, friction, and in imparting kinetic energy to the particles. The greater the rate at which the force is applied, the less effectively the energy is utilized and the higher is the proportion of fine material produced.

A flaw in a particle is any structural weakness that may develop into a crack under strain. The Griffith theory [4] of cracks and flaws assumes that all solids contain flaws and microscopic cracks, which increase as the applied force increases, according to the crack length and focus of the stress at the crack apex. A granule is an aggregation of particles that are held together by bonds of finite strength, and the ultimate strength of a wet granule depends on the surface tension of the granulating liquid and capillary forces. After drying, granules develop stronger bonds owing to the fusion and recrystallization of particles and curing of adhesives or binding the agent. The final strength of a granule depends on the base material, the type and the amount of granulating agent used, and the equipment employed.

A granule or particle may be subjected to one or more of the following four forces during milling:

1. Shear (cutting forces)
2. Compression (crushing force)
3. Impact (direct, high-velocity collision force)
4. Tension (the force that works to elongate or pull a particle apart)

The mechanism by which the sizing of dried granules occurs is similar to that of crystalline materials. Cleavage occurs at the weakest point or points in the granule, and it could be at [2]:

1. the binder–particle interface,
2. the bridge of binder between the individual ingredient particles being granulated,
3. flaws in the individual ingredient particles within the granules, or
4. a combination of any of the above.

Granules held together with lower binding-strength agents such as povidone will require less severe grinding conditions because the fractures take place primarily at the binder bridge or the binder–particle interface.

The milling process can be described mathematically [6–8]; however, its theory has not been developed to the point at which the actual performance of a mill can be predicted quantitatively. Three fundamental laws (Kick's Law, Rittinger's Law, and Bond's Law) have been proposed to relate size reduction to a single variable, the energy input to the mill. None of the energy laws apply well in practice [9]. Generally, laboratory testing is required to evaluate the performance of a particular piece of equipment; however, a work index and grindability index have been used to evaluate mill performance [5]. The efficiency of a milling process is influenced by the nature of the force, as well as by its magnitude. The rate of application of force affects comminution because there is a lag time between the attainment of maximum force and the fracture. Often, materials respond as a brittle material to fast impact and as a plastic material to a slow force.

20.3 PROPERTIES OF FEED MATERIALS AFFECTING THE SIZING PROCESS

The milling or sizing process is affected by a variety of factors and has a direct effect on the quality of the final product. The properties of feed material and the finished product specifications determine the choice of equipment to be used for the process of comminution. The properties of feed material include melting point, brittleness, hardness, and moisture content. The desired particle size, shape, and size distribution must also be considered in the selection of milling equipment.

Materials can be classified as hard, intermediate, soft, or fibrous materials (e.g., glycyrrhiza and rauwolfia) based on the Mohs' scale. Fibrous materials require cutting or chopping action and usually cannot be reduced in size effectively by pressure or impact techniques. Before selecting and optimizing a size-reduction process, one needs to know the properties of the material and the characteristics of a mill. The important material properties [5,10] are as follows:

1. Toughness: Toughness is the material's resistance to the propagation of cracks. Reduction of the particle size of tough material is difficult, but can sometimes be made easier by cooling the material, thereby diminishing its tendency to exhibit plastic flow and making it more brittle.
2. Brittleness: It is the opposite of toughness. Size reduction poses no problems except if the amount of fines is to be controlled.
3. Abrasiveness: This is an important factor because abrasive materials can wear mill parts and screens; hence, metal contamination may be a problem.
4. Cohesiveness/Adhesiveness: Particles sticking together or to machine surfaces are often dependent on moisture content and particle size. Problems with moisture content can be mitigated by drying the material or avoided by using a wet size-reduction process.
5. Melting point: This is critical because considerable heat is generated in size reduction. High temperatures generated can cause melting of the drug, blinding of the screen, or can degrade heat-sensitive materials.
6. Agglomeration: This can be counteracted by drying the material, either before or during size reduction. In some cases, mixing with other ingredients during milling might be helpful. Generally, materials having a strong tendency to agglomerate are wetted before milling.
7. Moisture: Moisture content above 5% can often lead to agglomeration or even liquefaction of the milled material. Hydrates will often release their water of hydration under high temperatures and may require cooling or low-speed milling.
8. Flammability and explosiveness: This is the measure of how readily a material will ignite or explode. Explosive materials must be processed in an inert gas atmosphere.
9. Toxicity: This has little influence on the selection of the mill itself; however, it must be considered in determining operator safety, containment, and setup for this type of material.
10. Reactivity: The possibility of materials chemically reacting with the materials of construction of the mill (including liners and gaskets) and cleaning solutions must be considered.

20.4 CRITERIA FOR SELECTION OF A MILL

The selection of equipment is determined by the characteristics of the material, the initial particle size, and the desired particle size of the milled product, that is, coarse, medium, or fine.

The criteria for selection of a mill include the following [4]:

1. Properties of feed material: Size, shape, moisture content, physical and chemical properties, temperature sensitivity, grindability, and material compatibility.
2. Product specifications: Size, particle-size distribution, and shape.
3. The versatility of operation: Wet and dry milling, rapid change of speed and screen, and safety features.
4. Scale-up: Capacity of the mill and production-rate requirements.
5. Repeatability: Ability to meter material to the mill to ensure a consistent process.
6. Product containment: Loss of costly drugs, health hazards, and contamination.
7. Batch or continuous operation: Mill can be used continuously or a minimum feed rate is required.

8. Sanitation: Ease of cleaning (clean in place, CIP) and sterilization (sterilization in place, SIP).
9. Auxiliary equipment: Cooling system, dust collectors, force-feeding, and stage reduction.
10. Safety: Electrical classification and inerting with nitrogen gas.
11. Economic factors: Equipment cost, power consumption, space occupied, and labor cost.

After consideration of the foregoing factors for a specific milling problem, it is suggested that a variety of mills should be evaluated for optimum product results such as the shape of granules and/ or scalability from development to commercial manufacturing. In addition to the standard adjustments of the milling process (e.g., screen, speed, rotor design, and feed rate), other techniques of milling may be considered for special materials. Hygroscopic materials can be milled in a closed system supplied with dehumidified air. As the bulk of the energy used in milling is converted into heat, heat-sensitive materials or hard materials that build up in the milling chamber may melt, decompose, or explode. A two- or multistep milling process can be used for harder and difficult-to-grind materials. Materials can be milled using a coarser screen, and the material can then be recycled by screening the discharge and returning the oversized material for second milling (closed-circuit mill). Alternatively, one may chill the air or gas (carbon dioxide or nitrogen) that transports the product, cool the product prior to processing, or cool the comminuting chamber through which the product passes. A chiller is necessary for all of these options and will add to the cost of processing [11]. If this is not sufficient to embrittle the material, it may be fed to the mill simultaneously with dry ice. For flammable/explosive dust, the equipment may be required to meet safety standards such as NEC/NFPA 70 (United States) or ATEX Directive 94/9/EC (Europe) and/or be inerted with nitrogen gas.

20.5   CLASSIFICATION OF MILLS

The majority of size-reduction equipment may be classified according to the way in which forces are applied, namely, impact, shear, attrition, and shear compression (Table 20.1). A given mill may operate successfully in more than one class: a hammer mill, with appropriate setup, may be used to wet mill a 16-mesh granulation and to dry mill a crystalline material to a 60-mesh powder.

The mills used for size reduction of the granules can be divided into two primary categories based on the energy input into the process. Even though there are several high-energy mills available for size reduction, only a few are used in the pharmaceutical industry for the wet or dry sizing process. Milling is an extremely inefficient unit operation with only 1% to 2% of the applied

---

TABLE 20.1
General Characteristics of Various Types of Mills

Mechanism of Action	Example	Product Size	Type of Material	Not Used for
Impact	Hammer mill	Moderate to fine	Brittle and dry material	Fibrous, sticky, low-melting substances
Shear	Extruder and hand screen	Coarse	Deagglomeration, wet granulation	Dry material, hard, abrasive materials
Attrition	Oscillating granulator	Coarse to moderate	Dried granulation	Wet granulation, abrasive materials
Compression	Conical-screening mill	Moderate to coarse	Wet, dry granulation	Abrasive materials

energy being utilized in the actual size reduction. Milling efficiency is dependent on the characteristics of the material used and the type of mill employed.

20.5.1 Low-Energy Mills

20.5.1.1 Hand Screen

- Size reduction using a hand screen occurs primarily by shear.
- They are typically made of stainless steel and consist of a woven wire cloth stretched in a circular or rectangular frame.
- They are available in sizes ranging from 4 to 325 mesh; however, for granulation, typically mesh sizes from 4 to 20 are used.
- They are most widely used for sieve analysis or for size reduction of wet and dry granules in the early stages of formulation development.

20.5.1.2 Oscillating or Rotary Granulator Mills

- Oscillating or rotary granulator mills consist of an oscillating bar passing closely to a woven wire screen. The material is forced through the screen by the motion of the bar (Figure 20.1a,b).
- Size reduction is primarily by shear with some attrition.
- Speed, rotary or oscillatory motion, and screen size are important variables to be considered during the sizing process.
- They are used primarily for size reduction of wet and dry granulations, and, to some extent, for milling tablets and compacts that must be reprocessed.
- The narrow size distribution and a minimum amount of fines are advantages during the size reduction of dry granulation [2].
- Heat-sensitive and waxy materials can be milled owing to the low heat generated during the sizing process.
- Low throughput rates and possible metal contamination from wearing down or broken screens are some of its limitations.
- Examples include the Frewitt Oscillowitt and Fitzmill with a bar rotor.

20.5.1.3 Low-Pressure Extruders

- Low-pressure extruders are primarily used for continuous wet granulation.

(a)   (b)

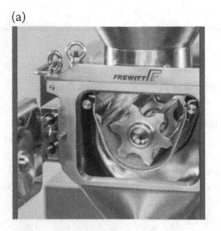
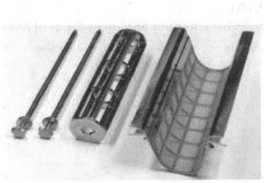

FIGURE 20.1 Oscillating Granulator: (a) Frewitt MF Line and (b) Rotor, Screen, and Tensioning Spindles. *Source*: From Frewitt USA.

- Wet material is forced through a screen and the extruded material is dried in a tray or fluid-bed dryer or can be spheronized to produce granules with a high degree of sphericity and then dried for controlled-release applications.
- Less dust generation and more uniform granules are some of the advantages.
- More information on extrusion may be found in Chapter 12.

20.5.2 HIGH-ENERGY MILLS

20.5.2.1 Hammer Mill

The hammer mill is one of the most versatile and widely used mills in the pharmaceutical industry. The principle of size reduction in the hammer mill is one of the high-velocity impacts between rapidly moving hammers mounted on a rotor and the powder particles (Figure 20.2a,b).

These mills can produce a wide range of particle sizes, even down to micrometer size. The particle shape, however, is generally sharper and more irregular than produced by compression methods [5]. The force imparted by the hammers and the screen opening size and shape controls the degree of particle-size reduction.

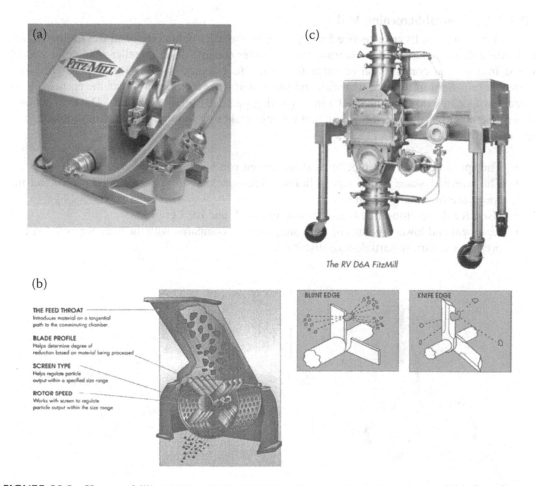

(a)

(c)

The RV D6A FitzMill

(b)

THE FEED THROAT
Introduces material on a tangential path to the comminuting chamber.

BLADE PROFILE
Helps determine degree of reduction based on material being processed.

SCREEN TYPE
Helps regulate particle output within a specified size range.

ROTOR SPEED
Works with screen to regulate particle output within the size range.

BLUNT EDGE

KNIFE EDGE

FIGURE 20.2 Hammer Mill: (a) Fitzmill Model L1A; (b) Principle of Operation, and (c) Containment Model with Nitrogen Inerting Capability.
Source: From The Fitzpatrick Company.

- They can be used for size reduction of wet or dry granulations and milling of raw materials.
- There is a wide range of interchangeable feed throats and variable feed-screw systems available to optimize the feed rate [12].
- Hammers can rotate horizontally or vertically, based on the rotor configuration, and at variable speeds.
- Hammers can be fixed or free-swinging.
- Hammers with blunt or impact edges are preferred for pulverizing, and knife or sharp edges are preferred for chopping or sizing of granules [12].
- Screen openings generally vary from 0.3 to 38 mm with round or square perforations, diagonal or straight slots, or with a rasping surface.
- Feed rate and dryness of the granules are important variables relative to the material.
- Type of hammers, rotor speed, screen type, thickness, and opening size are important variables relative to the machine.
- Ease of setup, clean-up, minimum scale-up problems, and ability to handle a wide variety of sizes and types of feedstock are some advantages.
- Heat build-up, screen wear, and potential clogging of screens are some of the limitations.
- Integrated designs are available for dust containment.
- Examples include the Granumill and Fitzmill.

20.5.2.2 Conical-Screening Mill

Conical-screening mills are effective for dry (deagglomeration/delumping) and wet milling of soft- to medium-hard materials. The comminution chamber consists of an impeller rotating at variable speed imparting a compression or shear forces inside a conical screen. The impeller imparts a vortex flow pattern to the feed material, and the centrifugal acceleration forces the particles to the screen surface and up the cone (360°) in a spiraling path [13] (Figure 20.3a,b). The dual action of conical-screening mills (size reduction and mixing) makes this equipment more desirable than the use of traditional oscillators [14,15].

- The space between the impeller and the screen can be adjusted.
- The size and shape of the screen holes, screen thickness, impeller configuration, and mill speed are important variables.
- Used for difficult-to-mill, heat-sensitive material, and hard granules.
- Low heat and lower amounts of fines are produced compared with the hammer mill; hence, it produces a narrow particle-size distribution.

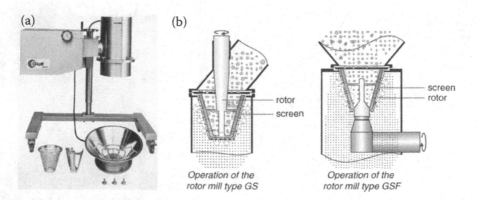

FIGURE 20.3 Conical-Screening Mill: (a) Glatt Model GSF 180 and the (b) Principle of Operation. *Source*: From Glatt Air Techniques.

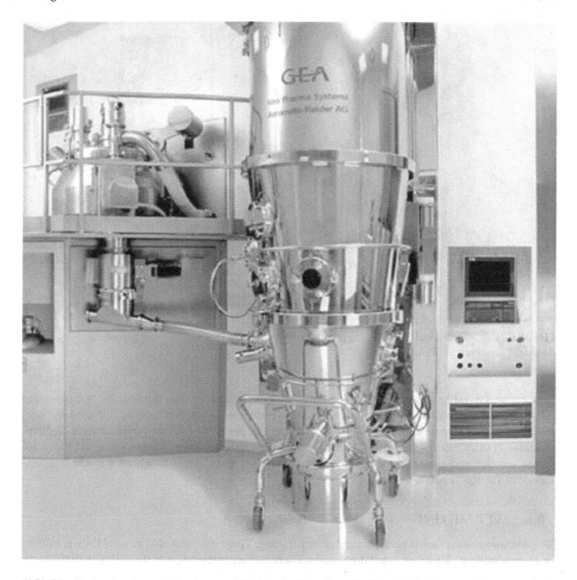

FIGURE 20.4 An integrated pharmaceutical manufacturing facility (high-shear granulator-conical-screening mill–fluid-bed drier).
Source: From GEA North America.

- The impeller does not touch the screen; hence, chances of screen breakage and metal contamination are greatly reduced compared with an oscillating granulator.
- Integrated designs available that are attached to a high-shear granulator discharge, which provides a deagglomerated, lump-free product for the dryer (Figure 20.4).
- Examples include the Quadro Comil and Glatt Rotor Sieve.

20.5.2.3 Centrifugal-Sifter Mills

Centrifugal-Sifter mills (Frewitt TurboWitt Figure 20.5) and sieves are useful to minimize the production of fine particles because their design combines sieving and deagglomeration into a single operation. Unlike the conical-screening mills, these consist of a nonrotating bar or stator that is fixed within a rotating sieve basket. This action produces a very low product agitation and

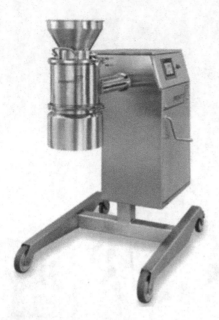 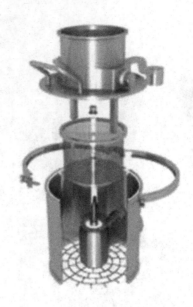

FIGURE 20.5 Centrifugal-Sifter Mill: Frewitt TurboWitt.
Source: From Frewitt USA.

impact; hence, no heat is generated. The particles that are smaller than the holes of the sieve can pass through the mill without comminution; however, the larger particles are directed by centrifugal force to impact the stator. Older designs are not preferred because the likelihood of sieve-to-stator contact can result in metal particulates in the product. Newer designs eliminate metal-to-metal contact and may include an integrated classifier to ensure the desired particle-size distribution for the product.

20.6 WET MILLING

The discussion thus far has been focused on dry milling. These mills can also be used for wet milling or coarse milling. There are several reasons for wet milling; these include the following [16]:

1. To increase surface area for more efficient drying
2. To improve size uniformity
3. To improve granule formation
4. To prevent large particles that will shatter to "fines" on dry milling
5. For further mixing or blending of ingredients

As discussed in low-energy mills, extruders can be used as a continuous wet granulation method. Wet milling is necessary with low-shear mixers, such as planetary, ribbon, or sigma mixers, but with high-shear mixers, the combination of high impeller speed and built-in choppers produces a product ready for drying. Also, integrated designs are available such that the wet-milling step is no longer a separate operation.

Finally, there are continuous granulators available such as Dome-EX COMBI (LCI) and ConsiGma (GEA) for product applications that do not require extensive kneading treatment and can be used for both batch and continuous operation. The wetted product is discharged in a continuous stream through an adjustable opening in the turbine cover. A homogeneous mix is produced in a few minutes and further milling may not be necessary.

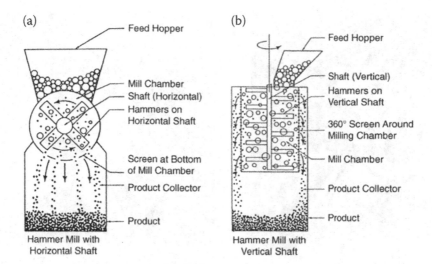

FIGURE 20.6 (a,b) Different Types of Hammer Mills.
Source: From The Fitzpatrick Company.

20.7 VARIABLES AFFECTING THE SIZING PROCESS

20.7.1 PROCESS VARIABLES

As discussed in the Introduction, the granule properties can dictate the properties of the final tablet. Some of the problems faced during the tableting process are the flow of granules, maintaining uniform density in the granule bed, and the particle-size distribution. Each of the stages of the granulation can be critical and can affect tableting. In addition to the wet granulation process, the sizing process can be critical for the particle-size distribution that, along with the number of fines, dictates the flow properties. These, in turn, influence the packing and density of the granules. The reproducibility of batches depends not only on the properties of the unmilled dry granules but also on the mill and milling parameters. Finally, the dry-milling stage is important because of the heat generated that might affect the stability of the final product.

The characteristics of the granules after size reduction depend mainly on the type of mill, impeller type, and speed, screen size, type, and thickness.

20.7.2 EQUIPMENT VARIABLES (TYPE OF MILL)

The type of mill chosen can affect the shape of the granules and throughput. The shape of the milled granules can affect the flow properties. An impact mill produces sharp, irregular particles that may not flow readily, whereas an attrition mill produces free-flowing spheroidal particles. An oscillating granulator uses shear and attrition as the main mechanisms for size reduction. The granules produced are more spheroidal because size reduction takes place by surface erosion. If the same material is subjected to impact by hammers in a hammer mill, the granules will shatter resulting in irregularly shaped particles. If a conical-screening mill is used for size reduction, it imparts some shear and compression between the rotating impeller and the screen, which may result in a narrower particle-size distribution than other types of mills.

20.7.2.1 Hammer Mill

There are a number of variables in a hammer mill that can influence comminution [12,17–19]. The following section discusses five operating variables in detail:

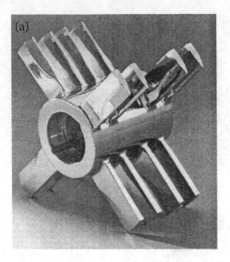
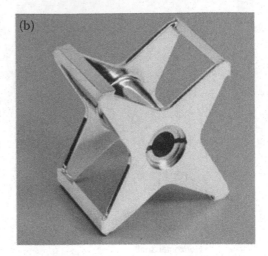

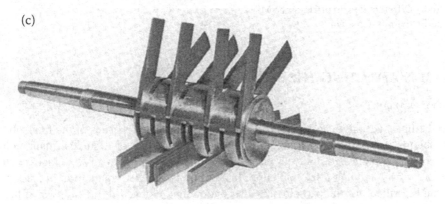

FIGURE 20.7   Different Types of Hammer-Mill Rotors (Fitzmill): (a) Cast Rotor, (b) Bar Rotor, and (c) Swing-Blade Rotor.
Source: From The Fitzpatrick Company.

1. Rotor shaft configuration: The hammers may be mounted on a vertical or horizontal shaft (Figure 20.6a,b). The vertical shaft mills (Stokes-Tornado mill) have feed inlets at the top, and material is fed perpendicular to the swing of the hammers. In the case of horizontal shaft mills (Fitzpatrick-Fitzmill), the material is fed tangentially to the hammer swing. Rotor configuration can influence the particle-size distribution of the granules. In the vertical configuration, the screen is placed 360° around the hammers, and this provides more screen open area and less product residence time in the milling chamber when compared with the horizontal shaft mills.
2. Material feed rate: The feed rate controls the amount of the feed material that enters the comminutor and prevents overfeeding (slugging) or underfeeding (starving) the milling chamber. Although both affect the particle-size distribution, overfeeding is relatively more detrimental. If the rate of feed is relatively slow, the product is discharged readily, and the amount of undersize material, or fines, is minimized. On the other hand, overfed material stays in the milling chamber for a longer time, because its discharge is impeded by the mass of material. This leads to a greater reduction of particle size, overloads the motor, and the capacity of the mill is reduced. The rule of thumb is to keep the feed rate equal to the rate of discharge. The feed rate can be controlled using variable-feed screws, vibratory feeders, or dischargers controlled by gravity. In addition to controlling the flow, the feed throat must allow the material to enter at a proper angle.

There are several feed-throat designs available that one needs to consider for optimizing the milling process. Most mills used in pharmaceutical operations are designed so that the force of gravity is sufficient to give free discharge, generally from the bottom of the mill.

3. Blade type: Please check formatting add period 3., 4., 5 Comminution is effected by the impact of the material with the fast-moving blades and attrition with the screen. Generally, the blades of a hammer mill have a blunt or flat edge on one side and a sharp or knife-edge on the other side. The desired particle-size range determines which blades to use. Many models of hammer mills have a rotor that may be turned 180° so that the blunt edges can be used for fine grinding or the knife-edge can be used for cutting or granulating. The blunt edge offers impact during milling, generating smaller granules. The knife-edge, because the sharper edge causes cutting of the granules, thereby generates larger granules. Individual blades (blunt, sharp, or reversible) are installed either fixed or swinging (Figure 20.7a–c). Fixed blades plow through the material being ground while swinging blades lie back and depend on the centrifugal force for movement. Fixed blades are preferred over swinging blades because they are easier to clean and work better than swinging blades at low rotor speeds, when grinding fibrous material, or if carefully controlled grinding is needed.

The material to be ground determines the configuration of the blades on the motor shaft, as well as the blade geometry. The shape of the blades (straight, stepped, sickle, or other) is largely a matter of designer preference. Little empirical evidence exists to establish the superiority of one shape over another. The size of the grinding chamber generally determines the number of blades (e.g., a 6-in. grinding chamber will have 16 blades).

4. Speed: The size of a product is markedly affected by the speed of the hammers. As a general rule, and with all other variables remaining constant, the faster the rotor's speed, the finer the grind. Changes in rotor speed are accomplished by variable-speed drive Usually, three-speed settings used are: slow (1000 rpm), medium (2500 rpm), and fast (4000 rpm). Rotor speeds of 2500 to 4000 rpm are typically used with blunt edges in fine grinding applications, whereas speeds of 1000 to 2500 rpm are typically used with knife-edges for coarse grinding. Particle-size distributions are wider at low speed than at medium and high speeds [12]. Below the critical rotor speed, material experiences attrition, rather than impact action, which causes more spheroidal granules and may result in overheating of the material.

5. Screen size and type: The screen is usually an integral part of the hammer mill and does not act as a sieve. The particle size of the product depends on the openings in the screen, the thickness of the screen, and the speed of the hammer. The particle size of the output granules will be much smaller than the size of the screen used, because particles exit at an angle, with high velocity. Screens can be perforated, woven wire type, or with a slot configuration. The screen openings may range in size and open area based on-screen configuration. Because of the large forces that the screens are subjected to, the perforated screens are preferred over the woven-type screens. However, if the raw material fuses from the heat generated, or if the material is difficult to mill, woven-type screens are preferred for their increased open area. The herringbone and cross-slot designs are preferred for grinding amorphous and crystalline materials (Figure 20.8a,b).

20.7.2.2 Conical-Screening Mill

Similarly, for conical-screening mills, the operating variables affecting particle-size distribution are the type of impeller, impeller speed, and screen size and type:

1. Material feed rate: In contrast to hammer mills, conical-screening mills perform with greater efficiency when the comminution chamber is kept relatively full. Underfeeding results in low efficiency and reduced throughput.

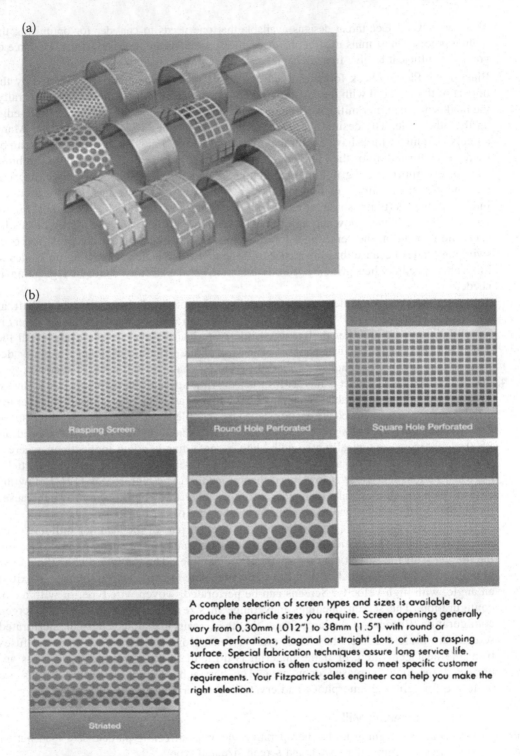

FIGURE 20.8 (a,b) Different Types of Hammer Mill Screens.
Source: From The Fitzpatrick Company.

(a)

(b)

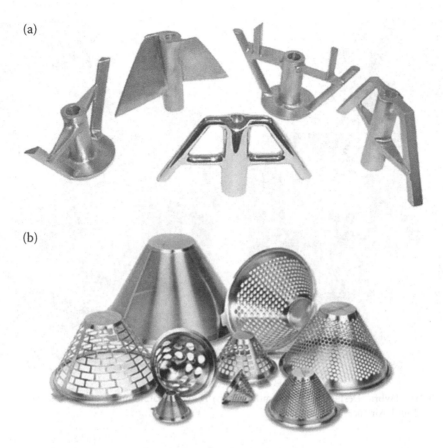

FIGURE 20.9 Conical-Screening Mill (Comil): (a) Impellers; (b) Screens.
Source: From Quadro Engineering Corp.

2. Impeller: There are several types of impellers available [13]; however, the four main types used frequently are as follows (Figure 20.9a):
Knife-edge: Its principal mode of operation is shear, and hence, it is used for compression-sensitive, heat-sensitive materials.
Round-edge: Its principal mode of operation is compression, and it provides high throughput and low retention. It is mainly used for wet or dry deagglomeration/delumping.
Round-edge with teeth: It is the same as the round-edge impeller except that it has teeth on one side, providing aggressive, high throughput. It reduces fines in milling compacted materials by pre-breaking with teeth and reducing retention time. It is often used for tablet rework.
Knife-edge low-intensity impeller: It is used where shear or cut is required; it gives a scissor-like action, for fibrous materials or capsule rework.
3. Speed: The speed of the impeller can affect the particle size of the product. Conical-screening mills available have variable or fixed-speed drives; however, revolutions per minute vary depending on the size of the impeller. When scaling up a milling process to achieve the same particle-size distribution, it is recommended to adjust the RPM to obtain the same linear tip velocity of the impeller.
4. Screen size and type: Screens are available in various sizes (Figure 20.9b), based on thickness, open area, and hole configuration such as round, square, slotted, or grater-type openings. Only perforated screens are available.

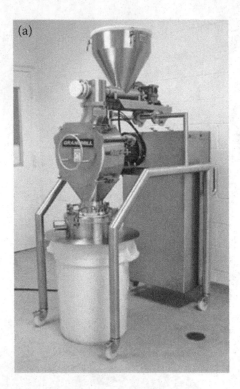
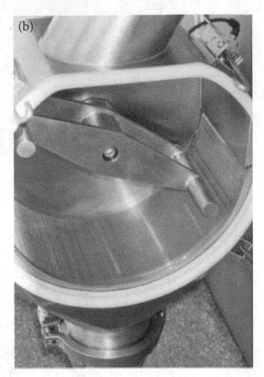

FIGURE 20.10 Hybrid Design: (a) Granumill and (b) Detail of Granumill Rotor and Screen.
Source: From Fluid Air Inc.

Various researchers have performed extensive studies of the effects of the foregoing variables on granulation and milling processes [20–22]. Motzi et al. [21], based on their observations of significant interaction effects, concluded that effects of mill speed, screen size, and impeller shape on particle-size distribution cannot be evaluated individually but must be evaluated at a level that is a combination of all three.

20.7.2.3 Hybrid Designs

Hybrid designs, such as the Granumill (Figure 20.10a,b), are now available, which utilize a one-piece cantilever rotor with heavy blades mounted parallel to the center shaft. Incorporating a variable-speed drive, these mills operate as screening mills when running at low speed, reducing fines, noise, heat, and dust, and as impact mills when running at high speed.

20.7.3 OTHER VARIABLES

Other variables can affect the sizing process, such as feed-material properties, granulation process, and drying process. The properties of materials have been discussed in section "Properties of Feed Materials Affecting the Sizing Process." The type of granulation, for example, dry (roller compaction), planetary, high shear, or fluid bed, can determine the strength of the granules, and hence, the sizing process. Furthermore, the drying process, whether tray or fluid bed, can also be important. Tray-dried granules are usually case-hardened and can be difficult to mill, whereas the fluid-bed process yields more porous and friable granules. Similarly, granules produced by high-shear granulators are harder, and they are therefore more difficult to mill than those manufactured using low-shear or fluid-bed processes.

20.8 SCALE-UP

20.8.1 HAMMER MILL

Table 20.2 shows the scale-up parameters for Fitzmills [12].

In addition to having the same screen size and type used on the lower scale, keeping the rotor tip speed constant is one of the most important considerations in the scale-up of a milling process. Vertical and horizontal rotor configurations may affect throughput and also particle-size distribution.

20.8.2 CONICAL-SCREENING MILL

Table 20.3 shows the scale-up parameters for various Comils [13]. In addition to having the same impeller type, screen size, and screen type used on the lower scale, the tip speed of the impeller is one of the key variables in scale-up; thus, it should be kept constant.

20.9 CASE STUDIES

20.9.1 COMPARISON OF FITZMILL VARIABLES

The variables that can be adjusted or easily changed to provide various different end results are [12] as follows:

- Rotor or tip speed of the blade (Figure 20.11a)
- Type of blade used (Figure 20.11b)

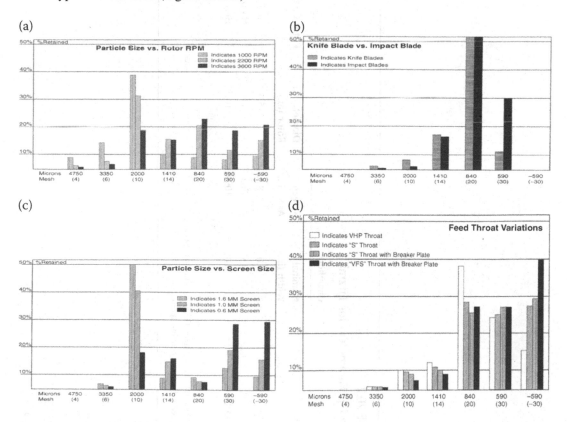

FIGURE 20.11 Particle-Size Distribution Milled Using a Fitzmill with Different (a) Rotor Speeds, (b) Blades, (c) Screens, and (d) Feed Throats.
Source: From Ref. [12].

TABLE 20.2
Scale-Up Parameters for Fitzmill

Model	Capacity[a] Factor		Chamber Nominal Width (in.)	Screen Area (in.²)	Diameter of Rotor (in.)	Rotor Configuration	No. of Blades	Tip Speed Factor[b]	Rotor Maximum rpm	Maximum Horsepower
L1A/MP	0.07×		1.0	8.5	5.4	Horizontal	4	1.42	9000/14000	0.5
M5A	0.7×		4.5	76.0	8.0	Horizontal	16	2.09	4600	3.0
D6A/DAS06	1.0×		6.0	109.0	10.5	Horizontal	16	2.75	4600	5.0/15.0

Source: From Ref. [12].
[a]Throughput relative to Model D6 at the same tip speed.
[b]Tip speed = factor × operating speed.

TABLE 20.3
Scale-Up Parameters for Comil

Model	Capacity Factor	Impeller Diameter (in.)	Screen Size (in.) A	B	C	Impeller Speed Scale-Up Comparison (rpm)						Motor Horsepower	Infeed Opening (in.)
197	1x	4.375	5	1.5	3	1200	2400	3600	4800	6000	7200	1 or 2	3 rounds
194	5x	7.625	8	2.5	5	700	1400	2100	2800	3500	4200	5600	5	6 rounds
196	10x	11.125	12	4	7	450	900	1350	1800	2250	2700	3600	10 or 15	8 rounds
198	20x	23.250	24	16	7	225	450	675	900	—	—	—	20	11 × 22 rectangular
199	40x	29.469	30	16		180	360	540					30	12 × 24 rectangular
Tip speed (ft/min)						1400	2800	4200	5600	7000	8400	11200		

Source. From Ref. [13].
A, screen upper diameter; B, screen lower diameter; C, screen height.

- Screen size and design (Figure 20.11c)
- Feed throat type and design (Figure 20.11d)

20.9.2 COMPARISON OF FITZMILL VS. COMIL

It is often difficult to predict the results from similar pieces of equipment having the same operating principle at two different scales, let alone using two pieces of equipment having different operating principles. Many times in the development of a pharmaceutical dosage form, the equipment used during formulation development and that used in production are quite different. Apelian et al. [22] studied the effect of particle-size distribution on chlorpheniramine maleate granules using a Fitzmill and a Comil. For the Fitzmill, various screens sizes (1, 2, 3, and so on) at medium speed were evaluated, and for the Comil, impellers (1601 and 1607) at two speeds (1680 and 3420 rpm) using various screen sizes (039, 045, 055, and 055 G) were studied. They reported that milling the granulation using a Fitzmill with a screen size of 2, at medium speed, gave a particle-size distribution similar to the granulation milled using a Comil (1601 impeller, 055 screen at 1680 rpm) (Figure 20.12). The results of this study suggest that, in making a major change in the milling process, one needs to optimize the critical processing variables to achieve a similar particle-size distribution.

20.9.3 COMPARISON OF HAND SCREEN VS. COMIL

The effect of changing the dry milling from a hand-screen operation to a conical-screening mill is shown in Figure 20.13. Naproxen granulations (0.5 and 4 kg) were manufactured in a fluid-bed granulator using PVP K-90 as a binder [23]. The particle-size distribution of granules (0.5 kg), passed manually through an 18-mesh screen, was much coarser than the granules (4 kg) that were milled using a Comil (Model 197 S). A flat-faced impeller (1607) at an impeller speed of 2500 rpm with a spacer setting 0.25 in. and screen number 2A055 (14-mesh) were used for the milling

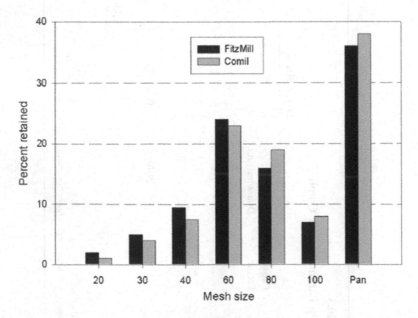

FIGURE 20.12   Particle-Size Distribution of Chlorpheniramine Maleate Granulations Milled Using Fitzmill and Comil.
Source: From Ref. [22].

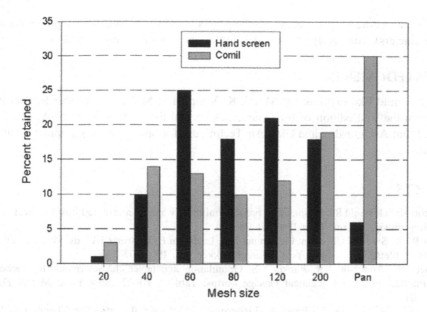

FIGURE 20.13   Particle-Size Distribution of Naproxen Granulations Milled Using Hand Screen and Comil. *Source*: From Ref. [23].

operation. Even though the granulations were prepared by the same procedure, the milling conditions drastically affected the particle-size distribution. As a general rule, during a switch over from a low-energy milling operation to a high-energy milling operation, the screen size should be coarser in the high-energy mill. The particle velocity is higher and therefore the size of the granule exiting out of the screen is much smaller than the screen opening. As seen from Figure 20.12, when the screen size was increased to 14-mesh for the conical-screening mill, the amount of fines generated was higher. Hence, during scale-up, optimization of milling conditions may be necessary to achieve the same particle-size distribution.

20.9.4   Modeling

Naik and Chaudhuri [24] recently published a review of experimental and modeling approaches for dry milling in pharmaceutical processing. With the ongoing initiative of the US FDA to encourage quality-by-design (QbD), the review is focused on some process analytical tools to characterize particle-size distribution as well as process modeling tools to simulate particle-size reduction. Finally, Leyva and Mullarney [25] in their publication have developed models for estimating powder-flow performance when only particle-size distribution data is available. All of these tools can be useful during new drug development, especially with regard to risk assessment when there is very little data available for a new API.

20.9.5   Scale-Up and Post -Approval Changes (SUPAC: Manufacturing Equipment Addendum)

In 2014, US FDA revised the SUPAC equipment addendum [26] for pharmaceutical unit operations (particle-size reduction, blending and mixing, granulation, etc.) providing general information and removing tables referencing specific equipment. When assessing manufacturing equipment changes from one class to another or from one subclass to another, it suggests a risk-based approach that includes a rationale and complies with the regulations, including the cGMP regulations. The guidance also recommends addressing the impact on the product quality attributes of equipment variations (via process parameters) when designing and developing the manufacturing process.

ACKNOWLEDGMENTS

The authors would like to thank Dr. Murali K. Vuppala of McNeil Consumer Healthcare for co-authorship on the first edition of this chapter. A special thanks to Frewitt USA, The Fitzpatrick Company, Fluid Air, Quadro, and Glatt Air Techniques for providing the equipment figures shown in this chapter.

REFERENCES

1. Prescott JK, Hossfeld RJ. Maintaining product uniformity and uninterrupted flow to direct-compression tableting presses. Pharm Tech 1994; 18:98–114.
2. Lantz RJ Jr. Size reduction. In: Lieberman HA, Lachman L, Schwartz JB, eds. Pharmaceutical Dosage Forms: Tablets. Vol. 2. New York: Marcel Dekker Inc., 1990:107–157.
3. Fonner DE, Anderson NR, Banker GS. Granulation and tablet characteristics. In: Lieberman HA, Lachman L, eds. Pharmaceutical Dosage Forms: Tablets. Vol. 2. New York: Marcel Dekker Inc., 1981:201.
4. Parrot EL. Milling. In: Lachman L, Lieberman HA, Kanig JL, eds. The Theory and Practice of Industrial Pharmacy. Philadelphia: Lea & Febiger, 1986:21–46.
5. O'Conner RE, Rippie ED, Schwartz JB. Powders. In: Gennaro AR, ed. Remington's Pharmaceutical Sciences. Easton: Mack Publishing Company, 1990:1615–1617.
6. Carstensen JT, Puisieux F, Mehta A, et al. Milling kinetics of granules. Int J Pharm 1978; 1:65–70.
7. Steiner G, Patel M, Carstensen JT. Effect of milling on granulation particle-size distribution. J Pharm Sci 1974; 63:1395–1398.
8. Motzi JJ, Anderson NR. The quantitative evaluation of a granulation milling process. III. Prediction of output particle-size. Drug Dev Indust Pharm 1984; 10:915–928.
9. Snow RH, Kaye BH, Capes CE, et al. Size reduction and size enlargement. In: Perry RH, Green D, eds. Perry's Chemical Engineers' Handbook. New York: McGraw-Hill Inc., 1984:8–20.
10. Prior MH, Prem H, Rhodes MJ. Size reduction. In: Rhodes MJ, ed. Principles of Powder Technology. New York: John Wiley & Sons, 1990:237–240.
11. Kukla RJ. Strategies for processing heat-sensitive materials. Powder Bulk Eng 1988; 2:35–43.
12. . Remove period. FitzMill Technical Bulletin. The Fitzpatrick Company, Waterloo, Canada.
13. Reove period. Comil Product Literature. Quadro Engineering Corp., Waterloo, Canada.
14. Poska RP, Hill TR, van Schaik JW. The use of statistical indices to gauge the mixing efficiency of a conical screening mill. Pharm Res 1993; 10:1248–1251.
15. Fourman GL, Cunningham DL, Gerteisen RL, et al. Improved color uniformity in tablets made by the direct compression method: a case study. Pharm Tech 1990; 14:34–44.
16. Schwartz JB. Theory of granulation. In: Kadam KL, ed. Granulation Technology for Bioproducts. Boca Raton: CRC Press, 1990:17.
17. Johnson C. Comminution variables and options. Powder Bulk Eng 1989; 3:40–44.
18. Owens JM. How to correct common hammermill problems. Powder Bulk Eng 1991; 5:38–43.
19. Hajratwala BR. Particle size reduction by a hammer mill I: Effect of output screen size, feed particle size, mill speed. J Pharm Sci 1982; 71:188–190.
20. Byers JE, Peck GE. The effect of mill variables on a granulation milling process. Drug Dev Indust Pharm 1990; 16:1761–1779.
21. Motzi JJ, Anderson NR. The quantitative evaluation of a granulation milling process. II. Effect of output, screen size, mill speed, and impeller shape. Drug Dev Indust Pharm 1984; 10:713–728.
22. Apelian V, Yelvigi M, Zhang GH, et al. Comparison of quadromill and Fitz mill used in the milling process of granulation. Pharm Res 1994; 11:8–142.
23. The University of Maryland at Baltimore (UMAB), School of Pharmacy/Food and Drug Administration (FDA) Collaborative Agreement RFP # 223–91–3401. On Scale-Up and Post-Approval Changes (SUPAC).
24. Naik S, Chaudhuri B. Quantifying dry milling in pharmaceutical processing: A review on experimental and modeling approaches. J Pharm Sci 2015; 8:2401–2413.

25. Leyva N, Mullarney MP. Modeling pharmaceutical powder-flow performance using particle-size distribution data. Pharm Tech 2009; 3:126–134.
26. Remove period Center for Drug Evaluation and Research. SUPAC: manufacturing equipment addendum. US FDA Guidance for Industry. 2014. https://www.fda.gov/drugs/guidance-compliance-regulatory-information/guidances-drugs.

LIST OF EQUIPMENT SUPPLIERS

1. Frewitt USA, Inc., Hillsborough, NJ, USA. http://www.frewitt.com.
2. The Fitzpatrick Company, Waterloo, Ontario, Canada. http://www.fitzmill-mpt.com.
3. Fluid Air, Inc., Naperville, IL, USA. http://www.fluidairinc.com.
4. Glatt Air Techniques Inc., Ramsey, NJ, USA. http://www.glatt.com.
5. GEA North America, Columbia, MD, USA. http://www.gea.com.
6. Quadro Engineering Corp., Waterloo, Ontario, Canada. http://www.quadro-mpt.com.
7. Hanningfield (North America) LLC, Hillsborough, NC USA. https://www.hanningfield.com/.
8. LCI Corporation, Charlotte, NC, USA. http://www.lcicorp.com.

21 Granulation Characterization

Cecil W. Propst

CONTENTS

21.1 INTRODUCTION

Physical property characterizations such as determination of particle size, surface area, and density are covered in more detail in Chapter 3 for active pharmaceutical ingredients (APIs) and excipients for granulating. Rather than repeating the testing detail, the information herein adds the characterization of the final granulations and applies the data to verification of both the granulation design and performance. Also, the discussion of chemical characterization and bioavailability of granulation properties needed for dissolution, permeation, and *in vivo–in vitro* correl`ations is covered in Chapter 22. In this chapter, we will deal with the chemical characterization of structure, location, and placement and its impact on content uniformity, compaction, and process-related issue of performance. Also as granulations are used as additives and processed into other dosage forms, the granulation designs' impact on the subsequent final product such as tablets, capsules, and final mixtures will be covered.

Characterization is divided into two parts: Structural design and performance characterization. Structural design targets the establishment of structural aspects to predict performance. Relating the design to performance is a major goal. To do this, the chapter is divided into three characterization areas:

1. Definitions of structure
2. Structural characterization
3. Granulation performance

Several terms will be used throughout the chapter as structural elements, and it is best to define these elements for clarity to apply these terms in characterization. Identifying the structural elements present in the granulation and verifying their influence on performance are initial tasks in characterization.

21.2 DEFINITIONS

A particle, as defined by United States Pharmacopeia (USP) < 776 >, is the smallest discrete unit of mass [1]. Thus, a particle does not need to be a stand-alone individual but must be discretely recognized. A primary particle is that same small discrete unit of mass bound into a granule or agglomerate. A granule is made up of primary particles that are firmly bonded together (will survive sieve testing). Bond former present in the transitional space is the "glue" holding the primary particles together. The transition's composition is normally a disordered region, a semi-solid and/or polymer boundary layer, that can extend to or be the surface of the granule. A "moving units" in a compressive process is a particle or particle fragment that is surviving the compression event [2]. "Moving units" as particles move through voidage during compression and remain intact. "Moving units" thus can be granules at low pressure, primary particles or fractured particles at higher pressures. Moving units can also be semisolids following under pressure. Voids in a granulation bed represent the volume or the space between particles in a granulation bed. As applied to granulation, the voids will be considered bed porosity. Bulk density as tested by USP <616> [3] is the mass of the granulation divided by the volume occupied, which includes voidage space between the particles and the porosity in the particles. Skeletal density considers the mass in the volume occupied by solid material including the volume in any closed pores within the granules (ASTM D3766). True density is mass in the volume that also excludes closed pores, thus it can be denser than skeletal density.

A granulation can contain particles as crystals or a combination of crystals and granules as is the case of the spray-dried lactose in Figure 21.1.

The arrowhead-shaped crystals may behave the same as the agglomerates when comparing flowability but may behave differently when comparing their compressive behavior. Note that the granules are made up of primary particles, crystals that are visible and relatively small compared to the non-agglomerated arrowhead-shaped crystals. Identifying structures and separately evaluating their influence on performance are important. Imaging methods used to identify types of structures present in a sample are visual, thermal, and/or analytical imagings. Visual imaging consists mainly of light obscuration methods, scanning electron microscope images (SEMs), and/or photomicrographs. Thermal analysis is a profile of bond energy and changes of state with temperature. Differential scanning calorimetry (DSC) can be used for structural identification. A review of thermal analysis applications is given by Duncan [4]. Analytical imaging is a set of morphological along with material composition and location data used to describe the granulation structure and/or composition.

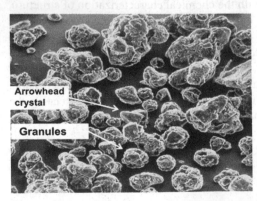

FIGURE 21.1   Spray-Dried lactose (from US patent 9358212; june 2016).

An example of using analytical data and SEM imaging to define granule structure was presented by Propst [5] for a granulated mannitol preparation. The granulation had a surface area, A_s, of 3800 cm^2/gm. Skeletal density of 1.481 gm/cm^3 along with melting point, heat of fusion, near infrared reflectance (NIR), and processing temperature confirmed a beta crystalline projection. This gave a relative volume to surface ratio, R_{sv}, of 1.77 μm using the skeletal density as the reference volume/mass to surface/mass ratio for this very porous granular structure. The true density ρ_t of the beta mannitol is 1.483 gm/cm^3. The close match of the skeletal density to true density indicated the particle is made up of open porosity with limited closed pores. If we assume a shape factor of 6 for an isometric particle with a 1.77 μm R_{sv}, the particle would have a diameter of 10.6 μm as a solid non-porous structure. Yet the particle size by laser diffraction centers at a d[50] of 446 μm. Along with the SEMs showing a highly porous filamentous particle, the analytical data supported the design description of a filamentous structure made up of ~1.77-μm-thick filaments having a continuous porosity with a 446-μm size made up mainly of a beta mannitol crystalline structure.

21.3 GRANULATION STRUCTURAL CHARACTERIZATION

The structural elements visible in the SEM of the spray-dried lactose example are crystals, agglomerates, smaller crystals as primary particles making up the agglomerates, and the potential for transitional "glue" holding the agglomerate structure together. In assay, the sample is mainly lactose and water, thus a form of lactose is the transitioning composition. A need to understand the impact of each of these structural elements on performance is evident.

1. Crystals versus agglomerates
2. Effect of primary particle size in the agglomerates
3. Effect of quantity and/or thickness of the transition material in the agglomerate structure.
4. The stability of the transition

Thus, defining the structures or determining the potential impact the structural differences have on performance is a characterization requirement.

Granulation can be characterized on the basis of at least four levels [6].

1. Molecular: Distribution and structure
2. Surface: Both as transitional surfaces and particle surface
3. Granular: The primary particle, transition, porosity, size, and shape
4. Granulation or bulk characteristics

The most important level to investigate depends on the final use of the granulations. The molecular level is important for content uniformity, stability, consolidation, dissolution, and other issues involving chemical makeup. The granular level is important also for content uniformity and ingredient placement (granule to granule), flow, compression, size of primary particles, and transitional issues. Surface characterization importance includes both the exterior and interior surfaces of granules but also transitional surfaces that can be exposed on compression. The bulk properties deal with in-process handling, segregation, die filling, flow rate, and bin and hopper designs. All levels of granulations must be accessed as part of the performance of the final dosage form, be it the granules themselves or as part of tablet or capsule products [7,8].

21.3.1 MOLECULAR LEVEL

Both the composition and thickness of the transition are important in molecular characterizations. Salpekar and Dent [9] characterized the film transition of an acetaminophen (APAP) granulation for direct compression as individual coated crystal made using a fluid-bed granulator. Seager et al.

did the same for roll-compacted, fluid-bed, and spray-dried granulations [10]. Armstrong et al. characterized the transition in dextrose monohydrate granulations as an amorphous dextrose transition [11]. Tillotson and Propst [2] described the transition on the surface of a spray-dried mannitol composition as a sorbitol–mannitol–maltitol fusion formed transition and defined the performance in tableting based on this composition. Three types of transition designs are possible.

1. Amorphous
2. Fusion Form
3. Polymeric

21.3.1.1 Amorphous Transitions

In the spray-dried lactose example, an amorphous lactose transition was found present and quantitated by Habib et al. [12] by differential vapor sorption (DVS). A ground sample was exposed to various levels of humidity, and weight gain of the sample was measured. Once 90% relative humidity (RH) was reached, the process of increasing the humidity was reversed, the sample was dried, and the weight loss was tracked.

The amount of moisture gained by the sample at an RH of 55% or higher and not lost on drying was related to the percent amorphous content of the sample converting to lactose monohydrate. The amorphous contents of four different marketed lactoses [Fast-Flo® (Foremost), Spray Dried® (Foremost), Pharmatose® DCL 11 (Crompton and Knowles), and Super-Tab® (Lactose Company of New Zealand)] and a crystalline α-lactose monohydrate (Foremost) were determined. The compaction properties of these lactoses were also studied by compressing each excipient to an in-die predetermined porosity of 20% using an Instron at a compression speed of 20 mm/min. The breaking force of these tablets was determined. The linear correlation of the amorphous content of the different lactoses with breaking force was greater than .98. The order of maximum breaking force reached was reported in the following order: Fast-Flo® > Spray Dried® > Super-Tab® > Pharmatose® DCL 11 > crystalline α-lactose monohydrate.

21.3.1.2 Fusion Form Transitions

Mannitol is an example of a material that can be processed to create fusion formed transitions with small amounts of other polyols. Bauer, Herkert, and Bartels [13] used DSC, X-ray, and near-infrared to characterize mannitol–sorbitol mixtures. If the amount of sorbitol is small, the sorbitol can be "fused" into the structure of the mannitol crystal matrix and does not melt as an independent peak in differential scanning calorimetry (DSC) but melts with the mannitol to lower the heat of fusion per mass of mannitol. This lower heat of fusion is an indication of the presence of lower bonding strength in the mannitol peak along with the presence of only a single peak in the DSC scan indicates the fusion form is mainly present. Sorbitol can be a surface deposit based on concentrations and solubility at process conditions. Placement of the fusion form on the surface can contribute to creating a pressure-activated bondable transition [2].

21.3.1.3 Polymer Transitions

Hydrophilic polymers such as starch paste, polyplasdone (PVP), hypermellose (HPMC), and maltodextrin are examples of film-forming polymers used as granulation transitions. These films hold residual moisture in their interior, and as a result, the polymer is plasticized. Thus, changes in the level of moisture in the film, especially if the polymer is close to its glass transition, will dramatically change the structure of the film. At room temperature (RT), PVP K-30 hydrated above 25% will be expanded and very soft and easily deformable with limited strength. Below 10% hydration, the PVP K-30 film will be very hard and brittle. A 5% PVP-based granulation hydrated to a 20% moisture level will plastically deform at RT. If only the film possesses moisture and none of the moisture is in the primary particles or core, the moisture in the total granulation will be 1% with PVP film hydrated at 20%. At 0.8% moisture content in the total granulation, the PVP hydration is 18%, will be more brittle, and may tend to crack. Film deposits by pouring the solution and drying at various temperatures and to various hydration levels and observing the films' consistency are recommended as part of design characterization [14].

The focus of moisture level control for hydrated binder film is twofold. First is to control the granulation process to build granules with the proper film hydration. Second is to obtain a final film hydration to create a non-brittle plastically deforming binder.

The Fox equation [Eq. (21.1)] is a modeling equation for the influence of moisture on the change in glass transition temperature (T_g) of the plasticized polymer system [15].

$$\frac{1}{T_g} = \frac{w_1}{T_{g1}} + \frac{w_2}{T_{g2}} \tag{21.1}$$

T_g is the glass transition temperature of the mixture, w_1, $T_{g1,}$ and w_2, and T_{g2} are weight fractions and glass transition temperature of components 1 and 2, respectively. Components are polymer and water.

Above the T_g, a polymeric system (film) is more rubbery. Below the glass transition temperature, the film is more solid and glassy. The presence of moisture, a miscible low molecular weight additive, increases the free volume of the system and subsequently lowers T_g, thus allowing the rubbery state and the plastic deformation and bonding desired at the in-process temperature of tableting.

An example in Figure 21.2 shows the effect of water added to PVP K-30 on the glass transition of the polymer system. If the temperature of the tableting environment during the compression is in the range of 30 to 38 °C, a 20% hydrated film with a T_g of 33 °C will be at or above its glass transition, and the film will be softer and more rubbery. After tablet ejection, the compact will cool to RT and the film will become more rigid, stronger, and glassy.

During granulating, polymer hydration is a key factor in granule growth and film structure. Thus during fluid-bed granulation, a range for moisture content as a target for in-process control is set up to prevent over-drying, lack of tackiness, and film cracking as well as to prevent over-wetting of the granules and lack of binder strength. An example is the granulation of a 95% acetaminophen (APAP) granulation with PVP. APAP neither contains nor adsorbs water during the granulation process. Thus, the loss on drying (LOD) of the bed is ~0% at the start. As the PVP film is sprayed onto the APAP, the amount of PVP in the granulation bed increases. To maintain the hydration level, the LOD of the granulation must be increased with the PVP in the granulation to maintain the film hydration at the target level. This safe range for hydration of the film is thus a design criteria developed to create a controlled granule growth, structure, and final film design.

Film surface stickiness in compression can hinder compression. Salpekar and Dent [9] reported an increase in packing density and hardness of tablets when the fluid-bed processed granulation was coated with 0.5% stearic acid. By using a surface lubricant, the hydration level of the final

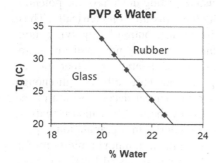

FIGURE 21.2   Plotted using fox equation.

granulation design could be increased to allow for more plasticity, and with the improved packing density, lower compression forces could be applied for the same tablet hardness, thus reducing the elastic loading of the APAP core.

21.3.1.4 Moisture Level and Location

Both the level and location of moisture are important factors for characterization. A roller compaction example is a dry powder blend with 0.6% moisture added and mixed into the dry ingredients before roll compaction compared to the same formula where the starch in the powder blend is made into a starch paste, granulated with the remaining ingredients, and then dried to a moisture content of 0.6%. The wetting of the roll-compacted dry powder premix makes more durable granules due to the wetting of the powder sugar in the dry mix. However, on tableting, tablets made with the wetted roll-compacted granulation harden with age. The same moisture level but with the moisture mainly in the starch polymer when tableted softened with age. Moisture wetting the powdered crystals of sucrose formed crystal bridges overtime in the tablets versus moisture in the starch polymer was bond into the polymer and the tablets softened with age.

Another example is a fluid-bed granulation containing dextrose monohydrate which was run with a warm up step prior to granulating. Lerk et al. [16] showed that bonding strength in tablets made with dextrose monohydrate increased with the level of dehydration temperature used to process the monohydrate. In this example, if at the start of the fluid-bed granulation process, a prewarming step to above 50°C is implemented prior to granulating, the water of hydration of dextrose monohydrate is removed. Thus, both the in-process water and final moisture can then reside in the water hydrating the polymer binder film. In a fluid-bed process with a bed temperature running at a product temperature of less than 40°C throughout the wetting and drying process, the hydrate is more preserved. Part of the moisture in the final granulation is then the water of hydration of dextrose to hydrate the polymeric binder. The final total LOD of the granulation must be higher, in the end, to maintain the polymer in the properly hydrated condition. The process choice to fully hydrate into dextrose, partially hydrate into dextrose, or fully hydrate into the polymeric binder can make a difference in process robustness and granulation performance.

Moisture on the completion of drying is often higher in larger granules than smaller ones as smaller granules dry faster [17]. If the API is added in the binder solution, then the active composition can vary based on granule particle size with the active composition also higher in granules with higher moisture content. Often the process over-dries the finer particles to obtain a satisfactory moisture level in the coarser fractions. Thus, a potential variation exists in hydrated compositions in coarse versus fines [14]. The binder concentration can also be higher on the surface of particles than in the particle core based on the drying temperature even though the total particle has the correct binder concentration [18]. This binder movement and relocation difference is due to binder as a solute migrating at a faster rate at higher drying temperatures versus the concentration gradient attempting to maintain a similar concentration in all areas. Location and amount of moisture are important in design characterization for both performance and physical stability.

Surface moisture can be measured using near infrared reflectance (NIR). NIR is both simple to apply and fast but requires calibration. Microwaves-based moisture testing units have the potential for deeper particle penetration. Capacitance techniques measure the moisture volumetrically. Thus, they have the potential of measuring surface to volume moisture distribution by applying more than one techniques [19]. Capacitance measures non-bound water and not total moisture. Measuring total moisture can be done with the proper setup and verification by either loss on drying (LOD) or Karl Fischer (KF) methods. Loss on drying methods require both high-enough temperatures and long-enough drying times, but weight loss from thermal decomposition of the sample needs to be avoided. A continuous tracing of moisture loss by thermal gravimetric analysis (TGA) is an LOD method that is useful in mapping the moisture energy in a granulation [4].

Zografi et al. [20] developed a predictive equation for calculating the minimum humidity for the storage of a granulation to prevent moisture adsorption using the materials tested for water vapor sorption energy. Badawy et al. [21] showed in a processing study that moisture content had the largest effect on the compressibility of the granulation compared with seven other process parameters. Within the tested levels, increasing moisture content increased the granulation compressibility. Armstrong et al. [11] studied the impact of moisture on the surface of anhydrous dextrose and dextrose monohydrate granulation. Water on dextrose anhydrous has a very complex relationship. As water is added to anhydrous dextrose, the surface gets tacky as shown by increased tensile strength for tablets made with the granulated powder with the small and increasing amount of water in a dextrose anhydrous granulation. The tensile strength increased with added moisture by adding up to 8.6% water. Above 9.2% moisture in the granulation, the tensile strength in the tablets formed from the granulation fell dramatically. Excess water, above 9.2%, is reported by Armstrong to be a physical barrier that prevents interparticulate bonding by hydrodynamic resistance to compression. Greonwold et al. [22] also suggested that excess water in sucrose granulation opposes the formation of strong bonds. Water-soluble carbohydrates are usually dried, "bone dry." Some residual water still remains, but always for most mono- and disaccharides, retaining less than 1% water is the target for granulation for chewable tablets. This low level of moisture is needed to set up a stable amorphous transition. A brittle fracture occurs at these transitions at low pressure, creating clean surfaces to allow at higher pressure close contact and crystal bond formation creating bonds.

21.3.2 SURFACE

Both physical and compositional surface differences can have a huge impact on functionality. An example of a chemistry difference on the granulation surface due to drying temperature was described by Ridgeway and Rubinstein for an ambient-dried 5% PVP granulation of magnesium hydroxide [18]. Scraping off surface samples and dissecting out the core for analysis, they reported that after drying at a 19.6 °C drying temperature, the surface contained less than 2% PVP. However, the same granulation dried at 59.6 °C the surface reached 13% PVP. Both drying conditions contained less than 2% PVP in the core even though the total granule contained 5% PVP.

An example of a physical difference in the porosity of the granule surface is a comparison of an ambient-dried versus a vacuum-dried granulation [14]. As in the Ridgeway and Rubinstein example, ambient drying increased the concentration of binder at the surface, but the same granulation vacuum-dried at a lower product temperature not only had a reduced binder concentration but also had a more porous and friable surface. With both higher porosity and less binder concentration, the granulation from the vacuum dried process was less compactable.

Seager et al. [10] went a bit further for acetaminophen granulated by the fluid bed with gelatin; after making a tablet, they cut the tablet in half, dissolved the active out of the granulation using acetone, and left the web of the protein S gelatin binder film to be observed. The structure of the web was shown to be both uniform in thickness and continuous across from one side of the tablet to the other in the fluid-bed processed product. The distribution of gelatin by roll compaction, spray-drying, and fluid-bed processing was also imaged [10].

Tillotson and Propst [2] characterized the images of the surface of ~140-μm spherical spray-dried mannitol preparation as a plate-like "solid layers," see Figure 21.3, whose layer thicknesses is less than 0.1 μm.

Material tableted to 12 kN and cross-sectioned (Figure 21.4) revealed fragments of less than 0.1-μm-thick plates from the fractured spray-dried mannitol product.

The image of the particle surface plate thickness corresponds closely to the image of fragmented thickness visible in the cross-sectioned tablet formed from the material. The fracturing transition is described as a deposit of mannitol with maltitol and sorbitol co-fused into the mannitol crystal surface. The ability of this material to develop at low compression forces in tableting of a low friability and maintain that low friability even at higher compressive forces without lamination was related to the very thin ~0.1-μm crystal fragments as "moving units" formed during early

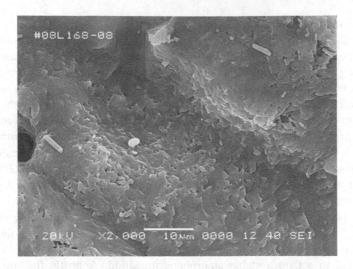

FIGURE 21.3   From US patent 9358212 (June 2016).

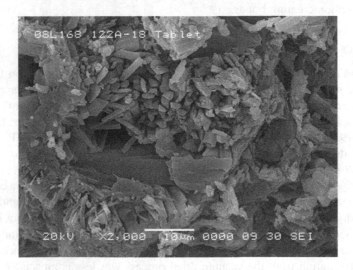

FIGURE 21.4   From US patent 9358212 (June 2016).

compression that easily migrated with pressure at higher compressive forces. Both the compression profile and compaction profile were linear with increase in compression pressure with little to no changes in friability.

21.3.3 Granular Level Characterization

Characterization on a granule level is a data set of placement, physical form, and porosity of the granule and visual imaging. An example of combining photo-micrographs for location and assay for confirmation is illustrated in a granulation core formation example [5]. Tablets made with the granulation laminated. The granulation was formed in a tumble blender and vacuum-dried. The same granulation composition when made using a batch continuous high-pressure granulating process did not laminate. The presence of a core was found by bisecting coarse granules of the tumble granulation process (Figure 21.5). The granulation was done with calcium carbonate, powder sucrose, and starch. By adding a lake color to the granulation formula, the core which did not take on the color was visible in the bisected granules. The non-core coating was of normal

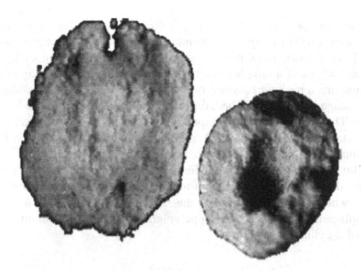

FIGURE 21.5 Calcium carbonate granulation core.

potency at 37% calcium carbonate. The core assayed to over 95% in calcium carbonate content. By removing the 600 μm and larger granules from the tumble granulated and vacuum-dried granulation, the material tableted normally. Adding back 15% or more of the 600 μm and larger granules to the granulation caused the tablets to become soft and laminate.

21.3.3.1 Granule Physical Structure

An example of controlling the physical form design was described by Hutton and Palmer [23] for a spray-dried lactose granulation. Using smaller crystals ~10 μm in size of lactose in the spray-dried lactose slurry, substantially 100% of lactose agglomerated and the agglomerates were much more spherical in structure. Any non-agglomerated crystals could be removed as fines and recycled.

The granule architecture for matrix granules was defined by Newitt and Conway-Jones [24] as pendular, funicular, capillary, and kneaded capillary. The authors used a granulation of sand with water of varying surface tensions using mixtures of ethanol and water from 0% to 100% to demonstrate the impact of structure on granule strength. The strength of the structures was determined by placing weights on a pan containing a layer of coarse granules under the pan and determining the weight needed to crush the granules. They found that granule strength increased linearly ($R^2 = 0.98$) with increasing surface tension of the wetting liquid. The authors defined the various granular structural designs based on the percent of porosity filled with solvent. With 0% porosity filled being dry sand with water added, pendular forming from >0% to ~22%, funicular forming between ~22% to ~80% and capillary from ~80% to ~120% of porosity filled with solvent. The amount of solvent determines not only granule strength but also granule size.

Compression, packing density, is a separate characterization of granule development from bonding strength. With % porosity filled with a binder a third granule design criteria. Thus, a key target for the development of a robust granulation is to achieve a similar granulation packing density. If packing is same, the granule strength is then controlled by the amount of binder in the porosity to hold the structure together. Confirmation of the final granulation porosity (packing density) and binder content, distribution, is therefore important in confirming design repeatability and robustness [5].

21.3.3.2 Granule Density and Porosity

To classify the granulation design type, the % porosity remaining needs to be determined along with granule density. To determine granule density, we need to determine the granular volume for a weight of the sample tested, the envelop volume. The envelope volume of a sample of granules can be determined by mixing the granules in a volumetric cylinder with very small latex microbeads [25]. Very small latex microbeads are added to a rotating cylinder filled with a known volume and weight of a sample to be tested. As the plunger is rotating in the cylinder, the plunger also maintains a packing pressure on the system. As the very small beads work themselves into the voidage in the granular bed, the total bed volume decreases and the plunger moves into the cylinder. The plunger force of compression is selectable (to not crush the granules) and therefore is repeatable from test to test. A preliminary compression cycle with only the displacement medium in the cell establishes a zero-volume h_o baseline. The granules are then placed in the cylinder with the dry latex medium, and the compression process is repeated. The difference in the distance, h_t, where the piston penetrates the cylinder during the test, and the distance, h_o, where it penetrates during the baseline procedure ($h = h_o - h_t$), is used to calculate the displacement volume or envelope volume (V_{EV}) of the medium, using the formula for the volume of a cylinder of height h:

$$V_{EV} = \pi r^2 h \qquad (21.2)$$

and

$$\rho_{EV} = \frac{m}{V_{EV}} \qquad (21.3)$$

The solid density can be skeletal density or the compressed density. The skeletal density of a granule can be determined using a helium pycnometer (AccuPyc 1330, Micromeritics Instrument Inc., Norcross, Georgia, USA). This device measures the volume of the space that helium gas can penetrate [25].

A dried granule porosity is calculated by dividing envelope density ρ_{ev} by the solid density ρ_s and subtracting from 1:

$$\%\text{Granule porosity} = \left[1 - \frac{\rho_{EV}}{\rho_s} \right] \cdot 100 \qquad (21.4)$$

Thus, porosity is generated as a calculation for relative density, the density of the granule relative to the density of the solids contained in the granule. The lower density of the granule versus the solid fraction is due to the porosity of the granule.

Instead of using skeletal density for the solid density, a compressed density can be used. Compressed density uses high-pressure compression of a weighed sample in a die cavity on a hydraulic press. This is meant to compress out all voids and both open and closed pores. The compressed density of the sample can be determined as the mass tested pressed to its minimum volume in the die cavity [4].

Paronen and Ilkka [26] have suggested that an increase in internal granular porosity increases the propensity of the granules to fragment, leading to the formation of stronger tablets. This is seen as a "crush in place" for increasing speed of deformation under load allowing for rapid deformation in high-speed tableting operations. For granulations that are less prone to fragmentation, Johansson et al. [27] showed that increased interior granular porosity increased the degree of deformation, resulting in higher densities at lower pressures during compression and stronger tablets.

21.3.4 GRANULATION LEVEL CHARACTERIZATION

Total porosity of a granulation bed is found using the following equation:

$$\%\text{Bed porosity} = \left[1 - \frac{\rho_{BD}}{\rho_s} \right] \cdot 100 \tag{21.5}$$

Where ρ_{BD} is the bulk density of the granulation obtained by measuring the volume occupied by a known weight of granulation [3]. We can use either the loose density or the tapped density for ρ_{BD}. By knowing the % bed porosity, we can track the status and change in porosity during processing. In a loose bed, the elimination of bed porosity reduces percolation segregation but can also cause failure to mix when using diffusive mixers such as tumbling type tote bins or double cone mixers.

21.4 GRANULATION PERFORMANCE

A common goal is to link structural characteristics to performance. Once linked, the design structure serves to justify performance. Changes in materials and processing are justified as safe if a similar structural design is obtained. If the change in performance is not explained by a change in design, then the characterization of the design is flawed and needs correction.

21.4.1 GRANULATION FLOWABILITY

An extension of the USP method for testing of bulk and tapped density [3] is the calculation of the Carr Index (Compressibility Index) [28]

$$\text{Carr index} = \frac{100 \times (P - A)}{P} \tag{21.6}$$

Where P is the tapped density (after vibration) and A is the bulk density (untapped). The higher the Carr index value, the poorer is the flowability. Values lower than 15 are considered a good flowing material for tableting. Values in the range of 25 to 30 are considered best for capsule filling [7]. As a compressibility index, the Carr Index value is a volume index. The amount of variability in bulk density possible in the granulation is estimated as the range of density from loose to packed density in feeding the material into a volumetric measuring system like a tablet die cavity. The higher the range between loose and packed density (higher Carr value), the more likely BD variability will affect weight. Thus, larger Carr Index values are more likely to cause tablet weight variation issues. Harwood and Pilpel describe a direct measurement of granulation flow rate as the "flow through an orifice" technique in great detail [29]. The test is a "use simulation test" and can use a hopper charged with the granules to be tested and flow the granules through an orifice. Hopper flow is important as most flow issues on tablet presses are hopper flow issues versus an issue with materials feeding out of the feeder into the die cavity. Time to discharge a fixed weight (300 to 500 gm) out of the funnel is measured. Another method discharges the material onto a scale for weighing [30]. Material discharges first hit a deflector to remove flow impact on the scale and then to the balance. The gain in weight is monitored with time intervals to track a fixed weight gain. The average and variation in the time needed for the fixed weight gain can then be used to calculate average weight gain and weight variation as average time and time variation to gain the fixed weight. Another variation in flow is measured through orifices of various diameters until the diameter is too small and flow is stopped [29].

Jenike [31] proposed a split ring shear cell measurement of the flow friction of granules under a normal load. The split cell is filled and packed with the sample to be tested. The upper ring of the two-piece split disk cell is pushed across the lower ring. The material filling the interior of split

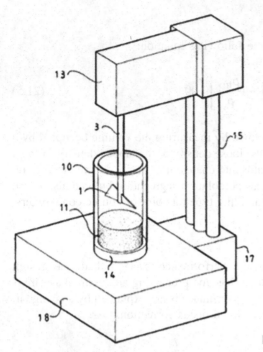

FIGURE 21.6   US patent 6481267B1 [32].

rings is sheared in this motion. The force required to push the upper ring is the resistance created in the granulation bed. The sample bed is normally loaded (packing weighted) to prevent bed expansion. The loading weight is also not enough to cause the bed to be compressed during shear. Thus, the flowing friction in the material is measured as the force needed to push the upper disk over a non-expanding or compressed lower bed. Values of friction are used to predict flow rates and storage bin design. Currently, rotating ring shear cells are favored as the units have unlimited rotary travel distances. This allows the ring shear tester to measure a complete yield locus without changing the sample or refilling the shear cell [32].

The powder rheometry measures flow resistance or friction as the energy to separate particles. An example of a powder flow rheometer is the Freeman FT4 Powder Rheometer (Figure 21.6) [33].

The Freeman rheometer consists of a specially designed agitator on a shaft placed in a cylinder. The agitator can be both rotated and lifted or lowered by the shaft at a fixed rate in the powder sample being tested. The agitator design is a special spiral curvature such that at a fixed rotational speed and a predetermined lift or lowering speed, the tip of the blade of the agitator will only slice through the material and not compress or lift the bed. At this specially balanced combination of paddle rotational speed and vertical speed, the granules in the sample are neither compressed nor expanded but only separated by the thickness of the blade as the paddle turns in the sample. The shaft is instrumented for torque. The resistance to the turning motion is a measure of the resistance to surface separation. At higher lift speed than the balanced speed, the sample can be fluidized or if lowered at higher speed compressed. Thus, we have a torque and a displacement curve generated. The test can be a torque displacement curve for a bed without density change, with an expanded bed, and with a compressed bed. Material conditioning is needed to obtain a uniform air voidage distribution in the sample, either loose or packed voidage, to develop a repeatable starting point [33,34].

The area under the torque displacement curve is the work done (mJ) by the paddle as it moves up or down the powder bed. That work required is related to the energy in the powder bed resisting the motion. Influence of humidity and amount of fines or additives can show a smaller or greater work required for particle separation.

21.4.2 GRANULATION DEFORMATION STRENGTH

Harwood and Pilpel [29] as did Newitt and Conway-Jones [24] measured granule strength by adding weights to a weighing pan placed over a narrow size cut of granules until the granules were crushed. This direct crushing approach was modified by both Ganderton and Hunter [35] and Gold et al. [36]. Gold et al.'s modification records the force required to crush the granule when a strain-gauged ring platen moving at a constant strain rate was used. Direct measurement of tensile strength is difficult for granules as the surface area forming in the break is hard to measure and the break is more of a crushing versus a straight plane break. These methods have inherent difficulties in measuring the strength of granules smaller than 40 mesh.

Granule attrition was measured by Mehta et. al. [37] using a ball mill to determine the durability of granules. A Roche Friability Tester was used by Serpelloni and Boonaertused [38] in determining granule friability. The unit is charged with a screen cut of granulation to be tested, a set of stainless steel spherical balls are added to the wheel, and friability is tested. The percentage loss of mass is the value that is represented as the granulation friability.

21.4.3 HIGH-PRESSURE CHARACTERIZATION

Both roll compaction and the tableting process compact powders. Compaction consists of two distinct processes: compression and consolidation. Compression is a loss in volume of the granulation bed. Consolidation is the formation of a solid body (bond formation). Compaction thus represents the decrease in voids and internal particle porosity, the increase in contact surface area (Acs), and the creation of bonds.

Compression is first repacking and at higher pressures the deformation of particles. The bed being compressed is losing porosity and is densifying. Starting at low pressures, the granules are rearranging and packing in the bed. This bed deformation is a "slip into place" mechanism where granule moves to occupy open spaces. Once lodged in a fixed position, the granule must deform. Another mechanism for volume loss is "crushing in place" [2]. In the crush, in place, the granule collapses, losing internal porosity. Hollow spray-dried particles such as spray-dried lactose are examples of a "crush in place" design. Crush in place is a brittle fracturing mechanism. Crush is fast and not a time-dependent deformation and suited for higher tableting speeds versus slip in place. Slip in place requires time for deformation. If the particle deforms to slip in place without breaking, the deformation is more plastic in nature. Plastic deformation is time-dependent. All materials elastically load to a greater or lesser degree, and as such if they do not yield, they can push back once the pressure is released and the compact is expanded [6].

Clean surfaces, such as semisolid transition, when brought in close contact, can form bonds. Semisolid transitions can also move under pressure and fill any open space and thus increase the contact surface. An example reported by Chirkot and Propst [39] of a low-shear granulation with limited binder distribution formed harder tablets with lower friability at lower compression pressures than fluid-bed granulations. At higher pressures, however, the fluid-bed granulations made harder tablets than the low-shear formulation, but friability was higher. This was said to be due to a more uniform binder distribution contained in a fluid-bed granulation versus the low-shear process.

Measuring the compression event and identify and quantitate the mechanisms of deformation and bonding requires the measurement of the pressure being applied and the displacement as well as the bond strength formed. For the compression event, a tablet simulator with force and displacement measurement abilities is used [25]. The information of force applied and displacement is used in calculating relative density [Eq. (21.7)], porosity [Eq. (21.8)], and degree of porosity reduction

[Eq. (21.9)]. These values are essential parameters for determining plasticity (Heckel equation), packing and deformation pressure, and relative densities using the Cooper–Eaton analysis.

$$D = \frac{\rho_a}{\rho_t} \tag{21.7}$$

$$\varepsilon = 1 - D \tag{21.8}$$

$$\varepsilon = 1 - \frac{\rho_a}{\rho_o} \tag{21.9}$$

In each equation, D is the relative density of a powder compact at pressure P, ρ_a is the apparent density of a powder compact at pressure P, ρ_t is the true density of a powder, ε is the porosity, and ρ_o is the bulk density of a powder.

21.4.3.1 Plastic Deformation

The Heckel equation [Eq. (21.10)] allows for the determination of the yield pressure needed to maintain plastic deformation. It is applied to medium- and high-pressure situations used in tablet making [27,40]:

$$\ln\left(\frac{1}{1 - D}\right) = kP + A \tag{21.10}$$

where D is the relative density of a powder compact at pressure P. Constant k is a measure of the $1/$(yield pressure) of a compressed material. Constant A is related to the die filling and particle rearrangement before deformation and bonding of the discrete particles [41]. Thus, a Heckel plot allows for the interpretation of the mechanism of deformation and the plasticity of the material. Asgharnejad and Storey [42] used the Heckel plasticity of materials and API to develop a formulation predictive strategy for very small samples of high-dose active ingredient using a tablet press simulator.

21.4.3.2 Repack and Deformation

The Cooper–Eaton equation [Eq. (21.11)] considers that powder compaction occurs in two steps. The first is the filling of the voids in the granulation by rearrangement of granules without any size change. The second proceeds into energies needed for the deformation of the granules by pressing them into pores smaller than their size [26,41].

$$\frac{|1/D_o - 1/D|}{1/D_o - 1} = a_1 \exp\left(-\frac{k_1}{P}\right) + a_2 \exp\left(-\frac{k_2}{P}\right) \tag{21.11}$$

where D_o is the relative density at zero pressure and D is the relative density at pressure P. Cooper–Eaton constants a_1 and a_2 describe the theoretical maximum densification that could be achieved by filling voids of the same size (a_1) and of a smaller size (a_2) than the actual particles. The value of $a_1 + a_2$ should equal unity for the equation to apply. The most probable pressures at which the respective densification processes would occur are described by k_1 and k_2 [41].

The bond strength (tensile strength) is the breaking force needed to rupture the compact divide by the area of the break. In tablets, this is determined by compressing a compact diametrically in a tablet hardness tester [Pharmatron tablet tester (model 6D, Dr. Schleuniger Pharmatron Inc., Manchester, New Hampshire, USA)]. The radial tensile strength of the compact is calculated from

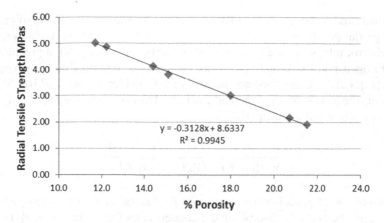

FIGURE 21.7 Redrawn from US Patent 9358212.

the compact breaking strength and tablet thickness using Eq. (21.12) of Fell and Newton [43], in which the radial tensile strength σ_t is given by Eq. (21.12).

$$\sigma_t = \frac{2F}{\pi dt_h} \tag{21.12}$$

Where σ_t is the tensile strength (MPa), F is the force required to cause failure in tension (N), d is the diameter of the compact (mm), and t_h is the thickness of the compact (millimeter).

If the surfaces come in close-enough contact, bonds will form. If all surfaces are in contact, compact porosity is zero and the tensile strength of the compact represents the bond strength per unit area. Thus, the strength of the compact formed is a combination of compression, the fraction of the total surface area bonding (A_b), times, consolidation, and the bond strength per unit area σ_b [Eq. (21.13)] [25].

$$\sigma_{TS} = \sigma_b \cdot \frac{A_b}{A_t} \tag{21.13}$$

Extrapolating total surface area (A_t) bonding as porosity remains at zero, the tablet tensile strength σ_b can be determined. This assumes a linear projection with no compaction failures [2].

An example of determining the bonding strength per unit area as a granulation design criteria is a spray-dried co-processed mannitol granulation by Tillotson and Propst [2]. The compaction profile plot in Figure 21.7 at seven compression pressures is plotted as compact porosity remaining versus the calculated tensile strength of compacts made from the granulation. The linear regression intercept is 8.6 Mpas and is the bonding strength per unit area for the granulation. This then becomes a design performance standard for the spray-dried product.

21.4.3.3 Focus on Granulation Surface

Three types of surface interfaces are present in granules: (i) the air to solid; (ii) the solid to solid; and (iii) solid to semisolid (or liquid) interfaces. Total air to solid surface is the sum of the outer surface of granule and the surface in the granular pores.

21.4.4 GRANULATION SURFACE AREA

The total air to solid surface area of granulation for outer surface and open pores can be measured by the Brunauer, Emmett and Teller Equation (BET) gas adsorption method. Developed by

Brunauer, Emmet, and Teller [44], the method features two ranges for the adsorption of gas. At lower relative partial pressures, range of $0.05 < P/P_0 < 0.35$, of nitrogen (the adsorption gas) to a carrier gas (helium), total surface area is measured. Higher than 0.35 partial pressures extends the test to measure open pores size and volume as well as pore size distribution per volume. In the BET equation [Eq. (21.14)], the slope and intercept are found for a plot of $1/V[(P_0/P) - 1]$ on the y axis and P/P_0 on the x axis. With slope and intercept known, the value for V_m (the volume of a monolayer of gas adsorbed) is calculated:

$$\frac{P}{V(P_0 - P)} = \frac{1}{V_m C} + \frac{(C - 1)P}{V_m C P_0} \tag{21.14}$$

Where V is the volume of gas adsorbed at pressure P, P is the partial pressure of adsorbate, C is a constant relating to the heats of adsorption and condensation for the material, P_0 is the saturation pressure of adsorbate at experimental temperature, and V_m is the volume of gas adsorbed as a monolayer on the surface.

Plots of $1/V[(P_0/P) - 1]$ on the y axis and P/P_0 on the x axis generates a straight line. V_m and C are calculated from both the slope and the intercept of this line. The specific surface area (SSA) in units of square meters per gram is calculated using Eq. (21.15):

$$\text{SSA} = \frac{(V_m N_0 A_{cs})}{M} \tag{21.15}$$

where N_0 is the Avogadro's number, A_{cs} is the cross-sectional area of adsorbate, and M is the mass of a solid sample.

21.4.4.1 Granule Size and Size Distribution

For a spherical particle, its diameter is a unique number that describes not only particle size but also surface area, shape, volume, and mass (if the density is known). Most particle size measurements are quoted relative to the equivalent diameter of a spherical particle.

21.4.5 EQUIVALENT DIAMETERS

Equivalent surface diameter can be calculated from a particle surface area using Eq. (21.16):

$$d_s = \sqrt{\frac{S}{\pi}} \tag{21.16}$$

Similarly, an equivalent volume diameter can be calculated using Eq. (21.17):

$$d_v = \sqrt[3]{\frac{6V}{\pi}} \tag{21.17}$$

If the particles consist of a single size and shaped rods with a diameter of 100 μm and height of 300 μm, the volume is 1.18×10^{-6} μm³:

$$V = \pi (50)^2 300 \tag{21.18}$$

The laser analysis sees the particle as a distribution with a size range of 100 and 300 μm.

The sphere of equivalent diameter for the volume of the particle is 160 μm found by Eq. (21.19):

$$\sqrt[3]{\frac{6V}{\pi}} \tag{21.19}$$

A single particle of non-spherical shapes like rods is seen by a laser analyzer as a distribution. Thus, it is important to know the particle shape when interpreting particle size data. Various ratios for number, surface, and volume as weighted mean diameters can be used to aid in interpreting the size data. Equation 20 is the surface-weighted mean diameter, $D[2,3]$.

$$D[2, 3] = \sqrt{\frac{\Sigma n_i d_i^3}{\Sigma n_i d_i^2}} \tag{21.20}$$

$D[2,3]$ is inversely related to the specific surface area, and as such, it is very useful in applications that involve surface, such as in coating application.

Equation 21.21 is the volume-weighted mean diameter, $D[3,4]$. $D[3,4]$ has its best uses in mixture studies as $D[3,4]$ gives a relationship of particle size as a mass size mean for comparison:

$$D[3, 4] = \sqrt{\frac{\Sigma n_i d_i^4}{\Sigma n_i d_i^3}} \tag{21.21}$$

For a spherical particle, the volume mean diameter and the surface-weighted mean diameter are the same. Thus, their ratio is 1 for spheres:

$$\sim 1 = \frac{D[2, 3]}{D[3, 4]} \text{for a sphere} \tag{21.22}$$

Thus, if the ratio of surface to volume-weighted mean diameters is not approximately 1, it is a good practice to obtain a visual image of the shape of the particles being tested.

Particle size can be measured by sieve analysis, laser light scattering, or optical microscopy as described in Chapter 3 in this book on drug substance and excipient characterization for granulating.

21.4.5.1   Sieve Analysis

Dry sieve analysis is a preferred method for measuring percent coarse particles in a sample. A small number of coarse particles by count can be a very large percentage in a mass distribution. Sieving allows for larger sample sizes to be tested and thus a greater chance of obtaining a better estimate of the coarse content. A sieve is a screen with normally square apertures (hole). The granulation is placed on top of a stack of five to six sieves, which have successively smaller-sized openings from top of the stack to the bottom. The stack is vibrated, rotated, and/or mallet shocked, or a combination of motions and the particles collected on top of the sieves. The data is usually represented in terms of percentage retained or percentage passing the sieve versus the screen size, or an accumulative distribution found on or through the sieve cut. It is always important to be sure that enough time is given to the sieving step and the sieve is not overloaded. It is also important to make sure that the sieve is not blinded. Due to the issue of blinding the smallest screen used in granulation, sieving has a 45-μm aperture [5].

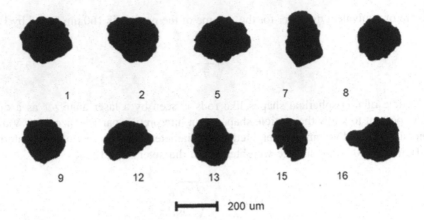

FIGURE 21.8 From EP 191635192.2 [47].

As part of sieve analysis, it is important in design characterization to assay the sieve cut for the content of API, binder, and moisture content.

21.4.6 Granulation Shape

Particle shape can be quantified by different methods. One easy way is the relationship of volume-weighted mean to surface-weighted mean in laser particle size analysis [45].

$$\Omega_L = \frac{[D\,[4,\,3]]}{[D\,[3,\,2]]} \tag{21.23}$$

If the particles are spherical, this ratio is equal to 1.

The effect of particle shape on bulk powder properties has been illustrated by Rupp [46]. The bulk volume increases as the shape becomes less spherical. The flow rate also drops with loss in a spherical shape.

Automated light obscuration imaging is a visual imaging tool that can be used for both analysis of particle size and particle shape. Dynamic imaging systems move particulates past the microscope optics while using high-speed flash illumination. A significant population of particles can be analyzed for both size and shape. In examining the shape characteristics of a spherical melt granule, Propst et. al. [47] examined samples of over 100,000 particles for shape characteristics.

Figure 21.8 shows ten actual particle images of a competitor's product from EP patent 191635192.2 [47]. The numbers are particle identification numbers. More than 100,000 particle images are stored and can be sorted and examined similarly by Yu and Handcock [48] for aspect ratio, circularity, convexity, solidity, and numerous other shape parameters.

Static imaging systems offer even more versatility in exploring the chemical composition of individual granules in the sample by Raman Spectroscopy [49]. In static imaging, the particulate is dispersed onto a stage where it remains fixed during analysis.

Classification of particles based on shape can also be done by physical separation based on shapes. A method that sorts particles by shape is described by Ridgeway and Rupp [50] in which the granulation is fed onto a vibrating triangular metal deck. Particles of different shape segregate on the deck and are collected for analysis by weight. Samples and data represent a weight distribution for spherical to non-spherical shapes.

21.5 ACTIVE PRINCIPLE CHARACTERIZATION

21.5.1 CRYSTALLINITY AND POLYMORPHISM

Understanding the effect of granulation on the form of the bulk drug has gained increasing attention in the past few years. A detailed description of X-ray diffraction is provided by Suryanarayanan and the references cited therein [51]. X-ray diffraction is mostly used to identify the crystalline form of a pure solid substance.

Modulated temperature X-ray powder diffraction (XRPD) is being used increasingly in the pharmaceutical industry at both preformulation and formulation stages. Airaksinen et al. [52] studied polymorphic transitions during drying using two methods: a multi-chamber microscale fluid-bed dryer or a variable temperature powder X-ray diffractometer. Relative amounts of different polymorphic forms of theophylline remaining in the dried granules were determined by XRPD. The authors concluded that metastable anhydrous theophylline predominated when the granules were dried at 40 °C to 50 °C. Temperature above 50°C produced mostly anhydrous theophylline, and more than 20% of the metastable form remained even at 90°C.

Morris et al. [53] reported polymorphic changes when hydroxymethylglutarate coenzyme A reductase inhibitor was wet-granulated with water. The starting material was in the anhydrous form, which was then converted into an amorphous form during the wet granulation process. The loss in crystallinity was experimentally determined using XRPD. Exposure of this granulation to an environment of greater than 33% RH caused a form conversion into its crystalline hydrate. This series of experiments demonstrated the usefulness of a sophisticated technique, such as XRPD, in the assessment of the physical stability of APIs during granulation.

21.5.2 HYDRATES

Approximately one-third of APIs are capable of forming hydrates. Hydrates can have a lower solubility rate. This tendency of materials to form hydrates can impact dissolution and stability. A hydrate screening study for nitrofurantoin using NIR/Raman Spectroscopy in an acetone/water system was reported by Aaltonen et al. [54]. Räsänen et al. [55] studied the polymorphic conversion of theophylline during wet granulation using NIR. The authors found that at a low level of granulation liquid (0.3 mol of water per mole of anhydrous theophylline), water absorption maxima in the NIR region occurred first at around 1475 and 1970 nm. These absorption maxima were identical to those of theophylline monohydrate. At higher levels of granulation liquid (1.3 ± 2.7 mol of water per mole of anhydrous theophylline), increasing absorption maxima occurred at 1410 and 1905 nm because of OH vibrations of free water molecules. Aaltonen et al. applied this to in-line NIR and Raman spectroscopy during fluid-bed drying to track the dehydration of theophylline monohydrate [56].

21.5.3 API UNIFORMITY

One of the benefits of granulating is the ability to generate a uniform dispersion of the API in all granular particles to assure content uniformity. Also, the lack of dust is an advantage in controlling cross-contamination and employee exposure. In the design to assure mode, it is the granulation consistency that needs to be verified.

In pharmaceutical delivery systems, it is the API dose that is being delivered and the target for the design to be assured. The dose (tablet weight times %API) delivered is variable based on the weight of the dosage form and its %API composition. It is important to separate the two, dose form weight variability from the variation in % composition during investigations and verification of process performance.

An example of the separation of the variability of weight versus compositional variation of the granulation is the weighing of 60 tablets for weight variation [5]. Weigh another set of ten tablets, and assay each tablet. If the dose per tablet is controlled only by the variability in the tablet weight, the mg/mg composition would be a fixed composition. All tablets would have the same % active. As tablet weight increases, the mg/mg concentration changes the granulation, making the tablet having a variable potency.

Besides the investigation into the composition of the granulation using the sieving approach discussed earlier, visual imaging can be used for investigations. An example of a Metoprolol Tartrate granulation with lactose using a PVP solution in a high-shear granulator was found to contain particles of different appearance. Based on assay as well as dissolution rates on a microscope slide, the less white and more cream-colored particles, which dissolved faster, were Metoprolol Tartrate clusters that survived both the granulation and drying process. The dry powder ingredients required premilling on charging to remove the API clusters to eliminate the problem as the use of chopper and higher agitator speeds alone was not enough to remove the clusters.

Drugs with high solubility in the granulation solvent have a higher tendency to migrate during drying creating a drug-rich surface on the drying particle [5]. Attrition or abrasion during subsequent handling leads to the formation of highly drug-concentrated fines relative to the larger particles. Kapsidou et al. [57] showed that drug migration increased with drug solubility and was projected to be a problem above a target range per granulation system.

Viscosity has a significant effect on drug migration. Drug migration increased from the pendular state (being dried) to the funicular state (being dried). Kiekens et al. [58] showed that a minimum liquid viscosity of 100 Mpas was needed to stop the migration of riboflavin in a-lactose using PVP K-90 as the wet binder.

REFERENCES

1. The United States Pharmacopeia. USP <776>. Rockville, MD, 2007.
2. Tillotson J., Propst C. Highly compactable and durable direct compression excipients and excipients systems. US patent 9358212 (June 7, 2016).
3. The United States Pharmacopeia. USP <616>. Rockville, MD, 2007.
4. Duncan C. The application of thermal analysis to pharmaceutical dosage forms. In: Augsburger L., ed. Pharmaceutical Dosage Forms – Tablets. 3rd ed. UK: Informa Publishing, 2008: 439–464.
5. Propst C. Characterization of granulation. In: Parikh D., ed. Handbook of Granulation. 23rd ed. New York: Informa Healthcare, 2009: 469.
6. Alderborn G., Wikberg M. Granule properties. In: Alderborn G., Nyström C., eds. Pharmaceutical Powder Compaction Technology. New York: Marcel Dekker Inc., 1996: 323–374.
7. Podczeck F. Powder, granule and pellet properties for filling of two piece capsules. In: Podczeck F., Jones B., eds. Pharmaceutical Capsules. London: Pharmaceutical Press, 2004: 101–118.
8. Hoag S., Lim H.-P. Particle and powder bed properties. In: Augsburger L., Hoag S., eds. Pharmaceutical Dosage Forms: Tablets. Unit Operations and Mechanical Properties. 3rd ed. Vol. 1. New York: Informa, 2008: 17–73.
9. Salpekar A., Dent L. Direct tableting acetaminophen compositions. US patent 4661521 (1987).
10. Seager H., Burt I., Ryder J., et al. The relationship between granule structure, process of manufacturing and tabletting properties of granulated products. Int J Pharm Technol Prod Manuf 1980; 1(2): 73.
11. Armstrong N., Patel A., Jones T., et al. The compression properties of dextrose monohydrate and anhydrous dextrose of varying water contents. Drug Dev Ind Pharm 1986; 12: 1885–1901.
12. Habib Y., Sprockel O. L., Abramowitz R. Evaluation of the amorphous content of currently marketed modified lactoses and its relationship to their compactibility. AAPS meeting in Nashville, TN, 1999.
13. Bauer H., Herkert T., Bartels M., et. al. Investigation on polymorphism of mannitol/sorbitol mixtures after spray-drying using differential scanning calorimetry, X-ray diffraction, and near-infrared spectroscopy. Pharm Ind 2000; 62: 231–235.
14. Propst C., Chirkot T. Drying. In: Augsburger L., Hoag S., eds. Pharmaceutical Dosage Forms – Tablets. 3rd ed. Taylor & Francis Group, Milton Park, Oxfordshire, 2008: 195–225.
15. Bicerano J. Prediction of Polymer Properties. New York: Marcel Dekker, 2002.
16. Lerk C. F., Zuurman K., Kussendrager K. Effect of dehydration on the binding capacity of particulate hydrates. J Pharm Pharmacol 1984; 36: 399.

17. Pitkin C., Carstensen J. T. Moisture content of granulations. J Pharm Sci 1973; 62(7): 1215.
18. Ridgeway K., Rubenstein M. H. Solute migration during granule drying. J Pharm Pharmacol 1974; 26(Dec suppl): 24S–29S.
19. Levin, M. Wet granulation: end-point determination and scale-up. Encyclopedia Pharm Technol 2006; 1(1): 4078–4098.
20. Zografi G., Grandofi G. P., Kontny M. J., et al. Prediction of moisture transfer in mixtures of solids: transfer via vapor phase. Int J Pharm 1988; 42: 77.
21. Badawy S., Menning M. M., Gorko M. A., et al. Effect of process parameters on the compressibility of granulation manufactured in a high-shear mixer. Int J Pharm 2000; 198: 51–61.
22. Greonwold H., Lerk C. F., Mulder R. J. Some aspects of the failure of sucrose tablets. J Pharm Pharmacol 1972; 24: 352–356.
23. Hutton J., Palmer G. Lactose product and method. US patent 363970A (May 1, 1970).
24. Newitt D., Conway-Jones J. A combination of theory and practice of granulation. Trans Inst Chem Eng 1958; 36: 422–442.
25. Amidon G. Physical and mechanical property characterization of powders. In: Brittian H., ed. Physical Characterization of Pharmaceutical Solids. New York: Informa Healthcare, 2007: 281.
26. Paronen P., Ilkka J. Porosity-pressure functions. In: Alderborn G., Nyström C., eds. Pharmaceutical Powder Compaction Technology. New York: Marcel Dekker Inc., 1996: 55–75.
27. Johansson B., Wikberg M., Ek R., et al. Compression behaviour and compactability of microcrystalline cellulose pellets in relation to their pore structure and mechanical properties. Int J Pharm 1995; 117: 57.
28. Carr R. Evaluating the flow properties of solids. Chem Eng 1965; 72: 163.
29. Harwood C. F., Pilpel N. Granulation of griseofulvin. J Pharm Sci 1968; 57: 478.
30. Gold G., Duvall R. N., Palermo B. T., Slater J. G. Powder flow studies III: factors affecting the flow of lactose granules. J Pharm Sci 1968; 57(4): 667–671.
31. Jenike A. W. Gravity Flow of Solids. Bulletin 108. Salt Lake City: Utah Engineering Experimental Station, University of Utah, 1961.
32. Shah R., Tawakkul M., and Khan M. Comparative evaluation of flow for pharmaceutical powders and granules. AAPS PharmSciTech 2008; 9(1): 250–258.
33. Freeman T. Powder or granulated material test appartusUS patent 10324010 (June 18, 2019).
34. Iles C. M., Bateson I. D., Walker J. A. Rheometer. US patent 6,481,267B1. Stable Microsystems Ltd (2002).
35. Ganderton D., Hunter B. M. A comparison of granules prepared by pan granulation and by massing and screening. J Pharm Pharmacol 1971; 23: 1S.
36. Gold G., Duvall R., Palermo B., et al. Granule strength as a formulation factor 1: instrumentation. J Pharm Sci 1971; 60: 922–925.
37. Mehta A., Zoglio M. A., Carstensen J. T. Ball milling as a measure of crushing strength of granules. J Pharm Sci 1978; 67: 905.
38. Serpelloni M., Boonaertused J. Pulverulent mannitol of moderate friability and process for its preparation. Roquette's US patent 5,573,777 (November 12, 1996).
39. Chirkot T., Propst C. Low-shear granulation. In: Parikh D, ed. Handbook of Granulation. 2nd ed. New York: Informa Healthcare, 2005: 229.
40. Heckel R. W. An analysis of powder compaction phenomena. Trans AIME 1961; 221: 1001–1008.
41. Cooper A. R., Eaton L. E. Compaction behavior of some ceramic powders. J Am Ceram Soc 1962; 45: 97–101.
42. Asgharnejad M., Storey D. Application of compaction simulator to the design of a high dose tablet formulation. Part I, Drug Dev Ind Pharm 1966; 22: 967–975.
43. Fell J., Newton J. M. The tensile strength of lactose tablets. J Pharm Sci 1971; 60: 628.
44. Brunauer S., Emmett P., Teller E. Adsorption of gases in multimolecular layers. J Am Chem Soc 1938; 60: 309.
45. Allen T. Particle Size Measurement. 4th ed. London: Chapman & Hill, 1990.
46. Rupp R. Flow and other properties of granulate. Boll Chim Farm 1977; 116: 251.
47. Propst C., Meadows M., Todd M. Crystalline microspheres and the process for manufacturing same. EP 191635192.2 ((June 7, 2019).
48. Yu W., Handcock B. Evaluation of dynamic image analysis for characterizing pharmaceutical excipient particles. Int J Pharm 2008; 361: 150–157.
49. Hickey J., Mansour H., Telko M., Xu Z., Smyth H., Mulder T., Mclean R., Langridge J., Papadopoulos D. Physical characterization of component particles included in dry powder inhalers. I. strategy review and static characteristics. J Pharm Sci 2007; 96: 1282–1301.

50. Ridgeway K., Rupp R. The effect of particle shape on powder properties. J Pharm Pharmacol 1969; 21: 30S.
51. Suryanarayanan R. X-Ray powder diffractometry. In: Brittian H., ed. Physical Characterization of Pharmaceutical Solids. New York: Informa Healthcare, 1995: 187.
52. Airaksinen S., Karjalainen M., Räsänen E., et al. Comparison of the effects of two drying methods on polymorphism of theophylline. Int J Pharm 2004; 276: 129.
53. Morris K. R., Newman A. W., Bugay D. E., et al. Characterization of humidity-dependent changes in crystal properties of a new HMG-CoA reductase inhibitor in support of its dosage form development. Int J Pharm 1994; 108: 195.
54. Aaltonen J., Strachan C. J., Pollanen K., et. al. Hydrate screening of nitrofurantoin using hyphenated NIR/Raman Spectroscopy. J Pharm Biomed Anal 2007; 44: 477–483.
55. Räsänen E., Rantanen J., Jergensen A., et al. Novel identification of pseudopolymorphic changes of theophylline during wet granulation using near-infrared spectroscopy. J Pharm Sci 2001; 90: 389–396.
56. Aaltonen J., Kogermann K., Strachan C. J., et al. Dehydration of theophylline monohydrate during fluid bed drying analyzed with inline NIR and Raman spectroscopy. Chem Eng Sci 2007; 62: 408–415.
57. Kapsidou T., Nikolakkis I., Malamataris S. Agglomeration state and migration of drugs in wet granulations during drying. Int J Pharm 2001; 227(1–2): 97–112.
58. Kiekens F., Zelko R., Remon J. P. Influence of drying temperature and granulation liquid viscosity on the inter- and intragranular drug migration in tray-dried granules and compacts. Pharm Dev Technol 2000; 5(1): 131–137.

22 Bioavailability and Granule Properties

Sunil S. Jambhekar

CONTENTS

22.1 INTRODUCTION

A high percentage of the drugs available in the market are administered via the oral route and via dosage forms like tablet, hard and soft gelatin capsule, suspension, and solution due to either convenience and/or its cost-effectiveness [1–4]. This route, compared to the intravenous as well as any other extravascular routes, is much more complex with respect to the physiological conditions existing at the absorption site. Additionally, the complexity in drug absorption via the oral route arises due to the different environment drug molecules encounter in the gastrointestinal tract as well as the nature of the membrane the drug molecules have to cross before reaching the general circulation. Therefore, the oral bioavailability of a drug becomes a primary focus and an important consideration for drug discovery of new chemical entities. It is well recognized that poor bioavailability and greater variability in bioavailability can result in poor therapeutics response and greater variability in therapeutic response, respectively. This becomes a greater concern for drugs that exhibit a narrow therapeutic range.

The oral bioavailability of a drug is influenced by several properties, including drug dissolution rate, solubility, intestinal permeability, and pre-systemic metabolism. Frequently, the rate-limiting step to drug absorption from the gastrointestinal tract is drug release and drug dissolution from the dosage form. Therapeutic agents with aqueous solubility lower than 100 µg/mL often present dissolution limitations to absorption. Physicochemical, formulation-related, process-related, and physiological factors can all influence drug dissolution.

For many drugs, pharmacological responses and therapeutic effects can be related to observed blood concentrations. This is based, essentially, on the following tenets, which collectively form the foundation for the validity of bioavailability testing. The first tenet is that drug concentration in the blood reflects, or is related to, its concentration at the site of action in any part of the body. The second assumption is that the intensity of the pharmacological activity of a drug is related to its concentration at the site of action. This assumption, however, does not hold true for certain drugs. In this case, a bioavailability study provides direct information only about drug concentration, but not the therapeutic response. Despite these limitations, bioavailability studies have proven to be extremely helpful in assessing the rate and extent of drug absorption and suggesting any modifications of drug formulation that may be required to optimize the product.

Oral bioavailability (F) of a drug is the product of a fraction of drug absorbed (F_a), a fraction of drug escaping intestinal metabolism (F_g), and a fraction of drug escaping liver metabolism (F_h) [5,6].

$$F = F_a \cdot F_g \cdot F_h \qquad (22.1)$$

Therefore, the oral bioavailability of a drug is largely a function of its solubility characteristics in gastrointestinal fluids, absorption into the systemic circulation, and metabolic stability. Oral absorption and the fraction of drug absorbed into the intestine are functions of a drug's solubility and permeability [7].

Historically, the concept of bioavailability from orally administered drugs is closely, if not exclusively, associated with dosage form performance. In particular, poor bioavailability is increasingly an issue in the drug discovery process [6]. In situations where different chemical entities are simultaneously under investigation, dosage form performance is just one of the possible contributing factors to the poor bioavailability. Other possible contributing factors may include diminished access for drug absorption due to chemical degradation, physical inactivation due to binding or complexation, microbial biotransformation, insufficient contact time in transit through the gastrointestinal tract, and poor permeability across the gastrointestinal mucosa. Drug dissolution and drug absorption processes and their consequential effects on bioavailability appear to be interdependent processes, which are influenced by the physicochemical properties of drugs, in particular for hydrophobic drugs.

22.2 DRUG DISSOLUTION

Drug dissolution is a prerequisite for drug absorption, which, in turn, influences the rate and extent at which the administered dose of a drug reaches the general circulation. For many drugs that cross intestinal mucosa easily, the onset of drug levels will be controlled by the time required for the dosage form to release its drug content and then for the drug to dissolve. Dissolution is a process by which a solid substance dissolves. As a fundamental property of a solid, it is controlled by the affinity between the solid and the liquid medium that surrounds it. The proliferation of interest in drug dissolution may be attributed, primarily, to drugs that tend to be very hydrophobic, because the rate-limiting step in the drug absorption process from the gastrointestinal tract is often drug dissolution from the solid dosage form. Approximately 40% of the compounds that enter the development phase fail to reach the market [8]. The main reason for failure is poor biopharmaceutical properties, which include low aqueous solubility, chemical instability, insufficient intestinal absorption, intestinal and/or hepatic metabolism, biliary excretion, and high systemic clearance. Even a highly potent compound can become not developable unless it manifests adequate pharmaceutical properties. For example, to be effective, an orally administered compound must be absorbable across the gastrointestinal mucosa. Consequently, a major challenge confronted by the medicinal chemists is the design of a potential therapeutic agent that exhibits desired physicochemical properties, including intestinal permeability.

Many theories describe the drug dissolution process. The most common theory for drug dissolution is the film theory, also known as the diffusion layer model; it espouses the assumption that the dissolution is determined by the transport process. The Noyes–Whitney [9,10] equation is probably the most frequently employed to describe the drug dissolution process and the physicochemical properties that play a pivotal role in influencing drug dissolution. Accordingly,

$$\frac{dX}{dt} = \text{Rate} = A \cdot \left(\frac{D}{h}\right) \cdot \left(C_s - \frac{X_d}{V}\right) \tag{22.2}$$

where dX/dt is the rate of dissolution, A is the available surface area, D is the diffusion coefficient or diffusivity, h is the thickness of the diffusion or boundary layer adjacent to the dissolving drug surface, C_s is the equilibrium or saturation solubility of the drug, X_d is the amount of the dissolving solid, and V is the volume of the dissolution fluid.

The oral bioavailability of a drug is determined by several properties, including drug dissolution rate, solubility, intestinal permeability, and pre-systemic metabolism. The literature reviews [11,12] reflect the overall importance of these properties in contributing to the success or failure of a potential therapeutic agent in clinical trials. This has provided an impetus for characterizing and estimating these properties in the drug discovery process.

Frequently, the rate-limiting step to drug absorption from the gastrointestinal tract is drug release and drug dissolution from the dosage form. Various drug dissolution models show that drug diffusivity, solubility in the gastrointestinal tract, the surface area of solid wetted by the luminal fluid, and the gastrointestinal fluid hydrodynamics all play critical roles in determining the *in vivo* dissolution rate. Solubility in the gastrointestinal fluid contents is determined by aqueous solubility, crystalline form, drug lipophilicity, solubilization, and pK_a of a drug concerning the gastrointestinal pH profile. Therapeutic agents with aqueous solubilities lower than 100 μg/mL often present dissolution limitations to absorption. Therefore, any factor that influences drug dissolution will likely influence drug absorption and bioavailability. These factors may be broadly classified as physicochemical, formulation-related, and physiological. Generally, any factor that will influence the equilibrium solubility [Eq. 22.2)] of a therapeutic agent will likely influence the dissolution rate and then it may be reflected in the bioavailability. Examples of these factors include particle size, the salt form of a weak acid or base, polymorphism, and complexation.

Recognizing the influential role of drug dissolution along with the permeability of a drug and other physical and chemical properties, Amidon et al. [7,13] proposed the biopharmaceutical classification system (BCS). Today, this classification serves as a guide for regulatory and industrial purposes to anticipate potential bioavailability problems by employing dose number, dissolution number, and absorption number. This is discussed further in the text of the chapter.

The most important property of a dosage form is its ability to deliver the active ingredient to the "site of action" in an amount sufficient to elicit the desired pharmacological response. This property of a dosage form has been variously referred to as its physiologic availability, biological availability, or bioavailability.

Bioavailability may be defined more accurately as the rate and extent of absorption of a drug from its dosage form into the systemic circulation. Accordingly, the absorption of a drug following intravenous administration is extremely rapid and complete. However, due to convenience and stability problems, drugs are often administered orally as a tablet or capsule dosage form. Therefore, their rate and extent of absorption in an individual must be known accurately. Furthermore, equally important is that the factors that influence the rate and extent of absorption of drugs be also known and understood by formulators.

The subject of bioavailability began to receive growing attention as studies showed that the therapeutic effectiveness of a drug from the dosage form depends, to a large extent, on the physiological availability of their active ingredient(s) and is a function of the drug concentration in the patient's blood or plasma. The importance of bioavailability in drug therapy, therefore, stems from the fact that the rate and extent of absorption of a drug from a dosage form can affect the patient's response to a drug. In light of these facts, the determination of bioavailability has become one of the ways to assess the *in vivo* performance of a dosage form following its formulation development. It must, however, be remembered that bioavailability studies, very often, are conducted in normal, fasted, and a small number of subjects, and therefore, the results of these studies may not always reflect the true efficacy relationship in patients under treatment conditions. For many years, it was assumed that if a dosage form contained the labeled amount of a drug, its performance could be taken for granted. However, it is now evident for some time that many factors acting individually or in concert may produce therapeutic failure.

22.3 BIOAVAILABILITY PARAMETERS

In assessing the bioavailability of a drug from a dosage form, three parameters are measured following the administration of a drug through a dosage form and obtaining the drug blood concentration–time profile (Fig. 22.1).

1. Peak concentration, $(C_p)_{max}$
2. Peak time (t_{max}), and
3. The area under the concentration-time curve, $(AUC)_0^{\infty}$

The parameters peak time (t_{max}) and peak concentration $\{(C_p)_{max}\}$ are the measures of the rate of absorption, and the area under the concentration–time curve, $(AUC)_0^{\infty}$, is a measure of the extent of absorption.

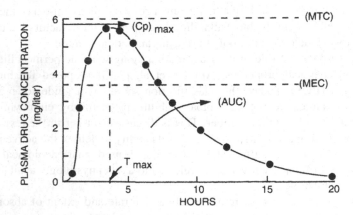

FIGURE 22.1 A graphical representation of plasma/serum drug concentration data following the administration of a drug by extravascular route.

22.3.1 PEAK TIME (T_{MAX})

This parameter represents the length of time required to attain the maximum concentration of drug in the systemic circulation. The parameter describes the onset of the peak level of the biological response and, hence, can be utilized as a measure of the rate of absorption. The faster the rate of absorption, the smaller is the value for the peak time and the quicker is the onset of action of the drug. The peak time is determined by using the following equation [Eq. 22.3]:

$$t_{max} = \frac{\ln(K_a/K)}{(K_a - K)} \tag{22.3}$$

where

K_a and K are the first-order absorption and elimination rate constants, respectively.

Equation 22.3 indicates that the larger the value of the absorption rate constant (K_a), the smaller is the value of peak time (t_{max}) and quicker is likely to be the onset of action.

The elimination rate constant (K) is constant for a drug in normal healthy individuals, and it changes when organs responsible for the elimination of the drug (i.e., kidney and liver) exhibit abnormalities. The absorption rate constant (K_a), on the other hand, depends on the route of administration, the dosage form, and the formulation of a drug. And, for hydrophobic drugs and/or when the absorption and dissolution rate is limited, the faster dissolution is generally reflected in the higher value for the absorption rate constant. Therefore, by changing the formulation of a drug or route of administration, one can alter the peak time and the rate of absorption and time for the onset of action.

22.3.2 PEAK PLASMA CONCENTRATION (C_P)$_{MAX}$

This parameter represents the highest drug concentration in the systemic circulation or the plasma concentration that corresponds to the peak time. Furthermore, this parameter is often associated with the intensity of the pharmacologic response of the drug. Therefore, the peak plasma concentration (Fig. 22.1) of a drug following the administration of a dosage form should be above the minimum effective concentration (MEC) and below the minimum toxic concentration (MTC). The peak plasma concentration can depend upon the absorption rate constant (K_a) and the fraction of the administered dose that eventually reaches the systemic circulation. The higher the absorption rate constant and the fraction that reaches the general circulation, the greater is the peak plasma concentration for the administered dose. The route of administration, the dosage form, and the formulation can, therefore, influence the peak plasma concentration. It is determined by using the following method:

$$(C_p)_{max} = K_a F(X_a)_0/V(K_a - K)(e^{-Kt_{max}} - e^{-Ka t_{max}}) \tag{22.4}$$

where,

F is the fraction of the dose that eventually reaches the systemic circulation, $(X_a)_0$ is the administered dose, V is the apparent volume of distribution of a drug, and t_{max} is the peak time.

Since the term $K_a F(X_a)_0/V (K_a - K)$ in Eq. (22.5) constitutes the intercept of the plasma concentrations against the time profile, Eq. (22.5) can be written as

$$(C_p)_{max} = I(e^{-Kt_{max}} - e^{-Ka t_{max}}) \tag{22.5}$$

Where I represents the intercept (mcg/mL) of the plasma concentrations against the time profile.

22.3.3 Area Under the Plasma Concentration–Time Curve $(AUC)_0^\infty$

This parameter represents the extent of absorption of a drug following the administration of a dosage form. The greater the fraction of the dose that reaches the general circulation, the greater is the extent of the absorption and, hence, $(AUC)_0^\infty$. The term $(AUC)_0^\infty$, expressed as mcg/mL.hr, for a drug following its administration by various extravascular routes or various dosage forms that are administered extravascularly is determined by employing the following equation [Eq. 22.6)]:

$$(AUC)_0^\infty = K_a F(X_a)_0 / V(K_a - K)[1/K - 1/Ka] \tag{22.6}$$

All the terms of Eq. (22.6) have been defined previously.

Equation (22.6) can further be reduced to

$$(AUC)_0^\infty = Intercept[1/K - 1/Ka] \tag{22.7}$$

The intercept in Eq. (22.7) is the intercept of the plasma concentration–time profile following the administration of a single dose of a drug. The extent of absorption can also be determined by using the following equation

$$(AUC)_0^\infty = F(X_a)_0 / VK \tag{22.8}$$

Where the term VK is the systemic clearance of the administered drug. This parameter being independent of the route of administration, the formulation, and the extravascularly administered dosage form, it is ostensible that the extent of absorption {i.e., $(AUC)_0^\infty$} is controlled by the product of the fraction of the administered dose reaching the general circulation and the administered dose [i.e., $F(X_a)_0$].

22.4   FACTORS AFFECTING THE BIOAVAILABILITY

There are several factors responsible for the variation in bioavailability. Broadly speaking, these factors can be classified as patient-related or dosage form related. Patient-related factors include age, disease state, abnormal genetic characteristics, and/or gastrointestinal physiology. The detailed discussion on these factors is beyond the scope of the objectives of this chapter.

Dosage form-related factors include formulation and manufacturing-related variables such as particle size, type and quantity of excipient used, method of manufacturing, compression pressure, derived properties of the powder, and many other factors.

The fact that the bioavailability of a drug may be significantly affected by its physical state and the dosage forms via which it is administered has been unequivocally demonstrated. And, because drugs are administered through dosage forms, these dosage forms should have adequate stability, uniform composition, and complete and consistent bioavailability.

Following the administration of a drug through a solid dosage form, a sequence of steps is required before the drug reaches the systemic circulation. As shown in Figure 22.2, an orally administered solid dosage form undergoes disintegration and deaggregation, followed by the dissolution of the drug. The dissolved drug molecules must penetrate the gastrointestinal membrane and reach the general circulation. Each of the steps involved may limit how fast the drug molecules reach the general circulation and, therefore, the site of action. The step that offers the maximum resistance is referred to as the rate-limiting step. Which step will be rate-limiting, on the other hand, will depend on the physicochemical properties of the dosage form and the physiology of the gastrointestinal tract. The focus of the discussion here, however, will be on the physicochemical properties of the dosage form.

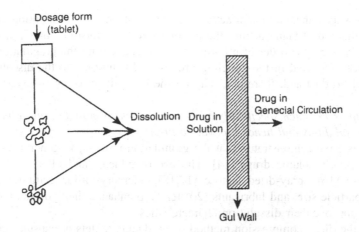

FIGURE 22.2   Schematic representation of the process of the drug dissolution and its entry into the general circulation.

As illustrated in Figure 22.2, the solid dosage form must disintegrate and/or deaggregate before much of the drug is available for absorption. Drug dissolution subsequently occurs from the resulting granules. Therefore, the properties of granules are important in understanding how dissolution is influenced by these properties. Following the ingestion of a solid dosage form, whether or not a drug is deaggregated, it will not be absorbed until it has dissolved into the luminal fluids of the gastrointestinal tract. Because of the effects of disintegration and deaggregation on the dissolution, the remaining discussion will focus on the factors influencing the dissolution of the drug.

22.5   DISSOLUTION AND GRANULE PROPERTIES

Among available dosage forms, compressed tablets are the most widely used dosage form. Tablets are generally prepared by using either wet granulation or direct compression process. The wet granulation process consists of mixing a drug with other powdered material and wetting the mixture with an aqueous and/or hydro-alcoholic solution of a suitable binder such as gelatin, starch, or polyvinylpyrrolidone. The damp mass is passed through the screens of 8 to 12 mesh and dried to produce cohesive granules. Each granule, in theory, is a blend of an active ingredient and excipients. The granules flow easily through the hopper into the tablet press and are easily compressed.

Many derived properties of the powder greatly influence the granule properties, which, in turn, influence the dissolution of an active ingredient from the dosage form. These derived properties include powder density, porosity, specific surface, particle morphology, and powder flow. These derived properties, in essence, are determined by the particle size and size distribution. Consequently, particle size and size distribution play a vital role in influencing the bioavailability of drugs, particularly, when dissolution is the rate-limiting step in the absorption process. The important role these properties play in influencing bioavailability must, therefore, be recognized and taken into consideration during optimization of formulation of a dosage form. For example, a smaller particle size is desirable, if a drug is hydrophobic, to improve the drug dissolution due to increased specific surface; however, too small a particle size may adversely affect the powder flow and content uniformity of a dosage form. Other derived powder properties like true and bulk density and particle size will play an important role in the mixing of powder blends, before the granulation and compression. Powder flow is another derived property of importance. The flow of the powder and/or granules can present difficulties in the manufacturing of a tablet dosage form, which, in turn, can affect the content uniformity of a drug and the bioavailability.

Many processes used in tablet manufacturing greatly influence the dissolution rates of an active ingredient. The method of manufacture, the granule size, the moisture content, age and the flow property of the granules, the order of mixing of ingredients during the granulation as well as the compression force employed in the tableting process, all contribute to the dissolution characteristics of the final product and, therefore, may be the bioavailability of a drug from the finished product.

(Refer to Chapter 17 which specifically addresses the poorly soluble drugs and how to process them to enhance solubility and hence bioavailability.)

Several studies have demonstrated that the granulation process, in general, enhances the dissolution rate of poorly soluble drugs [14]. The use of diluents and fillers such as starch [15], anhydrous lactose [16], spray-dried lactose [17,18], microcrystalline cellulose [19], and compression force, particle size, and lubricants [20] tends to enhance the hydrophilicity of the active ingredients and improve their dissolution characteristics.

Even though the direct compression method of producing tablets or capsules could give better dissolution results, the bioavailability which is dependent on the uniformity of a dosage form may not always be acceptable. However, newer tableting machines and excipients accompanied by careful formulation and proper mixing sequence will permit the preparation of tablets with good dissolution characteristics.

Marlow and Shangraw [21] reported that sodium salicylate tablets prepared by direct compression with spray-dried lactose uniformly exhibited more rapid and complete dissolution compared to those prepared by wet granulation. Furthermore, it was reported that the presence of disintegrant in the dry compression was essential for good dissolution. Finholt et al. [22] reported, in a separate comparative study utilizing phenobarbital tablets that were manufactured by both wet and dry granulation, that both procedures yielded comparable dissolution rates provided a disintegrate was incorporated and mixed with the drug before dry granulation. However, the incorporation of disintegrant following the dry granulation of a drug resulted in slower dissolution rates.

In the manufacturing of tablets by the conventional wet granulation method, many independent factors affect the granule properties and, therefore, the dissolution rate. Recent advances in granulation technology and the employment of high-shear mixers and fluid-bed granulating equipment have helped to identify several critical in-process variables, and the systematic control of variables such as the type and time of mixing of the granules, time and temperature of drying, blending time with lubricant, age of the granules, moisture content of the granules at the time of compression, and the tablet crushing strength is of importance to ensure the consistency in the dissolution and, hence, bioavailability.

In early studies on the physics of tablet compression, Higuchi et al. [23] recognized the influence of compressional forces employed in the tableting process on the apparent density, porosity, hardness, disintegration time, and average particle size of the compressed tablets. Hardness is a measure of the resistance of a dosage form to the mechanical deforming. It is a function of high compression force use in manufacturing, and it may change with the aging of granules. Higuchi et al. [23] reported a linear relationship between hardness and the logarithm of the compressional force, and the specific surface of the compressed tablets was found to undergo marked changes during the compressional process. The high compression may increase the specific surface and, hence, may enhance the dissolution. On the other hand, the high compression may also inhibit the wettability of a tablet due to the formation of a firmer and more effective sealing layer of the lubricant due to high pressure and temperature that accompany a strong compressional force. Levy et al. [15] reported that salicylic acid tablets, when prepared by a double compression, showed an increase in the dissolution with an increase in the pre-compression pressure due to fracturing of drug particles at higher pressure. The higher compression may also produce slower dissolution, at least in the initial period, due to an increased difficulty of fluid penetration into the compressed tablets. Luzzi et al. [24] and Jalsenjak et al. [25] observed the dissolution rate of sodium phenobarbital to be inversely proportional to the hardness from tablet and microcapsule, respectively.

Another important granule property that influences the dissolution of drugs is the moisture content of the granule at the time of compression. Chowhan et al. [26–30] studied the effect of moisture content and crushing strength on ticlopidine hydrochloride tablet's friability and dissolution. It was observed [29] that at the moisture content of 1 to 2%, the drug dissolution was inversely related to the tablet crushing strength. However, at the moisture content level of 3 to 4%, there was no clear relationship between the dissolution and the crushing strength.

In later studies by Chowhan et al. [27,30], it was reported that granules prepared by high-speed shear mixer were less porous than those prepared by planetary mixer, and the porosity of the tablet may improve the dissolution of the drug by facilitating solvent penetration provided the entrapment of air in the pores is minimized or avoided.

In yet another important study, Levy et al. [15] studied the effect of the granule size on the dissolution rate of salicylic acid tablets and found that the dissolution rate increased with a decrease in the granule size; the increase in dissolution rate, however, was not proportional to the increase in the apparent surface area of the granules. Furthermore, it was also reported that the dissolution rate decreased significantly with the increase in the age of the granules.

The chemical components of the formulation have also been shown to prolong disintegration time, which subsequently affects the drug dissolution and bioavailability. Inert fillers have been found to potentiate the chemical degradation of active ingredients causing an alteration in the disintegration and dissolution time of compressed tablets to change with storage. Alam and Parrott [31] have shown that hydrochlorothiazide tablets, granulated with acacia and stored at temperatures ranging from room temperature to 80 °C, increased in hardness with time. This was reflected in increased disintegration and dissolution time. On the other hand, tablets granulated with starch and polyvinylpyrrolidone did not show any change in disintegration and dissolution time.

(*Chapter 21 provides more comprehensive information on granulation characterization.*)

22.6   *IN VITRO–IN VIVO* CORRELATION

A key goal in the pharmaceutical development of dosage forms is a good understanding of the *in vitro* and *in vivo* performance of the dosage forms. One of the challenges of biopharmaceutics research is correlating *in vitro* drug release information of various drug formulations to the *in vivo* drug profiles (IVIVC). Such a tool shortens the drug development period, economizes the resources, and leads to improved quality. This is because the IVIVC includes *in vivo* relevance to *in vitro* dissolution specifications. It can also assist in quality control for certain Scale-up and Post-Approval Changes (SUPAC). This section of the chapter discusses the FDA guidance, various definitions of *in vitro–in vivo* correlations, various levels of correlations, and the use of such information in oral dosage forms, as biopharmaceutics classification systems (BCS).

The concept and application of the *in vitro–in vivo* correlation for pharmaceutical dosage forms have been a focus of the attention of the pharmaceutical industry, academia, and regulatory sectors. The optimization process may require alteration in formulation composition, manufacturing process, equipment, and batch sizes. Implementation of these requirements not only halts the marketing of the new formulation but also increases the cost of the optimization processes. Regulatory guidance for both immediate and modified-release dosage forms has, therefore, been developed by the FDA to minimize the need for bioavailability studies as part of the formulation design and optimization for generic drugs.

IVIVC can be used in the development of new pharmaceuticals to reduce the number of human studies during formulation development. It is to serve as a surrogate for *in vivo* bioavailability and to support biowaivers. They could also be employed to establish dissolution specifications and to support and/or validate the use of dissolution methods.

22.6.1 DEFINITIONS

Correlation is frequently employed within the pharmaceutical and related sciences to describe the relationship that exists between variables. Mathematically, the term correlation means interdependence between quantitative and qualitative data or the relationship between measurable variables and ranks. Two definitions of IVIVC have been proposed by the USP and by the FDA [32,33].

United States Pharmacopoeia (USP) definition

"The establishment of a rational relationship between a biological property, or a parameter derived from a biological property produced by a dosage form, and a physiochemical property or characteristic of the same dosage form [32]."

Food and Drug Administration (FDA) definition

"IVIVC is a predictive mathematical model describing the relationship between an in vitro property of a dosage form and a relevant in vivo response. Generally, the in vitro property is the rate or extent of drug dissolution or release while the in vivo response is the plasma drug concentration or amount of drug absorbed [33]."

22.6.2 CORRELATION LEVELS

Five correlation levels have been defined in the IVIVC FDA guidance [33]. The concept of correlation level is based upon the ability of the correlation to reflect the complete plasma drug level–time profile which will result from the administration of the given dosage form [32].

22.6.3 LEVEL A CORRELATION

This level of correlation is the highest category of correlation and represents a point-to-point relationship between *in vitro* dissolution rate and *in vivo* input rate of the drug from the dosage form [32]. Generally, the percent of drug absorbed may be calculated employing model-dependent techniques such as Wagner–Nelson procedure or Loo–Riegelman method or by model-independent numerical deconvolution [32]. These techniques represent a major advance over the single-point approach in that these methodologies utilize all of the dissolution and plasma level data available to develop the correlations [32].

The purpose of Level A correlation is to define a direct relationship between *in vivo* data such that measurement of *in vitro* dissolution rate alone is sufficient to determine the biopharmaceutical rate of the dosage form. An *in vitro* dissolution curve can serve as a surrogate for *in vivo* performance. Therefore, a change in manufacturing site, method of manufacture, raw material supplies, minor formulation modification, and even product strength using the same formulation can be justified without the need for additional human studies [32]. It is an excellent quality control procedure since it is predictive of the *in vivo* performance of a dosage form.

22.6.4 LEVEL B CORRELATION

A level B IVIVC utilizes the principles of statistical moment analysis. In this level of correlation, the mean *in vitro* dissolution time (MDT_{vitro}) of the product is compared to either *in vivo* mean residence time (MRT) or the *in vivo* mean dissolution time (MDT_{vivo}). MRT, MDT_{vitro}, and MDT_{vivo} will be defined where appropriate. Although a level B correlation uses all of the *in vitro* and *in vivo* data, it is not considered to be a point-to-point correlation, since there are many different *in vivo* curves that will produce similar mean residence time values [33]. A level B correlation does not uniquely reflect the actual *in vivo* plasma level curves. Therefore, one cannot rely upon a level B correlation alone to justify formulation modification, manufacturing site change, excipient source change, etc. In addition, *in vitro* data from such a correlation could not be used to justify the extremes of quality control standards [32].

22.6.5   LEVEL C CORRELATION

In this level of correlation, one dissolution time point ($t_{50\%}$, $t_{90\%}$, etc.) is compared to one mean pharmacokinetic parameter such as $(AUC)_0^\infty$, t_{max}, or C_{max}. Therefore, it represents a single point correlation and does not reflect the entire shape of the plasma drug concentration versus the time curve, which is a crucial factor that is a good indicator of the performance of modified-release products [32,33]. This is the weakest level of correlation as a partial relationship between absorption and dissolution is established. The usefulness of this correlation level is subject to the same caveats as a level B correlation in its ability to support product and site changes as well as justification of quality control standard extremes [32]. Level C correlations can be useful in the early stages of formulation development when pilot formulations are being selected. While the information may be useful in formulation development, the waiver of an *in vivo* bioequivalence study (biowaivers) is generally not possible [33].

22.6.5.1   Multiple Level C Correlation

A multiple level C correlation relates one or several pharmacokinetic parameters of interest $\{(C_{max}, (AUC)_0^\infty\}$ or any other suitable parameters to the amount of drug dissolved at several time points of the dissolution profile. A multiple point level C correlation may be used to justify a biowaiver, provided the correlation has been established over the entire dissolution profile with one or more pharmacokinetic parameters of interest. A relationship should be demonstrated at each time point at the same parameter such that the effect on the *in vivo* performance of any change in dissolution can be assessed [33].

22.6.6   LEVEL D CORRELATION

Level D correlation is a rank order and qualitative analysis and is not considered useful for regulatory purposes. It is not a formal correlation but serves as an aid in the development of a formulation or processing procedure [33,34].

22.6.7   SYSTEMATIC DEVELOPMENT OF A CORRELATION

An assumed IVIVR is essentially one that provides the initial guidance and direction for the early formulation development activity. This work sometimes results in revised *in vitro* targets and reformulation strategy and the same cycle of activity again.

22.6.7.1   Important Considerations in Developing a Correlation

When the dissolution is not influenced by factors such as pH, surfactants, osmotic pressure, mixing intensity, enzyme, and ionic strength, a set of dissolution data obtained from one formulation is correlated with a deconvoluted plasma concentration–time data set [33]. To demonstrate a correlation, fraction absorbed *in vivo* should be plotted against the fraction released *in vitro*. If this relationship becomes linear with a slope of 1, then curves are superimposable, and there is a 1:1 relationship which is defined as point-to-point or level A correlation. The correlation is considered general and could be extrapolated within a reasonable range for that formulation of the active drug entity.

   In a linear correlation, the *in vitro* dissolution and *in vivo* input curves may be directly superimposable or may be made to be superimposable by the use of appropriate scaling factor (time corrections) [32,33]. The time scaling factor should be the same for all formulations, and different time scales for each formulation indicate the absence of an IVIVC [33]. Non-linear correlation may also be appropriate [32,33].

In cases where the dissolution rate depends on the experimental factors mentioned above the deconvoluted plasma, concentration–time curves constructed following administration of batches of product with different dissolution rates (at least two formulations having significantly different behavior) are correlated with dissolution data obtained under the same dissolution condition. If there is no one-to-one correlation, other levels of correlation could be evaluated [32,33].

The in vitro dissolution methodology should be able to adequately discriminate between the study formulations. Once a system with the most suitable discrimination is developed, dissolution conditions should be the same for all formulations tested in the biostudy for the development of the correlation [33].

During the early stages of correlation development, dissolution conditions may be altered to attempt to develop a one-to-one correlation between the *in vitro* dissolution profile and the *in vivo* dissolution profile [33].

An established correlation is valid only for a specific type of pharmaceutical dosage form (tablets, gelatin capsules, etc.) with a particular release mechanism (matrix, osmotic system, etc.) and particular main excipients and additives. The correlation is true and predictive only if modifications of this dosage form remain within certain limits, consistent with the release mechanism and excipients involved in it [33].

Drugs are often taken just before, with, or after a meal. All of these factors may increase variability. A posterior correlation might be established using the patients' data only to increase the knowledge of the drug.

The release rates, as measured by percent dissolved, for each formulation studied, should differ adequately (e.g., by 10%). This should result in *in vivo* profiles that show a comparable difference, for example, a 10% difference in the pharmacokinetic parameters of interest $(C_p)_{max}$ or $(AUC)_0^{\infty}$ between each formulation [33].

22.7 BIOPHARMACEUTICS CLASSIFICATION SYSTEM (BCS)

The Biopharmaceutics Classification System (BCS) is a drug development tool that allows estimation of the contribution of three fundamental factors including dissolution, solubility, and intestinal permeability, which govern the rate and extent of drug absorption from solid oral dosage forms [13]. Permeability is referred to as the ability of the drug molecule to permeate through a membrane into the systemic circulation.

22.7.1 ABSORPTION NUMBER (A_N)

The Absorption Number (A_n) is the ratio of the Mean Residence Time (T_{res}) to the Mean Absorption Time (T_{abs}) and is calculated by using Eq. (22.9).

$$A_n = T_{res}/T_{abs} = (\Pi R_2\, L/Q)/R/P_{eff}) \tag{22.9}$$

22.7.2 DISSOLUTION NUMBER (D_N)

The Dissolution Number (D_n) is the ratio of Mean Residence Time (T_{res}) to Mean Dissolution Time (T_{diss}) and can be estimated by using Eq. (22.10).

$$D_n = T_{res}/T_{diss} = (\Pi R^2 L/Q)/\left(pr_o^2 /3DC_s^{min} \right) \tag{22.10}$$

22.7.3 DOSE NUMBER (D_o)

$$D_o = Dose/(V_o \times C_s^{min}) \qquad (22.11)$$

Where L = tube length, R = tube radius, $_{\Pi}$ = 3.14, Q = fluid flow rate, r_o = initial particle radius, D = particle acceleration, p = particle density, P_{eff} = effective permeability, V_0 is the initial gastric volume equal to 250 mL which is derived from typical bioequivalence study protocols that prescribe administration of a drug product to fasting human volunteers with a glass of water at the time of drug administration, and C_s^{min} is minimum aqueous solubility in the physiological pH range of 1–8 [13].

The dose, dose number, solubility, and estimated dissolution number for several drugs are reported [13] in the literature. The fraction dose absorbed could be estimated using these three major dimensionless parameters. However, the extent of solubilization and potential particle aggregation in the small intestine is unknown, and therefore the solubility dose and dissolution number of a drug *in vivo* are difficult to estimate precisely [13]. As drug dissolution and intestinal permeability are the fundamental parameters governing rate and extent of drug absorption, drugs could be categorized into high/low solubility and permeability classes.

Class I compounds such as metoprolol exhibit a high absorption (A_n) and a high Dissolution (D_n) number. The rate-limiting step to drug absorption is drug dissolution or gastric emptying rate if dissolution is very rapid [13]. This group of drugs is expected to be well absorbed unless they are unstable, form insoluble complexes, are secreted directly from the gut wall, or undergo first-pass metabolism [35]. For immediate-release products that release their content very rapidly, the absorption rate will be controlled by the gastric emptying rate, and no correlation of *in vivo* data with dissolution rate is expected [13].

When a class I drug is formulated as an extended-release product in which the release profile controls the rate of absorption and the solubility and permeability of the drug is site-independent, a level A correlation is most likely.

Class II drugs such as phenytoin have a high absorption number (A_n) but a low dissolution number (D_n). *In vivo* drug dissolution for Class II drugs is, therefore, a rate-limiting factor in drug absorption (except at very high dose number, D_o), and consequently, absorption is usually slower than Class I and takes place over a longer period of time [13]. The limitation can be *equilibrium* or *kinetic* in nature. In the case of an *equilibrium* problem, enough fluid is not available in the GI tract to dissolve the dose.

Class III drugs, such as cimetidine, are rapidly dissolving, and permeability is the rate-controlling step in drug absorption. Rapid dissolution is particularly desirable to maximize the contact time between the dissolved drug and absorption mucosa.

Class IV drugs are low-solubility and low-permeability drugs. This class of drugs exhibits significant problems for effective oral delivery. It is anticipated that inappropriate formulation of drugs falling in class IV, as in the case of class II drugs, could have an additional negative influence on both the rate and extent of drug absorption.

22.8 SUMMARY

Developing dependable and reproducible drug delivery via oral administration is probably the ultimate goal in the industry. Therefore, the design and formulation of such dosage forms will take into consideration many physiochemical, biopharmaceutical, and physiological factors. While solubility and permeability are fundamental parameters that determine and influence oral absorption, other factors like lipophilicity, hydrogen bonding, and a number of rotatable bonds also play a critical role in the transport of drug molecules across the biological membrane.

Drug availability to produce an effect, following the oral dosing, may be thought of as the result of the following steps:

1. Getting the drug from the dosage form into solution (dissolution)
2. Moving the drug molecules through the membrane of the gastrointestinal tract, and
3. Moving the drug away from the site of administration into the general circulation (absorption).

It is clear from the discussion that the bioavailability of drugs, particularly poorly soluble drugs, mainly depends on the ability of the drug to dissolve from the dosage form at the site of administration. Dissolution, in turn, especially from solid dosage forms such as tablets and capsules depends on several physicochemical properties of a therapeutic agent, granule properties, and the processing variables used in the manufacture of the dosage forms. The granule properties and other variables, which determine and influence the granule properties, will serve as major topics of discussion in subsequent chapters. Knowledge of the physicochemical properties such as particle size and size distribution, dissociation constant, equilibrium solubility, partition coefficient, dissolution rate, and specific permeability should be utilized as a guide for the potential bioavailability problems in the formulation of an optimum solid dosage form. These factors and their role in influencing the bioavailability of a drug, therefore, will allow the formulators to develop an optimum dosage form by selecting the process and preparation variables involved rationally.

REFERENCES

1. Lipinsky, C. A. Computational alerts for potential absorption problems: profiles of clinically tested drugs. Tools for oral absorption. Part II. Predicting human absorption. AAPS Meeting, Miami, FL, 1995.
2. Lipinsky, C. A. Drug-like properties and the causes of poor solubility and poor permeability. J. Pharmacol. Tox. Methods, 44 (1), 235–249, 2000.
3. Lipinsky, C. A., Lombardo, F., Dominy, B. W., and Feeney, P. J. Experimental and computational approaches to estimate solubility and permeability in drug discovery and development setting. Adv. Drug Deliv. Rev., 46 (1–3), 3–26, 2001.
4. Lipinsky, C. A. Solubility in water and DMSO: Issues and potential solutions. Pharmaceutical Profiling in Drug Discovery for Lead Selection AAPS, Washington DC, 2004.
5. Sun, D., Yu, L. X., Hussain, M. A., Wall, D. A., Smith, R. L., and Amidon, G. L. In-vitro testing of drug absorption for drug 'developability' assessment: forming an interface between in vitro preclinical data and clinical outcome. Curr. Opin. Drug Discovery Dev. 7, 75–85, 2004.
6. Kwan, K. C. Oral bioavailability and first pass effects. Drug Metab. Dispos., 25, 1329–1336, 1997.
7. Amidon, G. L., Sinko, P. J., and Fleisher, D. Estimating human oral fraction dose absorbed: a correlation using rat intestinal membrane permeability for passive and carrier- mediated compounds. Pharm. Res., 5, 651–654, 1988.
8. Brennan, M. B. Drug discovery: filtering out failures early in the game. Chem. & Eng. News, June 5, 63, 2000.
9. Noyes, A., and Whitney, W. J. The rate of solution of solid substances in their own solution. J. Am. Chem. Soc. 19, 930–934, 1897.
10. Noyes, A., and Whitney, W. J. Ueber Die Auslosungsgesch Wingdigkeit Von Festen Stossen In Ihern Eigenen Losungen. Z. Physik. Chem. 23, 689–692, 1897.
11. Caldwell, G. W. Compound optimization in early and late phase drug discovery: acceptable pharmacokinetics properties utilizing combined physicochemical, in-vitro and in vivo screens. Curr. Opin. Drug. Dis. Develop., 3, 30–41, 2000.
12. Venkatesh, S., and Lipper, R. A. Role of the development scientist in compound lead selection and optimization. J. Pharm. Sci. 89, 145–154, 2000.
13. Amidon, G. L., Lennernas, H., Shah, V. P., and Crison, J. R. A theoretical basis for a biopharmaceutics drug classification. The correlation of in vitro drug product classification and in vivo bioavailability. Pharm. Res., 12 (3), 413–419, 1995.

14. Solvang, S., and Finholt, P. Effect of tablet processing and formulation factors on dissolution rates of active ingredient in human gastric juice. J. Pharm. Sci., 59, 49–52, 1970.
15. Levy, G., Antkowiak, J., Procknal, J., and White, D. Effect of certain tablet formulation factors on dissolution rate of the active ingredient II: granule size, starch concentration, and compression pressure. J. Pharm. Sci., 52, 1047–1051, 1963.
16. Batuyios, N. Anhydrous lactose in direct tablet compression. J. Pharm. Sci., 55, 727–730, 1966.
17. Gunsel, W., and Lachman, L. Comparative evaluation of tablet formulations prepared by conventionally processed and spray dried lactose. J. Pharm. Sci., 52, 178–182, 1963.
18. Duvall, R., Koshy, K., and Dashiell, R. Comparative evaluation of dextrose and spray dried lactose in direct compression systems. J. Pharm. Sci., 54, 1196–1200, 1965.
19. Reier, G., and Shangraw, R. Microcrystalline cellulose in tableting. J. Pharm. Sci., 55, 510–514, 1966.
20. Iranloye, T., and Parrott, E. Compression force, particle size, and lubricants on dissolution rates. J. Pharm. Sci., 67, 535–539, 1978.
21. Marlow, E., and Shangraw, R. Dissolution of sodium salicylate from tablet matrices prepared by wet granulation and direct compression. J. Pharm. Sci., 56, 498–504, 1967.
22. Finholt, P., Pedersen, P., Solvang, R., and Wold, K. Effect of different factors on dissolution rate of drugs from powders, Granules and tablets II. Medd. Norsk Farm Selsk., 28, 238, 1966.
23. Higuchi, T., Rao, A., Busse, E., and Swintosky, J. The physics of tablet compression II: The influence of degree of compression on properties of tablets. Am. Pharm. Assoc., Sci. Ed., 42, 194–200, 1953.
24. Luzzi, L., Zoglio, M., and Maulding, H. Preparation and evaluation of the prolonged release properties of nylon microcapsules J. Pharm. Sci., 59, 338–341, 1970.
25. Jalsenjak, I., Nicolaidou, C., and Nixon, J. Dissolution from tablets prepared using ethycellulose microspheres J. Pharm. Pharmacol., 29, 169–172, 1977.
26. Chowhan, Z. T., and Palagyi, L. Hardness increase induced by partial moisture loss in compressed tablets and its effect on in vitro dissolution. J. Pharm. Sci., 67, 1385–1389, 1978.
27. Chowhan, Z. T. Moisture, hardness, disintegration and dissolution interrelationships in compressed tablets prepared by the wet granulation process. Drug Develop. Ind. Pharm., 5 (1), 41–62, 1979.
28. Chowhan, Z. T. Role of binders in moisture-induced hardness increase in compressed tablets and its effect on in vitro disintegration and dissolution. J. Pharm. Sci., 69, 1–4, 1980.
29. Chowhan, Z., Yang, I., Amaro, A., and Chi, L. Effect of moisture and crushing strength on tablet friability and in vitro dissolution. J. Pharm. Sci., 71, 1371–1375, 1982.
30. Chowhan, Z., and Chatterjee, B. A method for establishing in process variable controls for optimizing tablet friability and in vitro dissolution. Int. J. Pharm. Technol. Prod. Mfg., 5 (2), 6–12, 1984.
31. Alam, A. S., and Parrott, E. L. Effect of aging on some physical properties of hydrochlorothiazide tablets. J. Pharm. Sci., 60, 263–266, 1971.
32. United States Pharmacopoeia. In Vitro and In Evaluation of Dosage Forms. 27th edition. Mack Publishing Company, Easton, PA, 2004.
33. FDA, CDER. Guidance for industry, extended release oral dosage form: development, evaluation, and application of In Vitro-In Vivo correlations. FDA, CDER, 1997.
34. Sirisuth, N., and Eddington, N. D. In vitro-in vivo correlations, systemic methods for the development and validation of an IVIVC metoprolol and naproxen drug examples Int. J. Generic Drugs., 3, 250–258, 2002.
35. Dressman, J. B., Amidon, G. L., Reppas, C., and Shah, V. P. Dissolution testing as a prognostics tool for oral drug absorption: immediate release dosage forms. Pharm. Res., 12 (3), 413–419, 1998.

RECOMMENDED READING

1. Abdou, H. M. Dissolution, Bioavailability and Bioequivalence. Mack Publishing Company, Easton, PA, 1989.
2. Blanchard, J., Sawchuk, R., and Brodie, B. (Eds.) Principles and Perspectives in Drug Bioavailability. S. Krager AG, Basel, Switzerland, 1979.
3. Gibaldi, M. Biopharmaceutics and Clinical Pharmacokinetics. 4th Ed., Lea and Febiger, Philadelphia, PA, 1991.
4. Jambhekar, S. Micromeritics and Rheology, A Chapter in Theory and Practice of Contemporary Pharmaceutics. Ghosh T. K. and Jasti B. R. (Eds.), CRC Publication, Boca Raton, FL, 2005.
5. Leeson, L. J., and Carstensen, J. (Eds.) Dissolution Technology Academy of Pharmaceutical Sciences. APhA Publication, Washington DC, 1974.

6. Stavchansky, S. A., and McGinity, J. W. Bioavailability in Tablet Technology, A Chapter in Pharmaceutical Dosage Forms: Tablets. Lieberman, H. A., Lachman, L. and Schwartz, J. B. (Eds.). Volume 2. 2nd Ed., Marcel Dekker, Inc., New York, NY, 1990.

7. Emani, J. In vitro-in vivo correlations: from theory to applications. J. Pharm. Pharmaceut. Sci., 9 (2), 169–189, 2006.

8. Cardot, J. E., Beyssac, E., and Alric, M. In vitro-in vivo correlation: importance of dissolution in IVIVC. Dissolut. Technol., 15–19, 2007.

9. Galia, E., Nicolaides, E., Horter, D., Lotenberg, R., Reppas, C., and Dressman, J. Evaluation of various dissolution media for predicting in vivo performance of class I and class II drugs. Pharm. Res., 15 (5), 698–705, 1998.

10. Young, D., Devane, J. G., and Butler, J. (Eds.) In Vitro-In Vivo Correlations, Plenum Press, New York, NY, 1997.

11. Leeson, L. J. In vitro-in vivo correlations. Drug Inf. J., 29, 903–915, 1995.

12. Jung, H., Milan, R. C., Girard, M. E., Leon, F., and Montoya, M. A. Bioequivalence study of carbamazepine tablets: in vitro-in vivo correlations. Int. J. Pharm., 152, 37–44, 1997.

13. Rekhi, G. S., and Jambhekar, S. Bioavailability and in vitro/in vivo correlation for propranolol hydrochloride extended release bead products prepared using aqueous polymeric dispersions. J. Pharm. Pharmacol., 48, 1276–1284, 1996.

14. Jambhekar, S. Equilibrium Processes in Pharmaceutics, A Chapter in Pharmaceutics: Basic Principles and Application to Pharmacy Practice. Dash, A., Singh, S., and Tolman, J. (Eds.), Academic Press, Boston, USA, 2014.

15. Jambhekar, S., Physiochemical and Biopharmaceutical Properties of Drug Substances and Pharmacokinetics, A Chapter in Foye's Principles of Medicinal Chemistry. Lemke, T. L., and Williams, D. A. (Eds.). 7th Ed., Lippincott, Williams and Wilkins, Wolters Kluwer Health Company, Philadelphia, USA, 2012.

16. Jambhekar, S., and Breen, P. Drug dissolution: significance of physicochemical properties and physiological conditions. Drug Discov. Today, 18 (23/24), 1173–1184, 2013.

23 Granulation Process Modeling

Ian T. Cameron and Fu Y. Wang

CONTENTS

23.1 MODELING OF GRANULATION SYSTEMS

In this section, we introduce the background to granulation modeling by asking the questions, "Why model?" and "How can models be used in granulation systems applications?" The following sections seek to answer these questions and demonstrate the benefits that can flow from appropriate granulation process modeling.

23.1.1 MOTIVATION FOR MODELING

There are many motivations for modeling granulation systems that are common to all process-related issues. Process modeling is an area that has grown enormously over the last 50 years. Michaels [1] has pointed out that despite the change of particle technology from an underfunded and widely scattered research enterprise to a thriving globally recognized engineering discipline over the past 30 years, design and analysis of industrial particulate processes often remain rooted in empiricism. Without exception, granulation processes, like many solids handling operations, continue to be one of the least understood and hence inefficient operations in the process industries. Thus, granulation remained more of "an art than a science" until almost 20 years ago, as stated by Litster [2]. Granulation operations were performed by employing popular practice rather than through systematic scientifically-based strategies. The ineffectiveness of this approach led researchers into a quest to represent the dynamic or steady-state (SS) characteristics of systems through a deeper understanding of the relevant phenomena of the physicochemical mechanisms being studied. Granulation systems have benefited through a growing interest in the building of various models and their deployment to address a range of applications.

23.1.1.1   Benefits

The benefits from the use of modeling include:

- An increased understanding of the governing mechanisms through endeavoring to represent them in the model description.
- An increased understanding of the relative importance of mechanistic contributions to the outputs of the process.
- Capturing of insight and knowledge in a mathematically usable form.
- Documentation of research findings in accessible form for various applications.
- Application of models for improved control performance and process diagnosis.
- Potential reuse of model components for a variety of applications from design through to process diagnosis.
- As a vehicle for new, novel designs of processing equipment.
- As a means to direct further experimentation and process data generation.

23.1.1.2   Costs

There are several important and not insubstantial costs involved in process modeling, including:

- The time to plan, develop, test, and deploy models.
- Personnel with the requisite discipline background to generate effective models through insight and modeling skills.
- The effort in laboratory scale or plant scale trials to elucidate process behavior and the cost of doing so.
- The cost of poor modeling practice in terms of inadequate documentation through the modeling phases and loss of corporate memory.

23.1.2   PROCESS MODELING FUNDAMENTALS

Process modeling is purpose driven in that a model is developed for a particular application area. These application areas could include the following:

- Improved control performance through the use of process model-based control algorithms.
- Optimal performance of granulation systems through model-based optimization of production parameters such as shortest batch time or optimal product size distribution (PSD).
- Improved production scheduling using models to generate improved batch times estimates.
- Plant diagnosis for real-time plant operator guidance systems (OGS).
- Extraction of parameter estimates such as rate constants and granulation kernel parameters.
- Improved design of equipment or development of new designs based on better understanding and use of mechanistic phenomena.

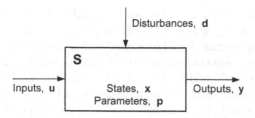

FIGURE 23.1 Schematic of a basic process system.

The resultant model must be "fit-for-purpose", and this is achieved by having clearly stated goals for the modeling that are used to help assess the appropriateness of the model form and the model fidelity required for the job. In particular, modeling requires a methodology that is generic in nature.

23.1.2.1 A Systems Perspective

Models need to be built on a systems engineering understanding of the process. A typical system schematic is seen in Figure 23.1. For the system (S), we need to clearly define the vectors of inputs (u) and disturbances (d) to our system as well as the outputs (y) and the states of interest (x). All these are multivariate functions of time t. Associated with the system are parameters ($\mathbf{p}$) that can be related to geometric aspects of the equipment design, kinetic parameters, growth and breakage constants, binder volume fraction, or heat transfer coefficients. Many parameters exist within the system.

The system S converts inputs and disturbances to outputs and is expressed as:

$$\mathbf{y} = S\,[\mathbf{u},\ \mathbf{d}] \tag{23.1}$$

In a similar manner, a model M is a representation of the system that transforms inputs to predicted outputs $\mathbf{y}^{(M)}$ in the form:

$$\mathbf{y}^{(M)} = M\,[\mathbf{u},\ \mathbf{d}] \tag{23.2}$$

How close y and $\mathbf{y}^{(M)}$ are is a key question in model validation.

Approaching modeling from a systems perspective provides a clear framework for developing models and identifying the key issues to be considered. The four principal classes of variables play particular roles in the modeling.

Inputs. The inputs u are the variables that are manipulated to "drive" the system or maintain its condition in the face of changes from disturbances. Typically, we consider such aspects as binder addition rate or mixing intensity as inputs that we can manipulate.

Disturbances. Disturbances d are variables over which we do not have clear control. They arise from raw material properties that might change from batch to batch. They could be environmental factors such as ambient temperature and humidity. They might be fluctuations in input voltage to motors or steam pressure that produce temperature disturbances in heated systems. Principal disturbances in all relevant categories need to be identified.

Outputs. The outputs y are the variables of interest for the designer, operator, or manager. They might be quality variables that are related to granule properties such as size distribution, granule moisture, or granule hardness. Other outputs of interest could be related to product temperature, flow rates, and composition. The outputs are necessarily measurable in some way, either directly online such as particle size distribution (PSD) and moisture, or via laboratory analysis such as composition.

States. The states x of the system are the internal variables that characterize the system behavior at any point in time.

Finally, the system S is a major consideration in modeling because of the variety of ways the real system can be represented by the model M of that system. Numerous forms of the model M are available. They can have a structure based on capturing fundamental phenomena from the physics and chemistry ("white box" models) to internal representations based on purely empirical approaches known as "black box" models. For black box models, the form is simply a convenient equation that captures the relationships among inputs, disturbances, and outputs. In reality, most models are "gray" in nature, being a combination of fundamental phenomena combined with empirical relationships.

23.1.2.2 Modeling Methodology and Workflow

Modeling should not be a haphazard activity. It is essential that a consistent and defensible methodology be adopted. One such methodology is given by Hangos and Cameron [3], and an update is seen in Figure 23.2. Each of the eight key steps is a vital part of any modeling activity, emphasizing that modern process modeling is not simply generating a set of equations, as it is a much more holistic activity. Documentation and model maintenance are also absolutely crucial. Modeling is iterative in nature as seen from Figure 23.2.

The key aspects can be summarized as follows:

- *Goal-set definition:* making clear the reasons for the modeling and the goals to be addressed in the modeling.
- *Model conceptualization:* clarifying the conserved quantities and the governing mechanisms to be included; clearly setting out the assumptions underlying the model.
- *Modeling data:* generating or referencing physical property data or plant data relevant to model building and model validation. Often more data is required for validation and calibration purposes.
- *Model building and analysis:* putting the model together and then analyzing the model for properties relevant to solution and dynamic properties.
- *Model solution:* solving the model numerically or in some limited circumstances analytically, which can be challenging.
- *Model verification:* the task of ensuring that the coded model in the simulation environment is correctly represented and bug-free.
- *Model calibration and validation:* performing parameter estimation and then validating the model against plant or laboratory data.
- *Model acceptance and deployment:* this is the actual use of the model in terms of control, optimization, or diagnosis. Many application areas exist.

A special mention is needed for an extensive documentation of the model. Without this, the maintenance of the model over a significant part of the life cycle becomes a major challenge and often leads to unnecessary rework and in some cases major financial impacts.

23.1.2.3 The Modeling Goal

The modeling goal plays a vital role in the development of the model. Here, we consider the most important general goals and briefly describe what is being achieved through use of the general process system illustrated in Figure 23.1.

Dynamic simulation problem. In this case, the model is developed to predict the system behavior in time. We want to predict the outputs y, given the inputs u, the disturbance pattern d, the model structure M, and the model parameters p. This is the most widely used goal.

Design problem. Here, we are interested in calculating certain parameters or design variables $\tilde{p}$ from the parameter set given for all the other inputs, model form and disturbances, and a set of desired outputs.

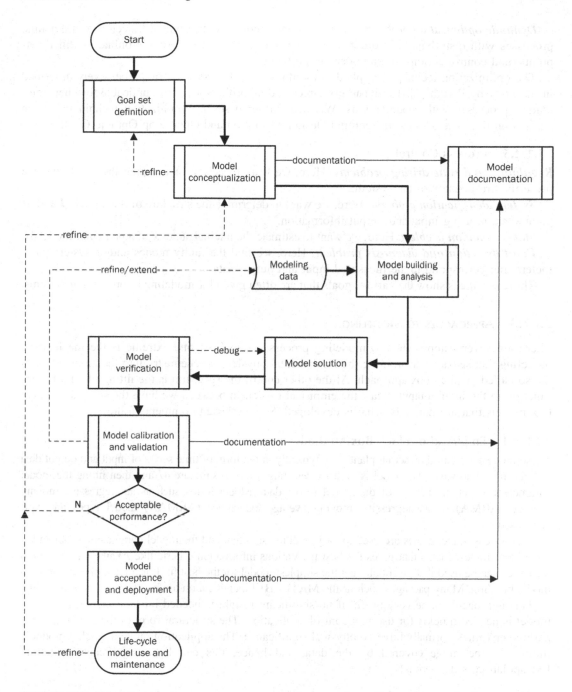

FIGURE 23.2 Modeling methodology and workflow.

23.1.2.4 System Optimization

Steady-state optimization problems. Here, we want to determine the optimal flowsheet, equipment structure and dimensions for the process design, and steady-state operational conditions as the set-points for the regulatory control system.

Dynamic optimization problem. Here, we want to compute the optimal trajectories of dynamic processes with disturbances in order to achieve online parameters, provide online modified set-points, and control actions for state-driving problems.

The optimization techniques applied to the fluid-bed processes are comprehensively described in the book by Parikh [4]. The basic principles and algorithms are also applicable to other granulation processes with modifications. We will further describe optimization techniques in the subsection titled "Modeling for Optimal Design, Operation and Open-loop Optimal Control".

23.1.2.5 Process Control

Regulation and state-driving problems. Here, we want to design or compute the inputs u for a prescribed response y of the system.

System identification problem. Here, we want to determine the structure of the model M and its parameters p, using input and output information.

State estimation problem. Here, we want to estimate the internal states x of a particular model M.

Fault detection and diagnosis problem. Here, we find the faulty modes and/or system parameters that correspond to the measured input and output data.

These key areas show the various goals that are often given for modeling of processing systems.

23.1.3 APPROACHES TO MODELING

There are several approaches to modeling process systems. At one extreme is the mechanistic modeling that seeks to incorporate the fundamental physics and chemistry into the model. This is the so-called "white" box approach. At the other end of the spectrum is the fitting of an arbitrary function to the input–output data—the empirical model. In between we have the so-called "gray" box models that are normally what is developed. Some relevant comments follow.

23.1.3.1 Empirical or Black Box Methods

These models are based on actual plant data, typically in the form of time series of input and output data at fixed time intervals. The model is built by selecting a model structure M and then fitting the model parameters to get the best fit of the model to the data. Model forms such as autoregressive moving average (ARMA) or autoregressive moving average exogenous (ARMAX) model types are typically used.

In most cases, techniques are used to vary both the structure and the model parameters to obtain the "best" or simplest model that gives the best fit. Various information criteria like Akaike's or Bayesian measures can be used that essentially get the simplest model for the best fit. It is a form of parsimony in model building. Many packages such as the MATLAB™ identification toolbox help in such modeling.

This approach can be very useful if no significant insight is needed into the model, but that a model is needed quickly for use in a control application. The structural form of the model and the parameter values normally have no physical significance. The application range of such a model is limited to the range covered by the data, and hence, this can be a significant limitation. Extrapolation is dangerous!

23.1.3.2 Mechanistic and Gray Box Models

Mechanistic models incorporate the underlying understanding of the physics and chemistry into the models. Typically, we can identify two major aspects in mechanistic modeling that cover conservation and constitutive aspects:

- Application of thermodynamic conservation principles for mass, energy, and momentum.
- Application of population balances that track PSDs as various particulate phenomena take place.
- Development of appropriate constitutive relations that define intensive properties, mass, and heat transfer mechanisms as well as particle growth and breakage mechanisms.

The development of mechanistic models is far more complex and time consuming than that of empirical models and is only justified when time permits or when the model is to be used over a wide operating range; and the relevant insight in establishing the constitutive relations is available.

As previously mentioned, even the best mechanistic models require some data fitting, leading to "gray" box models. This is normal practice in industrial modeling of such systems. It means that adequate data must be available to carry out the validation studies. This task is particularly difficult for validation of dynamic models.

23.1.4 QUALITY-BY-DESIGN APPROACH

In recent years, a quality-by-design (QbD) campaign has been witnessed in the pharmaceutical field to provide a systematic approach for understanding formation and process variable in drug design and manufacture [5]. A handbook focused on the theory and practice in a quality-by-design paradigm edited by Narang and Badawy [6] has appeared in the literature. In contrast to the conventional quality-by-testing (QbT) approach, QbD is a comprehensive approach targeting all phases of drug discovery, manufacture, and delivery simultaneously in order to achieve improved quality and reduced cost in a systematic manner. We are of the opinion that the fundamental methodology is to integrate the originally separated fields in science and engineering into a unified framework. These fields include, but are not limited to, granulation mechanisms, multiscale, multiform modeling, optimization, control, and risk analysis. Most of the issues will be addressed in the relevant section in this chapter. Selected topics, which are under the investigations by ourselves or collaborators, are outlined as follows:

Incorporation of Mechanisms in Modeling. Here, physical insights are used as an aid in drug design and manufacture. Models for *a priori* design and scaling up of wet granulation in pharmaceutical processing have been assessed by collaborators [7]. Regime maps, which are graphical representations of the physically based models, are used in the QbD approach. Both nucleation and coalescence regime maps are described and successfully applied to drug design and scaling in that review paper.

Design of experiments. Here, use is made of the Design of Experiment (DoE) method to identify the most important factors early in the experimentation phase when complete knowledge about the system is usually unavailable. It is recognized that Planckett–Burman and fractional factorial designs [5] are efficient screening methods to identify the active factors, using as few experimental runs as possible.

Integration of modeling, design, optimization and control. Here, we stress that all essential aspects in the QbD approach must be considered simultaneously. In particular, control schemes should be investigated in the design phase, and design parameters together with operational conditions should be determined using optimization techniques. Furthermore, dynamic optimization should be combined with closed-loop control. This is described in the "Control" section. All these efforts rely on suitable models. The integration of online parameter identification, dynamic optimization, and closed-loop control has been performed by the authors and is explained in the "Nonlinear Model Predictive Control" section in this chapter.

Development of hybrid models. Here, the intention is to incorporate particle-level behavior into the rate-based population balance models (PBM). To determine particle–particle, particle–equipment, and particle–droplet collisions, hybrid models combining PBM with discrete element method (DEM) and computational fluid dynamics (CFD) are useful. The combination of PBM with DEM has been studied by one of the authors [8] and is described in the section titled "Representing Granulation Processes through Population Balances".

Risk analysis. Here, we adopt the term "risk analysis" from the QbD literature [5], which is similar to the "failure tolerance analysis" in systems engineering. In this analysis, causes for the process and model failure, leading to the severe deterioration of product qualities, are identified. An example for diagnosing model failure using Ishikawa Fishbone Analysis (IFBA) is displayed in

"Application of Population Balance Modeling" section in this chapter on the basis of our experience.

23.2 KEY FACTORS IN GRANULATION MODELING

The modeling of granulation system from a mechanistic perspective inevitably means representing the conservation principles and the constitutive relations that reflect the key factors in granulation. We briefly consider these in turn but refer the reader to the relevant chapters in this handbook for detailed descriptions of the phenomena.

23.2.1 CONSERVATION PRINCIPLES

The conservation of mass, energy, momentum, and particle number can be important aspects of granulation modeling.

Mass conservation is crucial and is the fundamental concept for any granulation system. Key factors here will be solids or slurry feed rates, any outflows, and the addition of binders and additives to the granulation device. Accompanying the mass balance over the device, there will be the energy balance from which the intensive property of temperature can be estimated.

Of particular importance in granulation systems is the factor of particle populations. The PSD within granulation devices is crucial, and there are a number of mechanisms that simultaneously occur in the device, depending on the powder properties and operating regime. The challenge is in the description of these many mechanisms that are occurring. The following section outlines those mechanisms that require consideration. The section "Representing Granulation Processes Through Population Balances" deals in detail with the development of population balance representations and their variants.

23.2.2 THE PRINCIPAL CONSTITUTIVE MECHANISMS

There are three principal mechanisms that need to be considered.

23.2.2.1 Nucleation

Nucleation refers to the formation of initial aggregates that are typically a result of interaction between the binder spray droplets and the powder in the device. This mechanism provides the initial stage for further growth through a number of mechanisms. A number of nucleation models have been proposed in the literature [9–12].

23.2.2.2 Growth

Granule growth occurs through two key mechanisms that can be separated for discussion purposes. The topic is discussed more fully in the section on one-dimensional (1D) population balance models.

Layering. Layering refers to the take up of fine particles onto the surface of larger granules. It is often induced by rolling action and is a means of granule growth that creates hard, compact granules. A practical layering model is proposed in section "Optimization and Open-Loop Optimal Control Equations" for solving optimal control of granulation processes.

Agglomeration. Agglomeration or coalescence refers to the successful collision of two particles that result in a composite particle. The success of collisions can be a function of particle size, binder, and powder properties and operational factors such as bed height, powder velocity, and shear for mixer granulators (see section "Coalescence Kernels" for more details).

23.2.2.3 Breakage

Breakage in high-shear and drum granulation is a significant issue, being more important in high-shear devices. There are various forms of breakage from cleavage of particles to particle surface attrition where the granule is chipped by collision with other particles, the wall, or impeller. Complexity of breakage models extends from binary breakage models to full particle distributions represented by breakage and selection functions or empirical models [13–15].

The following sections now develop in detail some of the important aspects of granulation process modeling, through the use of population balances and alternative approaches.

23.3 REPRESENTING GRANULATION PROCESSES THROUGH POPULATION BALANCES

The particulate nature of solids is characterized by a number of properties, such as size, shape, liquid, gas content, porosity, composition, and age. These properties are denoted as internal co-ordinates, whereas the Euclidian coordinates, such as rectangular coordinates (x, y, and z), cylindrical coordinates (r, φ, and z), and spherical coordinates (r, θ, and φ), used to specify the locations of particles are defined as external coordinates.

The most important property for the characterization of particles is particle size. Randolph and Larson [16] have pointed out: "As no two particles will be exactly the same size, the material must be characterized by the distribution of sizes or particle-size distribution (PSD)". If only size is of interest, a single-variable distribution function is sufficient to characterize the particulate system. If additional properties are also important, multivariable distribution functions must be developed. These distribution functions can be predicted through numerical simulations using population balance equations (PBEs).

Ramkrishna [17] provided a brief explanation on the PBE: "The population balance equation is an equation in the foregoing number density and may be regarded as representing a number balance on particles of a particular state. The equation is often coupled with conservation equation for entities in the particles' environmental (or continuous) phase".

In this chapter, single-variable and multivariable population balances will be described. However, the emphasis will be placed on the single-variable PBEs with size as the only internal coordinate.

23.3.1 GENERAL POPULATION BALANCE EQUATIONS

A population balance for particles in some fixed subregion of particle phase space can be conceptually represented in natural words as follows:

$$
\begin{Bmatrix} \text{Density function change} \\ \text{in class, location, and time} \end{Bmatrix} = \begin{Bmatrix} \text{dispersion in} \\ \text{through boundary} \end{Bmatrix} - \begin{Bmatrix} \text{dispersion out} \\ \text{through boundary} \end{Bmatrix}
$$

$$
+ \begin{Bmatrix} \text{flow in} \\ \text{through boundary} \end{Bmatrix} - \begin{Bmatrix} \text{flow out} \\ \text{through boundary} \end{Bmatrix}
$$

$$
+ \begin{Bmatrix} \text{grow in} \\ \text{from lower classes} \end{Bmatrix} - \begin{Bmatrix} \text{grow out} \\ \text{from current class} \end{Bmatrix} \quad (23.3)
$$

$$
+ \begin{Bmatrix} \text{birth due to} \\ \text{coalescence} \end{Bmatrix} - \begin{Bmatrix} \text{death due to} \\ \text{coalescence} \end{Bmatrix}
$$

$$
+ \begin{Bmatrix} \text{breakup in} \\ \text{from upper classes} \end{Bmatrix} - \begin{Bmatrix} \text{breakup out} \\ \text{from current class} \end{Bmatrix}
$$

The superstructure of the general PBE can be represented as follows:

$$\frac{\partial}{\partial t}f(\mathbf{x}, \mathbf{r}, t) = \nabla_r \cdot \nabla_r [D_r f(\mathbf{x}, \mathbf{r}, t)] - \nabla_r \cdot \dot{R}f(\mathbf{x}, \mathbf{r}, t) - \nabla_x \cdot \dot{X}f(\mathbf{x}, \mathbf{r}, t)$$
$$+ B_c(\mathbf{x}, \mathbf{r}, t) - D_c(\mathbf{x}, \mathbf{r}, t) + B_b(\mathbf{x}, \mathbf{r}, t) - D_b(\mathbf{x}, \mathbf{r}, t) \tag{23.4}$$

where f is the multivariant number density as a function of properties and locations, r is the external coordinate vector (also known as spatial coordinate vector) for the determination of particle locations, x is the internal coordinate vector for the identification of particle properties, such as size, moisture content, and age, D_r is the dispersion coefficient, $\dot{R}$ is the velocity vector in the external coordinate system, $\dot{X}$ is the rate vector in the internal coordinate system, B_c and D_c are birth and death rates for coalescence, respectively, and B_b and D_b are birth and death rates for breakage, respectively. The first and second terms in the right-hand side of Eq. (23.4) represent dispersion and convection particle transport, respectively, whereas the third term quantifies the growth of particles with respect to various properties, such as size and moisture. The birth and death rates for coalescence are given by

$$B_c(\mathbf{x}, \mathbf{r}, t) = \int_{\Omega_x} dV_{x'} \int_{\Omega_r} \frac{1}{\delta}\beta(\tilde{\mathbf{x}}, \tilde{\mathbf{r}}; \mathbf{x}', \mathbf{r}')f(\tilde{\mathbf{x}}, \tilde{\mathbf{r}}, t)f(\mathbf{x}', \mathbf{r}', t)\frac{\partial(\tilde{\mathbf{x}}, \tilde{\mathbf{r}})}{\partial(\mathbf{x}, \mathbf{r})}dV_{r'},$$
$$D_c(\mathbf{x}, \mathbf{r}, t) = f(\mathbf{x}, \mathbf{r}, t)\int_{\Omega_x} dV_{x'} \int_{\Omega_r} \beta(\mathbf{x}', \mathbf{r}'; \mathbf{x}, \mathbf{r})f(\mathbf{x}', \mathbf{r}', t)dV_{r'}, \tag{23.5}$$

where β is the coalescence kernel, Ω_x and Ω_r are integration boundaries for internal and external coordinates, respectively; Vx' and Vr' are generalized representations of internal and external coordinates within the integral boundaries for particles with the original coordinates $[x', r']$ before collision; δ represents the number of times identical pairs have been considered in the interval of integration so that $1/\delta$ corrects for the redundancy, the term $\partial(\tilde{x},\tilde{r})/(\partial x,r)$ accounts for the co-ordinate transformation such that the colliding pair with original coordinates $[\tilde{x},\tilde{r}]$ and $[x',r']$, respectively, before collision should be identified by the coordinates $[x,r]$ after coalescence. Mathematically, this requires that the density with respect to coordinates $[\tilde{x}\,(x, r|x'r'), \tilde{r}(x, r|x'r')]$ must be transformed into one in terms of (x, r) by using the appropriate Jacobian of the transformation. Ramkrishna [17] showed that the determinant of the Jacobian of the transformation satisfies the following equation:

$$\frac{\partial(\tilde{\mathbf{x}}, \tilde{\mathbf{r}})}{\partial(\mathbf{x}, \mathbf{r})} = \begin{vmatrix} \frac{\partial \tilde{x}_1}{\partial x_1} & \cdots & \frac{\partial \tilde{x}_1}{\partial x_n} & \frac{\partial \tilde{x}_1}{\partial r_1} & \frac{\partial \tilde{x}_1}{\partial r_2} & \frac{\partial \tilde{x}_1}{\partial r_3} \\ \vdots & \vdots & \vdots & \vdots & \vdots & \vdots \\ \frac{\partial \tilde{x}_n}{\partial x_1} & \cdots & \frac{\partial \tilde{x}_n}{\partial x_n} & \frac{\partial \tilde{x}_n}{\partial r_1} & \frac{\partial \tilde{x}_n}{\partial r_2} & \frac{\partial \tilde{x}_n}{\partial r_3} \\ \frac{\partial \tilde{r}_1}{\partial x_1} & \cdots & \frac{\partial \tilde{r}_1}{\partial x_n} & \frac{\partial \tilde{r}_1}{\partial r_1} & \frac{\partial \tilde{r}_1}{\partial r_2} & \frac{\partial \tilde{r}_1}{\partial r_3} \\ \frac{\partial \tilde{r}_2}{\partial x_1} & \cdots & \frac{\partial \tilde{r}_2}{\partial x_n} & \frac{\partial \tilde{r}_2}{\partial r_1} & \frac{\partial \tilde{r}_2}{\partial r_2} & \frac{\partial \tilde{r}_2}{\partial r_3} \\ \frac{\partial \tilde{r}_3}{\partial x_1} & \cdots & \frac{\partial \tilde{r}_3}{\partial x_n} & \frac{\partial \tilde{r}_3}{\partial r_1} & \frac{\partial \tilde{r}_3}{\partial x_2} & \frac{\partial \tilde{r}_3}{\partial r_3} \end{vmatrix} \tag{23.6}$$

The birth and death rates for breakage are described as

$$B_b(\mathbf{x}, \mathbf{r}, t) = \int_{\Omega_r} dV_{r'} \int_{\Omega_x} b(\mathbf{x}', \mathbf{r}', t)P(\mathbf{x}, \mathbf{r}|\mathbf{x}', \mathbf{r}', t)S(\mathbf{x}', \mathbf{r}', t)f(\mathbf{x}', \mathbf{r}', t)dV_{x'}, \tag{23.7}$$

and

$$D_b(\mathbf{x}, \mathbf{r}, t) = S(\mathbf{x}, \mathbf{r}, t)f(\mathbf{x}, \mathbf{r}, t) \qquad (23.8)$$

where $b(\mathbf{x}', \mathbf{r}', t)$ is the average number of particles formed from the breakage of a single particle of state $(\mathbf{x}', \mathbf{r}')$ at time t, $P(\mathbf{x}, \mathbf{r}, |\mathbf{x}', \mathbf{r}', t)$ is the probability density function for particle from the breakage of state $(\mathbf{x}', \mathbf{r}')$ at time t that has state $(\mathbf{x}, \mathbf{r})$, and $S(\mathbf{x}, \mathbf{r}, t)$ is the selection function, which represents the fraction of particles of state $(\mathbf{x}, \mathbf{r})$ breaking per unit time.

Equations (23.5) and (23.6) involve three different locations: $\tilde{\mathbf{r}}$ and $\mathbf{r}'$ for the colliding pair of particles and $\mathbf{r}$ for the agglomerated particle. Although this treatment is general and mathematically rigorous, it could be unnecessarily complicated for engineering applications. A common practice is to assume that these three locations are very close to each other during the particle collision and granule formation. That is

$$\tilde{\mathbf{r}} \approx \mathbf{r}' \approx \mathbf{r} \qquad (23.9)$$

This assumption requires that the phenomenon of fast particle jumps in the system is not severe, which is achievable for most industrial granulation processes. If Eq. (23.9) holds, Eqs. (23.5) and (23.6) can be simplified considerably to obtain

$$
\begin{aligned}
B_c(\mathbf{x}, \mathbf{r}, t) &= \tfrac{1}{2} \int_{\Omega_x} \beta(\tilde{\mathbf{x}}, \mathbf{x}', \mathbf{r}) f(\tilde{\mathbf{x}}, \mathbf{r}, t) f(\mathbf{x}, \mathbf{r}, t) \frac{\partial(\tilde{x})}{\partial(x)} dV_{x'} \\
D_c(\mathbf{x}, \mathbf{r}, t) &= f(\mathbf{x}, \mathbf{r}, t) \int_{\Omega_x} \beta(\mathbf{x}', \mathbf{x}, \mathbf{r}) f(\mathbf{x}', t) dV_{x'}
\end{aligned}
\qquad (23.10)
$$

and

$$
\frac{\partial(\tilde{\mathbf{x}})}{\partial(\mathbf{x})} =
\begin{vmatrix}
\frac{\partial \tilde{x}_1}{\partial x_1} & \cdots & \frac{\partial \tilde{x}_1}{\partial x_n} \\
\vdots & \vdots & \vdots \\
\frac{\partial \tilde{x}_n}{\partial x_1} & \cdots & \frac{\partial \tilde{x}_n}{\partial x_n}
\end{vmatrix}
\qquad (23.11)
$$

Similarly, Eq. (23.7) becomes

$$B_b(\mathbf{x}, \mathbf{r}, t) = \int_{\Omega_x} b(\mathbf{x}', \mathbf{r}, t) P(\mathbf{x}|\mathbf{x}', \mathbf{r}, t) S(\mathbf{x}', \mathbf{r}, t) f(\mathbf{x}', \mathbf{r}, t) dV_{x'} \qquad (23.12)$$

In the following material, breakage effects have been considered negligible, and Eq. (23.9) is always assumed to be valid.

23.3.2 One-Dimensional Population Balance Models

One-dimensional (1D) population balance models for both batch and continuous systems are described in this section as special cases of the generalized population balance model stated in the previous section.

23.3.2.1 Batch Systems

For a well-mixed batch system with only one internal coordinate v (particle size), Eq. (23.4) is reduced to

$$
\begin{aligned}
\frac{\partial}{\partial t} n(v, t) = {}& -\frac{\partial}{\partial v}[Gn(v, t)] \\
& + \tfrac{1}{2} \int_0^v \beta(v - v', v') n(v - v', t) n(v', t) dv' - n(v, t) \int_0^\infty \beta(v, v') n(v', t) dv'
\end{aligned}
\qquad (23.13)
$$

where n is the 1D number density and G is known as the growth rate. For notational clarity, we use f and n to denote the multidimensional and 1D number density functions, respectively. Both notations bear the same physical significance. Through a comparison of Eq. (23.13) with Eqs. (23.4), (23.10), and (23.11), it is easy to observe the following membership relationships:

$$v \in \mathbf{x}, \; v' \in \mathbf{x}', \; (v - v') \in \tilde{\mathbf{x}},$$
$$G = \frac{dv}{dt} \in \dot{\mathbf{X}}, \; \frac{\partial (\tilde{\mathbf{x}})}{\partial (\mathbf{x})} = \frac{\partial (v - v')}{\partial v} = 1 \tag{23.14}$$

Equation (23.13) is more frequently applied to industrial granulation processes than its generalized format described by Eq. (23.4).

23.3.2.2 Continuous Systems

The PBE for continuous systems with internal and external coordinates is given by

$$\begin{aligned}
\frac{\partial}{\partial t} n(v, z, t) &= \frac{\partial}{\partial z}[\dot{Z} n(v, z, t)] - \frac{\partial}{\partial v}[Gn(v, z, t)] \\
&+ \frac{1}{2}\int_0^v \beta(v - v', v')n(v - v', z, t)n(v', z, t)dv' \\
&- n(v, z, t)\int_0^\infty \beta(v, v')n(v', z, t)dv'
\end{aligned} \tag{23.15}$$

where the special velocity is defined as

$$\dot{Z} = \frac{dz}{dt} \in \dot{\mathbf{R}} \tag{23.16}$$

Although continuous granulation processes are commonly encountered in the fertilizer and mineral processing industries, most granulation operations in the pharmaceutical industry are performed as batch processes employing either high-shear mixers or batch fluidized-bed granulators. Consequently, most modeling studies on pharmaceutical granulation have focused on batch processes. However, it is important to obtain a complete knowledge in both batch and continuous granulation processes for improved design and operations.

23.3.2.3 Coalescence Kernels

Conventional coalescence kernels. It is easy to see that a coalescence kernel is affected by two major factors: (i) collision probability of the specified pair of particles and (ii) successful coalescence or rebounding after collision. The first factor mainly depends on the particle sizes, granulator configurations, particle flow patterns, and operating conditions. The second issue has been intensively studied by Liu et al. [18] with the identification of the following five most important aspects affecting the success of coalescence: elastic–plastic properties, viscous fluid layer, head of collision, and energy balance. The authors have also observed that there are two types of coalescences distinguished by particle deformations. That is, the type I coalescence is not associated with any particle deformation during the collision, whereas the type II coalescence is accompanied by particle deformations. Liu and Litster [19] further proposed a new physically based coalescence kernel model based on the criteria developed earlier [18]. From these fundamental studies, it can be determined qualitatively that the coalescence kernels should depend on particle sizes, energy consumptions, particle deformability, and most importantly, the moisture content (viscous fluid layer). A historical summary of the proposed coalescence kernels is given in Table 23.1, which is an extension of the table originally presented by Ennis and Litster [20] with the new coalescence kernel developed by Liu and Litster [19] and another kernel from aerosol dynamics [21].

TABLE 23.1

A Summary of Conventional Coalescence Kernels in the Literature

Kernel	References
$\beta = \beta_0$	Kapur and Fuerstenau [22]
$\beta = \beta_0 \frac{(u+v)^a}{(uv)^b}$	Kapur [23]
$\beta = \beta_0 \frac{(u^{2/3} + u^{2/3})}{1/u + 1/u}$	Sastry [24]
$\beta = a(u+v)$	Golovin [25]
$\beta = a\frac{(u-v)^2}{u+v}$	Golovin [25]
$\beta = \begin{cases} k, \, t < t_s \\ a(u+v), \, t > t_s \end{cases}$	Adetayo et al. [26]
k: constant, t_s: switching time	
$\beta = \begin{cases} k, \, w < w_* \\ 0, \, w > w_* \end{cases}$	Adetayo and Ennis [27]
$w = \frac{(u+v)^a}{uv^b}$	
k, a, b: constants, w^*: critical granule volume	
$\beta = \beta_0 (1/u + 1/v)^{1/2} (u^{1/3} + v^{1/3})^2$	Friedlander [21]
$\beta = \beta_0 (u^{-1/3} + v^{-1/3})(u^{1/3} + v^{1/3})$	
$\beta\vert_{u,v} = \begin{cases} \beta_1 & \text{Types I and II without permanent deformation} \\ \beta_2 & \text{Type II with permanent deformation} \\ 0 & \text{rebound} \end{cases}$	Liu and Litster [19]

The rate processes of aggregation, consolidation, breakage, and nucleation that underlie the granulation process have been well-characterized over the years, as borne out by an exhaustive review by Iveson et al. [9]. The various mesoscale processes have been characterized in terms of dimensionless parameters, and regime charts have been developed. Although some of the kernels shown in Table 1 are physically based and inspired by the underlying process mechanisms, they are not truly mechanistic.

Mechanistic coalescence kernels. Immanuel and Doyle III [28] and Poon et al. [10] attempted the derivation of mechanistic kernels for the aggregation and nucleation processes. The mechanistic modeling of the aggregation kernels requires the identification of the net attraction potentials (energies) between the different particle pairs. In the granulation process, the kinetic energy of the particles constitutes the major potential of attraction between the granules ($1/2 \, mu_0^2$) [9,18,29]. The dissipation of the kinetic energy of the granules is primarily attributed to the viscous forces in the liquid-binder film. Other forces that contribute to the dissipation are the collision energy and the elastic energy of the granules, which come into play only when the particles are involved in an actual collision by overcoming the viscous dissipation. Different forces become important in different regimes of particle sizes, binder content, and operating conditions (mixing rates). The capillary repulsive forces between the particles are usually neglected in relation to the stronger viscous forces.

The particles that collide with each other as a result of their kinetic energy will either coalesce or rebound. Coalescence is classified into two types – type I and type II. Type I coalescence occurs when the viscous force is able to overcome the kinetic energy, causing the particles to coalesce before the occurrence of a collision, through the liquid bridge. Type II coalescence occurs when the particles actually collide and lose all the kinetic energy. The elastic energy causes the particles to rebound, being dissipated again in the viscous binder layer. If this dissipation is complete, then coalescence occurs either with or without complete recovery of the deformation. See study by Iveson [30] for further mechanistic details.

Net attractive potential for type I coalescence (balancing the kinetic energy with the viscous repulsion) is given by Eq. (23.17), where p_1 and p_2 are the two particles, m is the reduced mass of the particles, h is the separation distance between the particles, and u is the varying relative velocity of the particles as they approach each other. The velocity u is also defined in Eq. (23.17), wherein h_0 is the depth of the liquid-binder film on the surface, u_0 is the initial approach velocity of the particles (based on the mixing rates in the granulator), and St_v is the viscous Stokes number.

$$
\begin{aligned}
\Psi\left(p_1, p_2, h\right) &= \tfrac{1}{2}m\,[2u\,(h)^2] \\
u &= u_0 \text{ for } h > h_0 \\
&= u_0\left[1 - \frac{1}{St_v}\ln\left(\frac{h_0}{h}\right)\right] \text{ for } h < h_0
\end{aligned}
\tag{23.17}
$$

For type II coalescence, two different sequential processes are involved – the forward and the reverse paths. The process with the higher energetics is the rate-determining process. The net attractive potential for the two processes is defined in Eq. (23.18), where E_c is the energy lost during impact and deformation and u_1 is the velocity at impact. In this equation, u' is the net rebound velocity and δ'' is the permanent plastic deformation in the granules:

$$
\begin{aligned}
\Psi_{\text{forword}}\left(p_1, p_2, h\right) &= \tfrac{1}{2}m\,[2u\,(h)]^2 - E_c \\
\Psi_{\text{reverse}}\left(p_1, p_2, h\right) &= -\tfrac{1}{2}m\,[2u'\,(h)]^2 \\
E_c &= \tfrac{1}{2}m\,(2u_1)^2 \\
u'(h) &= u_2 - \frac{3\pi\mu\tilde{D}^2}{16\tilde{m}h^2}\left[(\delta'')^2\left(\frac{h^2}{h_a^2}-1\right) + 2h\delta''\left(\frac{h}{h_a}-1\right) + 2h^2\ln\left(\frac{h}{h_a}\right)\right] \text{ for } 0 < h < h_0 \\
&= u'(h_0) \text{ for } h < h_0 \\
\delta'' &= \left(\frac{8}{3\pi}\right)^{1/2}St_{\text{def}}^{1/2}\tilde{D}\left[1 - \frac{1}{St_v}\ln\left(\frac{h_0}{h_a}\right)\right]\left[1 - 7.36\frac{Y_d}{E^*}St_{\text{def}}^{-1/2}\right]\left[1 - \frac{1}{St_v}\ln\left(\frac{h_0}{h_a}\right)\right]^{-1/2}
\end{aligned}
\tag{23.18}
$$

These steady-state forces can be incorporated into a dynamic calculation of the aggregation rates and the aggregation kernel, as described in the emulsion polymerization literature [31]. This net attractive potential information can be employed in the Smoluchowski formulation as shown in Eq. (23.19). The Fuchs Stability Ratio W is defined in Eq. (23.20) for type I and type II aggregation, respectively. In these equations, r_i is the radius of particle p_i, k is the Boltzmann constant, T is the temperature, and c_1 is an adjustable constant.

$$
\beta\,(p_1, p_2) = c_1\frac{4\pi u_0\,(r_1 + r_2)^2}{W}
\tag{23.19}
$$

$$w = (p_1, p_2) = (r_1 + r_2) \int_{D=r_1+r_2}^{\infty} \frac{e^{\psi(p_1,p_2,D)/kT}}{D^2} dD$$

$$\frac{W(p_1,p_2)}{r_1+r_2} = \max\left(\int_{D=r_1+r_2}^{\infty} \frac{e^{-\psi\text{forword}(p_1,p_2,D-r_1-r_2)/kT}}{D^2} dD, \int_{D=r_1+r_2}^{\infty} \frac{e^{-\psi\text{reverse}(p_1,p_2,D-r_1-r_2)/kT}}{D^2} dD, \right) \tag{23.20}$$

23.3.3 MULTIDIMENSIONAL POPULATION BALANCE MODELS

23.3.3.1 Two-Dimensional Population Balance Models

In this section, we study a perfect mixing, batch granulation system [32,33] with two internal property coordinates: particle value v and liquid value v_L. Because of the perfect mixing feature, there is no spatial coordinate in the model. However, the proposed modeling strategy can easily be extended to continuous processes with both internal and external coordinates. The two-dimensional (2D) PBE for a batch granulation process is

$$\begin{aligned}
\frac{\partial}{\partial t}f(v, v_{L,t}) = &-\frac{\partial}{\partial t}\left[\frac{dv}{dt}f(v, v_{L,t})\right] - \frac{\partial}{\partial v_L}\left[\frac{dv_L}{dt}f(v, v_{L,t})\right] \\
&+ \frac{1}{2}\int_0^v \int^{\min(v_L, v-v')} \beta(v-v', v_L-v'_L, v'v'_L)f(v-v', v_L \\
&-v'_L, t)f(v', v'_L, t)dv'_L dv' \\
&-f(v, v_L, t)\int_0^\infty \int_0^{v_L} \beta(v, v_L, v', v'_L)f(v', v'_L, t)dv'_L dv'
\end{aligned} \tag{23.21}$$

The relationship between the bivariant number density function f and single-variant number density function n is determined as

$$n(v, t) = \int_0^v f(v, v_L, t)dv_L \tag{23.22}$$

For the aggregation-only processes, the first two terms on the right-hand side of Eq. (23.21) representing convective particle transport and particle growth by layering are negligible. Eq. (23.21) is reduced to

$$\begin{aligned}
\frac{\partial}{\partial t}f(v, v_L, t) = &+\frac{1}{2}\int_0^v \int_0^{\min(v_L, v-v')} \beta(v-v', v_L-v'_L, v', v'_L)f(v-v', v_L \\
&-v'_L, t)(v', v'_L, t)dv'_L dv' \\
&-f(v, v_L, t)\int_0^\infty \int_0^{v_L} \beta(v, v_L, v', v'_L)f(v', v'_L, t)dv'_L dv'
\end{aligned} \tag{23.23}$$

Under certain mathematical assumptions, a 2D PBE can be reduced to two single-dimension PBEs, which will be described in the next section.

23.3.3.2 Higher-Dimensional Population Balance Models

In consonance with the above study on 2D population balance models, Iveson [30] suggested that a 1D population balance model based on particle size is quite inadequate in accounting for the granulation process. As laid out previously, the three major contributing phenomena that have been identified in the granulation processes are wetting and nucleation; aggregation, layering, and consolidation; and breakage and attrition. Among these the major role played by consolidation is to reduce the porosity of the granules and thereby increase the fractional binder content and the chances of successful aggregation. The rate of aggregation itself is determined by both the size of the granules and its fractional binder content. Thus, at the least, the characterization of the binder content and porosity in addition to the granule size is important in the granulation processes. Iveson [30] also points out the importance of the heterogeneity at the macroscopic level in terms of binder distribution as well as size segregation effects that are required to be accounted for in a rigorous model of the granulation operation. He also points out that several applications also require the explicit characterization of the concentration of the granules.

$$\frac{\partial n(m, \varepsilon, w, x, t)}{\partial t} = B_{coal}(m, \varepsilon, w, x, t) - D_{coal}(m, \varepsilon, w, x, t)$$
$$+ C(m, \varepsilon, w, x, t) + W(m, \varepsilon, w, x, t)$$
(23.24)

where in m is the total mass of the granule particle, ε is the particle porosity, w is the fractional binder content (fraction of binder to solid mass), and x is the composition of the solid (drug vs. excipient). The terms "$B_{coal}(m, \varepsilon, w, x, t)$" and "$D_{coal}(m, \varepsilon, w, x, t)$" account respectively for the birth and death of particles due to coalescence events. "C" accounts for consolidation, and "W" accounts for wetting.

A similar multidimensional population balance model was also proposed by Verkoeijen et al. [34]. They extended the Iveson proposal in that they suggest the use of truly mutually independent particle properties as the internal variables. Thus, in a 3D formulation, they propose the use of the volumes of solid, liquid, and gas as the internal coordinates, rather than the particle total volume, binder content, and porosity, which are not mutually independent of each other. This approach results in elegantly separating the underlying mesoscopic processes of aggregation, consolidation, breakage, drying, and layering.

Immanuel and Doyle III [28] propose the following multidimensional formulation of the population balance model for the granulation process, using the individual volumes of solid, liquid, and air as the internal coordinates:

$$\frac{\partial}{\partial t}F(s, l, g, t) + \frac{\partial}{\partial g}\left(F(s, l, g, t)\frac{dg}{dt}\right) + \frac{\partial}{\partial s}\left(F(s, l, g, t)\frac{\partial s}{\partial t}\right) + \frac{\partial}{\partial l}\left(F(s, l, g, t)\frac{\partial l}{\partial t}\right)$$
$$= \Re_{aggre}(s, l, g, t) + \Re_{break}(s, l, g, t) + \Re_{nuc}(s, l, g, t)$$
(23.25)

where $F(s, l, g, t)$ is the population density function, defined such that $F(s, l, g, t)ds\,dl\,dg$ is the moles of granules of solid volume between s and $s + ds$, liquid volume between l and $l + dl$, and gas volume between g and $g + dg$. $\Re_{nuc}(s, l, g, t)$ accounts for the rate of nucleation of new granules. $\Re_{aggre}(s, l, g, t)$ accounts for the gain/loss of granules due to the aggregation process, while $\Re_{break}(s, l, g, t)$ comprises similar terms due to granule breakage. The partial derivative with respect to g on the left-hand side accounts for the consolidation phenomenon, wherein dg/dt is negative: there is a continuous decrease in the pore volume of the granules as they compact, while the solid and liquid content of each granule is left unaltered. The partial derivative term with respect to s accounts for any simultaneous crystallization and layering of the granule surface with the solid. The term with respect to l accounts for any drying effects. These latter two terms are usually restricted to certain special cases of granulation applications.

Further theoretical and experimental studies on 3D population balance model of granulation have been carried out collaboratively among a number of universities with fruitful outcomes [10,32,33].

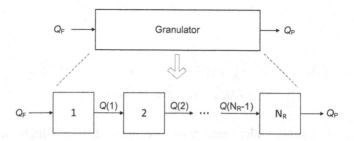

FIGURE 23.3 Concept of lumped regions in series.

23.3.4 REDUCED-ORDER MODELS

23.3.4.1 Reduced-Order Models Using the Concept of Lumped Regions in Series

When particle populations are spatial dependent, such as that in a long rotating drum granulator, the population balance model is described by Eq. (23.15) with spatial variable z included in the model equation. In many industrial applications, the concept of lumped regions in series is used to reduce the model order. By using this method, a whole granulator is divided into a number of sections with an assumption that perfect mixing can be achieved in each section. The basic idea is schematically depicted in Figure 23.3.

In Figure 23.3, Q denotes the number flow rate, the subscripts F and P represent the feed and product streams, respectively, and N_R is the total number of regions used to approximate the granulator. The reduced-order model for Eq. (23.15) using the method of lumped regions in series is given by

$$
\begin{aligned}
\frac{\partial}{\partial t}n(v, i, t) &= -\frac{\partial}{\partial v}[G_i n(v, i, t)] + Q(i-1)\frac{n(v, i-1, t)}{n_t(i-1, t)} - Q(i)\frac{n(v, i, t)}{n_t(i, t)} \\
&\quad + \frac{1}{2}\int_0^v \beta(v - v', v')n(v - v', i, t)n(v', i, t)dv' \\
&\quad - n(v, i, t)\int_0^\infty \beta(v, v')n(v', i, t)dv'
\end{aligned}
\tag{23.26}
$$

$$
i = 1, 2, \ldots, N_R
$$

where i represents the ith region, n_t is the total number density, and $Q(0) = Q_F$.

23.3.4.2 Model Order Reduction for Multidimensional Population Balances

Biggs et al. [35] developed a concept of binder size distribution (BSD) to correlate moisture content with particle size. On the basis of BSD, the mass of binder in the size range $(v, v + dv)$ is quantified as $dM = M(v)dv$ and

$$
M(t, v) = \rho_L \int_0^v v_L f(v, v_L, t)dv_L
\tag{23.27}
$$

where ρ_L is the binder density. They showed that given the assumption that at a given size all granules have the same liquid content, the 2D PBE given by Eq. (23.23) can be reduced to a set of two 1D equations described as follows:

$$
\begin{aligned}
\frac{\partial}{\partial t}n(v, t) &= \frac{1}{2}\int_0^v \beta(v - v', v')n(v - v', t)n(v', t)dv' \\
&\quad - n(v, t)\int_0^\infty \beta(v, v')n(v', t)dv
\end{aligned}
\tag{23.28}
$$

and

$$\frac{\partial}{\partial t} M(v, t) = \frac{1}{2} \int_0^v \beta(v - v', v') M(v - v', t) n(v', t) dv'$$
$$- M(v, t) \int_0^\infty \beta(v, v') n(v', t) dv$$

(23.29)

In their experiments, pharmaceutical materials were granulated in a high-shear mixer. Good agreement between experimental and simulation results was achieved enabling the granulation rates to be defined by two parameters: the critical binder volume fraction and the aggregation rate constant.

23.3.4.3 Reduced-Order Models Using the Method of Moments

The moments are defined as:

$$M_j = \int_0^\infty v^j n(v) dv$$
$$\mu_j = \frac{M_j}{M_0}$$
$$j = 0, 1, 2, \cdots$$

(23.30)

Because of the variety of coalescence kernels, it is impossible to develop a generalized structure for reduced-order models using the method of moments. A special kernel model is assumed in this work. The methodology can be extended to the development of moment models with different kernel structures. The example kernel model is assumed as

$$\beta(v, v') = \beta_0 \frac{v^b + v'^b}{(vv')^a} = \beta_0 \left[\frac{v'^{(b-a)}}{v^a} + \frac{v^{(b-a)}}{v'^a} \right]$$

(23.31)

The discretized format of Eq. (23.31) is given by

$$\beta_{i,j} = \beta_0 \left[\frac{v_j^{(b-a)}}{v_j^a} + \frac{v_j^{(b-a)}}{v_j^a} \right]$$

(23.32)

The 1D aggregation-only PBE described by Eq. (23.28) with the kernel model given by Eq. (23.32) can be reduced to a set of ordinary differential equations as follows:

$$\frac{d}{dt} M_0 = -\beta_0 (\mu_{(b-a)} \mu_{-a}) M_0$$
$$\frac{d}{dt} M_1 = 0$$
$$\frac{d}{dt} M = \frac{1}{2} \beta_0 \sum_{k=1}^{r-1} \binom{r}{k} \left[\mu_{(k-a)} \mu_{(r-k+b-a)} + \mu_{(k+b-a)} \mu_{(r-k-a)} \right] M_0^2, \quad r = 2, 3, \ldots$$

(23.33)

where μ is defined in Eq. (23.30), for example, by $\mu_{(k-a)} = M_{(k-a)}/M_0$. Equation (23.33) involves the determination of fractional and negative moments. If the type of PSD is more or less known, such as log-normal or Γ-distribution, Eq. (23.33) is solvable with the incorporation of interpolation and extrapolation techniques. For more general solution techniques, fractional calculus enabling the computation of fractional differentiations and integrations should be used, which exceed the scope of this chapter.

23.3.4.4 Multi Timescale Analysis

It is often the case that in an interconnected process situation where several processes are being simulated simultaneously, those processes operate on distinct timescales. Such is the case when combinations of pre-reaction units are combined with granulation devices, dryers, and screening in full process flowsheet simulations. It can also be the case within a particular processing unit that incorporates a range of mechanisms.

It can be observed that these processes often operate on different timescales covering the range of microseconds to minutes or even hours. This time separation in scales provides opportunity to make assumptions that can simplify the modeling by separating the phenomena into at least three classes.

- Slow modes (long time constant behavior)
- Medium modes
- Fast modes (short time constants)

When we do this analysis, we can often use qualitative methods based on our general understanding of the physics, chemistry, and the rate processes such as heat and mass transfer. As suggested by Robertson and Cameron, the alternative and more complex analytical approach is through the use of eigenvalue and eigenvector analysis that is based on the underlying models of the processes [36]. This analysis often allows us to simplify complex models when we model for particular goals by making the following assumptions:

- Slow modes can be treated as being constant over the timeframe of interest.
- Medium modes are modeled in detail.
- Fast modes are regarded as pseudo steady states, being represented by algebraic equations.

This timescale approach can simplify significantly the complexity of the process models depending on the timeframe of interest in the simulation, and the approach has general application to all forms of models.

23.3.4.5 Regime Separated Approach

In many cases, although a number of processes take place simultaneously, only one process is dominant with other processes to be identified as insignificant. In this case, a regime separate approach with a single process in one zone can be used to dramatically reduce the model complexity [37]. For example, the twin-screw wet granulator (TSWG) can be divided into mixing zone, wetting zone, and wet granulation zone [37], and a pulsed spray fluidized-bed granulator can be separated as a wetting and granulation zone, and a drying and breakage zone [38]. The simulation and experimental results show that the error tolerance levels are acceptable for both cases.

23.3.5 A Multiform Modeling Approach

A multiform modeling approach has been proposed by Wang and Cameron [39] in which the granulation process can be represented by a variety of model forms for different end uses. These include (i) the distributed parameter population balance model (DP-PBM) described by Eq. (23.15); (ii) the lumped parameter population balance model (LP-PBM) represented by Eq. (23.26); (iii) matrix representation with offline computed matrix elements; (iv) linear and local linear models that will be further explained in the section "Application of Population Balance Modeling"; (v) input–output, black box models, which will also be described in the same section; (vi) a variety of reduced-order models using various techniques, including method of moments and the dimension separation technique stated in the "Reduced-order Models". It can be shown through dynamic simulations that significant computing time reductions can be achieved with properly selected model forms. Since both open-loop optimal control and closed-loop model predictive control (MPC) rely on iterative dynamic optimization, overall computing time reduction makes online applications possible. Furthermore, the development of local linear models allows the applications of well-established linear system theory and techniques to process control, parameter identification, and model order reduction. The demonstrated advantages of the proposed multiform modeling approach imply a big step forward toward the industrial applications of model-based control for granulation processes.

23.3.6 HYBRID MODELS

23.3.6.1 Population Balance Model (PBM) Coupled with Discrete Element Method (DEM)

In order to accurately estimate the coalescence kernels, collision selection functions, and breakage functions in both size enlargement and reduction processes, evaluations of particle collision frequencies, velocities, deformation, and momentum transfer are essential. The PBM coupled with DEM provide a more efficient and accurate approach than the time-consuming and expensive experimentally based methods. The combination of PBM with DEM strategy has been successfully applied in the dense phase granulators, such as drum, high-shear, and twin-screw wet granulators [5,8].

23.3.6.2 Population Balance Model (PBM) Coupled with Computational Fluid Dynamics (CFD)

In the sparse phase granulators, such as top spray fluidized bed (TSFB) granulators, one needs to determine the particle transport between wetting zone with particle size enlargement and drying zone with particle size reduction. Furthermore, interactions between particles, particle and droplets, and particle and equipment are essential for the development of the coalescence kernels for size enlargement, selection function, and breakage function for size reduction processes in PBM. Particle transport and interactions can be computed by using CFD, so that PBM and CFD are hence combined together in an interactive manner [38].

23.4 SOLVING POPULATION BALANCES

In this section, we look at a number of important solution methods to solve PBEs. This covers conventional, well-established techniques as well as more recent and specialized approaches.

23.4.1 CONVENTIONAL DISCRETIZATION METHODS

Hounslow discretization. Hounslow et al. [11] developed a relatively simple discretization method by employing an M-I approach (the mean value theorem on frequency). The PBEs, such as Eq. (23.28), are normally developed using particle volume as the internal coordinate. Because of the identified advantages of length-based models, Hounslow et al. [11] performed the coordinate transformation to convert the volume-based model described by Eq. (23.28) to a length-based model as follows:

$$\frac{d}{dt}n(L, t) = \frac{L^2}{2}\int_0^L \frac{\beta[(L^3-\lambda^3)^{1/3},\lambda]n[(L^3-\lambda^3)^{1/3},t]n(\lambda,t)}{(L^3-\lambda^3)^{2/3},}d\lambda$$
$$- n(L, t)\int_0^\infty \beta(L,\lambda)n(\lambda, t)d\lambda \tag{23.34}$$

in which L and λ denote the characteristic length of particles. The Hounslow method is based on a geometric discretization, with the following ratio between two successive size intervals:

$$\frac{L_i + 1}{L_i} = \sqrt[3]{2}, \text{ or } \frac{v_i + 1}{v_i} = 2 \qquad (23.35)$$

where L and v represent the characteristic length and volume of particles, respectively, and the subscripts $i + 1$ and i denote the size classes. The continuous PBE described by Eq. (23.34) is converted into a set of discretized PBEs in various size intervals by using this technique. That is, the change of number density in the ith size interval is given by

$$
\begin{aligned}
\frac{d}{dt}n_i = \; & n_{i-1} \Sigma_{j=1}^{i-2} \left(2^{j-i+1} \beta_{i-1,j} n_j \right) + \tfrac{i}{2} \beta_{i-1,i-1} n_{i-1}^2 \\
& - n_i \Sigma_{j=1}^{i-1} \left(2^{j-i} \beta_{i,j} n_j \right) - n_i \Sigma_{j=1}^{i_{\max}} \left(\beta_{i,j} n_j \right)
\end{aligned}
\qquad (23.36)
$$

$$ i = 1, 2, \ldots, i_{\max} $$

The continuous BSD model described by Eq. (23.29) can also be discretized using a similar numerical scheme as follows (see Biggs et al. [35]):

$$
\begin{aligned}
\frac{d}{dt}M_i = \; & M_{i-1} \Sigma_{j=1}^{i-2} \left(2^{j-i+1} \beta_{i-1,j} n_j \right) + n_{i-1} \Sigma_{j=1}^{i-2} \left(2^{j-i+1} \beta_{i-1,j} n_j \right) \\
& + n_i \Sigma_{j=1}^{i-1} \left[(1 - 2^{j-i}) \beta_{i,j} M_j \right] + \beta_{i-1,i-1} n_{i-1} M_{i-1} \\
& - M_i \Sigma_{j=1}^{i-1} \left(2^{j-1} n_j \right) - -M_i \Sigma_{j=1}^{i_{\max}} \left(\beta_{i,j} n_j \right)
\end{aligned}
\qquad (23.37)
$$

$$ i = 1, 2, \ldots, i_{\max} $$

Kumar and Ramkrishna's Discretization Technique. Kumar and Ramkrishna [40] developed a discretization method by using a grid with a more general and flexible pattern with fine or coarse discretizations in different size ranges. The size range between two sizes v_i and v_{i+1} is called the ith section, and the particle size in this section is simply denoted by x_i (grid point) such that $v_i < x_i < v_{i+1}$ as seen in Figure 23.4.

A particle of size v in the size range x_i and x_{i+1} can be represented by two fractions $a(v, x_i)$ and $b(v, x_{i+1})$ associated with the two grid points x_i and x_{i+1}, respectively. For the conservation of two general properties $f_1(v)$ and $f_2(v)$, these fractions satisfy the following equations:

$$
\begin{aligned}
a(v, x_i)f_1(x_i) + b(v, x_{i+1})f_1(x_{i+1}) &= f_1(v) \\
a(v, x_i)f_2(x_i) + b(v, x_{i+1})f_2(x_{i+1}) &= f_2(v)
\end{aligned}
\qquad (23.38)
$$

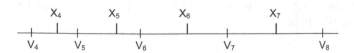

FIGURE 23.4 General grid used with Kumar and Ramkrishna [40] numerical technique.

By using this composition technique for particle properties, discrete equations for coalescence-only population balance model given by Eq. (23.22) have been formulated as follows:

$$\frac{dn_i}{dt} = \sum_{\substack{j,k \\ x_{i-1} \leq (x_j + x_k) \leq x_{i+1}}}^{j \geq k} \left(1 - \frac{1}{2}\delta_{j,k}\right)\eta\beta(j, k)n_j(t) - n_i(t) \sum_{k=1}^{i_{max}} \beta(i, k)n_k(t) \qquad (23.39)$$

In Eq. (23.39), n_i, β, and i_{max} are defined previously, $\delta_{j,k}$ is the Dirac delta function, and η is defined as follows:

$$\eta = \frac{x_{i+1} - v}{x_{i+1} - x_i}, \ x_i \leq v \leq x_{i+1}$$
$$\eta = \frac{v - x_{i-1}}{x_i - x_{i-1}}, \ x_{i-1} \leq v \leq x_i \qquad (23.40)$$

The first and second terms on the right-hand side of Eq. (23.39), respectively, represent the birth rate and death rate of particles in the ith size interval because of coalescence.

Attention should be paid to the selection of the internal coordinates. The original Kumar–Ramkrishna discretization [40] should be applied to volume-based models rather than length-based models. Although both are interconvertible, it is important to check the consistency in numerical computations.

23.4.2 Wavelet-Based Methods

Wavelet-based methods are relatively new numerical schemes for solving PBEs consisting of both differential and integral functions [41–44]. Again, the volume-based PBEs with particle volume as the internal coordinate are used to demonstrate the main characteristics of the wavelet methods. The most important advantage of these methods over other numerical techniques is their ability to effectively deal with steep-moving profiles. In this subsection, we only explain the basic algorithms of the wavelet-collocation method for practical applications using the Daubechies wavelets rather than to provide mathematical insights for general wavelet techniques.

Similar to other collocation methods, the coordinates should be normalized within the interval [0,1]. For the 1D PBE given by Eq. (23.13), this can be done by introducing the linear transformation $x = v/v_{max}$, where x is the dimensionless particle volume and v_{max} is the maximum particle size in the system. The original integral intervals $[0, v]$ and $[0, \infty]$ are transformed to $[0, x]$ and $[0, 1]$, respectively. Consequently, Eq. (23.13) becomes

$$\frac{\partial}{\partial t}n(x, t) = \frac{\partial}{\partial x}[G(x)n(x, t)]$$
$$+ \frac{v_{max}}{2}\int_0^x \beta(x - x', x')n(x - x', t)n(x', t)dx' \qquad (23.41)$$
$$- v_{max}n(x, t)\int_0^1 \beta(x', x')n(x', t)dx'$$

where $G(x)$ is defined as dx/dt rather than dv/dt. For a broad class of engineering problems, the approximate solution of a general function $w(x)$ with J-level resolution can be written in terms of its values in the dyadic points:

$$w_J(x) \approx \sum_m w_J(2^{-J}m)\theta(2^J x - m) \qquad (23.42)$$

where $\theta(x)$ is denoted as the autocorrelation function of scaling function. We first solve the coalescence-only PBE with $G(x) = 0$. If J-level wavelet method is used, the matrix representation at the ith dyadic point is given by

$$\frac{\partial n_i}{\partial t} = \frac{v_{max}}{2} [n_0 \quad n_1 \quad \cdots \quad n_{2^J}] \mathbf{M}^{3,i} \begin{bmatrix} n_0 \\ n_1 \\ \vdots \\ n_{2^J} \end{bmatrix} - v_{max} n_i \mathbf{M}_i^2 \begin{bmatrix} n_0 \\ n_1 \\ \vdots \\ n_{2^J} \end{bmatrix} \tag{23.43}$$

where n_i is the number density at the ith dyadic (collocation) point. The operational matrix $\mathbf{M}^{3,i}$ and vector $\mathbf{M}_i^2$ are constructed as follows. $\mathbf{M}^{3,i}$ are $(2^J + 1) \times (2^J + 1)$ operational matrices at volume point i represented as

$$\mathbf{M}^{3,i} = \begin{bmatrix} M_{0,0}^{3,i} & M_{0,1}^{3,i} & \cdots & M_{0,2^J}^{3,i} \\ M_{1,0}^{3,i} & M_{1,1}^{3,i} & \cdots & M_{1,2^J}^{3,i} \\ \vdots & \vdots & \ddots & \vdots \\ M_{2^J,0}^{3,i} & M_{2^J,1}^{3,i} & \cdots & M_{2^J,2^J}^{3,i} \end{bmatrix} \tag{23.44}$$

$\mathbf{M}_i^2$ are $1 \times (2^J + 1)$ operational vectors at volume point i described by

$$\mathbf{M}_i^2 = \begin{bmatrix} M_{i,0}^2 & M_{i,1}^2 & \cdots & M_{i,2^J}^2 \end{bmatrix}$$

Elements in the matrix $\mathbf{M}^{3,i}$ are developed as

$$M_{k_1,k_2}^{3,i} = \frac{1}{2^J} \sum_{l=0}^{2^J} \beta(x_i - x_l, x_l) \times \left[\Omega_{l-k_2, i-k_1-k_2}(i - k_2) - \Omega_{l-k_2, i-k_1-k_2}(-k_2) \right] \tag{23.45}$$

Elements in the operational vectors $\mathbf{M}_i^2$ are given by

$$M_{i,k}^2 = \frac{1}{2^J} \left[\sum_{l=0}^{2^J} \beta(x_i, x_l) H_{k-l}(k) \right] \tag{23.46}$$

The needed two-term integral of autocorrelation function $H_k(x)$ and three-term integral of autocorrelation function $\Omega_{j,k}(x)$ in Eqs. (23.45) and (23.46) are defined as

$$H_k(x) = \int_{-\infty}^{x} \theta(y - k)\theta(y)dy \tag{23.47}$$

and

$$\Omega_{j,k}(x) = \int_{-\infty}^{x} \theta(y - j)\theta(y - k)\theta(y)dy \tag{23.48}$$

The autocorrelation function $\theta(k)$ and its derivatives $\theta^{(s)}(k)$ are represented as follows:

$$
\begin{aligned}
\theta(k) &= \int_{-\infty}^{+\infty} \phi(x)\phi(x-k)dx \\
\theta^{(s)}(k) &= (-1)^s \int_{-\infty}^{+\infty} \phi(x)\phi^{(s)}(x-k)dx
\end{aligned}
\tag{23.49}
$$

where $\phi(x)$ is the scaling function. $\theta^{(s)}(k)$ can be evaluated by using the following recursive algorithm with $\theta(k) = \theta^{(0)}(k)$:

$$
\theta^{(s)}(2^{-J-1}k) = 2^s\theta^{(s)}(2^{-J}k) + 2^{s-1}\sum_{l=1}^{N} a_{2l-1}[\theta^{(s)}(2^{-J}k - 2l + 1) + \theta^{(s)}(2^{-J}k - 2l - 1)]
\tag{23.50}
$$

The differential operators in the PBE can also be evaluated at the collocation points as

$$
\begin{aligned}
\frac{\partial \mathbf{n}}{\partial x} &= \mathbf{A}(\theta^{(1)})\mathbf{n} \\
\frac{\partial^2 \mathbf{n}}{\partial x^2} &= \mathbf{B}(\theta^{(2)})\mathbf{n}
\end{aligned}
\tag{23.51}
$$

where $\mathbf{n} = [n_1 n_2 \cdots n_N]^T$ is a vector, in which n_i is the number density at the ith collocation point, $N = 2^J + 1$ is the number of collocation points, T stands for vector transpose, $\mathbf{A}$ and $\mathbf{B}$ are square matrices computed using the values $\theta^{(1)}(k)$ and $\theta^{(2)}(k)$, respectively. An algorithm for the computation of the matrices $\mathbf{A}$ and $\mathbf{B}$ was described in Liu and Cameron [43]. Consequently, the growth term in Eq. (23.41) can be approximated using Eq. (23.51).

It should be pointed out that after coordinate normalization, functions of interest are evaluated in the closed intervals [0,1] rather than [$-\infty$, ∞] or other intervals. In this case, some modified interpolation functions can be constructed to interpolate the values in dyadic points outside [0, 1] to the desired interval [42,43].

Three PBEs with different kernel models have been successfully solved by using the wavelet-collocation method [43,44]. These kernel models were (i) size-independent kernel $\beta = \beta_0 = $ constant, (ii) linear size-dependent kernel $\beta(x, x') = \beta_0(x + x')$, and (iii) nonlinear size-dependent kernel $Q(x, x') = \beta(x^{1/3} + x'^{1/3})(x^{-1/3} + x'^{-1/3})$. Simulation results have shown that the wavelet-collocation methods are able to achieve fast convergence with high accuracy if adequate resolution levels are selected. The methods are particularly effective for the processes with steep-moving profiles, which are difficult to solve by using other numerical schemes.

In this subsection, the emphasis has been placed on the introduction of basic techniques for the resolution of PBEs using wavelets, which requires to solve $2^J + 1$ ordinary equations for each PBE given by Eq. (23.41). Liu and Cameron [44] developed a new wavelet-based adaptive technique, which enables a dramatic reduction of the number of ordinary differential equations to be solved. Furthermore, this adaptive method allows the automatic selection of the minimum wavelet level J with acceptable accuracy. With the background knowledge described in this chapter, the readers may understand the adaptive technique through studies on the original papers without major difficulties.

The operational matrices $M^{3,i}$ and M_i^2, matrices $\mathbf{A}$ and $\mathbf{B}$, together with the integral functions H and Ω at various resolution levels are available from the authors.

23.4.3 HIERARCHICAL TWO-TIER TECHNIQUE

Another development in solution techniques has been presented by Immanuel and Doyle III [12]. This technique is based on a finite-element discretization of the particle population and tracks the

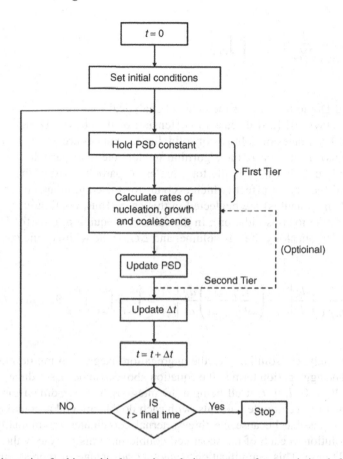

FIGURE 23.5 Schematic of a hierarchical two-tier solution strategy for population balance models.

total particles within each of the bins. The equation representing the total particles within each bin is derived from the PBE in a straightforward manner via partial analytical solution. The particle population in each bin is updated employing a hierarchical strategy, as depicted in Figure 23.5. The individual rates of nucleation, growth, and coalescence in each bin are computed in the first tier of the algorithm (at each time step), and the particle population is updated in the second tier. A simple predictor–corrector technique may be utilized for information exchange between the two tiers.

Employing the two-tier hierarchical solution strategy enables orders of magnitude improvement in the computation times. The improvement in computation times is achieved partly by a reduction of the stiffness of the system equations by a decomposition solution strategy for the nucleation, growth, and coalescence models. In effect, the PBE is reformulated in terms of the individual growth, aggregation, nucleation, and breakage events (as appropriate), thereby accommodating the differences in their timescales. The other major factor that contributes to this improvement in computation time is the offline analytical solution that is proposed for the aggregation quadratures. This results in casting the complex integrals in terms of simpler terms, major portions of which can be computed just once at the start, thereby leading to a substantial reduction in the computational load. These analytical solutions for the quadratures are derived based on an assumption of a uniform particle density within each element, although this assumption can be easily relaxed to enable larger finite elements. It also involves the assumption that the coalescence kernel for particles between any two bins is a constant [i.e., $\beta(V', V - V')$ in the following equation is constant for all particle coalescences between bins i and j].

$$\Re'_{formation}(V,\ t) = \frac{1}{2V_{aq}} \int_{V=V_{j-1}}^{V_j} \left[\int_{V'=V_{nuc}}^{V-V_{nuc}} \beta(V',\ V-V')F_V(V',\ t)F_V(V-V',\ t)dV' \right] dV$$

$$(23.52)$$

See Immanuel and Doyle III [12] for the detailed analytical solutions.

Immanuel and Doyle III [28] discuss the extension of the above 1D algorithm to the multi-dimensional case. The ranges of volumes of solid, liquid, and gas are divided into 3D grids (finite volumes or the bins). In this case, the algorithm models the total particle count within each of these bins, defined such that $F_{i,j,k}$ is the total moles of particles within the $(i,\ j,\ k)$th bin. The layering effect and the drying effect (which account for the continuous change in the solid and liquid contents of the granules) are neglected in this case. Thus, continuous growth is restricted to the gas volume (due to consolidation). In the following equation, g_k is the lower boundary of gas volume in the kth bin along the gas volume, and ΔG_k is the width of the kth bin along the gas volume.

$$\frac{d}{dt}F_{i,j,k} + \left(\frac{F_{i,j,k}}{\Delta G_{i,j,k}}\right)\frac{dg}{dt}\bigg|_k - \left(\frac{F_{i,j,k+1}}{\Delta G_{i,j,k+1}}\right)\frac{dg}{dt}\bigg|_{k+1} = \int_{s_{i-1}}^{s_i}\int_{l_{i-1}}^{l_i}\int_{g_{i-1}}^{g_i} \Re_{aggre}(s,\ l,\ g,\ t)ds\ dl\ dg$$

$$(23.53)$$

Extensions of the analytical solutions for the aggregation integrals to multidimensional cases are straightforward. The aggregation term in the equation above assumes a six-dimensional form in the current 3D case [$\Re_{aggre}(s,\ l,\ g,\ t)$ itself being a 3D integral]. This six-dimensional integral can be recast as a multiple of three double integrals, with each double integral accounting for one internal coordinate. This is possible because the three internal coordinates are mutually independent of each other. The solution to each of the separated double integrals is exactly the same as the ones derived for the 1D case. This simplification is another advantage of representing the population balance in terms of the volumes of solid, liquid, and gas in the granules, rather than in terms of the total particle size, binder content, and porosity.

The effectiveness of the technique has been further demonstrated by Pinto et al. [45] by solving higher-dimensional population balance models with breakage-division phenomena. The same authors [46] have extended the single-level discretization strategy to a multilevel discretization-based solution of multidimensional population balance models accounting for different fineness of discretization for the different rate processes of nucleation, growth, aggregation, and breakage as warranted by the particular rate process. Consequently, the computational efficiency has been significantly improved.

23.4.4 Solving Differential-Algebraic Equation Systems

Many of the previously mentioned numerical methods lead to large sets of differential equations coupled with sets of nonlinear algebraic equations. These are the so-called differential-algebraic equation (DAE) systems. A number of approaches are available to solve these equation sets, mainly based on implicit or semi-implicit methods such as the backward differentiation formulae (BDF) [41,47] or variants of Runge–Kutta methods [48,49].

The Mathworks package MATLAB also contains useful DAE solvers that are based primarily on implicit BDF formulae. Another widely used DAE solver, DASSL, uses BDF followed by the Newton method for updating the result through iterations [47]. Solution of these types of problems is generally straightforward. Some issues still remain in obtaining consistent initial conditions for the solution to commence and the solution of high-index problems.

23.4.5 MONTE CARLO METHODS

There is a long history in studies on the application of Monte Carlo methods to process engineering. The first serious research paper on a Monte Carlo treatment for systems involving population balances could be credited to Spielman and Levenspiel [50]. Since then, a significant number of publications have appeared in the literature on the resolution of PBEs using Monte Carlo methods [17]. Comprehensive Monte Carlo treatments are described in the literature [17,51]. Only selected issues on basic techniques will be addressed in this section.

23.4.5.1 Classification of Monte Carlo Methods

Monte Carlo methods can be used in two ways for engineering applications:

1. Direct evaluation of difficult functions. For example, the integral given by

$$I = \int_a^b f(x)dx \tag{23.54}$$

can be evaluated as

$$
\begin{aligned}
I &= E(Y) = E[(b-a)g(X)] = E[\bar{Y}(n)] \\
\bar{Y}(n) &= \cdots (b-a)\frac{\sum_{i=1}^n g(X_i)}{n}
\end{aligned}
\tag{23.55}
$$

where $X_1, X_2, \ldots, X_n$ are random variables defined in the closed interval $[a, b]$, and $E(Y)$ denotes the mathematical estimation of function Y.
2. Artificial realization of the system behavior [17]. This method is commonly applied to complex particulate processes, which will be described in some detail in the current section. In the artificial realization, the direct evaluation of integral and differential functions is replaced by the simulation of the stochastic behavior modeled by using a randomness generator to vary the behavior of the system [51]. It will be shown later that the important probabilistic functions in the original model equations, such as coalescence kernels for granulation processes, are still essential in Monte Carlo simulations.

Monte Carlo methods for the artificial realization of the system behavior can be divided into time-driven and event-driven Monte Carlo simulations. In the former approach, the time interval Δt is chosen, and the realization of events within this time interval is determined stochastically. In the latter case, the time interval between two events is determined on the basis of rates of processes. In general, the coalescence rates in granulation processes can be extracted from the coalescence kernel models. The event-driven Monte Carlo can be further divided into constant volume methods in which the total volume of particles is conserved and constant number method in which the total number of particles in the simulation remains constant. The main advantage of the constant number method for granulation processes is that the population remains large enough for accurate Monte Carlo simulations [52,53]. An additional advantage associated with the constant number methods is its ability to reduce the renumbering effort. Consequently, the constant number method is recommended and will be further explained.

23.4.5.2 Key Equations for Constant Number Monte Carlo Simulation

Key equations needed in Monte Carlo simulations include the interevent time Δt_q representing the time spent from $q-1$ to q Monte Carlo steps, coalescence kernel K_{ij}, normalized probability p_{ij} for a successful collision between particles i and j, and a number of intermediate variables. The coalescence kernel can be divided into particle property-independent part K_c and -dependent part $k_{ij}(X_i, X_j)$ as follows:

$$K_{ij} = K_c k_{ij}\left(\mathbf{X}_i, \mathbf{X}_j\right)$$
$$i, j = 1, 2, \cdots, N \tag{23.56}$$

where X denotes the vector of internal coordinates representing particle properties, such as size and moisture content, and N is the total number in the simulation system. It can be seen that Eq. (23.56) is similar to the coalescence kernel given by $\beta_{ij} = \beta_0 k_{ij}(v_i, v_j)$ described in the previous sections for 1D systems. However, it should be pointed out that i and j in Eq. (23.56) are used to identify the individual particles, whereas that in β_{ij}, $i, j = 1, 2 \ldots i_{max}$ are size classes rather than particle identity numbers. In order to avoid confusion, β_{ij} and β_0 are replaced by K_{ij} and K_c, respectively, in Monte Carlo simulations. The normalized probability for successful collision is given by

$$p_{ij} = \frac{k_{ij}}{k_{max}} \tag{23.57}$$

where k_{max} is the maximum value of the coalescence kernel among all particles. The final result of the interevent time is given by

$$\Delta t_q = \frac{2\tau_c}{\langle k_{ij} \rangle} \frac{1}{N}\left(\frac{N}{N-1}\right)^q \tag{23.58}$$

with

$$\tau_c = \frac{1}{K_c C_0} \tag{23.59}$$

and

$$\langle k_{ij} \rangle = \frac{\sum_{i=1}^{N} \sum_{j=1, i \neq j}^{N} k_{ij}}{N(N-1)} \tag{23.60}$$

In Eq. (23.59), C_0 is the total number concentration at $t = 0$ defined by $C_0 = N/V_0$, where V_0 is the volume of particles at the initial time. We have only presented the final results of needed equations here. The interested readers are referred to Smith and Matsoukas [52] for detailed mathematical derivations.

23.4.5.3 Simulation Procedure

The simulation procedure for the constant number Monte Carlo method applied to coalescence processes consists of the following key steps:

1. Initialization of the simulation system. This includes the determination of sample size (normally 10,000–20,000 particles) followed by assigning the identity number and properties to each particle. The properties must satisfy the initial property distributions, such as particle size and moisture distributions. Set $t_0 = 0$ and $q = 1$.

2. Acceptance or rejection of coalescence. In this step, two particles, i and j, are randomly selected, and the coalescence kernel k_{ij} with normalized probability p_{ij} given by Eq. (23.57) are computed, followed by the generation of a random probability p_{rq}. If $p_{ij} < p_{rq}$, the coalescence is rejected, and a new pair of particles is selected again to repeat the calculation until $p_{ij} > p_{rq}$, which implies a successful coalescence. When the coalescence is successful, the new agglomerated particle holds the identity number i, and another particle randomly selected from the rest of the system is copied as particle j and goes to step 3.

3. Computation of the interevent time. The interevent time for step q is computed using Eqs. (23.58)–(23.60). Total operational time is given by

$$t = t_0 + \sum_{m=1}^{q} \Delta t_m \tag{23.61}$$

Set $q = q + 1$ and return to step 2.

4. Simulation termination and result validation. As t reaches the prespecified termination time t_f, check the acceptance of simulation results. If acceptable, stop the simulation; otherwise, modify model parameters and start a new simulation process.

It can be seen that the Monte Carlo methods are applicable to both 1D and multidimensional coalescence processes without any theoretical and algorithmic hurdles. However most reported results with good agreement with experimental data are limited to 1D systems, except that reported by Wauters [53]. This is mainly due to the lack of reliable multidimensional kernel models rather than the applicability of Monte Carlo methods.

23.5 APPLICATION OF POPULATION BALANCE MODELING

Process systems modeling and applications in granulation have been comprehensively reviewed by Cameron et al. [54] and Cameron and Wang [55]. In this section, we consider the application of population balances to regulatory and optimal control of batch and continuous granulation systems. Models can also be applied to parameter estimation, process and equipment design, state estimation, and fault diagnosis.

23.5.1 Modeling for Closed-Loop Control Purposes

23.5.1.1 Development of Control Relevant, Linear Models

Since the linear control theory and techniques are better developed and easier to implement than their nonlinear counterparts, it is highly desirable to use linear models for control purposes. In process engineering, the nonlinear models are frequently linearized around certain operating points. The linearization technique is described briefly in this subsection.

Let the general nonlinear system be described as:

$$\begin{cases} \frac{d\mathbf{x}}{dt} = f(\mathbf{x}, \mathbf{u}) \\ y = h(\mathbf{x}) \end{cases} \tag{23.62}$$

where $\mathbf{x} = [x_1 x_2 \cdots x_p]^T$, $y = [y_1 y_2 \cdots y_q]^T$, and $\mathbf{u} = [u_1 u_2 \cdots u_s]^T$ are vectors of state, output, and control variables, respectively, and $f = [f_1 f_2 \cdots f_p]^T$ and $h = [h_1 h_2 \cdots h_q]^T$ are vectors of smooth functions, in which p, q, and s are dimensions of the vectors of state, output, and control variables, respectively. In the PBEs given by Eqs. (23.36), (23.39), and (23.53), $\mathbf{x} = [n_1 n_2 \cdots n_p]$, $p = i_{\max}$. The conventional linearization method is based on the first-order Taylor series expansion around certain operational points. The resulting linear model is given by:

$$\frac{d\delta x}{dt} = A\delta x + B\delta u$$

$$\delta y = C\delta x$$

$$A = \left.\frac{\partial f(x, u)}{\partial x^T}\right|_{\substack{x = x_o, \\ u = u_o}} \quad B = \left.\frac{\partial f(x, u)}{\partial u^T}\right|_{\substack{x = x_o, \\ u = u_o}} \quad C = \left.\frac{\partial h(x)}{\partial x^T}\right|_{\substack{x = x_o, \\ u = u_o}}$$

(23.63)

In the control literature, the symbol δ in front of x, y, and u is normally omitted for simplicity. The readers should be aware that in the models developed by this approach, x, y, and u denote deviations from their respective values at the specified operational point rather than the real values. That is, the linearized model used in control studies is represented as

$$\frac{dx}{dt} = Ax + Bu$$

$$y = Cx$$

(23.64)

The discretized PBEs given by Eqs. (23.36), (23.39), and (23.53), and the BSD model described by Eq. (23.37) can be linearized to obtain the models with the format given by Eq. (23.64). The control variables are normally connected with the coalescence kernels [56].

Instead of directly (numerically) linearizing the plant model, the linear model represented by Eq. (23.64) can also be determined by a subspace model identification method, as theoretically described by Ljung [57] and applied to MPC of a granulation process by Sanders et al. [58]. A Toolbox for the use of MATLAB is available for the implementation of system identification described by Ljung [57,59].

It should be pointed out that linear models are only applicable to systems with small deviations from steady states. If the variations of operational conditions exceed acceptable ranges, a piecewise linearization technique should be used, leading to the development of multiple linear models [39]. The multiple linear model approach has been applied to advanced control of nonlinear processes by the authors using mini–max optimization techniques, in which a quantitative measure, namely gap metric, is used for the determination of local linear regimes [60].

23.5.1.2 ARX and ARMAX Models for Linear Model Predictive Control

For MPC purposes, there are two commonly used black box models: ARX model with auto-regressive (AR) part and extra (X) input, and ARMAX model with additional moving average (MA) part accounting for disturbances. The method for the development of ARX and ARMAX models is well explained by Ljung [57]. The single input, single output ARX is given by

$$y(t) + a_1 y(t - 1) + \cdots + a_{n_a} y(t - n_a) = b_1 u(t - 1) + \cdots + b_{n_b} u(t - n_b) + e(t) \quad (23.65)$$

and the ARMAX model is represented as

$$\begin{aligned} y(t) + a_1 y(t - 1) + \cdots + a_{n_a} y(t - n_a) \\ = b_1 u(t - 1) + \cdots + b_{n_b} u(t - n_b) + e(t) + c_1 e(t - 1) + \cdots + c_{n_c} e(t - n_c) \end{aligned}$$

(23.66)

In Eqs. (23.65) and (23.66), y is the output (controlled) variable; u is the input (manipulative) variable; e is the disturbance; a, b, and c are time-varying coefficients identified online; and n_a, n_b, and n_c are defined as prediction, control, and disturbance horizons. The matrix formats for multivariable ARX and ARMAX models are described by

$$\mathbf{A}(q)\mathbf{y}(t) = \mathbf{B}(q)\mathbf{u}(t) + \mathbf{e}(t) \quad \text{(ARX)} \tag{23.67}$$

and

$$\mathbf{A}(q)\mathbf{y}(t) = \mathbf{B}(q)\mathbf{u}(t) + \mathbf{C}(q)\mathbf{e}(t) \quad \text{(ARMAX)} \tag{23.68}$$

In Eqs. (23.67) and (23.68), matrices A, B, and C are defined as

$$\begin{aligned}
\mathbf{A}(q) &= \mathbf{I}_{n_y} + \mathbf{A}_1 q^{-1} + \cdots + \mathbf{A}_{n_a} q^{-n_a} \\
\mathbf{B}(q) &= \mathbf{B}_0 + \mathbf{B}_1 q^{-1} + \cdots + \mathbf{B}_{n_b} q^{-n_b} \\
\mathbf{C}(q) &= \mathbf{I}_{n_y} + \mathbf{C}_1 q^{-1} + \cdots + \mathbf{C}_{n_c} q^{-n_c}
\end{aligned} \tag{23.69}$$

where q^{-k} is the delay operator representing "delayed by k time intervals", for example,

$$\mathbf{A}(q)\mathbf{y}(t) = \mathbf{y}(t) + \mathbf{A}_1 \mathbf{y}(t-1) + \cdots + \mathbf{A}_{n_a} \mathbf{y}(t-n_a) \tag{23.70}$$

The compact format of ARX and ARMAX models given by Eqs. (23.67) and (23.68) can easily be converted into more intuitive, expanded format exemplified by Eq. (23.70). With input (u and e) and output (y) data, the matrices A, B, and C can be readily identified employing the System Identification Toolbox for Use with MATLAB [59]. An ARX model for a pan granulation process was developed by Adetayo et al. [61], with a successful application to effective control of the plant.

23.5.1.3 Linear Model Predictive Control

Linear, control relevant models developed from nonlinear granulation processes are used for MPC. The basic idea of linear MPC is to determine the control actions through the minimization of a cost (objective) function. The objective function normally consists of the deviations between computed and desired outputs, and operational costs. The solution may depend on the weighting functions selected in the objective function to account for the relative importance among various terms. The MATLAB "Model Predictive Control Toolbox 2" [62] can be used to design the MPC. Two successful attempts for control of two different nonlinear granulation processes using MPC have been reported by Sanders et al. [58] and Glaser et al. [63]. Both have shown how linear model-predictive controller can be applied on nonlinear granulation processes.

23.5.1.4 Nonlinear Model Predictive Control Structure

Nonlinear model predictive control (NMPC) schemes consist of simultaneous determinations of manipulative variables and uncertain parameters. In some cases, the open-loop dynamic optimization is carried out for the determination of desired trajectories (set-points). This integrated control strategy was developed by Miller and Rawlings [64] in a study on model identification and control for batch cooling crystallizers, in which the population balance described by partial differential equation was reduced to a low-dimensional model using method of moments. That is, the control objective was average size rather than size distribution in Miller and Rawlings' work. Detailed studies on modeling and MPC of PSD in emulsion copolymerization processes using population balance models have been carried out by Immanuel and Doyle III [65] and Crowley et al. [66]. The reported research results have shown that the NMPC schemes using PBEs should also be applicable to pharmaceutical granulation processes due to the similar model structure. The main limitation of the conventional NMPC schemes is the difficulty in the determination of the

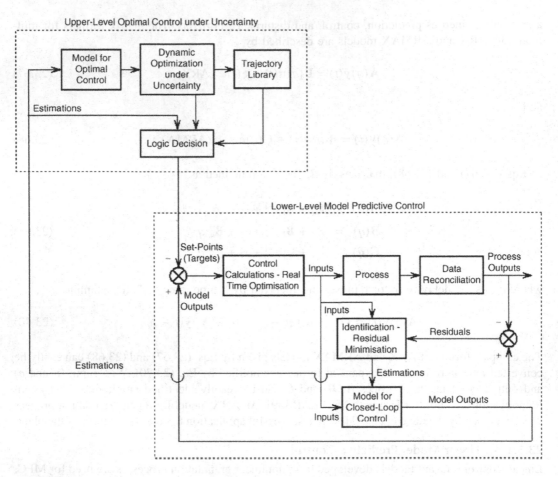

FIGURE 23.6   General structure of ML-NMPC using physically based models.

optimal set-points. In particular, the determination of the set-points under uncertainty remains as an unsolved problem. To fill this knowledge gap, a multilevel NMPC (ML-NMPC) scheme was proposed by Wang and Cameron [67] and Cameron and Wang [55]. The ML-NMPC scheme is shown in Figure 23.6, which depicts an integration of the modeling strategy originally proposed by Sanders et al. [68] with the model-based control scheme.

The upper-level optimal control employs dynamic optimization algorithm, which will be described in the section "Modeling for Optimal Design, Operation, and Open-Loop Optimal Control". The uncertainty issues can be addressed as follows. On the basis of the operational experience and simulation results, frequently encountered situations can be stored in the optimal control database. When online measurement data are available, the most suitable trajectories can be identified using logic rules. Since both control actions and uncertain parameters can be determined simultaneously using NMPC schemes based on dynamic optimizations, it is envisaged that the combination of upper-level optimal control with NMPC is scientifically justifiable. It can be seen from Figure 23.6 that two-way interactions between upper and lower control levels can be achieved for effective control of uncertain granulation processes.

A simulation study on ML-NMPC has been carried out by the authors with convincing results [67,69]. Since there exist measurement, information transfer, and computational delays, it could be more practical to implement the discrete-continuous scheme to handle the different time requirements for dynamic optimization and closed-loop control in industrial applications. That is, the closed-loop control system is operated continuously with the set-point corrections from dynamic optimization passed on to the lower-level control loop discretely. This can be defined as "near optimal" or "local optimal" strategy. Our early simulated study was carried out by Zhang et al. [56] to control an industrial scale fertilizer plant using a physically based model. The main limitation of the study was that the physically based population balance model was used to generate output data without real online measurements at that time. This implies that if a severe plant-model mismatch occurs, the proposed control strategy may fail. Further work has been reported by the authors with both simulation as well as measurement data [63]. The main limitation of the updated work is that we can only measure the product PSD using Opti-Sizer equipment without detailed information inside the granulator, which is required for the validation of the complete model.

23.5.1.5   Online Measurement-Based Control Schemes

In addition to model-based control schemes using PBEs, there are a number of practical control schemes in the pharmaceutical industry that do not rely on mathematical models. These include simple feedback control with or without feed-forward compensation, and fuzzy-logic control systems.

Simple feedback control with feed-forward compensation. One of the most important issues for the effective control of granulation processes is the development of fast and reliable measurement techniques for the characterization of particulate systems. Because of the difficulties associated with the direct measurement of particle characteristics, such as particle size distribution, moisture contents, and deformability, some indirect monitoring parameters have been adopted as the indicators of particle characteristics. A commonly accepted monitoring parameter in the pharmaceutical industry is the power consumption, which has been successfully used to control the particle size in high-shear mixers at the end-point [70,71]. On the basis of a series of investigations carried out by Leuenberger [70], the energy dissipated per unit volume in a high-shear mixer, dW/dV, can be approximately represented as

$$\frac{dW}{dV} = \mu \sigma_c K \propto \frac{1 - \varepsilon}{\varepsilon} \tag{23.71}$$

where W is the power consumption, V is the granulator volume, μ is the apparent coefficient of friction, σ_c is the cohesive stress, K is the dimensionless shear rate, and ε is the porosity of the powder mass. It is easy to show that the power consumption is related to the saturation level S defined as follows:

$$S = \frac{H(1 - \varepsilon)}{\varepsilon} \rho \tag{23.72}$$

where H is the mass ratio of liquids to solids and ρ is the density of the particle relative to the density of the liquid ($\rho = \rho_S/\rho_L$). Furthermore, Kristensen and Schaefer [72] pointed out that the saturation level defined by Eq. (23.72) could be related back to the average granule size. Consequently, the power consumption, the saturation level, and the granule particle size are interrelated, forming a technical basis to use power consumption as a monitoring parameter for the characterization of particles within the high-shear mixer. A detailed description of the control strategy using power consumption as the indicator of particle properties in high-shear mixers is also provided in Leuenberger [70].

Mort et al. pointed out that "with recent development in particle sizing technology, the agglomerate size distribution can be measured in-line at any number of points in the process" [73]. The main measurement technique is image analysis by mounting high-speed cameras and lighting systems in appropriate locations. Since the direct measurement data of particle sizes are available,

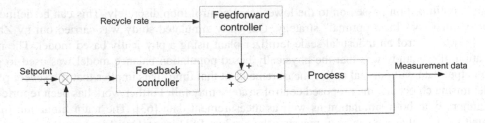

FIGURE 23.7 Simple feedback control scheme with feed-forward compensation.

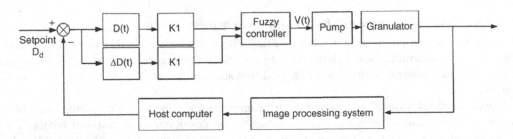

FIGURE 23.8 Block diagram of granule size control system.
Source: From Ref. [66].

the controller design can be based on these data without relying on the indirect indicators under the condition that the rate of binder addition is sufficiently slow to allow for image data to be collected, processed, and fed back. This concept has been used for batch granulation processes in fluidized beds. The same authors also proposed a feed-forward control strategy to compensate the fluctuation of the recycle rate. The simple feedback control with feed-forward compensation scheme is shown in Figure 23.7.

The measurement data in Figure 23.7 could be the indirect monitoring parameters [70], or the explicit PSD [65], depending on the relative speed of the measurement system and process dynamics.

Fuzzy-logic control of high-shear granulation. Watano et al. [74,75] developed a novel system to control granule growth in a high-shear mixer. The system basically consisted of image processing and a fuzzy controller as shown in Figure 23.8.

In Figure 23.8, $D(t)$ is the deviation between the desired value (D_d) and measured value (D_m) of granule size, and $\Delta D(t)$ denotes the change rate of measured values, which are mathematically represented as follows:

$$\begin{aligned} D(t) &= D_d - D_m(t) \\ \Delta D(t) &= D_m(t) - D_m(t-1) \end{aligned} \tag{23.73}$$

Other notations in Figure 23.8 are explained as follows. $V(t)$ is the result of fuzzy reasoning used to control the output power of the liquid feed pump; K_1 and K_2 represent gains of the input variables.

In the methodology developed by Watano et al. [74,75], four fuzzy variables were used, namely ZR (zero), PS (positive small), PM (positive medium), and PL (positive large). The values of $D(t)$, $\Delta D(t)$, and $V(t)$ were classified into these four categories. Ten rules were proposed to relate measured $D(t)$ and $\Delta D(t)$ with $V(t)$. Consequently, $V(t)$ can be quantified using the if–then statement. An example is given as follows:

If $D(t) = $ PS and $\Delta D(t) = $ PL, then $V(t) = $ ZR (rule 2 in Table 2 of Ref. 75).

In such a way, all the combinations of $D(t)$ and $\Delta D(t)$ can be connected with $V(t)$ for the effective control of the process. The technique can be considered as highly successful with the experimental justifications.

23.5.2 MODELING FOR OPTIMAL DESIGN, OPERATION, AND OPEN-LOOP OPTIMAL CONTROL

Process optimization and open-loop optimal control of batch and continuous drum-granulation processes are described in this section as another important application example of population balance modeling. Both steady-state and dynamic optimization studies are carried out, which consist of (i) construction of optimization and control relevant, population balance models through the incorporation of moisture content, drum rotation rate, and bed depth into the coalescence kernels; (ii) investigation of optimal operational conditions using constrained optimization techniques; and (iii) development of optimal control algorithms based on discretized PBEs.

The objective of steady-state (SS) optimization is to minimize the recycle rate with minimum cost for continuous processes. It has been identified that the drum rotation rate, bed depth (material charge), and moisture content of solids are practical decision (design) parameters for system optimization. The objective for the optimal control of batch granulation processes is to maximize the mass of product-sized particles with minimum time and binder consumption. The objective for the optimal control of the continuous process is to drive the process from one SS to another in a minimum time with minimum binder consumption, which is also known as the state-driving problem. It has been known for some time that the binder spray rate is the most effective control (manipulative) variable. Although other process variables, such as feed flow rate and additional powder flow rate, can also be used as manipulative variables, only the single-input problem with the binder spray rate as the manipulative variable is addressed here to demonstrate the methodology. It can be shown from simulation results that the proposed models are suitable for control and optimization studies, and the optimization algorithms connected with either SS or dynamic models are successful for the determination of optimal operational conditions and dynamic trajectories with good convergence properties.

It should be pointed out that only open-loop optimal control issues for granulation processes without uncertainty are addressed in this section. The integration of open-loop optimal control with closed-loop NMPC for uncertain processes has been reported elsewhere by the authors Wang and Cameron [67].

23.5.2.1 Statement of Optimization and Open-Loop Optimal Control Problems

A typical batch drum (e.g., pan) granulation process is schematically shown in Figure 23.9. There are two operational strategies: (i) premix the fine particles with the proper amount of liquid binder followed by the rotating operation until the desired size distribution is achieved; and (ii) simultaneous mixing and granulating by spraying liquid binder (and fine powders in some cases) on the moving surface of particles inside the rotating drum (pan). The first strategy involves system

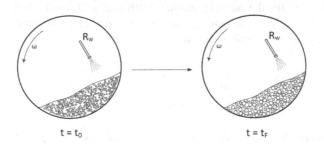

FIGURE 23.9 Schematic diagram of batch (e.g., pan) granulation.

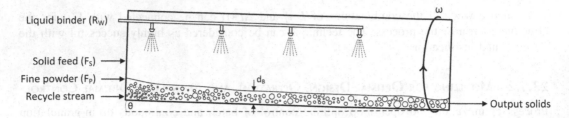

FIGURE 23.10 Schematic diagram of continuous rotating drum granulation.

optimization without any control action. The optimization problem can be stated as: to determine the optimal moisture content, initial size distribution, rotating rate (ω), and bed depth (drum charge) so that the desired size distribution can be obtained within a minimum time t_f. Optimal control techniques can be applied to the second strategy, which can be stated as follows: for the specified initial conditions, maximize the mass of product-sized particles in minimum time with minimum energy consumption by adjusting the manipulative variables, such as binder spray rate and drum-rotation speed. We will discuss the optimal control problem with the binder spray rate as the single manipulative variable in detail.

A slightly modified continuous drum-granulation process with an additional fine-powder stream is shown in Figure 23.10. As mentioned previously, the additional fine-powder stream is used to improve the controllability of the process, which is not seen in the conventional design. Our studies on continuous drum granulation include the steady-state optimization and optimal state driving from one steady state to another. The objective for steady-state optimization is to achieve minimum recycle rate with minimum cost through the determination of optimal operational conditions, such as rotating rate (ω), binder spray rate (R_W), feed flow rate (F_S), bed depth (d_B), and drum inclination angle (θ). The optimal state driving attempts to drive the system from one steady state to another in a minimum time with minimum energy consumption by adjusting the time-dependent manipulative variables, such as binder spray rate, feed flow rate, and optionally additional fine-powder flow rate (F_P).

23.5.2.2 Optimization and Open-Loop Optimal Control Equations

The optimization and open-loop optimal control equations consist of model equations and objective functions.

Optimization and control relevant model equations. The discretized PBE for batch system can be described as follows:

$$\frac{d}{dt}n_i = -\frac{\partial}{\partial L}(Gn_i) + B_i - D_i$$
$$i = 1, 2, \cdots, i_{\max}$$

(23.74)

where n_i, B_i, and D_i stand for the particle number, birth rate, and death rate in the ith size interval, respectively, $i = 1, 2,..., i_{\max}$, in which $i_{\max}$ is the total number of size intervals. Similarly, continuous processes can also be represented as

$$\frac{d}{dt}n_i = -\frac{\partial}{\partial L}(Gn_i) + B_i - D_i + F^{\text{in}}\frac{n_i^{\text{in}}}{n_t^{\text{in}}} - F^{\text{out}}\frac{n_i}{n_t}$$
$$i = 1, 2, \cdots, i_{\max}$$

(23.75)

where F is the number flow rate, the subscript t indicates the total value, and the superscripts identify the inlet and outlet streams. Using Hounslow's discretization methods, the relevant terms in the right-hand sides of Eqs. (23.74) and (23.75) are given by

$$B_i = n_{i-1} \sum_{j=1}^{i-2} \left(2^{j-i+1} \beta_{i-1,j} n_j \right) + \frac{i}{2} \beta_{i-1,i-1} n_{i-1}^2 \tag{23.76}$$

$$D_i = n_i \sum_{j=1}^{i-1} \left(2^{j-1} \beta_{i,j} n_j \right) - n_i \sum_{j=1}^{i_{\max}} \left(\beta_{i,j} n_j \right) \tag{23.77}$$

and

$$\frac{\partial G n_i}{\partial L} = -\frac{2G}{(1+r)L_i} \left(\frac{r}{r^2-1} n_{i-1} + n_i - \frac{r}{r^2-1} n_{i+1} \right)$$
$$r = \frac{L_{i+1}}{L_i} = \sqrt[3]{2} \tag{23.78}$$

where $\beta_{i,j}$ is equivalent to the representation $\beta(L_i, L_j)$. Consequently, an original PBE described by a partial differential–integral equation is converted into a set of ordinary differential equations. It is more convenient to convert the number-based PBEs described by Eqs. (23.74) to (23.78) to mass-based ones, which are demonstrated by the authors [69].

A control-relevant model was developed by Zhang et al. [56], in which the coalescence kernel is a function of the moisture content. In other developed kernel models reported by Balliu [76] and Wang et al. [69], in addition to moisture content, the bed depth and drum speed are also incorporated. Two kernel models, namely size-independent kernel and size-dependent kernel, are used in optimization and control simulations. The size-independent kernel is given by

$$\beta_{i,j} = \beta_0 = a_0 \cdot \left[(x_m)^{n_1} e^{-a_1 x_m} \right] \cdot \left[(B_d)^{n_2} e^{-a_2 B_d} \right] \cdot \left(S_d^{n_3} e^{-a_3 S_d} \right) \tag{23.79}$$

where x_m is the moisture content in particles, B_d is the bed depth, S_d is the drum-rotating rate, and $a_0 - a_3$ and $n_1 - n_3$ are constants determined through parameter identification techniques based on the measurement data. The size-dependent kernel is represented as [16]:

$$\beta_{i,j} = \beta_0 \frac{\left(L_i + L_j \right)^2}{L_i L_j} \tag{23.80}$$

where β_0 is also defined in Eq. (23.79).

Since the main mechanism determining the growth rate G in Eqs. (23.74) and (23.75) is layering of the fine powders on the surface of particles, it can be deduced that the growth rate is a strong function of the powder fraction and moisture content. The following correlation is used to calculate the growth rate:

$$G = G_m \cdot \frac{M_{\text{powder}}}{k \cdot \sum M_i + M_{\text{powder}}} \cdot \exp[-a(x_w - x_{wc})^2] \tag{23.81}$$

where G_m is the maximum growth rate, M_{powder} is the mass of fine powder below the lower bound of the particle classes, M_i is the mass of particles in the ith size class, x_{wc} is the critical moisture, and k and a are fitting parameters. Studies on powder mass balance lead to the following equation for batch processes:

$$\frac{dM_{\text{powder}}}{dt} = F_{\text{powder}}^{\text{in}} - 3G \int_0^\infty \frac{M(L)}{L} dL \tag{23.82}$$

and the following equation for continuous processes:

$$\frac{dM_{\text{powder}}}{dt} = F_{\text{powder}}^{\text{in}} - \frac{M_{\text{powder}}}{t_R} - 3G \int_0^\infty \frac{M(L)}{L} dL \tag{23.83}$$

where $F_{\text{powder}}^{\text{in}}$ represents the flow rate of additional powder stream in both batch and continuous cases. It can be used as an additional manipulative variable.

The liquid mass balance for batch processes is given by

$$\frac{dx_w}{dt} = \frac{1}{M_t} R_w \tag{23.84}$$

where M_t is the total mass of solids in the drum and R_w is the binder spray rate. Similarly, we can develop the liquid mass balance for the continuous process as

$$\frac{dx_w}{dt} = \frac{1}{M_t} [F_M^{\text{in}} x_w^{\text{in}} - F_M x_w + R_w] \tag{23.85}$$

where F_M^{in} and F_M are inlet and outlet mass flow rates, respectively, and x_w^{in} is the moisture content in the feed solids.

In summary, the equations in the control relevant model for batch systems are discretized PBEs given by Eq. (23.74), powder dynamics described by Eq. (23.82), and liquid dynamics represented by Eq. (23.84). The corresponding equations for continuous processes are Eqs. (23.75), (23.83), and (23.85). Both cases share the same kernel models given by Eqs. (23.79) and (23.80), and growth-rate model described by Eq. (23.81).

Objective functions for system optimization and open-loop optimal control. The objective function for system optimization of batch granulation is:

$$\underset{S_d, B_d, x_w}{\text{Minimize}} \left\{ J = \frac{-w_1 M_p(t_f)}{t_f} \right\} \tag{23.86}$$

Subject to equation (23.74)

The objective function for batch granulation with the binder spray rate as the only manipulative variable is given by:

$$\underset{R_w}{\text{Minimize}} \left\{ \frac{-w_1 M_p(t_f) + w_2 \int_0^{t_f} R_w dt}{t_f} \right\} \tag{23.87}$$

Subject to equations (23.74), (23.82), and (23.84)

In Eqs. (23.86) and (23.87), M_p is the mass of product-sized particles, and w_1 and w_2 are weighting functions.

The objective function for steady-state optimization of continuous granulation is:

$$\underset{S_d, B_d, F^{in}, R_w}{\text{Minimize}} \left\{ -w_1 F_p + w_2 R_w \right\} \tag{23.88}$$

Subject to equations (23.75), (23.83) and (23.85) and zero derivatives at final time

where F_p is the mass flow rate of product-sized particles.

For the state-driving study, we carry out steady-state (SS) optimizations for two different product specifications: the product range for SS1 is 2.0 to 3.2 mm, whereas that for steady state 2 (SS2) is 3.2 to 5.0 mm. The objective function for this optimal state-driving problem is described as

$$\underset{R_w}{\text{Minimize}} \left\{ J = \Sigma \left[w_{1,i} \left(M_i(t_f) - M_i^{SS2} \right)^2 \right] + w_2 \int_0^{t_f} R_w \, dt + w_3 t_f \right\} \tag{23.89}$$

Subject to equations (23.75), (23.83) and (23.85) and zero derivatives at final time

where $M_i(t_f)$ and M_i^{SS2} denote the mass of particles in the ith size interval at the final time and for SS2, respectively.

23.5.2.3 Dynamic Optimization Algorithm

It is not difficult to solve the steady-state optimization problems with constraints represented by algebraic equations by using commercial software packages. We mainly explain the dynamic optimization methods used in this work. The basic structure of the algorithm employed is shown in Figure 23.11.

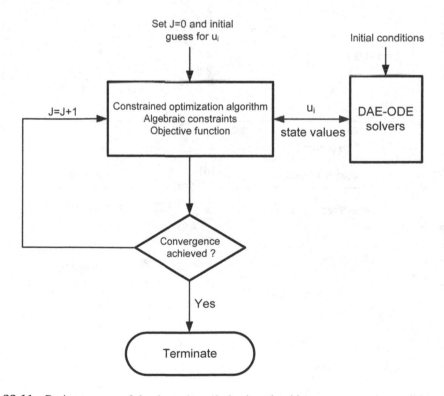

FIGURE 23.11   Basic structure of the dynamic optimization algorithm.

In the dynamic optimization algorithm depicted in Figure 23.11, a control parameterization technique [77] is used to discretize the originally continuous control variables. That is, a manipulative variable $u(t)$ is represented by a set of piecewise constants, u_i, $i = 1, 2,..., q$. These constants are treated as parameters to be determined by using dynamic optimization algorithms.

Since the MATLAB software packages with Optimization Toolbox provide both effective ordinary differential equation (ODE) solvers as well as powerful optimization algorithms, the dynamic simulations reported in this paper are carried out by using the MATLAB Optimization Toolbox [78].

23.5.2.4   Selected Simulation Results and Discussion

Simulations for both batch and continuous granulation processes are based on a pilot plant drum granulator with the following parameters: length = 2 m, diameter = 0.3 m, nominal hold up = 40 kg, rotation rate = 25 to 40 rpm, retention time range = 6 to 10 minutes. Other process parameters are available in the paper by Wang et al. [69].

The simulated optimal profiles for the batch processes are shown in Figure 23.12(a)–(c) with two data sets with and without constraints on control action. The control constraints restrict lower and upper bounds on the control variables (lower bound = 0 kg/sec, upper bound = 0. 015 kg/sec), as well as the gradient of the control actions ($|dR_w/dt| \leq 0.0003$ kg/sec^2). It can be seen from Figure 23.12(d) that if the normal constraints on the control variable are replaced by a high upper bound of control variable (0.036 kg/sec) as the only constraint, very high spray rates at the early

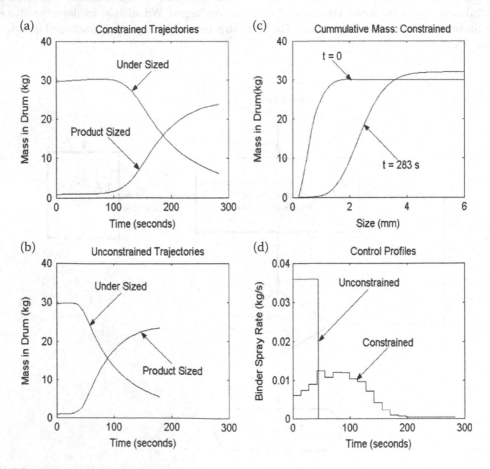

FIGURE 23.12   Optimal control of batch drum granulation.

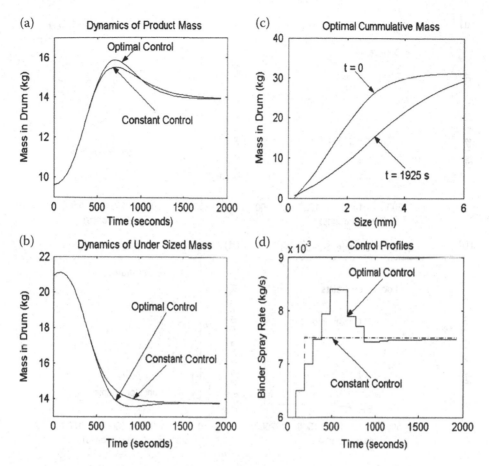

FIGURE 23.13 Optimal control of continuous drum granulation.

operating stage with very short spray time leads to the minimum objective function given by Eq. (23.87). However, if the normal constraints are activated, the control variable moves smoothly rather than suddenly with the price of a longer operational time. The difference between final times in the two cases is about 104 seconds (283–179 seconds), which is quite significant. The results clearly have implications on equipment design and specifications that could allow the constraints to be moved out, thus approaching the best operating policy.

Through steady-state optimizations using the objective function described by Eq. (23.88), optimal binder spray rates for two different specifications on product size ranges are obtained. These are $R_w = 0.050$ kg/sec for 2.0 to 3.2 mm as the product size range, and $R_w = 0.075$ kg/sec for 3.2 to 5.0 mm as the product size range. Figure 23.13(a), (b) show the profiles using an optimal control policy and a constant spray rate policy. The change of the cumulative mass between initial and final times under optimal control policy is shown in Figure 23.13(c). The control profiles are depicted in Figure 23.13(d). The optimal control policy leads to about 50% reduction on the objective function given by Eq. (23.89). The optimal spray policy can be stated as follows: "Gradually increase the spray rate from the first steady state (0.005 kg/sec) to achieve a relatively high spray rate (0.0084 kg/sec) followed by gradual reduction of the spray rate until the spray rate of the second SS value (0.0075 kg/ sec) is reached, which will be maintained for the rest of the operational period".

From Figure 23.13, the significance of optimal control studies can be demonstrated by observing the fact that the optimal profiles approach the second steady state faster, and the optimal control strategy is easy to implement with smooth movement. It should be pointed out that the

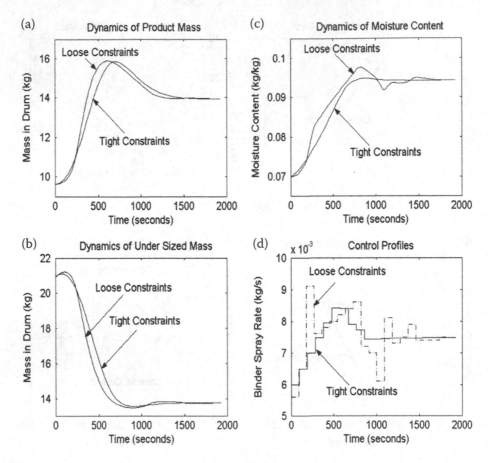

FIGURE 23.14 Effects of constraint tightness on optimal control of drum granulation.

small difference between two control policies shown in Figure 23.13 is due to little difference between two product specifications (product ranges from 2.0–3.2 mm to 3.2–5.0 mm). It can be predicted that if the two steady states are far away from each other, profound economic benefit can be achieved. Optimal control strategies are also particularly important to plant startup and shutdown operations.

Figure 23.14 shows the dynamic profiles of optimal state driving from SS1 to SS2 with different levels of constraints. Dynamic changes of product mass, undersized mass, and moisture content are shown in Figure 23.14(a)–(c), respectively, under two constraint levels. Figure 23.14(d) depicts control profiles for these two cases. In addition to the constraints on control actions, the final time constraints ensure the final SS status is imposed on the system. That is, the left-hand sides of Eqs. (23.75), (23.83), and (23.85) should be zero at the final time. However, it is not necessary to achieve zero exactly for the derivatives at the final time. We normally impose the final time constraints as $|dx(t_f)/dt| < \varepsilon$ in which x represents general state variables such as number of particles, mass of powder, and moisture content, and ε is a very small positive number for practical applications with the value depending on the tightness of constraints. The ε values are chosen as 10^{-6} and 10^{-3} for tight and loose constraints indicated in Figure 23.14, respectively.

It can be shown from Figure 23.14 that the control strategy with loose constraints leads to shorter operational time than that with tight constraints (1827 seconds vs. 1925 seconds). However, the moisture dynamics shows severe offset and oscillation. In optimization simulations, only final time constraints are changed for the two cases. It is interesting to note that the program with tight constraints leads to small and smooth controller movements even though the constraints on the control variable are not altered explicitly. It seems that the loose constraints allow too much manipulative variation that drives the system into a region ($x_w \approx 0.1$) where moisture variations have significant impact on the granulation performance. A marginal benefit identified by 5% time reduction is achievable using loose constraints with a price of process oscillations. Consequently, a control strategy with tight final time constraints is superior to that with loose constraints in this particular application.

Through an analysis on the simulation results, the following conclusions can be drawn.

1. Population balance modeling provides an important basis for optimal design and operations for both batch and continuous granulation processes.
2. The effects of liquid content, bed depth, and drum rotation rate on the coalescence behavior can be quantified through the development of new kernel models, with the structure described by Eqs. (23.79) and (23.80). The simulation results are qualitatively consistent with industrial experience in large-scale fertilizer production.
3. An optimal control strategy and algorithm using commercial optimization software packages connected to reliable DAE/ODE solvers are successful for the determination of optimal trajectories with good convergence properties. This implies that under certain conditions, the more complicated optimal control algorithms, such as that based on the well-known Pontryagin's maximum principle, could be avoided.
4. Since startup and shutdown operations are frequently encountered in granulation plants with huge financial impacts, studies on optimal control strategies can lead to significant economic benefits.

23.5.3 Sensitivity and Reliability Analysis

23.5.3.1 Sensitivity Analysis for Application of Multidimensional Models

A multidimensional PBM is applied to a pharmaceutical process by Shirazian et al. [79], in which microcrystalline cellulose is granulated in the twin-screw wet granulator (TSWG) with water as the binder. The internal coordinates are particle size and liquid content, and the external coordinate is the axial distance in the 2D PBM. Through an analysis of the experimental and simulation results, it can be seen that the model is robust for the prediction of the liquid distribution as a function of particle size. An important conclusion can be drawn that increasing screw speed and decreasing liquid to solid ratio (L/S) lead to more uniform liquid distribution. This conclusion indicates that the 2D PBM is useful for the granulator design. However, the results also show that liquid distribution is not very sensitive to the size variations with less than 15% deviations from the average moisture content in a broad size range. In other granulation processes using continuous or pulse spraying schemes, such as drum and fluidized-bed granulators, the liquid distribution is more significantly affected by the spray rate and method, particle location, and solid flow patterns rather than particle size. Consequently, we are of the opinion that in the simultaneous wetting and granulation processes without pre-wetting zone, applicability of 2D PBM should be further investigated. It could be more efficient to use 1D PBM coupled with moisture transport models such as the one described by Eq. (23.84) for batch and Eq. (23.85) for continuous process, respectively, in this chapter.

23.5.3.2 Reliability Analysis for Model Failure Diagnosis

Causes leading to failure in models as well as product quality are shown in an Ishikawa Fishbone Diagram depicted in Figure 23.15. Most parts of the figure are self-explanatory, and a few important points are stressed here based on our experiences. First of all, we would point out that there exists a disturbance amplification effect in continuous granulation processes with recycle streams.

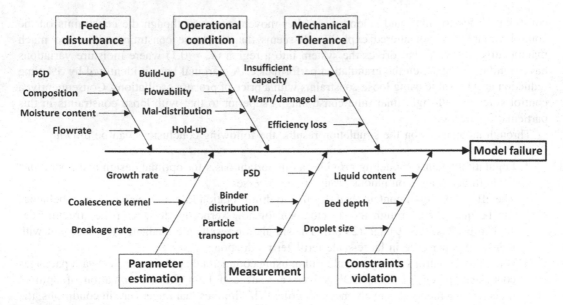

FIGURE 23.15   Ishikawa Fishbone diagram to track down model failure.

A minor disturbance in feed or operational conditions can lead to a major deviation in the output stream after a few recycles of the material. A typical example is that if the ratio of the difficult-to-agglomerate sized mass, such as "pin head" particles, is too high in the feed or recycle stream, this ratio will become increasingly higher in circuit operations without returning to the set-point. To model the disturbance amplification effect is still a challenging topic in granulation fields. Second, the PBM will become invalid with the violation of some constraints, which are defined as "hard constraints". Examples of hard constraints include moisture content, equipment hold-up, and ratio of difficult-to-agglomerate particles. Third, PBMs are developed based on specified solid flow patterns. Consequently, the development of hybrid models has become an important research area.

23.6   SUMMARY

It has long been realized that granulation is a very important process in pharmaceutical field as reviewed by Kristensen and Schaefer [72]. Granulation modeling is an area of design and operational importance. It continues to grow in importance and particularly so as companies push down the Industry 4.0 and Digitalization routes. Modeling practice is dominated by the population balance approach for developing mechanistic models. However, it requires an improved understanding of the key factors involved in particle nucleation, growth, coalescence, and breakage. It can be seen that much has been achieved over the last two decades through a comparison between the current article and the early review paper published by the authors in 2002 [80]. Also, the growing importance of particulate flow patterns is being addressed through approaches such as discrete element methods (DEM) and computational fluid dynamics (CFD) through the development of hybrid models, which will hopefully provide a microscale view of particle motions in the granulation device. The challenge is in addressing the multiscale nature of granulation modeling that spans the particle interactions length and timescales to individual plant equipment at the mesoscale and then up to macro-scale considerations of complete process operations.

The development of empirically based models has provided a simple means of quickly addressing a number of control-related applications. This will continue to be a useful approach for such problems.

Application of models to design, advanced control, and diagnosis will require mechanistic models that continue to incorporate the latest understanding of the underlying mechanisms. A number of mechanistic kernels have been reported in the literature and reviewed in this article. An integration of studies on granulation mechanisms, modeling, design of experiments (DoE), and risk analysis has been implemented in the pharmaceutical field through the Quality-by-Design (QbD) campaign, which can be classified as an area of process systems engineering.

The continued emphasis on Industry 4.0 initiatives with the intimate linking of physical and cyber assets, along with enhanced Digitalization activities, will only further drive the importance of an ecosystem of models that are used in real-time for operational decisions, process diagnostics, and risk management [81].

Much work is currently underway in these areas, and the incorporation into existing models of new insights will help extend the applicability of process models for granulation, thereby providing better design and increased performance across many industry sectors.

REFERENCES

1. Michaels JN. Toward rational design of powder processes. Powder Technol 2003; 138:1–6.
2. Litster JD. Scale-up of wet granulation processes: science not art. Powder Technol 2003; 130:5–40.
3. Hangos KM, Cameron IT. Process Modelling and Model Analysis. London: Academic Press, 2001, ISBN 0-12-156931-4.
4. Parikh DM. How to Optimize Fluid Bed Processing Technology. 1st ed. London: Academic Press, 2017, ISBN 978-0-12-804727-9.
5. Thapa P, Tripathi J, Jeong SH. Recent trend and future perspective of pharmaceutical wet granulation for better process understanding and development. Powder Technol 2019; 344:864–882.
6. Narang AS, Badawy SIF. Handbook of Pharmaceutical Wet Granulation: Theory and Practice in a Quality by Design Paradigm. USA: Elsevier, 2019, ISBN 978-0-12-810460-6.
7. Kayrak-Talay D, Dale S, Wassgren C, et al. Quality by design for wet granulation in pharmaceutical processing: assessing models for a priori design and scaling. Powder Technol 2013; 240:7–18.
8. Gantt JA, Cameron IT, Litster JD, et al. Determination of coalescence kernels for high-shear granulation using DEM simulations. Powder Technol 2006; 170:53–63.
9. Iveson SM, Litster JD, Hapgood K, et al. Nucleation, growth and breakage phenomena in agitated wet granulation processes: a review. Powder Technol 2001; 117:3–39.
10. Poon JM-H, Immanuel CD, Doyle III FJ, et al. A three-dimensional population balance model of granulation with a mechanistic representation of the nucleation and aggregation phenomena. Chem Eng Sci 2008; 63:1315–1329.
11. Hounslow MJ, Ryall RL, Marshall VR. A discrete population balance for nucleation, growth and aggregation. AIChE J 1988; 34(11):1821–1832.
12. Immanuel CD, Doyle III FJ. Computationally-efficient solution of population balance models incorporating nucleation, growth and coagulation. Chem Eng Sci 2003; 58(16):3681–3698.
13. Yekeler M, Ozkan A. Determination of the breakage and wetting parameters of calcite and their correlations. Part Syst Charact 2002; 19:419–425.
14. Salman AD, Fu J, Gorham DA, et al. Impact breakage of fertilizer granules. Powder Technol 2002; 130:359–366.
15. van den Dries K, de Vegt O, Girard V, et al. Granule breakage phenomena in a high shear mixer: influence of process and formulation variables and consequences on granule homogeneity. Powder Technol 2003; 130:228–236.
16. Randolph AD, Larson MA. Theory of Particulate Processes: Analysis and Techniques of Continuous Crystallization. 2nd ed. San Diego: Academic Press, 1988.
17. Ramkrishna D. Population Balances: Theory and Applications to Particulate Systems in Engineering. San Diego: Academic Press, 2000.
18. Liu LX, Litster JD, Iveson SM, et al. Coalescence of deformable granules in wet granulation processes. AIChE J 2000; 46(3):529–539.
19. Liu LX, Litster JD. Population balance modelling of granulation with a physically based coalescence kernel. Chem Eng Sci 2002; 57:2183–2191.

20. Ennis BJ, Litster JD. Size enlargement. In: Perry RH, Green DW, eds. Perry's Chemical Engineering Handbook. 7th ed. New York: McGraw-Hill, 1997.
21. Friedlander SK. Smoke, Dust and Haze. 1st ed. New York: Wiley, 1977; 2nd ed., New York: Oxford University Press, 2000.
22. Kapur PC, Fuerstenau DW. Coalescence model for granulation. Ind Eng Chem Proc Des Dev 1969; 8:56–62.
23. Kapur PC. Kinetics of granulation by non-random coalescence mechanism. Chem Eng Sci 1972; 27:1863–1869.
24. Sastry KVS. Similarity size distribution of agglomerates during their growth by coalescence in granulation or green pelletization. Int J Miner Process 1975; 2:187–203.
25. Golovin AM. The solution of coagulation equation for raindrops, taking condensation into account. Soviet Physics Dokl 1963; 8:191–193.
26. Adetayo AA, Litster JD, Pratsinis SE, et al. Population balance modelling of drum granulation of materials with wide size distribution. Powder Technol 1995; 82:37–49.
27. Adetayo AA, Ennis BJ. A unifying approach to modelling granulation processes coalescence mechanisms. AIChE J 1997; 43(1):927–934.
28. Immanuel CD, Doyle III FJ. Solution technique for multi-dimensional population balance model describing granulation processes. Powder Technol 2005; 156:213–225.
29. Ennis BJ, Tardos G, Pfeffer R. A microlevel-based characterization of granulation phenomena. Powder Technol 2001; 65:257–272.
30. Iveson SM. Limitations of one-dimensional population balance models of wet granulation processes. Powder Technol 2002; 124:219–229.
31. Immanuel CD, Cordeiro CF, Sundaram SS, et al. Population balance PSD model for emulsion polymerization with steric stabilizers. AIChE J 2003; 49(6):1392–1404.
32. Poon JM-H, Ramachandran R, Sanders CFW, et al. Experimental validation studies on a multi-dimensional and multi-scale population balance model of batch granulation. Chem Eng Sci 2009; 64:775–786.
33. Ramachandran R, Poon JM-H, Sanders CFW, et al. Experimental studies on distributions of granule size, binder content and porosity in batch drum granulation: inferences on process modeling requirements and process sensitivities. Powder Technol 2008; 188:89–101.
34. Verkoeijen D, Pouw GA, Meesters GMH, et al. Population balances for particulate processes—a volume approach. Chem Eng Sci 2002; 57:2287–2303.
35. Biggs CA, Sanders C, Scott AC, et al. Coupling granule properties and granulation rates in high-shear granulation. Powder Technol 2003; 130:162–168.
36. Robertson GA, Cameron IT. Analysis of dynamic process models for structural insight and model reduction. Part 1. Structural identification measures. Comput Chem Eng 1997; 21(5):455–473.
37. Shirazian S, Darwish S, Kuhs M, Crocker DM, Walker GM. Regime-separated approach for population balance modeling of continuous wet granulation of pharmaceutical formulation. Powder Technol 2018; 325;420–428.
38. Liu H, Li M. Two-compartment population balance modeling of a pulsed spray fluidized bed granulation based on computational fluid dynamics (CFD) analysis. Int J Pharm 2014; 475: 256–269.
39. Wang FY, Cameron IT. A multi-form modelling approach to the dynamics and control of drum granulation processes. Powder Technol 2007; 179:1–11.
40. Kumar S, Ramkrishna D. On the solution of population balance equations by discretization. I: a fixed pivot technique. Chem Eng Sci 1996; 51(8):1311–1332.
41. Liu Y, Cameron IT, Wang FY. The wavelet collocation method for transient problems with steep gradients. Chem Eng Sci 2000; 55:1729–1734.
42. Bertoluzza S. A wavelet collocation method for the numerical solution of partial differential equations. Appl Comput Harmonic Anal 1996; 3:1–9.
43. Liu Y, Cameron IT. A new wavelet-based method for the solution of the population balance equation. Chem Eng Sci 2001; 56:5283–5294.
44. Liu Y, Cameron IT. A new wavelet-based adaptive method for solving population balance equations. Powder Technol 2003; 130: 181–188.
45. Pinto MA, Immanuel CD, Doyle III FJ. A feasible solution technique for higher-dimensional population balance models. Comput Chem Eng 2007; 31:1242–1256.
46. Pinto MA, Immanuel CD, Doyle III FJ. A two level discretisation algorithm for the effective solution of higher-dimensional population balance models. Chem Eng Sci 2008; 63:1304–1314.

47. Petzold L. A description of DASSL: a differential-algebraic system solver. Proc IMACS World Congress, Montreal, Canada, 1982.
48. Cameron IT. Solution of differential-algebraic systems using diagonally implicit Runge-Kutta methods. IMA J Numer Anal 1983; 3:273–289.
49. Williams R, Burrage K, Cameron IT, et al. A four-stage index 2 diagonally implicit Runge-Kutta method. Appl Numer Math 2002; 40:415–432.
50. Spielman LA, Levenspiel O. A Monte Carlo treatment for reaction and coalescing dispersed systems. Chem Eng Sci 1965; 20:247.
51. Kaye BH. Powder Mixing. London: Chapman & Hall, 1997.
52. Smith M, Matsoukas T. Constant number Monte Carlo simulation of population balances. Chem Eng Sci 1998; 53(9):1777–1786.
53. Wauters PAL. Modelling and Mechanisms of Granulation. PhD thesis, The Delft University of Technology, The Netherlands, 2001.
54. Cameron IT, Wang FY, Immanuel CD et al. Process systems modelling and applications in granulation: a review. Chem Eng Sci 2005; 60:3723–3750.
55. Cameron IT, Wang FY. Process systems engineering applied to granulation. In: Agba S, Michael H, Jonathan S, eds. Handbook of Powder Technology. Amsterdam: Elsevier BV, 2006:499–552.
56. Zhang J, Lister JD, Wang FY, et al. Evaluation of control strategies for fertiliser granulation circuits using dynamic simulation. Powder Technol 2000; 108:122–129.
57. Ljung L. System Identification: Theory for the User. Upper Saddle River, NJ: Prentice Hall, 1987.
58. Sanders CFW, Hounslow MJ, Doyle III FJ. Identification of models for control of wet granulation. Powder Technol 2009; 188:255–263.
59. Ljung L. System Identification Toolbox for Use with MATLAB. Natick, MA: The Math Works, 2000.
60. Wang FY, Bahri PA, Lee PL, et al. A multiple model, state feedback strategy for robust control of nonlinear processes. Comput Chem Eng 2007; 31:410–418.
61. Adetayo AA, Pottman M, Ogunnaike B. Effective control of a continuous granulation process. Proceedings of the Control of Particulate Processes IV, 23–28, Engineering Foundation, New York, 1997.
62. Bemporad A, Morari M, Ricker NL. Model Predictive Control Toolbox 2 User Guide. MATLAB R2007a Version 7.4.0.287 (R2007a), 2007.
63. Glaser T, Sanders CF, Wang FY, et al. Model predictive control of continuous drum granulation. J Process Control 2009; 19:615–622.
64. Miller SM, Rawlings JB. Model identification and control strategies for batch cooling crystallisers. AIChE J 1994; 40(8):1312–1326.
65. Immanuel CD, Doyle III FJ. Hierarchical multiobjective strategy for particle-size distribution control. AIChE J 2003; 49(9):2383–2399.
66. Crowley TJ, Meadows ES, Kostoulas A, et al. Control of particle size distribution described by a population balance model of semi-batch emulsion polymerisation. J Process Control 2000; 10:419–432.
67. Wang FY, Cameron IT. Multi-level optimal control of particulate process with on-line identification. The 7th World Congress of Chemical Engineering (WCCE7), Glasgow, Scotland, July 10–14, 2005.
68. Sanders CFW, Willemse AW, Salman AD, et al. Development of a predictive high-shear granulation model. Powder Technol 2003; 138:18–24.
69. Wang FY, Ge X, Balliu N, et al. Optimal control and operation of drum granulation processes. Chem Eng Sci 2006; 61:257–267.
70. Leuenberger H. Moist agglomeration of pharmaceutical processes. In: Chulia D, Deleuil M, Pourcelot Y, eds. Powder Technology and Pharmaceutical Processes, Handbook of Powder Technology. Vol. 9. Amsterdam: Elsevier, 1994:337–389.
71. Faure A, York P, Rowe RC. Process control and scale-up of pharmaceutical wet granulation processes: a review. Eur J Pharm Biopharm 2001; 52:269–277.
72. Kristensen HG, Schaefer T. Granulation: a review on pharmaceutical wet granulation. Drug Dev Ind Pharm 1987; 13:803–872.
73. Mort PR, Capeci SW, Holder JW. Control of agglomerate attributes in a continuous binder agglomeration process. Powder Technol 2001; 117:173–176.
74. Watano S, Numa T, Koizumi I, et al. Feedback control in high shear granulation of pharmaceutical powders. Eur J Pharm Biopharm 2001; 52:337–345.
75. Watano S, Numa T, Koizumi I, et al. A fuzzy control system of high shear granulation using image processing. Powder Technol 2001; 115:124–130.

76. Balliu N. An Object Oriented Approach to the Modelling and Dynamics of Granulation Circuits. PhD thesis, School of Engineering, The University of Queensland, Australia, 2004.

77. Teo KL, Goh CJ, Wong KH. A Unified Computational Approach for Optimal Control Problems. New York: Longman Scientific and Technical, 1991.

78. Branch MA, Grace A. MATLAB Optimization Toolbox User's Guide. Natick: The Math Works Inc., 1996.

79. Shirazian S, Ismail HY, Singh M, Shaikh R., Crocker DM, Walker GM, Multi-dimensional population balance modeling of pharmaceutical formulations for continuous twin-screw wet granulation: Determination of liquid distribution. Int J Pharmaceutics 2019; 566: 352–360.

80. Wang FY, Cameron IT. Review and future directions in the modelling and control of continuous drum granulation. Powder Technol 2002; 124:238–253.

81. Alcacer V, Cruz V. Scanning the industry 4.0: a literature review for manufacturing systems, engineering science and technology. Int J 2019; 22: 899–919.

24 Scale-Up Considerations in Granulation

Yinghe He, Lian X. Liu, James Litster, and Defne Kayrak-Talay

CONTENTS

24.1 INTRODUCTION

Scale-up of any engineering process is a great technical and economic challenge. Scale-up of granulation processes, in particular, is difficult and often problematic because of the inherently heterogeneous nature of the materials used. However, recently improved understanding of the rate processes that control granulation improves our ability to do rational scale-up.

There are two situations where process scale-up is needed:

1. Commercialization of newly developed processes and/or products
2. Expansion of production capacities in response to increased market demand

TABLE 24.1
Scale-Up and Post-Approval Changes Level Component or Composition Change Levels

Excipient	Percent Excipient (w/w of Total Dosage Unit)		
	Level 1	Level 2	Level 3
Filler	±5	±10	>10
Disintegrant			
Starch	±3	±6	>6
Other	±0.5	±1	>1
Binder	±0.5	±1	>1
Lubricant			
Ca or Mg	±0.25	±0.5	>0.5
Stearate			
Other	±1	±2	>2
Glidant			
Talc	±1	±2	>2
Other	±0.1	±0.2	>0.2
Film coat	±1	±2	>2
Total drug recipient change (%)	5	10	n/a

Source: From Ref. [2].

For pharmaceutical applications, the challenge is almost always associated with new product development. Scale-up in the pharmaceutical industry is unique in that experiments at laboratory and pilot scales are also required to produce products of the desired specification for different stages of clinical trials. This gives additional constraints and challenges to engineers and technologists during scale-up.

A change in scale invariably impacts on process conditions and, consequently, on the product quality. For pharmaceutical industries, the Food and Drug Administration (FDA) ranks the impacts on the drug product arising from changes in process conditions including production scales into three levels as shown in Table 24.1 [1]. Level 1 is reserved for changes that are unlikely to have any detectable impact on the formulation quality and performance [2]. For all practical purposes, scale-up should aim to achieve an impact equivalent to or less than level 1.

In this chapter, we will first consider general scale-up approaches from a chemical engineering perspective. We will then look specifically at understanding pharmaceutical granulation scale-up through considering granulation as a combination of rate processes. Each rate process is affected by changes in the process during scaling, as well as by formulation decisions. Finally, we will present suggestions for the scaling of a fluid-bed, high-shear mixer, and twin-screw granulation processes that follow from this approach.

24.2 GENERAL CONSIDERATIONS IN PROCESS SCALE-UP: DIMENSIONAL ANALYSIS AND THE PRINCIPLE OF SIMILARITY

It is important to recognize that designing a commercial-scale operation via several stages of scale-up is, in one sense, an admission of failure. If we have a strong understanding of our processes, then the full-scale design can be performed using appropriate mathematical models, given feed formulation properties and clear required product specifications. Mature chemical engineering processes, such as distillation, are designed this way.

However, most solids' processing technologies do not have this level of maturity yet. In this case, scale-up studies reduce uncertainties in the design and operation of the scaled unit most economically. On this basis, the starting point in scale-up must be the commercial unit. In theory, once sufficient information for the commercial unit is known, scale-up can be done by applying similarity principles from data collected on a smaller unit. The similarity principle states [3]:

Two processes can be considered similar if they take place in similar geometric space and all dimensionless groups required to describe the processes have the same numerical values.

To establish the necessary dimensionless groups, a systematic dimensional analysis needs to be carried out during which the Buckingham Π theorem is used to reduce the number of dimensionless groups [4]. Assuming that a process can be described by k variables, we can express one variable as a function of the other $k - 1$ variable, that is,

$$x_1 = f(x_2, x_3, \ldots, x_{k-1}) \tag{24.1}$$

To conform to the dimensional homogeneity, the dimensions of the variable on the left side of the equation must be equal to those on the right side of the equation. With some simple mathematical rearrangements, equation (24.1) can be transformed into an equation of dimensionless groups (Π terms), that is,

$$\Pi_1 = \phi(\Pi_2, \Pi_3, \ldots, \Pi_{k-r}) \tag{24.2}$$

Equation (24.2) is a relationship among $k-r$ independent dimensionless products, where r is the minimum number of reference dimensions required to describe the variables. While the Buckingham Π theorem itself is straightforward, the development of a dimensionless expression for a process or a phenomenon requires a systematic dimensional analysis [4]. For most engineering problems, variables can be divided into three groups: (i) geometric variables, (ii) material property variables, and (iii) process variables. The reference dimensions are normally the basic dimensions such as mass (M), length (L), and time (T).

It is important to note that a systematic dimensional analysis can only be applied to processes where a clear understanding of the processes is established. The omission of any important variables of the process will lead to an erroneous outcome of the dimensional analysis, inevitably causing major problems in scale-up. Zlokarnik [3] divided the application of dimensional analysis into five general cases with different levels of understanding in each case.

1. The science of the basic phenomenon is unknown – dimensional analysis cannot be applied.
2. Enough is known about the science of the basic phenomenon to compile a tentative draft list – the resulting Π set is unreliable.
3. All the relevant variables for the description of the problems are known – application of dimensional analysis is straightforward.
4. The problem can be described by a mathematical equation – mathematical functions are better than Π relationships, which may help to reduce the number of dimensionless groups.
5. A mathematical solution of the problem exists – application of dimensional analysis is unnecessary.

Clearly, the more we understand a process or phenomenon, the better we can scale it up with confidence.

Full application of the similarity principle requires all the relevant Π groups to be measured at a small scale and kept constant during scale-up. Unfortunately, most industrial processes are very complex with many physical and chemical phenomena occurring. This leads to a large set of dimensionless groups required to fully characterize the process. This is particularly the case with processes involving particulate materials such as granulation. Maintaining all the dimensionless groups constant on the two scales is very difficult, if not impossible, because of constraints on the degrees of freedom in variables that can be changed on scale-up. In this case, scale-up can only be done based on partial similarity. That is, not all dimensionless numbers can be maintained the same on the two scales.

To scale-up based on partial similarity, experiments are carried out on a succession of types of equipment at different scales and results extrapolated to the final scale. That is, the scale-up ratio is kept low. With conflicting requirements on the dimensionless groups during scale-up, a common approach is to maintain one dimensionless group constant and check the effect of other dimensionless groups on the dependent variable by varying these dimensionless groups during experimentation. Once determined, only the dominant dimensionless number will be kept constant on scale-up. This partial similarity approach is often applied to granulation.

24.3   ANALYSIS OF GRANULATION RATE PROCESSES

Many of the required granule product attributes are directly related to the size, size distribution, and density of the granule product. These granule properties develop as a result of three classes of rate process in the granulator (Fig. 24.1):

1. Wetting and nucleation
2. Growth and consolidation
3. Breakage and attrition

Each of these processes is analyzed in depth by Litster and Ennis [5]. In this section, we will summarize each rate process in turn, particularly highlighting the main formulation properties and process variables. Where possible, we will define dimensionless groups that can be used in scale-up.

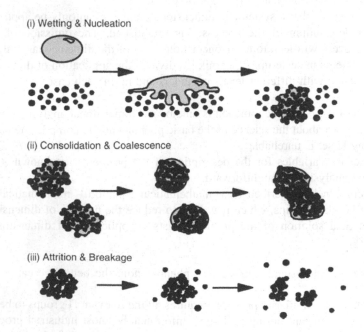

FIGURE 24.1   A classification of granulation rate processes.
Source: From Ref. [5].

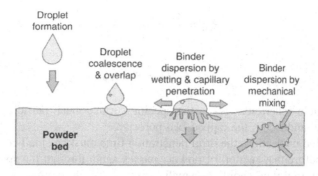

FIGURE 24.2   Wetting and nuclei formation in the spray zone of a granulator.

24.3.1   WETTING AND NUCLEATION

The first step in granulation is the addition of a liquid binder to the powder to form nuclei granules. Within the granulator, the key region for wetting and nucleation is the spray zone where liquid binder droplets contact the moving powder surface. The nucleation process is considered to consist of four stages (Fig. 24.2).

1. Droplet formation
2. Droplet overlap and coalescence at the bed surface
3. Drop penetration into the bed by capillary action
4. Mechanical dispersion of large clumps within the powder bed (only applicable to mixer granulators)

Poor wetting and nucleation lead to broad granule size distributions and poor distribution of the liquid binder, which increases substantially the chances of poor drug distribution. Despite the action of other rate processes, the broad size distributions and poor liquid distribution often persist throughout the granulation.

For ideal nucleation, the granulator should operate in the drop-controlled regime. Here, each drop that hits the powder bed penetrates into the bed to form a single nucleus granule. There is (almost) no drop overlap at the bed surface, and mechanical dispersion of large wet powder clumps is unnecessary.

To predict the required conditions for drop-controlled nucleation, we must understand

1. the thermodynamics and kinetics of drop penetration, largely controlled by formulation properties, and
2. the flux of drops onto the bed surface, largely controlled by process parameters.

The drop penetration time t_p can be estimated using a model that considers the rate at which liquid flows into the pores in the powder surface under capillary action [6].

$$t_p = 1.35 \frac{V_0^{2/3}}{\varepsilon_{eff}^2 R_{eff}} \frac{\mu}{\gamma_{LV} \cos \theta} \tag{24.3}$$

where V_0 is the drop volume, μ is the liquid viscosity, and $\gamma_{LV}\cos\theta$ is the adhesive tension between the liquid and the powder. The effective pore size R_{eff} and porosity ε_{eff} of the powder bed are given by

$$R_{eff} = \frac{\phi d_{3,2}}{3} \frac{\varepsilon_{eff}}{(1 - \varepsilon_{eff})} \tag{24.4}$$

$$\varepsilon_{eff} = \varepsilon_{tap}(1 - \varepsilon + \varepsilon_{tap}) \tag{24.5}$$

where ϕ is the particle sphericity, $d_{3,2}$ is the specific surface mean particle size, ε is the loose-packed bed porosity, and ε_{tap} is the tapped bed porosity.

For drop-controlled nucleation, the drop penetration time must be small compared with the bed circulation time t_c before that section of powder passes again through the spray zone, that is, the dimensionless penetration time should be small.

$$\tau_P = \frac{t_P}{t_c} < 0.1 \tag{24.6}$$

To avoid drop overlap on the bed surface and caking of the powder, the dimensionless spray flux ψ must also be kept small. ψ_a is the ratio of the rate of production of drop projected area by the nozzle to the rate at which powder surface area passed through the spray zone and is defined as

$$\Psi_a = \frac{3\dot{V}}{2\dot{A}d_d} \tag{24.7}$$

Figure 24.3 shows how the nuclei granule size distribution broadens as the spray flux increases. For drop-controlled nucleation, the dimensionless spray flux should be kept less than 0.2. For $\psi_a > 0.7$, the surface of the powder bed in the spray zone is effectively caked.

We can represent the nucleation behavior in a regime map (Fig. 24.4). Drop-controlled nucleation is achieved only when both ψ_a and τ_p are low. Figure 24.5 shows an example of full granulation data from a 25-L Fielder mixer granulator on this type of regime map. The granule size distribution is much narrower when nucleation is kept in the drop-controlled regime (lower left-hand corner). This illustrates that poor nucleation usually results in broad final granule size distributions despite the impact of other processes occurring in the granulator.

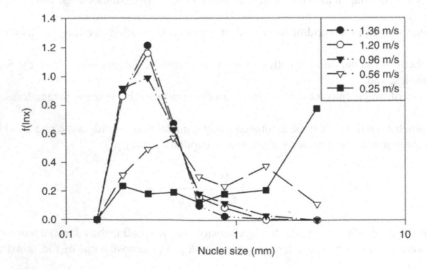

FIGURE 24.3 Effect of powder velocity on nuclei size distribution for lactose with water at 310 kPa. *Source:* From Ref. [6].

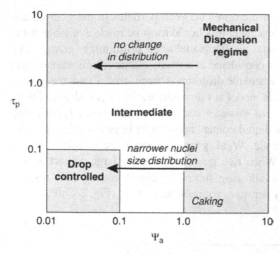

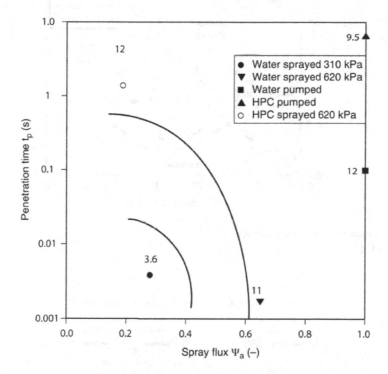

FIGURE 24.4 Nucleation regime map. For ideal nucleation in the drop-controlled regime, it must have (i) low ψ_a and (ii) low t_p. In the mechanical dispersion regime, one or both of these conditions are not met, and good binder dispersion requires good mechanical mixing.

FIGURE 24.5 Nucleation regime map in 25-L Fielder mixer at 15% liquid content. Merck lactose with water and hydroxypropyl cellulose (HPC) as liquid binders.
Source: From Ref. [6].

24.3.2 GROWTH AND CONSOLIDATION

Granule growth is very complex. The key question in establishing growth behavior is: will two granules that collide in a granulator stick together (coalesce) or rebound? To answer this question, it is useful to look at two extreme cases that cover most applications.

Deformable porous granules: These granules are typically formed by a nucleation process described above with the drop size of the same order or larger than the powder size.

Most of the liquid in the granule is contained in the pores between particles in the granule and held there by capillary action. For successful coalescence, this liquid must be made available at the contact point between colliding granules. This model is often suitable for drum mixer granulation.

Near elastic granules: Here, the wetted granule is considered as a nearly elastic sphere with a liquid layer on the surface. This is a good model for cases where the drop size is much smaller than the granule size and the granulator has simultaneous drying. This model is often suitable for fluid-bed granulation.

The different growth modes for *deformable porous granules* can be represented on a regime map (Fig. 24.6). For growth to occur by coalescence, the liquid content needs to be large enough to provide 85% to 105% saturation of the pores in the granule. Weak granules form large contact areas on collision and fall into the *steady growth* regime. When two granules collide, a large contact area is formed and liquid is squeezed to the contact area, allowing successful coalescence. In this regime, granules grow steadily and the growth rate is very sensitive to moisture content (Fig. 24.7a).

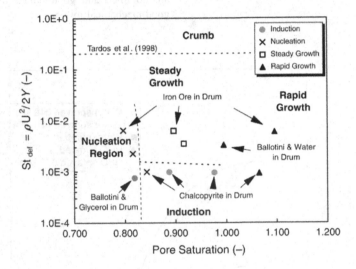

FIGURE 24.6   Granule growth regime map.
Source: From Ref. [7].

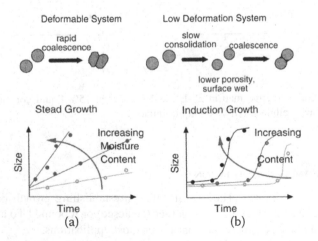

FIGURE 24.7   Coalescence growth modes for deformable granules.

Strong granules do not deform much on collision and granules rebound, rather than coalesce. However, as granules consolidate slowly, eventually the liquid is squeezed to granule surface, and this liquid layer causes successful coalescence. This is the *induction growth* regime (Figure 24.7b). At lower moisture contents, nuclei granules form and consolidate. Some growth by layering may occur, but there is insufficient liquid for growth by coalescence. This is the nucleation regime. Very weak granules simply fall apart and cannot sustain growth. This is the *crumb* regime.

Two dimensionless groups dictate the growth behavior, the Stokes deformation number, St_{def}, and the maximum pore saturation, S_{max}, which are defined as follows:

$$St_{def} = \frac{\rho_g U_c^2}{2Y} \tag{24.8}$$

$$S_{max} = \frac{w\rho_s(1 - \varepsilon_{min})}{\rho_l \varepsilon_{min}} \tag{24.9}$$

where ρ_g, ρ_s, and ρ_l are the granule, particle, and liquid densities; U_c is the effective granule collision velocity; Y is the granule yield strength; w is the liquid content (kg liquid/kg dry powder), and ε_{min} is the minimum granule porosity after complete consolidation.

Understanding where your system sits on the growth regime map is important for trouble-shooting and scale-up. Granules that grow in the induction regime are easy to scale with respect to granule size provided that the induction time is not exceeded. However, granule density often changes with scale because consolidation kinetics are important and these kinetics can change with scale. On the other hand, in the steady growth region, it is difficult to control granule size but granule density quickly settles to a minimum value and varies little with process parameters.

To make effective use of the granulation regime map, we need reasonable estimates of the effective collision velocity U_c (controlled by process conditions) and dynamic yield stress Y (a function of formulation properties). Table 24.2 gives estimates of the average and maximum collision velocities for different process equipment. In high-shear mixers, the difference between the average and maximum collision velocities can be very large.

The dynamic yield stress of the granule matrix is a function of strain rate due to the contribution of viscous dissipation to the granule strength. Therefore, it is dangerous to use static strength measurements to predict performance in the granulator. Iveson et al. [8] show how dynamic yield stress can be estimated from peak flow stress measurements in a high-speed load frame. They were able to correlate data for different formulations and strain rates in a single line when plotted as the dimensionless peak flow stress (Str*) versus the capillary number (Ca) (Figure 24.8). This line can be fitted by a simple empirical equation of the form

---

TABLE 24.2

Estimates of U_c for Different Granulation Processes

Type of Granulator	Average U_c	Maximum U_c
Fluidized beds	$\frac{6U_b d_p}{d_b}$	$\frac{6U_b d_p}{d_b \delta^2}$
Tumbling granulators	ωd_p	$d_b \delta^2$
		ωD_{drum}
Mixer granulators	$\omega_i d_p,\ \omega_c d_p$	$\omega_i D,\ \omega_c D_c$

Source: From Ref. [5].

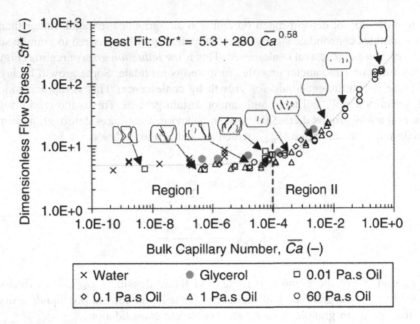

FIGURE 24.8 Dimensionless flow stress versus capillary number for widely sized 35-μm glass ballotini with six different binders.

$$Str^* = k_1 + k_2 Ca^z \tag{24.10}$$

where $Str^* = \sigma_{pk} d_p/\gamma cos\theta$ is the dimensionless peak flow stress, $Ca = \mu \dot{\varepsilon} \, d_p/\gamma cos\theta$ is the ratio of viscous to capillary forces, σ_{pk} is peak flow stress, $\dot{\varepsilon}$ is the bulk strain rate, and θ is the solid–liquid contact angle. k_1 gives the static strength of the pellets. k_2 determines the transition between strain rate-independent and strain rate-dependent behavior. z is an exponent that gives the power-law dependency of the flow stress on viscosity and strain rate. The best-fit value of z was found to be 0.58 ± 0.04, and the transition between strain rate-independent and strain rate-dependent flow stress occurred at $Ca \sim 10^{-4}$.

The rate of consolidation of granules can also be correlated with St_{def} in the form

$$k_c = \beta_c \exp(a \times St_{def}) \tag{24.11}$$

where β_c and a are constants and k_c is the consolidation rate constant for a first-order consolidation equation of the form

$$\frac{\varepsilon - \varepsilon_{min}}{\varepsilon_0 - \varepsilon_{min}} = \exp(-k_c t) \tag{24.12}$$

For *near elastic granules*, the conceptual model originally developed by Ennis et al. [9] considers the collision between two near elastic granules each coated with a layer of liquid (Figure 24.9). In this case, the key dimensionless group is the viscous Stokes number St_v.

$$St_v = \frac{4\rho_g U_c d_P}{9\mu} \tag{24.13}$$

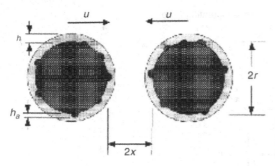

FIGURE 24.9 Two near elastic granules colliding – the basis for the coalescence/rebound criteria. *Source:* From Ref. [9].

St_v is the ratio of the kinetic energy of the collision to the viscous dissipation in the liquid layer. Successful coalescence will occur if St_v is less than some critical value St^*, and we can define three growth regimes as follows

1. *Noninertial growth* ($St_{v, max} < St^*$): The viscous Stokes number for all collisions in the granulator is less than the critical Stokes number. All collisions lead to sticking and growth by coalescence. In this regime, changes to process parameters will have little or no effect on the probability of coalescence.
2. *Inertial growth* ($St_{v, av} \gg St^*$): Some collisions cause coalescence, while others lead to a rebound. There will be steady granule growth by coalescence. The extent and rate of growth will be sensitive to process parameters, which will determine the proportion of collisions that lead to coalescence. Varying process parameters and formulation properties can push the system into either the noninertial or coating regimes.
3. *Coating regime* ($St_{v, min} > St^*$): The kinetic energy in most or all collisions exceeds viscous dissipation in the liquid layer. There is no coalescence. Granule growth will only occur by the successive layering of new material in the liquid phase (melt, solution, or slurry) onto the granule.

Figure 24.10 shows an example of granule growth in a fluidized bed where the growth regime changes as the granules grow. Glass ballotini are grown with two liquid binders of different viscosity. Initially, both systems grow steadily at the same rate (noninertial regime). When the granule size reaches approximately 800 μm, the polyvinylpyrrolidone (PVP) bound granule growth begins to slow, indicating a transition to the inertial growth regime (only some collisions are successful). Finally, the PVP granules level off at a maximum size of approximately 900 μm, showing the transition to the coating regime where no granule collisions are successful. In contrast, the more viscous carboxyl methylcellulose (CMC-M) granules grow steadily throughout the eight-hour experiment, that is, they remain in the noninertial regime for the whole experiment.

24.3.3 BREAKAGE AND ATTRITION

Breakage and attrition cover two separate phenomena.

1. Breakage of wet granules in the granulator
2. Attrition or fracture of dried granules in the granulator, drier, or subsequent handling

Breakage of wet granules will influence and may control the final granule size distribution. It is only an important phenomenon for high-shear granulators. Wet granule breakage is much less

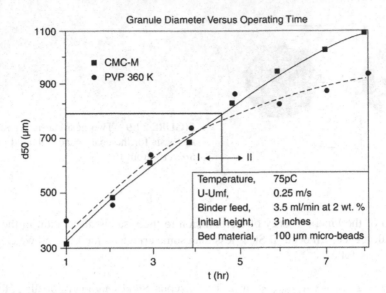

FIGURE 24.10   Growth of glass ballotini granules in a fluidized bed with binders of different viscosity. *Source*: From Ref. [9].

studied than nucleation and growth. There is very little quantitative theory or modeling available to predict conditions for breakage or the effect of formulation properties on wet granule breakage.

Tardos et al. [10] considered that a granule will break if the applied kinetic energy during an impact exceeds the energy required for breakage. This analysis leads to a Stokes deformation number criteria for breakage.

$$\mathrm{St}_{\mathrm{def}} > \mathrm{St}^*_{\mathrm{def}} \tag{24.14}$$

where $\mathrm{St}^*_{\mathrm{def}}$ is the critical value of Stokes number that must be exceeded for breakage to occur. However, this model is probably an oversimplification. Figure 24.8 shows the schematics of the failure mode of different formulations in dynamic yield strength measurements. Failure behavior varies widely from semibrittle behavior at low capillary numbers to plastic failure at high capillary numbers. We expect a purely plastic granule to smear rather than break when its yield stress is exceeded. At high impeller speeds, such materials will coat the granulator wall or form a paste. Semibrittle granules will break at high impact velocity, giving a maximum stable granule size or a weak crumb. Nevertheless, equation (24.14) provides a good starting point for quantifying wet granule breakage.

Liu et al. [11] developed a model to calculate the granule yield strength, which can then be used to calculate $\mathrm{St}_{\mathrm{def}}$ in equation (24.8). The model is a modified combination of two models introduced previously in the literature [12,13] for the static and dynamic contributions to granule strength, respectively. The model introduced by Liu et al. [11] takes into account both the effects of capillary force and the viscous force in liquid bridges when calculating the strength of the granule. It also incorporates liquid pore saturation. The model includes a particle shape factor that allows calculating the strength of granules made of nonspherical particles, and is given by the following equation:

$$Y = \mathrm{AR}^{-4.3} S \left[6 \frac{1 - \varepsilon_g}{\varepsilon_g} \frac{\gamma_{\mathrm{LV}} \cos\theta}{d_{3,2}} + \frac{9}{8} \frac{(1 - \varepsilon_g)^2}{\varepsilon_g^2} \frac{9\pi\mu v_{\mathrm{P}}}{16 d_{3,2}} \right] \tag{24.15}$$

where AR is the aspect ratio of the primary particles, S is the granule pore saturation, ε is the porosity of the granule, $d_{3,2}$ is the specific surface area diameter of the particles, and v_p is the relative velocity of the moving particle inside a granule after impact. Liu et al. [11] performed experiments in a "breakage-only granulator" for a wide range of formulations and determined the St^*_{def} as 0.2. If St_{def} is greater than 0.2, the granules are in the breakage regime. While breakage models remain very basic with simplistic descriptions of granule mechanical properties and many simplifying assumptions, models of the type described in equation (24.8) with an appropriate calculation of the granule strength [such as equation (24.15)] are immediately useful for scaling and troubleshooting.

Dry granule attrition is important where drying and granulation occur simultaneously (e.g., in fluidized beds) and in subsequent processing and handling of the granular product. We can consider dry granule breakage as a brittle or semibrittle phenomenon. The key granule properties that control the breakage are the granule fracture toughness K_c and the flaw or crack size c in the granule. K_c is set by formulation properties, while c is closely related to granule porosity controlled by the consolidation process in the granulator.

Dry granule breakage usually results in the production of fines by wear, erosion, or attrition brought about by diffuse microcracking. Within a fluid bed, there are a large number of low-velocity collisions between particles as they shear past each other. This process is analogous to abrasive wear. For abrasive wear of agglomerates, the volumetric wear rate V is given by Ref. 14:

$$V = \frac{d_i^{1/2}}{A^{1/4} K_c^{3/4} H^{1/2}} P^{5/4} l \tag{24.16}$$

where d_i is indentor diameter, P is applied load, H is the hardness of the particles, l is wear displacement of the indentor, and A is an apparent area of contact of the indentor with the surface. The number and relative velocity of the collisions depends on the number of bubbles in the bed and hence the excess gas velocity $(u - u_{mf})$. The applied pressure in a fluid bed depends on bed depth. Thus, the attrition rate B_w in a fluidized-bed granulator is

$$B_w = \frac{d_0^{1/2}}{K_c^{3/4} H^{1/2}} L^{5/4} (u - u_{mf}) \tag{24.17}$$

where d_0 is the distributor hole orifice size and L is the fluidized-bed height. Figure 24.11 shows the attrition rates of several formulations in a fluidized bed with a direct correlation between the attrition rate and the material properties grouping in equations (24.16) and (24.17).

Note that equations (24.16) and (24.17) only hold for breakage via a wear mechanism. For attrition during impact or compaction, there are different dependencies of the attrition rate on the properties of the material [5].

24.4 IMPLICATIONS FOR SCALE-UP

Table 24.3 summarizes the key controlling dimensionless groups for the rate processes described above and the main process parameters and formulation properties that impact on these groups.

In addition to these groups, there are dimensionless groups to describe [1] the geometry of the equipment and [2] the flow of the powder and granules in the granulator. Both these classes of controlling groups are very equipment dependent.

For scale-up using full-dimensional similarity, all these dimensionless groups need to be held constant. This is normally impossible because of the small number of degrees of freedom and a large number of constraints. In particular, for regulatory reasons, it is usually not possible

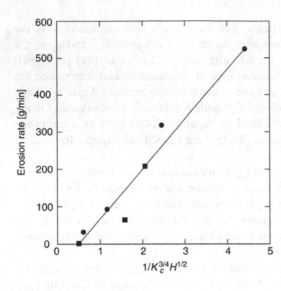

FIGURE 24.11 Erosion rates of agglomerate materials during attrition of granules in a fluidized bed. *Source:* From Ref. [15].

TABLE 24.3
Summary of Controlling Groups for Granulation Rate Processes

Rate Process	Controlling Groups	Key Formulation Properties	Key Process Parameters
Wetting and nucleation	Dimensionless spray flux Ψ Dimensionless penetration time τ_p	t_p, μ, $\gamma \cos \theta$, d_p, ε, ε_{tap}	$\dot{V}$, $\dot{A}$ (influenced by nozzle design and position, number of nozzles, and powder flow patterns)
Growth and consolidation	Stokes deformation number St_{def} Viscous Stokes number St_v Liquid saturation s	Y, ρ_g, μ, $\gamma \cos \theta$, d_p, ε_{tap}	U_c (influenced by powder flow patterns—see Table 24.2)
Attrition and breakage	Stokes deformation number St_{def}	K_c, H, Y, ρ_g, μ, $\gamma \cos \theta$, d_p, ε_{tap}	U_c, L, $u - u_{mf}$

to change formulation properties during scale-up except during the very early stages of process development. This leaves only a relatively small number of process parameters as degrees of freedom.

Therefore, a partial similarity approach for scale-up is recommended. The general steps are given below.

1. Maintain similar geometry throughout the scale-up process. For most pharmaceutical granulation equipment, this can be achieved from either 10- or 25-L nominal batch size to full scale. Be wary, however, in some cases, key geometric parameters do vary with scale in a particular design, for example, relative chopper size, and relative fill height. Manufacturers should be lobbied hard to provide geometrically similar designs at all scales.
2. Set key dimensionless groups to maintain similar powder flow during scale-up. In particular, avoid changes of flow regime during scale-up that make maintaining granule attributes during scale-up impossible.
3. Use your experience and an understanding of your process to decide which product attributes are most important and which granulation rate process is most dominant in controlling these

attributes. This is difficult to do *a priori*, but with a good characterization of your formulation and process, the regime map approaches described above are very useful.

4. Use your remaining degrees of freedom in the choice of process parameter values to keep the most important one or two rate process dimensionless groups constant.

This approach is most easily demonstrated on particular types of equipment (see sections "Scale-Up of Fluidized-Bed Granulators," "Scale-Up of High-Shear Mixer Granulators," and "Scale-up and Scale-Out of Twin-Screw Granulators").

24.5 SCALE-DOWN, FORMULATION CHARACTERIZATION, AND FORMULATION DESIGN IN PHARMACEUTICAL GRANULATION

In the development of a new pharmaceutical product, important decisions about the manufacturing process are made with a few grams or tens of grams of the formulation. To provide drug products for clinical trials and to provide the final design at a large scale, granulations are often conducted at several laboratory and pilot scales as well. Typical nominal batch sizes are 1, 10, 25, and 65 L scaling to commercial operation at 300 or 600 L.

Small-scale granulations up to 1 L are often done by hand and certainly performed in equipment that is very different from the equipment that will be used from scales of 10 L and larger. At this level, the general scale-up approach described in section "Implications for Scale-Up" does not hold. How do we *scale-down* to make the best use of data from the granulation of these small amounts?

The key is to consider granulation as a particle design process (Figure 24.12). During scaling from 10 L up, formulation properties cannot be varied. Only process parameters can be used to keep key granule attributes in the target range. Therefore, very small-scale experiments should target major *formulation design* decisions, and attempts to mimic completely different geometries at a larger scale should be avoided.

Table 24.3 summarizes the key formulation properties that should be measured. Most of these require relatively small amounts of material and can be measured at this level. By using this data to help estimate key controlling groups for the granulation rate processes in the larger-scale equipment, appropriate changes to the formulation can be made. This avoids major headaches at a later stage. Good communication between the technologists who design the formulations and the process engineers who scale the process and transfer the product to manufacturing is an essential part of this paradigm.

Some of the questions that can be addressed at this stage of formulation development and scale-up include the following:

1. Wetting and nucleation
   a. Contact angle: are the active and all the excipients easily wetted by the liquid binder?
   b. Drop penetration time: is the liquid phase too viscous, or the particle size too small to achieve fast drop penetration?

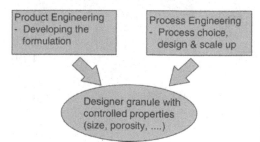

FIGURE 24.12 Granulation as an example of particle design. Both formulation properties and process parameters influence granule attributes.

2. Growth and consolidation
   a. What is the dynamic yield stress of the formulation?
   b. How much liquid binder is required for granule growth?
   c. What is the likely growth regime?
   d. What range of granule density is likely?

3. Attrition and breakage
   a. Will extensive granule breakage occur in the granulator?
   b. What is the dry granule strength (fracture toughness) and porosity?
   c. Are attrition and dust formation during handling likely?

4. Downstream processing issues
   a. Does the formulation compress well for tableting?
   b. Can desired dissolution profiles be met?

Details of how to measure key formulation properties are described in more detail by Litster and Ennis [5].

24.6 SCALE-UP OF FLUIDIZED-BED GRANULATORS

There are many different variations of fluidized-bed granulators including bubbling fluidized bed, draft tube fluidized beds, and spouted beds [5]. However, in this section, we limit ourselves only to the scale-up of the most commonly used fluidized-bed granulator, that is, bubbling fluidized-bed granulator. In particular, as most fluidized-bed granulators used in the pharmaceutical industry are operated in batch mode, we will concentrate on the scale-up of batch bubbling fluidized-bed granulators.

24.6.1 BED HYDRODYNAMICS AND SCALE-UP

Particle growth in a fluidized bed is closely related to the particle mixing and flow pattern in the bed. This dictates that the hydrodynamics of the scaled bed should be the same as the small unit, that is, hydrodynamic similarity. Basic fluidized-bed hydrodynamics are described in chapter 10.

In bubbling fluidized beds, bed expansion, solids mixing, particle entrainment, granule growth, and attrition are intimately related to the motion of bubbles in the bed (Fig. 24.13). The volume flow rate of bubbles in the bed Q_b, the bubble size d_b, and the bubble rise velocity u_b are the key parameters that characterize the bubbly flow. There are numerous correlations relating these bubble parameters to process conditions [16,17]. In general, Q_b is a strong function of the excess gas velocity $u - u_{mf}$. Growing granules are usually Geldart type B powders or perhaps type A powders at the start of the batch. For group B powders, d_b increases with bed height and is a function of excess gas velocity. The bubble rise velocity is directly related to d_b. For the simplest models for group B powders, we can write

$$Q_b = (u - u_{mf})\pi D_F^2 \tag{24.18}$$

$$u_b = 0.71\sqrt{gd_b} \tag{24.19}$$

$$d_b \propto (u - u_{mf})^{0.4}L^{0.8} \tag{24.20}$$

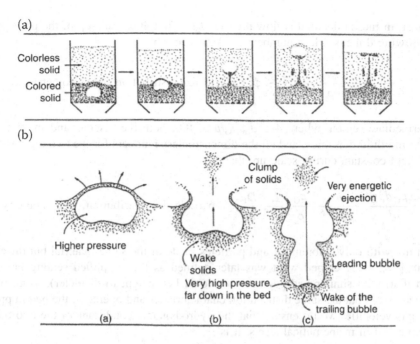

FIGURE 24.13 Effect of bubbles on (a) solid mixing and (b) solid entrainment.
Source: From Ref. [16].

Thus, the excess gas velocity $u - u_{mf}$ and the bed height L are the key process parameters that control bubbling behavior in the bed.

Several rules exist for scaling-up a bubbling fluidized bed under the condition of hydrodynamic similarity. Fitzgerald and Crane [18] proposed that the following dimensionless numbers be kept constant in scale-up.

- Particle Reynolds number based on gas density $d_p u \rho_G / \mu$
- Solid particle to gas density ratio ρ_s / ρ_G
- Particle Froude number $u/(g d_p)^{0.5}$
- The geometric similarity of distributor, bed, and particle L/d_p

where d_p is particle diameter, u is the fluidization velocity (superficial gas velocity), μ is the viscosity of fluidizing gas, ρ_G is the density of fluidizing gas, g is gravitational acceleration, and L is the fluidized-bed height.

In this approach, experiments on the smaller scale are performed with model materials, that is, model gas (different from the larger-scale one) and model solid particles (different particle density, size, and size distribution). For readers interested in following Fitzgerald's scale-up rules, a detailed calculation procedure can be found in Kunii and Levenspiel's book [16], illustrated with an example.

In a series of publications, Glicksman et al. [19–21] divided the scale-up into two regimes, namely, inertia-dominated and viscous-dominated flow regimes. In viscous-dominated flow regime, where particle Reynolds number based on fluid density is equal or less than 4, that is, when $d_p u \rho_G / \mu \leq 4$, the dimensionless numbers that need to be kept constant are

$$\frac{u}{(g d_p)^{0.5}}, \frac{d_p u \rho_s}{\mu}, \frac{L}{d_p}, \frac{D_F}{d_p}, \phi, \text{ particle size distribution, bed geometry} \tag{24.21}$$

where D_F is the fluidized-bed diameter.

In contrast, in inertia-dominated flow regime, $d_\mathrm{p}u\rho_\mathrm{G}/\mu \geq 400$, scale-up of the process demands that the following dimensionless numbers are kept constant.

$$\frac{u}{(gd_\mathrm{P})^{0.5}}, \frac{\rho_\mathrm{G}}{\rho_\mathrm{s}}, \frac{L}{d_\mathrm{P}}, \frac{D_\mathrm{F}}{d_\mathrm{P}}, \phi, \text{ particle size distribution, bed geometry} \qquad (24.22)$$

In the intermediate region, where $4 \leq d_\mathrm{p}u\rho_\mathrm{G}/\mu \leq 400$, both the viscous and inertial forces are important to the fluid dynamics, and all the dimensionless numbers for the two regions above will need to be kept constant during scale-up, that is,

$$\frac{\rho_\mathrm{s}\rho_\mathrm{G}d_\mathrm{P}^3 g}{\mu^2}, \frac{u}{(gd_\mathrm{P})^{0.5}}, \frac{\rho_\mathrm{G}}{\rho_\mathrm{s}}, \frac{L}{d_\mathrm{P}}, \frac{D_\mathrm{F}}{d_\mathrm{P}}, \phi, \text{ particle size distribution, bed geometry} \qquad (24.23)$$

Experimenting with only ambient air and particles made of the same material but different sizes, Horio et al. [22,23] developed what was later defined as the simplified scaling law. They demonstrated that, with similar bed geometry (ratio of bed height to diameter), using particles of different mean sizes but the same distribution characteristics and operating the bed in proportional superficial gas velocities would ensure that the hydrodynamic conditions of the two beds remain similar. Expressed in mathematical terms, it is

$$
\begin{aligned}
u_2 - u_\mathrm{mf2} &= \sqrt{m}\,(u_1 - u_\mathrm{mf1})\\
u_\mathrm{mf2} &= \sqrt{m}\,u_\mathrm{mf1}\\
m &= \frac{L_2}{L_1}\\
&\text{bed geometry}
\end{aligned}
\qquad (24.24)
$$

where 1 and 2 refer to the small-scale and large-scale beds, respectively.

Experimental results by Roy and Davidson [24] suggest that when $d_\mathrm{p}u\rho_\mathrm{G}/\mu < 30$, the criteria by Horio et al. [22,23] are sufficient to give similarity in behavior. However, when $d_\mathrm{p}u\rho_\mathrm{G}/\mu > 30$, the more restrictive approach of Fitzgerald and Crane has to be used.

Unfortunately, few of the above scaling rules for bubbling fluidized beds have been strictly followed for the scaling-up of fluidized-bed granulators. This is largely because the scaling rules require model materials to be used at a smaller scale, whereas in pharmaceutical granulation, the formulation is unchanged during scale-up. However, the simplified rules presented by Horio et al., combined with our understanding of granulation rate processes, do provide some guidance.

24.6.2 Granulation Rate Processes in Fluidized Beds

Figure 24.14 shows the rate processes occurring during fluidized granulation. Wetting, nucleation, and layered growth occur in the spray zone of the fluidized bed. Most consolidation and coalescence also occur in or near the spray zone because fluidized-bed granulators are also driers. The drying process "freezes" the granule structure and prevents further growth. Thus, the good design of the spray zone is very important, and the liquid flow rate is a critical process parameter. Beds should be designed to keep a dimensionless spray flux low (drop-controlled regime). If this is not done, the formation of large clumps leads to rapid wet quenching and defluidization with likely loss of the batch. Figure 24.15 shows how the product granule size distribution is closely related to the design of the spray zone. The x-axis variable (spray surface area per mass in granulator) is closely related to our definition of dimensionless spray flux.

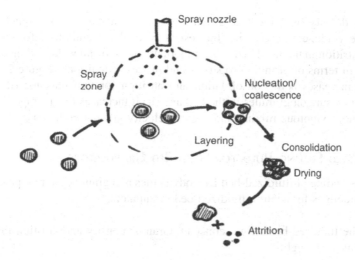

FIGURE 24.14 Important granulation processes in the fluidized bed.
Source: From Ref. [5].

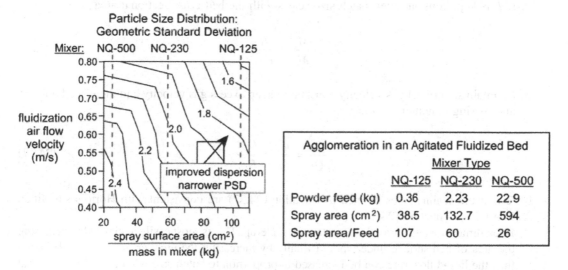

Agglomeration in an Agitated Fluidized Bed			
	Mixer Type		
	NQ-125	NQ-230	NQ-500
Powder feed (kg)	0.36	2.23	22.9
Spray area (cm²)	38.5	132.7	594
Spray area/Feed	107	60	26

FIGURE 24.15 Geometric standard deviation of granule size in an agitated fluid-bed granulator as a function of gas fluidization velocity and binder dispersion measured using spray surface area to mass in a mixer.
Source: From Ref. [10].

Because of the simultaneous drying, our consolidation and growth models for near elastic granules are usually appropriate and the viscous Stokes number is a key controlling group [equation (24.13)]. This model predicts that in batch granulation, granules will grow toward a maximum size corresponding to the critical Stokes number and transition to the coating regimes (e.g., Figure 24.10). The average and maximum granule collision velocities are set by the flow of bubbles in the fluid bed and are a function of bubble velocity and size (Table 24.3).

Fluidized beds produce porous granules because the consolidation time is limited to granule drying time, which is of the order of seconds, rather than minutes. Thus, process changes that reduce drying time (higher bed temperature, lower liquid flow rate, and smaller drop size) will decrease granule density (will increase granule porosity). Increasing the liquid binder viscosity decreases granule voidage by increasing the resistance of the granule to deformation.

Dry granule attrition in the fluid bed is an important source of fines. Equation (24.17) quantifies the attrition rate in terms of granule properties and process conditions (Figure 24.11). Increasing fluid-bed height increases both consolidation and attrition for two reasons: (i) it increases the effective "fluid" pressure on granules in the bed and (ii) it increases the average bubble size in the bed, leading to more vigorous mixing and higher-velocity granule collisions.

24.6.3 SUGGESTED SCALING RULES FOR FLUID-BED GRANULATORS

Given this understanding of fluidized-bed hydrodynamics and granulation rate process, we suggest the following guidelines for scaling fluidized-bed granulators.

1. Maintain the fluidized-bed height constant. Granule density and attrition rate increase with the operating bed height.

$$L_2 = L_1 \qquad (24.25)$$

2. If L is kept constant, then batch size scales with the bed cross-sectional area.

$$\frac{M_2}{M_1} = \frac{D_{F2}^2}{D_{F1}^2} \qquad (24.26)$$

3. Maintain superficial gas velocity constant to keep excess gas velocity and therefore bubbling and mixing conditions similar.

$$\frac{Q_2}{Q_1} = \frac{u_2}{u_1} = \frac{D_{F2}^2}{D_{F1}^2} \qquad (24.27)$$

Note that the scaling rules defined by equation (24.27) are consistent with Horio's simplified scaling rules [equation (24.24)].

4. Keep dimensionless spray flux constant on scale-up. This is most easily achieved by increasing the area of bed surface under spray (usually by increasing the number of nozzles). By doing this, the liquid flow rate can be increased in proportion to batch size without changing critical spray zone conditions. Thus, batch times at small and large scales should be similar.

$$\dot{V}_2 = \dot{V}_1 \qquad (24.28)$$

$$\frac{A_{spray,2}}{A_{spray,1}} = \frac{D_{F2}^2}{D_{F1}^2} \qquad (24.29)$$

5. Keep viscous Stokes number constant. By adhering to the scaling rules described above, St_v should automatically be similar at small and large scales, leading to similar consolidation and growth behavior.

There are also some cautionary notes relating to the minimum scale for the laboratory-scale studies. Slug flow, a phenomenon where single gas bubbles as large as the bed diameter form in regular patterns in the bed, significantly reduces solid mixing. It occurs in tall and narrow beds. Steward [25] proposed a criterion for the onset of slugging.

$$\frac{u - u_{mf}}{0.35\sqrt{gD_F}} = 0.2 \tag{24.30}$$

To ensure that the bed is operating in bubbling mode without risking slugging, the ratio in equation (24.30) must be kept below 0.2. In addition, both the bed height to bed diameter and particle diameter to bed diameter ratios should be kept low. For the pilot fluidized bed, the diameter should be greater than 0.3 m.

To avoid the gas entry effect from the distributor (gas jet), there is also a requirement on minimum fluidized-bed height. The jet length depends on the gas velocity and the size of the opening on the distributor. For the same opening size, jet length increases with gas velocity through the hole; for a given gas velocity through the hole, small holes give shorter jets but are accompanied by a larger pressure drop across the distributor. Even at a superficial gas velocity as low as 0.2 m/sec with a hole size of 9.5 mm in diameter, jet length as long as 0.6 m has been reported [26].

The amount of fluidization gas required to maintain constant fluidization velocity scales linearly with the cross-sectional area of the bed. However, for large fluidized beds, one of the major concerns is the even distribution of the fluidization gas across the whole area of the bed. In addition to the use of a plenum chamber and an even distribution of flow channels across the distributor, the distributor should be designed in such a way that the pressure drop across it is at least 20% of the total.

If these scaling rules are applied, there is a good chance to keep granule properties within the desired range on scaling. If fine-tuning is needed at a large scale, minor adjustments to the liquid spray rate can be used to adjust granule properties, as all the granulation rate processes in fluidized beds are very sensitive to this parameter.

24.7 SCALE-UP OF HIGH-MIXER GRANULATORS

Effective scale-up of mixer granulators is more difficult than fluidized beds. There are several reasons for this.

- The geometric and mechanical design of mixer granulators varies enormously, as do the powder flow patterns in the mixer. There is no such thing as a generic high-shear mixer, and caution is needed in transferring scaling rules from one design to another.
- Even with the same series from the same manufacturer, the geometric similarity is not always maintained between different scales, for example, impeller size in relation to bowl size.
- Powder flow in high-shear mixers is not fluidized, and powder flow patterns are much harder to predict than in a fluidized bed.
- All three rate processes, that is, wetting and nucleation, growth and consolidation, and breakage and attrition, take place simultaneously in the mixer granulator of all scales. However, the relative dominance of each of the rate processes can vary significantly on different scales of the same series, let alone in granulators of different series.

In this section, we will focus mainly on vertical shaft mixers, for example, Fielder and Diosna designs. Some of the suggested approaches may be used with caution for other mixer designs.

24.7.1 GEOMETRIC SCALING ISSUES

For a simple vertical mixer design, the key dimensions are the impeller diameter D, which is usually equal to the bowl diameter, the chopper diameter D_c, and the fill height H_m. The dimensionless groups that need to be held constant for geometric similarity are

$$\frac{D_c}{D}, \frac{H_m}{D}$$

In addition, the shape and positioning of the impeller and chopper should be the same on scale-up. Unfortunately, manufacturers do not always adhere to these rules. It is common for the absolute size of the chopper to be invariant, meaning its relative influence is much larger in the small-scale granulator.

Relative fill height is also often varied with scale. This often reflects the small-sized batches required for early-stage clinical trials and the desire to maximize production rate (by maximizing batch size) at full scale. Varying relative fill height is very dangerous, as it can have a major impact on powder flow patterns.

24.7.2 Powder Flow Patterns and Scaling Issues

There are two flow regimes observed in a vertical shaft mixer granulator, namely, bumping and roping regimes [27]. At low impeller speeds in the bumping regime, the powder is displaced only vertically as the blade passes underneath, leading to a slow, bumpy powder motion in the tangential direction. There is almost no vertical turnover of the powder bed, as shown in Figure 24.16a.

At higher impeller speed in the roping regime, material from the bottom of the bed is forced up the vessel wall and tumbles down at an angle of the bed surface toward the center of the bowl. There is both a good rotation of the bed and good vertical turnover (Figure 24.16b).

The transition from bumping to roping is due to a change in the balance between centrifugal force and gravity. The centrifugal force, which is caused by the rotational movement of the powder from the spinning of the blades, pushes the powder outward toward the wall of the bowl, while gravity keeps the powder tumbling back toward the center of the bowl from the buildup at the wall region. This balance between rotational inertia and gravity is given by the Froude number:

$$Fr = \frac{DN^2}{g} \tag{24.31}$$

where N is the impeller speed and g is the gravitational acceleration.

When the Froude number exceeds a critical value, a transition from bumping to roping takes place.

$$Fr > Fr_c \tag{24.32}$$

Fr_c will be a function of relative fill height (H_m/D), impeller design (size and geometry), and powder flow properties.

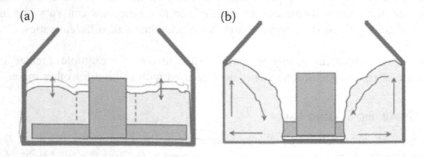

FIGURE 24.16 Powder flow regimes in Fielder mixer granulators: (a) bumping and (b) roping.

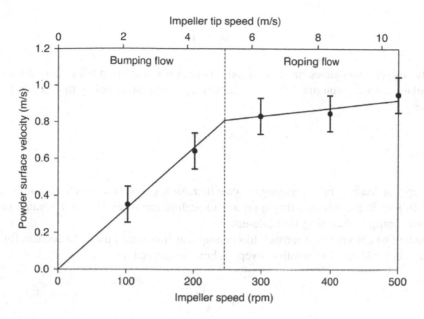

FIGURE 24.17 Powder surface velocities as a function of impeller tip speed.
Source: From Ref. [27].

Roping flow is more difficult to achieve as relative fill height increases because the centrifugal force is only imparted to powder in the impeller region. This region becomes a smaller fraction of the total powder mass as fill height increases. Schaefer [28] also showed that impeller design had a significant effect on both Fr_c and bed turnover rates.

Cohesive powders transfer to roping at lower values of Fr because the momentum from the spinning impeller is more effectively transferred into the powder mass. Note that powder flow properties generally change with the addition of the liquid binder, and therefore, flow patterns will probably change significantly during a batch granulation.

Figure 24.17 shows dry lactose powder surface velocity data in a 25-L Fielder granulator [27]. In the bumping flow regime, the powder surface velocity increases in proportion to the impeller speed. In the roping regime, the surface velocity stabilizes and is less sensitive to impeller speed. In all cases, the surface velocity of the powder is only of the order of 10% of the impeller tip speed. Knight et al. [29] showed that dimensionless torque T is a direct function of Froude number and effective blade height h_{eff}:

$$T = T_0 + k Fr^{0.5} \text{ where } k = \beta \left(\frac{2h_{eff}}{D} \right)^b \tag{24.33}$$

Thus, to maintain a similar powder flow pattern during scale-up, the Froude number should be kept constant, that is,

$$\frac{N_2}{N_1} = \sqrt{\frac{D_1}{D_2}} \tag{24.34}$$

In addition, the dimensionless bed height should also be kept constant, that is, the same fraction of the bowl is filled at all scales.

$$\frac{Hm_2}{Hm_1} = \frac{D_2}{D_1} \tag{24.35}$$

Historically, mixer granulators have been more commonly scaled up using constant tip speed or constant relative swept volume [28,30]. Maintaining constant impeller tip speeds leads to the scaling rule

$$\frac{N_2}{N_1} = \frac{D_1}{D_2} \tag{24.36}$$

This scale-up rule leads to Fr decreasing as scale increases. Combined with the common practice of overfilling full-scale granulators, this approach to scaling can often lead to a change in operating regime from roping to bumping on scale-up.

The constant swept volume approach to scale-up was introduced partly to account for variations in geometry on scale-up. The relative swept volume is defined as

$$\dot{V}_R = \frac{\dot{V}_{imp}}{V_{mixer}} \tag{24.37}$$

where $\dot{V}_r$ is the relative swept volume, $\dot{V}_{imp}$ is the rate of swept volume of the impeller, and V_{mixer} is the mixer volume.

On scale-up,

$$\dot{V}_{R,1} = \dot{V}_{R,2} \tag{24.38}$$

This approach is useful for comparing granulators where geometry changes with scale. For geometrically similar granulators, (24.38) is equivalent to scale-up with constant tip speed [(24.36).

In addition to constant tip speed, constant Froude number, and constant swept volume approaches, a new approach was introduced for scale-up of high-shear mixer granulators, where shear rate is kept constant across all scales [31]. Provided that the bowl and impeller geometries are similar, constant shear stress leads to the scaling rule

$$\frac{N_2}{N_1} = \left(\frac{D_1}{D_2}\right)^{0.8} \tag{24.39}$$

In summary, in all approaches mentioned above, the main impeller speed (N) is varied according to the following equation.

$$N D^n = constant \tag{24.40}$$

where the scaling index "n" equals to 0.5, 0.8, and 1 in constant Fr, constant shear rate, and constant tip speed cases, respectively.

24.7.3 GRANULATION RATE PROCESSES AND RELATED SCALING ISSUES

In high-shear mixer granulation, all three classes of rate process can have a significant effect on the granule size distribution. Section "Wetting and Nucleation" describes conditions for good nucleation in the drop-controlled regime and uses examples from mixer granulation. For good nucleation, the granulator should be operated in the roping regime for good bed turnover and the dimensionless spray flux Ψ_a should be kept low. This implies a careful choice of the liquid flow rate, nozzle design, and positioning in the granulator.

To maintain similar nucleation behavior and equivalent liquid distribution, the dimensionless spray flux Ψ_a should be kept constant on scale-up. If spray drop size in the full-scale granulator is similar to that in the small-scale granulator, this implies

$$\frac{\dot{V_2}}{A_2} = \frac{\dot{V_1}}{A_1} \Rightarrow \frac{\dot{V_2}}{\dot{V_1}} = \frac{A_2}{A_1} \tag{24.41}$$

A common scale-up approach is to keep the same total spray time and still use a single nozzle at a large scale. Thus, $\dot{V}$ is proportional to D^3. Even though the powder area flux will increase slightly with scale, this approach generally leads to a substantial increase in dimensionless spray flux. To keep dimensionless spray flux constant, multiple spray nozzles and/or longer spray times should be used at a large scale.

It should be noted that consolidation, growth, and breakage processes are controlled by St_{def}. This can lead to quite complicated growth behavior in mixer granulators. Figure 24.18 illustrates some of the complex behaviors [30]. Both decreasing liquid viscosity and increasing impeller speed *increase* the rate of granule growth but *decrease* the final equilibrium granule size. Both of these effects increase St_{def}. In the early stage of granulation, this increases the probability of successful coalescence. However, as the granules grow, the critical value of Stoke's number for breakage may be exceeded – at least near the impeller blade leading to a balance of breakage and growth and an equilibrium granule size. This example also highlights that most high-shear mixers have a very wide range of collision velocities in different parts of the bed. Granule coalescence will occur in regions of low collision velocity, while breakage and consolidation are more likely near the impeller. To properly quantify and predict this behavior, we need more sophisticated models that divide the granulator into at least two regions and incorporate a better understanding of powder flow than we currently have.

Nevertheless, we can make some intelligent comments with regard to scale-up. In a mixer granulator, the maximum collision velocity for a granule will be of the order of the impeller tip

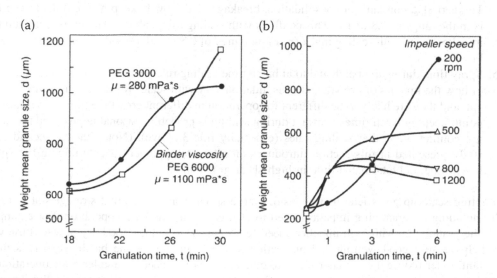

FIGURE 24.18 Variations in granule growth rate and extent of growth in a mixer granulator with changes to (a) binder viscosity and (b) impeller speed.
Source: From Ref. [30].

speed. To maintain constant St_{def}, the impeller tip speed should be kept constant, that is, (24.36). If a constant Fr rule is used [Eq. (34)],

$$\frac{St_{def,2}}{St_{def,1}} = \frac{U_{c,2}^2}{U_{c,1}^2} = \frac{N_2^2 D_2^2}{N_1^2 D_1^2} = \frac{D_2}{D_1} \tag{24.42}$$

Thus, St_{def} increases with scale. This will lead to an increase in the maximum achievable granule density and a decrease in the maximum achievable particle size. The actual granule density and size may also depend on the kinetics of consolidation and growth and are difficult to predict without more sophisticated quantitative modeling. As such, the variation in St_{def} with scale potentially leads to changes in granule attributes that are difficult to predict.

The liquid saturation S [Eq. (9)] should be kept constant on scaling. This implies a similar liquid content on a kg/kg dry powder basis *provided the granule density does not change with scale*. For operation in the steady growth regime, this is a reasonable assumption. However, for operation in the induction growth regime, the change in density with scale is harder to predict.

24.7.4   RECOMMENDED SCALING RULES FOR HIGH-SHEAR MIXER GRANULATORS AND CASE STUDY EXAMPLES

The complexity of powder flow and granulation rate processes makes it impossible to recommend a single definitive set of scaling rules. It is important to know which granule attribute is of most importance during scaling and the main granulation rate process that controls this attribute.

Overall, we recommend the following approach:

1. Keep granulators geometrically similar during scale-up where manufacturer's designs allow. In particular, keep dimensionless fill height constant during scale-up [Eq. (35)].
2. To ensure similar powder mixing, keep Froude number constant during scale-up by adjusting the impeller speed according to Eq. (34). At the very least, make sure $Fr > Fr_c$ at all scales.
3. To achieve good binder distribution, Ψ_a should be kept constant on scale-up. This is likely to mean multiple spray nozzles at a large scale to give sufficient spray zone area [(24.41)].
4. To keep St_{def} constant for consolidation, breakage, and growth, keep ND^n constant, where n is in the range of 0.8 to 1.0. This conflicts with scaling rule 2 above. Therefore, scale-up the impeller speed with scaling index (n) in the range of 0.8 to 1.0, provided that at a large scale $Fr > Fr_c$.
5. Spray time during the batch and total batch time scaling rules require a sound understanding of how the kinetics of growth and consolidation vary with scale. We do not know these rules yet, and they are likely to be different for operation in different growth regimes. As a starting point, keeping batch times constant during scaling is probably reasonable provided this does not conflict with other scaling rules (especially rule 3 above). (Note that the second case study presented in this section introduces an alternate approach in determining the spray batch time and total batch time in high-shear granulation.)

Conflicting scale-up goals lead us to consider more sophisticated operating strategies at a large-scale including programming impeller speed to change during the batch operation. For example, begin the granulation with high impeller speed (constant Fr) to induce good dry powder turnover. This helps ensure good wetting and nucleation at the beginning of the batch when it is most important. Later reduce the impeller speed to give a similar tip speed to smaller-scale operation to control granule density or size. As the powder mass is now wet, it will be more cohesive, and operation above the critical Froude number for rolling flow will be easier to maintain.

TABLE 24.4
Case Study 1: Operating Conditions for the 25-L Granulator

Parameter	Value
Nominal volume (L)	25
Powder charge (kg)	5
Impeller speed (rpm)	330
Spray time (min)	8
Drop size (μm)	100
ε_{min}	0.3
W	0.15
$\dot{V}$ (m^3/sec)	1.6×10^{-6}
Spray width W (m)	0.13
Powder surface velocity (m/sec)	0.85
Ψ_a	0.22

Litster and Ennis [5] give a case study for scale-up of a lactose granulation that is useful for illustrating these scaling rules and conflicts. It is represented in the next section.

Case Study 1: Scale-up of a lactose granulation from 25 to 300 L

A lactose-based granulation in a 25-L granulator has given granules with acceptable properties. The operating conditions for the 25-L granulator are summarized as follows (Table 24.4):

The dimensionless spray flux Ψ_a above was calculated by Eq. (7)

$$\Psi_a = \frac{3\dot{V}}{2\dot{A}d_d}$$

This granulation is to be scaled to 300 L using the following rules and heuristics:

- Keep Fr constant.
- Keep spray time constant.
- Spray from a single nozzle on a large scale.

How do Ψ_a and St_{def} change on scale-up? What are the implications of granulation rate processes at a full scale?

Scaling to 300-L granulation

Assuming geometric similarity,

$$\frac{D_2}{D_1} = 12^{1/3}$$

Keeping Fr constant,

$$N_2 = \left(\frac{D_1}{D_2}\right)^{0.5} N_1 = 218\,\text{rpm}$$

Assume spray width scales with impeller diameter.

$$W_2 = \left(\frac{D_2}{D_1}\right)W_1 = 0.3\,\text{m}$$

Powder surface velocity scales with tip speed.

$$v_2 = \left(\frac{D_2 N_2}{D_1 N_1}\right)v_1 = 1.28\,\text{m/sec}$$

Keeping spray time constant with one nozzle,

$$\dot{V}_2 = 12\dot{V}_1$$

Thus, the dimensionless spray flux at 300 L is

$$\psi_{a,2} = \frac{3\dot{V}_2}{2W_2 v_2 d} = \frac{3(12\dot{V}_1)}{2.\,(12^{1/3}W_1)\,12^{1/6}v_1 d} = 3.41\psi_{a,1} = 0.75$$

There has been a substantial increase in Ψ_a on scale-up taking the granulation from nearly drop-controlled into the mechanical dispersion regime. This could result in a much broader granule size distribution on a large scale. A similar spray flux could be achieved by using an array of four nozzles spaced at 90° intervals around the granulator (all positioned so that the spray fan is at right angles to the direction of powder flow).

We cannot calculate the value of St_{def} because the dynamic yield stress Y for the lactose/binder system is not given. However, if we neglect changes in Y because of the larger strain rate, then St_{def} will increase as

$$St_{def,2} = \frac{U_{c,2}^2}{U_{c,2}^1}St_{def,1} = \frac{(D_2 N_2)^2}{(D_1 N_1)^2}St_{def,1} = 2.3St_{def,1}$$

There is a significant increase in St_{def} with scale-up that could impact on the granule density and maximum size. It is not possible to scale with constant St_{def} while simultaneously maintaining constant Fr. A scale-up summary data is tabulated in Table 24.5.

Case Study 2: Scale-up of a conventional pharmaceutical formulation granulation from 2 to 25 and 300 L

Michaels et al. [32] demonstrated a new approach to high-shear granulation scale-up, which is named.as "steady states in granulation." In a steady-state approach, the liquid binder is introduced to the powder very slowly to ensure drop-controlled nucleation, and also long time is allowed for wet massing in order to eliminate the effects of both steps on the granule properties. When the wet powder is mixed for a sufficiently long time, simultaneous growth and breakage take the granules to a steady state, where the granule properties do not change anymore. In this approach, during scale-up, the only variable that needs to be adjusted is the impeller speed. The authors applied constant shear stress rule for the impeller speed scale-up, that is, ND^n = constant and $n = 0.8$ [(24.39)]. The heuristics and rules applied in this scale-up are tabulated in Table 24.6.

- The geometric similarity was maintained across all scales.
- The fill ratio was kept constant during the scale-up.

TABLE 24.5
Case Study 1: Scale-Up Summary Data

Parameter	25 L	300 L
Nominal volume (L)	25	300
Powder charge (kg)	5	60
Impeller speed (rpm)	330	218
Spray time (min)	8	8
Drop size (μm)	100	100
ε_{min}	0.3	0.3
W	0.15	0.15
$\dot{V}$ (m³/sec)	1.6×10^{-6}	19.2×10^{-6}
Spray width W (m)	0.13	0.3
Powder surface velocity (m/sec)	0.85	1.28
Ψ_a	0.22	0.75
$St_{def}/St_{def,25L}$	1	2.3

- The fluid level was held constant.
- Spray rate and wet mixing time were kept constant during scale-up; however, their durations were much longer compared with the conventional granulation practices (steady-state approach).
- The main impeller speed was varied according to the constant shear stress rule.

The process conditions at each scale are summarized in Table 24.6.

The exact Ψ_a and St_{def} cannot be calculated for this study because of the lack of necessary information, but it can be deduced that both Ψ_a and St_{def} increase during scale-up when the scaling rules mentioned above are used (i.e., single spray, constant spray rate, and constant shear stress rule). However, it should also be noted that the increases in Ψ_a and St_{def} are less in this case compared with the constant Fr number case presented in the previous section. Increases in both Ψ_a and St_{def} would cause differences in granule properties in conventional high-shear granulation practices where the wet massing time is limited to a few minutes, that is, the rate processes are at transient state. Michaels et al. [32] showed that by applying the constant shear rule and steady-state

TABLE 24.6
Case Study 2: Process Conditions at Each Scale

Parameter	2 L	25 L	300 L
Granulator type	Fukae Powtec	Fielder PMA25	Fielder PMA25
Nominal volume (L)	2	25	300
Powder charge (kg)	0.4	5	70
Fluid level (%)	24, 28, 32	24, 28, 32	24, 28, 32
Spray rate (g/min)	8	100	1400
Impeller speed (rpm)	600, 800, 1000	296, 395, 494	146, 194, 242
Chopper speed (rpm)	2000	3000	1000
Wet massing time (min)	30–40	30–40	30–40

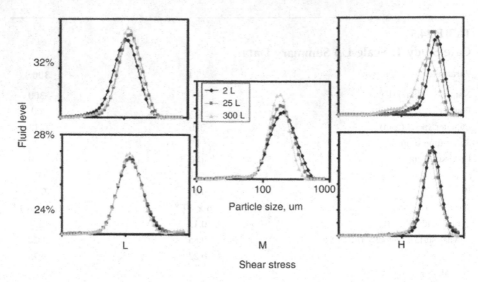

FIGURE 24.19   Granule size distribution for steady-state granulation at three scales (2, 25, and 300 L) for three levels of shear stress (low, medium, and high) and three levels of fluid amount (24%, 28%, and 32%). *Source:* From Ref. [32].

approach, it is possible to get similar granule properties as you scale-up. Their results showed that at the lowest liquid level and lowest shear rate, the granule mean particle sizes for 25 and 300 L deviated only 1% from the mean particle size of the granules produced in a 2-L granulator. The worst case was obtained for the highest liquid level and highest shear rate combination (31%). At all other conditions, the results were within 18% or better agreement. Figure 24.19 shows the particle size distribution of the granules from all three scales at different fluid levels and shear stresses. The main concern with a steady-state approach might be getting too dense granules that may be a problem in tableting and disintegration. Although the authors did not perform an extensive study on tablet performance, they showed that the dissolution profiles of tablets made by granules from conventional and steady-state granulation were comparable.

24.8   SCALE-UP OF TWIN-SCREW GRANULATORS

Twin-screw granulators (TSG) have gained popularity increasingly in the pharmaceutical industry in the past decade or so due to their mode of continuous operation and advantages in process efficiency, control, and economy [33]. In the twin-screw granulation process, the powder blend is continuously fed from one end, then mixed and kneaded while being transported through the barrel of the TSG by the screw elements, producing the required product granules at the other end of the barrel. Figure 24.20 is a schematic that illustrates the principle components of a twin-screw granulation process with online monitoring and control capabilities [34].

Depending on the binding mechanisms, TSGs can be categorized into three types, namely, twin-screw wet granulators (TSWGs), twin-screw dry granulators (TSDGs), and twin-screw melt granulators (TSMGs). In a TSWG, a liquid binder is added to the dry feed powder blend to aid the granulation process. In a TSDG, a polymeric binder with a glass transition temperature much lower than the melting temperature of the active pharmaceutical ingredients (API) is often used, and the granulation is performed at a temperature near or above the glass transition temperature of the binder but below the melting point of the API. With TSMG, a solid binder is added to the feed powder blend and granulation is performed at a temperature near or above the melting point of the binder [34]. In this section, we focus our attention mainly on the most common process of wet granulation but will include some limited discussions on the general scaling rules for TSDGs and TSMGs.

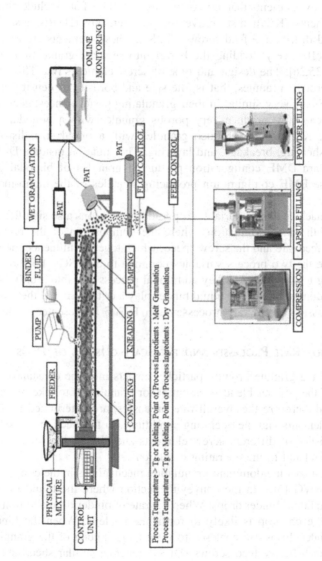

Process Temperature > Tg or Melting Point of Process ingredients : Melt Granulation
Process Temperature < Tg or Melting Point of Process ingredients : Dry Granulation

FIGURE 24.20 A schematic of continuous twin-screw granulation with monitoring and control.
Source: From Ref. [34].

24.8.1 Characteristics of TSG Processes

TSG technology is adopted from the continuous hot-melt extrusion process employed in the plastic and food industry. One of the distinct characteristics of TSGs is the availability of a wide range of screw elements and the flexibility in the configurations of the screw elements in the construction of TSGs. This can be both an advantage and a disadvantage. The advantage is that each TSG can be customized to suit one's purpose. The disadvantage is that it makes it difficult, if not totally impossible, to develop generic scaling rules for TSGs [35].

Several types of screw elements that are commonly used in a TSG include conveying elements (CEs), kneading elements (KEs), distributive mixing elements (DMEs, also known as comb mixing elements), and distributive feed screws (DFSs). These elements are assembled along the length of the barrel, effectively dividing the barrel into separate granulation zones of different growth mechanisms [35,36]. The design and type of screw elements in a TSG strongly influence the attributes of the product granules, that is, the size and porosity or density of the granules. In general, CEs and DFSs are very similar in their granulating performances, generating a relatively low shear, and thus can only produce very porous granules with a bimodal granule size distribution. In contrast, KEs usually produce granules with a broad size distribution from the combined actions of shearing, breakage, and layering. The situation inside a DME block is more complex with a forward DME configuration producing granules of bimodal granule size distribution and a reverse DME configuration producing granules of the mono-modal granule size distribution [37].

In addition to the machine design variables, operating conditions also significantly influence the granule attributes. With each formulation, where the composition of the powder blend is determined, the powder feed rate and the screw speed, which together influence the level of fill in the barrel of the TSG, are the two process variables common to all TSGs. For both the TSDGs and TSMGs, the operating temperature is a key additional process variable. For TSWGs, in contrast, the quantity and the addition rate of the liquid binder play a critical role in the granulation process. A more detailed discussion on the rate processes in a TSWG is presented in the next section.

24.8.2 Granulation Rate Processes and the Scaling Issues of TSGs

To enable nucleation and granule growth, particle contacts must be constantly renewed; that is, continuous mixing of the powder blend is essential for granulation to take place. For a TSG, the mixing behaviors, and therefore the overall rate processes, are determined by both the physical design of the screw elements and the operating conditions. In this section, we will summarize the granulation characteristics of different screw elements and discuss the scaling process using dimensionless numbers related to the operating conditions.

Figure 24.21 summarizes the dominant granulation mechanisms in the conveying and kneading compartments of a TSWG [38]. In the conveying section where the liquid binder is added, nucleation occurs around liquid binder drops. When the rate of binder drop addition is low relative to the powder feed rate, each drop is likely to form one nucleus. When the binder addition rate becomes too high, binder drops can coalesce to form larger nuclei of the granules. Although not shown in the figure, distributive feed screws (DFSs) generate similar shear and mixing environments to the powder blend. As such, granule growth mechanisms in the DFS compartment are expected to be similar to those in the CE compartment. In the kneading compartment, which is usually located after conveying compartment, two dominant granulation rate processes are taking place, namely, breakage followed by layering. In addition, the design of the kneading elements significantly impacts on the morphology of the resultant granules from the breakage. Obviously, the elongated, flake-like granules from the reverse configuration of the KEs are likely to have a poor flow property, which will cause powder-handling problems downstream and should, therefore, be avoided.

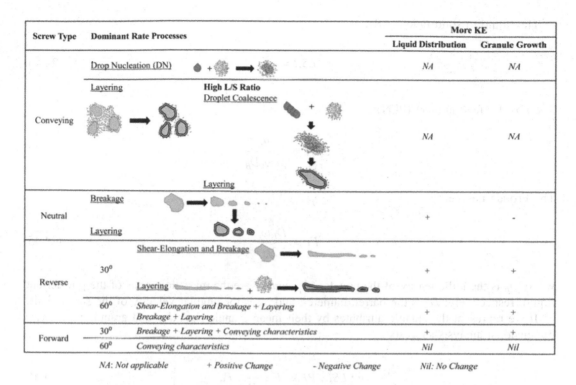

Screw Type	Dominant Rate Processes	More KE	
		Liquid Distribution	Granule Growth
Conveying	Drop Nucleation (DN)	NA	NA
	Layering / High L/S Ratio Droplet Coalescence / Layering	NA	NA
Neutral	Breakage / Layering	+	-
Reverse 30°	Shear-Elongation and Breakage / Layering	+	+
60°	Shear-Elongation and Breakage + Layering / Breakage + Layering	+	+
Forward 30°	Breakage + Layering + Conveying characteristics	+	+
60°	Conveying characteristics	Nil	Nil

NA: Not applicable   + Positive Change   - Negative Change   Nil: No Change

FIGURE 24.21 Summary of granulation rate processes in the conveying and kneading compartments of a TSWG.
Source: from Ref. [38].

Screw Type	Dominant Rate Processes	
DME - Forward	Breakage	Layering
DME - Reverse	Breakage	Layering

FIGURE 24.22 Summary of granulation rate processes in the DME compartment of a TSG.
Source: From Ref. [37].

The dominant granulation rate processes in the DME compartment are shown in Figure 24.22. Overall, liquid distribution and the morphology of granules produced in the DME compartment, irrespective of the orientation of the DMEs, are better than those from other screw elements. In general, granules from the DME compartment are more spherical in shape and have a monomodal granule size distribution without the oversize lumps, which could potentially negate the milling requirement downstream.

Key process variables for TSGs include powder feed rate $\dot{m}_p$ and screw speed ω_s. Additionally, there is also, for a TSWG, liquid binder feed rate $\dot{m}_l$, and for both TSDG and TSMG, operating temperature, T, of the granulating section. Taking the same general approach of dimensional analysis to the scaling-up of TSGs, the following dimensionless numbers can be defined for a TSWG:

The liquid to solid ratio (LSR):

$$LSR = \frac{\dot{m}_l}{\dot{m}_p} \tag{24.43}$$

The powder feed number (PFN):

$$PFN = \frac{\dot{m}_p}{\rho_b \omega_s D_B^3} \tag{24.44}$$

The Froude number:

$$Fr = \frac{D_B \omega_s^2}{2g} \tag{24.45}$$

where ρ_b is the bulk density of the powder; $\dot{m}_p$ and $\dot{m}_l$ are the mass flow rates of the powder and liquid, respectively; D_B is the barrel diameter; and ω_s is the angular velocity of the screw shaft.

If we represent the granule attributes by their mean granule size, d_{50}, and granule porosity, ε, dimensional analysis suggests:

$$\frac{d_{50}}{D_B} = g_1 \left(LSR, \ PFN, \ Fr, \ \frac{L_B}{D_B}, \ F_1, \ F_2, \ \dots \right) \tag{24.46}$$

and

$$\varepsilon = g_2 \left(LSR, \ PFN, \ Fr, \ \frac{L_B}{D_B}, \ F_1, \ F_2, \ \dots \right) \tag{24.47}$$

where L_B is the barrel length after wetting addition of liquid, and $F_1, F_2, \dots$ are a series of geometric ratios that describe the geometry of the individual screw elements and the screw configurations.

LSR has a profound effect on the granule size and its distribution [35]. Increasing the LSR increases the proportion of larger granules of the bimodal granule size distribution, as shown in Figure 24.23. In contrast, PFN and Fr have little influence on the key granule attributes, as demonstrated by the median granule size, d_{50}, in Figure 24.24(a) and (b).

Figure 24.24(c) reveals a critical characteristic of the TSGs, that is, the median granule size increases with the barrel size of the TSG. In other words, it is impossible to produce granules with the size and size distribution from TSGs of different scales. This is because, for geometrically similar, noncustom-designed TSGs (e.g., the same L_B/D_B for the whole TSG and for each screw element), the clearance between the screw elements and the barrel, as well as the gap between the intermeshing screw elements, scales almost linearly with the diameter of the barrel of the TSG. These gaps have a strong impact on the size of large granules (e.g., d_{90}) and the spread of the granule size distribution; d_{90} scales almost linearly with the diameter of TSGs, while the spread of the granule size distribution also increases with the barrel size of the TSG [35]. This is to be expected as the smallest gap between the intermeshing screw elements determines the largest granule size because the granules have to traverse the length of the TSG unbroken during the granulation process. Consequently, without modifications to the physical construction of the TSGs, in particular, maintaining the same absolute gap size between the screw elements for the TSGs of

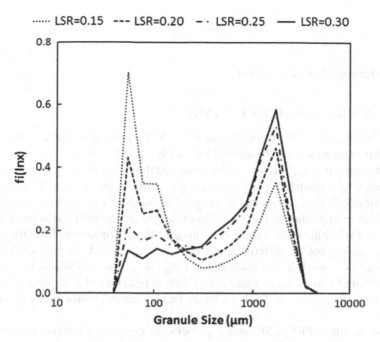

FIGURE 24.23 Effect of LSR on granule size distribution.
Source: From Ref. [35].

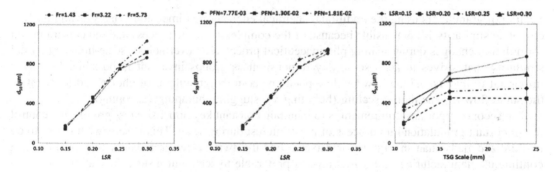

FIGURE 24.24 Median granule size (d_{50}) change with (a) Fr and LSR; (b) PFN and LSR; and (c) LSR and TGS scale.
Source: From Ref. [35].

different scales, it is not possible to achieve the same granule size distribution of product granules from TSGs of different scales.

For TSDGs and TSMGs, in addition to the operating temperature of the granulating section, the granule attributes are determined by the residence time of the powder blend, t_r, and the specific mechanical energy consumption, E_m, which are defined in equations (24.48) and (24.49), respectively [34,39].

$$t_r = \frac{D_B^2 L_B \rho_b \cdot \% \, of \, fill}{\dot{m}_p}$$

(24.48)

$$E_m = \frac{\tau \omega_s}{\dot{m}_p} \qquad\qquad (24.49)$$

where τ is the torque of the screw shaft.

24.8.3 Suggested Scaling Rules for TSGs

As mentioned before, one of the main advantages of TSGs is the continuous manufacturing mode that allows them to increase their throughput by simply extending the duration of the operation. In addition, the throughput of a TSG can also be increased through increasing the speed of screws and powder feed rate while maintaining other operating conditions constant (i.e., maintaining both LSR and PFN constant). Within a reasonable range, this method can increase the production rate without significantly impacting on the attributes of the product granules. This method of increasing throughput of a TSG, which has widely been used in the pharmaceutical industry, is defined by researchers as "scaling out" to differentiate it from the increase of the physical size of the granulator [35]. Whenever possible, the preferred scaling choice for all TSGs is to scale out.

When the required throughput increase can no longer be achieved with increased operating time or increased screw speed, that is, TSGs of larger barrel diameters must be used, we only suggest the following:

For TSWGs: maintain PFN, LSR, and gaps between the screw elements invariant.

For TSDGs and TSMGs: maintain granulation temperature, E_m and t_r invariant.

24.9 CONCLUDING REMARKS

Scaling of granulators using the traditional chemical engineering dimensional analysis approach of complete similarity is not possible because of the complexity of the process and the constraints on formulation changes during scaling pharmaceutical processes. Nevertheless, scale-up using partial similarity that strives to keep some key dimensionless groups invariant is possible. It is very important to understand the powder flow phenomena in the granulator of choice and to maintain the same flow regime during scaling (bubbling vs. slugging, bumping vs. roping).

The second important requirement is to maintain constant key dimensionless groups that control the important granulation rate process of most interest during scale. This is somewhat easier to do in fluidized beds than in high-shear mixers. For the twin-screw granulators that operate in a continuous manufacturing mode, it is always preferable to scale out instead of scaling-up.

Very small-scale tests, which have no geometric similarity to pilot and full scale, should be used to focus on formulation design and measurement of key formulation properties that influence the granulation rate processes.

Insightful understanding of the granulation processes is essential for the identification of key variables and parameters for the dimensional analysis and scale-up considerations. While the development of definitive mathematical models for the granulation processes is incomplete, the scaling approaches recommended in this chapter help reduce the uncertainty during new product development and transfer to industrial scales.

NOMENCLATURE

a	constant in equation (24.11)
A	apparent area of contact of the indentor with the surface
$\dot{A}$	area flux of powder through the spray zone
AR	Aspect Ratio of particles
b	constant in equation (24.33)

B_w	attrition rate
Ca	capillary number
d_o	distributor hole orifice size
$d_{3,2}$	specific surface mean particle size
d_b	bubble size
d_d	liquid drop size (diameter)
d_i	indentor diameter
d_p	particle or granule size
D_{drum}	drum granulator diameter
D	impeller diameter of mixer granulators
D_B	diameter of TSG barrel
D_c	chopper diameter of mixer granulators
D_f	fluidized-bed diameter
E_m	specific mechanical energy consumption in TSG
Fr	Froude number
Fr_c	critical Froude number
G	gravitational acceleration
h_{eff}	effective blade height
H	hardness of granules
H_m	fill height of mixer granulators
L	wear displacement of the indentor
L	characteristic length of a fluidized bed
L_B	length of TSG barrel
K	constant in equation (24.33)
k_1, k_2	constants in (24.10)
k_c	consolidation rate constant
K_c	fracture toughness of granules
M_1, M_2	mass of particles in the fluidized bed
M	scaling ratio
$\dot{m}_p$	mass flow rate of powder
$\dot{m}_l$	mass flow rate of liquid binder
N	impeller speed
N	scaling index
P	load
Q_b	volume flow rate of bubbles in the fluidized bed
S	granule pore saturation
S_{max}	granule pore saturation at ε_{min}
St*	critical Stokes number
St_{def}	Stokes deformation number
St_v	viscous Stokes number
Str*	dimensionless peak flow stress
T	dimensionless torque
T_o	extrapolated intercept value of dimensionless torque at an impeller speed of zero
t_p	drop penetration time
t_r	residence time
U	superficial fluidization velocity
u_1	fluidization velocity on the smaller bed
u_2	fluidization velocity on the larger bed
u_{mf1}	minimum fluidization velocity on the smaller bed
u_{mf2}	minimum fluidization velocity on the scaled bed
u_b	bubble rise velocity
U_c	particle collision velocity
v_p	relative velocity of a particle inside a granule after impact
$\dot{V}_r$	relative swept volume
$\dot{V}_{imp}$	rate of swept volume of impeller

V_{mixer}	mixer volume
$\dot{V}$	volumetric spray rate
W	liquid to solid mass ratio
W	spray zone width
Y	yield stress of granules
Z	exponent in (24.10)
B	constant in equation (24.33)
β_c	constant in equation (24.11)
γ_{LV}	liquid surface tension
Δ	dimensionless bubble space, defined as the ration of bubble space over bubble radius
ε	powder bed porosity
ε_g	bulk strain rate
ε_g	granule porosity
ε_{min}	minimum porosity of granule
ε_{tap}	bed tap density
Θ	solid-liquid contact angle
μ	viscosity of binder
ρ_b	bulk density of powder
ρ_g	granule density
ρ_G	density of fluidizing gas
ρ_s	particle density
ρ_l	binder liquid density
σ_{pk}	peak flow stress
Φ	particle sphericity
Ψ_a	dimensionless spray flux
τ	torque of TSG
Ω	drum peripheral speed
ω_i	impeller peripheral speed
ω_c	chopper peripheral speed
ω_s	angular velocity of the screw shaft

REFERENCES

1. Hileman G. A. Regulatory issues in granulation processes. In: Parikh D. M., ed. Handbook of Pharmaceutical Granulation Technology. New York: Marcel Dekker, Inc., 1997.
2. Skelly J. P., Van Buskirk G. A., Savello D. R., et al. Scaleup of immediate release oral solid dosage forms. Pharm Res 1993; 10:2–29.
3. Zlokarnik M. Dimensional Analysis and Scale-up in Chemical Engineering. Berlin: Springer-Verlag, 1991.
4. Munson B. R., Young D. F., Okiishi T. H. Fundamentals of Fluid Mechanics. 2nd ed. New York: John Wiley & Sons, Inc., 1994.
5. Litster J. D., Ennis B. The Science and Engineering of Granulation Processes. Dordrecht: Kluwer Academic Publishers, 2004.
6. Hapgood K. P., Litster J. D., Smith R. Nucleation regime map for liquid bound granules. AIChE J 2003; 49(2):350–361.
7. Iveson S. M., Wauters P. A. L., Forrest S., et al. Growth regime map for liquid-bound granules: further development and experimental validation. Powder Technol 2001; 117(1–2):83–97.
8. Iveson S. M., Beathe J. A., Page N. W. The dynamic strength of partially saturated powder compacts: the effect of liquid properties. Powder Technol 2002; 127:149–161.
9. Ennis B. J., Tardos G. I., Pfeffer R. A microlevel-based characterization of granulation phenomena. Powder Technol 1991; 65:257–272.
10. Tardos G. I., Irfran-Khan M., Mort P. R. Critical parameters and limiting conditions in binder granulation of fine powders. Powder Technol 1997; 94:245–258.

11. Liu L. X., Smith R., Litster J. D. Wet granule breakage in a breakage only high-shear mixer: Effect of formulation properties on breakage behavior. Powder Technol 2009; 189:158–164.

12. Rumpf H. The strength of granules and agglomerates. In: Kneper W. A., ed. AIME Agglomeration. New York: Interscience, 1962:379–418.

13. Van den Dries K., Vromans H. Relationship between inhomogeneity phenomena and granule growth mechanisms in a high-shear mixer. Int J Pharm 2002; 247:167–177.

14. Evans A. G., Wilshaw T. R. Quasi-static solid particle damage in brittle solids, I. Observations, analysis and implications. Acta Metall 1976; 24:939–956.

15. Ennis B. J., Sunshine G. On wear mechanism of granule attrition. Tribology Int 1993; 26:319–927.

16. Kunii D., Levenspiel O. Fluidization Engineering. 2nd ed. Boston: Butterworth-Heinemann, 1991.

17. Sanderson J., Rhodes M. Hydrodynamic similarity of solids motion and mixing in bubbling fluidized beds. AIChE J 2003; 49:2317–2327.

18. Fitzgerald T. J., Crane S. D. Cold fluidized bed modelling. Proc Int Conf Fluidized Bed Combustion, 1985 3:85–92.

19. Glicksman L. R. Scaling relationships for fluidized beds. Chem Eng Sci 1984; 39:1373–1379.

20. Glicksman L. R. Scaling relationships for fluidized beds. Chem Eng Sci 1987; 43:1419–1421.

21. Glicksman L. R., Hyre M., Woloshun K. Simplified scaling relationships for fluidized beds. Powder Technol 1993; 77:177–199.

22. Horio M., Nonaka A., Sawa Y., et al. A new similarity rule for fluidized-bed scale-up. AIChE J 1986; 32:1466–1482.

23. Horio M., Takada M., Ishida M., et al. The similarity rule of fluidization and its application to solid mixing and circulation control. Proc Fluidization V Engineering Foundation, New York, 1986:151–156.

24. Roy R., Davidson J. F. Similarity between gas-fluidized beds at elevated temperature and pressure. Proc Fluidization V Engineering Foundation, New York, 1986:293–299.

25. Steward P. S. B., Davidson J. F. Slug flow in fluidised beds. Powder Technol 1967; 1:61–80.

26. Werther J. Influence of the distributor design on bubble characteristics in large diameter gas fluidized beds. In: Davidson J. F. and Keairns D. L., eds. Fluidization. New York: Cambridge University Press, 1978.

27. Litster J. D., Hapgood K. P., Michaels J. N., et al. Scale-up of mixer granulators for effective liquid distribution. Powder Technol 2002; 124:272–280.

28. Schaefer T. PhD thesis, The Royal Danish School of Pharmacy, 1977.

29. Knight P. C., Seville J. P. K., Wellm A. B., et al. Prediction of impeller torque in high shear powder mixers. Chem Eng Sci 2001; 56:4457–4471.

30. Kristensen H. G., Schaefer T. Granulation: a review on pharmaceutical wet-granulation. Drug Dev Ind Pharm 1987; 13:803–872.

31. Tardos G. I., Hapgood K. P., Ipadeola O. O., et al. Stress measurements in high-shear granulators using calibrated "test" particles: application to scale-up. Powder Technol 2004; 140:217–227.

32. Michaels J. N., Farber L., Wong G. S., et al. Steady states in granulation of pharmaceutical powders with application to scale-up. Powder Technol 2009; 189:295–303.

33. Li J., Pradhan S. U., Wassgren C. R. Granule transformation in a twin screw granulator: Effects of conveying, kneading, and distributive mixing elements. Powder Technol 2019; 346:363–372.

34. Bandari S., Nyavanandi D., Kallakunta V. R., et al. Continuous twin screw granulation – An advanced alternative granulation technology for use in the pharmaceutical industry. Int J Pharm 2020; 580:119215.

35. Osorio J. G., Sayin R., Kalbag A. V., et al. Scaling of continuous twin screw wet granulation. AIChE J 2017 63:921–932.

36. Liu H., Ricart B., Stanton C., et al. Design space determination and process optimization in at-scale continuous twin screw wet granulation. Comput Chem Eng 2019; 125:271–286.

37. Sayin R., El Hagrasy A. S., Litster J. D. Distributive mixing elements: towards improved granule attributes from a twin screw granulation process. Chem Eng Sci 2015; 125:165–175.

38. El Hagrasy A. S., Litster J. D. Granulation rate processes in the kneading elements of a twin screw granulator. AIChE J 2013; 59:4100–4115.

39. Maniruzzaman M., Nokhodchi A. Continuous manufacturing via hot-melt extrusion and scale up: regulatory matters. Drug Discovery Today 2017; 22:340–351.

25 Advances in Process Controls and End-Point Determination

Kevin A. Macias and M. Teresa Carvajal

CONTENTS

25.1 INTRODUCTION

Granulation is a manufacturing-enabling technology where fine particles are agglomerated together to improve drug product manufacturing and performance. The most common agglomeration mechanisms used in pharmaceutical granulation are dry pressure agglomeration and wet binder-assisted granulation. Many factors should be considered during process selection to avoid unwanted chemical, solid-state, or functional changes that may occur in the presence of moisture, solvents, or pressure [1–3]. After the appropriate process is selected, it is necessary to identify the granulation attributes responsible for improved downstream drug product performance. To achieve this, it is necessary to correlate the measured values of these attributes with desired downstream improvements.

To begin correlating process improvements with the attributes, it is first necessary to identify the process improvements gained by performing granulation. Desirable downstream process and drug product improvements include enhanced flow, the formation of strong tablets, uniform drug product mass, consistent *in vivo* drug substance exposure, dose release profiles, and absence of tablet defects such as sticking, picking, and delamination. These qualitative and quantitative improvements are then empirically correlated to the values of one or more granulation attributes. The next step to correlate process improvements with the attributes is to select the attributes.

Two conventional critical attributes of granulation are particle size and density. Granulations with increased particle size typically flow better, have reduced dusting, reduced potential for ingredient segregation, and improved compactibility, and may have reduced sticking to process equipment. It is important to recognize, however, that particle size enlargement, taken to an extreme, could erode downstream processes. Particle size also governs the packing arrangement in the filling of tablets and capsules and directly affects final product weight variation [4,5]. Some authors suggest, as a rule of thumb, that the size of the granules should ideally be matched to the size of the tablet dies or capsules to minimize weight variation [6,7]. Solid dosage forms suitable for pediatric patients, mini-tablets and sprinkle capsules, have also recently motivated a deeper understanding between the optimum size of granular materials and the physical size of tablets and capsules [8–10]. The balance between enhanced flow and acceptable weight uniformity is in dynamic tension, and empiricism is required to inform the optimum value of particle size.

Following particle size, another attribute often correlated to downstream process improvement is the arrangement of primary particles within the granule, collectively known as density. Increased density has long been correlated with improved flow properties of granulations [11]. Granules prepared through pressure agglomeration have mechanical properties that correlate well with density. For granules prepared by wet binder agglomeration, density and binder adhesion to the primary particles provide a more complete representation of mechanical properties. It is important to recognize, however, that increased granule density, taken to an extreme, could erode downstream processes. The dynamic tension of density occurs between flow improvement while minimizing attrition or breakage during handling and assuring that the granules can be compressed into tablets and subsequently dissolves to release the drug in the body. Decreased porosity, which represents increased density, of tablets and granules has been reported to negatively impact disintegration and dissolution [12–14]. On the opposite extreme of high density, granules having low density are often weak and friable. These weak granules may break down to the original ungranulated materials prematurely and will not contribute to downstream process improvement.

In addition to particle size and density, many other critical attributes contribute to improved drug product manufacturing and performance including particle shape, the fraction of fines, chemical homogeneity, wet bulk density, and air permeability. Due to a large number of considerations for process improvement and critical attributes, no universal particle size distribution or optimal granule density has been identified that once met ensures the desired product performance. In the absence of these metrics and the improbability that such metrics could be identified, the process to identify critical attributes requires a trial-and-error approach to correlating the measurements of these attributes to the desired downstream performance to establish the desired endpoint [15]. With the concept of how critical attributes affect downstream performance in mind, attention shifts to the quantitative measurement of critical granulation attributes.

So far, the discussion on the impact of critical attributes on downstream performance has been qualitative: increased particle size and density have led to increased flow and are associated with poor weight uniformity and drug release when the granulations are too large or too dense. To define an end-point, it is necessary to identify value, or magnitude, of the critical attribute that is highly correlated with the optimum downstream performance metric or metrics. Attribute measurements can be direct or indirect. Direct measurements of critical attributes provide a value or distribution of values that represent the granulation. These values can then be attempted to be correlated to granulation performance. The optimum value of the attribute that is associated with the improved performance represents the granulation end-point. Common direct particle size measurements are mesh or sieve analysis and laser diffraction. Density is often directly measured using mercury intrusion porosimetry (MIP) or other displacement technologies such as GeoPyc. While these methods to determine particle size and density are direct and their values easily correlate with performance, they also almost always occur after the granulation process is over. Since these offline measurements take place after the process is over, there is no chance to control the process to meet the desired end-point. This means that if the value of the attributes happens to be different from the desired end-point value, the downstream performance will be negatively affected. An additional drawback of these offline techniques is that they are often destructive since the sample is consumed during the test. The effect of not meeting granulation end-point is illustrated in Figure 25.1, the root cause of which was not divulged.

Since offline measurements cannot detect the end-point during granulation, attempts have been made to measure the critical attributes during the process. Measuring attributes during the process provides insight into how the attributes form and provide the ability to stop the process once the optimum values of the critical attributes have been reached. Online techniques currently used by the pharmaceutical industry to obtain wet granulation end-points are listed in Table 25.1.

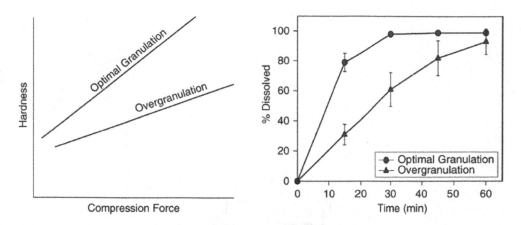

FIGURE 25.1 Effect of compaction and dissolution.
Source: Courtesy of W. Phuapradit, H. Ahmed, and N. Shah, Hoffman LaRoche.

TABLE 25.1

Examples of Techniques Used to Measure Critical Properties During Wet Granulation

Technique	Granulation Property Measured
Boots Diosna probe	Granule density and size
Capacitance	Granule moisture and saturation
The conductivity of the damp mass	Uniformity of liquid distribution, packing density
Impeller torque	End-point determination and scale-up (more sensitive to high-frequency oscillation than power)
Impeller tip speed	Corresponds to shear rate. Some benefit in scale-up for geometrically similar mixers
Power consumption (kW)	Widely used for end-point determination and scale-up
Probe/bowl vibration	Granulation adhesiveness/cohesiveness monitoring and end-point determination
Torque rheometer	An offline technique for measuring mechanical properties of the granulation
FBRM	Chord length distribute, correlated to the particle size distribution

One common drawback of online measurements is that they are almost always an indirect measure of the critical granulation attributes. For example, impeller torque and power consumption require correlation to direct offline measurement attributes like particle size and density that are further correlated to downstream improvement. Adding another level of correlation, between the online and offline attributes, increases the empiricism required to determine granulation end-point in real-time. Despite the additional complexity and empiricism, online measurements invaluably provide opportunities to understand granulation mechanisms and determine granulation end-point during the process. To take it one step further, an ideal online measurement system would directly measure the values of critical attributes in real-time to enable end-point determination and enable process control. The goal beyond merely stopping granulation at its end-point is to assure downstream performance by manipulating process variables and steering the critical attributes to values consistent with the end-point. To achieve this ultimate level of process control, it is necessary to measure or otherwise predict the critical attributes in real-time and have an actionable control framework that links process parameters to the formation of the desired granulation attributes. Figure 25.2 outlines progress that has been made toward developing a high-shear wet granulation control framework.

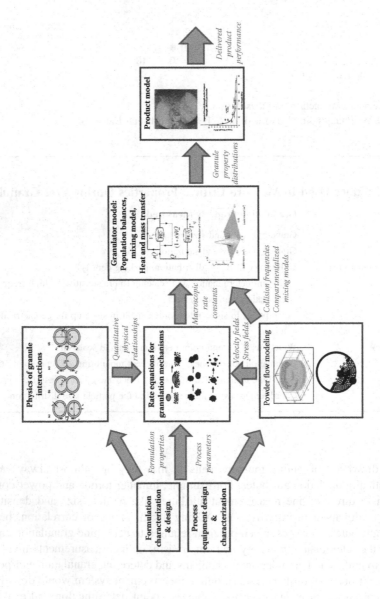

FIGURE 25.2 Modern holistic approach to modeling granulation.
Source: Courtesy of Professor James Litster, The University of Sheffield.

This type of holistic modeling framework is established over time by forming testable hypotheses and conducting experimental studies to test the hypotheses. Eventually, the modeling framework provides full connectivity between input material properties, process variables, critical attributes, granulation rate phenomena, downstream improvement, and final drug product performance. By adopting, testing, and continually verifying the structured relationships within the model, it can be used to inform process levers capable of controlling the granulation process. For relationships that are incompletely described, the framework guides the systematic application of new measurement and modeling technologies capable of more deeply understanding wet granulation. In cases where the framework completely explains all granulation phenomena, it can be implemented in real-time to consistently achieve the end-point.

The rest of this chapter will discuss advances that have been made in the pharmaceutical industry to measure and model critical granulation attributes and their formation during the process. Examples of offline, online, direct, and indirect granulation attribute measurements that have been applied to end-point determination and control of roller compaction, fluid-bed granulation, dense-phase wet granulation, and twin-screw granulation will be shared. This chapter will close by highlighting exciting emerging trends that will shape the future of granulation technologies.

25.2 ROLLER COMPACTION

Roller compaction starts by feeding a well-mixed blend through counter-rotating rolls. The geometry of the rolls physically reduces the volume of the blend and compresses the powdered blend into a solid ribbon. The ribbon is subsequently milled into granules that have a larger particle size, higher density, and better flow characteristics compared to the original well-mixed blend that was fed through the roller compactor. Roller compaction transforms a small amount of material over an extended period. Attributes are monitored continuously, or at time intervals, and process changes can be made in case of deviation from desired attributes. The continuous nature of roller compaction has also made it an ideal candidate to be incorporated within continuous manufacturing operations.

Ribbon density, particle size, and bulk granulation density are common critical attributes that correlate strongly with the downstream process and product improvement. Ribbon density is often directly measured using offline displacement methods such as mercury intrusion porosimetry and GeoPyc [16]. Online and indirect real-time approaches to measuring ribbon attributes include acoustic relaxation emission techniques and using near-infrared (NIR) spectroscopy [17,18]. The intensity of acoustic relaxation was correlated to the relative degree of ribbon consolidation through the roller compaction force. NIR spectra were found to be correlated to multiple ribbon attributes including density, Young's modulus, and tensile strength using this measurement approach. Even though these methods indirectly measure critical attributes, both approaches have the potential to become real-time methods for process control. Another indirect measurement technique capable of predicting mechanical properties of ribbons is using instrumented roll technology [19]. In this real-time and indirect approach, the force experienced during roller compaction is measured using load cell sensors embedded in the roll. The force distribution is then related through material compactibility to predict the ribbon properties. It is not always necessary to measure the critical attributes to obtain its quantitative value. Ribbon density values, for example, have been reported in real-time using a novel modeling approach by Nkansah et al. who proposed a model for deriving the average ribbon density, without taking measurements of ribbon samples [20]. This indirect modeling method requires the mass of ribbons produced during a steady-state time interval to be divided by the volume through which that mass passed in the same time interval. In this model, the volume is calculated by multiplying the average roll gap by the roll width and ribbon length as determined by the roll diameter and number of revolutions that occurred during the steady-state interval. Due to the fixed roller compactor geometry and the well-controlled roll gap and roll speed, very constant ribbon density predictions are produced by only measuring the mass of the collected product. This simple and highly effective model to measure ribbon density opens a new path to control the process in real-time by manipulating roll force and gap to achieve the desired ribbon density.

Quantifying particle size is also of great interest for roller compaction. Silva et al. provide a thorough review of offline and online as well as direct and indirect particle-sizing techniques [21]. Some of the online and direct particle-sizing techniques that have been successfully applied to roller compaction include digital image analysis using EyeCon analyzer [16]. An attribute that is derived from particle size is process efficiency. Process efficiency, defined by percentage of uncompressed particles, needs to be minimized to optimize granules size and assure in-spec tablets are produced after roller compaction [22]. In the report, am Ende et al. reported the modeling structure between percentage of fines, roll gap, and roll force. With a control framework in mind for this product, a measured decrease in efficiency might be corrected by reducing the roll gap by increasing roll force. As more of these interactions between roller compaction settings, intermediate granulation attributes, and final product performance are elucidated, control frameworks can be established, tested, and used to meet process efficiency requirements and produce the desired granulation size.

25.3   FLUID-BED GRANULATION

Fluidized-bed granulation starts by passing heated air through a well-mixed powder bed at a sufficient velocity to overcome gravity. Fluid-bed granulators have a narrow chamber at the bottom and a tapered expansion chamber at the top. As the powder meets the level of the expansion chamber, the air velocity drops and the fluidized powder falls under the influence of gravity back toward the narrow section of the fluid bed. As this cyclical pattern continues, a liquid polymer-containing solution is added to the powder bed. As the liquid binder spreads over the powder, the particles are gathered together and form wet agglomerates. In addition to binder–formulation interactions that are reliant on the thermodynamics of wetting parameters, binder solution viscosity and binder solution quantity determine granule growth kinetics. During the spraying process, the heated fluidization air drives off moisture to form solid polymer bridges between the particles, thereby creating permanent granules. The simultaneous processes of liquid addition, agglomeration, and drying work together to produce granulations having increased particle size, high porosity, improved flow, and uniform shape.

Granule formation during fluid-bed granulation relies on steady-state moisture content that is comprised of balancing liquid binder addition and simultaneous evaporation. For this reason, it is desirable to understand and control the dynamic process of drying and wetting during fluid-bed granulation by constantly measuring critical granule attributes including particle size, density, and moisture content. Offline and direct measurement of moisture content is usually completed by loss on drying. In this method, a sample from the wet granulation is heated while the mass of the sample is recorded. The mass lost during heating, compared to the original sample mass, represents the quantity of moisture contained in the sample. With the sample that is now dry, it is common to measure other attributes including particle size, density, and attrition. By completing these tests at time intervals during the granulation process, the quality of granulation attributes can be assessed and an end-point can be determined.

To enable continuous measurement, rather than in discrete intervals, of the moisture present during processing, near-infrared (NIR) spectroscopy has been applied to indirectly determine moisture content to guide granulation and determine the end-point of drying [23,24]. In addition to moisture, another critical attribute that has been indirectly measured in real-time is particle size. In one application, particle size was predicted from multivariate data analysis of microwave

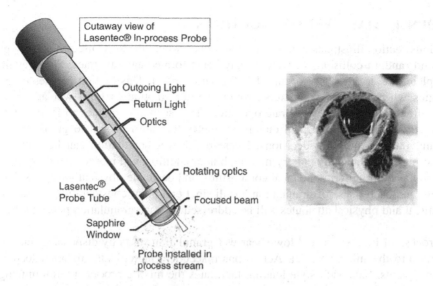

FIGURE 25.3   Cutaway view of Lasentec FBRM® probe showing various parts.
Source: Courtesy of Mettler Toledo Autochem, Inc.

resonance spectra and used to monitor granulation size progression [25]. In another substantial publication, success was reported in monitoring both moisture and mean particle size indirectly with NIR spectroscopy [24,26]. As useful as these indirect methods are, they still require a large amount of work to correlate the offline granulation attributes to the online signals. The next advance in the end-point determination of fluid-bed granulation comes in the form of directly measuring particle size during the process.

The focused beam reflectance method (FBRM®) directly measures particles and has been successfully used at-line to assess the progression of fluid-bed granulation with respect to particle growth [27]. While this is a great step forward and eliminates the need for drying before sizing, it still required samples to be extracted from the granulator. Techniques, such as FBRM and particle vision and measurement (PVM®) microscopy, both allow real-time direct measurement of granule size without sampling or extracting product. Figure 25.3 shows the FBRM cutaway view of the probe that tracks the effect of changing critical process conditions and quickly detects undersized and oversized granule distributions.

Another direct method, image analysis has successfully monitored the change in granule size during processing [28,29]. For systems that measure only particle size, other critical attributes are not measured and may need to be verified after the process is complete. While particle size does not tell the whole story, it has still been a very useful quality attribute and has been used for real-time control of granulation processes. Watano has demonstrated the ability to control the process of fluid-bed granulation using direct particle size image analysis and fuzzy logic combined with delay terms to help prevent overgranulation [30]. Reimers et. al. implemented a closed-loop feedback control system by measuring real-time particle size directly with spatial filtering technique [31]. In the absence of a critical attribute measurement system, Hu et al. incorporated thermodynamic models of wetting and evaporation to enable moisture prediction prior to granulation [32]. The authors illustrated success in controlling moisture during granulation by using the process models to modulate the temperature of the air entering and fluidizing the granulation. Successfully implementing a modeling framework to predict moisture indicates that fluidized-bed granulation has become well-understood, and a generalized control framework may soon become available.

25.4 DENSE-PHASE WET GRANULATION

The previous section illustrates a granulation approach where the air is used to convey particles in a vessel and random collisions of wetted ingredients formed agglomerates. When agglomeration was complete, the drying phase occurred in the same vessel. This section focuses on granulation technologies where mechanical mixers provide particle motion to form wet agglomerates and drying is often completed in a separate operation. This section continues to focus on measuring, either directly or indirectly, critical quality attributes that are required to guide the granulation process and inform end-point decisions. Dense-phase wet granulation can be broken into four subphases: ingredient loading and dry-mixing, binder addition, wet massing, and drying. The ideal granulation has both uniform chemical composition and desirable physical attributes that facilitate processing, and each phase of granulation has distinct end-point considerations. The end-point of both chemical and physical attributes will be addressed for each granulation phase in the following sections.

The process of high-shear and low-shear wet granulation starts by dispensing and loading dry ingredients into the mixing vessel. Active pharmaceutical ingredients are often loaded between bulking excipients. Sandwich-style loading facilitates the mixing process by minimizing material adherence to the mixing vessel. The dry ingredients are mechanically agitated using impellers and/ or choppers until the end-point of dry-mixing is reached, and all ingredients are acceptably uniform. Ingredient uniformity can be assessed by directly measuring samples offline using wet chemistry or non-destructive spectroscopy. Instead of thief sampling for offline analysis, some investigators have used indirect measurement online tools such as near-infrared (NIR) spectroscopy, Raman spectroscopy, and hyperspectral imaging to assess blend uniformity during the dry-mixing phase of granulation. When uniformity end-point is achieved at this stage, there is less risk of meeting content uniformity requirements of the final drug product.

The second phase of wet granulation consists of adding a liquid binder to the well-mixed and mechanically agitated dry ingredients. Dense-phase wet granulation, just like fluid-bed granulation, uses polymeric binders to hold granules together. Selecting which binder to use has become a well-understood science, and many publications discuss wettability, spreading coefficients, viscosity, and desired granule strength to guide binder selection [33,34]. Polymeric binders can be added to granulations in the liquid or solid state. With dry binder addition, the polymer is added to the vessel with the other dry ingredients, and water or other solvent is added to activate the binder by hydration or solvation. With wet binder addition, a prehydrated or presolvated binder solution is prepared and sprayed or poured onto the mechanically mixed ingredients. Hapgood et al. have shown that the rate of water uptake is an important step in the formation of granule nuclei [35]. The formation of nuclei can be directly measured offline using laser diffraction or sieve analysis of samples taken during the early binder addition phase [36,37]. After nuclei form, binder addition continues until the granules have grown to a sufficiently large size and have sufficient binder saturation to form acceptably strong granules. Most traditional measurements to determine binder requirements aim to monitor the dynamic transitions between physical states of the wet mass during binder addition. Determining the optimal quantity of binder required for a granulation has historically been completed using sensory techniques such as squeeze tests, and hearing increased granulator load during binder addition. Non-biased techniques to determine binder quantity have been sought to ensure products are manufactured reproducibly while minimizing exposure of operators to drug products. Many characterization techniques to assess binder addition and the resulting granules are available (Table 25.2).

Boots Diosna Probe, impeller torque, power consumption, conductivity, and capacitance are online and indirect measurements that describe binder addition end-point that are indirectly related to the particle size and the relative degree of binder saturation within granules. Variations measured by power consumption and torque during granulation are indirectly attributed to the evolution of wet agglomerate strength and granule size. Despite the research that has attempted to

TABLE 25.2
Review of Various Characterization Techniques

Technique	Pros	Cons	Comment
Sieve analysis	Simple technique	Must dry granules	A feasible method to find granulation growth rates
Malvern	Fast	The offline technique, data is not reliable	The current model is not appropriate
Lasentec FBRM	Online method	The information does not correlate to other techniques. The new prototype will be tested	Need further understanding of obtained information
NIR	Online method	Combined particle size and density information	Information is currently not useful for distribution
Optical microscopy	Direct method	Small sample size	Not feasible to measure the entire batch
Sympatec	Fast, reliable method	Offline method	A feasible method to find granulation growth rates

Source: From David Ely, Carvajal's research group.
Abbreviation: NIR, near-infrared.

predict the optimal quantity of binder, the requirements remain empirically determined [38–40]. While useful information is gained by using surrogate transition states of granulation, recent measurements of end-point research aim to directly measure granule attributes responsible for improved downstream functionality including particle size and density. Decoupling the signals into individual critical attributes allows for better understanding and provides mechanisms for process control decisions. In addition to mesh analysis and laser scattering, at-line focused beam reflectance methods have been useful to directly measure granule growth during binder addition. Attempts have been made to automate the real-time diversion of material during granulation to enable measurement by laser diffraction equipment but are not well documented in the open literature. One of the obstacles to enabling the automated diversion is the blocking of sampling streams due to adhesive properties of the wet mass. The adhesive nature of binder-soaked material has also limited the implementation of laser backscattering techniques [41]. One of the hurdles to monitoring wet granulations is the fouling of probes, and several recent efforts have tried to address this issue. Figure 25.4 shows the results of various levels of moisture addition in a high-shear mixer, and the resulting particle size increases due to different water addition and different massing time measured by Lasentec FBRM and PVM.

Material adherence to the probe has been reported as a drawback to this probe technology. To mitigate material adherence to a probe, an FBRM with an integrated wiper became commercially available and was applied to directly measure granule growth during wet granulation [42,43]. This same style of FBRM with wiping technology has been used to monitor binder addition during granulation and found success as a real-time end-point technique [44–46]. Granule density is most often measured offline using mercury intrusion porosimetry (MIP) [11,47]. Measurements of torque have been correlated to particle size and density. Recently a direct strain probe technique has shown promise [48–52]. This optical-based sensor measures probe deflection and has been correlated with the density and kinetic energy of the granules. This new measurement shows promise to determine wet mass transition states of binder addition directly at the individual granule level. A final critical attribute that affects the downstream process and product improvement is binder uniformity. Proper selection of binder, optimum spray flux, and consistent granule growth

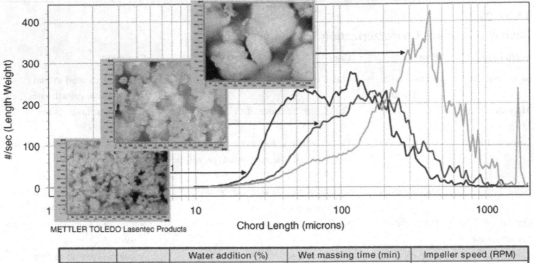

		Water addition (%)	Wet massing time (min)	Impeller speed (RPM)
―――	1	20	4	542
―――	2	25	2.5	542
·····	3	30	4	542

FIGURE 25.4 Three levels of moisture addition and massing times with the resultant granule growth measured by Lasentec FBRM® and PVM®.
Source: Courtesy of Mettler Toledo Autochem, Inc.

should translate into uniform binder distribution throughout the granulation. To check for homogeneity, binder uniformity has been directly measured offline with PVP extraction and loss on drying as well as indirectly online using spectroscopy [36,53,54].

After the binder addition phase is complete, mechanical agitation of the wet mass continues for a period of time. The wet massing phase of wet granulation helps further distribute the liquid binder, consolidate granules, and form final granule size and shape. As was true during binder addition, sensory techniques have traditionally been used to determine granulation progress in the wet massing phase. Arising from the experienced-based squeeze test are the technologies of direct probe strain [55] and indirect vibration analysis [56,57] that have provided indirect measures of particle size, density, and liquid saturation. To displace hearing the granulator, torque, power consumption, and direct impeller torque have been tested simultaneously to test the predictive capability of a low-shear wet granulation to indirectly assess subsequent tablet manufacture [58]. More recently, indirect methods using passive acoustic technology have been successful in determining granulation end-point with respect to particle size and granules properties [59–63]. In general, particle size and density remain the primary critical attributes to determine the end-point of wet massing. As such, the same measurements used to assess binder addition are applied to understand and ultimately control wet massing. Figure 25.5 illustrates a correlation that was found between the wet mass consistency measured during granulation and the relative flow of the granulation [64].

This very important publication by Faure et al. demonstrates that it is possible to draw correlations between wet mass properties and dry granulation behavior. The authors took it a step further and described the ability of the granules to maintain their attributes during downstream processing by introducing the friability test. Granules having low friability are able to withstand processing and thereby enable correlation between wet and dry granulation attributes. In Figure 25.6, the relative friability of granulations is reported for granulations in which the wet

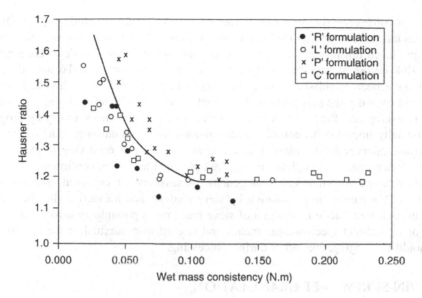

FIGURE 25.5 Hausner ratio determined for granulations in which the wet mass was characterized in terms of wet mass consistency.
Source: From Ref. 64.

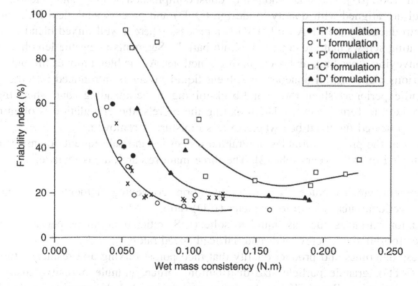

FIGURE 25.6 Friability determined for granulations in which the wet mass was characterized in terms of wet mass consistency.
Source: From Ref. 64.

mass was characterized prior to drying [64]. This key wear-resistance attribute assures that the desired level of flow will be maintained until the final product is manufactured.

Now that critical attributes have been formed through dry-mixing, binder addition, and wet massing, the final phase of wet granulation is to remove the excess binding liquid by drying. There are many drying options available including fluidized-bed drying, tray drying, and microwave drying. The end-point of drying has been reached with the moisture or solvent that has reached a low and acceptable level. The moisture level is often monitored by a combination of bed temperature and direct measurement of moisture content using the loss-on-drying (LOD) technique from samples taken from the fluidized-bed dryer. In a quasi-continuous process, over-dry granules have been produced during start-up. It was found that the over-dry granules were a result of the large heat sink before steady-state, evaporative-cooling operation [65]. To negate over-drying, approaches have been established where the temperature has been controlled to ramp the temperature to not over-dry the first portion of the continuous manufacturing drying system. It is also common to develop real-time NIR moisture models to constantly measure drying progress. This trend is especially important to embrace as continuous wet granulation production lines strive to reduce operator intervention by manual sampling and offline loss-on-drying analysis.

With the entire process complete, and desired physical attributes confirmed, the final granulation is often tested for chemical homogeneity. Assessment of chemical composition can be evaluated by fractionating the granulation by sieve analysis and measuring the chemical composition within each size fraction. Analysis of sieve fractions is possible by direct testing using wet chemistry or by indirect spectroscopic means and is used to contextualize the risk to blend uniformity should any segregation occur during processing.

25.5 TWIN-SCREW WET GRANULATION

Continuous twin-screw wet granulation (TSG) is well established in food, detergent, and polymer industries [66]. Its adoption is owed to its potential to improve process efficiency through continuous processing. TSG is gaining interest in the pharmaceutical industry since first patented and introduced in 2002 [67]. The small footprint, robust equipment assembly, and potential for closed-loop control are aligned with quality-by-design (QbD) and process analytical technology (PAT) concepts introduced by the FDA [68]. TSG is a process where a well-mixed blend is fed through dual co-rotating screws that are confined within barrels. Segments along the length of the screws perform conveying, kneading, and back-mixing functions. As the blend moves through the screws, and the various elements, an aqueous or solvent liquid binder is introduced into the blend. The wetted blend experiences shear forces and back-mixing in the kneading zone where the binder is uniformly mixed to form granules. Upon exiting the barrels, the granulation is often discharged directly into a heated fluidized bed where excess moisture is removed.

The effect of the process variables on granule properties and subsequent downstream behavior has been studied over the years [68–72]. The three main research areas include:

1. Equipment which includes: screw configuration, conveying elements, kneading elements, cross-sectional area, length to diameter (L/D) ratio;
2. Operation variables such as liquid to solid (L/S) ratio, material properties (excipient and binder formulation), screw and material feed speed rates;
3. Process outcomes and product quality that incorporate mixing and residence time distribution (RTD), granule particle size distribution, torque, granule porosity/density, and final tablet properties. Research has been undertaken on the characterization for equipment geometry, operation variables and product quality/outcomes [69–71,73,74], or the lack thereof in the case of formulation and materials [72,73,75,75,76].

The same critical attributes, particle size, density, shape, and flow, that were important to fluidized-bed and dense-phase granulation are important to measure and control in TSG. Particle size is often measured by offline and direct techniques with relatively few successful examples of online measurements. Near-infrared spectra, which were previously correlated to offline particle size, were able to measure particle size in real-time [77]. Image analysis has directly measured particle size and has been implemented in closed-loop control of particle size for TSG [78]. Other imaging systems, including EyeCon, have been successfully used to measure particle size during TSG [79].

To measure moisture content, researchers have qualified the use of an inline torque method that measured the energy uptake of the system [80]. In the Consigma-25, NIR, Raman, and photometric imaging were shown to correlate to quality attributes of granule moisture content, tapped and bulk density, and flowability [81]. The drying process after extrusion is also very amenable to moisture measurement by indirect means of NIR spectroscopy [82].

Material traceability is used to evaluate the residence time during wetting, kneading, and densification. Many times spectroscopy can be used to monitor tracer studies that are required for RTD parameterization. Successful examples of traceability with positron emission particle tracking (PEPT) experiments have allowed the visualization of powder flow in high-shear granulators and residence time distribution (RTD) measurement of twin-screw granulators [83]. Material flow tracking and better links between the granulation process and final quality attributes have been enabled by modeling and control systems [84]. Once the desired screw configuration is established, TSG has few levers to control, increase, or decrease the powder feed rate, slow down or speed up the screws, and add more or less binder to increase or decrease the liquid to solid ratio [74,85]. A digital tool called flowsheet modeling has formed the modeling framework that connects material attributes, equipment parameters, and downstream performance of continuous operations [86]. Automation has also enabled the rapid development of mechanistic and model-based analysis for TSG [87]. By combining the flowsheet modeling framework with automated recipe execution, the framework-guided experiments can quantitatively inform the modeling relationships very quickly, sometimes in a matter of hours. In situations where model-based control is required, techniques using advanced process control have been established [88]. Eventually, these frameworks might be so well understood that they form the basis of control strategies or become a useful digital twin that informs major effects on critical attributes through sensitivity analysis.

25.6 EMERGING APPROACHES

25.6.1 SURFACE CHEMISTRY AND ENERGETICS IN GRANULATION

The next level of understanding fluid-bed, dense-phase, and TSG involves understanding the thermodynamics, kinetics, and physics of the concurrent processes occurring during granulation. It is known in wet granulation that the wettability of granular solids such as pharmaceutical materials depends on particle inherent chemistry and physical properties such as particle morphology (size distribution, shape, and surface roughness), binder addition (spray flux), composition, and spreading of the liquid in the bed powder [89–91]. The study of these characteristics helps to predict the behavior of the material between granulation and compression. More recently, the surface chemistry of materials has slowly gained interest as an important attribute that affects the performance of various unit operations (milling, granulation, spray-drying, or freeze-drying) during manufacture [92–94]. The surface chemistry characterization has proven to help in the understanding of powder behavior, physical performance (flowability, water repellency), and stability of the materials that were subjected to secondary processing [94,95].

Studies on the powder surface chemistry and its effect on particle cohesion-adhesion and wettability of powders are anticipated to play an important role during its use in producing agglomerates for formulations during new product development. The comprehensive characterization of powder surface properties is necessary to facilitate the manufacture of granules by adding appropriate binder solutions and for controllable critical attributes. The surface characterization can analytically be obtained for surface energetics via inverse gas chromatography (iGC) measurements [96–98] and surface composition via X-ray Photoelectron Spectroscopy (XPS) or electron spectroscopy for chemical analysis (ESCA) measurements [94,99]. With complete understanding, empirically driven screening studies to perform binder selection and binder quantity could become obsolete.

25.6.2 Measurements and Controls

Despite the excellent benefits provided by end-point determination and process control, there are common roadblocks to technology adoption routinely encountered. Investment of PAT for drug product manufacturing can be difficult for pharmaceutical companies due to the lack of commercially available "PAT-Ready" equipment. Although there are a few equipment vendors that allow for easy integration, for the vast majority of equipment, a PAT-focused team must develop a bespoke system and integrate it into the equipment. This includes mechanical interfacing, assurance of equipment integrity, assurance of intrinsic safety, having complete confidence in the information being collected, and maintaining the data that must be reported in the batch record. Connections between the bespoke system and the equipment controls must also be completed and maintained. Too often, this scenario is viewed as too much of an investment of time and resources. There are a few commercially available options for directly measuring granule attributes. Examples include fluid-bed drying equipment that can be delivered with PAT ports for NIR and microwave sensing technologies.

The introduction of continuous manufacturing has increased the adoption rate of direct and indirect methods to monitor and control the critical attributes. These methods have taken the form of soft sensors and traditional PAT measurement methods. The exponential growth of sensors has enabled many projects under the broad Industrial Internet of Things (IIoT) umbrella. Not only are there more sensors available, but they are available in smaller form factors and with higher reproducibility. With time, these highly capable and robust sensors might be integrated by pharmaceutical equipment manufacturers.

Autonomous systems have emerged in many fields such as robotics and automobiles. Faster development, faster and more robust systems, and better yields are exceptional value propositions for the adoption of autonomous continuous processing systems. Now that meaningful pharmaceutical frameworks exist and there is technology available to measure critical attributes, the final level of sophistication is to measure the quality attributes and then control the quality attributes by a closed feedback loop with automated decision-making. With this significant migration, there will be an emphasis placed on reducing operator exposure and improving the overall process robustness with remote operation. The same infrastructure also allows the removal of non-conforming materials from the process line during planned process deviations in the case of startup and shutdown and unplanned deviations of unknown origin. These new technologies, coupled with emerging telepresence technologies, will continue to reveal a deeper understanding of granulation and guide formulation and process decisions using the science-based approach with the goal of having unsupervised control loops. Ultimately, these technologies could become useful to increase transparency between stakeholders including regulatory agencies. With the adoption of these technologies, there is hope for continued compliance assurance between audits and potential frameworks that continually track the risk of drug shortages [100,101].

REFERENCES

1. Bauer, J., et al., Ritonavir: an extraordinary example of conformational polymorphism. Pharmaceutical Research, 2001. 18(6): p. 859–866.
2. Shefter, E. and T. Higuchi, Dissolution behavior of crystalline solvated and nonsolvated forms of some pharmaceuticals. Journal of Pharmaceutical Sciences, 1963. 52(8): p. 781–791.
3. Morris, K. R., et al., Theoretical approaches to physical transformations of active pharmaceutical ingredients during manufacturing processes. Advanced Drug Delivery Reviews, 2001. 48(1): p. 91.
4. Podczeck, F., et al., The filling of granules into hard gelatine capsules. International Journal of Pharmaceutics, 1999. 188(1): p. 59–69.
5. Podczeck, F. and G. Lee-Amies, The bulk volume changes of powders by granulation and compression with respect to capsule filling. International Journal of Pharmaceutics, 1996. 142(1): p. 97–102.
6. Banker, G. and N. Anderson, Tablets. 3rd ed. In The Theory and Practice of Industrial Pharmacy, L. Lachman, H. Lieberman, and J. Kanig, Editors. 1986, Philadelphia, PA: Lea and Febiger.

7. Marks, A. M. and J. J. Sciarra, Effect of size on other physical properties of granules and their corresponding tablets. Journal of Pharmaceutical Sciences, 1968. 57(3): p. 497–504.
8. Mitra, B., et al., Feasibility of mini-tablets as a flexible drug delivery tool. International Journal of Pharmaceutics, 2017. 525(1): p. 149–159.
9. Mitra, B., et al., Decoding the small size challenges of mini-tablets for enhanced dose flexibility and micro-dosing. International Journal of Pharmaceutics, 2020. 574: p. 118905.
10. Zhao, J., et al., Understanding the factors that control the quality of mini-tablet compression: flow, particle size, and tooling dimension. Journal of Pharmaceutical Sciences, 2018. 107(4): p. 1204–1208.
11. Zoglio, M. A. and J. T. Carstensen, Physical aspects of wet granulation III. Effect of wet granulation on granule porosity. Drug Development and Industrial Pharmacy, 1983. 9(8): p. 1417–1434.
12. Cruaud, O., et al., Correlation between porosity and dissolution rate constants for disintegrating tablets. Journal of Pharmaceutical Sciences, 1980. 69(5): p. 607–608.
13. Higuchi, T., Mechanism of sustained-action medication. Theoretical analysis of rate of release of solid drugs dispersed in solid matrices. Journal of Pharmaceutical Sciences, 1963. 52(12): p. 1145–1149.
14. Ertel, K., et al., Physical aspects of wet granulation. IV - Effect of kneading time on dissolution rate and tablet properties. Drug Development And Industrial Pharmacy, 1990. 16(6): p. 963–981.
15. Leuenberger, H., et al., Manufacturing pharmaceutical granules: Is the granulation end-point a myth? Powder Technology, 2009. 189(2): p. 141–148.
16. McAuliffe, M. A. P., et al., The use of PAT and off-line methods for monitoring of roller compacted ribbon and granule properties with a view to continuous processing. Organic Process Research & Development, 2015. 19(1): p. 158–166.
17. Gupta, A., et al., Real-time near-infrared monitoring of content uniformity, moisture content, compact density, tensile strength, and young's modulus of roller compacted powder blends Journal of Pharmaceutical Sciences, 2005. 94(7): p. 1589–1597.
18. Salonen, J., et al., Monitoring the acoustic activity of a pharmaceutical powder during roller compaction. International Journal of Pharmaceutics, 1997. 153(2): p. 257–261.
19. Nesarikar, V. V., et al., Instrumented roll technology for the design space development of roller compaction process. International Journal of Pharmaceutics, 2012. 426(1): p. 116–131.
20. Nkansah, P., et al., A novel method for estimating solid fraction of roller compacted ribbons. Drug Development and Industrial Pharmacy, 2008. 34(2): p. 142–148.
21. Silva, A. F. T., et al., Particle sizing measurements in pharmaceutical applications: comparison of in-process methods versus off-line methods. European Journal of Pharmaceutics and Biopharmaceutics, 2013. 85(3, Part B): p. 1006–1018.
22. am Ende, M. T., et al., Improving the content uniformity of a low-dose tablet formulation through roller compaction optimization. Pharmaceutical Development & Technology, 2007. 12(4): p. 391–404.
23. Wildfong, P. L. D., et al., Accelerated fluid bed drying using NIR monitoring and phenomenological modeling: method assessment and formulation suitability. Journal of Pharmaceutical Sciences, 2002. 91(3): p. 631–639.
24. Frake, P., et al., Process control and end-point determination of a fluid bed granulation by application of near infra-red spectroscopy. International Journal of Pharmaceutics, 1997. 151(1): p. 75.
25. Lourenço, V., et al., Combining microwave resonance technology to multivariate data analysis as a novel PAT tool to improve process understanding in fluid bed granulation. European Journal of Pharmaceutics and Biopharmaceutics, 2011. 78(3): p. 513–521.
26. Nieuwmeyer, F. J. S., et al., Granule characterization during fluid bed drying by development of a near infrared method to determine water content and median granule size. Pharmaceutical Research, 2007. 24(10): p. 1854–1861.
27. Hu, X., et al., Study growth kinetics in fluidized bed granulation with at-line FBRM. International Journal of Pharmaceutics, 2008. 347(1): p. 54–61.
28. Närvänen, T., et al., A new rapid on-line imaging method to determine particle size distribution of granules. AAPS PharmSciTech, 2008. 9(1): p. 282–287.
29. Watano, S. and K. Miyanami, Image processing for on-line monitoring of granule size distribution and shape in fluidized bed granulation. Powder Technology, 1995. 83(1): p. 55.
30. Watano, S., Direct control of wet granulation processes by image processing system. Powder Technology, 2001. 117(1–2): p. 163.
31. Reimers, T., et al., Implementation of real-time and in-line feedback control for a fluid bed granulation process. International Journal of Pharmaceutics, 2019. 567.
32. Hu, X., et al., Understanding and predicting bed humidity in fluidized bed granulation. Journal of Pharmaceutical Sciences, 2008. 97(4): p. 1564–1577.

33. Zhang, D., et al., Wettability of pharmaceutical solids: its measurement and influence on wet granulation. Colloids and Surfaces A: Physicochemical and Engineering Aspects, 2002. 206(1–3): p. 547.

34. Keningley, S. T., et al., An investigation into the effects of binder viscosity on agglomeration behaviour. Powder Technology, 1997. 91(2): p. 95.

35. Hapgood, K. P., et al., Nucleation regime map for liquid bound granules. AIChE Journal, 2003. 49(2): p. 350–361.

36. Holm, P., et al., End-point detection in a wet granulation process. Pharmaceutical Development & Technology, 2001. 6(2): p. 181–192.

37. Holm, P., Effect of impeller and chopper design on granulation in a high speed mixer. Drug Development and Industrial Pharmacy, 1987. 13(9–11): p. 1675–1701.

38. Kristensen, H. G., Particle agglomeration in high shear mixers. Powder Technology, 1996. 88(3): p. 197.

39. Bouwman, A. M., et al., The effect of the amount of binder liquid on the granulation mechanisms and structure of microcrystalline cellulose granules prepared by high shear granulation. International Journal of Pharmaceutics, 2005. 290(1): p. 129–136.

40. Kristensen, H. G. and T. Schaefer, Granulation. Drug Development And Industrial Pharmacy, 1987. 13(4&5): p. 803–872.

41. Macias, K. and T. Carvajal, An assessment of techniques for determining particle size during high-shear wet granulation. Tablets & Capsules, 2008. 6(1): p. 32–40.

42. Arp, Z., et al., Optimization of a high shear wet granulation process using focused beam reflectance measurement and particle vision microscope technologies. Journal of Pharmaceutical Sciences, 2011. 100(8): p. 3431–3440.

43. Huang, J., et al., A PAT approach to improve process understanding of high shear wet granulation through in-line particle measurement using FBRM C35. Journal of Pharmaceutical Sciences, 2010. 99(7): p. 3205–3212.

44. Narang, A. S., et al., Resolution and sensitivity of inline focused beam reflectance measurement during wet granulation in pharmaceutically relevant particle size ranges. Journal of Pharmaceutical Sciences, 2016. 105(12): p. 3594–3602.

45. Narang, A. S., et al., Application of in-line focused beam reflectance measurement to brivanib alaninate wet granulation process to enable scale-up and attribute-based monitoring and control strategies. Journal of Pharmaceutical Sciences, 2017. 106(1): p. 224–233.

46. Narang, A. S., et al., Chapter 14 - Inline Focused Beam Reflectance Measurement During Wet Granulation, in Handbook of Pharmaceutical Wet Granulation, A.S. Narang and S.I.F. Badawy, Editors. 2019, London, United Kingdom: Academic Press. p. 471–512.

47. Badawy, S. I. F., et al., A study on the effect of wet granulation on microcrystalline cellulose particle structure and performance. Pharmaceutical Research, 2006. 23(3): p. 634–640.

48. Sheverev, V., et al., Chapter 15 - Principles of Drag Force Flow Sensor, in Handbook of Pharmaceutical Wet Granulation, A.S. Narang and S.I.F. Badawy, Editors. 2019, London, United Kingdom: Academic Press. p. 513–538.

49. Narang, A. S., et al., Process analytical technology for high shear wet granulation: wet mass consistency reported by in-line drag flow force sensor is consistent with powder rheology measured by at-line FT4 Powder Rheometer®. Journal of Pharmaceutical Sciences, 2016. 105(1): p. 182–187.

50. Narang, A. S., et al., Chapter 19 - Wet Mass Consistency Reported by In-Line Drag Force Flow Sensor Compared With Powder Rheology and Shaft Amperage, in Handbook of Pharmaceutical Wet Granulation, A.S. Narang and S.I.F. Badawy, Editors. 2019, London, United Kingdom: Academic Press. p. 651–664.

51. Narang, A. S., et al., Chapter 16 - Real-Time Assessment of Granule Densification and Application to Scale-up, in Handbook of Pharmaceutical Wet Granulation, A.S. Narang and S.I.F. Badawy, Editors. 2019, London, United Kingdom: Academic Press. p. 539–567.

52. Narang, A. S., et al., Real-time assessment of granule densification in high shear wet granulation and application to scale-up of a placebo and a brivanib alaninate formulation. Journal of Pharmaceutical Sciences, 2015. 104(3): p. 1019–1034.

53. Harwood, C. F. and N. Pilpel, Granulation of griseofulvin. Journal of Pharmaceutical Sciences, 1968. 57(3): p. 478–481.

54. Oka, S., et al., Analysis of the origins of content non-uniformity in high-shear wet granulation. International Journal of Pharmaceutics, 2017. 528(1): p. 578–585.

55. Kay, D. and P. C. Record, Automatic wet granulation end-point control system. Manufacturing Chemist and Aerosol News, 1978(49): p. 45–46.

56. Staniforth, J. N. and S. M. Quincey, Granulation monitoring in a planetary mixer using a probe vibration analysis technique. International Journal of Pharmaceutics, 1986. 32(2): p. 177–185.

57. Staniforth, J. N., et al., Granulation monitoring in a high speed mixer/processor using a probe vibration analysis technique. International Journal of Pharmaceutics, 1986. 31(3): p. 277–280.

58. Kopcha, M., et al., Monitoring the granulation process in a high shear mixer/granulator: an evaluation of three approaches to instrumentation. Drug Development & Industrial Pharmacy, 1992. 18(18): p. 1945–1968.

59. Briens, L., et al., Monitoring high-shear granulation using sound and vibration measurements. International Journal of Pharmaceutics, 2007. 331(1): p. 54–60.

60. Daniher, D., et al., End-point detection in high-shear granulation using sound and vibration signal analysis. Powder Technology, 2008. 181(2): p. 130–136.

61. Papp, M. K., et al., Monitoring of high-shear granulation using acoustic emission: predicting granule properties. Journal of Pharmaceutical Innovation, 2008. 3(2): p. 113–122.

62. Whitaker, M., et al., Application of acoustic emission to the monitoring and end point determination of a high shear granulation process. International Journal of Pharmaceutics, 2000. 205(1–2): p. 79.

63. Rudd, D., The use of acoustic monitoring for the control and scale-up of a tablet granulation process. The Journal of Process Analytical Technology, 2004. 1(2): p. 8–11.

64. Faure, A., et al., Process control in a high shear mixer-granulator using wet mass consistency: the effect of formulation variables. Journal of Pharmaceutical Sciences, 1999. 88(2): p. 191–195.

65. Leuenberger, H., Scale-up in the 4th dimension in the field of granulation and drying or how to avoid classical scale-up. Powder Technology, 2003. 130(1): p. 225–230.

66. Kittikunakorn, N., et al., Processes, challenges, and the future of twin-screw granulation for manufacturing oral tablets and capsules. AAPS News Magazine, March 2018.

67. Ghebre-Sellassie, I., et al., Continuous production of pharmaceutical granulation, in Google Patents.

68. Seem, T. C., et al., Twin screw granulation — A literature review. Powder Technology, 2015. 276: p. 89–102.

69. Keleb, E. I., et al., Twin screw granulation as a simple and efficient tool for continuous wet granulation. International Journal of Pharmaceutics, 2004. 273(1): p. 183–194.

70. Vercruysse, J., et al., Impact of screw configuration on the particle size distribution of granules produced by twin screw granulation. International Journal of Pharmaceutics, 2015. 479(1): p. 171–180.

71. Dhenge, R. M., et al., Twin screw granulation using conveying screws: effects of viscosity of granulation liquids and flow of powders. Powder Technology, 2013. 238: p. 77–90.

72. El Hagrasy, A. S., et al., Twin screw wet granulation: Influence of formulation parameters on granule properties and growth behavior. Powder Technology, 2013. 238: p. 108–115.

73. Saleh, M. F., et al., Twin screw wet granulation: effect of process and formulation variables on powder caking during production. International Journal of Pharmaceutics, 2015. 496(2): p. 571–582.

74. Meier, R., et al., Impact of fill-level in twin-screw granulation on critical quality attributes of granules and tablets. European Journal of Pharmaceutics and Biopharmaceutics, 2017. 115: p. 102–112.

75. Cartwright, J. J., et al., Twin screw wet granulation: loss in weight feeding of a poorly flowing active pharmaceutical ingredient. Powder Technology, 2013. 238: p. 116–121.

76. Khorsheed, B., et al., Twin-screw granulation: understanding the mechanical properties from powder to tablets. Powder Technology, 2019. 341: p. 104–115.

77. Pauli, V., et al., Real-time monitoring of particle size distribution in a continuous granulation and drying process by near infrared spectroscopy. European Journal of Pharmaceutics and Biopharmaceutics, 2019. 141: p. 90–99.

78. Madarász, L., et al., Real-time feedback control of twin-screw wet granulation based on image analysis. International Journal of Pharmaceutics, 2018. 547(1): p. 360–367.

79. Kumar, A., et al., Evaluation of an in-line particle imaging tool for monitoring twin-screw granulation performance. Powder Technology, 2015. 285: p. 80–87.

80. Köster, M. and M. Thommes, In-line dynamic torque measurement in twin-screw extrusion process. Chemical Engineering Journal, 2010. 164(2): p. 371–375.

81. Fonteyne, M., et al., Prediction of quality attributes of continuously produced granules using complementary pat tools. European Journal of Pharmaceutics and Biopharmaceutics, 2012. 82(2): p. 429–436.

82. Dahlgren, G., et al., Continuous twin screw wet granulation and drying—control strategy for drug product manufacturing. Journal of Pharmaceutical Sciences, 2019. 108(11): p. 3502–3514.

83. Lee, K. T., et al., Twin screw wet granulation: the study of a continuous twin screw granulator using

Positron Emission Particle Tracking (PEPT) technique. European Journal of Pharmaceutics and Biopharmaceutics, 2012. 81(3): p. 666–673.

84. Pauli, V., et al., Predictive model-based process start-up in pharmaceutical continuous granulation and drying. Pharmaceutics, 2020. 12(1): p. 67.

85. Dhenge, R. M., et al., Twin screw wet granulation: granule properties. Chemical Engineering Journal, 2010. 164(2): p. 322–329.

86. Dosta, M., et al., Flowsheet simulation of solids processes: current status and future trends. Advanced Powder Technology, 2019. 31(3): p. 947–953.

87. Kumar, A., et al., Model-based analysis of a twin-screw wet granulation system for continuous solid dosage manufacturing. Computers & Chemical Engineering, 2016. 89: p. 62–70.

88. Pereira, G. C., et al., Combined feedforward/feedback control of an integrated continuous granulation process. Journal of Pharmaceutical Innovation, 2019. 14(3): p. 259–285.

89. Hapgood, K. P., et al., Drop penetration into porous powder beds. Journal of Colloid and Interface Science, 2002. 253(2): p. 353.

90. Hapgood, K. P., et al., Dimensionless spray flux in wet granulation: Monte-Carlo simulations and experimental validation. Powder Technology, 2004. 141(1–2): p. 20.

91. Litster, J. D., et al., Liquid distribution in wet granulation: dimensionless spray flux. Powder Technology, 2001. 114(1–3): p. 32.

92. Burnett, D. J., et al., Effect of processing route on the surface properties of amorphous indomethacin measured by inverse gas chromatography. AAPS PharmSciTech, 2012. 13(4): p. 1511–1517.

93. Chamarthy, S. P. and R. Pinal, Plasticizer concentration and the performance of a diffusion-controlled polymeric drug delivery system. Colloids and Surfaces A: Physicochemical and Engineering Aspects, 2008. 331(1): p. 25–30.

94. Chávez Montes, B. E., et al., A surface characterization platform approach to study flowability of food powders. Powder Technology, 2019. 357: p. 269–280.

95. Kim, E. H. J., et al., Surface characterization of four industrial spray-dried dairy powders in relation to chemical composition, structure and wetting property. Colloids and Surfaces B: Biointerfaces, 2002. 26(3): p. 197–212.

96. Ho, R., et al., Role of surface chemistry and energetics in high shear wet granulation. Industrial & Engineering Chemistry Research, 2011. 50(16): p. 9642–9649.

97. Martinez-Alejo, J. M., et al., Quantifying the surface properties of enzymatically-made porous starches by using a surface energy analyzer. Carbohydrate Polymers, 2018. 200: p. 543–551.

98. Mora, C. P., et al., Molecular and physical characterization of octenyl succinic anhydride-modified starches with potential applications in pharmaceutics. International Journal of Pharmaceutics, 2020. 579: p. 119163.

99. Pinal, R. and M. T. Carvajal, Integrating particle microstructure, surface and mechanical characterization with bulk powder processing. KONA Powder and Particle Journal, 2020. 37: p. 195–213.

100. Musazzi, U. M., et al., New regulatory strategies to manage medicines shortages in Europe. International Journal of Pharmaceutics, 2020. 579: p. 119171.

101. U.S. Drug and Food Administration. Drug Shortages: Root Causes and Potential Solutions. Full Report, Oct. 2019 Report, Updated Feb. 2020.

Section V

Optimization Strategies, Tools, and Regulatory Considerations

26 Use of Artificial Intelligence and Expert Systems in Pharmaceutical Applications

Metin Çelik

CONTENTS

26.1   INTRODUCTION

Artificial intelligence (AI) can be defined as the attempt to make machines achieve human-like capabilities, such as seeing, hearing, and thinking. Expert Systems (ES) are a subset of AI projects that attempt to achieve expert-level results in solving tough problems.

The idea of inanimate objects coming to life as intelligent beings has been around for a long time. The ancient Greeks had myths about robots, and Chinese and Egyptian engineers built automatons. The beginnings of modern AI can be traced to classical philosophers' attempts to describe human thinking as a symbolic system [1]. But the field of AI wasn't formally founded until a summer conference which was formally proposed by McCarthy et al. [2]. Their proposal stated: "We propose that a 2-month, 10-man study of artificial intelligence be carried out during the summer of 1956 at Dartmouth College in Hanover, New Hampshire. The study is to proceed on the basis of the conjecture that every aspect of learning or any other feature of intelligence can in principle be so precisely described that a machine can be made to simulate it" marks the debut of the term "artificial intelligence" (AI). But achieving an artificially intelligent being wasn't so simple. After several reports criticizing progress in AI, government funding and interest in the field dropped off – a period from 1974 to 1980 that became known as the "AI winter." The field later revived in the 1980s when the British government started funding it again in part to compete with efforts by the Japanese. The field experienced another major winter from 1987 to 1993, coinciding with the collapse of the market for some of the early general-purpose computers, and reduced government funding. But research began to pick up again after that, and in 1997, IBM's Deep Blue became the first computer to beat a chess champion when it defeated Russian grandmaster Garry Kasparov. And in 2011, the computer giant's question-answering system Watson won the quiz show "Jeopardy!" by beating reigning champions Brad Rutter and Ken Jennings [1,3].

The history of ESs has played an integral part in the development of its structure and components. ESs did not begin as a known program with defined components and relationships. Instead, ES was preceded by the general development of AI. ESs have been defined in various ways, but all the definitions share a common thread, suggesting that ESs are artificial means to emulate how human (domain) experts solve problems. A definition of such systems that may be appropriate for the applications in pharmaceutical science would be "ES is a computer program capable of making recommendations, decisions or predictions based on knowledge gathered from the experts and/or experimental data obtained in the field" [4].

Experts, or in other words domain experts, can solve difficult problems, explain the result, learn, restructure knowledge, and determine relevance, and they know what they don't know. So, a domain expert can be defined as a person who possesses the skill and knowledge to solve a specific problem in a manner superior to others. The human experts are not 100% reliable in different domains, which can be taken into consideration as the advantages and benefits of all accomplished things, but they may disagree with each other or forget to take into account a crucial parameter before making a decision. A human expert can have unsurpassed knowledge in the field and can gain as much knowledge as possible but be hopeless explaining that to someone else.

ESs mimic the first – the ability to solve problems – most successfully. Most systems also are able to explain themselves by backtracking through the logic used to arrive at a question or conclusion, and some ESs have rudimentary learning capabilities as well. In addition to the characteristics of expert performance, an ES should be able to provide a high-level explanation of its results. Not only should the system obtain the performance of a domain expert, but it should also explain results like the human expert. This necessarily implies a sequence of reasoning similar to that of the human expert whose expertise is being modeled. Thus, this would exclude most purely statistical models, mathematical simulations, and numerical approximation methods.

Functional areas of ESs include, but are not limited to, control, design, diagnosis, instruction, interpretation, monitoring, planning, prediction, prescriptions, selection, and simulation. ESs are being used in many disciplines such as agriculture, business, chemistry, communications, computers, education, electronics, engineering, environment, geology, image, information, law, manufacturing, mathematics, medicine, meteorology, military, science, space, and transformations. The literature reported less than 50 ESs in use in 1985; this number increased to more than 12,000 in about seven years [5]. According to AI Index 2018 Annual Report, the number of AI/ES-related publications increased from about 1000 per year to about 50,000 within the last two decades [6].

The pharmaceutical industry has entered the 21st century, a new era that will be far more scientific, technological, and sophisticated than anyone would have imagined just a quarter of a century ago when it was still a tradition to develop formulation and processes mostly based on the trial-and-error method. However, nowadays, the awareness of and the use of AI-based ESs [such as rule-based systems, fuzzy logic, genetic algorithm (GA), artificial neural networks (ANNs), simulations, etc.] in the areas of preformulation, formulations and process development, regulatory affairs, new drug delivery system development, project management, and all other areas of pharmaceutical science seem to be slowly growing [4,7]. Even though problems faced in the pharmaceutical industry are not necessarily more complicated than some of the problems encountered in the area of non-pharmaceutical fields, the number of ESs used in pharmaceutical science is still negligibly low despite the recent slow increases. One of the reasons for the insignificant use of ESs in pharmaceutical applications is the challenge facing ES developers in terms of their verification and validation (V&V) processes, in part because of the FDA's interest in the V&V of all types of software. However, the main reason is that pharmaceutical scientists prefer to use well-established concepts. Many in the industry will let somebody else try a new concept first, and if it works, then join the crowd. It is a safe approach to use an established system, but it does not provide us with the immediate benefits of being on the technological edge. On the other hand, it is always risky to try a new concept, even though the outcome may prove to be rewarding for both the scientist(s) and the company [4].

The future success in all areas of pharmaceutical science will depend entirely on how fast pharmaceutical scientists will adapt to the rapidly changing technologies (such as shifting toward continuous manufacturing and implementation of new industry 4.0-based manufacturing concepts in Pharma 4.0™ which requires alignment of expectations, interpretation, and definitions with the pharmaceutical regulation) and more strict regulatory requirements [such as FDA's quality-by-design (QbD)/process analytical technology (PAT) initiative which requires an understanding and control the manufacturing process to demonstrate that quality was not tested into the product but was built in or by design]. AI applications and ESs will inevitably be the major contributors to the future success or even survival of many companies in the pharmaceutical industry.

26.2 BUILDING AN EXPERT SYSTEM

In the introduction, the definition of an ES appropriate for pharmaceutical science was made as a computer program capable of making recommendations, decisions, or predictions based on knowledge gathered from the experts and/or experimental data obtained in the field [4].

In order to build an ES, first, a development team (task force) should be formed. Three vital members of this task force, as shown in Figure 26.1, are (i) domain expert(s), (ii) knowledge engineer(s), and (iii) user(s). To build an ES successfully, the full participation of all three contributors is essential. Let's elaborate on this by explaining its contributors and components and briefly.

26.2.1 Who Is a Domain Expert?

A domain expert possesses the knowledge and skill to solve a specific problem in a manner superior to the others. There may be a need for more than one domain expert depending on the

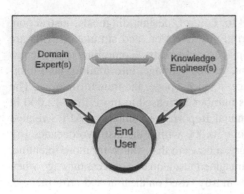

FIGURE 26.1 Three essential members of an ES development team.

specific problem to be addressed in the ES. The domain experts are expected to have expert knowledge and efficient problem-solving skills, and they should be able to communicate the relevant knowledge consistently and completely to the knowledge engineer. Also, the domain experts should be able to devote time and should not be hostile to the ES. An ES with irrelevant, incomplete, or inconsistent knowledge is bound to prove the junk-in junk-out principle.

26.2.2 Who Is a Knowledge Engineer?

The knowledge engineer transforms the expert's highly specialized knowledge to the knowledge-based component of an AI-based program. This person has a dual task; therefore, in addition to having the knowledge engineering and ES programming skills to match the problem to the appropriate software, the knowledge engineer should have good communication skills to be able to elicit knowledge from the expert, gradually gaining an understanding of an area of expertise. Intelligence, tact, empathy, and proficiency in specific techniques of knowledge acquisition are all required of a knowledge engineer. Knowledge-acquisition techniques include conducting interviews with varying degrees of structure, protocol analysis, observation of experts at work, and analysis of cases.

On the other hand, the knowledge engineer must also select a tool appropriate for the project and use it to represent the knowledge with the application of the knowledge acquisition facility.

26.2.3 Who Is the End-User?

As the name suggests, the end-users are the people who will run the ES to perform the tasks. They can also help define the interface specifications and can aid in knowledge acquisition.

26.2.3.1 Why Build an Expert System?

In general, the reasons for the development of an ES can be listed as follows, although every company may have different motivations:

Improved Productivity: The system is expected to be capable of improving the quality of decisions, to reduce the time to reach a decision, and/or to provide expertise to locations within the organization where this capability is lacking.

Reduced Costs of Product Development: The system is expected to improve the use of materials during manufacturing and/or to reduce labor costs by allowing a time-consuming task to be completed quickly or act in place of a highly paid expert.

Improved Quality: The system is expected to improve the quality of the final product or the services supplied by the organization and/or to provide training to personnel that improves their work activities.

Improved Image: The system is expected to improve the organization's image as a leader and innovator.

Justification of Decision: The system is expected to provide a step-by-step explanation and/or justification for all advises it gives.

Training of Newcomers: The system is expected to be used in the training of the newcomers without compromising their productivity. ESs result in a faster learning curve for novices.

Assisting an Expert: The system is expected to assist an expert to improve productivity in some routine tasks, to manage the complex projects effectively, to access information that is difficult to recall, and to free the expert's time to be used in other tasks.

Replacement of an Expert: The system is expected to make the expertise available anywhere/anytime, even in a hostile environment, or in the absence of the expert due to illness, resignation, or retirement.

Corporate Memory: ESs can become a vehicle for building up organizational knowledge, as opposed to the knowledge of individuals in the organization.

The above-given list also explains the advantages of the ESs over human experts. The advantages of the ESs are related to knowledge, decisions, safety, and cost. The knowledge of an ES is permanent and easy to transfer, while the human expert's knowledge is perishable and difficult to transfer from one worker to another. The decisions made by human experts can be unpredictable and difficult to document. In contrast, the ES decision process is consistent and easy to document. In an unsafe or hostile environment, an ES is replaceable, while the human expert is definitely irreplaceable. When cost is an issue, the ES services are often more affordable than those of the human expert.

When compared with human experts, ESs have the following advantages: An ES's knowledge is permanent and can be easily transferrable. The decision process is fast and consistent, therefore predictable, and it is easily documented. Despite these advantages, ESs are not intended to take the place of formulation scientists. They must be considered as vital tools to be used by formulators for the rapid, cost-effective, and scientifically sound development of a dosage form as well as useful for training inexperienced scientists.

However, there are some factors that favor the human expert as opposed to an ES. These factors are much more difficult to quantify but can often be important to a project. A human expert is creative and adaptive and uses sensory experiences. The computer ES is uninspired, needs to be directed, and uses only symbolic input. A human expert has a broad focus and may be able to use knowledge from another field or experience to aid in problem-solving, whereas an ES has a narrow focus constrained to the domain knowledge. Lastly, the human expert can use common sense knowledge, while the ES can only use technical knowledge.

26.2.3.2 Phases of an Expert System Development Process

Many articles and textbooks are addressing the strategies and/or tools employed in building ESs in-depth [5,8–11]. A typical ES development process is schematically shown in Figure 26.2, and the following should be considered only as a general overview of the phases involved in the development of an ES.

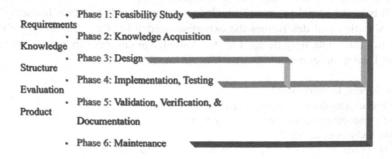

FIGURE 26.2   A typical ES development process.

26.2.4   FEASIBILITY STUDY

A project team assesses whether an ES can or should be developed for a specific problem or project. The team evaluates the motivation for the development of the ES in terms of improving productivity, quality, and image as well as cost reduction. The team must also consider the problem and the people-related feasibility issues very carefully. Some of the important questions that must be answered positively are as follows:

Is the problem solvable?
Are the problem-solving steps definable?
Is the problem stable and well-focused and its complexity reasonable?
Does the task not require common sense?
Does the task require only cognitive skills?
Can experts articulate their methods?
Do genuine experts exist?
Do the experts agree on solutions?
Is the task reasonably manageable?
Is the task clearly understood?
Is the management supportive of the project, receptive to change, and not skeptical, and does it have reasonable expectations?

If all the answers to these questions are in the affirmative, then the next step is to justify the ES development by considering the following:

Task solution has a high payoff
Human expertise being lost
Human expertise scarce
Expertise needed in many locations
Expertise needed in a hostile environment

After the ES development is justified, ES Task Force should continue to evaluate the other problem – the deployment-related issues concerning the development of the ES for that particular problem or project.

If and when a decision is made in favor of the development of the ES, the project team defines the features and specifications of each component of the ES and develops flow charts for each specific problem.

26.2.5   CONCEPTUALIZATION AND ACQUISITION OF THE KNOWLEDGE

The next phase of ES development, conceptualization, involves designing the proposed program to ensure that specific interactions and relationships in the problem domain are understood and defined. The key concepts, relationships between objects and processes, and control mechanisms are determined. This is the initial stage of knowledge acquisition. It involves the specific characterization of the situation and determines the expertise needed for the solution of the problem.

The following questions may be used by the knowledge engineer to help understand what the expert does and what the expectations from the ES would be [9,12]:

Who are the experts to work with?
Exactly what decisions does the expert make?
Who are the prospective users of the expert system?
What are the decision outcomes?
Which outcomes require greater reflection, exploration, or interaction?
What resources or inputs are required to reach a decision?

Are there any relevant textbooks?

What conditions are present when a particular outcome is decided?

How consistently do these conditions predict a given outcome?

At what point after exposure to influential inputs is a decision made?

Given the particulars of a specific case, will the outcome predictions of the knowledge engineering team be consistent with those of the expert?

If it is possible, is it justified in the particular circumstances?

Does the problem show characteristics that make expert system development appropriate?

What are the boundaries of the domain?

What is the language of the domain?

What hardware and software are available for use?

Is expert system development possible?

Has any similar research been reported in the literature?

The objective of knowledge acquisition is to compile a body of knowledge on the problem of interest that can then be encoded into the ES. The major difficulties with the knowledge gathering from the human experts lie in the fact that some domain experts may be unaware of or unable to verbalize the knowledge or may provide irrelevant, incomplete, or inconsistent knowledge.

One of several, or combinations of several, knowledge acquisition methods is used. Additional details are provided in the Knowledge Acquisition module.

There are different types of knowledge and different methods of obtaining them. Some of these types of knowledge are as follows:

1. Declarative (e.g., facts, objects)
2. Procedural (e.g., rules, strategies)
3. Heuristic (rule of thumb)
4. Structural (e.g., rule sets concept relationship)

Declarative Knowledge, also known as Descriptive knowledge, is thought of as "knowledge about" or the answers to the what, where, when, or who types of questions, rather than the "how." Facts or rules for mathematical equations are all examples of declarative knowledge. Declarative knowledge is also usually explicit knowledge, meaning that you are consciously aware that you understand the information.

Procedural Knowledge, also known as Interpretive knowledge, is the type of knowledge in which it clarifies how a particular thing can be accomplished. It's basically "how" you know to do something. The difference between procedural and declarative knowledge is presented in Table 26.1.

Heuristic knowledge is representing knowledge of some experts in a field or subject. It is basic rule of thumb based on previous experiences, awareness of approaches, and which are good to work but not guaranteed.

Structural knowledge is basic knowledge to problem-solving. It describes relationships between various concepts such as kind of, part of, and grouping of something. It also describes the relationship that exists between concepts and objects.

26.2.6 DESIGN OF THE EXPERT SYSTEM

The knowledge engineer determines which software to use to transform the acquired knowledge into a coded program for the development of the ES. Some of the AI tools (knowledge representation techniques) used alone or in combinations in the development of an ES include decision trees, object–attribute–value (OAV) triplets, rules (if–then–because statements) with forward and/or backward chaining, fuzzy logic, GA, case-based reasoning (CBR), and ANNs. A successful ES is usually developed by combining more than one AI technique.

TABLE 26.1

Difference Between the Procedural and Declarative Knowledge

Procedural knowledge	Declarative knowledge
It is also known as Interpretive knowledge.	It is also known as Descriptive knowledge.
Procedural Knowledge means how a particular thing can be accomplished.	While Declarative Knowledge means basic knowledge about something.
Procedural Knowledge is generally not used, that is, it is not more popular.	Declarative Knowledge is more popular.
Procedural Knowledge can't be easily communicated.	Declarative Knowledge can be easily communicated.
Procedural Knowledge is generally process-oriented in nature.	Declarative Knowledge is data-oriented in nature.
In Procedural Knowledge, debugging and validation are not easy.	In Declarative Knowledge, debugging and validation are easy.
Procedural Knowledge is less effective in competitive programming.	Declarative Knowledge is more effective in competitive programming.

26.2.7 IMPLEMENTATION, TESTING THE MODULES AND DEVELOPMENT OF THE PROTOTYPE, AND TROUBLESHOOTING OF THE FINAL PROGRAM

Case studies with known results are used to test the ability of the rules, databases, and programming to perform properly.

In addition to the case studies, untested materials and parameters are also used to verify the proper operation of the program and to troubleshoot any additional problems identified.

During the implementation stage, the formalized knowledge is mapped or coded into the framework of the development tool to build a working prototype. The contents of knowledge structures, inference rules, and control strategies established in the previous stages are organized into a suitable format.

The testing phase involves considerably more than finding and fixing syntax errors. It covers the verification of individual relationships, validation of program performance, and evaluation of the utility of the software package. How the sequence of questions and output is presented to the end-user may have as much to do with acceptance and use as does the accuracy of the recommendations. The lessons learned from human engineering cannot be ignored if the program is to be successful.

26.2.8 VERIFICATION AND VALIDATION (V&V) OF AN EXPERT SYSTEM

Verification of an ES determines whether the system is developed according to its specifications. Validation of an ES determines whether the system meets the purpose for which it was intended. Verification and validation must occur during the entire development process. Verification proves that the models within the program are true relationships. It ensures that the knowledge is accurately mimicked by having the domain expert operate the program for all possible contingencies. Perhaps the most difficult aspect of testing is accurately handling the uncertainty that is incorporated in most ES in one way or another. Certainty factors are one of the most common methods for handling uncertainty. Verification of the certainty factors assigned to the knowledge base is largely a process of trial and error, refining the initial estimates by the domain expert until the program consistently provides recommendations at a level of certainty that satisfies the expert. To ensure program accuracy, all possible solution paths must be painstakingly evaluated.

An effective validation procedure is critical to the success and acceptance of the program. During validation, the following areas are of concern: (i) correctness, consistency, and completeness of the rules; (ii) ability of the control strategy to consider the information in the order that corresponds to the problem-solving process; (iii) appropriateness of the information about how conclusions are reached and why certain information is required; and most critical (iv) agreement of the computer program output with the domain expert's corresponding solutions.

Validation is an ongoing process requiring the output recommendations to be accurate for a specific user's case. Validation is enhanced by allowing others to review critically and recommend improvements. A formal project evaluation is helpful to establish whether the system meets the intended original goal. The evaluation process focuses on uncovering problems with credibility, acceptability, and utility. This can be determined from the program accuracy that is determined from comparisons with the real-world environment. Included are the understanding and flexibility of the program, ease of use, adaptability of the design, and the correctness of solutions.

Very critical differences exist between an ES and conventional systems in terms of V&V. An ES is both a piece of software and a domain model, and there may not be a unique, correct answer to a problem given to an ES. An ES can adapt itself by modifying its behavior in relation to changes in its internal representation of the environment.

An ES should be considered correct when it is complete, consistent, and satisfies the requirements that express expert knowledge about how the system should behave. If a system has hundreds of rules, however, it may require thousands of distinct decision paths, and this makes the aspect of correctness hard to establish. This is not, of course, a problem in a conventional programming technique.

These differences between the AI and conventional programming tools provide flexibility and special capabilities to an ES, but these differences also make the use of traditional V&V of an ES difficult. This is one of the problems slowing the development and acceptance of ESs in a regulated industry like pharmaceuticals. Experts do not agree on how to accomplish the V&V of ESs. One of the impediments to a successful V&V effort for ESs is the nature of ESs themselves. They are often used for working with incomplete and uncertain information or ill-structured situations. Because the ES specifications often do not provide precise criteria against which to test, there is a problem in verifying and validating them according to the definitions. This is unavoidable. If there are precise enough specifications for a system, there would not be any need to use an AI tool to develop the system, and a conventional programming language would be sufficient for the development of a piece of software for that system.

In reality, the first part of V&V, that is, verification of an ES, is not so difficult to establish because it is possible, and also highly recommended, to build small modules (sub-ESs) for each problem within a system. This is a significant help to the verification process of the whole system. This is true even if the ES is developed by combining more than one system.

The main problem is the second part of V&V, that is, validation. ESs will make a recommendation on the basis of the domain knowledge. If the domain knowledge is inaccurate, then the recommendation of the ES will naturally be inaccurate. How can someone validate the correctness of knowledge provided by a domain expert, or if two domain experts have conflicting views over a problem-solving process, who will decide which is correct?

FDA's requirements for the submission of the software code can also add an additional burden to the software validation of an ES. This is a serious obstacle because only a few AI tool providers and ES developers will be willing to share the code. As some of the AI tools may cost more than tens of thousands of dollars, no one could blame the software providers for not wishing to share the code.

26.2.9 Training of Users

A user acceptance questionnaire is used during the implementation of the program.

26.2.10 MAINTENANCE AND UPGRADE OF THE PROGRAM

Depending on the availability of the new knowledge and/or the data in the field of a particular ES, an upgrade may be needed to ensure that the ES will evolve continuously to overcome new challenges concerning that specific project or problem. Therefore, the knowledge base should be extensively documented as it is coded. The potential for later misunderstanding and confusion should be minimized wherever possible. Furthermore, extensive justifications and explanations should be included to assist the end-user in fully understanding questions posed to them by the program, so that the user can effectively use the program output, and to show the user, on-demand, how the recommendation was logically derived.

26.2.11 MANAGE EXPECTATIONS

As exciting and promising as ESs are, overenthusiasm can sometimes lead to unfounded assumptions and unrealistic expectations. A typical claim is that expert systems help companies "clone experts." That claim is overblown. Problem-solving is only a small part of what an expert does in a company. The best ESs to date capture only a portion of the expert's knowledge. Moreover, even the most advanced expert systems do not replace experts but rather augment their capabilities or allow less-experienced individuals to perform better. Generally speaking, humans are supported by – not replaced by – expert systems. Moreover, as mentioned above, expert systems are regularly, if not continually, monitored and updated by humans.

ESs are not 100% correct 100% of the time. People tend to expect much higher and more consistent performance from a computer program than they would ever expect from a human expert, but such lofty expectations court disaster. One can expect consistency from an ES, but ESs mimic the strengths of human judgment. Besides, assessing whether an answer is "correct" is often a matter of opinion. This is true in credit authorization as well as in computer configuration. Many configurations will work, but choosing the best one is a matter of judgment [13].

26.2.11.1 Expert System Components

An ES has typically five *basic components:* knowledge base, working memory, inference engine, and user interface. These components can be found in many types of AI programs including decision trees, ANNs, GAs, and fuzzy logic. In addition, many of the AI tools have a fifth component, an explanation facility, providing the reason for the decision or recommendation of the ES. How the essential components of an ES are integrated and how does an ES work to mimic the way a human expert thinks is illustrated in Figure 26.3.

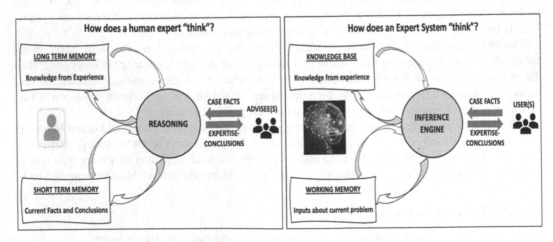

FIGURE 26.3 General description for human expert versus the expert system.

26.2.12 KNOWLEDGE BASE

The knowledgebase contains the factual and empirical domain knowledge in a particular subject area and all the facts, rules, and procedures, which are important for problem-solving. The domain knowledge can be acquired from literature and/or experts in the field and is in an electronic form that can be searched and updated easily. The knowledge base is similar to human long-term memory or experience.

One typical way of representing the knowledge in an ES is the rules. In its very basic form, a rule is an *if/then* structure that logically relates information contained in the *if* part to the other information contained in the *then* part. Some derivations of such a structure could also include *else* and/or *because* parts as well.

For example, the following rule represents the knowledge for the selection of a plasticizer to be used with a film-forming polymer:

if
The selected polymer is HPMC only.
and
There is no regulatory restriction for the use of PEG 400 in that country.
then
Recommend PEG 400.
because
PEG 400 is compatible with HPMC, and it is efficient in its functionality.

26.2.13 WORKING MEMORY

The working memory contains facts about the problem discovered during the problem-solving session. This component is similar to human short-term memory or current experience. Knowledge in the working memory can be inferred by the system, or it can be obtained by user input. Knowledge inferred by the system is obtained by matching user input with knowledge in the knowledge base to produce new facts.

26.2.14 INFERENCE ENGINE

The inference engine is the component that models the human reasoning process. It matches facts in the working memory with domain knowledge in the knowledge base and conclusion. It works by searching the database for a match between its contents and the information in the working memory. If a match is found, the conclusion from the match is added to the working memory and the inference engine continues to scan the database for additional matches.

The inference engine simulates the problem-solving strategy of a human expert, represents the logical unit by means of which conclusions are drawn from the knowledge base according to a defined problem-solving method, controls the execution, which questions to ask and in what order, and simulates the problem-solving process of human experts. Functions of the inference engine are to determine which actions are to be executed between individual parts of the expert system, how they are executed, and in what sequence, to determine how and when the rules will be processed and to control the dialogue with the user.

26.2.15 EXPLANATION FACILITY

A unique feature of an ES is its ability to explain the reasoning used to conclude. The following part of the example rule given above represents the explanation facility of the ES.

because
PEG 400 is compatible with HPMC, and it is efficient in its functionality.

Because an ES can explain why user input was requested or how a conclusion was reached, the system developer can use this component to uncover errors in the system's knowledge and the user can benefit from the transparency provided into the system's reasoning.

26.2.16 User interface

The user interface employs natural language for dialogues with the user whenever possible. Questions posed such as "how should questions be answered by the user?", "how will system responses to these questions will be formulated?", and "what info is to be graphical?" must be easy to use, erroneous errors kept to a minimum, and questions and answers must be understandable. Figure 26.3 provides a graphical description for human expert versus the expert system.

26.2.16.1   Knowledge Representation

Several techniques represent the knowledge [5,14–18] including, but not limited to,

> OAV triplets,
> semantic networks (SN),
> frames,
> rule-based systems,
> fuzzy logic,
> ANNS,
> GA, and
> others: decision trees, hybrid systems (e.g., neurofuzzy systems), case-based reasoning, etc.

These techniques will be briefly described in the following sections. The most successful ES applications integrate more than one technique. For example, the rule-based systems are very good in providing the reasoning for how and why they reach a decision, but they are not best in automated learning (without updating their knowledge base) or recognizing patterns in a large amount of data. This gap can be filled by integrating ANNs, which are very powerful in automated learning, although they lack in justifying their predictions. Therefore, combining these two techniques can bring the strength of both approaches while eliminating their weaknesses.

26.2.17   Object–Attribute–Value Triplets

OAV triplets provide a particularly convenient way to represent certain facts within a knowledge base. Each OAV triplet is concerned with some specific (conceptual) entity or (physical) object. For example, our object of interest may be a granule (particle). Associated with every object is a set of attributes. Using the granule as an example (i.e., object), some of the attributes include the following: particle size, particle shape, particle density, particle porosity, surface roughness, moisture content, etc.

For each attribute, there is an associate value or set of values. For example, in the granule example, the particle size attribute can have the values of large, small, fine, etc. Please note that values could be numerical as well.

Most OAV triplet systems also have a confidence factor associated with each specific triplet. Confidence factors, or certainty factors, refer to a numerical weight given to a fact or a relationship to indicate the confidence one has in that fact or relationship (Figure 26.4). There are two kinds of confidence: "expert confidence" (the confidence that an expert feels when suggesting a rule) and "user confidence" (the confidence that a user feels when answering a question).

In a typical ES programming language, there are several ways of handling the uncertain data such as confirmatory (yes/no) system, numerical range (-1 to 1, 0 to 10, -100 to 100, etc.),

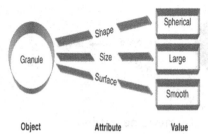

FIGURE 26.4 An example of an object–attribute–value triplet fuzzy variables, shape, size, and surface.

systems, increment/decrement system, custom formula systems, and fuzzy logic. In many instances, the user may have to answer a question to determine the confidence factor. In the numerical approach, this is achieved by asking the trueness (definitely false, almost false, probably false, unknown, probably true, almost definitely true, and true) or sureness of a fact or value (Figure 26.5). The ES inference engine then converts the answer to a numerical value that computers understand.

26.2.18 SEMANTIC NETWORKS

A semantic network (SN) may be thought of as a network that is composed of multiple OAV triplets in a network and characterizes their interrelationships. An advantage of this method is its flexibility to add new objects whenever needed.

SNs are an alternative of predicate logic for knowledge representation. In SNs, we can represent our knowledge in the form of graphical networks. This network consists of nodes representing objects and arcs which describe the relationship between those objects. Such networks can categorize the object in different forms and can also link those objects. Semantic networks are easy to understand and can be easily extended. This representation consists of mainly two types of relations:

IS-A relation (Inheritance)
Kind of relation

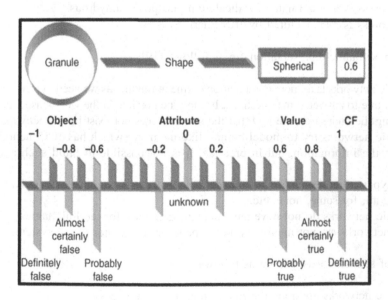

FIGURE 26.5 An example of an object–attribute–value triplet with confidence factors.

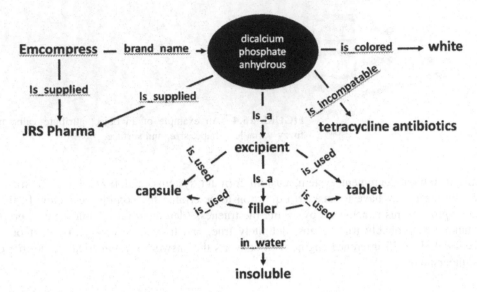

FIGURE 26.6   An example for Semantic Networks.

The following example is a set of some statements which are represented in the form of nodes and arcs in Figure 26.6 in which each object is connected with another object by some relation.

Statements:
1. Dicalcium phosphate anhydrous is an excipient.
2. Dicalcium phosphate anhydrous is a filler.
3. Dicalcium phosphate anhydrous is insoluble in water.
4. Dicalcium phosphate anhydrous is used in tablets.
5. Dicalcium phosphate anhydrous is used in capsules.
6. Dicalcium phosphate anhydrous is incompatible with tetracycline antibiotics.
7. Emcompress is a brand name for dicalcium phosphate anhydrous.
8. Emcompress is manufactured by JRS Pharma.

Drawbacks in Semantic representation are as follows [19]:

1. Semantic networks take more computational time at runtime as we need to traverse the complete network tree to answer some questions. It might be possible in the worst-case scenario that after traversing the entire tree, we find that the solution does not exist in this network.
2. Semantic networks try to model human-like memory (which has 1015 neurons and links) to store the information, but in practice, it is not possible to build such a vast semantic network.
3. These types of representations are inadequate as they do not have any equivalent quantifier, e.g., for all, for some, none, etc.
4. Semantic networks do not have any standard definition for the link names.
5. These networks are not intelligent and depend on the creator of the system.

Advantages of semantic network are as follows:

1. Semantic networks are a natural representation of knowledge.

2. Semantic networks transparently convey meaning.

3. These networks are simple and easily understandable.

26.2.19 FRAMES

A frame contains an object plus slots for any and all information related to the object. The contents of slots are typically the attributes, and the attribute values, of a particular object. Therefore, a frame is a natural extension of the semantic networks.

Facets: The various aspects of a slot is known as Facets. Facets are features of frames that enable us to put constraints on the frames. Example: IF-NEEDED facts are called when data of any particular slot are needed. A frame may consist of any number of slots, and a slot may include any number of facets and facets that may have any number of values. A frame is also known as slot-filter knowledge representation in artificial intelligence.

Frames are derived from semantic networks and later evolved into our modern-day classes and objects. A single frame is not much useful. Frames system consist of a collection of frames that are connected. In the frame, knowledge about an object or event can be stored together in the knowledge base. The frame is a type of technology that is widely used in various applications including material processing and machine visions. Table 26.2 is an example of a frame for an excipient that can be recommended by an ES as a directly compressible formulation.

Advantages of frame representation:

The frame knowledge representation makes the programming easier by grouping the related data.

The frame representation is comparably flexible and used by many applications in AI.

It is very easy to add slots for new attributes and relations.

It is easy to include default data and to search for missing values.

Frame representation is easy to understand and visualize.

Disadvantages of frame representation:

In the frame system, inference mechanism is not be easily processed.

The inference mechanism cannot be smoothly proceeded by frame representation.

Frame representation has a much-generalized approach.

TABLE 26.2
An Example of a Frame for an Excipient

Slots	Filter
Generic name	Dibasic calcium phosphate
Grade	Anhydrous
Brand name	Emcompress
Manufacturer	JRS Pharma
Category	Excipient
Function	Filler
Solubility in water	Insoluble
Bulk density, g/mL	0.709
Tapped density, g/mL	0.768
Absolute density, g/mL	2.808
Angle of repose	29.4
Mass flow, g/sec	5.2
Surface area, m^2/g	1.5

TABLE 26.3
Examples of Fuzzy Variables with Typical Values

Fuzzy variables	Typical values
Size	Fine, small, large, coarse
Shape	Oval, spherical, needle
Temperature	Hot, warm, cold
Tablet strength	Hard, soft
Pressure	High, low

26.2.20 FUZZY LOGIC

Fuzzy logic is mainly concerned with quantifying and reasoning about vague or fuzzy terms that appear in our daily lives. In fuzzy logic, these terms are referred to as linguistic variables or fuzzy variables. Some examples of fuzzy variables that are encountered in pharmaceutical applications are given in Table 26.3.

Fuzzy sets. The classical set theory establishes systematic relation among objects within a set as well as between elements of various sets. A set is a collection of any number of definite, well-distinguished objects, called the elements of the set that share common properties. Thus, an object may either belong to the set or be completely excluded. In other words, if A is a set and x is an element to the set, then x belongs to A, if and only if x satisfies all the membership requirements if A; otherwise, x does not belong to A.

The fuzzy set theory differs from classical set theory in one critical aspect. An element can belong to the fuzzy set, be completely excluded from the fuzzy set, or can belong to the fuzzy set to any intermediate degree between these two extremes. The extent to which an element belongs to a given fuzzy set is called the grade of membership or degree of membership. It can be said, therefore, that classical set theory is a special case of fuzzy sets.

Fuzzy sets can be obtained to reflect the general opinion of the scientists or experts in the files, for example, in Figure 26.7, where fuzzy sets are shown in a piecewise linear form for the issues of three different categories (small, medium, and large) of the size of granule(s). In this fuzzy subset, a granule particle with a size of 0.25 mm is a member of medium size with a membership value of about 1, and at the same time a member of small and large sizes with a value of about 0.15 and 0.25, respectively.

26.2.21 RULE-BASED SYSTEMS

The most common way of representing knowledge is found in rule-based systems (RBS), which employ rules to represent the experts' knowledge. Such rules are typical of if–then variety. However, in some instances, this is extended to include if–then–else or if–then–else–because type or rules. In a rule-based system, the uncertainty of the knowledge is handled using the method of confidence factors, as described above in the OAV triplets.

In the RBSs, two main inference techniques are used: forward chaining and backward chaining (Figure 26.8).

Forward chaining is a "data-driven" way to run the rules and is about the knowledge base searched for rules that match the known facts, and the action part of these rules is performed. The rules are simply tested in the order they occur based on available data. If information is needed, other rules are not invoked. Instead, the user is asked for information. Consequently, forward chaining systems are dependent on the order of the rules, and the process continues until a goal is reached and puts the symptoms together to conclude.

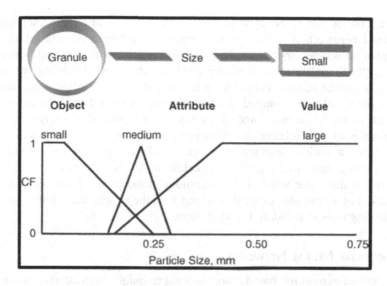

FIGURE 26.7 An example of a fuzzy set with confidence factors. Fuzzy variables, particle size; fuzzy values, small, medium, and large.

Backward chaining is a term used to describe running the rules in a "goal-driven" way, that is, in this technique, there is always a "goal" or "conclusion" to be satisfied and a specific reason why rules are tested and it is by far the most common strategy used in the simple RBSs, and A "goal" is an attribute for which the ES tries to establish a value. In backward chaining, if a piece of information is needed, the program will automatically check all the rules to see if there is a rule that could provide the needed information. The program (inference engine) will then "chain" to this rule before completing the first rule. This new rule may require information that can be found in yet another rule. The program will then again automatically test this new rule. The logic of why the information is needed goes backward through the chain of rules. Backward chaining is much slower than forward chaining since in the latter technique, all of the rules do not have to be fired every time to determine whether the information can be derived.

In control by hybrid backward and forward chaining, the basic approach is data-driven, but the information needed by rules is derived through backward chaining.

Another technique is to divide an ES to subsets of rules and run some in the forward chaining and some in backward chaining.

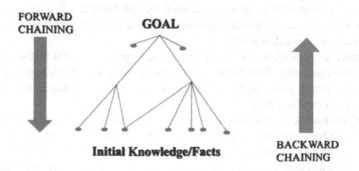

FIGURE 26.8 Forward chaining and backward chaining techniques in rule-based systems. *Source*: From Ref. 10.

The construction of rule-based systems can be based on both expert knowledge and data. Knowledge-based construction follows a traditional engineering approach, which is in general domain-dependent. It is necessary to have knowledge or requirements acquired from experts at first and then to identify the relationships between attributes (features). Modeling, which is the most important step, is further to be executed in order to build a set of rules. Once the modeling is complete, then the simulation is started to check the model toward the fulfillment of systematic complexity such as model accuracy and efficiency. Finally, statistical analysis is undertaken to validate whether the model is reliable and efficient in an application. On the other hand, data-based construction follows a machine learning approach, which is in general domain-independent [20].

Backward chaining starts from a goal, the conclusion. All the rules that contain this conclusion are then checked to determine whether the conditions of these rules have been satisfied. For example, the doctor has an end idea of what is wrong with the patient, though they must prove it by going from the diagnosis and finding the symptoms.

26.2.22 ARTIFICIAL NEURAL NETWORKS

ANNs can be defined as machine-based computational techniques that attempt to simulate some of the neurological processing abilities of the human brain. In the human brain, neurons are the information carriers. In the same way, ANNs are composed of interconnected simulated neurons capable of pattern recognition or data analysis. The human brain, on the other hand, has a unique characteristic of creating transient states through neurons in between the sensory organs and the brain (decision-taking unit). Hence, the probabilistic interim state brings out a factor of randomness, which brings out what we call "Creativity." In ANN or rather all machine learning algorithms, we build some kind of transient states, which allows the machine to learn in a more sophisticated manner. Processing of the data using pattern recognition produces classification of the data, while data analysis produces numerical output. One of the most powerful characteristics of ANNs is the ability to find complex and latent patterns in the information being processed. Unlike a most statistical experimental design, analysis of data using ANN does not require a specific number of experiments. Also, neural networks can generate hypotheses that can be tested by other scientific methods, and the outputs of one network can become the inputs to a subsequent network.

Artificial neural network elements. ANNs can be represented by a neuron model like the one found in Figure 26.9. As seen in this model, an ANN is composed of interconnected processing elements (PE) or neurons. The interconnections represent weights or weighing factors applied to the input values of the neuron as the information is passed forward through the network. These weights are sometimes referred to as synaptic weights since the interconnections are similar to the synapses of the human brain. Output values from each neuron are passed forward to the next layer through its interconnections or used as part of the final output of the network. The architecture of a network is defined by the number of layers in the network, the number of neurons in each layer, the configuration of their interconnections, and how the weights of the interconnections are calculated.

Network types. Generally, there are three basic types of neural networks, feed-forward, feedback, and self-organizing. The network type to be utilized depends on the task to be accomplished. The following paragraphs will describe the network architectures and types of input data suitable for each network type.

Feed-forward networks. Feed-forward networks, also called error backpropagation or backprop networks, contain the basic network components described in the neuron model. A feed-forward network is designed by defining its number of layers and the number of neurons in each layer. The number of neurons in the input and output layers is equal to the number of independent and dependent variables, respectively. The input layer serves as a distribution point for the data to the first hidden layer and can only scale the data, not calculate weighting factors. The purpose of scaling the data is to normalize it to a

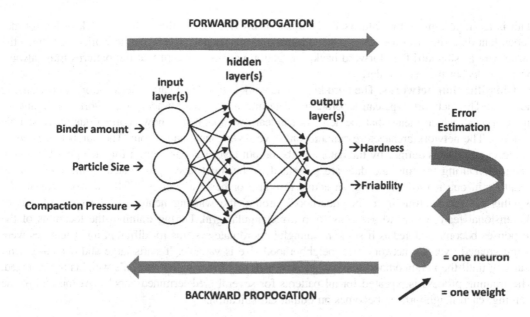

FIGURE 26.9 An example of a neuron model with feed-forward and feed-backward networks.

constant numerical range, such as 0 to 1 or −1 to +1. Scaling can be performed using linear or non-linear scaling functions. The number of hidden layers is based on personal preference and rules of thumb. The purpose of the hidden layers is to provide a balance between network accuracy and network generalization. A higher number of hidden layers leads to a narrow, accurate network with a decreased ability to predict outside the boundaries of its original data. Fewer hidden layers will produce a more generalized robust network but may smooth the curve between the data points too much. The balance required between network accuracy and generalization depends on the purpose of the network.

Once the network is designed, it is ready to be trained. Training is the process of tuning the synaptic weights to minimize the difference between the actual output and the network output values. The next step is the error backpropagation step or learning step. Learning in this context does not imply the human qualities of understanding, consciousness, or intelligence. Instead, it simply implies the use of data for tuning a set of parameters or, in this case, the tuning of the synaptic weights. Once the network training is complete, the network does not store or refer to the training data. Instead, the trained network is an independent summary of the data. With the weights established by training, the network is capable of producing outputs for input data not originally contained in the training data set. The use of a data set to train a network is called supervised learning and requires that the output data corresponding to the input data be available during training. For example, if the effect of binder amount, particle, and compaction pressure on the hardness and friability will be modeled using an ANN, there should be enough "input" data for the binder amount, particle size, and compaction pressure as well as enough corresponding "output" measurements (Figure 26.9). As a rule of thumb, for each input parameter, 10 input–output data set is recommended. In this example, $10 \times 3 = 30$ sets of data with binder amount, particle size and compaction pressure inputs, and hardness and friability measurements would be recommended. Then, a portion (usually 80–90%) of that data set would be used for training, and the remaining data sets would be used for validation.

Feedback networks. Feedback networks (also called recurrent networks) are similar in structure to the feed-forward networks. The difference between the two types is an additional layer. This layer contains one layer's information from the previous training pass. This extra layer, or context layer, allows the network to see knowledge about previous inputs and is sometimes called the network's long-term memory. The result of this additional layer is that the network responds to the same input differently at different times depending on the previous patterns. The result is that the sequence of the data is as important as the data itself. This use of previous data allows the network to learn time-dependent data such as time-series data and financial market data. Recurrent networks are trained the same way as standard feed-forward backpropagation networks except that the patterns must always be presented in the same order.

Classification networks. The third kind of network is the classification network or self-organizing network. This network type can separate the data into a specified number of categories. It is always unsupervised, which means that the network can learn without being shown correct outputs in sample patterns. The network architecture contains only two layers, input and output. The number of neurons in the input layer is defined by the data, and the output layer has one neuron for each possible output category. During training, the data are presented to the input layer, propagated to the output layer resulting in one neuron providing an active response or being a "winner." The network adjusts the weights for the neurons in a "neighborhood" around the winning neuron on the basis of a two-dimensional feature map whose cells form a rectangular grid. During training, the locations of the responses become ordered as if some meaningful coordinate systems for different input features were being created over the network. The neighborhood size is variable. It starts large and decreases with learning until the neighborhood approaches zero and only the winning neuron's weights are changed. The training process is repeated for all patterns for several predetermined epochs. At the end of the training, each neighborhood becomes an output classification.

26.2.23 GENETIC ALGORITHMS (GA)

GAs are mathematical tools that solve optimization problems. This type of problem is usually composed of several variables that control a process or outcome, and formula or algorithm, which combines these variables to fully model the process. The goal of the problem is then to find the values of the variables, which optimize the model in some way, usually by minimizing or maximizing one of the dependent variables. While many mathematical methods can solve optimization problems, these traditional methods tend to break down when the problem is more complex. Examples of complex problems include combinatorial problems or problems where the fitness function is not a smooth, continuous mathematical formula, such as a neural network function.

GAs optimize these complex problems using the methods of evolution, specifically, the survival of the fittest. Much of the terminology used to describe GAs is partially based on concepts from biology; however, some terms may have different names depending on the author. In this case, "survival of the fittest" means that the GA solves the problem by allowing the less fit individuals in the population to die and selectively breeding the most fit individuals, that is, those who solve the problem best.

The use of GA in combination with neural networks for the optimization of process parameters has been investigated by Cook et al.[1] In this example, a neural network model was developed to predict the effect of several processes' operating parameters and conditions on the internal bond strength of particleboard. A GA was applied to this neural network model to determine the process parameters that would result in the optimal strength for a given set of operating conditions. This ANN GA system was successful in predicting the process parameters, which allowed the manufacturer to achieve optimal levels of board strength based on the current, variable operating conditions. The ANN portion was used to model the process parameters, while the GA utilized this model to obtain the optimal processing parameters under actual manufacturing conditions.

26.2.24 OTHER METHODS OF KNOWLEDGE REPRESENTATION

Decision trees. A decision tree takes as input an object or situation described by a set of properties and outputs a yes/no decision. Decision trees, therefore, represent Boolean functions. Functions with a larger range of outputs can also be represented. Decision trees are considered to be auxiliary tools in ES development and are usually incorporated with other systems as the case in the spray-drying ES example that is described later in this chapter.

Case-based reasoning. Case-based reasoning (CBR) is the technique which involves the process of solving new problems based on the solutions of similar past problems, that is, it works based on previously experienced and stored problem–solution case set. Retrieve, Reuse, Revise, and Retain are the four key steps involved in the CBR process to solve or predict an optimal solution for new problems or cases [21].

CBR does not require an explicit domain model and so elicitation becomes a task of gathering case histories; implementation is reduced to identifying significant features that describe a case, an easier task than creating an explicit model; by applying database techniques, large volumes of information can be managed; and CBR systems can learn by acquiring new knowledge as cases, thus making maintenance easier.

Neurofuzzy logic. In the field of AI, neurofuzzy refers to combinations of ANNs and fuzzy logic. Neurofuzzy hybridization results in a hybrid intelligent system that synergizes these two techniques by combining the human-like reasoning style of fuzzy systems with the learning and connectionist structure of neural networks [22,23].

Because fuzzy logic allows objectives to be expressed in simple terms, it complements neural network modeling. In the case of neurofuzzy logic (NFL), as the name suggests, the fuzzy logic is tightly coupled with a neural network. Neurofuzzy logic combines the ability of neural networks to learn from data with fuzzy logic's ability to express complex concepts intuitively. This creates a degree of transparency for the otherwise "black box" neural network models, leading to the term "grey box modeling" being applied for these methods. Neurofuzzy logic has proved to be exceptionally suited to data mining since it not only can develop good models from data, but it also has the capability of expressing these as linguistic IF ... THEN rules. The neurofuzzy architecture is in essence a neural network with two additional layers for fuzzification of inputs and defuzzification of outputs. The modeling capabilities of neurofuzzy systems depend on the number, shape, and distribution of the fuzzy membership input functions. In the simplest case, only two, LOW and HIGH, would suffice. In some cases, it is appropriate to add more; for example, a problem showing a quadratic dependency would require at least LOW, MEDIUM, and HIGH so that it be properly represented. Where data are scarce, relatively few membership functions should be used. As the number and complexity of the inputs increase, the rules become more complicated, and this can make them difficult to understand.

26.2.25 HYBRID SYSTEMS

Hybrid systems combining two or more AI techniques such as fuzzy logic, neural networks, genetic algorithms, and expert systems are proving their effectiveness in a wide variety of real-world problems. Every intelligent technique has particular computational properties (e.g., ability to learn, explanation of decisions) that make them suited for particular problems and not for others. For example, while neural networks are good at recognizing patterns, they are not good at explaining how they reach their decisions. Fuzzy logic systems, which can reason with imprecise information, are good at explaining their decisions, but they cannot automatically acquire the rules they use to make those decisions. These limitations have been a central driving force behind the creation of intelligent hybrid systems where two or more techniques are combined in a manner that overcomes the limitations of individual techniques. Hybrid systems are also important when considering the varied nature of application domains. Many complex domains have many different component problems, each of which may require different types of processing. If there is a complex application that has two distinct subproblems, say a signal processing task and a serial reasoning task, then a neural network and an expert system respectively can be used for solving these separate tasks. The use of intelligent hybrid systems is growing rapidly with successful applications in many areas including medical diagnosis, cognitive simulation, process control, engineering design, product development, and troubleshooting [23].

26.3 AN EXAMPLE TO EXPERT SYSTEMS: SPRAYEX, A SPRAY-DRYING EXPERT SYSTEM

The example of ES, SPRAYex, was developed by PTI, Inc. [24]. Briefly, the current version of the system evaluates the spray ability of a given substance alone with no additives involved. This function is implemented using decision trees, rules, and fuzzy logic. Another function of the system is to predict the process conditions to obtain a product with the desired properties in terms of particle size, moisture content, and bulk density by utilizing several trained ANNs simultaneously. The system also has mathematical modeling predicting the interactions between numerous process variables. Finally, the system has a comprehensive database containing material characteristics of six model materials and process conditions for over 150 spray-drying experiments. The following sections describe the development strategies or functions of the system in more detail.

26.3.1 SPRAY-DRYING FEASIBILITY DECISION TREES

The user interface of this system helps the user to input material characteristics and makes a decision by incorporating several decision trees to determine the feasibility of a material to be spray-dried [25].

The sequence of the execution of the decision trees (Figure 26.10) was chosen based on the order required to prepare the feed. First, the material is evaluated based on its melting point. Next, the feed type feasibility is determined based on the DSC scans obtained. Once the feed is determined, it is screened for particle size, viscosity, and sedimentation potential. The analysis of the physical characterization data for the selected model materials using these decision trees resulted in the generation of a confidence factor that represented the ability of the proposed material to be spray-dried as a percentage value. These confidence factors were then integrated into a decision-making process. In addition, the generated confidence factors were also stored as part of the database for future reference.

An example of such sequences was based on the melting points (Figures 26.11 and 26.12). Melting point data provide information about the ability of the material to withstand the inlet air temperature of the spray-drying process. If the melting point is low, the material may only be able to be processed in a countercurrent configuration, or it may not be able to be spray-dried. It is well known that the minimally acceptable melting point for a material to be processed in a spray dryer is dependent on the spray configuration of the dryer. The melting point decision tree in Figure 26.11 incorporates a critical melting point to represent this concept. In this tree, materials having a melting point higher than the critical temperature have a confidence level of 100% for this variable, which means that the material is 100% feasible for the spray-drying process in terms of melting point. The confidence level for a material with a melting point lower than the critical temperature is determined using an equation representing the probability of success. This equation and a graphical representation of the function are shown in Figure 26.12. This probability, which increases using a second-order function with increasing melting point, is employed because there is no single melting point above which the material is 100% feasible and below which the material is 100% unfeasible. If the melting point is less than the critical temperature, a confidence factor is determined using this equation.

The critical temperature is designed to be flexible based on dryer configuration. Since the only configuration used during this experimentation was cocurrent product airflow, a single critical temperature was employed. In the cocurrent configuration, the inlet air comes into direct contact with the feed at the point of atomization and flows in the same direction as the feed. If a material that is atomized in the feed melts at a temperature lower than the vaporization temperature of the

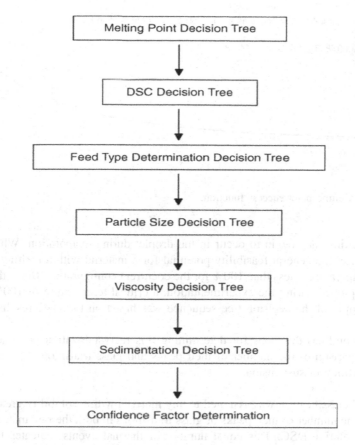

FIGURE 26.10 Decision tree sequence.

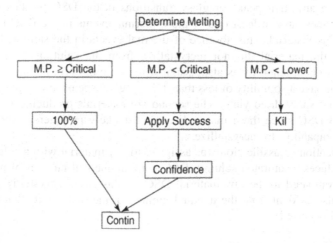

FIGURE 26.11 Melting point decision tree.

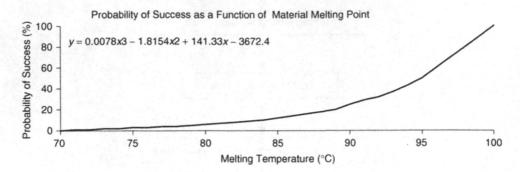

FIGURE 26.12   Melting point success function.

solvent, then melting may begin to occur in the droplet during evaporation. While this may not always be the case, the general feasibility potential for a material with a melting point under the vaporization temperature is less than 100% for the cocurrent configuration. Since the water was the only solvent employed during the experimentation, a critical temperature of 100°C was chosen.

Another example of the decision tree sequence was based on the DSC results (Figures 26.13 and 26.14).

Figure 26.13 outlines the steps for determining this recrystallization classification, which is based on a comparison of the number of melt peaks and glass transitions between DSCs of the solid and the solution or suspension.

    a. The "Yes" classification was assigned to any material with a solubility greater than 1% that has the same number of melt peaks or glass transitions in both the raw material DSC and the saturated solution DSC. This equal number of thermal events indicates that the material recrystallized from the solution during the evaporation process. However, since the temperatures of these thermal events were not considered by the decision tree, polymorphs could be present.

    b. The "No" classification was assigned to any material with a solubility greater than 1% that does not have any melt peaks or glass transitions in the DSC produced by the saturated solution but does have at least one of these thermal events in the DSC produced by a suspension of this material. This absence of thermal events in the saturated solution DSC indicated that the material did not recrystallize from the solution during the evaporation process. This classification was also assigned to two other types of materials. The first are materials that have a solubility of less than 1% since a suspension will be required to produce any significant spray-dried yield. The second are materials producing no melt peaks in the raw material DSC since these materials are most likely polymers without any crystalline structure or capability to recrystallize.

    c. The "Modification" classification was assigned to any material with a solubility greater than 1% that produces a saturated solution DSC with an unequal number of melt peaks or glass transitions compared to the raw material DSC. In this case, recrystallization had occurred, and it was also evident from the unequal number of thermal events that a crystalline modification had occurred.

Figure 26.14 uses the material classifications to determine the feasible feed types. If the material is classified as "Yes," then it will recrystallize from a saturated solution. In addition, a suspension is also feasible since it is composed of a saturated solution with additional undissolved solids. If the classification is "No," then the saturated solution does not recrystallize, and the only feasible feed type is a suspension. Lastly, materials classified as "Modification" also recrystallize from a

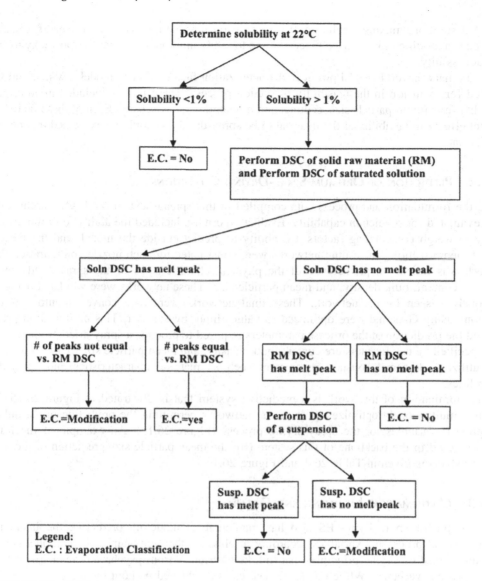

FIGURE 26.13 DSC decision tree.

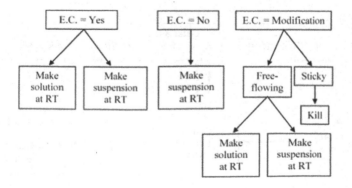

FIGURE 26.14 Decision tree for feed type.

saturated solution, making a solution or a suspension feasible feed type. However, if a material undergoes a modification from 100% crystalline to 100% amorphous, it may be too sticky to spray dry successfully.

In summary, several critical physical characterization factors of each model raw material were selected for inclusion in the feasibility prediction process. These factors included melting point, solubility, maximum particle size, sedimentation potential, and viscosity. Each of these factors had a direct effect on the ability of the material to be spray-dried that could be expressed in a decision tree format.

26.3.2 PREDICTION OF OPTIMUM SPRAY-DRYING CONDITIONS

Using the formulation and process data compiled in this spreadsheet, several ANN architectures were evaluated for prediction capability. Evaluation criteria included the ability to fit the data, the ability to weigh contributing factors, the ability to predict outside the model, and the tendency toward memorization. Three final networks were constructed for each nozzle configuration. Each network was trained to predict one of the physical characteristics of the spray-dried powder, moisture content, bulk density, and mean particle size. These networks were validated using data previously unseen by the network. These final networks were then converted into predictive functions using GAs and were optimized to values input by the user. This optimization process allowed the prediction of the process parameters required to produce a spray-dried product having user-specified values for moisture content, bulk density, and mean particle size. This optimization also utilizes additional constant parameters such as material characteristics and spray-dryer capabilities.

The culmination of this work is a predictive system that is illustrated in Figure 26.15. This system simultaneously optimizes three neural networks permitting the prediction of formulation and process variables for the spray-drying process (Figure 26.16). An example of the trained networks used in the backbone of this system (for the mean particle size prediction of the spray-dried product) is given in Table 26.4 and Figure 26.17.

26.3.3 MATHEMATICAL MODELING AND DATABASE

The example of spray-drying ES also has mathematical modeling predicting the interactions among several processing variables according to classical thermodynamics. This model contains equations based on drying principles that link key attributes from psychrometric charts to spray-drying process variables. While this same task can be achieved without the aid of mathematical modeling, these models provide process settings in a user-friendly format without the tedious calculations required for converting psychrometric terms such as adiabatic saturation temperature,

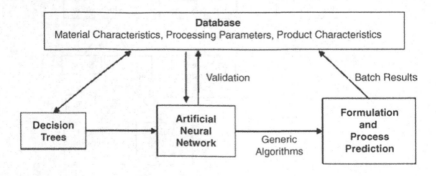

FIGURE 26.15 Predictive system diagram.

(a)

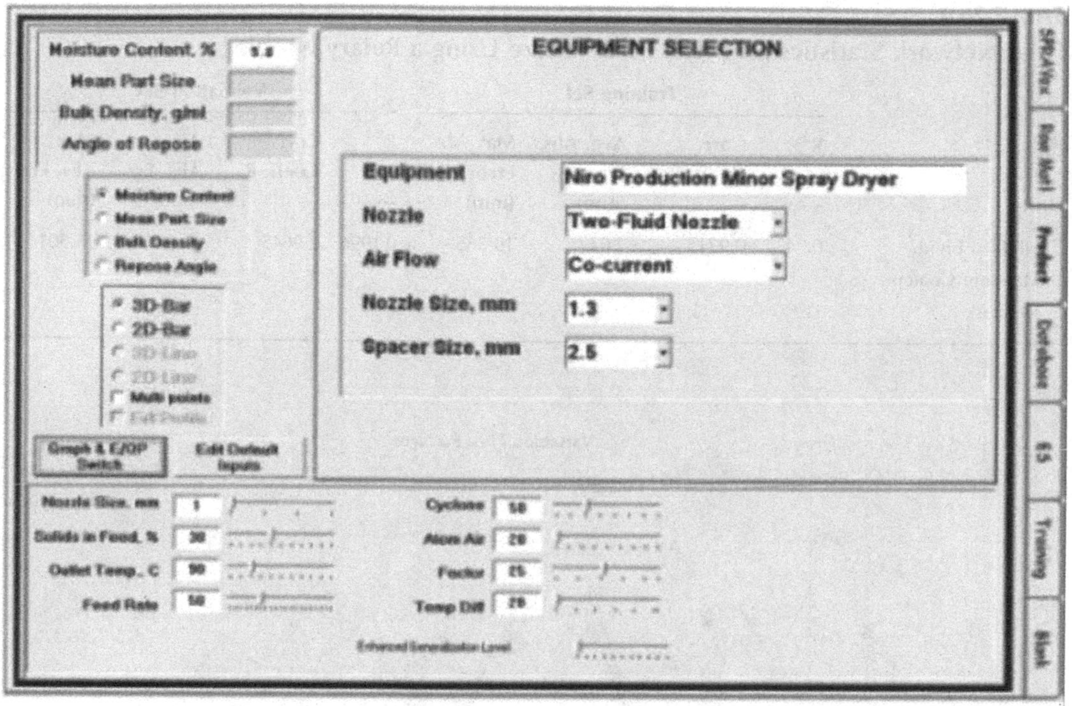

(b)

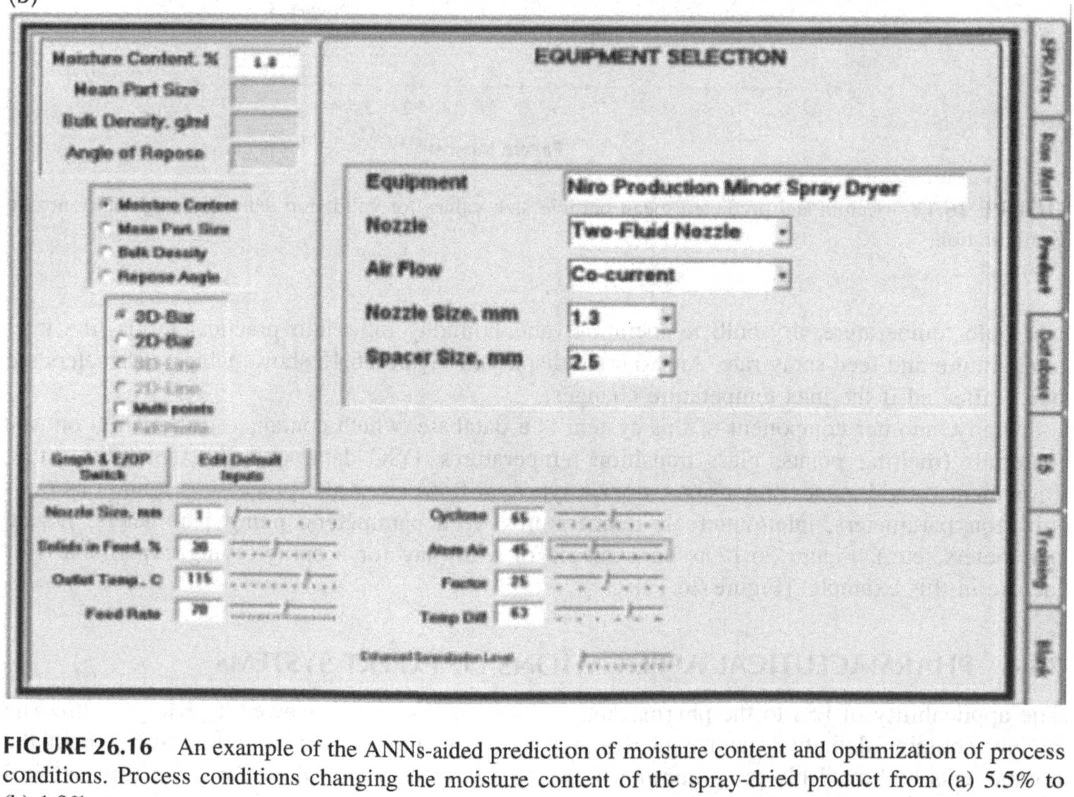

FIGURE 26.16 An example of the ANNs-aided prediction of moisture content and optimization of process conditions. Process conditions changing the moisture content of the spray-dried product from (a) 5.5% to (b) 1.8%.

TABLE 26.4

Final Network Statistics for Mean Particle Size Using a Rotary Nozzle

	Training Set				Validation Set			
	R^2	Corr. Coeff. R	Avg. Abs. Error	Max Abs. Error	R^2	Corr. Coeff. R	Avg. Abs. Err.	Max Abs. Err.
Units	---	---	(mm)	(mm)	---	---	(mm)	(mm)
Final Two Fluid Moisture Content Network	0.9437	0.9715	2.044	19.565	0.1996	0.9645	5.632	11.501

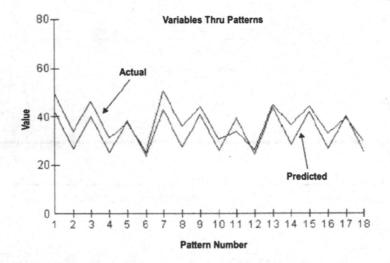

FIGURE 26.17   Actual and predicted mean particle size values for validation data set using rotary nozzle configuration.

wet bulb temperature, dry-bulb temperature, and humidity ratio into practical terms like inlet temperature and feed spray rate. An example display in Figure 26.18 shows which parameters are being affected if the inlet temperature changes.

Finally, another component of this system is a database, which contained information on raw materials (melting points, glass transition temperatures, DSC data, viscosity, solubility, etc.), equipment (brand name, dimensions, nozzle types, airflow, etc.), and processing conditions (atomization parameters, inlet/outlet air temperatures, feed parameters, pump parameters, nozzle parameters, etc.). Figure 26.17 is an example of a display for a spray-drying experiment (for lactose in this example) (Figure 26.19).

26.4   PHARMACEUTICAL APPLICATIONS OF EXPERT SYSTEMS

The applicability of ESs to the pharmaceutical industry has been reviewed by Klinger [26]. The review contains definitions and explanations of AI and ESs as well as information about the components and available programming languages. Possible applications for the pharmaceutical industry outlined include pathological evaluation, molecular modeling, biological activity

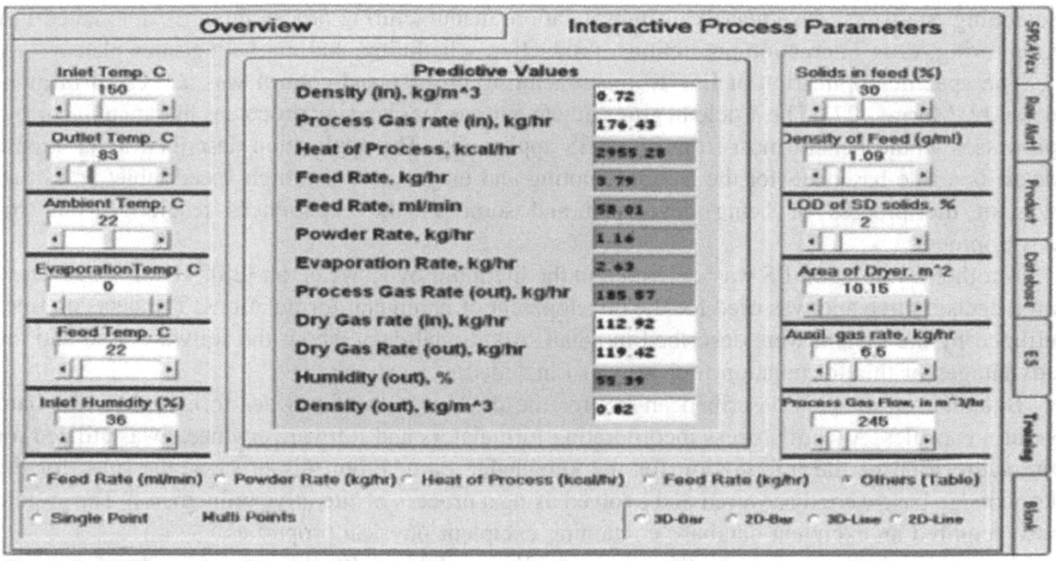

FIGURE 26.18 Mathematical modeling showing the processing variables (dark gray background) affected by the changes in outlet temperature.

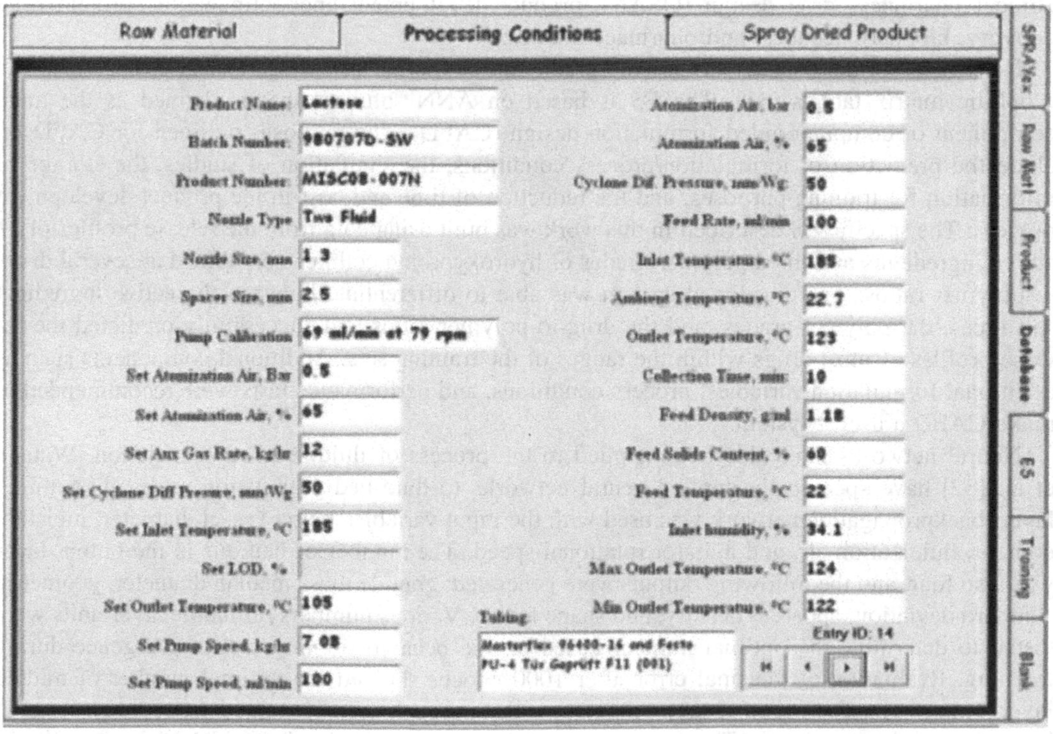

FIGURE 26.19 Database component showing the processing conditions for spray-drying lactose.

screening, statistical design/analysis/interpretation, manufacturing process/control, automated QA monitoring, drug interaction predictions, production scheduling, and marketing/sales plans.

The specific application of ESs to manufacturing process and control was addressed in more detail by Murray [27]. The article begins with an outline for choosing processes that manufacturing processes would benefit most from in an ES application. The application described in additional detail is a rule-based ES for the troubleshooting and diagnostics of a high-speed tablet press that was in the process of being developed and some of the experiences resulting from this development.

Another formulation ES was described in the literature by Rowe et. al. [28]. This ES was based on a decision tree and was used for the development of parenteral formulations. The decision trees utilized by the system were described in detail. Additional detail about the software used and the advantages of this formulation tool was also included.

Bateman et. al. [29] described an ES for the development of powder formulations for hard gelatin capsules. A team process incorporating formulators and software engineers was utilized for the acquisition of the information for the knowledge base. From this process, the rules for the knowledge base were discovered and evolved using a process of "iterative refinement." The system also required an excipient database containing excipient physical properties.

A comprehensive review of the commercially available software for use in developing intelligent systems was provided by Rowe [30]. Rowe divided the software into five types describing the applications, advantages, and disadvantages of each type as well as diagramming the operation processes. Software tool names and supplier information are also provided.

Within the pharmaceutical literature, ANNs have been applied to several areas. These include clinical pharmacy, drug design (QSAR), product development and optimization, protein drug delivery, biopharmaceutics, and pharmacokinetics.

Hussain et al. describe an ES for the prediction of the *in vitro* drug release profile from hydrophilic matrix tablets [31]. The ES is based on ANN software that is defined as the main component of computer-aided formulation design (CAFD). The purposes outlined for CAFD include the prediction of formulation/process conditions, the simulation of studies, the storage of information for training purposes, and the reduction of time and cost in the product development process. The specific ES described in this work was built using data from the release profiles of 11 active ingredients and three polymer grades of hydroxypropyl cellulose combined at several drug-to-polymer ratios. The developed system was able to differentiate between the active ingredient salt types, the polymer grades, and the drug-to-polymer ratios and successfully predicted the release profiles of most drugs within the ranges of the training sets. Additional components such as additional formulation variables, process conditions, and performance tests were recommended to make CAFD a useful system.

Neural networks have also been applied to the process of fluidized-bed granulation. Watano et al. [32] have specifically applied neural networks to fluid-bed granulation scale-up. A three-layer, backpropagation network was used with the input variables being vessel diameter, moisture content, fluidization air, and agitator rotational speed. The number of neurons in the output layer was also four, and the following outputs were generated: granule mass median diameter, geometric standard deviation, apparent density, and shape factor. Various numbers of middle layer units were tested to determine the optimal number based on the behavior of the error convergence during learning. Evaluation of the final error after 1000 epochs showed the optimal number of middle layer units to be four. The data used to train the network were obtained from three sizes of laboratory-scale granulators. The trained network was used to predict the granule characteristics of material produced using commercial-scale equipment. These granulations were produced, the actual granule data were compared with the predicted values, and an excellent correlation was observed. Additional networks using the same architecture were also trained by the authors using fewer data points in the training set. From this investigation, it was shown that the training data could be decreased while retaining good accuracy. However, the authors noted that when the number of training sets was less than 13, the accuracy of the predictions decreased.

Murtoniemi et al. have also used ANN to model the fluid-bed granulation process [33]. In their work, three input variables, inlet air temperature, atomizing air pressure, and binder solution amount, were varied at three levels. The output variables, mean granule size, and granule friability, were measured. This training data were processed using a modified backpropagation algorithm in a basic feed-forward architecture containing one or two hidden layers. The number of neurons in each hidden layer was varied from 3 to 15. In all, 36 networks were trained. Evaluation of the training data revealed that the number of hidden neurons did not greatly affect the average error except when the networks were small and contained only three or four hidden neurons. The data produced by the optimal network were also compared with the data calculated using a regression model. For both outputs, the ANN data were closer to the experimental values than the regression data. In a second article by the same authors, the topology and the training endpoint of this network were investigated further [34]. The purpose of this study was to optimize the ability of the ANN to generalize by varying the number of hidden layer neurons and the training endpoint. The results again showed that the number of hidden neurons did not affect the ability of the network to generalize. However, the training endpoint had a significant effect on generalization and the number of iteration epochs required.

In a review of neural network computing in the pharmaceutical literature published in 1993, Erb comprehensively described the backpropagation architecture by citing much of the original neural network literature as well as additional helpful books [35].

The prediction of *in vitro* dissolution as a function of formulation variables was also the goal of the work performed by Ebube et al. [36]. This study demonstrated the importance of optimizing the number of hidden layers and the number of iterations or epochs. The developed network had two inputs, the level of polymers 1 and 2, and one output, the percentage dissolved in one hour. Optimization of the network resulted in three neurons for the hidden layer and an optimal number of iterations, which varied from 81 to 671 depending on the number of formulations in the training set. The authors also found that the network predicted data outside the training set less accurately than data bounded by the training set. However, the predictive capability of the network was improved using replicate input and output data.

As indicated earlier in this chapter, the application of AI in the pharmaceutical industry increased during the last few decades. When it comes to granulation and tablet production, AI methods such as ANN, cubist model, random forest method, k-NN, and the combination of neurofuzzy logic (NFL) and gene expression programming (GEP) were found to be capable of not only predicting the potential problem but also finding a suitable solution for it [37].

Continuous pharmaceutical processing is designed to overcome this drawback and therefore offers more advantages compared to batch processing. In order to develop continuous pharmaceutical manufacturing, each unit operation in the manufacturing line should be interconnected appropriately. Continuous processing has a great deal of potential to address issues of agility, flexibility, cost, and robustness in the development of pharmaceutical manufacturing processes. Over the past decade, there have been significant advancements in science and engineering to support the implementation of continuous pharmaceutical manufacturing. These investments along with the adoption of the QbD paradigm for pharmaceutical development and the advancement of PAT for designing, analyzing, and controlling manufacturing have progressed the scientific and regulatory readiness for continuous manufacturing. The FDA supports the implementation of continuous manufacturing using science- and risk-based approaches [38].

A powerful tool for the development of continuous pharmaceutical manufacturing is model predictive control (MPC), which is considered as an advanced control strategy. MPC considers each unit operation and takes a holistic view of the manufacturing line. Therefore, each unit operation should be specified, and its model needs to be developed to implement MPC for the manufacturing line. There are different processes in the manufacturing of solid-dosage drugs such as milling, mixing, granulation, drying, and coating. Granulation is the key step in manufacturing pharmaceutical formulations, in which granules are produced from a fine powder including an active pharmaceutical ingredient (API) and an excipient. Moreover, wet granulation is the most complex unit operation in pharmaceutical manufacturing since many mechanisms are involved in the formation of granules from fine powder [39]. Recently, twin-screw granulation has gained a lot of attention over other granulation methods due to its unique characteristics. The main advantage of twin-screw granulation is that it is an intrinsic continuous process that can promote the development of continuous pharmaceutical manufacturing [40]. Some theoretical and experimental work using twin-screw extruder has been carried out to simulate continuous wet granulation. Several researchers have investigated predictive modeling of wet granulation by using Population Balance Model (PBM) and Discrete Element Model (DEM) [41–43]. They developed a multi-dimensional population balance model for the prediction of granule properties in a twin-screw granulation. The lumped parameter and compartment approach were used for the numerical solution of population balance equations. This model was found to be able to predict the granule size, liquid content, and porosity as a function of process parameters. The results of mechanistic models developed for twin-screw granulation revealed that these mechanistic models are quite slow for the use of MPC in the development of continuous pharmaceutical manufacturing. However, these mechanistic models can be used for process design and optimization. The main disadvantage of the aforementioned mechanistic models is that it is not fast enough to be used as a model for the development of the MPC approach in continuous manufacturing. In MPC, the model of the process should be able to run within a few seconds in order to predict the future behavior of the process. Therefore, these mechanistic models fail to be applied for MPC, and in fact, faster models are required for industrial applications. Recently, some researchers have tried to reduce the solution time for the mechanistic model by coupling PBM and ANN for describing wet granulation. The main aim of a hybrid model is to make the solution time faster. The results showed that ANN is capable of simulation for the wet granulation process, although it does not look at the mechanisms associated with the granulation. A list of different mechanistic and hybrids models applicable to wet granulation is also reported [39,44]. In a recent study [45], computational modeling of twin-screw granulation was conducted by using an ANN approach. The experimental work consists of wet granulation of microcrystalline cellulose using a twin-screw extruder. Process parameters including liquid to solid ratio, screw speed, and powder flow rate were considered as inputs. On the other hand, particle size distribution parameters of d10, d50, and d90 were selected as outputs. Linear and non-linear activation functions were taken into account in the simulations, and more accurate results were obtained for non-linear function in terms of prediction. The most accurate prediction was obtained by the two hidden layers with two nodes per layer and three-fold cross-validation method. The developed modeling methodology was found to be fast and reliable and could be used for the implementation of model predictive control in developing continuous pharmaceutical manufacturing.

Landin [46] demonstrated the potential of AI tools for predicting the endpoint of the granulation process in high-speed mixer granulators of different scales from 25 L to 600 L. In this work, the combination of neurofuzzy logic and gene expression programming technologies was used for the modeling of the impeller power as a function of operating conditions and wet granule properties, establishing the critical variables that affect the response and obtaining a unique experimental polynomial equation (transparent model) of high predictability ($R^2 > 86.78\%$) for all size equipment. Gene expression programming allowed the modeling of the granulation process for granulators of similar and dissimilar geometries and can be improved by implementing additional characteristics of the process, as composition variables or operation parameters (e.g., batch size, chopper speed). The principles and the methodology proposed were claimed to be applied to understand and control the manufacturing process, using any other granulation equipment, including continuous granulation processes.

Studies utilizing the QbD approach and machine learning modeling for scale-up of wet granulation processes often use either process parameters or formulation factors [47]. Furthermore, responses being observed are usually related to granule properties (particle size distribution [48], porosity [49], size, and bulk density [50]). In studies conducted by Aikawa et al. [51] and Badawy et al. [52], the analyzed responses were tablet properties. Those studies, however, did not utilize machine learning techniques. Previous studies with machine learning modeling involved testing of the prediction capability of developed methods on either laboratory [53] or pilot scale runs [54]. In this study, for the first time, the developed models were tested using a large data set obtained from both pilot and commercial-scale runs. We also utilized and compared multiple machine learning techniques (regression, regularization, decision tree, and ensemble algorithms). Both formulation and process parameters were used as input variables. Analyzed responses are quality attributes of granules and tablets relevant in the context of the complex system of the wet granulation process scale-up – compatibility [55], compressibility, and manufacturability. Millen et al. [56] provided an extensive example of how different machine learning techniques could be utilized to determine significant variables (both categorical and numerical) and the magnitude of their influence on tablet critical quality attributes (CQAs).

As industries across the world reaping the benefits of Industry 4.0 and its technologies, the pharma industry has taken a nimble step toward embracing and adopting the change commonly referred to as Pharma 4.0. The move is aimed at the digital transformation of the two most important areas of pharma, namely, product development and regulatory operations. A recent article addressed how Pharma 4.0 would have an impact on product development, regulatory operations, and how Pharma 4.0 functionalities will focus on the areas of drug research and development, clinical research, manufacturing, and quality management [57]. Needless to say, AI and ES applications will be an indispensable part of Pharma 4.0.

26.5 CONCLUSION

The future success in all areas of pharmaceutical science will depend entirely on how fast pharmaceutical scientists will adapt to the rapidly changing technologies (such as shifting toward continuous manufacturing and implementation of new industry 4.0-based manufacturing concepts in Pharma 4.0™) and more strict regulatory requirements [such as FDA's Quality by Design (QbD)/Process Analytical Technology (PAT) initiative]. AI applications and ESs will inevitably be the vital tool for the pharmaceutical scientist to develop scientifically sound dosage forms and to overcome the challenges of new technologies, regulatory requirements, and new era such as Pharma 4.0. In any case, sooner or later, all of us will be happily using AI and ESs. Those who use them sooner will enjoy being the pioneers in their fields. They will also have the personal satisfaction of contributing to pharmaceutical science by catching up with the rest of the world in the application of such useful tools, even though it is a highly complicated process to develop an ES to the full satisfaction of the users, domain experts, company, FDA, etc.

ACKNOWLEDGMENT

I would also like to thank Dr. Susan C. Wendel for her contribution to the last edition of this chapter. The Spray Drying Expert System, which was presented in the current chapter, was mainly based on her Ph.D. work. In any case, any errors are my own and should not tarnish the reputation of my esteemed former student.

NOTE

1 Cook DF, Ragsdale CT, Major RL. Combining a neural network with a genetic algorithm for process parameter optimization. Eng Appl Artif Intell 2000; 13:391–396.

REFERENCES

1. Lewis T A Brief History of Artificial Intelligence. 2014. Available from: https://www.livescience.com/49007-history-of-artificial-intelligence.html#:~:text=The%20beginnings%20of%20modern%20AI,%22artificial%20intelligence%22%20was%20coined.
2. McCarthy J, Minsky M, Rochester N, Shannon C A Proposal for the Dartmouth Summer Research Project on Artificial Intelligence. 1955. Available from: http://wwwformal.stanford.edu/jmc/history/dartmouth/dartmouth.html.
3. Lewis T Jeopardy!'-Winning Computer Now Crunching Data for Science. 2014. https://www.livescience.com/47591-ibm-watson-science-discoveries.html.
4. Çelik M Catching up with ES. Pharm Technol 2001: 25(7), 122–124.
5. Durkin J Introductions to expert systems. Expert systems design and development. Eaglewood Cliffs, New Jersey, US: Prentice Hall. 1994: 1–25.
6. Artificial Intelligence Index. 2018. Available from: http://cdn.aiindex.org/2018/AI%20Index%202018%20Annual%20Report.pdf.
7. Çelik M The past, present and future of tableting technology. Drug Dev Ind Pharm 1996: 22(1), 1–10.
8. Kastner JK, Hong SJ A review of expert systems. Eur J Oper Res 1984: 18(3), 285–292. doi:10.1016/0377-2217(84)90150-4.
9. Neale IM. First generation expert systems: a review of knowledge acquisition methodologies. Knowl Eng Rev 1988: 3(02), 105. doi:10.1017/s0269888900004288.
10. Vizureanu P Introductory Chapter: Enhanced Expert System - A Long-Life Solution, Enhanced Expert Systems. London, United Kingdom: IntechOpen, 2019. DOI: 10.5772/intechopen.85704. Available from: https://www.intechopen.com/books/enhanced-expert-systems/introductory-chapter-enhanced-expert-system-a-long-life-solution.
11. Judson P Knowledge-Based Expert Systems in Chemistry Artificial Intelligence in Decision Making. 2nd Edition. Cambridge, United Kingdom: Royal Society of Chemistry, 2019.
12. Jones DD, Barrett JR Building expert systems. In: Barrett JR, Jones DD (eds). Knowledge Engineering in Agriculture. ASAE Monograph No. 8, St. Joseph, MI, ASAE, 1989.
13. Leonard-Barton D, Sviokla J Putting expert systems to work. Harvard Business Review, 1988.
14. Harmon P, Sawyer B Creating Expert Systems for Business and Industry. New York, USA. John Wiley & Sons, Inc., 1990.
15. Ignizio JP Introduction to Expert Systems: The Development and Implementation of Rule-Based Expert Systems. New York, USA. McGraw-Hill, Inc., 1991.
16. Schneider M, Kandl A, Langholz G, Chew G Fuzzy Expert System Tools. Chichester, UK. John Wiley & Sons., 1996.
17. Swingler K Applying Neural Networks: A Practical Guide. London, UK. Academic Press, 1996.
18. Rowe C, Roberts RJ Intelligent Software for Product Formulation. London, UK. Taylor & Francis, 1998.
19. https://www.javatpoint.com/ai-techniques-of-knowledge-representation.
20. Liu H, Gegov A, Stahl F Categorization and construction of rule-based systems. In: Mladenov V, Jayne C, Iliadis L (eds). Engineering Applications of Neural Networks. vol 459. Cham. Springer, 2014. Available from: https://doi.org/10.1007/978-3-319-11071-4_18.
21. Sharma M, Sharma C A review on diverse applications of case-based reasoning. In: Sharma H, Govindan K, Poonia R, Kumar S, El-Medany W (eds). Advances in Computing and Intelligent Systems. Algorithms for Intelligent Systems. Singapore. Springer, 2020. Available from: https://doi.org/10.1007/978-981-15-0222-4_48.
22. Fuller R Fuzzy logic and neural nets in intelligent systems. Available from: https://pdfs.semanticscholar.org/89b7/4b349f90846de6c550bff1996055f6f7de54.pdf.
23. Fuller R Introduction to Neuro-Fuzzy Systems. New York City, USA: Springer-Verlag Berlin Heidelberg, 2000, p. 171.
24. SPRAYex. Available from: http://www.pt-int.com/Sprayex.html.
25. Wendel SC The prediction of spray drying formulations and processes for pharmaceutical powders. Ph.D. Thesis, 2001.
26. Klinger DE Expert systems in the pharmaceutical industry. Drug Inf J 1988: 22, 249–258.
27. Murray FJ The application of expert systems to pharmaceutical processing equipment. Pharm Technol 1989: 13(3), 100–110.

28. Rowe RC, Wakerly MG, Roberts RJ, Grundy RU, Upjohn NJ Expert systems for parenteral development. PDA J Pharm Sci Technol 1995: 49, 257–261.
29. Bateman SD, Verlin J, Russo M, Guillot M, Laughlin SM The development and validation of a capsule formulation knowledge-based system. Pharm Technol 1996: 20(3), 174–184.
30. Rowe RC Intelligent software systems for pharmaceutical product formulation. Pharm Technol 1997: 21(3), 178–188.
31. Hussain AS, Shivanand P, Johnson RD Application of neural computing in pharmaceutical development: computer-aided formulation design. Drug Dev Ind Pharm 1994: 20(10), 1739–1752.
32. Watano S, Takashima H, Miyanami K Scale-up of agitation fluidized-bed granulation by neural-network. Chem Pharm Bull 1997: 45(7), 1193–1197.
33. Murtoniemi E, Yliruusi J, Kinnunen P, Merkku P, Leiviska K The advantages by the use of NN in modeling the fluidised bed granulation process. Int J Pharm 1994: 108, 155–164.
34. Murtoniemi E, Merkku P, Kinnunen P, Leiviska K, Yliruusi J Effect of NN topology and training endpoint in modeling the fluidised bed granulation process. Int J Pharm 1994: 110, 101–108.
35. Erb RJ Introduction to backpropagation neural network computation. Pharm Res 1993: 10, 165–170.
36. Ebube NK, McCall T, Chen Y, Meyer MC Relating formulation variables to in vitro dissolution using an ANN. Pharm Dev Technol 1997: 2(3), 225–232.
37. Sokolović N, Ajanović M, Badić S, Banjanin M, Brkan M, Čusto N, Stanić B, Sirbubalo M, Tucak A, Vranić E Predicting the outcome of granulation and tableting processes using different artificial intelligence methods. Proceedings of the International Conference on Medical and Biological Engineering, 16–18 May 2019, Banja Luka, Bosnia and Herzegovina, 499–504.
38. Lee SL, O'Connor TF, Yang X, Cruz CN, Chatterjee S, Madurawe RD, Moore CMV, Yu LX, Woodcock J Modernizing pharmaceutical manufacturing: from batch to continuous production. J Pharm Innov 2015: 10, 191–199.
39. Rogers A, Hashemi A, Ierapetritou M Modeling of particulate processes for the continuous manufacture of solid-based pharmaceutical dosage forms. Processes 2013: 1, 67.
40. Seem TC, Rowson NA, Ingram A, Huang Z, Yu S, de Matas M, Gabbott I, Reynolds GK Twin-screw granulation- a literature review. Powder Technol 2015: 89–102.
41. Barrasso D, Ramachandran R Multi-scale modeling of granulation processes: bi-directional coupling of PBM with DEM via collision frequencies. Chem Eng Res Des 2015: 93, 304–317.
42. Barrasso D, Tamrakar A, Ramachandran R A reduced-order PBM—ANN model of a multi-scale PBM—DEM description of a wet granulation process. Chem Eng Sci 2014: 119, 319–329.
43. Barrasso D, El Hagrasy A, Litster JD, Ramachandran R Multi-dimensional population balance model development and validation for a twin-screw granulation process. Powder Technol 2015: 270, 612–621 Part B.
44. Kumar A, Gernaey KV, Beer TD, Nopens I Model-based analysis of high shear wet granulation from batch to continuous processes in pharmaceutical production—a critical review. Eur J Pharm Biopharm 2013: 85, 814–832.
45. Shirazian S, Kuhs M, Darwish S, Croker D, Walker GM Artificial neural network modelling of continuous wet granulation using a twin-screw extruder. Int J Pharm 2017: 521, 102–109.
46. Landin M Artificial intelligence tools for scaling up of high shear wet granulation process. J Pharm Sci 2017: 106(1), 273–277.
47. Pandey P, Badawy S A quality by design approach to scale-up of the high-shear wet granulation process. Drug Dev Ind Pharm 2016: 42(2), 175–189.
48. Chaudhury A, Barrasso D, Pandey P, Wu H, Ramachandran R Population balance model development, validation, and prediction of CQAs of a high-shear wet granulation process: towards QbD in drug product pharmaceutical manufacturing. J Pharm Innov 2014: 9(1), 53–64.
49. Barrasso D, Eppinger T, Pereira FE, Aglave R, Debus K, Bermingham SK, Ramachandran R A multi-scale, mechanistic model of a wet granulation process using a novel bi-directional PBM–DEM coupling algorithm. Chem Eng Sci 2015: 123, 500–513.
50. Luo G, Xu B, Sun F, Cui X, Shi X, Qiao Y Quality by design based high shear wet granulation process development for the microcrystalline cellulose. Acta Pharm Sinica B 2015: 50(3), 355–359.
51. Aikawa S, Fujita N, Myojo H, Hayashi T, Tanino T Scale-up studies on high shear wet granulation process from mini-scale to commercial scale. Chem Pharm Bull (Tokyo) 2008: 56(10), 1431–1435.
52. Badawy SI, Narang AS, LaMarche KR, Subramanian GA, Varia SA Mechanistic basis for the effects of process parameters on quality attributes in high shear wet granulation. In: Narang A, Badawy S (eds). Handbook of Pharmaceutical Wet Granulation. Amsterdam, Netherlands. Elsevier, 2019. p. 89–118.
53. Aksu B, Paradkar A, de Matas M, Özer Ö, Güneri T, York P A quality by design approach using

artificial intelligence techniques to control the critical quality attributes of ramipril tablets manufactured by wet granulation. Pharm Dev Technol 2013: 18(1), 236–245.

54. Kayrak-Talay D, Dale S, Wassgren C, Litster J Quality by design for wet granulation in pharmaceutical processing: assessing models for a priori design and scaling. Powder Technol 2013: 240, 7–18.

55. Sonnergaard JM Quantification of the compactibility of pharmaceutical powders. Eur J Pharm Biopharm 2006: 63(3), 270–277.

56. Millen N, Kovačević A, Khera L, Djuriš J, Ibrić S Machine learning modelling of wet granulation scale-up using compressibility, compactibility and manufacturability parameters. Hem Ind 2019: 73(3), 155–168.

57. Krishnamurthy S Pharma 4.0: Redefining Product Development and Regulatory Operations. Pharmaexec.com, 2019. Available from: https://www.pharmexec.com/view/pharma-4-0-redefining-product-development-and-regulatory-operations.

Leading Next-Generation Manufacturing

Prasad Kanneganti

CONTENTS

27.1   INTRODUCTION

The pharmaceutical industry is one of the most regulated consumer industries today. Concerned with the safety of its citizens, governments across the world have set up regulations that govern the manufacturing and distribution of finished pharmaceuticals for human consumption. Like the industry, the regulations are also evolving to meet current business needs and emerging technological developments. Current Good Manufacturing Practices (cGMPs) are now widely used across the world. Globalization of the pharmaceutical industry has taken place rapidly in recent times, fueled by mergers and acquisitions within the industry and also by economic, political, and regulatory drivers. The industry today is supported by a complex global supply chain that feeds raw materials and packaging components to manufacturers and delivers finished drug products to patients around the world. The rapid rise of Asian economies such as China and India contributed significantly to the flow of goods and services between East and West. These economies are not only major manufacturers of Active Pharmaceutical Ingredients (APIs) but also major consumers of finished pharmaceuticals. Consequently, they are attracting increasing attention from health authorities checking for compliance with cGMPs. Regulatory harmonization initiatives at the global and regional levels are making some progress. Harmonization has become challenging with more health authorities from emerging economies coming on board. In recent years, regulatory agencies in the United States and European Union have encouraged the use of new modalities and technologies for manufacturing. This is leading to a paradigm shift in how pharmaceutical processes are controlled and how product quality is defined and managed.

27.2 PHARMACEUTICAL QUALITY MANAGEMENT

Quality management is that aspect of management function that establishes and implements the quality policy formally authorized by senior management. The fundamental elements of quality management are an appropriate infrastructure or quality system and systematic actions known as quality assurance taken to ensure adequate confidence that the product or service will satisfy established requirements for quality. Thus, quality assurance is a management tool covering all matters that individually or collectively influence the quality of a product. It incorporates cGMP as well as other factors such as product design and development. Quality control is a subset of cGMP and concerns mainly with sampling, specifications, and testing of raw materials and finished pharmaceutical products. The concepts of quality assurance, cGMP, and quality control are thus interrelated aspects of quality management.

27.2.1 CURRENT GOOD MANUFACTURING PRACTICES

cGMP is that part of the quality assurance system that ensures that medicinal products are consistently produced and controlled to the quality standards appropriate to their intended use and as required by the marketing authorization provided by the regulatory agencies. The production of pharmaceutical products involves some risks, for example, cross-contamination, label mix-ups, etc., that cannot be prevented entirely through end product testing, and cGMPs diminish such risks. This quality assurance element is mandated by law around the world for the manufacturing, storage, and distribution of pharmaceuticals. Although the standards set by the U.S. Food and Drug Administration (FDA) [1,2] are well recognized as an industry benchmark, standards from other countries and regions are also well accepted [3–6].

One of the cGMP standards that has gained worldwide recognition is the one setup by the Pharmaceutical Inspection Cooperation Scheme (PIC/S). It is a non-binding, informal co-operative arrangement between regulatory authorities in the field of Good Manufacturing Practice (GMP) of medicinal products for human or veterinary use and is open to any authority having a comparable GMP inspection system [3]. PIC/S aims at harmonizing inspection procedures worldwide by developing common standards in the field of cGMP and by providing training opportunities for Inspectors. It also aims at facilitating co-operation and networking between competent authorities, regional and international organizations, thus increasing mutual confidence. PIC/S became operational in November 1995, and as of December 2020, PIC/S had 53 participating authorities spread across five continents.

In the United States, cGMP requirements were established to be flexible to allow each manufacturer to decide individually how best to implement the necessary controls by using scientifically sound design, processing methods, and testing procedures. Regulations were made flexible to encourage companies to use modern technologies and innovative approaches to achieve higher quality through continual improvement. FDA issued guidance on a significant new initiative, Pharmaceutical cGMPs for the 21st Century [7]. This initiative was aimed at modernizing FDA regulations to support the early adoption of new technological advances and state-of-the-art manufacturing science by the pharmaceutical industry. In addition, the industry was encouraged to implement an integrated quality system and a risk-based approach for managing production processes and quality assurance [8].

27.2.2 INTERNATIONAL COUNCIL FOR HARMONIZATION

The International Council for Harmonization (ICH), formerly the International Conference on Harmonization (ICH), held the inaugural assembly meetings on 23 October 2015 establishing ICH as an international non-profit association under Swiss law. This step built upon a 25-year track record of successful delivery of harmonized guidelines for global pharmaceutical development as well as their regulation, and a long-standing recognition of the need to harmonize [9]. ICH was initially set up as a project that brought together the regulatory authorities of Europe, Japan, and the United States and experts from the pharmaceutical industry in these regions to discuss scientific and technical aspects of drug registration. Since its inception in 1990, ICH has gradually evolved to address the needs of globalization of drug development activity. Its mission now is to achieve greater harmonization worldwide to ensure that safe, effective, and high-quality medicines are developed and registered in the most resource-efficient manner. Harmonization is achieved through the development of ICH Guidelines via a process of scientific consensus with regulatory and industry experts working together.

Guidelines issued by ICH are very useful reference documents for both the industry and regulatory bodies. The topics for these guidelines are divided into four major categories, each with a specific topic code.

- Quality Topics (Q), for example, Stability Testing (Q1), Impurity Testing (Q3)
- Safety Topics (S), for example, Carcinogenicity Testing (S1), Genotoxicity Testing (S2)
- Efficacy Topics (E), for example, Dose-Response Studies (E4), Good Clinical Practices (E6)
- Multidisciplinary Topics (M), for example, Medical Terminology (M1), The Common Technical Document (CTD) (M4)

There is no specific ICH guideline covering the topic of pharmaceutical granulations; however, guidelines such as the CTD highlight the requirements for specifications, testing, impurities, stability, and validation in drug product regulatory submissions. Because of the wide international acceptance of these guidelines, it would be prudent to check compliance with requirements specified in them while putting together documentation dossiers to support regulatory filings or product/technology transfers.

27.2.3 ISO 9000 STANDARDS

The International Organization for Standardization (ISO) is the world's largest developer of standards and is an independent, non-governmental international organization. ISO's principal activity is the development of technical standards. These are very useful to the industry, regulatory bodies, trade officials, suppliers, and customers of products and services. With its Central Secretariat in Geneva, Switzerland, ISO coordinates a network of the national standard institutes of 164 countries [10]. Each country is represented by one member that, unlike in the case of the United Nations, need not be a delegation of the national government. Through its members, it brings together experts to share knowledge and develop voluntary, consensus-based, market-relevant International Standards that support innovation and provide solutions to global challenges.

ISO has gained wide acceptance internationally as a commonly understood baseline for quality, safety, and environmental standards. It ensures fair play and facilitates cross-border trade. ISO standards are voluntary, and being a non-governmental organization, it has no legal authority to enforce its implementation. This is an essential difference with cGMPs that have been legislated into law in several countries.

One of the most popular standards is the ISO 9000 family, which is a generic management system standard that has become an international reference for quality requirements in business-to-business dealings. The latest standard in this series is ISO 9001–2015 which sets out the criteria for a quality management system and is the only standard in the family that can be certified to. The requirements are generic and are intended to apply to any organization, regardless of its type or size, or the products and services it provides. Today, there are over one million companies and organizations in over 170 countries certified to ISO 9001. The quality management principles embedded in this standard represent a strong customer focus, the motivation and implication of top management, the process approach, and continual improvement.

Several excipients used in pharmaceutical granulations may be common substances that are also used in the food and cosmetic industries. For manufacturers of such substances, if cGMP is not mandated by law, compliance with ISO 9000 is generally expected as a minimum by pharmaceutical manufacturers as part of their supplier management program.

27.3 MANUFACTURING SCIENCE

The pharmaceutical industry today is facing many challenges. The cost of drug research has increased steeply, and at the same time, R&D productivity is waning. Patent expiry and loss of exclusivity are resulting in decreasing revenues. Manufacturers are thus being forced to improve efficiencies and reduce costs. This is affecting the way manufacturing is carried out, with greater emphasis on the use of science-based tools and quality risk management to improve operational performance and to focus on elements that are critical to product quality.

Manufacturing science encompasses knowledge about products and processes, the technology used to manufacture and control these processes, and the underlying foundation of a robust quality system at the manufacturing site. This results in the manufacture of medicinal products in a reproducible manner and mitigates risk to the patient.

27.3.1 REGULATORY OUTLOOK

Dr. Janet Woodcock, who is currently the U.S. FDA Director of Center for Drug Evaluation and Research (CDER), once stated, "Industry must reinvent itself and its relationship with FDA to deal with a future that promises to be very different from today. Archaic regulatory practices that have stifled innovation and made the industry inefficient cannot continue. Part of the problem was that we didn't know what influenced product quality. We treated everything the same, every deviation was a threat to product quality but if your processes are under control and well understood, we can do things very differently." This is a clear indication to the industry to strive for process understanding based on science and to unburden pharmaceutical manufacturing based on this understanding.

Another senior FDA official, Dr. Mark McClellan, who was a former FDA Commissioner, once remarked, "Pharmaceutical companies must catch up with potato chip and soap flake manufacturers by modernizing operations and applying technology effectively." This remark has often been quoted in the media and at various conferences as a wake-up call to the industry to adopt new technologies and eliminate waste.

In 2002, the Food and Drug Administration (FDA) announced a significant new initiative, Pharmaceutical Current Good Manufacturing Practices (cGMPs) for the 21st Century, to enhance and modernize the regulation of pharmaceutical manufacturing and product quality. This resulted in the release in September 2004 of FDA guidance on Pharmaceutical cGMPs for the 21st Century

[7] that encourages the use of manufacturing science as a basis for innovation and continuous improvement. Following this guidance, there commenced a period of sharing of knowledge between manufacturers and regulators and the application of regulatory processes proportional to the level of risk and applied manufacturing science demonstrated by a manufacturer.

27.4 PROCESS ANALYTICAL TECHNOLOGY

In September 2004, alongside the guidance on Pharmaceutical cGMPs for the 21st Century, the FDA issued another significant guidance on process analytical technology (PAT). This guidance [11] considers PAT to be a system for designing, analyzing, and controlling manufacturing through real-time measurement of critical quality and performance attributes of raw/in-process materials and processes, to ensure final product quality. The goal of PAT is to enhance the understanding and control of the manufacturing process.

Most pharmaceutical processes have traditionally been controlled based on time-defined endpoints, for example, blending for ten minutes. Such an approach does not always address variation in physical attributes such as particle size and shape for raw materials and differences arising during the process. The PAT toolkit consists of process analyzers, multivariate tools, process control tools, and continuous improvement and knowledge management tools. These tools can be used in combination for a single-unit operation or an entire manufacturing process and its quality assurance to gain a thorough understanding of the process. Process analyzers provide voluminous non-destructive test data gathered at-line, on-line, or in-line. Within the PAT framework, the completion of a process step, for example, granulation endpoint, is not a fixed time period but the achievement of the desired material attribute.

Process analyzers are well suited for granulation process equipment and can provide real-time data on critical process parameters (CPPs) and critical quality attributes (CQAs). Granulation endpoint measurements using transducers, motor current, torque, etc. have been standard fixtures on equipment used for pharmaceutical manufacturing for a long time. What has changed now is the data gathering and data processing capability and the availability of statistical data analysis tools such as multivariate analysis that provide a process signature in real-time. Over a period of time, manufacturers are able to leverage on assimilated knowledge to develop a set of process attributes defining an ideal batch known sometimes as the "golden batch."

The FDA's PAT team worked with the American Society for Testing and Materials (ASTM) [12] to establish the Technical Committee E55 on the pharmaceutical application of PAT. This committee developed several guidelines covering PAT terminology, system management, and system implementation/practice.

A more detailed discussion on PAT and process control instrumentation can be found in chapter 25 of this book.

27.5 QUALITY RISK MANAGEMENT

The new paradigm shift in pharmaceutical manufacturing includes the use of risk management and risk tools. What is risk? It is a combination of exposure and hazard. This is also sometimes referred to as probability and severity. What is the probability of a certain event such as a product failure due to equipment malfunction occurring, and when does it occur? What is the severity or impact on product quality and patient risk?

The ICH trio consists of pharmaceutical development (Q8) [13], quality risk management (QRM) (Q9) [14], and pharmaceutical quality systems (Q10) [15]. Combined together, these three guidance documents provide a structured way to define critical quality attributes and design space supporting the development of a robust manufacturing process with appropriate control strategies.

Q8 provides guidance on the content of the pharmaceutical development section for the CTD filed for drug products. The manufacturing process development program is expected to identify

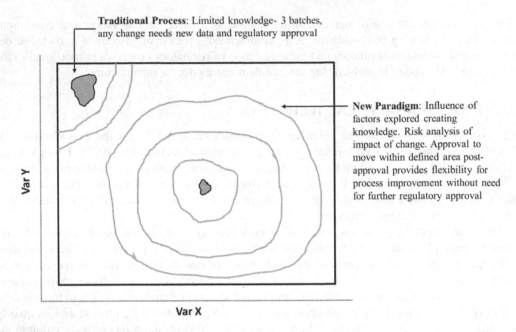

FIGURE 27.1   Design space.

CPPs that should be monitored or controlled to ensure that the product is of the desired quality. Granulation endpoint monitoring is provided as an example. The collection of process monitoring data during the development phase enhances process understanding. The design space is a multidimensional combination and interaction of input variables, for example, material attributes and process parameters that have been demonstrated to provide assurance of quality. Figure 27.1 shows a schematic representation of the design space and compares it with the conventional approach to controlling processes. Working within the design space is not considered as a change, while movement out of the design space is considered to be a change requiring postapproval regulatory filing.

Q9 offers a systematic approach to quality risk management. It is an independent document that complements other ICH quality documents and enables effective and consistent risk-based decisions by both regulators and industry. It states the following primary principles:

1. The evaluation of the risk to quality should be based on scientific knowledge and ultimately linked to the protection of the patient.
2. The level of effort, formality, and documentation of QRM should be commensurate with the level of risk.

Thus, the element of risk is assessed based on a scientific understanding of the process and quantified where possible. It is important to link the risk to the protection of the patient. Risk assessment documentation is essential; however, this is not just a paper exercise. The effort put in must be in line with the level of risk. Annex I of Q9 provides a list of risk assessment tools.

Q10 describes a comprehensive model for an effective pharmaceutical quality system that is based on ISO quality concepts and cGMPs and complements Q8 and Q9. It can be implemented throughout the different stages of a product life cycle. Figure 27.2 shows how the ICH trio contributes to risk reduction.

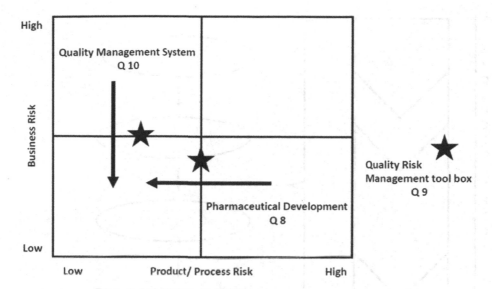

FIGURE 27.2 How Q8, Q9, and Q10 contribute to risk reduction.

The risk tools described in Q9 can be used to reduce product and process risk during pharmaceutical development, as described in Q8. Similarly, the risk toolkit can be used to reduce the risk to the quality system, as described in Q10. This ultimately benefits the organization as a whole.

In November 2009, FDA issued a revised guidance on ICH Q8, adding an annex that clarifies the original document and adds the principle of quality by design (QbD) [16]. Guidance for industry critical quality attributes, defined in the document as elements that could affect strength, purity, release, and stability, and their impact on development are covered in more detail in the revised guidance. The revised guidance also covers how risk assessment tools can be used to identify and rank parameters, such as process, equipment, and ingredients based on their potential to impact product quality. Other topics covered in the guidance include design space, life cycle management, and quality target product profiles (QTTP).

The product life cycle starts from development through commercial manufacturing and ultimately, product discontinuation (Figure 27.3).

During the development phase, QRM is used to identify what to monitor and measure. Risk assessments supported by laboratory-scale data generated from the design of experiments (DOE) are used to establish what material attributes and granulation process parameters are critical to product quality. The methodology used for monitoring the critical attributes, for example, off-line testing of moisture content of granulations or use of on-line/in-line NIR devices for content uniformity, is established at the pilot phase. At the manufacturing phase, on-line data generated is analyzed in real-time using statistical tools. This facilitates timely corrective actions to be taken for any adverse trends observed.

ICH also issued a new guideline on technical and regulatory considerations for pharmaceutical product life cycle management (Q12) [17]. This guideline addresses the commercial phase of the product life cycle, and it complements and adds to the flexible regulatory approaches to post-approval changes described in Q8 and Q10. The focus is on increased product and process knowledge to support change management through a better understanding of risk to product quality.

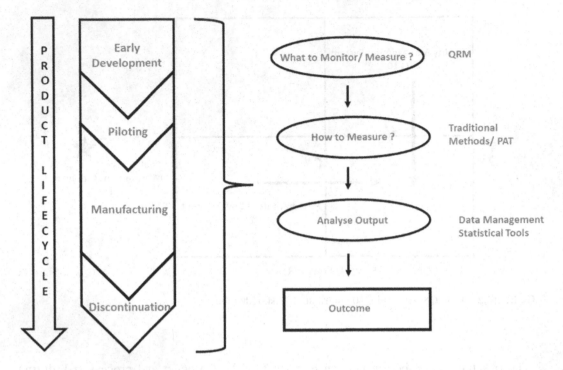

FIGURE 27.3 Product/process monitoring.

27.6 CONTINUOUS MANUFACTURING

Continuous manufacturing (CM) is an innovation that can reduce manufacturing and scale-up costs and make unit operations easy to transfer between plants and sites. Manufacturing start-up up costs are also lower as a continuous process skid occupies a smaller footprint than a typical batch processing plant. These skids are also portable and can be moved around easily and made operational after hooking up to required utilities and services. The concept of CM has been in practice in the specialty chemical and food industries for quite a while. However, embedding the concept of CM into commercial operations for pharmaceuticals has been a challenge due to the lack of harmonized regulatory guidance. Some companies started experimenting with CM approaches over ten years back as the current regulatory framework allows for the commercialization of products using CM technology. However, this concept was still new for both manufacturers and regulators who initially looked at continuous processes through a batch process lens. This resulted in a lot of expectations with an additional burden for process monitoring and control. The regulatory filing complexity also discouraged manufacturers to develop continuous processes for new products. The advantages of CM are now getting recognized as leading to next-generation manufacturing, and industry forums have started working with regulatory bodies to develop new guidance.

In February 2019, FDA issued draft guidance on quality considerations for CM in the pharmaceutical industry [18]. This guidance reflects the FDA's current thinking on the quality considerations for CM of small molecule, solid oral drug products. It describes several key quality considerations and provides recommendations for how manufacturers should address these considerations in new drug applications (NDAs), abbreviated new drug applications (ANDAs), and supplemental NDAs and ANDAs, for small molecule, solid oral drug products that are produced via a CM process.

The FDA considers CM to be a process in which the input material(s) are continuously fed into and transformed within the process, and the processed output materials are continuously removed from the system. This guidance applies to manufacturing operations wherein a continuous process is applied to two or more unit operations linked together. It addresses scientific and regulatory considerations unique to CM, for example, process dynamics, batch definition, control strategy, scale-up, stability, and bridging of existing batch manufacturing to CM.

Granulation process steps are quite suitable for integration with continuous plant operations. Continuous fluid-bed granulations whereby input materials are added and granulated material is harvested simultaneously is a good example. Another example is dry granulations using roller compactors. Even in the case of batch process wet granulations, it is possible to integrate such batch steps into a continuous process that starts with the feed of input material for mixing at one end and the collection of compressed tablets at another end.

ICH also got interested in the harmonization of CM concepts and published in November 2018 a final concept paper on the continuous manufacturing of drug Substances and drug Products (Q13) [19]. The plan is to develop a new guideline on CM within three years. This was a recognition by ICH that their current guidelines do not sufficiently address technical and regulatory requirements that are unique to CM. A harmonized regulatory guideline issued by ICH is expected to benefit industry and regulators and improve access to medicines for patients. It is also expected to facilitate uniform implementation, regulatory approval, and life cycle management, particularly for products intended for commercialization internationally.

27.7 DATA INTEGRITY

In recent years, data integrity within pharmaceutical manufacturing has become a key quality and regulatory compliance concern. We are now seeing increasing use of electronic records with electronic signatures to capture cGMP data in plants and QC laboratories. The storage, retrieval, and integrity of vast amounts of electronic data have become a challenging task. This data control has not been of the same rigor as that for paper records used erstwhile. During manufacturing site inspections, the FDA has increasingly observed cGMP violations involving data integrity. This resulted in regulatory actions, including warning letters, import alerts, and consent decrees.

The FDA issued new guidance in December 2018 on data integrity and compliance with drug cGMP that defines terminology and answers several questions regarding paper and electronic data [20]. FDA emphasizes that all cGMP data should be reliable and accurate, and the guidance clarifies the role of data integrity to achieve this. Complete, consistent, and accurate data should be attributable, legible, contemporaneously recorded, original or a true copy, and accurate (ALCOA). Metadata is the contextual information required to understand data. A data value is by itself meaningless without additional information about the data, and hence, metadata is often described as data about data. As an example, if CPPs such as mixing and granulation time for wet granulation or inlet/outlet air temperature for fluid-bed granulation are data, the date/time stamp of when such data was generated and the name/identity of operator collecting such data are considered as metadata. Another key focus area is audit trail which means a secure, computer-generated, time-stamped electronic record that allows for the reconstruction of the course of events relating to the creation, modification, or deletion of an electronic record. As an example, a record for a granulation process step should include details of the recipe used, operator identity, equipment used, the identity of material inputs, measures for CPPs, timestamp and duration for individual process steps, process interruptions, a second person check for critical process steps, etc. Data once generated needs to stay in its original form, and the audit trail keeps track of amendments made if permitted by the procedure. Regular and independent review of audit trails is a requirement.

27.8 POSTAPPROVAL CHANGE CONSIDERATIONS

Scale-up of manufacturing is required during the transfer of production processes from drug product development laboratories to commercial manufacturing centers or between manufacturing centers. During the manufacture of clinical batches, the amount of active ingredient available is limited, and the process equipments available are often scaled-down versions of those used for the production of commercial batches. Batch sizes are thus smaller than those used during the manufacture of routine commercial batches. Process scale-up and commercial manufacturing are expedited as the industry attempts to maximize the commercial benefits afforded by patent protection for new drug molecules. Most companies formally record the scientific data that is generated into product development reports. These form the basis for establishing the manufacturing process, specifications, in-process controls, and validation acceptance criteria used during the commercial production of the drug product. Product development reports also provide a link between the bio batch/clinical batch and commercial process through development and scale-up. Information from the development phase is used to prepare the chemistry, manufacturing, and controls (CMC) section of an application such as a new drug application (NDA) filed with the FDA [21]. Where applicable, reference is also provided to other documents such as drug master files (DMFs) submitted earlier to the FDA by the manufacturer or their suppliers of excipients and product contact equipment components such as gasket/seal elastomers [22].

The FDA, with input from the industry, developed guidance for scale-up postapproval changes (SUPAC) for oral dosage forms. SUPAC covers components or composition, site of manufacture, the scale of manufacture, and manufacturing process/equipment. These guidelines represent the agency's current thinking on the topic and are not binding on the industry or agency with alternative approaches being acceptable. These guidance documents have been well received by the pharmaceutical industry as they enhance their ability to plan and implement change and manage resources efficiently.

The scale-up postapproval changes immediate-release (SUPAC-IR) guidance for immediate-release solid oral dosage forms [23] provides recommendations to sponsors of NDAs, abbreviated new drug applications (ANDAs), and abbreviated antibiotic applications (AADAs) who intend, during the postapproval period, to make changes. This guidance was the result of a workshop on the scale-up of immediate-release products conducted by the American Association of Pharmaceutical Scientists (AAPS) in conjunction with the U.S. Pharmacopeia Convention (USP) and the FDA [24]. It defines the levels of change, recommended CMC tests for each level of change, *in vitro* dissolution tests, and/or *in vivo* bioequivalence tests for each level of change and filing documentation that should support the change (Figures 27.4 and 27.5).

Notification to FDA of postapproval changes to NDAs is made using change documentation known as supplements [25]. The regulations describe the type of changes that require prior approval from the FDA before the change can be implemented (preapprovable changes). Under some circumstances, changes can be made before approval from FDA (changes being affected or CBEs) or described in the annual report to the FDA. In the case of CBE supplements, the FDA may, after a review of the information submitted, decide that the changes are not approvable. The SUPAC guidance documents list information that should be provided to the FDA to assure that product quality and the performance characteristics of the drug products are not adversely affected by the changes proposed to be carried out.

27.8.1 COMPONENT AND COMPOSITION CHANGES

The SUPAC guidance focuses on changes in excipients in the drug product. Changes in the amount of drug substance are not addressed by this guidance. The changes are categorized into three levels according to the increasing impact on product quality and performance expected.

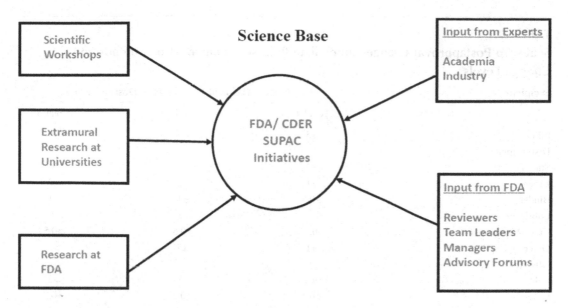

FIGURE 27.4   Developments of scale-up postapproval change guidance documents.

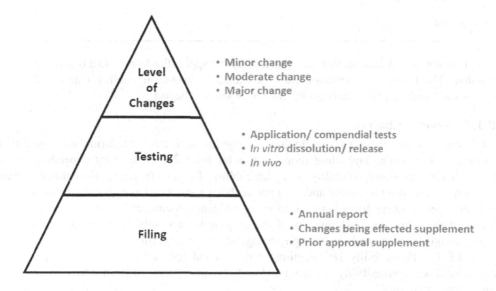

FIGURE 27.5   Formats of scale-up postapproval change guidance documents.

27.8.1.1   Level 1 Changes

Level 1 changes are those that are unlikely to have any detectable impact on formulation quality and performance. Examples of such changes are deletion or partial deletion of an ingredient intended to affect the color or flavor of the drug product, changes in the composition of the printing ink to another approved ingredient, etc. Changes in excipients expressed as percentages (w/w) of the total formulation, less than or equal to the percent range shown in Table 27.1, are also level 1 changes. The total additive effect of all excipient changes should not be more than 5%.

The documentation necessary to support this type of change is application/compendial release requirements and stability data for one batch on long-term stability. No *in vivo* bioequivalence data or

TABLE 27.1

Scale-Up Postapproval Changes Immediate Release: Component or Composition Change Levels

Excipient	Percent Excipient (w/w of Total Dosage Unit)		
	Level 1	Level 2	Level 3
Filler	±5	±10	>10
Disintegrant			
Starch	±3	±6	>6
Other	±1	±2	>2
Binder	±0.5	±1	>1
Lubricant			
Ca or Mg stearate	±0.25	±0.5	>0.5
Other	±1	±2	>2
Glidant			
Talc	±1	±2	>2
Other	±0.1	±0.2	>0.2
Film coat	±1	±2	>2
Total drug excipient change (%)	5	10	n/a

Source: From Ref. 23.

additional dissolution data other than that required by the application/compendia is necessary for this submission. The entire documentation package including long-term stability data for the level 1 change is filed with the FDA through the annual report mechanism.

27.8.1.2 Level 2 Changes

Level 2 changes are those that could have a significant impact on formulation quality and performance. The testing and filing requirements for level 2 changes vary depending on three factors – therapeutic range, solubility, and permeability. Therapeutic ranges are defined as narrow or non-narrow, and drug solubility and drug permeability are defined as either low or high. A list of narrow therapeutic range drugs is provided in the guidance document. Solubility is calculated on the basis of the minimum concentration of the drug, milligram/milliliter (mg/mL), in the largest dosage strength, determined in the physiological pH range (pH 1 to 8) and temperature ($37\,^{\circ}\text{C} \pm 0.5\,^{\circ}\text{C}$). Permeability [$P_e$, centimeter per second (cm/sec)] is defined as the effective human jejunal wall permeability of a drug and includes an apparent resistance to mass transport to the intestinal membrane.

An example of a level 2 change is the change in the technical grade of an excipient, for example, Avicel PH102 versus Avicel PH200. Changes in excipients expressed as a percentage (w/w) of the total formulation, greater than those listed earlier for level 1 change but less than or equal to a percent range representing a twofold increase over level 1 changes (Table 27.1), are also deemed as level 2 changes. The total additive effect of all excipient changes should not be more than 10%.

The documentation necessary to support this type of change is application/ compendial release requirements, batch records, and stability data for one batch with three months' accelerated stability data in supplement and one batch on long-term stability. Dissolution data requirements depend on three scenarios known as cases that cover a high/low permeability and a high/low drug solubility, as shown in Table 27.2. No *in vivo* bioequivalence data is necessary for this submission if the situation falls within one of the cases shown in Table 27.2. A prior approval supplement that

TABLE 27.2

Scale-Up Postapproval Changes Immediate Release: Dissolution Testing Categories

Category	Nature of Drug	Dissolution Medium	Time Points (min)	Specification
Case A	High permeability High solubility	0.1 N HCl	15	≥85%
Case B	Low permeability High solubility	As stated in application/ compendia	15, 30, 45, 60, 120, or until an asymptote is reached	Dissolution profile similar to the current formulation
Case C	High permeability Low solubility	Water, 0.1 N HCl, USP buffer media at pH 4.5, 6.5, and 7.5 (plus surfactant if justified)	15, 30, 45, 60, 120	90% or an asymptote is reached. Profile similar to the current product

Source: From Ref. 23.

contains all information including accelerated stability data is to be filed. The long-term stability data is filed through the annual report mechanism.

27.8.1.3 Level 3 Changes

Level 3 changes are those that are likely to have a significant impact on formulation quality and performance. Similar to level 2 changes, the testing and filing documentation requirements vary depending on therapeutic range, solubility, and permeability. Examples of level 3 changes are any qualitative and quantitative excipient changes to a narrow therapeutic drug beyond the ranges stated for level 1 changes (Table 27.1) and all drugs not meeting the dissolution criteria listed for level 2 changes (Table 27.2).

A change in granulating solution volume is not covered under SUPAC-IR as it is a minor change to a normal operating procedure and should be included in the batch record after undergoing validation and manufacturer's site change control procedure. A change in the granulating solvent, for example, from alcohol to water, can be expected to alter the composition of the drug product even though it may be removed during manufacturing, and hence, it is a level 3 change that requires a prior approval supplement.

The documentations required to support level 3 changes are application/compendial release requirements and batch records. If a significant body of information is available, one batch with three months' accelerated stability data is to be included in the supplement and one batch on long-term stability data is to be reported in the annual report. Where a significant body of information is not available, up to three batches with three months' accelerated stability data are to be included in the supplement and one batch on long-term stability data is to be reported in the annual report.

Dissolution data requirements for level 3 changes are as specified for case B in Table 27.2. In addition, a complete *in vivo* bioequivalence study is required. This study may be waived if an acceptable *in vivo/in vitro* correlation has been verified. A prior approval supplement that contains all information including accelerated stability data is to be filed.

27.8.2 SITE CHANGES

Site changes consist of changes in the location of the site of manufacture for both company-owned and contract manufacturing facilities. These do not include any scale-up changes, changes in the manufacturing process and/or equipment, or changes in components or composition. The new manufacturing locations are expected to have a satisfactory cGMP inspection. Similar to those for component and composition changes, site changes are also categorized into three different levels that require a differing depth of test and filing documentation. Level 1 changes are site changes within a single facility, while level 2 changes are site changes within the same campus. Level 3 changes consist of a change in manufacturing site to a different campus, that is, the facilities are not on the same original contiguous site or in adjacent city blocks. These requirements are summarized in Table 27.3.

27.8.3 CHANGES IN BATCH SIZE

Postapproval changes in the size of a batch (scale-up/scale-down) from the pivotal/pilot scale biobatch material to a larger or smaller production batch require additional information to be submitted with the change application. Scale-down below 100,000 dosage units is not covered by the SUPAC guidance. All scale-up changes are required to undergo suitable process validation and are to undergo regulatory inspection. There are two levels of batch size changes that cover batch size increases up to and including a factor of 10 times the size of the pilot/ biobatch and increases beyond a factor of 10 times, respectively (Table 27.3).

27.8.4 MANUFACTURING EQUIPMENT/PROCESS CHANGES

Equipment changes consist of changes from non-automated or non-mechanical equipment to automated or mechanical equipment or changes to alternative equipment of either the same or different design and operating principle or of a different capacity. Process changes include changes such as mixing time and operating speeds either within or outside application/validation ranges. A change in the type of process used in the manufacture of the drug product, that is, change from wet granulation to direct compression of dry powder, is also included. Table 27.3 provides a summary of the documentation requirements to file changes to manufacturing equipment and process.

27.8.5 MODIFIED-RELEASE SOLID DOSAGE FORMS

Modified-release solid dosage forms include both delayed- and extended-release drug products. The delayed-release is the release of a drug (or drugs) at a time other than immediately following oral administration. Extended-release products, on the other hand, are formulated to make the drug available over an extended period after ingestion so that a reduction in the dosing frequency compared with an immediate-release dosage form is achieved.

Following the successful release of the guidance document for immediate-release solid oral dosage forms (SUPAC-IR), the FDA issued specific guidance, the scale-up postapproval changes modified release (SUPAC-MR) for scale-up and postapproval changes affecting modified-release solid dosage forms [26,27] in 1997. This guidance covers postapproval changes for modified-release solid oral dosage forms that affect components and composition, scale-up/scale-down, manufacturing site change, and manufacturing process or equipment changes. It permits less burdensome notice of certain postapproval changes within the meaning of Changes Being Effected (CBE) supplement (21CFR 314.70).

In the case of components and composition, SUPAC-MR covers changes in non-release controlling excipients and release controlling excipients separately. The criticality of an excipient to drug release is to be established and appropriate justifications are to be provided if an excipient is claimed as a non-release controlling excipient in the formulation of the modified-release solid dosage form. The change level classification, therapeutic range, test and filing documentation for components and composition changes, site changes, changes in batch size (scale-up/scale-down), and manufacturing equipment changes and manufacturing process changes for extended-release solid dosage forms and delayed-release solid dosage forms are summarized in this guidance document.

TABLE 27.3

Scale-Up Postapproval Changes Immediate Release: Site Equipment and Process Change Requirements by Category

Type/Level	Change Permitted	Exclusions	Chemistry	Documentation Dissolution	Bioequivalence	Filing
Component/composition						
Level 1	Table 27.1 total change ≤ 5%	No change beyond approved target ranges	LTSS commitment	Application/ compendial only	None	Annual report
Level 2	Table 27.1 total change ≤10%	No narrow therapeutic range drugs	Accelerated stability data plus LTSS commitment	Varies, see Table 27.2	None	Prior approval supplement
Level 3	Table 27.1	None	Accelerated stability data plus LTSS commitment	Case B, see Table 27.2	Full	Prior approval supplement
Site change						
Level 1	Single facility	No scale or process changes	None	Application/ compendial only	None	Annual report
Level 2	Contiguous campus	No scale or process changes	None	Application/ compendial only	None	Changes being effected supplement
Level 3	Different campus	No scale or process changes	Accelerated stability data and LTSS commitment	Case B, see Table 27.2	None	Change being effected supplement
Scale-up/scale-down						
Level 1	≤10-fold increase in batch size	No change in site, controls, or equipment	LTSS commitment	Application/ compendial only	None	Annual report

(continued)

TABLE 27.3 (Continued)

Type/Level	Change Permitted	Exclusions	Chemistry	Documentation Dissolution	Bioequivalence	Filing
Level 2	>10-fold increase in batch size	No change in site, controls, or equipment	Accelerated stability data and LTSS commitment	Case B, see Table 27.2	None	Change being effected supplement
Manufacturing equipment						
Level 1	Non-automated to automated/non-mechanical to mechanical; new equipment design w/w same capacity	No change in operating principle	LTSS commitment	Application/compendial only	None	Annual report
Level 2	New design or operating principle	None	Accelerated stability data and LTSS commitment	Case C, see Table 27.2	None	Prior approval supplement with change justification
Manufacturing process						
Level 1	Operating within validation ranges	None	None	Application/compendial only	None	Annual report
Level 2	Operating outside validation ranges	None	LTSS commitment	Case B, see Table 27.2	None	Changes being affected
Level 3	The new process (e.g., wet-to-dry granulation)	None	Accelerated stability data and LTSS commitment	Case B, see Table 27.2	Full	Prior approval supplement with change justification

Abbreviation: LTSS, long-term stability study. *Source*: From Ref. 23.

27.8.6 Changes to Granulation Equipment

The FDA released in January 1999 another guidance document that specifically addressed documentation requirements for filings addressing changes to pharmaceutical manufacturing equipment [28]. This is the manufacturing equipment addendum developed with the assistance of the International Society of Pharmaceutical Engineering (ISPE) and is used in conjunction with the SUPAC-IR and SUPAC-MR guidance documents. It includes a representative list of equipment commonly used in the industry but does not include equipment modified by a manufacturer to meet specific needs. Definitions and classification for broad categories of unit operations such as blending and mixing, drying, particle size reduction/separation, granulation, unit dosage, coating, printing, and soft gelatin encapsulation are provided. For each unit operation, a table categorizing process equipment by class (operating principle) and subclass (design characteristics) along with examples of commercially available equipment is presented.

In December 2014, the FDA issued new guidance for industry covering the manufacturing equipment addendum [29] that superseded the earlier guidance issued in January 1999 [28]. This guidance was recommended to be used in conjunction with the SUPAC guidance for industry covering immediate-release solid oral dosage forms [23] and modified-release solid oral dosage forms [26], respectively. The list of manufacturing equipment was removed in this new guidance as the tables referencing specific equipment in the earlier guidance were misinterpreted by manufacturers as equipment required by the FDA. There was a concern that such a misunderstanding could discourage the implementation of innovation and technology advancements.

Granulation is defined as the process of creating granules either by using a liquid that causes particles to bind through capillary forces or by dry compaction forces. Granulation is stated to impact one or more of the powder properties such as enhanced flow; increased compressibility; densification; alteration of physical appearance to attain more spherical, uniform, or larger particles; and/or enhanced hydrophilic surface properties.

The operating principles listed in the SUPAC manufacturing equipment addendum [29] are as follows:

1. Dry granulation
   Dry powder densification and/or agglomeration by direct physical compaction.
2. Wet high-shear granulation
   Powder densification and/or agglomeration by the incorporation of a granulation fluid into the powder with a high power per unit mass through rotating high-shear forces.
3. Wet low-shear granulation
   Powder densification and/or agglomeration by the incorporation of a granulation fluid into the powder with low power per unit mass through rotating low-shear forces.
4. Low-shear tumble granulation
   Powder densification and/or agglomeration by the incorporation of a granulation fluid into the powder with low power per unit mass through rotation of the container vessel and/or intensifier bar.
5. Extrusion granulation
   Plasticization of solids or wetted mass of solids and granulation fluid with linear shear through a sized orifice using a pressure gradient.
6. Rotary granulation
   Spheronization, agglomeration, and/or densification of a wetted or non-wetted powder or extruded material. This is accomplished by centrifugal or rotational forces from a central rotating disk, rotating walls, or both. The process may include the incorporation and/or drying of a granulation fluid.
7. Fluid-bed granulation
   Powder densification and/or agglomeration with little or no shear by direct granulation fluid

atomization and impingement on solids while suspended by a controlled gas stream, with simultaneous drying.

8. Spray-dry granulation

A pumpable granulating liquid containing solids (in solution or suspension) is atomized in a drying chamber and rapidly dried by a controlled gas stream, producing a dry powder.

9. Hot-melt granulation

An agglomeration process that utilizes a molten liquid as a binder(s) or granulation matrix in which the active pharmaceutical ingredient (API) is mixed and then cooled down followed by milling into powder. This is usually accompanied in a temperature-controlled jacketed high-shear granulating tank or using a heated nozzle that sprays the molten binder (s) onto the fluidizing bed of the API and other inactive ingredients.

10. Melt Extrusion

A process that involves melting and mixing API and an excipient (generally a polymer) using low- or high-shear kneading screws followed by cooling and then milling into granules. Thermal energy for melting is usually supplied by the electric/water heater placed on the barrel. Materials are either premixed or fed into an extruder separately. Melt extruder subclasses primarily are distinguished by the configuration of the screw – Single screw extruder or Twin-screw extruder.

The classification of granulation equipment in the SUPAC manufacturing equipment addendum [29] is as follows:

1. Dry granulator

Dry granulator subclasses are primarily distinguished by the densification force application mechanism.
- Slugging
- Roller compaction

2. Wet high-shear granulator

Wet high-shear granulator subclasses are primarily distinguished by the geometric positioning of the primary impellers; impellers can be top, bottom, or side driven.
- Vertical (top or bottom driven)
- Horizontal (side driven)

3. Wet low-shear granulator

Wet low-shear granulator subclasses are primarily distinguished by the geometry and design of the shear-inducing components; shear can be induced by rotating impeller, reciprocal kneading action, or convection screw action.
- Planetary
- Kneading
- Screw

4. Low-shear tumble granulator

Low-shear tumble granulators may differ from one another in vessel geometry and type of dispersion or intensifier bar.
- Slant cone
- Double cone
- V-blender

5. Extrusion granulator

Extrusion granulator subclasses are primarily distinguished by the orientation of extrusion surfaces and driving pressure production mechanism.
- Radial or basket

- Axial
- Ram
- Roller, gear, or pelletizer

6. Rotary granulator

   Rotary granulator subclasses are primarily distinguished by their structural architecture. They have either open-top architecture, such as a vertical centrifugal spheronizer, or closed-top architecture, such as a closed-top fluid-bed dryer.
   - Open
   - Closed

7. Fluid-bed granulator

   Although fluid-bed granulators may differ from one another in geometry, operating pressures, and other conditions, no fluid-bed granulator subclasses have been identified.

8. Spray-dry granulator

   Although spray-dry granulators may differ from one another in geometry, operating pressures, and other conditions, no spray-dry granulator subclasses have been identified.

9. Holt-melt granulator

   Although hot-melt granulator may differ from one another in primarily melting the inactive ingredient (particularly the binder or other polymeric matrices), no subclasses have been identified at this time.

The SUPAC manufacturing equipment addendum [29] contains general information on SUPAC equipment and no longer references specific manufacturing equipment from listed suppliers. When assessing manufacturing equipment changes from one class to another or from one subclass to another, manufacturers are recommended to follow a risk-based approach that includes a rationale and complies with cGMP regulations. The impact on the product quality attributes of equipment variations needs to be evaluated by reviewing process parameters when designing and developing a manufacturing process.

SUPAC guidance is to be referred to determine the filing requirements for equipment changes. In assessing the change notification, FDA considers the types of equipment changes and the availability of scientific data and risk-based rationale. Equipment within the same class or subclass would be considered to have the same design and operating principle under SUPAC-IR and SUPAC-MR. As an example, a change from one type of wet high-shear granulator (e.g., vertical type from manufacturer *A*) to another type of wet high-shear granulator (e.g., vertical type from manufacturer *B*) generally would not represent a change in operating principle and would, therefore, be considered to be the same under either SUAPC-IR or SUPAC-MR.

A change from equipment in one class to equipment in a different class would usually be considered a change in design and operating principle. Thus, a change from a wet high-shear granulator to a fluid-bed granulator demonstrates a change in the operating principle from powder densification by wet agglomeration using high shear to powder densification with little or no shear. Such a change would be considered to be different under either SUPAC-IR or SUPAC-MR.

The FDA advises change applicants to carefully consider and evaluate on case-by-case basis changes in equipment that are in the same class but different subclasses. For example, a change from a horizontal (side-driven) wet high-shear granulator to a vertical (top- or bottom-driven) wet high-shear granulator represents a change within a class and between subclasses. This change would not require a preapproval supplement provided the manufacturing process with the new equipment is validated. The data and rationale used to make this determination can be reviewed by the FDA at its discretion. In the event, a single piece of equipment is capable of performing multiple discrete unit operations, for example, mixing, granulation, drying, etc., and the unit was evaluated solely for its ability to granulate.

27.9 INTERNATIONAL CHANGE NOTIFICATION

The manufacturing process and equipment change notification outside the United States varies from region to region. A brief description of the manufacturing process is required as part of the filing requirements for marketing a drug product. Some countries require master batch records to be filed, but most others do not require much detail. In addition, a site master file that provides information on the production and control of the manufacturing operations including major process equipment at the site is sometimes required [30].

Regulatory agencies in countries that form the European Community (EC) have adopted a common approach to the procedures for variations to the terms of a marketing authorization as defined by EC regulations (EC) No 1234/2008 [31]. Variations can be by notifications that are categorized as minor and major variations that fulfill the conditions outlined in the regulations. A minor variation of Type IA means a variation which has only a minimal impact, or no impact at all, on the quality, safety, or efficacy of the medicinal product concerned. Examples of Type IA variations are deletion of a manufacturing site, change of specification to comply with updated pharmacopeia monograph, voluntary tightening of specifications, etc. Extension of a marketing authorization or "extension" means a variation which is listed in Annex I of the EC regulation and fulfills the conditions laid down therein [31]. An example of extension is change or addition of a new pharmaceutical form, for example, tablets to capsules.

A major variation of Type II means a variation which is not an extension and which may have a significant impact on the quality, safety, or efficacy of the medicinal product concerned. This includes variations related to substantial changes to the manufacturing process, formulation, specifications, or impurity profile of the active substance or finished medicinal product. A minor variation of type IB means a variation which is neither a minor variation of type IA nor a major variation of type II nor an extension.

In Japan, the Pharmaceutical and Food Safety Bureau of the Ministry of Health, Labor, and Welfare (MHLW) issued a guideline [32] for describing the manufacturing method in the marketing approval application form. In the manufacturing method description section, it is stated that for process parameters that serve as target values/set values, ranges intended to be addressed as minor change notification are enclosed in "square brackets" ([]) and those that are addressed in a partial change approval application are to be enclosed in "arrow brackets" (<>). Process descriptions other than target values/set values that are to be addressed in a minor change notification are to be enclosed in "inverted commas" (""), and everything else is to be addressed in a partial change approval application. Critical processes are defined to include process conditions, tests, and other related parameters that need to be controlled within predetermined control values to ensure that the product meets specifications. Examples of critical processes are blending, granulation, particle size reduction, tableting, etc.

In China, the National Medical Products Administration (NMPA) issued Article 113 of SFDA Order No. 28 [33] which states that for any supplementary application to amend the drug registration specifications, change excipients for pharmaceutical use in the drug formulation, or modify the manufacturing process that affects the drug quality, etc., the drug regulatory department of the province, autonomous region, or municipality directly under the Central Government shall provide a review opinion, report it to the State Food and Drug Administration for review and approval, and inform the applicant at the same time.

27.10 LIFE CYCLE MANAGEMENT

ICH issued in March 2020 the final version of guidance on technical and regulatory considerations for pharmaceutical product life cycle management (Q12) [17]. This guideline provides a framework for the management of postapproval CMC changes. The ICH trio of Q8, Q9, and Q10 discussed earlier cover science and risk-based approaches for use in drug development. This information is valuable in the development of the CMC content of regulatory dossiers and essentially covers the early stages of the product life cycle, that is, product development, registration, and launch. Q12, on the other hand, addresses the commercial phase of the product life cycle and complements the ICH trio. Increased product knowledge and process understanding gained during the commercial supply of a product contribute toward understanding which postapproval changes require a regulatory submission and the level of reporting for such changes. The expectation is that many CMC changes can be managed effectively under a company's Pharmaceutical Quality System with less need for extensive regulatory oversight before implementation. Continual improvement of processes will make them robust, and the regulatory burden will also be reduced due to fewer postapproval submissions to the Market Authorization Application (MAA).

27.11   VALIDATION OF GRANULATION PROCESSES

Validation is defined by the FDA as establishing documented evidence, which provides a high degree of assurance that a specific process will consistently produce a product meeting its predetermined specifications and quality attributes [34]. Process validation is required both in general and specific terms by cGMPs for finished pharmaceuticals – 21 CFR Parts 210 and 211. The WHO defines validation as a collection and evaluation of data, from the process design stage through to commercial production, which establishes scientific evidence that a process is capable of continuously delivering the finished pharmaceutical product meeting its predetermined specifications and quality attributes [35].

For a manufacturing facility, process knowledge is provided through technology transfer dossiers. Granulation is a critical process step that has a direct impact on the quality of the drug product manufactured and hence requires validation. The overall validation activity at a manufacturing facility is detailed in a document known as the validation master plan (VMP). The validation of the granulation process is described in the VMP. CPPs for granulation such as the rate and amount of granulation fluid added, impeller and chopper speed, and mixing time are identified, and in-process controls such as moisture content and granulation endpoint measurement are established during the product development phase.

27.11.1   Equipment/Utilities Qualification

The qualification of the manufacturing equipment and control instrumentation is a prerequisite to the qualification of the granulation process. Critical utilities are product contact utilities such as purified water, compressed air, gaseous nitrogen, etc., required for granulation, that are also validated to ensure that they meet the required quality specification at the point of delivery to the granulation process.

The qualification of granulation equipment is carried out sequentially beginning with design qualification (DQ), followed by installation qualification (IQ) and operational qualification (OQ), respectively (Figure 27.6). The quality of process equipment depends on the effort put into its design, and DQ provides evidence that quality is built into the design of the equipment. Quite often a design rationale instead of a DQ is prepared. This document addresses why a specific piece of equipment was chosen, highlighting its quality and safety considerations, and provides evidence of the assessment carried out to judge its suitability for the manufacturing of the drug product.

IQ provides documented evidence that the equipment is installed as designed and specified and correctly interfaced with other systems such as electrical supply and utilities. During this phase of qualification, equipment manuals/drawings, specifications, manufacturers' test records, etc., together with installation documents and "as-built" drawings, are compiled and verified. Calibration of instrumentation and maintenance checks are also established. OQ is a documented demonstration of the fact that the process equipment as installed operates well. At this stage, generally, a manufacturing process simulation is carried out using a placebo formulation instead of the actual

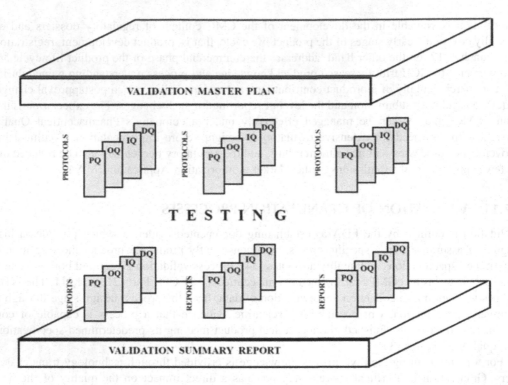

FIGURE 27.6 Documentation hierarchies for pharmaceutical process validation.

drug product recipe. For each qualification phase, a protocol detailing the activity and acceptance criteria is prepared. After the testing activity, a summary report that discusses the results and the readiness to proceed to the next phase of qualification is issued.

27.11.2 PERFORMANCE QUALIFICATION

Performance qualification (PQ) is a documented program that demonstrates that the granulation process when carried out within defined parameters will consistently perform its intended function to meet its pre-established acceptance criteria. Thus, PQ is dynamic testing that combines the equipment, utilities, and manufacturing process to produce the product under routine operational conditions. Product specifications that become the basis for the acceptance criteria at the PQ stage are established during the development of the process with the biobatch or pivotal clinical batch serving as the reference batch. Prospective validation of the granulation process is generally carried out for new products and the data included in regulatory submissions, if necessary. The norm is to manufacture at least three consecutive PQ batches; however, a process capability study can establish the actual number of batches required based on the natural variability of a process [36]. Revalidation may be required after process changes are made that significantly impact product quality or at scheduled intervals.

An FDA field inspection guide for validation of oral solid dosage forms lists granulation/mix analysis as a major area for investigation [37]. It discusses various types of mixers and granulation equipment and highlights their design features as well as problems associated with their efficiency and validation. Blending validation and content uniformity failures due to poor mixing is of main concern for most conventional mixers (Table 27.4). This guide also compares dryers and notes that the fluid-bed dryer is superior to the oven dryer as it yields a more uniform granulation with spherical particles.

TABLE 27.4

Typical Problems Associated with Mixing Equipment

Mixer Type	Design Feature	Limitations/Problems
Planetary (pony pan)	Open pan/pot horizontal blending	• Dusty operation. • Cross-contamination problem. • Poor vertical mixing. • Segregation or unmixing of components. • Difficult to validate.
Ribbon blender	Top loading Horizontal and vertical blending Discharge valve Blade clearance	• Moderately dusty operation. • Cross-contamination problem. • "Dead spot/zone" at the discharge valve. • Poor mixing at ends of the center horizontal mixing bar and shell wall. • Cleaning problems with seals/packing. • Risk of overfill leading to poor mixing.
Tumble blender	Twin shell/double cone Mild mixing action	• Mild mixing action. • Powder lumps will not break up. • Low humidity results in static charge build-up. • High humidity leads to lumping.
High shear	High-energy chopper	• Different mixing time compared with conventional mixers. • Drug substance may partially dissolve or recrystallize. • Charring due to heat generation. • Cleaning requires disassembly of a chopper.

Source: From Ref. 37.

27.11.3 COMPUTER VALIDATION

Granulation equipment is supported by computer control systems that are getting increasingly sophisticated. Most commercial equipments have programmable logic controllers (PLCs) or embedded microprocessors. International forums with representation from users and the vendors of equipment and software have been set up to address the software life cycle documentation requirements. Good Automated Manufacturing Practice (GAMP) 5 is a globally accepted guidance document developed by ISPE and the GAMP Forum to address computer validation [38]. The PIC/S Guide to Good Practices for computerized systems in regulated "GXP" environments developed by international regulatory agencies is also a useful reference document for manufacturers and other users [39].

Electronic records and electronic signatures that have cGMP implications are generally expected by regulatory agencies to be equivalent to paper records and handwritten signatures executed on paper [40]. The guidance that represents FDA's thinking on electronic records and electronic signatures was released in August 2003 [41]. The agency took a narrower interpretation of the requirements stated in 21 CFR Part 11 following feedback from the pharmaceutical industry and vendors that the regulations could stifle technological advances by restricting the use of electronic technology and increasing the cost of compliance. PIC/S also requires the regulated user to validate the system for storage of the information electronically for the required time and to ensure that the data is protected from damage or loss and can be easily retrieved in a legible form [39].

27.11.4 CURRENT GUIDANCE FOR PROCESS VALIDATION

The FDA issued in May 1987 guidance on general principles of process validation. Over the years, this has been a key reference document for manufacturers carrying out process validation [34]. Subsequently, a Compliance Policy Guide was released to explain the enforcement policy regarding the timing of the completion of certain process validation activities for drug products and active pharmaceutical ingredients subject to premarket approval [42]. Recognizing the role of emerging technologies in the area of process validation, the FDA commenced work on new guidance for process validation to replace the 1987 guidance. This revised guidance [43] was issued in January 2011 and replaced the May 1987 guidance. It conveys the FDA's current thinking on process validation and is consistent with basic principles first introduced in the 1987 guidance. It is aligned with Pharmaceutical cGMPs for the 21st Century, the use of technological advances in manufacturing, and the implementation of risk management.

The new guidance defines process validation as the collection and evaluation of data, from the process design state throughout production, which establishes scientific evidence that a process is capable of consistently delivering quality products. Process validation activities take place over the life cycle of a product and are carried out in three stages.

- Stage 1: Process Design: The commercial process is defined during this stage based on knowledge gained through development and scale-up activities.
- Stage 2: Process Qualification: During this stage, the process design is confirmed as being capable of reproducible commercial manufacturing.
- Stage 3: Continued process verification: Ongoing assurance is gained during routine production that the process remains in a state of control.

REFERENCES

1. 21 CFR Part 210. Current good manufacturing practice in manufacturing, processing, packing, or holding of drugs, general. Available at: https://www.fda.gov.
2. 21 CFR Part 211. Current good manufacturing practice for finished pharmaceuticals. Available at: https://www.fda.gov.
3. Pharmaceutical Inspection Cooperation Scheme (PIC/S). Guide to good manufacturing practice for medicinal products (PE 009–14), January 1, 2018. Available at: http://www.picscheme.org.
4. World Health Organization. WHO expert committee on specifications for pharmaceutical preparations, 48th report, Good manufacturing practices for pharmaceutical products: main principles (Annex 2), Geneva, 2014. Available at: http://www.who.int.
5. Brazil Agência Nacional de Vigilância Sanitária (ANVISA). RDC 17/2010 Drug Product GMP. Available at: https://portal.anvisa.gov.br.
6. Japan Pharmaceuticals and Medical Devices Agency (PMDA). Ministerial ordinance No. 136, 2004 on standards for quality assurance for drugs, quasi-drugs, cosmetics and medical devices. Available at: https://www.pmda.go.jp.
7. Food and Drug Administration. Guidance on pharmaceutical cGMPs for the 21st century—a risk-based approach, September 2004.
8. Food and Drug Administration. Quality systems approach to pharmaceutical current good manufacturing practice regulations, September 2006.
9. International Conference on Harmonization (ICH). Available at: http://www.ich.org.
10. International Organization for Standardization (ISO). Available at: http://www.iso.org.
11. Food and Drug Administration. Guidance for industry on PAT—a framework for innovative pharmaceutical development, manufacturing, and quality assurance, September 2004.
12. American Society for Testing and Materials (ASTM). Available at: http://www.astm.org.

13. International Conference on Harmonization. Guideline on pharmaceutical development Q8 (R2), step 4 version, August 2009.
14. International Conference on Harmonization. Guideline on quality risk management Q9, step 4 version, November 9, 2005.
15. International Conference on Harmonization. Guideline on pharmaceutical quality system Q10, step 4 version, June 4, 2008.
16. Food and Drug Administration. Guidance for industry Q8 (R2) pharmaceutical development, November 2009.
17. International Conference on Harmonization. Guideline on technical and regulatory considerations for pharmaceutical product lifecycle management Q12, Step 5 version, March 4, 2020.
18. Food and Drug Administration. Quality considerations for continuous manufacturing guidance for industry (Draft), February 2019.
19. International Conference on Harmonization. Final Concept Paper ICH Q13: continuous manufacturing of drug substances and drug products, November 14, 2018.
20. Food and Drug Administration. Data integrity and compliance with drug cGMP- Questions and answers guidance for industry, December 2018.
21. Food and Drug Administration. Guideline for the format and content of the chemistry, manufacturing, and controls section of an application, February 1987.
22. Food and Drug Administration. Guideline for drug master files, September 1989.
23. Food and Drug Administration. Guidance for industry: scale-up and post approval changes for immediate release solid oral dosage forms, November 1995.
24. Skelly JP, Van Buskirk GA, Savello DR, et al. Workshop report: scale up of immediate release oral solid dosage forms. Pharm Res 1993; 10(2):313–316.
25. 21 CFR Part 314.70. Supplements and other changes to an approved application. Available at: https://www.fda.gov.
26. Food and Drug Administration. Guidance for industry: scale-up and post approval changes for modified release solid oral dosage forms, September 1997.
27. Skelly JP, Van Buskirk GA, Arbit HM, et al. Workshop report: scale up of oral extended-release dosage forms. Pharm Res 1993; 10(12):1800–1805.
28. Food and Drug Administration. Guidance for industry: scale-up and postapproval changes for immediate release and modified release solid oral dosage forms (manufacturing equipment addendum), January 1999.
29. Food and Drug Administration. SUPAC: manufacturing equipment addendum guidance for industry, December 2014.
30. Health Sciences Authority (Singapore). Guidance notes on the preparation of a site master file, May 1999.
31. European Commission regulation (EC) No. 1234/2008, November 24, 2008.
32. Japan Pharmaceutical and Food Safety Bureau, Ministry of Health, Labour and Welfare. Guideline for description of application forms for marketing approval of drugs, etc. under the revised pharmaceutical law—PSSB/ELD Notification No. 0210001, February 10, 2005.
33. National Medical Products Administration (China). Provision for drug registration, SFDA Order No. 28, July 25, 2019.
34. Food and Drug Administration. Guideline on general principles of process validation, May 1987.
35. World Health Organization. WHO expert committee on specifications for pharmaceutical preparations, 49th report, Guidelines on good manufacturing practices: validation, Appendix 7: non-sterile process validation (Annex 3), Geneva, 2015.
36. Kieffer R, Torbeck L. Validation and process capability. Pharm Technol 1998; 22(6):66–76.
37. Food and Drug Administration. Guide to inspections of oral solid dosage forms pre/post-approval issues for development and validation, January 1994.
38. International Society of Pharmaceutical Engineering (ISPE). Good automated manufacturing practice guide (GAMP 5), February 2008. Available at: http://www.ispe.org.
39. Pharmaceutical Inspection Cooperation Scheme. Guide to good practices for computerized systems in regulated "GXP" environments (PE 011–3), September 25, 2007.
40. 21 CFR Part 11. Electronic records; electronic signatures. Available at: https://www.fda.gov.

41. Food and Drug Administration. Guidance for industry on Part 11, electronic records; electronic signatures—scope and application, August 2003.
42. Food and Drug Administration. Compliance policy guide (CPG 7132c.08) on process validation requirements for drug products and active pharmaceutical ingredients subject to pre-market approval, December 2004.
43. Food and Drug Administration. Guidance on process validation: general principles and practices, January 2011.

28 QbD and PAT in Granulation

Shivang Chaudhary

CONTENTS

28.1 INTRODUCTION

Quality by design (QbD) is a systematic approach for pharmaceutical product development first established by the quality pioneer Dr. Joseph M. Juran [1]. Dr. Juran anticipated that quality should be designed into a product and that most quality crises and problems relate to how a product was designed in the first place. Dr. Woodcock [2] defined a high-quality drug product as a medicinal product free of contamination and reliably delivering the therapeutic benefit promised in the label to the consumer, that is, patient. The U.S. Food and Drug Administration (USFDA) issued guidance documents and regulations for risk-based approaches and the adoption of Quality by Design (QbD) principles in drug product formulation development, manufacturing process optimization, scale-up process, and post-approval changes. FDA's emphasis on QbD began with the recognition that increased testing does not necessarily improve product quality. Quality cannot be *tested into the product* but must be *built into the product* by designing and planning.

In the former Quality by Testing (QbT) system, overall pharmaceutical development is mainly empirical entire developmental research often conducted through one variable at a time (OVAT). In that QbT, manufacturing processing parameters are fixed, and process validation is also done primarily based on initial full-scale batches, which focuses only on reproducibility. In that process, controls are also finalized through in-process off-line analytical tests primarily for go/no go decisions. In the QbT system, the control strategy for drug product quality control is primarily implemented based on in-process materials, and end-product testing and product specifications are the primary means of controls fixed based on batch data available at the time of registration. In that testing-based developmental system, product lifecycle management is mainly reactive, in which problems during commercial manufacturing are mainly solved through corrective action taken for a particular ingredient or processing unit operation.

The International Council for Harmonisation of Technical Requirements for Pharmaceuticals for Human Use (ICH) has advanced pharmaceutical QbD with the issuance of ICH Q8 (R2) (Pharmaceutical Development), ICH Q9 (Quality Risk Management), and ICH Q10 (Pharmaceutical Quality System) guidance [3–5]. Additionally, ICH Q1WG on Q8, Q9, and Q10 Questions and Answers; the ICH Q8/Q9/Q10 Points to Consider document; and ICH Q11 (Development and Manufacture of Drug Substance) have been issued, as having the conclusions of FDA-EMA's harmonization and parallel assessment of QbD elements of marketing applications [6–9]. These documents provide high-level guidelines concerning the scope and definition of QbD as it applies to the pharmaceutical industry. But there is confusion among industry scientists-technocrats, academic professors-students, and regulators despite recent publications for implementation of QbD. This chapter is projected to describe the objectives of pharmaceutical QbD in detail, its concept, and elements along with tools and tactics for implementation.

In QbD system, overall pharmaceutical development is based on the systematic multivariate Design of Experiments (DoE) to build a mathematical relationship between critical material attributes and process parameters to drug product Critical Quality Attributes (CQA)s for the establishment of flexible design space. In QbD, manufacturing processing parameters are adjustable within flexible design space, and statistical process control methods and Process Analytical Technology (PAT) tools are utilized for tracking and trending the process to support post-approval continuous improvement efforts as well as for controlling the process with appropriate feedforward and feedback controls. In QbD, drug product quality is ensured by a risk-based control strategy in which quality controls are shifted upstream, with the possibility of real-time release testing or reduced end-product testing and product specifications are also part of the overall quality control strategy. In this design-based developmental system, product lifecycle management is primarily based on continuous improvement of the commercial manufacturing process.

28.2   DEFINITION AND OBJECTIVES OF QUALITY BY DESIGN

Pharmaceutical QbD is a systematic approach to product development that begins with predefined objectives in the form of Quality Target Product Profile (QTPP) and emphasizes product and process understanding in the form of Critical Material Attributes (CMAs), Critical Processing Parameters (CPPs), Critical Quality Attributes (CQAs), and their controls based on sound science and quality risk management (3) to ensure the following objectives [10]:

1. To increase product development and manufacturing process efficiencies with multivariate DoE and PAT.
2. To reduce product variability and defects and to increase process performance and capability by improving product and process design, understanding, and control.
3. To achieve significant product quality and performance specifications that are based on clinical performance in vivo.
4. To ease up regulatory submission, approval, and post-approval change management from both applicant and reviewer prospective
5. To speed up root-cause analysis for any variation(s) or defect(s) observed during commercial manufacturing batches.

With QbD, these objectives can be repeatedly achieved by linking product quality to the desired clinical performance and by designing a robust formulation and process at the time of development to consistently deliver the desired quality product during commercial manufacturing. QbD uses a systematic multivariate approach to product development, so it enhances development capability and speed. Moreover, QbD transfers resources from a downstream corrective mode to an upstream proactive mode. So, it increases product development and manufacturing efficiencies.

To increase process performance and capability, and reduce product variability that frequently leads to product defects, rejections, and product recalls, robustly designed product formulation and manufacturing processes are required. Besides, an improved product and process understanding achieved through QbD can facilitate the identification and control of factors, that is, CMAs and CPPs affecting the drug product quality and performance attributes. Detailed idea through DoE-developed model will help in predicting how the product will behave with changes in each CMAs or CPPs within design space along with PAT, increased process capability, and reduced product variability during manufacturing. After regulatory approval, efforts should be continued to improve the process to reduce product variability, defects, rejections, and product recalls.

With the initiation of pharmaceutical QbD, the FDA has made significant progress in achieving the third objective, that is, performance-based quality specifications. Some examples of FDA policies include assayed potency limits for narrow therapeutic index drugs and some of the physical attributes of generic drug products, that is, tablet scoring [11] and bead sizes in capsules labeled for sprinkle [12]. FDA is also putting more development of discriminative and bio-relevant dissolution method development based on *In-Vitro In-Vivo Correlationship* (IVIVC) for modified release formulations and BCS Class II or IV immediate-release formulations [13–14].

Drug product application review and approval process will become easier and faster for reviewers, as QbD defines product and process controls based on stepwise systematic quality risk management. Moreover, design space developed through DoE/QbD will provide regulatory flexibility for post-approval change management for applicants [15–17]. Root-cause analysis for process variability or batch failure will become faster and easier at the commercial stage as the risk assessment report at the development stage is available through QbD.

28.3 PHASES AND ELEMENTS OF QUALITY BY DESIGN (QbD)

An enhanced, systematic quality by design approach to pharmaceutical product development should include the following elements as represented by step-by-step algorithm in Figure 28.1:

1. *Defining the Quality Target Product Profile (QTPP)* as it relates to quality, safety, and efficacy, considering the route of administration, dosage form, bioavailability, strength, and stability.
2. *Identification of potential Critical Quality Attributes (CQAs)* of the drug product, so that those product characteristics having an impact on product quality can be studied and controlled; then relevant prior knowledge about the drug substance, potential excipients, and process operations should be gathered to establish a knowledge space.
3. *Identification of all risk factors, that is, Critical Material Attributes (CMAs) and Critical Process Parameters (CPPs)* that can affect product CQAs thorough risk assessment with systematic identification, analysis, and evaluation for refining and prioritizing of the formulation material attributes and manufacturing process parameters based on prior knowledge, scientific rationale, and initial experimentations.
4. *Design of Experiments for* establishing the functional model relationships that link CMAs and CPPs to product CQAs through Multivariate Data Analysis for development of design space, that is, multidimensional flexible ranges of CMAs or CPPs within which all the CQAs will be met with their predefined specifications.
5. *Implementing Control Strategy for each and every CMAs, CPPs* to ensure batch-to-batch consistency in in-process and finished product CQAs during commercial manufacturing, considering expected scale-up changes.
6. *Continuous Improvement of the process with* a continuous trend analysis of CMAs, CPPs, CQAs, and update in the process to assure consistent quality throughout the product lifecycle.

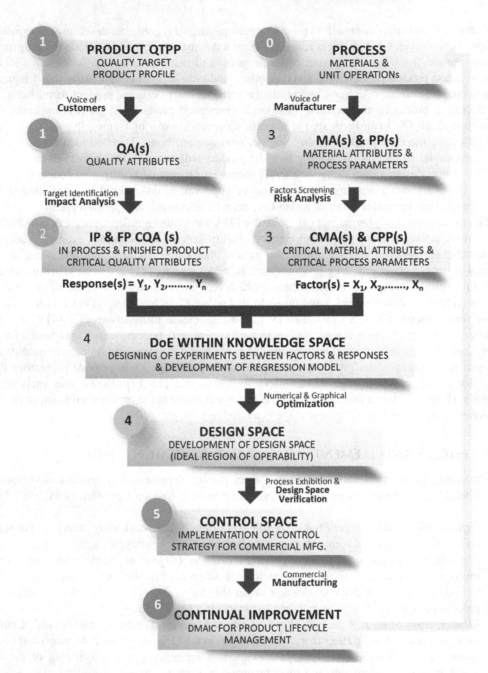

FIGURE 28.1   Quality by Design (QbD) algorithm for formulation and process development.

28.3.1   Definition of Quality Target Product Profile (QTPP)

During the implementation of the QbD system; "What we want?" should be defined from the very first as TPP, which records the voice of the customers. Because quality does not happen accidentally, it must be designed by planning. By beginning with the end in mind, the result of development is a robust formulation and manufacturing process with a control strategy that ensures the performance of the drug product. QTPP is a prospective summary of the quality characteristics of a drug product that *ideally* will be achieved to ensure the desired quality, taking into account the safety and efficacy of the drug product. The quality target product profile forms the basis of design for the development of the product. For Abbreviated New Drug Applications (ANDAs) of generic drug products [18], the QTPP will be defined early in the development based on the (i) properties of the drug substance (DS), (ii) characterization of the Reference Listed Drug (RLD) product or comparator product, and (iii) consideration of the RLD label or Patient Information Leaflet (PIL) of comparator product and intended patient population. Depending upon the characterization and review of these components, QTPP will be defined in the form of the voice of the customers:

a. Requirements of Pharmacist: Product Quality and Performance Attributes with Stability
b. Requirements of Physician: Patient Safety and Efficacy - Bioavailability
c. Requirements of Patient: Acceptance and Compliance

Table 28.1 summarizes all the elements of QTPP in the form of target customers' requirements (Specifications with Ranges, Targets) with justifications of each and every prerequisite (Therapeutic Equivalence = Pharmaceutical Equivalence + Bio-Equivalence) of the generic drug product for innovator or comparator reference drug product.

28.3.2 Determination of Critical Quality Attributes (CQAs)

Out of all the QAs of QTPP, CQAs are determined, as summarized in Table 28.2, based on the following [19]:

1. "Impact Analysis by a change in formulation &/or process variables" (i.e., what's the impact of change in any formulation or process variable on a quality attribute?) and
2. "Severity of harm to a patient" (i.e. How severe its consequences on patient health?) resulting from failure to meet that quality attribute of the drug product. CQAs are generally associated with the drug substance, excipients, intermediates (in-process materials), and drug products.

CQAs are physical, chemical, biological, or microbiological properties or characteristics that can be impacted by a change in formulation or process variables that should be within an appropriate limit, range, or distribution to ensure the desired product quality considering the severity of its harm on patient's health (3). Potential drug product CQAs derived from the quality target product profile or prior knowledge is used to guide the product and process development. The list of potential CQAs can be modified when the formulation and manu-facturing process is selected and as product knowledge and process understanding increase. Potential relevant CQAs can be identified and prioritized by an iterative process of quality risk management and experimentation that assesses the extent to which their variation can have an impact on the quality of the drug product.

28.3.3 Risk Assessment of Material Attributes (MAs) and Process Parameters (PPs)

After determination of all in-process and finished product CQAs, risks related to individual MAs or PPs will be identified, analyzed, and evaluated [4]. Risk assessment tools can be used to identify and rank parameters (e.g., process, equipment, and input materials) with the potential to have an impact on product quality, based on prior knowledge and initial experimental data [19]. During the risk assessment, first of all, the input MAs and PPs involved in different processes as listed out in Tables 28.3A–28.3E are mapped out in line with individual unit operations through process mapping for output CQAs. Process mapping maps a process at a high level and identifies feedback and feed-forward loops gaps between customers, suppliers, and the process' it jump-starts the team to begin thinking in terms of cause and effect in the same light.

TABLE 28.1
Definition of QTPP with Customer's Specifications

QTPP Elements	Target (Customers' Requirements)	Justification
Pharmaceutical Equivalence		
Dosage Form	Tablet	Pharmaceutical equivalence: *same dosage form*
Dosage Design	Immediate Release Dosage Form	Immediate release design needed to meet *label claims*
Route of Administration	Oral	Pharmaceutical equivalence: *same route of administration*
Dosage Strength	XX mg	Pharmaceutical equivalence requirement: *same strength*
Drug Product Quality	Pharmaceutical equivalence requirement: Must meet the same compendia or other applicable reference standards, that is, Appearance, Assay, Impurities, Uniformity, Friability, Dissolution, Water Content, Residual Solvent, Microbial Limits	Pharmaceutical equivalence requirement: should meet same compendia or other applicable reference standards attributes for quality
Bio-Equivalence		
Drug Product Performance – PK / PD	*In vitro* dissolution profiling should meet with that of reference product; *In vivo* bioequivalence requirement: Fasting BE study with reference Product: 90% CI of the PK parameters, AUC0-t, AUCt-24, AUC0-∞ and Cmax, should fall within BE limits of 80–125	Bioequivalence required to ensure *rapid onset and efficacy*
Patient Acceptance-Compliance		
Primary and Secondary Packaging	Container and closure system should be qualified as suitable for a drug product with desired compatibility and stability. Should protect products from external heat, moisture, oxygen, carbon dioxide, and light and microbial attack	Required to achieve the *target shelf-life* and to ensure tablet integrity during shipping
Target Shelf Life	At least 24-months of Long-Term Shelf-Life is required at room temperature. At least three months of in-use shelf life is required during routine use of the multi-dose product	*Equivalent to or better than* Reference Product Shelf-life
Patient Acceptance and Compliance	Should possess acceptable taste/flavor/odor (if any) and color most probably as similar to Reference Product. Can be easily administered similarly with Reference Product labeling	Required to achieve the desired patient acceptability to his senses with suitable compliance

After identification of all MAs and PPs; all the MAs of active(s), inactive ingredient(s), and PPs are analyzed by relative risk-based matrix analysis. As analyzed in Table 28.4, for relative risk-based matrix analysis of MAs and PPs through brainstorming sessions; all of the formulation attributes and process variables are categorized into three grades of risks concerning

TABLE 28.2

Impact Analysis for Determination of CQAs

Quality Attributes of Drug Product	1. Whether Change in Formulation or Process Variables will impact this Quality Attribute?	2. Whether failure to meet this Quality Attribute severely harm to Patients?	Is this a CQA?	Justification
Physical Attributes	Yes	No	No	Not linked to safety and efficacy, but it may impact patient acceptability concerning Reference Product.
Identification	No	Yes	Yes*	Identification is critical, but it should be effectively controlled at the drug substance release stage itself.
Assay	Yes	Yes	Yes	Assay variability may directly impact product efficacy & patient safety.
Impurities	Yes	Yes	Yes	Impurities may directly impact safety and must be controlled to limit patient exposure.
Particle Size Distribution	Yes	Yes	Yes	PSD may impact dissolution which will impact bioavailability-efficacy.
BD/TD/Flow Property	Yes	Yes	Yes	Flow property may impact uniformity which may impact safety-efficacy.
Weight/ Content Variation	Yes	Yes	Yes	Weight Variation or Content Variability may directly impact content uniformity, which will impact safety & efficacy
Tablet Hardness/ Friability	Yes	Yes	Yes	Thickness & Hardness may indirectly impact dissolution, which will impact bioavailability-efficacy.
Disintegration/ Dissolution	Yes	Yes	Yes	Failure to meet the dissolution specs may severely impact bioavailability-efficacy.
Water Content	Yes	Yes	Yes	Moisture Content may generate impurities & which may impact patient safety.
Residual Solvent	No	Yes	Yes*	Residual Solvents is critical to safety, but it should be controlled at the raw material release stage (if not added during manufacturing).
Microbial Limits	No	Yes	Yes*	Microbial Load is critical to safety, but it should be controlled at the raw material release stage itself as well as during processing.
No	This CQA will not be investigated and discussed in detail in formulation &/or process development			
Yes*	This CQA remains a target element of the release stage due to its severity of harm to the patient's health, but it will not be discussed in detail during development.			
Yes	This CQA will be investigated & discussed in detail in the formulation &/or process development			

its impact on individual CQA according to prior knowledge and preliminary research work, that is, (i) high, (ii) medium, and (iii) low, (13, 14). Independent formulation variables, that is, physicochemical properties of active(s) and excipient(s) most likely affecting CQAs of semi-finished or finished drug products are termed as *Critical Material Attributes* (CMA). Whereas, independent processing parameters most likely to affect the CQAs of an intermediate or

TABLE 28.3A
Risk Factors Identification of Dry Mixing Process

Input Material Attributes	Input Process Parameters	Quality Attributes
☐ Particle size distribution (fines/oversize)	☐ Type and geometry of mixer	☐ Blend uniformity
☐ Moisture content	☐ Mixer load level	☐ Assay (potency)
☐ Particle shape	☐ Order of addition	☐ Particle size distribution
☐ Bulk/tapped density	☐ Number of revolutions (time and speed)	☐ Bulk/tapped density
☐ Cohesive/adhesive properties	☐ Agitating bar (on/off pattern)	☐ Flow properties
☐ Electrostatic properties	☐ Discharge method	☐ Cohesive/adhesive properties
	☐ Holding time	☐ Powder segregation
	☐ Environment temperature and RH	☐ Electrostatic properties
		☐ Moisture content

TABLE 28.3B
Risk Factors Identification of Dry Granulation-Roller Compaction Process

Input Material Attributes	Input Process Parameters	Quality Attributes
☐ Particle size distribution (Fines/oversize)	☐ Type of roller compactor	☐ Ribbon appearance (edge attrition, splitting, lamination, color, etc.)
☐ Solid form/polymorph	☐ Auger (feed screw) type	☐ Ribbon tensile strength/breaking force
☐ Particle shape	☐ Auger design (Horizontal/Vertical/Angular)	☐ Ribbon thickness
☐ Cohesive/adhesive properties	☐ Deaeration (e.g., Vacuum)	☐ Ribbon density (e.g., envelop density)
☐ Electrostatic properties	☐ Auger (feed screw) speed	☐ Ribbon porosity/solid fraction
☐ Hardness/Plasticity/Elasticity	☐ Roller shape (cylindrical/interlocking)	☐ API polymorphic form and transition
☐ Bulk/Tapped density	☐ Roll surface design (smooth/knurled/serrated/pocketed)	☐ Throughput rate
☐ Viscoelasticity	☐ Roll gap width (flexible / fixed)	
☐ Brittleness	☐ Roll speed	
	☐ Roll pressure	
	☐ Roller Temperature	
	☐ Fines recycled (Yes / No, no. of cycles)	

finished drug product, as represented in Figure 28.2, required to be monitored or controlled to ensure the process produces the desired quality product are termed as *Critical Process Parameter* (CPP) (3).

Risk assessment is typically performed early in the pharmaceutical development process development and is repeated as more information becomes available and greater knowledge is obtained. The list can be refined further through experimentation to determine the significance of individual variables and potential interactions. Once the significant parameters are identified, they can be further studied (e.g., through a combination of design of experiments, mathematical models, or studies that lead to mechanistic understanding) to achieve a higher level of process understanding.

TABLE 28.3C

Risk Factors Identification of High-Shear Wet Granulation Process

Input Material Attributes	Input Process Parameters	Quality Attributes
☐ Particle size distribution (fines/ oversize)	☐ Type of granulator (high/low shear, top/bottom drive)	☐ Blend uniformity
☐ Solid form/polymorph	☐ Fill level percentage	☐ Assay (potency)
☐ Particle shape	☐ Pre-granulation mixing time	☐ Moisture content
☐ Moisture content	☐ Granulating liquid or solvent quantity	☐ Particle size and distribution
☐ Cohesive/adhesive properties	☐ Impeller speed, tip speed, configuration, location, power consumption/torque	☐ Granule size and distribution
☐ Electrostatic properties	☐ Chopper speed, configuration, location, power consumption	☐ Bulk/tapped density
☐ Hardness/Plasticity/Elasticity	☐ Spray nozzle type and location	☐ Flow property
☐ Bulk/Tapped density	☐ Method of binder excipient addition (dry/wet)	☐ Granule strength and uniformity
☐ Viscoelasticity	☐ Method of granulating liquid addition (spray or pump)	☐ Solid form/polymorph
☐ Brittleness	☐ Granulating liquid temperature	☐ Cohesive/adhesive properties
	☐ Granulating liquid addition rate and time	☐ Electrostatic properties
	☐ Post-granulation wet mixing time)	☐ Granule brittleness / elasticity
		☐ Endpoint measurement

28.3.3.1 Risk Assessment of Dry Mixing-Blending Process

In dry mixing, particles are reoriented in relation to one another when they are placed in random motion and inter-particular friction is reduced as the result of bed expansion (usually within a rotating container), also known as tumble blending to achieve the blend uniformity. During dry mixing, it is imperative to optimize the blending time to minimize the variability and thus bioavailability and subsequently the content uniformity challenges [20].

28.3.3.2 Risk Assessment of Dry Granulation-Roller Compaction Process

The dry granulation process is used to form granules without using a liquid solution because the product to be granulated may be sensitive to moisture and heat. Forming granules without moisture requires compacting and densifying the powders. Roller compactors use counter-rotating rollers to densify dry powder into sticks or sheets or ribbons. As the material flows from the hopper, a variable-speed screw forces it between the two rollers. One roller is usually fixed, while the other moves, enabling an operator or PLC to maintain the size of the gap between them and to apply the desired force. Upon discharge, the compacts pass through a built-in comminutor or they are collected and subsequently milled.

During roller compaction granulation, if roller pressure is higher than optimum or roller gap is lower than optimum or roller speed is lower than optimum, then the ribbon density may get increased affecting the dissolution and bioavailability and hence the efficacy [20]. If roller pressure is lower than optimum or roller gap is higher than optimum or roller speed is higher than optimum, it may result in a softer and friable ribbon with lower density impacting particle size distribution (PSD), bulk tapped density, flowability, uniformity, compressibility, and friability of tablets [21].

TABLE 28.3D
Risk Factors Identification of Fluid Bed Granulation Process

Input Material Attributes	Input Process Parameters	Quality Attributes
☐ Particle size distribution (fines/ oversize)	☐ Type of fluid bed	☐ Blend uniformity
☐ Solid form/polymorph	☐ Inlet air distribution plate	☐ Assay (potency)
☐ Particle shape	☐ Spray nozzle (tip size, type/quantity/ pattern/ configuration/position	☐ Moisture content
☐ Moisture content		☐ Particle size and distribution
☐ Cohesive/Adhesive properties	☐ Filter type and orifice size	☐ Granule size and distribution
☐ Electrostatic properties	☐ Fill Level percentage	☐ Bulk/Tapped density
☐ Hardness/Plasticity/Elasticity	☐ Bottom screen size and type	☐ Flow property
☐ Bulk/Tapped density	☐ Preheating temperature/time	☐ Solid form/polymorph
☐ Viscoelasticity	☐ Method of drug and binder addition (dry/wet)	☐ Cohesive/Adhesive properties
☐ Brittleness	☐ Granulating liquid temperature	☐ Electrostatic properties
	☐ Granulating liquid quantity	☐ Granule brittleness / elasticity
	☐ Granulating liquid concentration/ viscosity	☐ Granule strength and uniformity
	☐ Granulating liquid spray rate	☐ Endpoint measurement
	☐ Inlet air volume	
	☐ Inlet air temperature	
	☐ Inlet air dew point	
	☐ Atomization air pressure	
	☐ Product and filter pressure differentials	
	☐ Product temperature	
	☐ Exhaust air temperature, flow	
	☐ Filter shaking interval and duration	

During integrated milling, if mill speed and sieve size is not optimized, it will create variability in physical attributes of milled granules and impact subsequent processing.

28.3.3.3   Risk Assessment of High-Shear Wet Granulation Process

The granulating process in a High-Shear Granulator (HSG) or Rapid Mixer Granulator (RMG) incorporates liquid binder in a bowl of powder to be granulated. The main impeller and chopper in the unit agglomerate by applying high shear as the binder liquid is added and high energy imparted by the impeller densifies the granules. The chopper assists in preventing larger lumps from being formed. During wet granulation, If the pre-granulation mixing rate is not optimized, then variability in the blend or content uniformity may result in affecting the efficacy of the granulated product [22–23]. A higher spray rate or higher impellor rate will densify granules resulting in higher bulk density and longer disintegration and or dissolution. A lower rate of binder addition or lower impeller speed may result in softer granules, with a higher amount of fines affecting its subsequent processing [24–25].

   (Please refer to chapter 9 for detailed information on wet granulation using HSG/RMG.)

28.3.3.4   Risk Assessment of Fluid Bed Granulation Process

In top spray fluid bed granulation, powder densification or agglomeration occurs with little or no shear spraying of liquid binder on the fluidized powder bed in the unit while the conditioned hot air

TABLE 28.3E
Risk Factors Identification of Extrusion-Spheronization Process

Input Material Attributes	Input Process Parameters	Quality Attributes
☐ Particle size distribution (fines/ oversize)	☐ Type of extruder (Screw or basket)	Extrudate
☐ Solid form/polymorph	☐ Screw length, pitch, and diameter	☐ Density
☐ Particle shape	☐ Screw channel depth	☐ Length/Thickness/Diameter
☐ Cohesive/Adhesive properties	☐ Screw blade configuration	☐ Moisture content
☐ Electrostatic properties	☐ Number of screws (single/dual)	☐ API polymorphic form and transition
☐ Hardness/Plasticity/Elasticity	☐ Die or screen configuration (e.g., radial or axial)	☐ Content uniformity
☐ Bulk/Tapped density	☐ Die length/Diameter ratio	☐ Throughput
☐ Viscoelasticity	☐ Roll diameter (mm)	☐ Pellets after spheronization
☐ Brittleness	☐ Screen opening diameter (mm)	☐ Pellets size and distribution
	☐ Screw speed (rpm)	☐ Pellets shape factor (e.g., aspect ratio)
	☐ Feeding rate (g/min)	☐ Bulk/Tapped density
	☐ Type and scale of spheronizer	☐ Flow properties
	☐ Spheronizer load level	☐ Brittleness
	☐ Plate geometry and speed	☐ Elasticity
	☐ Plate groove design (spacing and pattern)	☐ Mechanical strength
	☐ Air flow	☐ Friability
	☐ Residence time	

concurrently drying the product. As soon as the desired size of the agglomerates is achieved, spraying is stopped and the residual liquid is evaporated. The structures created by the liquid bridges are then maintained by solid binder bonds between the primary particles.

During the granulation in fluid bed granulator, a higher spray rate in relation to lower evaporation rate will result in denser and larger granules affecting disintegration and dissolution [26]. In contrast, if the spray rate is too low and the evaporation rate relatively is too high, improper granules will be formed which will be soft, friable, and affecting further processing.

(Please refer to chapter 10 for detailed information on fluid bed granulation.)

28.3.3.5   Risk Assessment of Extrusion-Spheronization Process

Extrusion/spheronization is a process capable of producing spherical particles that have many uses in the preparation of pharmaceutical dosage forms. Extrusion-spheronization is a multi-step process typically requiring several units of operations. The wet mass is forced through the required size orifice to form extrudates, which are subsequently spheronized in a spheronizer to form round pellets, and then dried in a fluid bed dryer or the oven.

During the extrusion process, if the feeding and extrusion screw speed is increased, it will cause extrudate surface impairments, such as roughness and shark-skinning, which leads to pellets with lower quality because the extrudate will break up unevenly during the initial stages of the spheronization process, resulting in several fines and wide particle-size distribution [26]. Pellet quality is also dependent on spheronizer load, which affects the particle-size distribution,and bulk and tap density of the final pellets. The increase in the spheronizer speed and a low spheronizer load will result in wider particle size distribution with less yield of pellets, whereas it increases

TABLE 28.4

Relative Risk Matrix Analysis of Different Granulation Processes

Granulation Process	Co-sifting	Dry Mixing	Dry Granulation	High Shear Wet Granulation	Fluid Bed Granulation	Extrusion	Spheronization	Fluid Bed Drying	Milling & Sifting	Blending & Lubrication	Tablet Compression
1. Dry Mixing – Direct Compression	☑	☑							☑	☑	☑
2. Dry Granulation – Roller Compaction	☑	☑	☑						☑	☑	☑
3. High Shear Wet Granulation	☑	☑	☑	☑				☑	☑	☑	☑
4. Top Spray Fluid Bed Granulation	☑	☑			☑			☑	☑	☑	☑
5. Extrusion-Spheronization	☑	☑		☑		☑	☑	☑	☑	☑	☑

In Process or Finished Product CQAs	Co-sifting	Dry Mixing	Dry Granulation	High Shear Wet Granulation	Fluid Bed Granulation	Extrusion	Spheronization	Fluid Bed Drying	Milling & Sifting	Blending & Lubrication	Tablet Compression
Appearance (Physical Attributes)	L	L	H	H	H	M	H	L	M	H	H
Assay	L	M	M	H	H	L	L	L	L	L	L
Impurities / Related Substances	L	L	M	H	H	L	L	H	M	L	L
PSD / BD / TD / Flow Property	L	L	H	H	H	H	H	L	H	L	L
Weight/ Content Variation	M	M	M	H	H	L	L	L	H	H	M
Hardness / Friability	L	L	L	L	L	L	H	L	L	L	H
Disintegration Time / % Drug Dissolution	L	L	H	H	H	L	H	L	H	H	H
Water Content	L	L	L	H	H	L	L	H	L	L	L

L = Low Risk	Broadly acceptable risk. No further investigation is needed.
M = Medium Risk	Risk is acceptable. Further investigation may be needed to reduce the risk.
H = High Risk	Risk is unacceptable. Further investigation is needed to reduce the risk.

☑ Symbol indicates "whether that particular unit operation is involved in that particular Granulation Process or not?"

with extended spheronization time at a higher spheronizer load. If the spheronizer speed increases, then bulk and tap density increases and the size of the pellets decreases. If spheronizer load decreases, then the roundness, hardness, and friability of pellets increases significantly [27]. If

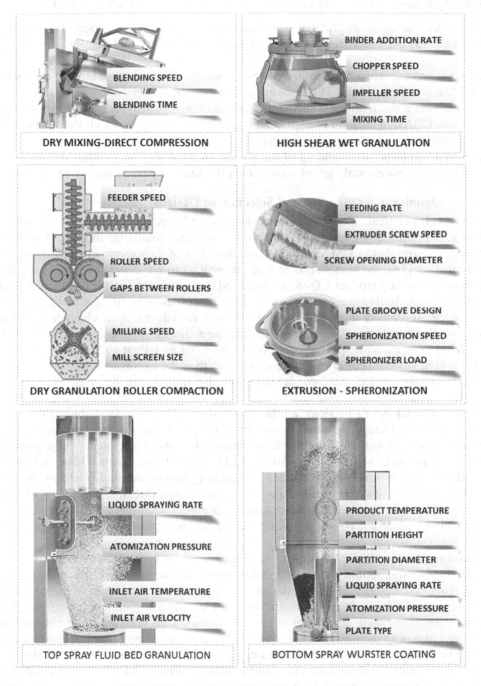

FIGURE 28.2 Critical processing parameters involved in different types of granulations.

spheronization speed is too slow, then it will produce no significant shape changes in the extrudate, and if spheronization speed is too high, then it will result in a size reduction of the extrudate particles.

(Please refer to chapter 12 for detailed information on the Extrusion/spheronization process.)

28.3.4 DESIGNING OF EXPERIMENTS (DoE) AND DEVELOPMENT OF DESIGN SPACE

After Risk Assessment of all Material Attributes and Process Parameters concerning CQAs, DoE should be carried out as a systematic series of experiments as follows [3]:

1. Experiments in which purposeful changes are made to input factors to identify causes, that is, CMAs and CPPs, for significant changes in the output responses, that is, CQAs
2. Determining the relationship between factor(s), that is, CMAs and CPPs and response(s), that is, CQAs, in the form of regression model equation, to evaluate all the potential factors simultaneously, systematically and speedily
3. With a complete understanding of the process to assist in better product development and subsequent process scale-up with pretending the finished product quality and performance

28.3.4.1 Definition of Objective and Selection of Designs

In DoE, several critical risk factors should be finalized depending upon risk assessment on the basis of preliminary experiments or prior arts. After finalizing the list of *critical independent factors*, that is, CMAs or CPPs and *objective* of the experiment, that is, screening or optimization [28], the next step is to find out which *critical dependent responses*, that is, in-process or finished product CQAs, are required to be measured and how to measure them. Identifying "quantitative" responses is one of the most important steps of a successful DoE. Response measurements should be sensitive enough to reflect minute changes in the factor levels [29]. For "qualitative" responses, one can use a *"rating"* or *"ranking"* system, that is, a scale of 1–5. For example, product quality can be rated as 1-Poor to 5-Excellent. This will require having several people rate the product and then the average rating can be used as a primary response or the standard deviation of the ratings can be used as a secondary response.

Through **brainstorming** sessions, all the factors should be grouped into categories such as – easily controllable factors and difficult to control factors. From this list, one can decide how many and which factors are required to be included in the experiment. Only controllable factors are required to be considered during the Design of Experiments. Other factors should be decided if they will be held constant, continuously monitored, or ignored as such. After finalization of the factors to be studied, ranges for each factor, that is, "level," must be decided. The range should be large enough so that one can expect to observe a difference in the response, but it should not be so large that can be fallen off the edge and couldn't get any measurable results [30].

According to the (i) Objective of the Experiment and (ii) Numbers of the Factors, *Experimental Design* should be selected. After selection of any experimental design out of all the experimental designs [31] summarized in Table 28.5, dependent responses (CQAs) should be measured for all experimental runs for a different combination of independent factors settings and their actual observed values should be measured and inserted in the respective column in the design table. Before measurement of responses, Randomization of runs can be done by mixing up of planned experimental runs in such a way that they follow no particular pattern to cancel the effects of a hidden variable, which is not included in the experiment, but which changes with time, for example, temperature and humidity, and influences the dependent response [32]. However, blocking can be also implemented as a group of trials based on common nuisance factors to reduce the noise in the experiment and improves the sensitivity to the other effects. For example, if all the experiments cannot be conducted in one day or using one batch of raw material, the experimental points can be grouped or divided in such a way that the blocked effect is eliminated before the computation of the model. Blocking is advantageous when there is a known nuisance factor that may influence the experimental result, but the effect is not of interest [33].

TABLE 28.5

Experimental Designs with Levels, Runs, and Applications with Advantages and Disadvantages

Design	Levels	No of Experimental Runs	Diagrammatic Representations	Description
Screening Designs				
Plackette Burmann Design	2 Levels: (−1, +1)	4n for Factors up to 4n-1	PB design in 12 runs for an experiment containing up to (12−1 =) 11 factors	Economical screening design for numerous factors, when only *main effects* are concerned of interest, assuming all other interactions negligible.
Fractional Factorial Design	2 Levels: (−1, +1)	L^{F-f} Where,L = No of LevelsF = No of Factorsf = No. of Fractions	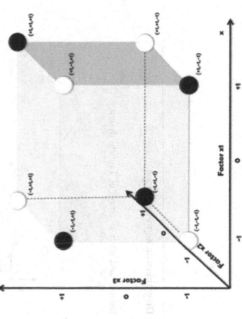 Design points are at the Alternate Corner of Cube	A better choice for screening of four or more factors in which only an adequately chosen *fraction of the full factorial combinations* are selected to be run. In general, a fraction such as ½, ¼, of full factorial, etc. of the runs has been picked up for fractional factorial. Here the ability to evaluate the effect of 3FI has to be sacrificed.

TABLE 28.5 (Continued)

Design	Levels	No of Experimental Runs	Diagrammatic Representations	Description
Taguchi Design	2 Levels: (−1, +1)		Inner 2^3 and outer 2^2 arrays of Taguchi design	Used to develop the products or processes as robust amidst natural variability. The design is also referred to as experimental design as "off-line quality control" because it is a method of ensuring good performance in the development of products or processes.

Optimization Designs

Full Factorial Design

2 Levels: (−1, +1)3 Levels: (−1, 0, +1)

L^F Where, L = No of LevelsF = No of Factorsf = No. of Fractions

Design points are at the CORNER of Square

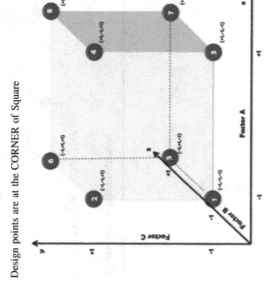

Efficient screening design for 3 or fewer factors and when only *main effects and interaction* are of interest, assuming all curvature effects negligible.

(Continued)

TABLE 28.5 (Continued)

Design	Levels	No of Experimental Runs	Diagrammatic Representations	Description
Central Composite RSM Design	3 Levels: (−1, 0, +1)5 Levels: (−α, −1, 0, +1, +α)	L^F + SP + CPWhere,L = No. of LevelsF = No. of Factorsf = No. of FractionsSP = No. of Star PointsCP = No. of Center Points	Factorial CUBE within Star SPHERE 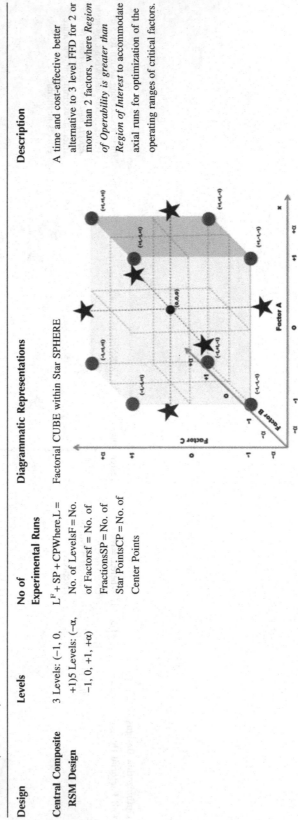	A time and cost-effective better alternative to 3 level FFD for 2 or more than 2 factors, where *Region of Operability is greater than Region of Interest* to accommodate axial runs for optimization of the operating ranges of critical factors.

Box-Behnken RSM Design

3 Levels: (−1, 0, +1)

MP + CP = 12 + 3 = 15 Where, MP = No. of Mid Points CP = No. of Center Points

Design Points are at the MIDPOINTS of edges of the process space and at the CENTER

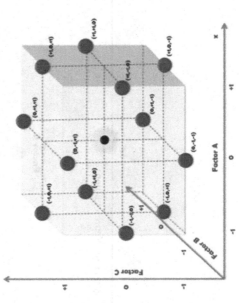

An economic alternate choice of CCD for fitting quadratic models that require three levels of each factor, where *Region of Interest and Region of Operability nearly the same*. Provides strong coefficient estimates near the center of the design space (where the presumed optimum is), but weaker at the corners of the cube (where there weren't any design points).

(*Continued*)

TABLE 28.5 (Continued)

Design	Levels	No of Experimental Runs	Diagrammatic Representations	Description
Simplex Mixture Design		$(q + m-1)! / (m!(q-1)!) = 6$ {q components, m degree} = {3,2}	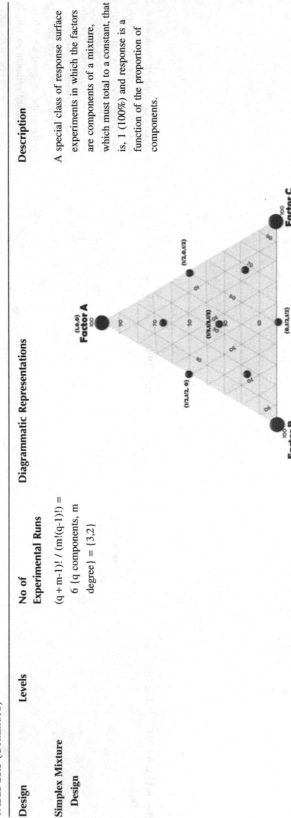	A special class of response surface experiments in which the factors are components of a mixture, which must total to a constant, that is, 1 (100%) and response is a function of the proportion of components.

Constrained Mixture Design

$$xi = Li + (1 - L) xi^*$$

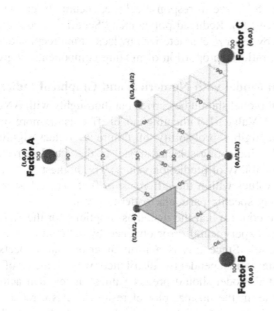

When the domain is irregular in shape, optimal designs can be used. These are the non-classic custom designs generated by the exchange algorithm using a computer. In general, such custom designs are generated based on specific optimality criteria, such as D-, A-, G-, I- and, V- optimality.

28.3.4.2   Types of Regression Models for Analysis of Responses

After running all the experiments, a mathematical equation is required that can relate factors with a response. *Model* is that mathematical relationship between factors (independent variables) and response (dependent variables), which can assist in calculations and future predictions for any design, represent different shapes of response behavior as represented in Figure 28.3.

First order *Linear* model terms modeling slopes of a straight line or flat plane, used for screening of significant factors for identification of main effects (A, B, C) and interactions (AB, AC, BC). Second order *Quadratic* model terms modeling curvatures of the eclipse, used for identification of curvature (A², B², C²) and optimization of critical factors for estimating true behavior of response surface. Third order *Cubic* model terms (ABC, A²B, A²C, AB², A^3, B^3, C^3) modeling inflected asymmetry like "S" curve in response eclipse, accurately giving the adequate view of asymmetric response surface [34]. Reduced polynomial "Scheffe" model depends on the number of components symbolized by letter q, characterized by lack of intercept and lack of square and cube terms for optimization of ratio or proportion of mixture components (ingredients).

28.3.4.3   Analysis of Regression Model with Numerical and Graphical Indicators

After selection of model, analysis of model should be carried out thoroughly with ANOVA [35] for testing of (i) significance of model (F Value »1 (indicating model effect is far more significant than a residual error) and $p < 0.05$ (negligible probability of failure to detect significant effect); (ii) insignificant lack of fit ($p > 0.1$ – indicating selected model fit the actual response behavior); (iii) adequate precision > 4 (reproducibility of prediction values); (iv) highest R^2 unadjusted value with R^2 adjusted and R^2 predicted values within the difference of 0.2; (v) well-behaved residuals (actual-predicted values) with no any specific particular pattern or trend.

Residual Analysis is required to confirm that the model assumptions for the ANOVA are met because, Residuals ($e_i = y_i - \hat{y}_i$) are experimental error obtained by subtracting the observed responses from the predicted responses. Since this is a form of error, one expects them to be (roughly) normal and (approximately) independently distributed with a mean of 0 and some constant variance [36]. Thus selected model should predict values higher than actual and lower than actual with equal probability as in the normal plot of residuals. Also, residuals should be independent of when the observation occurred as in the study as in residual versus the run plot or the size of the observation being predicted as in residual versus predicted plot. Model graphs give a clear picture of how the response will behave at different levels of factors at a time through the prediction model: (a) One factor *Main Effect plot* shows the linear effect of changing the level of a single factor, while interaction plot reveals interaction occurs with two nonparallel cross lines (b) *2D Contour plot* reveals the effect of two independent factors on one response at a time (c) *3D Response Surface plot* reveals the effect of two independent factors on one response at a time (d) *Cube plot* reveals the effect of 3 independent factors on 1 response at a time, while holding the magnitude of response and other factors as constant [37].

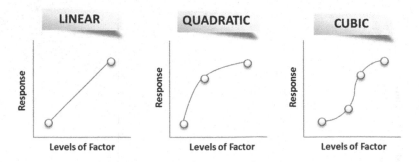

FIGURE 28.3   Different types of regression models.

28.3.4.4 Numerical and Graphical Optimization for Development of Design Space

After analysis of responses, design space – which is a multidimensional combination and interaction of input variables, that is, CMAs and CPPs, where all the specifications for the individual responses, that is, CQAs met to the predefined targets – will be developed to assure quality. Movement within the design space is not considered as a change. Movement out of the design space is considered to be a change and would initiate a regulatory post-approval change process [3].

For numerical optimization, the best combination of multiple responses is found out by a geometric mean function called the "Overall Desirability." In this method, depending upon the goals, the values of each response for a given combination of factors is first translated to a number between 0 and 1 known as individual desirability (di) and then the overall desirability (D) is calculated by taking the geometric mean of all individual desirabilities [38–40].

$$\text{Composite Desirability (D)} = (d_1^{r1} \times d_2^{r2} \times \ldots\ldots\ldots \times d_n^{rn})^{1/\Sigma ri} = \left(\prod_{i=1}^{n} d_i^{ri}\right)^{1/\Sigma ri}$$

Where, d_i = "individual desirability", n = the number of responses,

$$r_l = \text{"Importance" priorities from 1 (+) to 5 (+++++)}$$

$$D = 0 \rightarrow \text{one or more responses fall outside acceptable limits}$$

$$D = 1 \rightarrow \text{all the goals are satisfied.}$$

For Graphical Optimization, contour plots of individual responses are superimposed or overlaid on top of each other concerning their set specifications to get a sweet spot in overlay plot [41], where all the responses simultaneously meet with their set specifications as predefined in QTPP as represented in Figure 28.4.

28.3.4.5 Verification of Design Space concerning Prediction Intervals (PI) and Confidence Interval (CI)

After the development of design space, a minimum of three confirmatory runs should be conducted within design space for verification of the design space through the correlation between observed results with model-predicted results utilizing Prediction Intervals (PI) [42–43].

The 95% CI (confidence interval) is the range in which you can expect the process average to fall into 95% of the time.

$$95\% \text{ CI} = Y_{bar} \pm t-\text{value} * SE_{mean}$$

where the t value is for alpha = 0.05 and the df that correspond to the problem.

$$SE_{mean} = 1 + \sqrt{(\text{"}X^T(X^TX)^{-1}X * \text{"})}$$

The 95% PI (prediction interval) is the range in which you can expect any individual value to fall into 95% of the time.

$$95\% \text{ PI} = Y_{bar} \pm t - \text{value} * SE_{pred}$$

where the t-value is for alpha = 0.05 and the df that correspond to the problem.

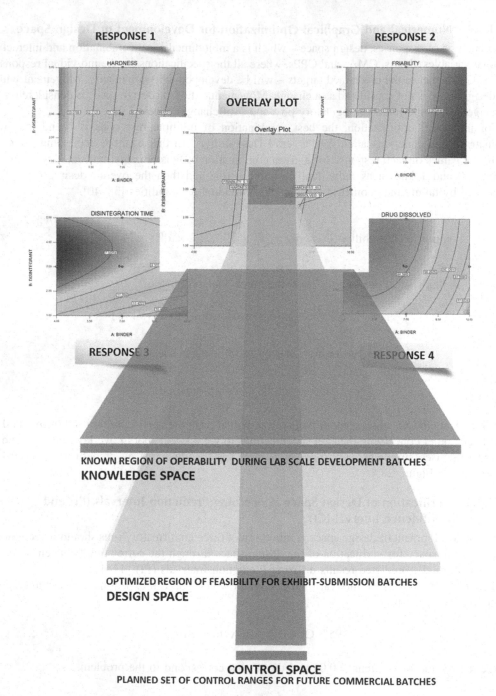

FIGURE 28.4 Graphical optimization by overlaying Contour plots of all responses on top of each other with respect to their target specifications.

$$SE_{pred} = 1 + \sqrt{(``1 + X^T(X^TX)^{-1}X_*")}$$

The prediction interval will be larger (a wider spread) than the confidence interval as more scatter is expected within individual values than in averages. A design space can be developed on any scale. The applicant should justify the relevance of a design space developed at a small or pilot scale to the proposed production-scale manufacturing process and discuss the potential risks in the scale-up operation. It's not recommended to extrapolate outside design space because there is no idea what may be out there beyond their initial set ranges.

28.3.5 Implementation of Control Strategy

Based on prior art, scientific rationale and One Factor at Time (OFAT)/DoE-based proven acceptable ranges and design space for different CMAs and CPPs, the control strategy for each and every CMAs and CPPs are proposed for future commercial manufacturing to ensure batch-to-batch consistency in product quality. A control strategy is a planned set of controls derived from the current product and process understanding during the lab-scale developmental stage, the scale-up exhibit-submission stage that ensures consistent process performance and product quality during commercial manufacturing.

The controls can include [3]:

1. Control of ***input material attributes*** (e.g., drug substance, excipients, primary packaging materials) based on an understanding of their impact on processability or product quality;
2. Controls for ***processing parameters of unit operations*** that have an impact on downstream processing or product quality (e.g., the impact of drying on degradation, the particle size distribution of the granulate on dissolution, the impact of machine speed on weight variation, and the impact of blending or mixing time on content uniformity);
3. ***In-process or real-time*** release testing instead of end-product testing (e.g., measurement and control of CQAs during processing);
4. A ***monitoring program*** (e.g., full product testing at regular intervals) for verifying multivariate prediction models;
5. ***Finished product specification(s)*** (e.g., Product name and descriptions, physical attributes, Identification, and assay values of active ingredient(s), storage conditions, etc.)

A control strategy can include different elements. For example, one element of the control strategy could rely on end-product testing, whereas another could depend on real-time release testing. The rationale for using these alternative approaches should be described in the submission.

The control strategy is built upon the outcome of extensive product and process understanding studies. These studies investigated the material attributes and process parameters that were deemed high risk to the CQAs of the drug product during the initial risk assessment. In some cases, variables considered medium risk were also investigated. All variables ranked as high risk, that is, critical in the initial risk assessment, are included in the control strategy because the conclusion of the experiments was dependant on the range(s) studied and the complex multivariate relationship between variables. Thus, the control strategy is an integrated overview of how quality is assured based on the current process and product knowledge.

For finalizing and implementation of a control strategy for each and individual CMAs or CPPs, ranges studied at lab-scale developmental stage will be reviewed with pilot plant scale-up and pivotal-scale exhibit batches to ensure batch-to-batch consistent quality and performance of a finished product during commercial manufacturing as summarized in Table 28.6. Thus, a control strategy is an integrated overview of how quality is assured for commercial batches based on the current process and product knowledge gained from the QbD-DoE-PAT system. Individual ranges of CMAs of API and excipients and CPPs of manufacturing processes are reviewed and ranges for commercial batches are proposed for the batch-to-batch consistency of respective CQAs. All the ranges are tabulated systematically with purpose, that is, *(i) ranges studied at laboratory scale, (ii) ranges studied during exhibit batches, and (iii) ranges proposed for commercial batches* [13–14].

TABLE 28.6
Control Strategies for CPPs involved in Unit Operations of Granulation Processes

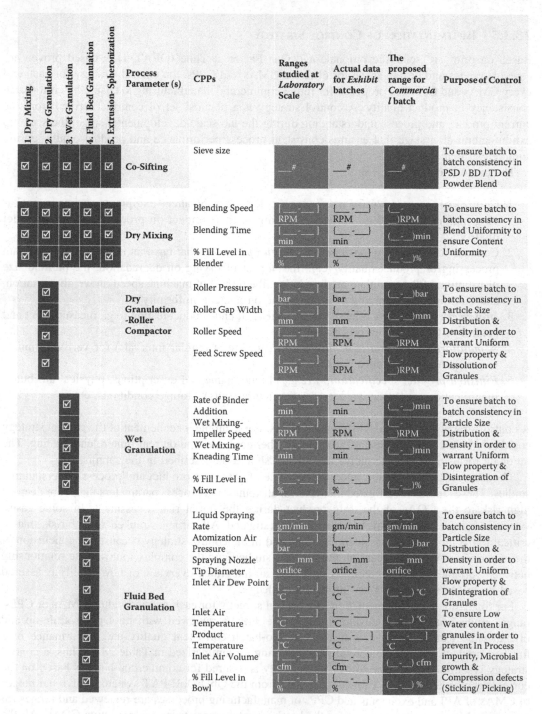

1. Dry Mixing	2. Dry Granulation	3. Wet Granulation	4. Fluid Bed Granulation	5. Extrusion- Spheronization	Process Parameter (s)	CPPs	Ranges studied at *Laboratory* Scale	Actual data for *Exhibit* batches	The proposed range for *Commercial* batch	Purpose of Control
☑	☑	☑	☑	☑	**Co-Sifting**	Sieve size	_#	_#	_#	To ensure batch to batch consistency in PSD / BD / TD of Powder Blend
☑	☑	☑	☑	☑	**Dry Mixing**	Blending Speed	[_-_] RPM	{_-_} RPM	(_-_)RPM	To ensure batch to batch consistency in Blend Uniformity to ensure Content Uniformity
☑	☑	☑	☑	☑		Blending Time	[_-_] min	{_-_} min	(_-_)min	
☑	☑	☑	☑	☑		% Fill Level in Blender	[_-_] %	{_-_} %	(_-_)%	
	☑				**Dry Granulation -Roller Compactor**	Roller Pressure	[_-_] bar	{_-_} bar	(_-_)bar	To ensure batch to batch consistency in Particle Size Distribution & Density in order to warrant Uniform Flow property & Dissolution of Granules
	☑					Roller Gap Width	[_-_] mm	{_-_} mm	(_-_)mm	
	☑					Roller Speed	[_-_] RPM	{_-_} RPM	(_-_)RPM	
	☑					Feed Screw Speed	[_-_] RPM	{_-_} RPM	(_-_)RPM	
		☑			**Wet Granulation**	Rate of Binder Addition	[_-_] min	{_-_} min	(_-_)min	To ensure batch to batch consistency in Particle Size Distribution & Density in order to warrant Uniform Flow property & Disintegration of Granules
		☑				Wet Mixing- Impeller Speed	[_-_] RPM	{_-_} RPM	(_-_)RPM	
		☑				Wet Mixing- Kneading Time	[_-_] min	{_-_} min	(_-_)min	
		☑				% Fill Level in Mixer	[_-_] %	{_-_} %	(_-_)%	
			☑		**Fluid Bed Granulation**	Liquid Spraying Rate	[_-_] gm/min	{_-_} gm/min	(_-_) gm/min	To ensure batch to batch consistency in Particle Size Distribution & Density in order to warrant Uniform Flow property & Disintegration of Granules
			☑			Atomization Air Pressure	[_-_] bar	{_-_} bar	(_-_) bar	
			☑			Spraying Nozzle Tip Diameter	_ mm orifice	_ mm orifice	_ mm orifice	
			☑			Inlet Air Dew Point	[_-_] °C	{_-_} °C	(_-_) °C	
			☑			Inlet Air Temperature	[_-_] °C	{_-_} °C	(_-_) °C	To ensure Low Water content in granules in order to prevent In Process impurity, Microbial growth & Compression defects (Sticking/ Picking)
			☑			Product Temperature	[_-_] °C	[_-_] °C	[_-_] °C	
			☑			Inlet Air Volume	[_-_] cfm	{_-_} cfm	(_-_) cfm	
			☑			% Fill Level in Bowl	[_-_] %	{_-_} %	(_-_) %	

(Continued)

TABLE 28.6 (Continued)

					Unit Operation	Parameter				Justification
		☑		☑		Type of Extruder	Screw	Screw	Screw	
		☑		☑		Feeding Rate (g/min)	[__-__] gm/min	{__-__} gm/min	(__-__) gm/min	
		☑		☑	**Extrusion**	Screw Speed (rpm)	[__-__] RPM	{__-__} RPM	(__-)RPM	To ensure batch to batch consistency in the plasticity of Extrudates to control the losses & to ensure batch to batch consistency in Particle Size Distribution, Bulk Density & True Density to warrant Uniform Flow property, Hardness, Friability, Disintegration & Dissolution of Sphere- Granules
		☑		☑		Screen Opening Diameter (mm)	[__-__] mm	{__-__} mm	(__-)mm	
		☑		☑		Die or Screen Configuration	Radial	Radial	Radial	
		☑		☑		Plate Groove Design (pattern)	Radial	Radial	Radial	
		☑		☑	**Spheronization**	Spheronizer Plate Geometry	grooves running radially from the center of the disc	grooves running radially from the center of the disc	grooves running radially from the center of the disc	
		☑		☑		Spheronizer Plate Speed	[__-__] RPM	{__-__} RPM	(__-)RPM	
		☑				Residence Time	[__-__] min	{__-__} min	(__-) min	
		☑		☑		Spheronizer %Fill Level	[__-__] %	{__-__} %	(__-) %	
	☑	☑	☑			Inlet Air Temperature for Drying	[__-__] °C	{__-__} °C	(__-) °C	To ensure batch to batch consistency in Low Water content in granules to prevent In Process impurity, Microbial growth & Compression defects (Sticking/ Picking)
	☑	☑	☑		**Drying**	Inlet Air Volume for Drying	[__-__] cfm	{__-__} cfm	(__-)cfm	
	☑	☑	☑			%Fill Level in Bowl for Drying	[__-__] %	{__-__} %	(__-) %	
	☑	☑	☑	☑	**Sizing**	Mill Speed for Sizing	[__-__] RPM	{__-__} RPM	(__-__) RPM	To ensure consistency in PSD, BD, TD of granules
	☑	☑	☑	☑		Screen Size for Sizing	[__-__] mm	{__-__} mm	(__-_) mm	
☑	☑	☑	☑	☑		Blending Speed	[__-__] RPM	{__-__} RPM	(__-_) RPM	To ensure batch to batch consistency in Blend Uniformity & Dissolution
☑	☑	☑	☑	☑	**Lubrication**	Blending Time	[__-__] min	{__-__} min	(__-_) min	
☑	☑	☑	☑	☑		%Fill Level in Blender	[__-__] %	{__-__} %	(__-_) %	
☑	☑	☑	☑	☑		Compression-Turret Speed	[__-__] RPM	{__-__} RPM	(__-_) RPM	To ensure batch to batch consistency in Hardness, Weight & Disintegration to ensure Minimum %Friability Loss, Maximum CU & Desired Dissolution without any Compression defects (Capping/ Lamination)
☑	☑	☑	☑	☑		Compression- Feed Frame Paddle Speed	[__-__] RPM	{__-__} RPM	(__-_) RPM	
☑	☑	☑	☑	☑	**Compression**	Compressed Tablet Thickness	[__-__] mm	{__-__} mm	(__-_) mm	
☑	☑	☑	☑	☑		Pre Compression Force	[__-__] kN	{__-__} kN	(__-_) kN	
☑	☑	☑	☑	☑		Main Compression Force	[__-__] kN	{__-__} kN	(__-_) kN	
☑	☑	☑	☑	☑		%Fill Level in Hopper	[__-__] %	{__-__} %	(__-_) %	
☑	☑	☑	☑	☑	**Environmental Conditions**	Environmental Temperature	[__-__] °C	{__-__} °C	(__-_) °C	To ensure batch to batch consistency in Physical & Chemical Stability
☑	☑	☑	☑	☑		Environmental Relative Humidity (%RH)	[__-__] %RH	{__-__} %RH	(__-_) %RH	

☑ The symbol indicates "whether that particular unit operation & associated processing parameters are required to be included in Control Strategy for that particular Granulation Processor not?"

The control strategy may be further refined based on additional experience gained during the commercial lifecycle of the product. However, any post-approval changes should be reported to the agency per CFR 314.70 and should follow steps as outlined by guidance used for scale-up and post-approval changes.

Understanding sources of variability and their impact on downstream processes or processing, in-process materials, and drug product quality can provide an opportunity to shift controls upstream and minimize the need for end-product testing. Product and process understanding, in combination with quality risk management [4], will support the control of the process such that the variability (e.g., of raw materials) can be compensated for in an adaptable manner to deliver consistent product quality. This process understanding can enable an alternative manufacturing paradigm where the variability of input materials could be less tightly constrained. Instead, it can be possible to design an adaptive process step (a step responsive to the input materials) with appropriate process control to ensure consistent product quality.

Enhanced understanding of product performance can justify the use of alternative approaches to determine that the material is meeting its quality attributes. The use of such alternatives could support real-time release testing. For example, disintegration could serve as a surrogate for dissolution for fast-disintegrating solid forms with highly soluble drug substances. Unit dose uniformity performed in-process (e.g., using weight variation coupled with near-infrared [NIR] assay) can enable real-time release testing and provide an increased level of quality assurance compared to the traditional end-product testing using compendia content uniformity standards [44]. Real-time release testing can replace end-product testing but does not replace the review and quality control steps called for under GMP to release the batch.

28.3.6 CONTINUOUS IMPROVEMENT AND PROCESS CAPABILITY

Throughout the product lifecycle, companies should evaluate innovative approaches to improve product quality, through the improvement of the process continuously. Process performance can be monitored to ensure that it is working as anticipated to deliver product quality attributes as predicted by the design space. This monitoring could include a trend analysis of the manufacturing process as additional experience is gained during routine commercial manufacturing. For certain design spaces using mathematical models, periodic maintenance could be useful to ensure the model's performance. Model maintenance is an example of an activity that can be managed within a company's internal quality system, provided the design space is unchanged. Expansion, reduction, or redefinition of the design space could be desired upon gaining additional process knowledge.

Upon approval, the manufacturing process will be validated using the lifecycle approach that employs risk-based decision-making throughout the drug product lifecycle as defined in the FDA process validation guidance. *Process Validation* is defined as the collection and evaluation of data, from the process design stage through commercial production, which establishes scientific evidence that a process is capable of consistently delivering a quality product. Process validation involves a series of activities taking place over the lifecycle of the product and process. This guidance describes process validation activities in three stages [45].

- **Stage 1 – Process Design:** The commercial manufacturing process is defined during this stage based on knowledge gained through development and scale-up activities. The QbD approach taken during pharmaceutical development facilitated product and process understanding relevant to stage 1 (Process Design) of process validation.
- **Stage 2 – Process Qualification:** During this stage, the process design is evaluated to determine if the process is capable of reproducible commercial manufacturing. The manufacturing facility will be designed according to cGMP regulations on building and facilities. Activities will be performed to demonstrate that utilities and equipment are suitable for their intended use and perform properly. The protocol for process performance qualification (with

Sampling points and Acceptance Criteria) will be written, reviewed, approved, and then executed to demonstrate that the commercial manufacturing process performs as expected.

- **Stage 3 – Continued Process Verification:** Ongoing assurance is gained during routine production that the *process remains in a state of control* (the validated state) during commercial manufacture by *continual trend analysis in control charts*. Throughout the product lifecycle, the manufacturing process stability, *process performance, and process capability* will be continuously measured, monitored, and evaluated to ensure that it is working as anticipated to deliver the product with desired quality attributes. If any unexpected process variability is detected, appropriate actions will be taken to correct, anticipate, and prevent future problems so that the process remains in control. The additional knowledge gained during routine manufacturing will be utilized for adjustment of process parameters as part of the continual improvement of the drug product.

The control chart is a graph used to study how a process changes over time. Data are plotted in time order. During trend analysis of CMAs or CPPs concerning CQAs, process behavior over time was observed using control charts. If all the points fall within the control limits and if they are randomly distributed on both sides of the central line, then the process is said to be *under control* [46]. This indicates the presence of only common chance causes of variation. *Variation due to common chance* causes is due to many minor noise factors that behave randomly. This type of variation is permissible and indeed inevitable in manufacturing. When the variation present in a production process is confined to chance causes only, the process is said to be in a state of statistical control. Such common variation can be the result of several factors such as inappropriate procedures/ SOP, poor design and poor maintenance of machines, poor working conditions substandard raw materials, measurement error, vibration in industrial processes, ambient temperature/ humidity, insufficient training, normal wear and tear, variability in settings, and computer response time. If one or more points fall outside the control limits, or there are longer runs (falling of consecutive points on the same side), the process is said to be *out of control* with respect to average. This indicates the presence of assignable special causes of variation. *Variation due to special assignable causes* may be attributed to some special non-random causes. This type of variation is serious and it cannot be overlooked. When the variation present in a production process is due to assignable causes, the process is said to be *out of control*. These causes should be detected and removed and the process should be brought under control. Such special variation can be the result of several factors such as absent operator, poor adjustment of equipment, machine malfunction, a poor batch of raw material, operator falls asleep, faulty controllers, fall of ground, computer crash, or power surges.

Before the commencement of regular commercial batches, "Whether Commercial Process will be Capable and Acceptable to perform Consistently and Closely within Process Specification Limits or not?" is required to be evaluated. Process capability measures the inherent variability of a stable process that is in a state of statistical control with the established acceptance criteria. Process capability terms Cp and Cpk are used once the process is already mature and stable enough (in a state of statistical control) to predict its capability and acceptability for future commercial batches [47]. Table 28.7 covers the definition, calculation formula, and application of Cp and Cpk.

In a non-QbD approach, common cause variation is more likely to be discovered during commercial production and may interrupt commercial production and it will require a root-cause analysis. In a QbD development process, the product and process understanding gained during pharmaceutical development should result in early identification and mitigation of potential sources of common cause variation via the control strategy. The manufacturing process will move toward a state of statistical control, once the manufacturer continues to improve the process capability by either reducing or removing some of the random causes present and/or by adjusting the process mean toward the preferred target value, so the quality of the product improves, benefiting the patient.

TABLE 28.7
Cp and Cpk: Process Capability Indices for Continuous Improvement

Cp (Process Spreads)

Cp: is an indication that *predicts* either any mature process is capable to meet within process specification limits (Customer Tolerance) in the future or not? Assuming the process is already under statistical control (=stable)

Cp is used, when a mature process is under statistical control, to predict its *capability* concerning process variation.

Cpk (Process Centering)

Cpk is an index, which *predicts* how close any mature process mean to nearest of process specification limits (Customer's Target) in future. Assuming the process is already under statistical control (=stable)

Cpk is used, when a mature process is under statistical control, to predict its *acceptability* concerning Process variation and centralization.

Use Cp and Cpk once the process is *already mature and stable enough* (in a state of statistical control)

$Cp = (USL - LSL) / 6\sigma$

Where,

USL = Upper Specification Limit

LSL = Lower Specification Limit

USL-LSL = Specification Spread = Voice of the Customer/ Client

σ = Process Standard deviation

= $\bar{R}$/d2 or $\bar{s}$ / C4

= Process Spread = Voice of the Process

$Cpk = Min (Cpu, Cpl)$

Where,

Cpu = (USL – Process Population Mean μ) / (3* Process Standard Deviation σ)

Cpl = (Process Population Mean μ– LSL)/ (3*Process Standard Deviation σ)

Cp and Cpk are used for computing the index for the subgrouping of your data into a group *within* different shifts, machines, operators, etc.

Continuous improvement is a set of activities to enhance its ability to meet requirements. Continual improvements typically have five phases (*DMAIC*) as follows [48]:

1. ***Define*** the problem and the project goals, specifically.
2. ***Measure*** key aspects of the current process and collect relevant data.
3. ***Analyze*** the data to investigate and verify cause-and-effect relationships. Determine what the relationships are, and attempt to ensure that all factors have been considered. Seek out the root cause of the defect or variability if any.
4. ***Improve or*** optimize the current process based upon data analysis using techniques such as Design of Experiments to create a new future state process. Set up pilot runs to establish process capability.
5. ***Control*** the future state process to ensure that any deviations from the target are corrected before they result in defects. Implement control systems such as statistical process control, production boards, visual workplaces, and continuously monitor the process.

Process capability can be used to measure process improvement through continuous improvement efforts that focus on removing sources of inherent variability from the process operation conditions and raw material quality. Ongoing monitoring of process data for Cp/Cpk will also identify when any special variations occur that need to be identified and corrective and preventive actions implemented. Also, continuous improvement can apply to already-approved legacy products, which have a large amount of historical manufacturing data. Using multivariate data analysis could uncover major disturbances in the form of variability in raw materials and process parameters. Continuous improvement could be achieved by reducing and controlling this variability. Design space facilitates continuous process improvement since applicants will have regulatory flexibility to move within the design space.

28.4 PAT DEFINITION AND GOALS

PAT is a system for designing, analyzing, and controlling manufacturing through timely measurements (i.e., during processing) of critical quality and performance attributes of raw and in-process materials and processes to ensure final product quality [49]. Thus through PAT, On-line/In-line/At-line Analyzing system for the individual in process or finished product CQAs can be developed with feedback or feed-forward controlling system for relevant CMAs or CPPs at the individual unit operation of the manufacturing process.

A desired goal of the PAT framework is to design and develop well-understood processes that will consistently ensure a predefined quality at the end of the manufacturing process. Such procedures would be consistent with the basic tenet of quality by design and could reduce risks to quality and regulatory concerns while improving efficiency. Through the implementation of PAT system along with QbD, gains in quality, safety and efficiency will vary depending on the process and the product, and are likely to come from:

- reducing production cycle times by using on-, in-, or at-line measurements and establishing real-time controls;
- facilitating real-time release (parametric release) ability to ensure the in-process or final product quality based on in-process measurements;
- increasing process automation, which can improve operator safety and reduce human errors;
- improving energy and material use and increasing capacity;
- reducing or prevent product rejections, scrap, and re-processing; and
- facilitating continuous processing with the use of a dedicated series of small-scale equipment to eliminate certain scale-up issues and to improve efficiency and manage variability.

28.5 PAT PHASES AND TOOLS

A process is generally considered well understood when

1. all critical sources of variability are identified and explained;
2. variability is managed by the process; and
3. product quality attributes can be accurately and reliably predicted over the design space established for materials used, process parameters, manufacturing, environmental, and other conditions. The ability to predict reflects a high degree of process understanding.

Even though retrospective process capability data (Pp and Ppk) are indicative of a state of control, these alone may be insufficient to estimate or communicate process understanding. A focus on process understanding can reduce the burden for validating systems by providing more options for justifying and qualifying systems intended to monitor and control material attributes and processing parameters.

The main difference between Pp and Cp on one side and Ppk and Cpk on the other side is whether we use a complete set of data for calculation (Pp and Ppk) where we calculate the real performance of the system, or we use sample (pre-production, batch, and logical subgroups) where we calculate capability of the process. In the equation for Pp and Ppk, we use standard deviation based on studied data (whole population), and in the equation, for calculating Cp and Cpk, we use sample deviation or deviation mean within rational subgroups.

The biggest difference between Cp and Pp is how the standard deviation is determined. In Pp, we use sampling and have to calculate an estimated standard deviation of the sample. In Cp, we assume a stable process and are likely have enough data to calculate a true standard deviation.

Even though retrospective process capability data (Pp and Ppk) are indicative of a state of control, these alone may be insufficient to estimate or communicate process understanding. A focus on process understanding can reduce the burden for validating systems by providing more options for justifying and qualifying systems intended to monitor and control material attributes and processing parameters.

When process knowledge is not available during proposing a new process analyzer, the test-to-test comparison between an on-line or in-line process analyzer and a conventional analytical test method on collected samples may be the only available validation option. Transfer of laboratory methods to on-, in-, or at-line methods may not necessarily be PAT. Existing regulatory guidance and compendia approach to analytical method validation should be considered. Structured product and process development on a small-scale using experimental design and on- or in-line process analyzers to collect data in real-time can provide increased insight and understanding for process development, optimization, scale-up, technology transfer, and control. Moreover, continuous learning over the life cycle of a product is important when material attributes with respect to different suppliers and environmental processing parameters change over time.

Formulation design strategies are not generalized and it's almost based on the experience of an individual formulator, and the quality of these formulations can be evaluated only by testing in-process and finished drug product samples. Currently, these tests are performed off-line after preparing collected samples for analysis. Different tests, each for a particular quality attribute, are needed because such tests only address one attribute of the active ingredient following sample preparation. During sample preparation, other valuable information of the formulation matrix is often lost. Several new technologies are now available that can acquire information on multiple attributes with minimal or no sample preparation. These technologies provide an opportunity to assess multiple attributes, often non-destructively.

At present, most pharmaceutical processes are based on time-defined endpoints (e.g., blending for 15 minutes). Yet, in some cases, these time-defined endpoints do not consider the effects of physical differences in raw materials. Processing difficulties can arise that result in the failure of a finished product to meet specifications, even if certain raw materials conform to established pharmacopoeial specifications, which generally address only chemical identity and purity. Appropriate use of PAT tools and principles can provide relevant information relating to physical, chemical, and biological attributes of in-process and finished drug products. The process understanding gained from this information will enable process control and optimization, address the limitation of the real-time defined endpoints, and improve process efficiency.

There are many tools available that enable process understanding for scientific, risk-managed pharmaceutical development, manufacture, and quality assurance. In the PAT framework, these tools can be categorized according to the phases as represented in Figure 28.5, as follows:

1. **Designing Phase:** Multivariate tools for design, data acquisition, and analysis
2. **Analyzing Phase**: Process analyzers
3. **Controlling Phase:** Process control tools

An appropriate combination of some, or all, of these tools may apply to a single-unit operation, or an entire manufacturing process and it's quality assurance.

28.5.1 DESIGNING PHASE WITH MULTIVARIATE TOOLS FOR DESIGN, DATA ACQUISITION, AND ANALYSIS

Pharmaceutical products and processes are complex multi-factorial systems concerning the physical, chemical, or biological perspective of critical quality attributes. The knowledge base acquired in these development programs can help to support and justify flexible regulatory pathways for innovation in manufacturing and post-approval changes. A knowledge-base can be of most advantageous when it consists of scientific understanding of the relevant multi-factorial relationship between formulation attributes, process parameters, and quality attributes. This multi-factorial relationship can be achieved through the use of multivariate mathematical approaches, such as the

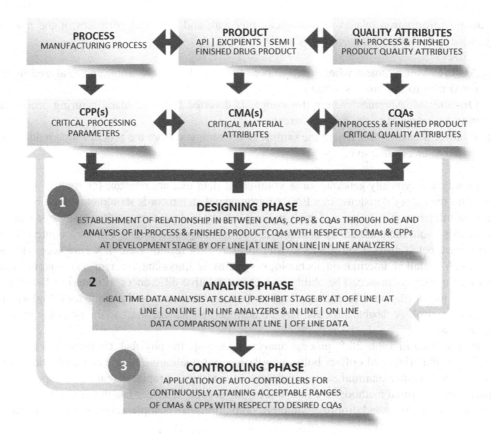

FIGURE 28.5   Phases for development of Process Analytical Technology (PAT).

statistical design of experiments, response surface methodologies, process simulation, and pattern recognition tools, in combination with knowledge management systems.

The applicability and reliability of knowledge in the form of model, that is, mathematical relationships between CMAs, CPPs and CQAs, can be assessed by statistical evaluation of model predictions. Information from such structured experiments supports the development of a knowledge system for a particular product and its processes. This information, along with information from other development projects, can then become part of an overall institutional knowledge base. As this institutional knowledge base grows then it will cover a large range of variables and different scenarios and data density, which can be extracted to determine the useful patterns for future development projects. These experimental databases can also support the development of process simulation models, which can contribute to continuous learning and help to reduce overall development time. When used appropriately, these tools enable the identification and evaluation of product and process variables that may be critical to product quality and performance. These tools may also identify potential failure modes and mechanisms and quantify their effects on product quality.

28.5.2   ANALYSIS PHASE WITH PROCESS ANALYZERS

Process analysis tools have been advanced and evolved from those univariate process measurements, such as pH, temperature, and pressure, to those that measure multivariate biological, chemical, and physical attributes. Some process analyzers provide non-destructive measurements that contain information related to biological, physical, and chemical attributes of the materials being processed. These measurements can be

i. **At-line:** Measurement where the sample is removed, isolated from, and analyzed in close proximity to the process stream.
ii. **On-line:** Measurement where the sample is diverted from the manufacturing process and may be returned to the process stream.
iii. **In-line:** Measurement where the sample is not removed from the process stream and can be invasive or noninvasive.

Process analyzers typically generate large volumes of data that are relevant for routine quality assurance and regulatory decisions. In a PAT environment, batch records should include scientific and procedural information indicative of high process quality and product conformance. For example, batch records could include a series of charts depicting acceptance ranges, confidence intervals, and inter-and intra-batch distribution plots showing measurement results. Ease of secure access to these data through installed information technology systems is important for real-time manufacturing control and quality assurance. The ability to measure relative differences in materials before (e.g., within a lot, lot-to-lot, and different suppliers) and during processing will provide useful information for process control. A flexible process may be designed to manage the variability of the materials being processed.

As summarized in Table 28.8, process analyzers measure the physical, chemical and biological properties of materials and collect both quantitative and qualitative data. Data collection can be nondestructive, require minimal sample preparation, and have a rapid or real-time response when compared to traditional methods. On-line and in-line process analyzer has the greatest potential to reduce operating costs and improve quality; both minimize sample requirements and sample

TABLE 28.8

PAT Tools used in Analyzing Phase for Drug Products Manufacturing

Unit Operations	In- Process, or Finished Product CQAs	NIR	Raman	FT-IR	FBRM
API & Excipients Release	Particle Size Distribution				☑
	The purity of API & Excipients	☑	☑	☑	
	Particle Polymorphism	☑	☑	☑	
Granulation	Particle Size Distribution				☑
	Particle Polymorphism	☑	☑	☑	
	Moisture Determination	☑		☑	
Drying	Particle Size Distribution				☑
	Impurities / Related Substances	☑		☑	
Milling	Particle Size Distribution				☑
	Impurities / Related Substances	☑		☑	
Blending	Blend Uniformity	☑		☑	
Compression	Content Uniformity	☑		☑	
Coating	Color Shade Variation		☑		
Packaging	Identification	☑	☑	☑	

☑ Symbol indicates "whether that particular PAT analyzer is useful for that CQA or not?"

handling compared to their at-line and off-line counterparts. Near-Infrared (NIR) and Fourier Transform Infrared (FT-IR) analyzers can be used for in-line/on-line analysis of assay, related substances, blend uniformity, content uniformity, and moisture content of semi-finished or finished products [50–51]. Focused Beam Reflectance Measurement (FBRM) analyzer is used for in-line or on-line for particle size distribution during different stages of the granulation process [52]. Raman spectroscopy analyzer can be used in-line or on-line for coating integrity, coating uniformity, thickness, color shade variation, and packaging material identification [53] as well as characterizing fluid bed granulation.

Comprehensive statistical and risk analyses of the process are generally necessary to assess the reliability of predictive mathematical relationships. Based on the estimated risk, a simple correlation function may need further support or justification, such as a mechanistic explanation of causal links among the process, material measurements, and target quality specifications. For certain applications, sensor-based measurements can provide a useful process signature that may be related to the underlying process steps or transformations. Based on the level of process understanding, these signatures may also be useful for process monitoring, control, and endpoint determination when these patterns or signatures relate to product and process quality.

28.5.3 CONTROLLING PHASE AND PROCESS CONTROL TOOLS

It is important to emphasize that a strong link between product design and process development is essential to ensure effective control of all critical quality attributes. Process monitoring and control strategies are intended to monitor the state of a process and actively manipulate it to maintain the desired state. Strategies should accommodate the attributes of input materials, the ability and reliability of process analyzers to measure critical attributes, and the achievement of process endpoints to ensure consistent quality of the output materials and the final product.

In a PAT framework, validation can be demonstrated through continuous quality assurance where a process is continually monitored, evaluated, and adjusted using validated in-process measurements, tests, controls, and process endpoints. Figure 28.6 represents PAT integrated high-shear wet granulation system, which simultaneously analyzes in-process and finished product CQAs and controls relevant associated CMAs and CPPs with the goal of continuously ensuring the quality of in-process materials and finished product. Thus, PAT will ensure the quality of the product during manufacturing, when no one is looking.

28.6 APPLICATIONS OF QBD AND PAT

Quality by Design offers multiple applications for different departments of the pharmaceutical industry. This methodical approach to development predefines target product profile and implements control strategy for each and every critical CMAs and CPPs based on sound science and quality risk management principles. Through DoE, a systematic and mechanistic model describing the effect of changes in factor(s) – that is, CMAs and CPPs on the response(s), that is, CQAs – can be established. With the help of that regression model, design space, that is, where all the response CQAs meet with set specifications simultaneously, can be obtained, which will assure successful development and scale-up from formulation R&D (FR&D) to production. Design space will provide regulatory flexibility for post-approval change management for the applicant. Through QbD-derived controls, meaningful product quality specifications can be achieved that is based on clinical performance.

Detailed idea through DoE-developed model will help in predicting how the product will behave with changes in each CMAs or CPPs within design space along with PAT, increase process capability, and reduce product variability during manufacturing. Root-cause analysis for process variability or batch failure will become faster and easier for the quality assurance team, as risk assessment report at the development stage will be available through QbD.

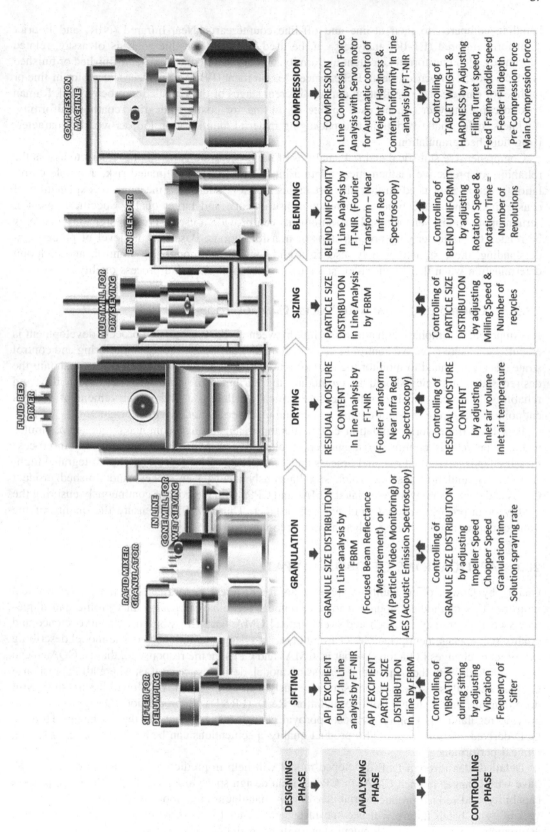

FIGURE 28.6 Process analytical technology tools for high-shear wet granulation process.

PAT can be applied as an integral part of the control strategy [28]. PAT can continuously analyze CMAs, CPPs, or CQAs through in-line or on-line tools to make go-forward/ not-go decisions to demonstrate that the process is maintained within the design space. In a more robust process, PAT can actively control CMAs or CPPs, and timely adjustment of the operating parameters if a variation or defects in the CQAs or input materials that would adversely impact the drug product quality will be observed or detected.

28.7 SUMMARY AND CONCLUSION

The modern philosophy for pharmaceutical drug product development and manufacturing begins with the identification of core regulatory documents that define cGMPs for the 21st-century process analytical technology (PAT), and quality by design (QbD) as shown in this chapter. QbD-based formulation and process development requires, first of all, the determination of CQAs according to predefined goals of QTPP, followed by the identification of all the risk factors (CMAs or CPPs) according to its impact analysis and then a mathematical model can be established in between CMAs, CPPs, and CQAs to develop design space within which all the CQAs should be confirmed using risk assessment tools. Establishing the design space, along with proven acceptable ranges and edges of failures, control strategies can be proposed for each and every CMAs and CPPs to ensure batch-to-batch consistency in CQAs during commercial manufacturing. Thus, QbD is entirely based on sound science and quality risk management principles, which results in a clear understanding of the impact of identified risk factors on the manufacturing process. The resulting formulation and manufacturing process developed through QbD will be more robust along with many other benefits including better product quality, reduced process variability, reduced product defects, enhanced process understanding, higher process capability, comparatively faster approvals, regulatory flexibility, fewer regulatory queries, fewer post-launch issues, more rapid resolution of post-approval change management, and increased flexibility to implement continuous improvement changes. QbD approaches based on PAT also facilitate real-time release testing. This gives companies earlier information on product quality and means that any manufacturing problem can be dealt with faster, in a more informed manner. Adopting QbD and PAT principles for new product development makes sense not only from a regulatory compliance perspective but also for sound financial reasons.

REFERENCES

1. Juran J. M. Juran on quality by design: the new steps for planning quality into goods and services. New York: The Free Press, 1992.
2. Woodcock J. The concept of pharmaceutical quality. Am Pharm Rev 2004: 1–3.
3. U.S. Food and Drug Administration. Guidance for industry: Q8 (R2): Pharmaceutical development. 2009.
4. U.S. Food and Drug Administration. Guidance for industry: Q9: Quality risk management. 2006.
5. U.S. Food and Drug Administration. Guidance for industry: Q10: Pharmaceutical quality system. 2009.
6. U.S. Food and Drug Administration. Guidance for industry: Q8,Q9, and Q10 questions and answers. 2011.
7. ICH Quality Implementation Working Group. Points to consider. ICH-endorsed guide for ICH Q8/Q9/ Q10 implementation. 2011.
8. U.S. Food and Drug Administration. Guidance for industry: Q11 development and manufacture of drug substance. 2012.
9. U.S. Food and Drug Administration. FDA-EMA parallel assessment of quality-by-design elements of marketing applications. https://www.ema.europa.eu/en/documents/other/european-medicines-agency-food-drug-administration-pilot-programme-parallel-assessment-quality_en.pdf Accessed on June1, 2020.
10. Yu L.X, Amidon G, Woodcock J., et al. Understanding pharmaceutical quality by design. AAPS J 2014, 16(4):771–783.

11. U.S. Food and Drug Administration. Guidance for industry: Tablet scoring: Nomenclature, labeling, and data for evaluation. 2013.
12. U.S. Food and Drug Administration. Guidance for industry: Size of beads in drug products labeled for sprinkle. January, 2011.
13. U.S. Food and Drug Administration. Quality by design for ANDAs: An example for immediate-release dosage forms. 2012. https://www.fda.gov/media/83664/download Accessed on July1, 2020.
14. U.S. Food and Drug Administration. Quality by design for ANDAs: An example for modified-release dosage forms. 2012. https://www.fda.gov/media/82834/download Accessed on June3, 2020.
15. U.S. Food and Drug Administration. Guidance for industry: Immediate release solid oral dosage forms scale-up and post approval changes: Chemistry, manufacturing, and controls, in vitro dissolution testing, and in vivo bioequivalence documentation. 1995.
16. U.S. Food and Drug Administration. Guidance for industry: modified release solid oral dosage forms scale-up and post approval changes: Chemistry, manufacturing, and controls, in vitro dissolution testing, and in vivo bioequivalence documentation. 1997.
17. U.S. Food and Drug Administration. Guidance for industry: CMC postapproval manufacturing changes to be documented in annual reports. 2014.
18. Lionberger R., Lee S., Lee L., Raw A., Yu L. X. Quality by design: Concepts for ANDAs. AAPS J 2008, 10: 268–276.
19. Yu L.X. Pharmaceutical quality by design: product and process development, understanding, and control. Pharm Res. 2008, 25: 781–791.
20. Csordas K, Wiedey R, Kleinebudde P. Impact of roll compaction design, process parameters, and material deformation behavior on ribbon relative density. Drug Development and Industrial Pharmacy 2018, 44(8): 1295–1306.
21. Omar C.S, Hounslow M.J, Salman A.D. Implementation of an online thermal imaging to study the effect of process parameters of roller compactor. Drug Delivery and Translational Research 2018 8: 1604–1614.
22. Pandey P, Badawy, SIF. Chapter 18 – A quality by design approach to scale-up of high shear wet granulation process. Handbook of pharmaceutical wet granulation theory and practice in a quality by design paradigm, Academic Press, 2019, 615–650.
23. Faure A, York P, Rowe R.C. Process control and scale-up of pharmaceutical wet granulation processes: a review. European Journal of Pharmaceutics and Biopharmaceutics 2001, 52(3): 269–277.
24. Tao J, Pandey P, Bindra D.S et al. Evaluating scale-up rules of a high-shear wet granulation process pharmaceutics. Drug Delivery and Pharmaceutical Technology 2015, 104(7): 2323–2333.
25. Huang J, Kaul G, Hernandez H et al. A PAT approach to improve process understanding of high shear wet granulation through in-line particle measurement using FBRM C35. J Pharm Sci. 2010, 99(7): 3205–3212.
26. Désiré A, Paillard B, Bougaret J et al. Extruder scale-up assessment in the process of extrusion–spheronization: Comparison of radial and axial systems by a design of experiments approach. Drug Development and Industrial Pharmacy 2013, 39(2): 176–185.
27. Trivedi N.R, Gerald R, James J et al. Pharmaceutical approaches to preparing pelletized dosage forms using the extrusion-spheronization process. Critical Reviews in Therapeutic Drug Carrier Systems 2007, 24(1):1–40.
28. "Objectives and design options":- StatEase: Design-Expert. https://www.statease.com/docs/v11/getting-started/objectives/ Accessed on July1, 2020.
29. "Identify responses":- StatEase: Design-Expert. https://www.statease.com/docs/v11/contents/getting-started/identify-responses/ Accessed on July1, 2020.
30. "Identify Factors and Levels": - StatEase: Design-Expert. https://www.statease.com/docs/v11/contents/getting-started/identify-factors-and-levels/ Accessed on July1, 2020.
31. "How do you select an experimental design?":- Engineering Statistics Handbook. https://www.itl.nist.gov/div898/handbook/pri/section3/pri33.htm Accessed on July1, 2020.
32. "What is randomization?":- Minitab. https://support.minitab.com/en-us/minitab/18/help-and-how-to/modeling-statistics/doe/supporting-topics/basics/what-is-randomization/ Accessed on July1, 2020.
33. "What is a block?":- Minitab. https://support.minitab.com/en-us/minitab/18/help-and-how-to/modeling-statistics/doe/supporting-topics/basics/what-is-a-block/ Accessed on July1, 2020.
34. "Response surface designs":- Engineering Statistics Handbook. https://www.itl.nist.gov/div898/handbook/pri/section3/pri336.htm Accessed on July1, 2020.
35. "ANOVA Output":- StatEase: Design-Expert. https://www.statease.com/docs/v11/contents/analysis/anova-output/ Accessed on July1, 2020.

36. "Diagnostics plots":- StatEase: Design-Expert. https://www.statease.com/docs/v11/contents/analysis/diagnostics/diagnostics-plots/#diagnostics-plots Accessed on July1, 2020.

37. "Model graphs":- StatEase: Design-Expert. https://www.statease.com/docs/v11/contents/analysis/model-graphs/ Accessed on July1, 2020.

38. "Multiple responses: The desirability approach":-Engineering Statistics Handbook. https://www.itl.nist.gov/div898/handbook/pri/section5/pri5322.htm Accessed on July1, 2020.

39. "Individual & composite desirability":- Minitab. https://support.minitab.com/en-us/minitab/18/help-and-how-to/modeling-statistics/using-fitted-models/how-to/response-optimizer/methods-and-formulas/individual-desirabilities/ and https://support.minitab.com/en-us/minitab/18/help-and-how-to/modeling-statistics/using-fitted-models/how-to/response-optimizer/methods-and-formulas/composite-desirability/ Accessed on July1, 2020.

40. "Numerical optimization": - StatEase: Design-Expert. https://www.statease.com/docs/v11/navigation/numerical-optimization/ Accessed on July 1, 2020.

41. "Graphical optimization":- StatEase: Design-Expert. https://www.statease.com/docs/v11/navigation/graphical-optimization/ Accessed on July1, 2020.

42. "Confirmation":- StatEase: Design-Expert. https://www.statease.com/docs/v11/contents/analysis/confirmation/#confirmation Accessed on July 1, 2020.

43. "How to confirm DOE results (confirmatory runs)":- Engineering Statistics Handbook. https://www.itl.nist.gov/div898/handbook/pri/section4/pri46.htm Accessed on July1, 2020.

44. Near-infrared assay and content uniformity of tablets. Pharmaceutical Technology 2007, 31(4). http://www.pharmtech.com/near-infrared-assay-and-content-uniformity-tablets Accessed on July1, 2020.

45. U.S. Food and Drug Administration. Guidance for industry: Process validation: General principles and practices. January 2011.

46. "What are control charts?":- Engineering Statistics Handbook https://www.itl.nist.gov/div898/handbook/pmc/section3/pmc31.htm Accessed on July 1, 2020.

47. "Process capability (Cp, Cpk) and process performance (Pp, Ppk) – what is the difference?":- Engineering Statistics Handbook https://www.isixsigma.com/tools-templates/capability-indices-process-capability/process-capability-cp-cpk-and-process-performance-pp-ppk-what-difference/ Accessed on July 1, 2020.

48. De Feo JA. Barnard W. JURAN Institute's six sigma breakthrough and beyond: Quality performance breakthrough methods. India: Tata McGraw-Hill Publishing Company Limited, 2005.

49. U.S. Food and Drug Administration. Guidance for industry: PAT – A framework for innovative pharmaceutical development, manufacturing, and quality assurance, 2004.

50. Bakri B., Weimer M., Hauck G. et al. Assessment of powder blend uniformity: Comparison of real-time NIR blend monitoring with stratified sampling in combination with HPLC and at-line NIR chemical imaging. European Journal of Pharmaceutics and Biopharmaceutics 2015, 97(Pt A): 78–89.

51. Abatzoglou N. Real-time NIR monitoring of pharmaceutical blending processes with multivariate quantitative models https://www.europeanpharmaceuticalreview.com/article/732/real-time-nir-monitoring-of-pharmaceutical-blending-processes-with-multivariate-quantitative-models/

52. Vijay Kumar, Michael KT, Mehrotra A et al. Real-time particle size analysis using focused beam reflectance measurement as a process analytical technology tool for a continuous granulation–drying–milling process. AAPS PharmSciTech 2013, 14(2): 523–530.

53. Müller J, Knop K, Thies J et al. Feasibility of Raman spectroscopy as PAT tool in active coating. Drug Dev Ind Pharm 2010, 36(2): 234–243.

ABBREVIATIONS USED IN THE CHAPTER

API	Active Pharmaceutical Ingredient
CI	Confidence Interval
CMA	Critical Material Attribute
CPP	Critical Process Parameter
CQA	Critical Quality Attribute
DoE	Design of Experiments
OFAT	One Factor at Time
OVAT	One Variable at a Time

PAT   Process Analytical Technology
PI   Prediction Intervals
QbD   Quality by Design
QbT   Quality by Testing
QTPP   Quality Target Product Profile

Index

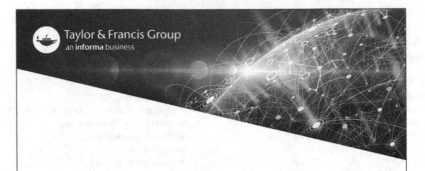